MyNursingLab®

www.mynursinglab.com

Learn more about and purchase access to MyNursingLab.

MyNursingApp™

www.mynursingapp.com

MyNursingApp puts all the information you need in the palm of your hand.

myPEARSONstore

www.mypearsonstore.com

Find your textbook and everything that goes with it.

Fourth Edition

Maternal & Child Nursing Care

Marcia L. London, RN, MSN, APRN, CNS, NNP-BC
Senior Clinical Instructor and Ret. Director of Neonatal Nurse Practioner Program
Beth-El College of Nursing and Health Sciences, University of Colorado, Colorado Springs, Colorado

Patricia A. Wieland Ladewig, RN, PhD
Provost
Regis University, Denver Colorado

Michele R. Davidson, RN, PhD, CNM, CFN
Associate Professor of Nursing and Women's Studies
Coordinator of the School of Nursing PhD Program
George Mason University, Fairfax, Virginia

Jane W. Ball, RN, CPNP, DrPH
Consultant
American College of Surgeons, Gaithersburg, Maryland

Ruth C. McGillis Bindler, RNC, PhD
Professor Emeritus
Washington State University, College of Nursing, Spokane, Washington

Kay J. Cowen, RN-BC, MSN
Clinical Professor
University of North Carolina at Greensboro School of Nursing, Greensboro, North Carolina

PEARSON

Boston   Columbus   Indianapolis   New York   San Francisco   Upper Saddle River
Amsterdam   Cape Town   Dubai   London   Madrid   Milan   Munich   Paris   Montreal   Toronto
Delhi   Mexico City   São Paulo   Sydney   Hong Kong   Seoul   Singapore   Taipei   Tokyo

Library of Congress Cataloging-in-Publication Data

London, Marcia L., author.

Maternal & child nursing care / Marcia L. London, Patricia A. Wieland Ladewig, Michele R. Davidson, Jane W. Ball, Ruth C. Bindler, Kay J. Cowen.—Fourth edition.

p. ; cm.

Maternal and child nursing care

Preceded by: Maternal & child nursing care / Marcia L. London . . . [et al.]. 3rd ed. c2011.

Includes bibliographical references and index.

ISBN-13: 978-0-13-304600-7

ISBN-10: 0-13-304600-1

I. Title. II. Title: Maternal and child nursing care.

[DNLM: 1. Maternal-Child Nursing—methods. 2. Pediatric Nursing—methods. WY 157.3]

RG951

618.2′0231—dc23

2013032544

Publisher: Julie Levin Alexander
Publisher's Assistant: Regina Bruno
Program Manager: Melissa Bashe
Editorial Assistant: Erin Rafferty
Development Editors: Lynda Hatch and Mary Cook
Project Management Team Lead: Patrick Walsh
Project Manager: Maria Reyes
Interior Designer: Mary Siener
Cover Designer: Eva Ruutopold
Cover Art Direction: Mary Siener
Director of Marketing: David Gesell
Executive Marketing Manager: Phoenix Harvey
Marketing Specialist: Michael Sirinides
Media Project Managers: Karen Bretz/Tanika Henderson
Manufacturing Manager: Maura Zaldivar-Garcia
Composition: S4Carlisle Publishing Services
Production Editor: Lynn Steines, S4Carlisle Publishing Services
Printer/Binder: Courier/Kendallville
Cover Printer: Lehigh-Phoenix Color/Hagerstown
Cover Image: Shutterstock: Andresr

Notice: Care has been taken to confirm the accuracy of information presented in this book. The authors, editors, and the publisher, however, cannot accept any responsibility for errors or omissions or for consequences from application of the information in this book and make no warranty, express or implied, with respect to its contents.

The authors and publisher have exerted every effort to ensure that drug selections and dosages set forth in this text are in accord with current recommendations and practice at time of publication. However, in view of ongoing research, changes in government regulations, and the constant flow of information relating to drug therapy and drug reactions, the reader is urged to check the package inserts of all drugs for any change in indications of dosage and for added warnings and precautions. This is particularly important when the recommended agent is a new and/or infrequently employed drug.

10 9 8 7 6 5 4 3 2
ISBN-13: 978-0-13-304600-7
ISBN-10:   0-13-304600-1

About the Authors

MARCIA L. LONDON Marcia L. London received her BSN and School Nurse Certificate from Plattsburgh State University in Plattsburgh, New York, and her MSN in pediatrics as a clinical nurse specialist from the University of Pittsburgh in Pennsylvania. She worked as a pediatric nurse and began her teaching career at Pittsburgh Children's Hospital Affiliate Program. Mrs. London began teaching at Beth-El School of Nursing and Health Science in 1974 (now part of the University of Colorado, Colorado Springs) after opening the first intensive care nursery at Memorial Hospital of Colorado Springs. She has served in many faculty positions at Beth-El, including assistant director of the School of Nursing. Mrs. London obtained her postmaster's Neonatal Nurse Practitioner certificate in 1983 and subsequently developed the Neonatal Nurse Practitioner (NNP) certificate and the master's NNP program at Beth-El. She is active nationally in neonatal nursing and was involved in the development of National Neonatal Nurse Practitioner educational program guidelines. Mrs. London pursued her interest in college student learning by taking doctoral classes in higher education administration and adult learning at the University of Denver in Colorado. She feels fortunate to be involved in the education of her future colleagues and teaches undergraduate education. Mrs. London and her husband, David, enjoy reading, travel, and hockey games. They have two sons. Craig, who lives in Florida with his wife, Jennifer, works with Internet companies. Matthew works in computer teleresearch. Both are more than willing to give Mom helpful hints about computers.

PATRICIA A. WIELAND LADEWIG Patricia A. Wieland Ladewig received her BS from the College of Saint Teresa in Winona, Minnesota; her MSN from Catholic University of America in Washington, D.C.; and her PhD in higher education administration from the University of Denver in Colorado. She served as an Air Force nurse and discovered her passion for teaching as a faculty member at Florida State University. Over the years, she taught at several schools of nursing. In addition, she became a women's health nurse practitioner and maintained a part-time clinical practice for many years. In 1988, Dr. Ladewig became the first director of the nursing program at Regis College in Denver. In 1991, when the college became Regis University, she became academic dean of the Rueckert-Hartman College for Health Professions. Under her guidance, the School of Nursing has added a graduate program. In addition, the college has added a School of Physical Therapy and a School of Pharmacy. In 2009 Dr. Ladewig became Vice President for Academic Affairs, and in 2012 she became Provost at Regis University. She and her husband, Tim, enjoy skiing, baseball games, and traveling. However, their greatest pleasure comes from their family: son Ryan, his wife Amanda, and grandchildren Reed and Addison Grace; and son Erik, his wife Kedri, and grandchildren Emma and Camden.

MICHELE R. DAVIDSON Michele R. Davidson completed her ADN degree from Marymount University and worked in multiple women's health specialty areas including postpartum, newborn nursery, high-risk nursery, labor and delivery, reproductive endocrinology, gynecology medical-surgical, and oncology units as a registered nurse while obtaining a BSN from George Mason University. Dr. Davidson earned her MSN and a nurse-midwifery certificate at Case Western Reserve University and continued to work as a full-scope nurse-midwife for 16 years. She has delivered over 1,000 babies during her career as a nurse-midwife. She completed her PhD in nursing administration and healthcare policy at George Mason University (GMU) and began teaching at GMU in 1999 while continuing in her role as a nurse-midwife. Dr. Davidson serves as the Coordinator for the PhD program in the School of Nursing. She has an interest in women's mental health and focuses her research on perinatal and postpartum mood and anxiety disorders. Dr. Davidson also has an interest in the care of individuals with disabilities and serves as a member of the Loudoun County Disability Advisory Committee and is a disability advocate in her community. She was a member of the American College of Nurse-Midwives Certification Council, the body that writes the national certification examination for certified nurse-midwives. She is a member of numerous editorial and advisory boards and has a passion for writing. In 2000, Dr. Davidson developed an immersion clinical experience for GMU students on a remote island in the Chesapeake Bay. In 2003, she founded the Smith Island Foundation, a nonprofit organization in which she served as executive director for eight years. Dr. Davidson has also completed certifications in lactation consulting, forensic nursing, and surgical first assistant. In 2012, her book, *A Nurse's Guide to Women's Mental Health*, won an American Journal of Nursing Book Award. In her free time, she enjoys spending time with her mother, writing, gardening, Internet surfing, and spending time on Smith Island with her nurse-practitioner husband, Nathan, and their four active children, Hayden, Chloe, Caroline, and Grant. Dr. Davidson and her family love the Eastern Shore of Maryland and continue to be part-time residents of Smith Island.

JANE W. BALL Jane W. Ball graduated from The Johns Hopkins Hospital School of Nursing, and subsequently received a BS from The Johns Hopkins University. She worked in the surgical, emergency, and outpatient units of the Johns Hopkins Children's Medical and Surgical Center, first as a staff nurse and then as a pediatric nurse practitioner. Thus began her career as a pediatric nurse and advocate for children's health needs. Jane obtained both a master of public health and doctor of public health degree from the Johns Hopkins University Bloomberg School of Public Health with a focus on maternal and child health. After graduation she became the chief of child health services for the Commonwealth of Pennsylvania Department of Health. In this capacity she oversaw the state-funded well-child clinics and explored ways to improve education for the state's community health nurses. After relocating to Texas, she joined the faculty at the University of Texas at Arlington School of Nursing to teach community pediatrics to registered nurses returning to school for a BSN. During this time she became involved in writing her first textbook, *Mosby's Guide to Physical Examination,* which is currently in its eighth edition. After relocating to the Washington, D.C., area, she joined the Children's National Medical Center to manage a federal project to teach instructors of emergency medical technicians from all states about the special care children need during an emergency. Exposure to the shortcomings of the emergency medical services system in the late 1980s with regard to pediatric care was a career-changing event. With federal funding, she developed educational curricula for emergency medical technicians and emergency nurses to help them provide improved care for children. A textbook entitled *Pediatric Emergencies, A Manual for Prehospital Providers* was developed from these educational ventures. She served as the executive director of the federally funded Emergency Medical Services for Children National Resource Center for 15 years, providing consultation and resource development for state health agencies, health professionals, families, and advocates to improve the emergency healthcare system for children. Dr. Ball is a consultant for the American College of Surgeons, assisting states to develop and enhance their trauma systems. She is also the managing investigator on an Emergency Medical Services for Children grant to evaluate the implementation of an emergency department recognition program for pediatric care in Delaware.

RUTH C. MCGILLIS BINDLER Ruth Bindler received her BSN from Cornell University–New York Hospital School of Nursing in New York. She worked in oncology nursing at Memorial–Sloan Kettering Cancer Center in New York, and then moved to Wisconsin and became a public health nurse in Dane County. Thus began her commitment to work with children as she visited children and their families at home, and served as a school nurse for several elementary, middle, and high schools. As a result of this interest in child healthcare needs, she earned her MS in child development from the University of Wisconsin. A move to Washington State was accompanied by a new job as a faculty member at the Intercollegiate Center for Nursing Education in Spokane, Washington, now the WSU College of Nursing. Dr. Bindler has been fortunate to be involved for 38 years in the growth of this nursing education consortium, which is a combination of public and private universities and offers undergraduate and graduate nursing degrees. She has taught theory and clinical courses in child health nursing, cultural diversity, graduate research, pharmacology, and assessment; served as lead faculty for child health nursing; was the first director of the PhD program; and most recently served as Associate Dean for Graduate Programs, which includes Master of Nursing, Post-Masters certificates, and PhD and Doctor of Nursing Practice (DNP) programs. She recently retired from this position and serves the college and profession as a professor emeritus, continuing work with graduate students and research. Her first professional book, *Pediatric Medications*, was published in 1981, and she has continued to publish articles and books in the areas of pediatric medications and pediatric health. Her research was focused in the area of childhood obesity, type 2 diabetes, and cardiovascular risk factors in children. Ethnic diversity and interprofessional collaboration have been other themes in her work. Dr. Bindler believes that her role as a faculty member and administrator has enabled her to learn continually, to foster the development of students in nursing, and to participate fully in the profession of nursing. In addition to teaching, research, publication, and leadership, she enhances her life by service in several professional and community activities, and by outdoor activities with her family.

KAY J. COWEN Kay Cowen received her BSN degree from East Carolina University in Greenville, North Carolina, and began her career as a staff nurse on the pediatric unit of North Carolina Baptist Hospital in Winston Salem. She developed a special interest in the psychosocial needs of hospitalized children and preparing them for hospitalization. This led to the focus of her master's thesis at the University of North Carolina at Greensboro (UNCG) where she received a Master of Science in Nursing Education degree with a focus in maternal child nursing. Mrs. Cowen began her teaching career in 1984 at UNCG, where she continues today as Clinical Professor in the Parent & Child Nursing Department. Her primary responsibilities include coordination of the pediatric nursing course, teaching classroom content, and supervising a clinical group of students. Mrs. Cowen shared her passion for the psychosocial care of children and the needs of their families through her first experience as an author of the chapter "Hospital Care for Children" in *Child Health Nursing: A Comprehensive Approach to the Care of Children and Their Families*, published in 1993. In the classroom Mrs. Cowen realized that students learn through a variety of teaching strategies, and she became especially interested in the strategy of gaming. She led a research study to evaluate the effectiveness of gaming in the classroom and subsequently continues to incorporate gaming in her teaching. In the clinical setting Mrs. Cowen teaches her students the skills needed to care for patients and the importance of family-centered care, focusing on not only the physical needs of the child but also the psychosocial needs of the child and family. During her teaching career, Mrs. Cowen has continued to work part time as a staff nurse, first on the pediatric unit of Moses Cone Hospital in Greensboro and then at Brenner Children's Hospital in Winston Salem. In 2006 she became the part-time pediatric nurse educator in Brenner's Family Resource Center. Through this role she is able to extend her love of teaching to children and families. Through her role as an author, Mrs. Cowen is able to extend her dedication to pediatric nursing and nursing education. She is married and the mother of twin sons.

Thank You!

We are grateful to all the nurses, both clinicians and educators, who reviewed the manuscript of this text. Their insights, suggestions, and eye for detail helped us prepare a more relevant and useful book, one that focuses on the essential components of learning in the fields of maternal, newborn, and child health nursing.

Mike Aldridge, MSN, RN, CNS, CNE
Concordia University Texas
Austin, TX

Stacee Bertolla, MSN, RN, CPNP
University of South Alabama
Fairhope, AL

Amy Bigham, DNP, MSN, FNP, ANCC, BSN
Samford University
Birmingham, AL

Ann Bowling, PhD, CPNP
Wright State University
Dayton, OH

Karen Breitkreuz, EdD, MSN, CNS, RN
Boise State University
Boise, ID

Susan Buchholz-Jones, MS, RN
Plymouth State University
Plymouth, NH

Nancy Caddy, RN, BC
Cone Health
Greensboro, NC

Mary Ann Cantrell, PhD, RN, CNE
Villanova University
Villanova, PA

Tonya Chapin, RN, MSN
Colorado Mesa University
Grand Junction, CO

Kate Chappell, MSN, APRN, CPNP
University of South Carolina
Columbia, SC

Kelly Conner, MS, RN
Boise State University
Boise, ID

Margot De Sevo, PhD, RNC
Adelphi University
Garden City, NY

Holly Diesel, PhD, RN
Barnes-Jewish College
St. Louis, MO

Karen Dublin, MEd, RN
Tyler Junior College
Tyler, TX

Crystal Edds, RN, MS, CPNP
Georgia Southern University
Statesboro, GA

JoAnne Flagg, DNP, CPNP, IBCLC
Johns Hopkins University
Baltimore, MD

Ali Marie Galindo, MSN, ARNP-FP
Florida International University
Miami, FL

Barbara Gross, ARNP, DNP
University of Central Florida
Orlando, FL

Karen Hessler, PhD, FNP-C
University of Northern Colorado
Greeley, CO

Ozzie Hunter, RN, MSN
Southern Illinois University
Edwardsville, IL

Gina Idol, RN, BSN, CPN
Brenner Children's Hospital
Winston-Salem, NC

Cindy Jarrett-Pulliam, BSN, MSN
University of North Carolina
Greensboro, NC

Susan Kennel, PhD, ARNP
University of South Florida
Tampa, FL

Mary Kishman, PhD, RN
College of Mount St. Joseph
Cincinnati, OH

Meredith Krutar, MSN, FNP-BC
Carroll College
Helena, MT

Robyn Leo, RN, MS
Worcester State University
Worcester, MA

Angela Lukomski, RN, DNP, CPNP
Eastern Michigan University
Ypsilanti, MI

Valerie O'Dell, DNP, RN
Youngstown State University
Youngstown, OH

Sharon Rappold, MSN, RN, BC
Wharton County Junior College
Wharton, TX

Maria Ronquillo, MS, RNC-OB, C-EFM
Samuel Merritt University
San Francisco, CA

Aissa Scott, MS, ARNP, CNM
St. Petersburg College
Pinellas Park, FL

Cordia Starling, RN, EdD
Dalton State College
Dalton, GA

Brenda Tanner, MSN, RNC-OB
Greenville Technical College
Greenville, SC

Karen Urban, RN, MSN
Colorado Mesa University
Grand Junction, CO

Sheila Whitworth, DNP, MSN, RN
University of South Alabama
Fairhope, AL

Barbara Wilford, MSN, MBA, RN
Lorain County Community College
Elyria, OH

Judy Williams, RN, MSN
Colorado Mesa University
Grand Junction, CO

Melissa Williams, RN, BSN, MSN, EdS
Augusta State University
Augusta, GA

Cynthia Zeller, MSN, CPNP, IBCLC
Frederick Community College
Frederick, MD

Dedication

Throughout the ages, nurses have cared for families, fathers, mothers, and their children—treating, healing, soothing, educating, and advocating.

And so we dedicate this book to nurses—

> For their wisdom, expertise, and compassion
> For their willingness to challenge the system when necessary
> For their ability to remain strong during times of difficulty and stress
> And for their unfailing commitment to the families they assist.

And to nursing students everywhere—

> For seeking to serve others when so many have become self-serving
> For committing their minds and talents to a proud profession
> For accepting the challenges posed by the changes in health care
> And for daring to envision a brighter tomorrow.

Then, too, as always, we honor our beloved families—

> David London, Craig, Jennifer, and Matthew
> Tim Ladewig, Ryan, Amanda, Reed and Addison Grace; Erik, Kedri, Emma, and Camden
> Nathan Davidson, Hayden, Chloe, Caroline, and Grant
> Ronald Ball
> Julian Bindler, Dana and Brady, Ross and Cami
> Fred Cowen III, Benjamin and Marcia, Michael and Caroline

Preface

Faculty and students in today's maternity and pediatric nursing courses face a wide variety of issues and challenges. Courses are increasingly shortened, clinical experiences are more limited, and patients in hospitals are often more seriously ill. Time is precious for both students and faculty, and competence in nursing practice is essential. Changes in healthcare delivery stem from the Affordable Care Act, and new regulations offer challenges to the student and faculty member. The primary goal in this edition is to present key content in an accurate, readable format that helps students and faculty focus on what is important. This textbook helps students develop the skills and abilities they need now and in the future in an ever-changing healthcare environment. This is done through the Learning Outcomes and the Critical Concept Review feature at the end of each chapter, through the illustrations and photographs that clarify concepts more efficiently than words can do, and through the electronic resources at www.nursing.pearsonhighered.com, which depicts clinical situations and requires students to engage in critical thinking. In its structure, format, and delivery, this text provides a concise look at maternal–newborn, women's health, and pediatric nursing.

ORGANIZATION

The organization of the text also reflects a time-saving approach. As educators and nurses, we know how difficult it is to teach everything that students need to learn in so little time. Consequently, we sought to reduce duplication in the text by carefully integrating maternity and pediatric nursing topics. For example, two introductory chapters address concepts important for maternal, newborn, and child nursing. Chapter 1 discusses introductory concepts of family-centered care, health promotion, community and home care, evidence-based practice, legal issues, as well as the complex ethical considerations related to reproductive decisions, cord blood banking, stem cell research, terminating life-sustaining treatment, and organ transplantation issues. Chapter 2 addresses concepts that are important for culturally appropriate care for the entire family, such as cultural norms related to childbearing and childrearing, cultural assessment, and complementary and alternative therapies. Throughout the text we cross-reference to other chapters to avoid the duplication of content, and we have worked to eliminate potentially conflicting information.

Subsequent chapters focus on reproductive issues and women's health, pregnancy, birth processes, postpartum care, and newborn management. The maternal–newborn chapters begin with basic theory followed by nursing assessment and nursing care for essentially healthy women or infants. Complications of a specific period appear in the last chapter or chapters of each section. The second half of the text transitions into the pediatric care chapters. The pediatric chapters begin with introductory concepts, such as growth and development, nutrition, assessment, health promotion for children ranging from newborn to adolescents, and care of the child in the community and hospital settings. Chapters 45 through 58 cover the nursing care of children with various disorders, organized by body system.

IMPORTANT THEMES IN THIS EDITION

Central to this edition are several key themes that are increasingly evident in nursing care of childbearing and childrearing families.

Family-Centered Nursing Care

Nursing care for pregnant women and children is a family-centered process, and it is essential to providing culturally competent care. The underlying philosophy of *Maternal & Child Nursing Care* is simple: We believe that family members are co-participants in care during pregnancy and childbirth. Parents must be integrated into the care of an infant or child at any stage of development, as they are the central influence on the child's life. Families experience the excitement and exhilaration of welcoming a healthy infant into their home, but they also experience sorrow and concern when a health problem occurs. Nurses play a pivotal role in helping families celebrate the normal life processes associated with birth, in promoting the health of the family and child, in fostering the child's growth and development from infancy through adolescence, and in caring for the child with any health condition. We are committed to providing a text that integrates the needs of families across the continuum from conception through adolescence.

Health Promotion

As nurses and educators, we are supportive of the goals and objectives of *Healthy People 2020*. This science-based effort provides a 10-year agenda for improving the health and well-being of the nation. Throughout the text, we have incorporated content reflecting the objectives of the project as they relate to childbearing families, infants, children, and adolescents.

We also subscribe to the paradigm that all childbearing and childrearing families and children need health promotion and health maintenance interventions, no matter where they seek health care or what health conditions they may be experiencing. Families may visit offices or other community settings specifically to obtain health supervision care. Nurses may also integrate health promotion and health maintenance into the care for childbearing and childrearing families and for children with acute and chronic illness in a variety of inpatient and outpatient settings. The inclusion of *Healthy People 2020* initiatives throughout the text integrates the national public health efforts to improve healthcare outcomes and assists nursing students and nurses with integrating healthcare policy into practice. This textbook provides health promotion and health maintenance content throughout, most visibly in four chapters: Chapter 5, *Health Promotion for Women*; Chapter 35, *Health Promotion and Maintenance: General Concepts, the Newborn, and the Infant*; Chapter 36, *Health Promotion and Maintenance: The Toddler, the Preschooler, and the School-Age Child*; and Chapter 37, *Health Promotion and Maintenance: The Adolescent*.

In addition, a feature entitled **Health Promotion** summarizes the needs of women from preconception to postpartum, newborns, and children with specific chronic conditions, such as asthma or diabetes. These overviews teach the student to look at the child with a chronic illness like any other child, with health maintenance needs for prevention, education, and basic care.

Nursing Care in the Community

Most maternity and pediatric nursing care occurs in the community setting, especially since most children and pregnant women are healthy and have only episodic acute health conditions. Even women with high-risk pregnancies and children with serious chronic health conditions are receiving more care in their homes and in the community. This textbook integrates community and home care throughout, including information on long-term management of complex health conditions, which are especially challenging to manage in community settings.

Five chapters provide a theoretical perspective and important tools in caring for childbearing and childrearing families in the community setting: Chapter 10, *Antepartum Nursing Assessment*; Chapter 11, *The Expectant Family: Needs and Care*; Chapter 30, *The Postpartum Family: Early Care Needs and Home Care*; Chapter 38, *Family Assessment and Concepts of Nursing Care in the Community*; and Chapter 39, *Nursing Considerations for the Child and Family with a Chronic Condition*. In addition, Community-Based Nursing Care is a special heading used throughout this text.

Patient and Family Education

Patient and family education remains a critical element of effective nursing care, one that we emphasize in this text. Nurses teach their patients during all stages of pregnancy and the childbearing process, during the child's health visits, and while providing care for specific conditions. Throughout the book, we include **Teaching Highlights** that present a special healthcare issue or problem and the related key teaching points for the family.

Clinical Reasoning

Nurses are faced with the responsibility to manage care for multiple families with diverse healthcare needs, and to work collaboratively with other health professionals to enhance care. Thus, nurses must be able to think critically, communicate well, and problem solve effectively.

To promote the development of clinical reasoning skills that will support nurses in challenging situations, **Clinical Reasoning** boxes provide brief scenarios that ask students to determine the appropriate response. Students can test their own decision-making skills by submitting answers to these questions on the text's website, where the feature also appears. The instructor can then grade their answers using the suggested answers provided in the Instructor's Manual, which is replicated on the website. Students can access a variety of critical thinking exercises and case studies on the textbook's website at www.nursing.pearsonhighered.com.

Another feature that emphasizes these skills is the **Clinical Reasoning in Action** feature. This case study at the end of each chapter introduces a patient situation along with questions to enable the student to decide which nursing actions are appropriate. Answers are provided at www.nursing.pearsonhighered.com. In addition, some of the exercises tied to the patient situation ask the student to create a **Concept Map** using the interactive template found on the text's website. The use of concept maps is an exciting trend in nursing care management. Concept maps are visual depictions of the relationships that exist among a variety of concepts and ideas related to a patient's specific health problems. The relationship "picture" created by the map allows the nurse to plan interventions that can address multiple problems more effectively. To help students understand how concept maps can influence care planning, we have included a sample concept map in Chapter 1.

The Instructor's Resource Manual has more suggestions for clinical reasoning exercises for both the classroom and the clinical setting.

Evidence-Based Practice

Healthcare professionals are increasingly aware of the importance of using evidence-based practice approaches as the foundation for planning and providing skilled, effective care. The approach of evidence-based practice draws on information from a variety of sources, including nursing research. To help nurses become more comfortable integrating new knowledge into their nursing practice, a brief discussion of evidence-based practice is included in Chapter 1.

A feature entitled **Evidence-Based Practice** further enhances the approach of using research to determine nursing actions. It describes a particular problem or clinical question and investigates the evidence that suggests solutions to the problem. In these features, we provide an interpretation explaining the implications of the studies and then invite the student to apply clinical reasoning skills to further identify nursing care approaches.

Developing Cultural Competence

The influence of a family's culture on health beliefs and healthcare practices cannot be underestimated. Chapter 1 briefly introduces cultural issues relevant to maternity and child nursing care. Additionally, we include Chapter 2, *Culture and the Family,* to directly and specifically address cultural issues.

We also emphasize cultural competence throughout the text. We highlight specific cultural issues and their application to nursing care in the **Developing Cultural Competence** features.

Other New or Expanded Concepts in This Edition

Many other important concepts are emphasized throughout this text:

- *Assessment* is an essential and core role in nursing management. Several chapters are dedicated to helping the student perform an assessment during the pregnancy continuum, including the fetus and newborn, and later through the stages of childhood. In addition, body system assessment guidelines are provided in many of the pediatric chapters.

- *Communication* is one of the most important skills that students need to learn. Effective communication is the very fiber of nursing practice. This book integrates communication skills in an applied manner where students can most benefit. It is an essential part of the **Clinical Tip** and **Teaching Highlights** boxes. The importance of communication with families and other health professionals underscores the Collaborative Care sections of this text.

- *Ensuring appropriate nutrition* during pregnancy, the newborn period, infancy, and childhood is important to promote growth, development, and health. A growing national focus on healthy nutrition patterns underscores the importance of this information. Chapters 12, 26, 29, and 33 address nutrition for pregnant women, newborns, and children.

- *Patient safety* is an essential element of effective patient care. It is the focus of the Joint Commission and one of the key elements of the Quality and Safety Education for Nurses (QSEN) project, which is discussed in Chapter 1. To help keep safety in the forefront, a new feature called **SAFETY ALERT!** has been added. This feature calls attention to issues that could place a patient (or a nurse) at risk. Another feature, **Clinical Tip**, relates to patient safety and many other nursing concepts by providing readers with concrete suggestions for safe, effective practice.

- *Pain* is now considered the fifth vital sign, and pain management is a priority in healthcare settings. All of the chapters in Part 4, *Birth and the Family*, address pain assessment and management, and it is the primary focus in Chapter 20, *Pharmacologic Pain Management*. Pain assessment and management is also a focus in five chapters (Chapters 24, 26, 27, 30, and 31) of Part 5, *The Postpartum Family and the Newborn*. In Part 6, Chapter 40 addresses pain assessment and management in the nursing care plan, and it is the primary subject of Chapter 41, *Pain Assessment and Management in Children*. We discuss applicable pain management when appropriate in other chapters, including each of the chapters in Part 7, *Caring for Children*

with Alterations in Health Status. Current research is used as the basis for pain discussions and nursing management throughout the text.

- *End-of-life care* has rightfully gained prominence as a critical component of nursing care. Expanded focus on the care of the family and the child who is dying has been added to Chapter 42, *The Child with a Life-Threatening Condition and End-of-Life Care*. Grief and loss associated with miscarriage are addressed in Chapter 16, *Pregnancy at Risk: Gestational Onset*. Care of the family experiencing perinatal loss is presented in Chapter 22, *Childbirth at Risk: Labor-Related Complications*.

TOOLS THAT FOCUS STUDENT REVIEW TO MAXIMIZE TIME

Both instructors and students value learning aids that unify the objectives and concepts of a chapter as well as reinforce the overall themes in a text. In keeping with our theme of family-centered care, each chapter begins with a **Family Quote** that helps personalize and set the stage for content that follows from the family's perspective. This is followed by a list of **Learning Outcomes** and **Key Terms** with page numbers to identify the place where the term first appears in the chapter. An **Audio Glossary** of these terms commonly used in the field of maternal–newborn and child nursing can be found on the book's website, with audio pronunciations of the terms as well as printed definitions.

Critical Concept Review

This feature is a direct response to instructors' and students' requests that the text provide more opportunities for review. Each chapter ends with a **Critical Concept Review**, a feature designed to help students retain the most important concepts from a chapter in a short period of time. This visual tool isolates the essential content in a chapter by means of a flowchart that links **Learning Outcomes** to their corresponding **Concepts**. Students save time by having the important concepts identified for them, allowing them to use more of their study time for reviewing the concepts themselves.

Explore Pearson Nursing Student Resources

The last section of each chapter includes a list of references and an invitation to visit Pearson Nursing Student Resources at www.nursing.pearsonhighered.com. This encourages students to use the additional chapter-specific NCLEX-RN® review questions and other interactive exercises that appear on the website. These online offerings will further enhance the student's learning experience, build on knowledge gained from this textbook, prepare students for the NCLEX-RN®, and foster clinical reasoning. In addition, throughout the chapters themselves, thumbtabs appear along the edges of the pages that point the reader to supplements on www.nursing.pearsonhighered.com that relate to a topic discussed near the thumbtab. The thumbtabs cross-reference specific animations, case studies, activities, and other materials that will assist students in understanding key concepts.

APPLICATION OF THE NURSING PROCESS

NURSING MANAGEMENT

The nursing process is emphasized throughout the nursing care chapters. The heading **Nursing Management** highlights nursing assessment, actions, and evaluation. In chapters with frequently seen or high-risk health issues or conditions, the expanded section on nursing management helps students understand and apply care principles more completely. The expanded section includes the headings Nursing Assessment and Diagnosis, Planning and Implementation, and Evaluation.

In keeping with changing approaches to nursing care management, we feature **Nursing Care Plans** throughout the text. The Nursing Care Plans address nursing care for patients who have complications, such as a woman with preeclampsia or a child with otitis media. We designed this feature to help students approach care from the nursing management perspective. Care plans integrate nursing diagnoses, Nursing Intervention Classifications (NIC), and Nursing Outcome Classifications (NOC).

VISUALS THAT TEACH

The conviction that art can teach is evident throughout the book. There are hundreds of contemporary photographs of childbearing and childrearing families and children in healthcare and related settings throughout the textbook, as well as illustrations, all of which serve to display conditions, compare developmental stages, and depict concepts.

Pathophysiology Illustrated

In particular, **Pathophysiology Illustrated** figures allow the student to see into the body and to visualize the causes and effects of conditions on childbearing women, newborns, and children. Each Pathophysiology Illustrated feature box begins with a head like the one shown here.

As Children Grow

As Children Grow illustrations help the student visualize the important anatomic and physiologic differences between a child and an adult. These features illustrate how the child progresses through developmental stages and the important ways in which a child's development influences healthcare needs and how the child progresses through developmental stages. Each As Children Grow feature box begins with a head like the one shown here.

Nursing is facing many new challenges: an ongoing nursing shortage, dramatic advances in healthcare knowledge, implementation of the Affordable Care Act, revisioning of nursing education needs and approaches, and natural and human-made disasters that create a critical need for skilled nurses. We believe that nursing is becoming reenergized and is facing these issues and challenges with enthusiasm and commitment. Many people feel a strong desire to choose professions that make a difference—professions such as nursing. We, like you, know that expert nurses can have a tremendous impact on the lives of childbearing and childrearing families. Our goal in writing this text is to help prepare nurses with the skills and knowledge to make a difference—one family at a time.

Marcia L. London
Patricia W. Ladewig
Michele R. Davidson
Jane W. Ball
Ruth C. Bindler
Kay J. Cowen

Features That Help You Use This Textbook Successfully

Instructors and students alike value the in-text learning aids that we include in our textbooks. The following guide will help you use the features and resources from *Maternal & Child Nursing Care*, Fourth Edition, to be successful in the classroom, in the clinical setting, on the NCLEX-RN® examination, and in nursing practice.

Each chapter begins with **Learning Outcomes** and a chapter opening **Quote**. These personal stories illustrate the diversity of cultures, parental concerns, and family situations that nurses will encounter throughout the course of their careers.

CHAPTER 26

The Normal Newborn: Needs, Care, and Feeding

When our daughter was laid in my arms right after birth she was so delicate. I had not dared to hope that we would be blessed with a girl because there were so few girls in my husband's family. Our 2-year-old niece was the first girl in 107 years, so I had pretty much decided that another boy would be just fine. But here she was, right here in my arms. —Catherine, 32

LEARNING OUTCOMES

26.1 Summarize essential information to be obtained about a newborn's birth experience and immediate postnatal period.

26.2 Explain how the physiologic and behavioral responses of the newborn during the first 4 hours after birth (admission and transitional period) determine the nursing care of the newborn.

26.3 Explain the advantages and disadvantages of breastfeeding and formula-feeding in determining the nursing care of both mother/family and newborn.

26.4 Formulate guidelines for helping both breast- and formula-feeding mothers to feed their newborns successfully in hospital and community-based settings.

26.5 Identify activities that should be included in a daily care plan for a normal newborn.

26.6 Describe the common concerns of families regarding their newborn.

26.7 Identify opportunities to individualize parent teaching and enhance each parent's abilities and confidence while providing infant care in the birthing unit.

26.8 Explain the influence of cultural values on infant care, especially feeding practices.

583

KEY TERMS

Circumcision, 591
Colostrum, 596
Foremilk, 596
Hindmilk, 596
Letdown reflex, 596
Mature milk, 596
Newborn screening tests, 617
Oxytocin, 596
Parent–newborn attachment, 588
Prolactin, 596
Transitional milk, 596

At the moment of birth, numerous physiologic adaptations begin to take place in the newborn's body. Because of these dramatic changes, newborns require close observation to determine how smoothly they are making the transition to extrauterine life. Newborns also require specific care that enhances their chances of making the transition successfully.

The two broad goals of nursing care during this period are (1) to promote the physical well-being of the newborn, and (2) to support the establishment of a well-functioning family unit. To meet the first goal, the nurse provides comprehensive care to the newborn in the mother-baby unit. To meet the second goal, the nurse teaches family members how to care for their new baby and supports their efforts so that they feel confident and competent. Thus, the nurse must be knowledgeable about necessary family adjustments as well as the healthcare needs of the newborn. It is important that the family return home confident, knowing that they have the support, information, and skills to care for their newborn. Equally important is the need for each member of the family to begin a unique relationship with the newborn. The cultural and social expectations of individual families and communities affect the ways in which normal newborn care is carried out.

The previous two chapters presented an informational database of the physiologic and behavioral changes occurring in the newborn and the pertinent nursing assessments that are needed. This chapter discusses nursing management while the newborn is in the birthing unit and feeding methods for the full-term, healthy infant.

NURSING CARE DURING ADMISSION AND THE FIRST FOUR HOURS OF LIFE

Immediately after birth, the baby is formally admitted to the healthcare facility.

Nursing Diagnoses

Physiologic alterations of the newborn form the basis of many nursing diagnoses, as does the family members' incorporation of them in caring for their newborn. Nursing diagnoses are based on an analysis of the assessment findings. As discussed in Chapter 24 ❂, the newborn's physiologic adaptation to extrauterine life occurs rapidly and all body systems are affected. Therefore, many of these nursing diagnoses and associated interventions must be identified and implemented in a very short period.

Nursing diagnoses that may apply to newborns include the following (NANDA-I © 2012):

- *Airway Clearance, Ineffective*, related to presence of mucus and retained lung fluid
- *Body Temperature, Imbalanced, Risk for*, related to evaporative, radiant, conductive, and convective heat losses
- *Pain, Acute*, related to heel sticks for glucose or hematocrit tests, vitamin K injection, or hepatitis B immunization

Nursing Plan and Implementation
Initiating Admission Procedures
After birth, the newborn is formally admitted to the healthcare facility. The admission procedures include a review of prenatal and birth information for possible risk factors, a gestational age assessment, and an assessment to ensure that the newborn's adaptation to extrauterine life is proceeding normally. This evaluation of the newborn's status and risk factors must be done no later than 2 hours after birth (American Academy of Pediatrics [AAP] Committee on Fetus and Newborn & American College of Obstetricians and Gynecologists [ACOG] Committee on Obstetrics, 2012).

584

On the second page of each chapter is a list of **Key Terms** that will be introduced in the chapter. Page numbers are included with each key term to identify the place where the term first appears in the chapter.

Media thumbtabs in each chapter remind you to use the accompanying supplemental materials found on the text's companion website, www.nursing.pearsonhighered.com. These thumbtabs cross-reference additional information or specific activities related to the concepts introduced on that page in the textbook. These resources enhance learning and provide an application beyond the textbook experience. For example, you can see a video of breastfeeding in Chapter 26.

As Children Grow boxes illustrate the anatomic and physiologic differences between children and adults. These features illustrate how the child progresses through developmental stages and the important ways in which a child's development influences healthcare needs.

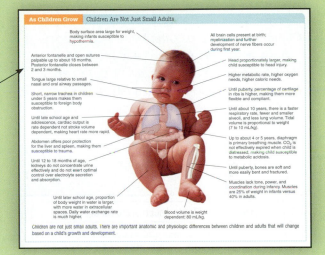

Assessment Guides, found in the maternal–newborn chapters, assist you with diagnoses by incorporating physical assessment and normal findings, alterations and possible causes, and guidelines for nursing interventions. Assessment guides within several chapters of Part 7, *Caring for Children with Alterations in Health Status*, provide a system-oriented approach to assessing the child's health condition.

Clinical Reasoning boxes provide brief case scenarios that ask students to determine the appropriate response.

Clinical Reasoning Glucose Intolerance

Patti Chang, a 35-year-old G3P2, is a well-educated, active Chinese American woman with no history of glucose intolerance. Her two children were born healthy at 36 weeks' gestation. She receives the usual 50-g glucose tolerance test at 26 weeks' gestation, and her plasma level is 160 mg/dL. She seems irritated and frustrated when her obstetrician tells her that it would be best to perform a 3-hour fasting glucose tolerance test. After the physician leaves the room, Patti asks you the following questions: "Will the glucose hurt my baby? What will the treatment be?" How will you answer the questions? Why does Patti seem so upset?
See www.nursing.pearsonhighered.com for possible responses.

Clinical Reasoning in Action

Ann Nelson, a 28-year-old, G2P0010 at 41 weeks' gestation, is admitted to the birthing unit where you are working. She is here for cervical ripening and induction of labor due to postdate pregnancy and decreased amniotic fluid volume. A review of her prenatal chart reveals a pertinent history of infertility (Clomid-induced pregnancy) and asthma (treated with inhalers on a PRN basis). The Doppler picks up a fetal heart rate of 120 beats/min. You place Ann on the electronic fetal monitor and obtain the following data: BP 126/76, T 98°F, P 82, R 16; vaginal exam reveals a 20% effaced cervix, 1 cm dilatation in the posterior position, and vertex at −2 station. The fetal monitor shows a fetal heart rate baseline of 120 to 128 with occasional variable decelerations, accelerations to 140 with fetal activity. No contractions are noted on the monitor or palpated. Ann asks you what to expect with "cervical ripening" using prostaglandin gel.

1. Discuss the action of prostaglandin gel.
2. Ann asks you why cervical ripening and induction of labor are recommended for her and her baby. How would you best respond to her?
3. Ann asks how she will know if she is getting contractions. How would you answer her?
4. Discuss the difference between mild, moderate, and strong contractions.
5. Describe the latent phase of labor.
6. Create a concept map for Ann's care based on the need for cervical ripening and induction of labor due to postdate pregnancy and decreased amniotic fluid volume. Ann also has a history of asthma that warrants consideration in her plan of care.

See www.nursing.pearsonhighered.com for possible responses and an interactive template for a concept map.

Clinical Reasoning in Action features at the end of each chapter propose a real-life scenario and a series of clinical reasoning questions so that you can apply to the clinical setting what you learned in class.

Clinical Tip features offer hands-on suggestions and clinical tips. These are placed at locations in the text that will help you apply them. They include topics such as legal and ethical considerations, nursing alerts, and home and community care considerations.

Clinical Tip

With a sleepy baby, unwrap the baby, encourage lots of skin-to-skin contact between the mother and baby, and have the mother rest with her baby near her breast so that the baby can feel and smell the breast. Encourage the mother to watch for feeding cues, such as hand-to-mouth activity, fluttering eyelids, vocalization (but not necessarily crying), and mouthing activities.

Complementary Care Acupressure During Labor

Acupressure is an ancient Chinese medical treatment that involves using the fingers to press key pressure points on the surface of the skin. This pressure ultimately stimulates the immune system to promote healing by triggering the release of endorphins, reducing stress through muscle relaxation, and promoting circulation. The specific acupressure point used in laboring women is the San Yin-Jiao (SP-6) acupressure point. The SP-6 acupressure point is located on the medial side of the leg, in the calf region, approximately 3 cm (1.2 in.) superior to the prominence of the inner malleus. The use of acupressure in labor has been associated with shorter labors and lower subjective and objective pain scores. Women who receive acupressure typically use less pain medication than those who do not receive acupressure (Simpkin, Bolding, Keppler, et al., 2010).

Complementary Care boxes present information and critiques research about commonly used alternative and complementary measures to treat or provide comfort for various conditions.

Developing Cultural Competence boxes highlight specific cultural issues and their application to nursing care.

Developing Cultural Competence
Birth Choices

Sometimes nurses make the mistake of assuming that a pregnant woman will make the same decisions about the birth experience as the nurse would have. However, the choices a woman and her family make are influenced by many factors, including ethnic background, culture, and religious beliefs. These factors may profoundly influence decisions such as care provider (male or female), birth setting, labor support person(s), use of medications for analgesia, position during birth, saving the placenta, dietary practices immediately postpartum, and a host of other issues. There is no one right way to give birth.

Drug Guides for selected medications commonly used in maternal–newborn and child nursing aid you in correctly administering the medications and evaluating their actions.

Evidence-Based Practice boxes present recent nursing research, discuss implications, and challenge you to incorporate this information into your nursing practice through nursing actions.

Growth and Development boxes, found exclusively in the pediatric chapters, provide information about the different responses of children at various ages to health conditions.

A feature entitled **Health Promotion** summarizes the needs of children with specific chronic conditions, such as asthma or diabetes. These overviews teach you to look at the child with a chronic illness like all children, with health maintenance needs for prevention, education, and basic care.

A **Medications Used to Treat** feature in tabular format provides an overview of the types of medications that can be used for a specific condition and nursing considerations associated with their use.

Also provided are **Nursing Care Plans** that address nursing care for women who have complications such as preeclampsia or diabetes mellitus, as well as for high-risk newborns and children. We designed this information to enhance your preparation for the clinical setting.

Pathophysiology Illustrated boxes feature unique drawings that illustrate conditions on a cellular or organ level, and may also portray the step-by-step process of a disease. These images visually explain the pathophysiology of certain conditions to increase your understanding of the condition and its treatment.

The *SAFETY ALERT!* features present essential information that calls attention to issues that could place a patient or a nurse at risk and provide guidance on maintaining a safe environment for all patients and healthcare providers.

> **SAFETY ALERT!**
> Observe the child continuously for inability to swallow, absence of voice sounds, increasing degree of respiratory distress, and acute onset of drooling. A change in the child's level of consciousness—from anxiety to lethargy to stupor—occurs as hypoxia increases. If any of these signs occur, get medical assistance immediately. The quieter the child, the greater the cause for concern.

Teaching Highlights present special healthcare issues or problems and the related key teaching points to address with the family.

Each chapter ends with a **Critical Concept Review** that outlines the main points of the chapter as they relate to each Learning Outcome, a list of **References**, and directions to link to www.nursing.pearsonhighered.com for additional resources.

In addition, **cross-reference** icons help you to easily locate related information in other chapters. Important **laboratory values** are highlighted in a different color as a tool for you to assess your patients' conditions. Where relevant, SKILLS found in the companion book, *Clinical Skills Manual for Maternal & Child Nursing Care* (ISBN 0133145824), are cited.

Acknowledgments

Nursing is a dynamic, exciting healthcare profession. As curricula develop, many nursing programs have begun to teach nursing of childbearing families and nursing of children together in a single course. This combined format requires that faculty approach these two fields with a similar framework and philosophy, and with similar teaching methods, so that students can maximize learning. With this fourth edition, we have created a tool that will enable students to master these two critical areas of nursing—the care of childbearing families and the care of children. Creating a dynamic and integrated text would not be possible without the skill and dedication of a host of people.

We are grateful to Janet Houser, PhD, RN, for developing the Evidence-Based Practice boxes that are presented in the women's health and maternal–newborn sections of this textbook.

We would personally like to thank several people. Our thanks go to Julie Levin Alexander, our publisher. Julie is committed to excellence and creativity. She is the driving force behind the exciting changes occurring at Pearson Health Science and is truly a creative futurist in publishing.

For this edition we have been blessed to have two developmental editors who worked together astonishingly well: Lynda Hatch for the maternal–newborn chapters and Mary Cook for the pediatric chapters. Lynda and Mary challenged us creatively, ensured consistency, and kept us on track. They have been supportive, innovative, and unflappable during the long months of hard work. Thank you both for all you have done!

Special thanks to the people of S4Carlisle Communications, especially Lynn Steines, for coordinating production and moving things forward so effectively.

Finally we all wish to thank our other co-authors. As six individuals, but two teams, we came together with our own ideas, writing styles, and vision for this book. Over four editions we have grown closer in our collaboration, with productive discussions of important issues that have ultimately resulted in a new and different text for maternal, newborn, and child health nursing. We hope that this book and associated learning aids will be a useful tool for legions of nursing students to come.

Marcia L. London
Patricia W. Ladewig
Michele R. Davidson
Jane W. Ball
Ruth C. Bindler
Kay J. Cowen

Detailed Contents

CHAPTER
1

Contemporary Maternal, Newborn, and Child Health Nursing

Justin Pumfrey/Getty Images

My younger son turned 21 today—officially a man now. I remember so well the night he was born in a birthing room at our local hospital. I watched my husband rock our baby and talk to him just minutes after his birth. Over the years we sought emergency health care for our son several times—when he was diagnosed with asthma as a high school freshman, when he fell skateboarding and needed surgery to put three pins in his wrist, when he fell snowboarding and dislocated his shoulder. Active kids do get their share of bumps! It is easy to take good health care for granted, but we shouldn't. It can make all the difference. —Marjorie, 47

LEARNING OUTCOMES

1.1 Identify the nursing roles available to maternal-newborn and pediatric nurses.

1.2 Summarize the use of community-based nursing care in meeting the needs of childbearing and childrearing families.

1.3 Summarize the current status of factors related to health insurance and access to health care.

1.4 Relate the availability of statistical data to the formulation of further research questions.

1.5 Delineate significant legal and ethical issues that influence the practice of maternal-child nursing.

1.6 Discuss the role of evidence-based practice in improving the quality of nursing care for childbearing families.

Skilled nurses care for people, care about people, and use their expertise to help people care for themselves. This is the essence of nursing. Most nurses experience special moments professionally, times in which they know that they have practiced the essence of nursing and, in doing so, have touched the lives of others. For nurses who work with childbearing families or with children and their families, the rewards that come from skilled nursing practice can be especially rich.

This chapter focuses on introductory concepts related to the nurse and childbearing families, infants, children, and adolescents.

NURSING ROLES IN MATERNAL-CHILD NURSING

Traditionally, **maternal-child nursing** refers to the care of women during pregnancy, birth, and postpartum, as well as the care of infants, children, and adolescents. However, this label is somewhat misleading because it fails to acknowledge clearly the consideration due to fathers, partners, and family members. As nurses who work with families quickly learn, a holistic, inclusive approach is crucial to effective nursing care.

The nursing process provides the framework for delivery of direct nursing care. The nurse assesses the patient—whether childbearing woman, infant, child, or adolescent—and identifies the nursing diagnoses that describe the responses of the individual and family to the condition or area of needed knowledge. The nurse then implements and evaluates nursing care. This care is designed to meet specific physical and psychosocial needs. For children the care is tailored to the individual developmental stage, giving the child additional responsibility for self-care with increasing age.

Nurses play a major role in minimizing the psychologic and physical stress experienced by childbearing families and by children and their families. This often involves listening to concerns, being present during stressful or emotional experiences, and implementing strategies to help the individual and family members cope. Nurses help families by suggesting ways to support their loved one in the hospital, in community settings, and in the home. Nurses also suggest ways to support families with informational resources, family support groups, referral for healthcare services, and, in some cases, respite care.

Patient education is a major component of maternal-child nursing. During pregnancy, nurses provide anticipatory guidance to prepare the woman and her partner, if he or she is involved, for the changes that each month brings. For example, the woman is taught self-care measures to relieve discomforts and learns to identify the warning signs that she should report. Both partners receive information on the psychologic changes of pregnancy that they may experience. Education for the laboring woman focuses on activities that help her deal successfully with a challenging experience—childbirth—whereas postpartum teaching addresses the needs of the woman and her newborn to prepare them for discharge.

In pediatric nursing, education is especially challenging because nurses must be prepared to work with children at various levels of understanding and to include family members in all aspects of care. As patient educators, nurses help children adapt to the hospital setting and prepare them for procedures.

When a child is ill, most hospitals encourage a parent to stay with the child and to provide much of the direct and the supportive care under the guidance of a nurse. Nurses teach parents to watch for important signs and responses to therapies, to increase the child's comfort, and even to provide advanced care. Taking an active role during hospitalization helps prepare the parent to assume total responsibility for care after the child leaves the hospital.

Nurses also serve as advocates, acting to safeguard and advance the interests of families. To be an effective advocate, the nurse must be aware of the individual's needs, the family's needs and resources, and the healthcare services available in the hospital and the community. The nurse can then assist the family to make informed choices about these services and to act in their best interests. Nurses must also ensure that the policies and resources of healthcare agencies meet the psychosocial needs of childbearing women and of children and their families.

Developing Cultural Competence
Adapting the Reading Level of Patient Education Materials

Among U.S. adults, 20% read at a fifth-grade level or below, and 90 million people have difficulty using and understanding health information (Hawkins, Kantayya, & Sharkey-Asner, 2010). Healthcare materials need to be provided in the appropriate language and at the appropriate reading level. Printed materials to educate children and families about a health condition might be readily available, but they often are written at too high a reading level. The recommended reading level for educational materials is fifth or sixth grade equivalency (Hawkins et al., 2010). Even though printed material may be available in the primary language of the patient and family, do not assume that the family has reading skills in that language.

In developing patient education materials with a lower reading level:

- Use short, familiar words with one or two syllables and short sentences.
- Substitute simple language for a medical term.
- Use pictures or graphics to give directions when possible.
- Use lists and tables to simplify content.
- Use "must" to express a requirement.
- Divide the content into small sections and use headers.
- Color code information to help readers understand its importance.
- Use a computer program to evaluate the reading level of materials you develop.

Collaborative practice is a comprehensive model of health care that uses a multidisciplinary team of health professionals to provide high-quality, cost-effective care. In maternal-newborn settings the team generally includes certified nurse-midwives (see later discussion), physicians, nurse practitioners, nurses, and other health specialists such as pharmacists, lactation consultants, or childbirth educators. Similarly, the multidisciplinary team assembled when a child has a significant health problem or handicapping condition may include physicians, nurses, pediatric nurse practitioners, social workers, physical and occupational therapists, and other specialists. The team's goal is to create an interdisciplinary plan designed to meet the child's medical, nursing, developmental, educational, and psychosocial needs. Because nurses spend large amounts of time providing nursing care for the patient and family, they often are better informed than other healthcare professionals about the family's wishes and resources. As a member of the team, the nurse serves as an advocate to ensure that the plan of care considers the family's wishes and contains appropriate services.

Case management is a process of coordinating the delivery of healthcare services in a manner that focuses on both quality and cost outcomes. This is often a collaborative practice with other healthcare providers designed to promote continuity of care. The nurse case manager has control over the use of healthcare resources that are considered appropriate for the patient's condition and links the patient and family to these services. The goal is to help the individual and family have the best healthcare outcome and decrease fragmentation of care, while controlling the cost of healthcare services. In maternal-child nursing, case management is often used for a complicated high-risk pregnancy and for long-term care of children with chronic conditions.

Discharge planning is a form of case management. Effective discharge planning promotes a smooth, rapid, and safe transition into the community and improves the results of treatment begun in the hospital. To be a discharge planner, the nurse needs to know about community medical resources, appropriate home care agencies and community resources, reliable Internet sites, educational interventions, and services reimbursed by the individual's health plan or other financial resources.

In addition, several advanced-practice roles are available to maternal-child nurses with additional education. A **nurse practitioner (NP)**, who has specialized education in a doctor of nursing practice (DNP) program or a master's degree program, often provides ambulatory care services to pregnant women, newborns, children, adolescents, and families. The area of specialization determines the NP's title, so there are family nurse practitioners, neonatal nurse practitioners, pediatric nurse practitioners, women's health nurse practitioners, and so forth. NPs focus on physical and psychosocial assessments, including history, physical examination, and certain diagnostic tests and procedures. They make clinical judgments and begin appropriate treatments, seeking physician consultation when necessary. **Clinical nurse specialists (CNSs)** have a master's degree and specialized knowledge and competence in a specific clinical area. They often are found on mother-baby units, on pediatric units, and in intensive care units assisting staff to provide excellent, evidence-based care. The **certified nurse-midwife (CNM)** is educated in the two disciplines of nursing and midwifery and is certified by the American College of Nurse-Midwives. The CNM is prepared to manage independently the care of women at low risk for complications during pregnancy, birth, and the postpartum period, as well as the care of healthy newborns (Figure 1–1 ●).

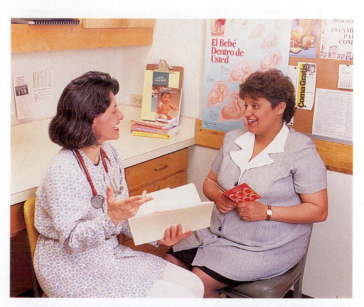

● **Figure 1–1**   A certified nurse-midwife confers with her patient.

The **nurse researcher** has an advanced doctoral degree, typically a Ph.D., and assumes a leadership role in generating new research. Nurse researchers are typically found in university settings although more and more hospitals are employing them to conduct research relevant to patient care, administrative issues, and the like.

FAMILY-CENTERED MATERNAL-CHILD CARE

Contemporary childbirth is family centered—that is, characterized by an emphasis on the family and the family's choices about their birth experience. Consequently, today the concept of family-centered childbirth is accepted and encouraged. Fathers and partners are active participants, not simply bystanders; siblings are encouraged to visit and meet the newest family member, and they may even attend the birth.

New definitions of family are evolving. For example, the family of a single mother may include her mother, her sister, another relative, a close friend, a same-sex partner, or the father of the child. Many cultures also recognize the importance of extended families, and several family members may provide care and support. See Chapter 2 🔗 for an in-depth discussion of family and culture.

In pediatric settings, *family-centered care* is a dynamic, deliberate approach to building collaborative relationships between health professionals and families that is respectful of their diversity and beliefs about the nature of children's health conditions and ways to manage them. It is designed to meet the emotional, social, and developmental needs of children and families seeking health care. The family is the principal caregiver and center of strength and support for the child (Figure 1–2 ●). As partners in the child's care, the family needs to learn about the child's condition and participate in decisions regarding his or her care. The Society of Pediatric

Nurses and the American Nurses Association have established practice guidelines for family-centered care. See Table 1–1 for concepts of family-centered care.

Contemporary Childbirth

Contemporary childbirth is characterized by an increasing number of choices about the birth experience. The family can make choices about the primary caregiver (physician, certified nurse-midwife [CNM], or certified midwife); the use of a *doula* to provide labor support (see Chapter 8 🔗 for more information about doulas); and birth-related experiences such as the method of childbirth preparation, position for birth, and use of analgesia and anesthesia, as well as breastfeeding and childcare choices.

Many women elect to have their pregnancy and birth managed by a CNM. Some women choose to receive care from a direct-entry certified midwife or even a lay midwife, who is an unlicensed or uncertified midwife trained through an informal

Table 1–1	Concepts of Family-Centered Care

- The family is acknowledged as the constant in the child's life and a partner in the child's health care.
- The family, child, and health professionals work together in the best interest of the child and the family. Over time, the child assumes a partnership role in his or her healthcare.
- Health professionals listen to and respect the skills and expertise that the family brings to the relationship.
- Trust is a fundamental element of the relationship between the family, child, and health professionals.
- Communication occurs in an open, unbiased manner and is ongoing.
- Families, children, and health professionals make decisions regarding the child's care in a collaborative manner in all health-care settings and for all types of health care needed (e.g., health promotion, health maintenance, acute care, chronic condition care, and end-of-life care). Negotiation may be involved in collaborative decision making.
- The child is supported to learn about and participate in his or her health care and decision making. The adolescent is supported to assume a partnership role in his or her health care and in the transition to adult health care.
- The racial, ethnic, cultural, and socioeconomic background of the family and child, as well as family traditions, are honored. Health professionals work to integrate these values and the preferences of the family and child when planning and providing health care.
- Family-to-family and peer support is encouraged.
- Healthcare settings develop policies, procedures, practices, and systems that are family friendly and family centered; they support the choices the family and child will make regarding care.
- Health information for children and families is available and provided to match the range of cultural and linguistic diversity in the community as well as the health literacy levels.

Source: Data from Goode, T., & Jones, W. (2006). *A guide for advancing family-centered and culturally and linguistically competent care.* Washington, DC: National Center for Cultural Competence, Georgetown University Center for Child and Human Development; Lewandowski, L. A., & Tesler, M. D. (Eds.). (2003). Family-centered care: Putting it into action. *The SPN/ANA Guide to Family-Centered Care.* Washington, DC: American Nurses Association; Committee on Hospital Care, & Institute for Patient and Family-Centered Care. (2012). Patient- and family-centered care and the pediatrician's role. *Pediatrics, 129*(2), 394–404.

● **Figure 1–2** Many facilities now encourage family visitation for children with health problems who require long-term hospitalization. Extended family visits enable parents to learn about the child's care and provide siblings with opportunities to interact with the hospitalized child.

route such as apprenticeship or self-study rather than a formal educational program (Midwives Alliance of North America [MANA], 2009). Midwives who complete a direct-entry midwifery education program that meets the standards established by the American College of Nurse-Midwives (ACNM) may take a certification exam to become a *certified midwife (CM)* (ACNM, 2009).

The North American Registry of Midwives (NARM) is also a certification agency. Midwives certified through NARM may become midwives through a formal educational program at a college, university, or midwifery school, or through apprenticeship or self-study. They are eligible to use the credential *certified professional midwife (CPM)* (MANA, 2009).

The place of birth is an important decision. Birthing centers and special homelike labor-delivery-recovery-postpartum (LDRP) rooms in hospitals have become increasingly popular. Some women choose to give birth at home, although healthcare professionals do not generally recommend this approach. Most professionals are concerned that, in the event of an unanticipated complication, delay in receiving emergency care might jeopardize the well-being or even the life of the mother or her infant. Some CNMs do attend home births; however, the majority of home births are attended by CMs, CPMs, or lay midwives. In 2006, just over half of 1% (0.59%) of births occurred at home. Of those, 61% were attended by midwives. Of the midwife-attended home births, only one fourth (27%) were done by CNMs (MacDorman, Menacker, & Declerq, 2010).

Contemporary Care of Children

As of the 2010 national census, an estimated 83.3 million children and youth under 20 years of age live in the United States, and they account for approximately 27% of the population (U.S. Census Bureau, 2011). (See Figure 1–3 ● for a distribution of the population by age group.)

Pediatric nursing is a specialized area of nursing that focuses on caring for children in many different settings within the hospital and the community. These settings include the following:

■ Various hospital units, such as pediatric units, intensive care units, emergency departments, radiology, rehabilitation units, and specialty care clinics

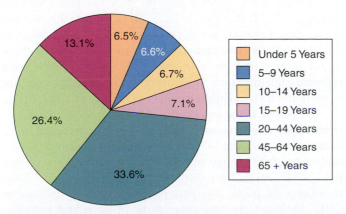

● Figure 1–3 In 2010, children from birth to 19 years of age accounted for approximately 27% of the total population of the United States.

■ Physician offices, healthcare centers, clinics

■ Schools, childcare centers, homeless shelters, and camps

■ The child's home

Pediatric health care occurs along a continuum that reflects not only the various settings of care, but also the complexity and range of care needed by individual children and their families. For example, all children need health promotion and health maintenance care, but some children need care for chronic conditions, acute illnesses and injuries, and even end-of-life care. See Figure 1–4 ● for the model of pediatric health care used in this textbook.

Managing the child's transition from the hospital to another setting involves planning the discharge, implementing interdisciplinary plans, ensuring that the family understands the aspects of care they need to provide, helping the family to develop an emergency care plan in the event their child has an unexpected healthcare crisis, and collaborating with a broad range of healthcare professionals.

● Figure 1–4 The Bindler-Ball Continuum of Pediatric Health Care for Children and Their Families. The outer bars represent the family, cultural, and community influences on the care that the child receives, either through the services sought by the family or the services provided in the community. Cultural influences include the family's values and beliefs, and the cultural competence of the nurse in caring for a child and family.

The inner categories represent the range of health care needed by children. All children need health promotion and health maintenance services, represented by the base of the triangle. Notice the arrows representing the upward and downward movement between the levels of care as the child's condition changes.

Children may be healthy with episodic acute illnesses and injuries. Some children develop a chronic condition for which specialized health care is needed. A child's chronic condition may be well controlled, but acute episodes (such as with asthma) or other illnesses and injuries may occur, and the child also needs health promotion and health maintenance services. Some children develop a life-threatening illness and ultimately need end-of-life care. A healthy child may also experience a catastrophic injury leading to death and the family needs supportive end-of-life care.

Source: Bindler & Ball, 2007.

Maternal-Child Care in the Community

Primary care is the focus of much attention as caregivers search for a new, more effective direction for health care. Primary care includes a focus on health promotion, illness prevention, and individual responsibility for one's own health. These services are best provided in community-based settings. Healthcare payers are beginning to recognize the importance of primary care in containing costs and maintaining health. Community-based healthcare systems that provide primary care and some secondary care are becoming available in schools, workplaces, homes, churches, clinics, transitional care programs, and other ambulatory settings.

The growth and diversity of health payer plans offer both opportunities and challenges for women's and children's health care. Opportunities for improved delivery of screening and preventive services exist in community-based models of coordinated and comprehensive well-woman and well-child care. A challenge that health payer plans face is how to relate to essential community providers of care, such as family-planning clinics, women's health centers, and child health centers, that offer a unique service or serve groups of women and children with special needs (adolescents, women and children with disabilities, and ethnic or racial minorities).

Community-based care remains an essential element of health care for uninsured or underinsured individuals, as well as for individuals who benefit from programs such as Medicare, Medicaid, or the Children's Health Insurance Program (CHIP). Some of these programs are broad based, such as those offered through public health departments, while others, such as parenting classes for adolescents, are geared to the needs of a specific population.

Maternal-child nurses are especially sensitive to these changes in healthcare delivery because the vast majority of health care provided to childbearing and childrearing families takes place outside of hospitals in clinics, offices, and community-based organizations. In addition, maternal-child nurses offer specialized services such as childbirth preparation classes, sibling classes, and parenting classes.

Healthcare reform has increased the emphasis on the need for individuals to have a *medical home* or *healthcare home*—a continuous, comprehensive, family-centered, and compassionate source of health care. This is especially important for children throughout their developmental years. Criteria for a medical or healthcare home for children include being well known by a physician or nurse who provides the usual source of sick care and having access to specialty care and other services or therapies. In addition, the healthcare provider spends adequate time communicating clearly with the family, provides help with care coordination when needed, respects the family's values and partners with the family in the child's care, and provides interpreters when necessary. An estimated 57.5% of U.S. children have a healthcare home that meets these criteria (Health Resources and Services Administration, 2009).

The current trend toward shorter hospital stays can end in the discharge of individuals who still require support, assistance, and teaching. Health care provided in a patient's home helps fill this gap. Home care also enables infants, children, and women to remain at home with conditions that formerly would have required hospitalization.

Nurses are major providers of home care services. Home care nurses perform direct nursing care and also supervise unlicensed assistive personnel who provide less skilled levels of service. In a home setting, nurses use their skills in assessment, intervention, communication, teaching, problem solving, and organization to meet the needs of childbearing and childrearing families. They also play a major role in coordinating services from other providers, such as physical therapists or lactation consultants.

Postpartum and newborn home visits help ensure a satisfactory transition from the birthing center to the home. This positive trend meets the needs of childbearing families and should become standard practice. See Chapter 30 🔗 for discussion of home care and guidance about making a home visit. Information on home care is also provided as appropriate throughout this text.

Many children with serious chronic conditions and disabilities assisted by technology are now cared for at home by families rather than by long-term hospitalization. After studies in the 1980s found that home health care was substantially less expensive than hospital care, Congress amended laws to permit payment of home care services with federal funds, such as through Medicaid. Children with conditions considered fatal 15 years ago are thriving with home care and are participating in family, community, and school life. See Chapter 39 🔗.

Complementary Care

Interest in complementary care, previously termed complementary and alternative therapies (CAM), continues to grow nationwide and affects the care of childbearing and childrearing families. Complementary care includes a wide array of therapies, such as acupuncture, acupressure, therapeutic touch, biofeedback, massage therapy, meditation, herbal therapies, and homeopathic remedies. Concepts related to the use of complementary care by families are presented in more detail in Chapter 2 🔗 and in special boxed features throughout the text.

ACCESS TO HEALTH CARE

In 2009, healthcare expenditures in the United States were $2.5 trillion, a 4% increase over the previous year (National Center for Health Statistics [NCHS], 2011). Despite this increase in spending, however, not all pregnant women and children in the United States have access to health care. In 2010, 18.2% of people in the United States, or roughly 48.3 million people, were without health insurance. This includes 22.3% of adults under age 65 years and 8.3% of children under age 19 years (NCHS, 2011).

For people living in poverty, Medicaid and the Children's Health Insurance Program (CHIP) are the most prevalent forms of insurance, covering 17% of the population under age 65, including pregnant women who fall into specified income categories (NCHS, 2011). More than two thirds of uninsured children are eligible for public insurance programs such as Medicaid or CHIP. Medicaid provides coverage to children and individuals with disabilities who meet income level qualifications set by

Clinical Tip

The federal poverty rate is used to determine eligibility for many health and welfare services. The rate is a sliding scale based on the number of people in the family, and it is updated annually. For example, the poverty rate for a family of four in 2011 was $22,350 (Centers for Medicare and Medicaid Services, 2011).

the state. Children covered under the Temporary Assistance to Needy Families (TANF) program are usually eligible.

For women who become pregnant, early prenatal care is one of the most important approaches available to reduce adverse pregnancy outcomes. In 2008, 70.7% of pregnant women in the United States who had live births began prenatal care in the first trimester. However, these percentages vary significantly among groups, with black or African American, Hispanic or Latina, and Native American women less likely to receive early and adequate prenatal care than white and Asian women (NCHS, 2011).

Uninsured children often do not have a usual source of health care and have difficulty obtaining basic preventive health care, including immunizations or care for chronic conditions. When children are enrolled in CHIP, their health care improves with significantly increased access to care, and their families experience fewer financial burdens (Smith-Campbell & Pile, 2010).

Healthy People 2020 Goals

For 30 years the federal government's *Healthy People* program has been providing science-based, national agendas for improving the health of all Americans. "The Healthy People initiative is grounded in the principle that setting national objectives and monitoring progress can motivate action, and indeed, in just the last decade, preliminary analyses indicate that the country has either progressed toward or met 71 percent of its *Healthy People* targets" (U.S. Department of Health and Human Services, 2011, p. 1). In December 2010 the next 10-year effort, *Healthy People 2020*, was launched. *Healthy People 2020* is grouped by topic area and objectives. Maternal-newborn, pediatric, and women's health nurses focus directly on many of the topics, including these:

- Maternal, infant, and child health
- Adolescent health (new to the list)
- Family planning
- Injury and violence prevention
- Lesbian, gay, bisexual, and transgender health (new)
- Sexually transmitted infections

Because of the role women play in maintaining their family's health, many other topics may also be of importance to women, such as immunization and infectious diseases, diabetes, and nutrition and weight status, to name but a few. Nurses of all disciplines will find it helpful to become familiar with the 2020 topics and objectives, which may be found at the *Healthy People* website.

Culturally Competent Care

The population of the United States daily becomes more diverse. Approximately 46% of all children younger than 18 years of age are from families of minority populations (Federal Interagency Forum on Child and Family Statistics, 2012). Thus, it is vitally important for a nurse who cares for women and children to recognize the importance of a family's cultural values and beliefs, which may be quite different from those of the nurse.

Specific elements that contribute to a family's value system include the following:

- Religion and social beliefs
- Presence and influence of the extended family, as well as socialization within the ethnic group
- Communication patterns
- Beliefs and understanding about the concepts of health and illness
- Permissible physical contact with strangers
- Education

When the family's cultural values are incorporated into the care plan, the family is more likely to accept and comply with the needed care, especially in the home care setting. It is important for nurses to avoid imposing personal cultural values on the families and children in their care. By learning about the values of the different ethnic groups in the community, nurses can develop an individualized nursing care plan for each child and family.

Because of the importance of culturally competent care, this topic is discussed in more depth in Chapter 2 🔗 and throughout the book in special boxed features.

STATISTICAL DATA AND MATERNAL-CHILD CARE

Health-related statistics provide an objective basis for projecting patient needs, planning the use of resources, and determining the effectiveness of specific treatments. Statistics are used to help identify certain healthcare trends and high-risk target groups. The following sections discuss descriptive statistics that are particularly important to maternal-child health care.

Developing Cultural Competence
Cultural Conflicts

Conflicts can occur within a family when the traditional rituals and practices of the family do not conform with current healthcare practices. Nurses need to be sensitive to these potential conflicts when managing a child's health care, especially after the child has been discharged from the hospital. When cultural values are not part of the nursing care plan, parents may be forced to decide whether the family's beliefs should take priority over the healthcare professional's guidance.

Birth Rate

Birth rate refers to the number of live births per 1000 people in a given population. Worldwide, birth rates vary dramatically as Table 1–2 indicates. In the United States in 2010, the total number of births declined by 3% to 3,999,386. This is significant because it is the largest absolute decrease since 1971–72. Birth rates decreased for women in all age groups under 40. The rate for women ages 40 to 44 increased and the rate for women ages 45 to 49 was unchanged (Martin et al., 2012).

Statistics also indicate that the caesarean birth rate in 2010 was 32.8%, down from the record high of 32.9% in 2009. This rate has increased by nearly 60% from 20.7 in 1996 (Martin et al., 2012).

The statistics do raise questions. For example: What is the impact of cultural differences and changing societal values on birth rates? Do birth rates change when access to information on contraception increases? What role does government policy, such as China's legislation limiting births to one child per family, play?

Maternal Mortality

The **maternal mortality rate** is the number of deaths from causes related to or aggravated by pregnancy or the management of pregnancy during the pregnancy cycle (including the 42-day postpartum period) per 100,000 live births. It does not include deaths of pregnant women due to external causes such as accidents, homicides, and suicides. The maternal mortality rate in the United States in 2007 was 12.7 deaths per 100,000 live births. However, black women have a significantly higher risk of maternal death than white women. The maternal mortality rate for black women was 26.5 deaths per 100,000 live births as compared to 10 deaths for white women. The maternal mortality rate for Hispanic women is cited as 8.9, but inconsistencies in reporting Hispanic origin on death certificates and on censuses and surveys make this number less precise (Xu, Kochanek, Murphy, et al., 2010).

Factors influencing the long-term decrease in maternal mortality include the increased use of hospitals and specialized healthcare personnel by maternity patients, the establishment of care centers for high-risk mothers and infants, the prevention and control of infection with antibiotics and improved techniques, the availability of blood products for transfusions, and the lowered rates of anesthesia-related deaths. Additional factors may be identified by asking the following research questions: Is there a correlation between maternal mortality and age? Is there a correlation between maternal mortality and availability of health care? Economic status?

Infant Mortality

The **infant mortality rate** is the number of deaths of infants under 1 year of age per 1000 live births in a given population. *Neonatal mortality* is the number of deaths of infants less than 28 days of age per 1000 live births, *perinatal mortality* includes both neonatal deaths and fetal deaths per 1000 live births, and *fetal death* is death in utero at 20 weeks or more gestation.

Table 1–2	Live Birth Rates and Infant Mortality Rates for Selected Countries (2012 est.)	
Country	Birth Rate*	Infant Mortality Rate**
Afghanistan	39.3	121.6
Argentina	17.3	10.5
Australia	12.3	4.6
Cambodia	25.2	54.1
Canada	10.3	4.9
China	12.3	15.6
Egypt	24.2	24.2
Germany	8.3	3.5
Ghana	32	41
India	20.6	46.1
Iraq	28.2	40.3
Japan	8.4	2.2
Mexico	18.9	16.8
Russia	12.3	7.3
Somalia	42.1	103.7
United Kingdom	12.3	4.6
United States	13.7	6

*The number of live births per 1000 people in a given population.
**The number of deaths to all infants less than 1 year of age per 1000 live births.
Source: Data from *The World Fact Book 2012.* Washington, DC: The Central Intelligence Agency.

In 2009, the infant mortality rate in the United States was 6.39 per 1000 live births. This rate varied widely by the race of the mother. Infant mortality rates were highest among non-Hispanic black or African American women (12.64 per 1000 live births). This compares with 5.3 among non-Hispanic white women (Kochanek, Xu, Murphy, et al., 2011). Infant mortality rates are higher among infants born in multiple births, infants born prematurely, and those born to unmarried mothers; rates are also higher for infants of teen mothers (9.59) and mothers ages 40 and older (8.07) (Mathews & MacDorman, 2012).

Figure 1–5 ● identifies the five leading causes of infant death (Heron, 2012).

The U.S. infant mortality rate continues to be an area of concern because the United States has fallen to 30th place in infant mortality rankings among industrialized nations. Much of this

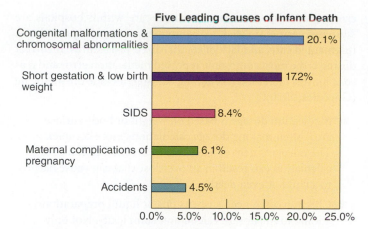

Five Leading Causes of Infant Death

Cause	%
Congenital malformations & chromosomal abnormalities	20.1%
Short gestation & low birth weight	17.2%
SIDS	8.4%
Maternal complications of pregnancy	6.1%
Accidents	4.5%

● **Figure 1–5** Of the five leading causes of infant death, nearly 40% can be attributed to pregnancy or birth-related problems including congenital malformations and chromosomal abnormalities, short gestation and low birth weight, and maternal complications of pregnancy.

Source: National Center for Health Statistics, 2011.

rate can be attributed to the high percentage of preterm births in the United States (MacDorman & Mathews, 2009). Healthcare professionals, policy makers, and the public continue to stress the need for better prenatal care, coordination of health services, and provision of comprehensive maternal-child services in the United States.

Table 1–2 identifies infant mortality rates for selected countries. As the data indicate, the range is dramatic among the countries listed. Information about birth rates and mortality rates is limited for some countries because of a lack of organized reporting mechanisms.

The information raises questions about access to health care during pregnancy and after birth and about standards of living, nutrition, and sociocultural factors. Additional factors affecting the infant mortality rate may be identified by considering the following research questions: What are the leading causes of infant mortality in each country? Why do mortality rates differ among racial groups?

Pediatric Mortality

The most common cause of death in 2010 for U.S. children between 1 and 19 years of age was unintentional injury. For children ages 1 to 9 years, other leading causes of death include congenital anomalies, cancer, homicide, and diseases of the heart. For older children and adolescents ages 10 to 19 years, other leading causes of death include cancer, homicide, suicide, congenital anomalies, and diseases of the heart (NCHS, 2011).

Motor vehicle traffic-related crashes were the major cause of unintentional injury in all children ages 5 to 19. In children ages 1 to 4, the leading cause of unintentional injury was drowning, followed by pedestrian-related injuries, fires and burns, and motor vehicle crashes. In children ages 5 to 9 and 10 to 14, pedestrian accidents followed motor vehicle transportation-related injuries as the most common cause of unintentional death. However, for youth ages 15 to 19 years, poisoning was the next most common cause of unintentional

injury (National Center for Health Statistics, National Vital Statistics System, 2011).

Pediatric Morbidity

Morbidity—an illness or injury that limits activity, requires medical attention or hospitalization, or results in a chronic condition—also varies according to the age of the child. In 2009, there were 6.4 million hospital discharges for children in the United States between birth and 17 years of age. Approximately 72% of hospitalizations were for infants under age 1 year, which includes newborns (Yu, Wier, & Elixhauser, 2011). Respiratory diseases are a leading cause of hospitalization in children of all ages. Injury and poisoning are also a leading cause of hospitalization. Mental disorders were the leading cause of hospitalization in children between 10 and 17 years of age. Pregnancy and childbirth were the leading causes of hospitalization for female adolescents between 15 and 21 years of age (Agency for Healthcare Research and Quality, 2011).

Implications for Nursing Practice

Nurses can use statistics in a number of ways. For example, they can use statistical data to:

- Determine populations at risk.
- Assess the relationship between specific factors.
- Help establish databases for specific patient populations.
- Determine the levels of care needed by particular patient populations.
- Evaluate the success of specific nursing interventions.
- Determine priorities in caseloads.
- Estimate staffing and equipment needs of hospital units and clinics.
- Apply for funding to support health needs.

Nurses who use statistical information are better prepared to promote the health needs of maternal, newborn, and pediatric patients and their families.

LEGAL CONSIDERATIONS IN MATERNAL-CHILD NURSING

Scope of Practice

The *scope of practice* is defined as the limits of nursing practice set forth in state statutes. Although some state practice acts continue to limit nursing practice to the traditional responsibilities of providing patient care related to health maintenance and disease prevention, most state practice acts cover expanded practice roles that include collaboration with other health professionals in planning and providing care, physician-delegated diagnosis and prescriptive privilege, and the delegation of direct care tasks to other specified licensed and unlicensed personnel. A nurse must function within the scope of practice or risk being accused of practicing medicine without a license.

Standards of Nursing Care

Standards of care establish minimum criteria for competent, proficient delivery of nursing care. Such standards are designed to protect the public and are used to judge the quality of care provided. Legal interpretation of actions within standards of care is based on what a reasonably prudent nurse with similar education and experience would do in similar circumstances.

The American Nurses Association (ANA) has published standards of practice for maternal-child health. ANA, the National Association of Pediatric Nurse Practitioners, and the Society of Pediatric Nurses (2008) collaborated on the development of standards for pediatric clinical nursing practice. The ANA and the National Association of Neonatal Nurses also published the scope and standards of practice for neonatal nursing (2004). Specialty organizations such as the Association of Women's Health, Obstetric and Neonatal Nurses (AWHONN) continue to set the standards of professional nursing practice in the care of women and newborns. Agency policies, procedures, and protocols also provide appropriate guidelines for care standards. For example, **clinical practice guidelines** and critical pathways are comprehensive interdisciplinary care plans for a specific condition that describe the sequence and timing of interventions that should result in expected patient outcomes. Clinical practice guidelines or critical pathways are adopted within a healthcare setting to reduce variation in care management, to limit costs of care, and to evaluate the effectiveness of care.

While standards of care do not carry the force of law, they have important legal significance. Any nurse who fails to meet appropriate standards of care invites allegations of negligence or malpractice. Practicing within the guidelines established by an agency or following local or national standards decreases the potential for litigation.

Patient Safety

The Joint Commission, a nongovernmental agency that audits the operation of hospitals and healthcare facilities, has identified patient safety as an important responsibility of healthcare providers and provides an annual list of specific patient safety goals. Specific criteria that healthcare facilities must meet for accreditation can be found on the Joint Commission website.

Safety is a major focus of nursing education programs. The Quality and Safety Education for Nurses (QSEN) project, established in 2005, is designed "to meet the challenge of preparing future nurses who will have the knowledge, skills and attitudes (KSAs) necessary to continuously improve the quality and safety of the healthcare systems within which they work" (p. 1) (QSEN, 2011). The project focuses on competencies in six areas: (1) patient-centered care, (2) teamwork and collaboration, (3) evidence-based practice, (4) quality improvement, (5) safety, and (6) informatics. To support the efforts of the Joint Commission and to draw special attention to the importance of the QSEN project's emphasis on safety, key issues related to safety are noted throughout this text with the words *SAFETY ALERT!* in red. See page 32 for an example.

Infants and children are at a higher risk for medical error than others and also may be more vulnerable to harm from errors made. Most errors in medical care within hospitals are "systems" errors related to equipment, complex procedures, fragmented care, and lack of standardized procedures. Incorrect dosing is the most commonly reported medication error and reasons for this increased risk among children include the following (Gonzales, 2010):

- Medication dosage is based on weight or body surface area, often making dosage calculations more complex. The misplacement of a decimal in the medication dosage calculation can result in an overdose that can cause harm to a child or even death.

- Children often need suspensions or liquid preparations, adding to the dosage calculation complexity. Not only must the correct dose be calculated, but also the amount of liquid preparation with that dose. Some medications are in concentrations that require dilution, further complicating the accurate medication dosage calculation. See Chapter 41 ⊘ in the text and Chapters 11 and 12 in the *Clinical Skills Manual* SKILLS for more information about medication administration to children.

- Medications not yet approved for use in children by the U.S. Food and Drug Administration (FDA) are sometimes prescribed before pediatric dosage guidelines have been established.

- Young children cannot communicate well if they are having a reaction to the medication.

Limited English proficiency may also be a potential source of medical error for childbearing women and children. In such cases a risk exists for errors in interpretation—either of what the health professional says or what the family member understands. Healthcare facilities are actively working to implement strategies that will reduce medical errors in all child patients.

Informed Consent

Informed consent is a legal concept that protects a person's right to autonomy and self-determination by specifying that no action may be taken without that individual's prior understanding and freely given consent. Although this policy is actively enforced for major procedures, surgery, or regional anesthesia, it pertains to any nursing, medical, or surgical intervention. To touch a person without consent (except in an emergency) constitutes *battery* (Foederer, 2007). Consent is not informed unless the patient, or parent in the case of a child, understands the recommended procedures or treatments, their rationales, the benefits of each, alternative treatments, and any associated risks. When possible, it is important to have translators available for non–English-speaking women and families.

The person, usually the physician, who is ultimately responsible for the treatment or procedure should provide the information necessary to obtain informed consent. In such cases the nurse's role is to witness the patient's signature (or the parent's signature for a child) giving consent. The nurse may also serve as a witness if parents give verbal consent by telephone. If the nurse determines that the individual does not understand the procedure or risks, the nurse must notify the physician, who must then provide additional information to ensure that the consent is informed. The nurse also responds to questions asked by adult patients or by parents and children. Anxiety, fear, pain, and medications that alter consciousness may influence an individual's ability to give informed consent. An oral consent is legal, but written consent is easier to defend in a court of law.

Children under 18 or 21 years of age, depending on state law, can legally give informed consent in the following circumstances (American Academy of Pediatrics, 2011):

- The minor is a parent or is pregnant.

- The adolescent is a legally **emancipated minor** (self-supporting adolescents under 18 years of age, not living at home, married, or on active duty in the military). In most states, a pregnant teen is considered emancipated.

- In some states, **mature minors** (14- to 18-year-old adolescents who are able to understand treatment risks) can give independent consent for treatment or refuse treatment for some limited conditions such as testing and treatment for sexually transmitted infections, family planning, drug and alcohol abuse, blood donation, and mental health care (Figure 1–6 ●) (Levetown & Committee on Bioethics, 2008).

Refusal of a treatment, medication, or procedure after appropriate information is provided also requires that the individual sign a form releasing the doctor and clinical facility from liability resulting from the effects of such a refusal. Jehovah's Witnesses' refusal of blood transfusions is an example of such refusal.

Nurses are responsible for educating patients about any nursing care. Before each nursing intervention, the maternal-child nurse lets the individual and/or family know what to expect, thus ensuring cooperation and obtaining consent. Afterward the nurse documents the teaching and the learning outcomes in the person's record. The importance of clear, concise, and complete nursing records cannot be overemphasized. These records are evidence that the nurse obtained consent, performed prescribed treatments, reported important observations to the appropriate staff, and adhered to acceptable standards of care.

Because children are not considered competent to make healthcare decisions, parents, as the legal custodians of minor children, are customarily requested to give informed consent on behalf of a child. Both children and parents must understand that they have the right to refuse treatment at any time. In an emergency, consent for treatment to preserve life or limb is not required. When parents are divorced, some states limit the parental rights to give informed consent to the parent with custody. When parents have joint custody, in most cases either may give consent. The nurse should obtain legal advice from the facility's designated legal experts for complex family issues related to guardianship, divorced parents disagreeing over care, or a caregiver who is not the legal guardian.

Parents or guardians have absolute authority to make choices about their child's health care except in certain cases. Specifically:

- When the parents' choice of treatment does not permit lifesaving treatment for the child

- When there is a potential conflict of interest between the child and parents, such as with suspected child abuse or neglect

In some cases the court may be requested to appoint a proxy decision maker for the child or to determine that the child is capable of making a major treatment decision.

Children should become more actively involved in decision making about treatment procedures as their reasoning skills develop. Children too young to give informed consent can be given age-appropriate information about their condition and asked about their care preferences. Their parents, however, make ultimate decisions about their care.

With regard to children's participation in research, federal guidelines state that children 7 years of age and older must receive information about a research project and give assent (the voluntary agreement to participate in a research project or to accept treatment) before they are enrolled. Children should be given adequate time to ask questions and be told that they have the right to refuse to participate in the study. The child is then asked if he or she wishes to participate. If the child assents, parents then provide signed permission for the child to participate in the research project.

● **Figure 1–6** Marvin, a 15-year-old boy with acute nonlymphocytic leukemia, has definite opinions about his treatment. His parents have a difficult time accepting his opinions when they differ from their own. At what age can children make an informed decision about whether to accept or refuse treatment?

● Growth and Development

By 7 or 8 years of age, a child is able to understand concrete explanations about informed consent for research participation. By age 11, a child's abstract reasoning and logic abilities are advanced. By age 14, an adolescent can weigh options and make decisions regarding consent as capably as an adult.

Right to Privacy

The *right to privacy* is the right of a person to keep his or her person and property free from public scrutiny. To protect this right for patients and families, only those responsible for their care should conduct an examination or discuss their case.

The right to privacy is protected by state constitutions, statutes, and common law. The ANA, the National League for Nursing (NLN), and the Joint Commission have adopted professional standards protecting the privacy of patients. Healthcare agencies should also have written policies dealing with patient privacy. The Health Insurance Portability and Accountability Act of 1996 (HIPAA), which was fully implemented in 2002, also has a provision to guarantee the security and privacy of health information.

Laws, standards, and policies about privacy specify that information about an individual's treatment, condition, and prognosis can be shared only by health professionals responsible for his or her care. Information considered vital statistics (name, age, occupation, and so on) may be revealed legally, but is often withheld because of ethical considerations. The patient should be consulted as to what information may be released and to whom.

Clinical Tip

Concerns about privacy and the fear of disclosure of sensitive information to parents is a major reason why adolescents do not seek health care (Shapiro, 2010). Breaching confidentiality is a potential problem for adolescents, who are just learning whom they can trust in the healthcare system. Make sure you openly discuss the limits of confidentiality for such things as mandatory reporting requirements with the patient and family. Inadvertent disclosure of personal information may lead to psychologic, social, or physical harm in some patients.

Patient Self-Determination Act

The federal Patient Self-Determination Act directs healthcare institutions to inform hospitalized patients about their rights, which include expressing a preference for treatment options and making **advance directives** (writing a living will or authorizing a durable power of attorney for healthcare decisions on the individual's behalf). Nurses often discuss these issues with patients and their families. Minor children and their parents should also be informed of their rights. Adolescents with serious acute or chronic conditions with a higher risk of death should be encouraged to talk with their parents about their healthcare wishes and to prepare advance directives jointly.

Do-not-resuscitate (DNR) (or *allow natural death [AND]*) orders have become more common for children with terminal illnesses in which no further aggressive treatments are available or desired. In many cases these children are cared for at home or in a hospice program. Implementation of DNR orders for such children then becomes a community issue, to ensure that resuscitation measures are not initiated by any emergency care provider when the child has a life-threatening event. State health policies must be developed so children with these signed orders are easily identified and appropriate documentation of the orders is on file.

ETHICAL ISSUES IN MATERNAL-CHILD NURSING

Although ethical dilemmas confront nurses in all areas of practice, those related to pregnancy, birth, newborns, and children seem especially difficult to resolve.

Maternal-Fetal Conflict

Until fairly recently the fetus was viewed legally as a nonperson. Mother and fetus were viewed as one complex patient—the pregnant woman—of which the fetus was an essential part. However, advances in technology have permitted the physician to treat the fetus and monitor fetal development. The fetus is increasingly viewed as a patient separate from the mother. This focus on the fetus intensified in 2002 when President George W. Bush announced that "unborn children" would qualify for government healthcare benefits. This move was designed to promote prenatal care, but it represented the first time that any U.S. federal policy had defined childhood as starting at conception.

Most women are strongly motivated to protect the health and well-being of their fetus. In some instances, however, women have refused interventions on behalf of the fetus, and forced interventions have occurred. These include forced cesarean birth, coercion of mothers who practice high-risk behaviors such as substance abuse to enter treatment, and, perhaps most controversial, mandated experimental in utero therapy or surgery in an attempt to correct a specific birth defect. These interventions infringe on the autonomy of the mother. They may also be detrimental to the baby if, as a result, maternal bonding is hindered, the mother is afraid to seek prenatal care, or the mother is herself harmed by the actions taken.

Attempts have also been made to criminalize the behavior of women who fail to follow a physician's advice or who engage in behaviors (such as substance abuse) that are considered harmful to the fetus. This raises two thorny questions: (1) What practices should be monitored? and (2) Who will determine when the behaviors pose such a risk to the fetus that the courts should intervene?

The American College of Obstetricians and Gynecologists (ACOG) Committee on Ethics has affirmed the fundamental right of pregnant women to make informed, uncoerced decisions about medical interventions and has taken a direct stand against coercive and punitive approaches to the maternal-fetal relationship (ACOG, 2005).

Both ACOG and the American Academy of Pediatrics recognize that cases of maternal-fetal conflict involve two patients, both of whom deserve respect and treatment. Such cases are best resolved by using internal hospital mechanisms, including counseling, the intervention of specialists, and consultation with an institutional ethics committee. Court intervention should be considered a last resort, appropriate only in extraordinary circumstances.

Abortion

Since the 1973 Supreme Court decision in *Roe v. Wade*, elective abortion has been legal in the United States. Abortion can be performed until the period of viability, that is, the point at which the fetus can survive independently of the mother. After that time, abortion is permissible only when the life or health of the mother is threatened. Before viability, the rights of the mother are paramount; after viability, the rights of the fetus take precedence.

Personal beliefs, cultural norms, life experiences, and religious convictions shape people's attitudes about abortion. Ethicists have thoughtfully and thoroughly argued positions supporting both sides of the question. Nevertheless, few issues spark the intensity of response seen when the issue of abortion is raised.

At present the decision about abortion is to be made by the woman and her physician. Nurses (and other caregivers) have the right to refuse to assist with the procedure if abortion is contrary to their moral and ethical beliefs. However, if a nurse works in an institution where abortions may be performed, the nurse can be dismissed for refusing to assist. To avoid being placed in a situation contrary to personal ethical values and beliefs, it is important to identify the practices of an institution before going to work there. A nurse who refuses to participate in an abortion because of moral or ethical beliefs has a responsibility to ensure that someone with similar qualifications is available to provide appropriate care for the patient. Patients must never be abandoned, regardless of a nurse's beliefs.

Intrauterine Fetal Surgery

Intrauterine fetal surgery, an example of therapeutic research, is a therapy for anatomic lesions that can be corrected surgically and are incompatible with life if not treated. Examples include surgery for myelomeningocele and some congenital cardiac defects. The procedure involves opening the uterus during the second trimester (before viability), performing the planned surgery, and replacing the fetus in the uterus. The risks to the fetus are substantial, and the mother is committed to cesarean births for this and subsequent pregnancies (because the upper, active segment of the uterus is entered). The parents must be informed of the experimental nature of the treatment, the risks of the surgery, the commitment to cesarean birth, and alternatives to the treatment.

As in other aspects of maternity care, caregivers must respect the pregnant woman's autonomy. The procedure involves health risks to the woman, and she retains the right to refuse any surgical procedure. Healthcare providers must be careful that their zeal for new technology does not lead them to focus unilaterally on the fetus at the expense of the mother.

Reproductive Assistance

Assisted reproductive technology (ART) is the term used to describe highly technologic approaches used to produce pregnancy. *In vitro fertilization* and *embryo transfer (IVF-ET)*, a therapy offered to selected infertile couples, is perhaps the best known ART technique.

Multifetal pregnancy may occur with ART because the use of ovulation-inducing medications typically triggers the release of multiple eggs that, when fertilized, produce multiple embryos, which are then implanted. Multifetal pregnancy increases the risk of miscarriage, preterm birth, and neonatal morbidity and mortality. It also increases the mother's risk of complications, including cesarean birth. To help prevent a high-level multifetal pregnancy, the American Society for Reproductive Medicine (ASRM) has issued guidelines to limit the number of embryos transferred. These guidelines are designed to decrease risk while allowing for individualized care (ASRM & Society for Assisted Reproductive Technology, 2009). This practice raises ethical considerations about the handling of the unused embryos. However, when a multifetal pregnancy does occur, the physician may suggest that the woman consider fetal reduction, in which some of the embryos are aborted to give the remaining ones a better chance for survival. Clearly this procedure raises ethical concerns about the sacrifice of some so that the remainder can survive.

Prevention should be the first approach to the problem of multifetal pregnancy. It begins with careful counseling about the risks of multiple gestation and the ethical issues that relate to fetal reduction. No physician who is morally opposed to fetal reduction should be expected to perform the procedure; however, physicians should be aware of the ethical and medical issues involved and be prepared to respond to families in a professional and ethical manner (ACOG, 2007).

Surrogate childbearing is another approach to infertility. Surrogate childbearing occurs when a woman agrees to become pregnant for a childless couple. She may be artificially inseminated with the male partner's sperm or a donor's sperm or may receive a gamete transfer, depending on the infertile couple's needs. If fertilization occurs, the woman carries the fetus to term and releases the infant to the couple after birth.

These methods of resolving infertility raise ethical issues about candidate selection, responsibility for a child born with a congenital defect, and religious objections to artificial conception. Other ethical questions include the following: What should be done with surplus fertilized oocytes? To whom do frozen embryos belong? Who is liable if a woman or her offspring contracts HIV from donated sperm? Should children be told about their conception?

Embryonic Stem Cell Research

Human stem cells can be found in embryonic tissue and in the primordial germ cells of a fetus. Research has demonstrated that in tissue cultures these cells can be made to differentiate into other types of cells such as blood, nerve, or heart cells, which might then be used to treat problems such as diabetes, Parkinson and Alzheimer diseases, spinal cord injury, or metabolic disorders. The availability of specialized tissue or even organs grown from stem cells might also decrease society's dependence on donated organs for organ transplants.

Positions about embryonic stem cell research vary dramatically, from the view that any use of human embryos for research is wrong to the view that any form of embryonic stem cell research is acceptable, with a variety of other positions that fall somewhere in between these extremes. Other questions also arise: What sources of embryonic tissue are acceptable for research? Is it ever ethical to clone embryos solely for stem cell research? Is there justification for using embryos remaining after fertility treatments?

The question of how an embryo should be viewed—with status in some way as a person or in some sense as property (and, if property, whose?)—is a key question in the debate. Ethicists recognize that it is not necessary to advocate full moral status or personhood for an embryo to have significant moral qualms about the instrumental use of a human embryo in the "interests" of society. The issue of consent, which links directly to an embryo's status, also merits consideration. In truth, the ethical questions and dilemmas associated with embryonic stem cell research are staggeringly complex and require careful analysis and thoughtful dialogue.

Making Treatment Decisions for Children

Technology makes it possible to sustain the lives of children who previously would have died, thus creating many ethical issues. Conflict often arises between health professionals and parents when parents choose to withhold therapy or to request aggressive therapy on behalf of their child and the health professionals have a different opinion about treatment. Nurses often face ethical dilemmas when providing care to such a child, especially as they witness parents struggling to decide among treatment options.

When making treatment decisions in pediatrics, healthcare professionals need to determine whether their responsibility is limited to the child or includes the interests of the parents. The healthcare institution's ethics committee often plays a role in resolving conflicts about treatment decisions. Courts should make ethical decisions only when healthcare professionals and parents are unable to agree about providing or withholding treatment.

Terminating Life-Sustaining Treatment

Federal "Baby Doe" regulations were developed to protect the rights of infants with severe defects. The Child Abuse and Treatment Act of 1984, also known as the Baby Doe regulations, defines the withholding of medically indicated treatment as child abuse, except when care is futile (Curtin, 2008). Parents of such infants are usually the ultimate decision makers about the child's care. Factors important to parents in making their decision include the child's quality of life, degree of pain and suffering, likelihood for improvement, and physician recommendations. Physicians may believe treatment will help the child and improve the quality of life (sometimes defined as a meaningful existence or an ability to develop human relationships). Physicians are not obligated to offer interventions that cause extreme pain and suffering when there is limited or no potential benefit. Treatments that only prolong life represent a misuse of expensive healthcare resources. Federal regulations require a formalized ethical decision-making process before physicians accept or reject a parent's wishes.

The ethics committee members consider all options according to their individual beliefs and their perceptions of the value of specific interventions for an individual child, using ethical theory to guide decision making. There may be no right or wrong answer—and a plan of action may result that is a compromise about which neither the health professionals nor family is totally happy.

Organ Transplantation Issues

The death of a child can benefit another child through organ transplantation. Children between 11 and 17 years of age account for nearly 45% of all children waiting for a transplant (Health Resources and Services Administration & Organ Procurement and Transplant Network, 2011). The National Organ Transplant Act (PL 98-507) generated laws, regulations, and guidelines for organ collection and transplantation. The limited supply of organs has created numerous ethical issues: Which individuals on a waiting list should receive the organs available? Should a child with multiple congenital anomalies or abnormal chromosomes be eligible for a transplant? Should families be permitted to pay donor families for organs? Should the family's ability to pay for an organ transplant give a child higher priority for an organ? Should parents conceive another child hoping that the new baby is a potential stem cell donor for a child with an illness? If so, what pressures does this knowledge place on each child as he or she grows older?

Genetic Testing of Children

Genetic testing and screening of children are now possible for detection of carrier status or for presymptomatic detection of a specific condition, such as Duchenne muscular dystrophy. When genetic testing is considered, both the risks and benefits of receiving the results of the genetic test should be discussed when seeking informed consent. Genetic screening of newborns, such as for inborn errors of metabolism, cystic fibrosis, sickle cell disease, and other conditions, routinely occurs. In this case, the early identification of the genetic condition will have a clear benefit to the child, a system is in place to confirm the diagnosis, and treatment and follow-up are available for affected newborns. See Chapter 7 🕖 for more information on genetic testing.

EVIDENCE-BASED PRACTICE IN MATERNAL-CHILD NURSING

Evidence-based practice—that is, nursing care in which all interventions are supported by current, valid research evidence—is emerging as a force in health care. It provides a useful approach to problem solving and decision making and to self-directed, patient-centered, lifelong learning. Evidence-based practice builds on the actions necessary to transform research findings into clinical practice by also considering other forms of evidence that can be useful in making clinical practice decisions. These other forms of evidence may include statistical data, quality measurements, risk management measures, and information from support services such as infection control.

As practicing clinicians, nurses need to meet three basic competencies related to evidence-based practice:

1. Recognize which clinical practices are supported by sound evidence, which practices have conflicting findings as to their effect on patient outcomes, and which practices have no evidence to support their use.

2. Use data in their clinical work to evaluate outcomes of care.

3. Appraise and integrate scientific bases into practice.

Nurses need to know what data are being tracked in their workplaces and how care practices and outcomes are improved as a result of quality improvement initiatives. However, there is more to evidence-based practice—competent, effective nurses learn to question the very basis of their clinical work.

Throughout this text we have provided *snapshots* of evidence-based practice related to childbearing women and families, such as the one on page 31. We believe that these *Evidence-Based Practice* features will help you understand the concept more clearly and may challenge you to question the usefulness of some of the routine care you observe in clinical practice. That is the impact of evidence-based practice—it moves clinicians beyond practices of habit and opinion to practices based on high-quality, current science.

CONCEPT MAPS AND CLINICAL REASONING

It can be challenging to use evidence, analyze information, and make sound decisions that result in safe, effective patient care.

A new tool that aids in this process is the *Concept Map*. The use of concept maps is an exciting trend in nursing care management. Concept maps are visual depictions of the relationships that exist among a variety of concepts and ideas related to a patient's specific health problems. The relationship "picture" created by the map allows the nurse to plan interventions that can address multiple problems more effectively. An example of a concept map is shown below.

Scenarios provide a realistic way of enabling students to apply concepts. The *Clinical Reasoning in Action* feature at the end of every chapter in this text presents a patient scenario and asks clinical reasoning questions to help students formulate how they would handle the issues raised and how they would apply concepts they have learned in the chapter. To help students understand how concept maps can influence care planning, many of the *Clinical Reasoning in Action* features ask students to visit the text's website and use the interactive, e-template provided to create their own concept maps for a particular patient problem.

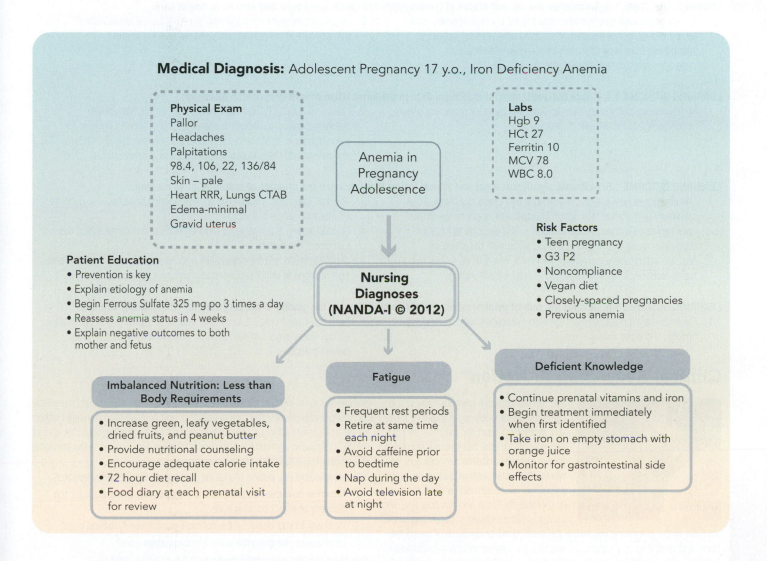

Medical Diagnosis: Adolescent Pregnancy 17 y.o., Iron Deficiency Anemia

Physical Exam
Pallor
Headaches
Palpitations
98.4, 106, 22, 136/84
Skin – pale
Heart RRR, Lungs CTAB
Edema-minimal
Gravid uterus

Labs
Hgb 9
HCt 27
Ferritin 10
MCV 78
WBC 8.0

Anemia in Pregnancy Adolescence

Risk Factors
• Teen pregnancy
• G3 P2
• Noncompliance
• Vegan diet
• Closely-spaced pregnancies
• Previous anemia

Patient Education
• Prevention is key
• Explain etiology of anemia
• Begin Ferrous Sulfate 325 mg po 3 times a day
• Reassess anemia status in 4 weeks
• Explain negative outcomes to both mother and fetus

Nursing Diagnoses (NANDA-I © 2012)

Imbalanced Nutrition: Less than Body Requirements
• Increase green, leafy vegetables, dried fruits, and peanut butter
• Provide nutritional counseling
• Encourage adequate calorie intake
• 72 hour diet recall
• Food diary at each prenatal visit for review

Fatigue
• Frequent rest periods
• Retire at same time each night
• Avoid caffeine prior to bedtime
• Nap during the day
• Avoid television late at night

Deficient Knowledge
• Continue prenatal vitamins and iron
• Begin treatment immediately when first identified
• Take iron on empty stomach with orange juice
• Monitor for gastrointestinal side effects

Critical Concept Review

LEARNING OUTCOME 1.1: Identify the nursing roles available to maternal-newborn and pediatric nurses.

1. Registered nurse:
   - Provides nursing care to both inpatient and outpatient women with childbearing or reproductive issues as well as newborns and children.
2. Nurse practitioner:
   - Provides ambulatory care services to expectant families and to children.
   - Provides care in some acute care, high-risk units such as neonatal intensive care units.

- Focuses on physical and psychosocial assessments and orders diagnostic tests and procedures.
- Makes clinical judgments and orders appropriate care.
3. Certified nurse-midwife:
   - Manages the care of a woman who is at low risk for complications during pregnancy and childbirth.

LEARNING OUTCOME 1.2: Summarize the use of community-based nursing care in meeting the needs of childbearing and childrearing families.

Community-based care is important in meeting the needs of the childbearing and childrearing family because the vast majority of care takes place outside of hospitals and in such places as:

1. Clinics
2. Offices
3. Community-based organizations
4. Private homes

LEARNING OUTCOME 1.3: Summarize the current status of factors related to health insurance and access to health care.

1. Community-based care remains an essential element of health care for uninsured or underinsured individuals, as well as for individuals who benefit from programs such as Medicare, Medicaid, or state-sponsored, health-related programs.

2. Healthcare insurers are beginning to recognize the importance of primary care in containing costs and maintaining health.

LEARNING OUTCOME 1.4: Relate the availability of statistical data to the formulation of further research questions.

1. Health-related statistics provide an objective basis for projecting patient needs and planning the use of resources.

2. Statistical data can also reveal trends that require research to determine cause, to analyze the implications of specific findings for given populations, to explore relationships between specific factors, and to evaluate the success of specific nursing interventions.

LEARNING OUTCOME 1.5: Delineate significant legal and ethical issues that influence the practice of maternal-child nursing.

1. The abortion debate is especially difficult and raises questions about maternal rights versus fetal rights. Abortion can legally be performed until the fetus reaches the age of viability. The decision to have an abortion is made by a woman in consultation with her physician.
2. Assisted reproductive technology (ART) is a term that describes the highly technologic approaches used to produce pregnancy.

3. Federal "Baby Doe" regulations were developed to protect the rights of infants with severe defects.
4. Genetic testing is available for children with conditions for which there is no current treatment.
5. Organ donation and transplantation ethical issues involve selection and qualifications of donor recipients and payment for organs.

LEARNING OUTCOME 1.6: Discuss the role of evidence-based practice in improving the quality of nursing care for childbearing families.

1. Evidence-based practice refers to clinical practice based on research findings and other available data.

2. Evidence-based practice increases nurses' accountability to integrate current knowledge and research into practice and results in better patient outcomes.

Clinical Reasoning in Action

You are working as a prenatal nurse in a local clinic. Before entering a patient's room, you review the chart for pertinent information such as cultural background, significant family members, weeks of gestation, test results, birth plan, and education for health promotion. You greet each patient and family member by name and ask how they are coping with the pregnancy. Depending on the trimester of the pregnancy, you review the discomforts or concerns of the mother/ family and what they may expect. You examine the mother, including fundal height, fetal heart rate and fetal position if appropriate, maternal blood pressure, weight gain, and urine analysis. With each patient, you discuss the community resources available such as prenatal classes, lactation consultants, and prenatal exercise/yoga classes. Based on the information you obtain, you might refer the mother to social services or the WIC program as appropriate. At the end of the clinic session, you review the status of the patients you saw with the collaborating physician.

1. How would you define the terms *family* and *family-centered care*?
2. Describe how the nursing process provides the framework for the delivery of direct nursing care.
3. How would you describe the concept of community-based care?
4. How would you describe culturally competent care?

See www.nursing.pearsonhighered.com for possible responses.

References

Agency for Healthcare Research and Quality. (2011). *HCUP kids' inpatient database, 2009: Patient and hospital characteristics for ICD-9-CM principal diagnosis code.* Retrieved from http://hcupnet.ahrq.gov

American Academy of Pediatrics (AAP). (2011). Policy statement: Consent for emergency medical services for children and adolescents. *Pediatrics, 128*(2), 427–433.

American College of Nurse-Midwives (ACNM). (2009). *Position statement: Mandatory degree requirements for entry into midwifery practice.* Retrieved from http://www.midwife.org/siteFiles/position/Manadatory_Degree_Req_for_Entry_Midwifery_Practice_7_0.pdf

American College of Obstetricians and Gynecologists (ACOG). (2005). *Maternal decision making, ethics, and the law* (Committee Opinion No. 321). Washington, DC: Author.

American College of Obstetricians and Gynecologists (ACOG). (2007). *Multifetal pregnancy reduction* (Committee Opinion No. 369). Washington, DC: Author.

American Nurses Association & National Association of Neonatal Nurses. (2004). *Neonatal nursing: Scope and standards of practice.* Washington, DC: American Nurses Association.

American Nurses Association, National Association of Pediatric Nurse Practitioners, & Society of Pediatric Nurses. (2008). *Pediatric nursing: Scope and standards of practice.* Silver Spring, MD: Nurses books.org.

American Society for Reproductive Medicine (ASRM) and the Society for Assisted Reproductive Technology. (2009). Guidelines on number of embryos transferred. *Fertility and Sterility, 92*(Suppl. 5), 1518–1519.

Bindler, R. C., & Ball, J. W. (2007). The Bindler-Ball healthcare model: A new paradigm for health promotion. *Pediatric Nursing, 33*(2), 121–126.

Centers for Medicare and Medicaid Services. (2011). *2011 poverty level guidelines.* Retrieved from http://www.cms.gov/MedicaidEligibility/downloads/POV11Combo.pdf

Committee on Hospital Care, & Institute for Patient and Family-Centered Care. (2012). Patient- and family-centered care and the pediatrician's role. *Pediatrics, 129*(2), 394–404.

Curtin, L. (2008). The Babies Doe: Finding middle ground. *American Nurse Today, 3*(1), 7–10.

Federal Interagency Forum on Child and Family Statistics. (2012). *America's children: Key national indicators of well-being, 2012: Demographics.* Retrieved from http://www.childstats.gov/americaschildren/demo.asp

Foederer, A. A. (2007). Appropriately navigating through treacherous medicine: Health care decision making panels for vulnerable minors. *Journal of Nursing Law, 11*(2), 108–117.

Gonzales, K. (2010). Medication administration errors and the pediatric population: A systematic search of the literature. *Journal of Pediatric Nursing, 25,* 555–565.

Goode, T., & Jones, W. (2006). *A guide for advancing family-centered and culturally and linguistically competent care.* Washington, DC: National Center for Cultural Competence, Georgetown University Center for Child and Human Development.

Hawkins, A. O., Kantayya, V. S., & Sharkey-Asner, C. (2010). Health literacy: A potential barrier in caring for underserved populations, *Disease A Month, 56,* 734–740.

Health Resources and Services Administration, Maternal and Child Health Bureau. (2009). *The National Survey of Children's Health 2007.* Rockville, Maryland: U.S. Department of Health and Human Services. Retrieved from http://www.mchb.hrsa.gov/nsch/07emohealth/index.html

Health Resources and Services Administration & Organ Procurement and Transplant Network. (2011). *Transplants in the U.S. by recipient age, and current U.S. waiting list by age.*

Heron, M. (2012). Deaths: Leading causes for 2009. *National Vital Statistics Reports, 61*(7), 1–96.

Kochanek, K. D., Xu, J., Murphy, S. L., Miniño, A. M., & Kung, H. C. (2011). Deaths: Final data for 2009. *National Vital Statistics Reports, 60*(3), 1–117.

Levetown, M., & Committee on Bioethics. (2008). Communicating with children and families: From everyday interactions to skill in conveying distressing information. *Pediatrics, 121*(5), e1441–e1460.

Lewandowski, L. A., & Tesler, M. D. (Eds.). (2003). Family-centered care: Putting it into action. *The SPN/ANA Guide to Family-Centered Care.* Washington, DC: American Nurses Association.

MacDorman, M. F., & Mathews, T. J. (2009). Behind international rankings of infant mortality: How the United States compares with Europe. *NCHS Data Brief,* No. 23.

MacDorman, M. F., Menacker, F., & Declerq, E. (2010). Trends and characteristics of home and other out-of-hospital births in the United States, 1990–2006. *National Vital Statistics Reports, 58*(11), 1–14.

Martin, J. A., Hamilton, B. E., Ventura, S. J., Osterman, M. J. K., Wilson, E. C., & Mathews, T. J. (2012). Births: Final data for 2010. *National Vital Statistics Reports, 61*(1), 1–72.

Mathews, T. J., & MacDorman, M. F. (2012). Infant mortality statistics from the 2008 period linked birth/infant death data set. *National Vital Statistics Report, 60*(5), 128.

Midwives Alliance of North America (MANA). (2009). *Definitions.* Retrieved from http://www.mana.org/definitions.html

National Center for Health Statistics (NCHS). (2011). *Health, United States, 2011. With Special Feature on Socioeconomic Status and Health.* Hyattsville, MD: Author.

National Center for Health Statistics, National Vital Statistics System. (2011). *Leading causes of injury deaths by age group highlighting unintentional injury deaths, United States—2008.* Retrieved from http://webapppa.cdc.gov/cgi-bin/broker.exe

Quality and Safety Education for Nurses (QSEN). (2011). *About QSEN.* Retrieved from www.qsen.org/about_qsen.php

Shapiro, N. A. (2010). Confidentiality and access to adolescent health care services. *Journal of Pediatric Health Care, 24*(2), 133–136.

Smith-Campbell, B., & Pile, D. (2010). Children's Health Insurance Program and pediatric nurses. *Journal of Pediatric Nursing, 25,* 138–141.

U.S. Census Bureau. (2011). Age and sex composition: 2010. *2010 Census Briefs.* Retrieved from http://www.census.gov/prod/cen2010/briefs/c2010br-o3.pdf

U.S. Department of Health and Human Services. (2011). *Healthy People 2020.* Retrieved from http://www.healthypcople.gov/2020/about/default.aspx

U.S. Department of Health and Human Services. (2010). News Release: HHS announces the nation's new health promotion and disease prevention agenda. Retrieved from http://www.hhs.gov/news/press/2010pres/12/20101202a.html

Xu, J., Kochanek, K. D., Murphy, S. L., & Tejada-Vera, B. (2010). Deaths: Final data for 2007. *National Vital Statistics Reports, 58*(19), 1–135.

Yu, H., Wier, L. M., & Elixhauser, A. (2011). *Hospital stays for children, 2009* (HCUP Statistical Brief No. 118). Rockville, MD: Agency for Healthcare Research and Quality. Retrieved from http://www.hcup-us.ahrq.gov/reports/statbriefs/sb118.pdf

Culture and the Family

Ken Usami/Photodisc RF/Getty Images

My parents came here from China when I was three. They wanted the chance to make a better life and they wanted another child. Needless to say, although I have always felt loved and cherished, I know how thrilled they were when my brother was born. Sometimes I feel as though I am walking a line between their ways and the ways I have learned growing up in this country. My husband is Chinese but he, too, grew up here. We are expecting our second baby in a few months. We talk often about which Chinese ways we want to retain and which new ways make more sense. I am not sure that my parents will under-stand, however. To them the old ways are always best. —Li Wei, 29

LEARNING OUTCOMES

2.1 Compare the characteristics of different types of families.

2.2 Identify the stages of a family life cycle.

2.3 Identify prevalent cultural norms related to childbearing and childrearing.

2.4 Summarize the importance of cultural competency in providing nursing care.

2.5 Discuss the use of a cultural assessment tool as a means of providing culturally sensitive care.

2.6 Identify key considerations in providing spiritually sensitive care.

2.7 Differentiate between complementary and alternative therapies.

2.8 Determine the benefits and risks of complementary and alternative therapies.

2.9 Summarize complementary therapies appropriate for the nurse to use with childbearing and childrearing families.

Individuals do not live in isolation. Their values, beliefs, behaviors, decisions, attitudes, and biases are shaped by many factors, including their families, their culture, and their religious beliefs. Nurses who provide effective, holistic care recognize this reality and seek to learn about and care for the entire family.

This chapter begins with a brief discussion of family types, functioning, and assessment. It then addresses the impact of culture on the family and concludes with a brief examination of some of the complementary and alternative therapies a family might use.

THE FAMILY

The U.S. Census Bureau defines a **family** as two or more individuals who are joined together by marriage, birth, or adoption and live together in the same household (U.S. Census Bureau, 2012). More broadly, however, families are generally characterized by bonds of emotional closeness, sharing, and support.

Families are guided by a common set of values or beliefs about the worth and importance of certain ideas and traditions. These values often bind family members together, and these values are greatly influenced by external factors including cultural background, social norms, education, environmental influences, socioeconomic status, and beliefs held by peers, coworkers, political and community leaders, and other individuals outside the family unit. Because of the influence of these external factors, a family's values may change considerably over the years.

Types of Families

Families are diverse in structure, roles, and relationships. Various types of families—both those considered traditional and nontraditional—exist in contemporary American society. This section identifies common types of family structures.

- In the *nuclear family,* children live in a household with both biologic parents, and no other relatives or persons. One parent may stay home to rear the children while one parent works, but more commonly, both parents are employed by choice or necessity. Two-income families must address important issues such as childcare arrangements, household chores, and how to ensure quality family time. *Dual-career/dual-earner families* are now considered the norm in modern society.

- The *child-free family* is a growing trend. In some cases, a family is child free by choice; in other cases, a family is child free because of issues related to infertility.

- In an *extended family,* a couple shares household and childrearing responsibilities with parents, siblings, or other relatives. Families may reside together to share housing expenses and child care. However, in many cases, the child may be residing with the grandparent and one parent because of issues associated with unemployment, parental separation, parental death, or parental substance abuse. Grandparents may raise children due to the inability of parents to care for their own children.

- An *extended kin network family* is a specific form of an extended family in which two nuclear families of primary or unmarried kin live in proximity to each other. The family shares a social support network, chores, goods, and services.

- The *single-parent family* is becoming increasingly common. In some cases, the head of the household is widowed, divorced, abandoned, or separated. In other cases, the head of the household, most often the mother, remains unmarried. Single-parent families often face difficulties because the sole parent may lack social and emotional support, need assistance with childrearing issues, and face financial strain (Figure 2–1 ●).

● **Figure 2–1** Single-parent families account for nearly one third of all U.S. families. What types of challenges do single-parent families face?
Source: © Phase4Photography/Fotolia.

- The *blended or reconstituted nuclear family* includes two parents with biologic children from a previous marriage or relationship who marry or cohabitate. This family structure has become increasingly common due to high rates of divorce and remarriage. Potential advantages to the children may include better financial support and a new supportive role model. Stresses can include lack of a clear role for the stepparent, lack of acceptance of the stepparent, financial stresses when two families must be supported by stepparents, and communication problems.

- A *binuclear family* is a postdivorce family in which the biologic children are members of two nuclear households, with co-parenting by the father and the mother. The children alternate between the two homes, spending varying amounts of time with each parent in a situation called co-parenting, usually involving joint custody. Joint custody is a legal situation in which both parents have equal responsibility and legal rights, regardless of where the children live. The binuclear family is a model for effective communication. It enables both biologic parents to be involved in a child's upbringing and provides additional support and role models in the form of extended family members.

- A *heterosexual cohabitating family* describes a heterosexual couple who may or may not have children and who live together outside of marriage. This may include never-married individuals as well as divorced or widowed persons. While some individuals choose this model for personal reasons, others do so for financial reasons or to seek companionship.

- *Gay and lesbian families* include those in which two adults of the same sex live together as domestic partners with or without children, and those in which a gay or lesbian single parent rears a child. Children in these families may be from a previous heterosexual union, or be born to or adopted by one or both member(s) of the same-sex couple. A biologic child may be born to one of the partners through artificial

insemination or through a surrogate mother. Children who are adopted or born into lesbian and gay families are highly valued, as with heterosexual families. Small studies that evaluated children reared by same-sex couples found no significant differences in childrearing or in the children's adjustment compared to children reared in other types of families. These children have been found to do as well emotionally, behaviorally, and socially as those born into heterosexual families (Chamberlain, Miller, & Bornstein, 2008).

Family Development Frameworks

Family development theories use a framework to categorize a family's progression over time according to specific, typical stages in family life. These are predictable stages in the life cycle of every family, but they follow no rigid pattern. Duvall's (1977) eight stages in the family life cycle of a traditional nuclear family have been used as the foundation for contemporary models of the family life cycle that describe the developmental processes and role expectations for different family types. Table 2–1 lists Duvall's eight stages to illustrate important developmental transitions that occur at some point in most families.

Other family development models have been developed to address the stages and developmental tasks facing the unattached young adult, the gay and lesbian family, those who divorce, and those who remarry. Textbooks on families and developmental psychology provide further information on this topic.

Family Assessment

The nurse's understanding of a family's structure helps provide insight into the family's support system and needs. A *family assessment* is a collection of data about the family's type and structure, current level of functioning, support system, sociocultural background, environment, and needs.

To obtain an accurate and concise family assessment, the nurse needs to establish a trusting relationship with the woman or child, and the family. Data are best collected in a comfortable, private environment, free from interruptions.

Basic information should include the following:

- Name, age, sex, and family relationship of all people residing in the household

- Family type, structure, roles, and values

- Cultural associations, including cultural norms and customs related to childbearing, childrearing, and infant feeding

Table 2–1	Eight-Stage Family Life Cycle
Stages	**Characteristics**
Stage I	Beginning family, newly married couples*
Stage II	Childbearing family (oldest child is an infant through 30 months of age)
Stage III	Families with preschool children (oldest child is between 2.5 and 6 years of age)
Stage IV	Families with schoolchildren (oldest child is between 6 and 13 years of age)
Stage V	Families with teenagers (oldest child is between 13 and 20 years of age)
Stage VI	Families launching young adults (all children leave home)
Stage VII	Middle-aged parents (empty nest through retirement)
Stage VIII	Family in retirement and old age (retirement to death of both spouses)

*Keep in mind that this was the norm at the time the model was developed, but today families form through many different types of relationships.
Source: Adapted from Duvall, E. M. (1977). *Marriage and family development* (5th ed.). Philadelphia, PA: Lippincott; Duvall, E. M., & Miller, B. C. (1985). *Marriage and family development* (6th ed.). New York, NY: Harper Row; Friedman, M. M., Bowden, V. R., & Jones, E. G. (2003). *Family nursing: Research, theory, and practice* (5th ed.). Upper Saddle River, NJ: Prentice Hall; Gedaly-Duff, V., Nielsen, A., Heims, M. L., & Pate, M. D. (2010). Family child health nursing. In J. R. Kaakinen, V. Gedaly-Duff, D. P. Coehlo, & S. M. H. Hanson, *Family health care nursing: Theory, practice, and research* (4th ed., pp. 332–378). Philadelphia, PA: F. A. Davis.

- Religious affiliations, including specific religious beliefs and practices related to childbearing
- Support network, including extended family, friends, and religious and community associations
- Communication patterns, including language barriers

The nurse also gathers information about the health of individual family members because health status can have a major impact on family functioning. When possible, it is helpful to have information about the family's home environment as well. In many cases this information is gathered during patient interviews. However, a home visit provides far more data about family relationships, roles, needs, and preparation for a new baby. See Chapter 38 🔴 for more information about family assessment.

CULTURAL INFLUENCES AFFECTING THE FAMILY

When caring for families, it is critical to consider the influence of culture, which may affect how a family responds to health-related issues. **Culture** has many definitions and is currently described as:

the combination of a body of knowledge, a body of belief and a body of behavior. It involves a number of elements, including personal identification, language, thoughts, communications, actions, customs, beliefs, values, and institutions that are often specific to ethnic, racial, religious, geographic, or social groups. (National Institutes of Health [NIH], 2012)

Culture is characterized by certain key elements, including the following:

- *Culture is based on shared values and beliefs.* Each culture identifies and articulates its shared values and beliefs. Expected behaviors and roles emerge that are consistent with those values and beliefs. A belief system suggests what preventive health measures and treatment for diseases are sought and accepted. It may also state the importance of children, of the family, of other individuals, and of the collective group, all of which can influence the choices people in the culture make regarding health.

- *Culture is learned and dynamic.* A child is born into a culture and starts learning the beliefs and practices of the group from birth. Children who are members of two cultural groups, such as African and immigrant, learn about both groups as they grow and develop. Immigrants may face challenges when integrating the rules of the dominant culture. Children who have family members from two or more cultural groups integrate parts of the worldview from each group. Therefore, although culture is connected with groups, each individual's manifestation of his or her own cultural background will be unique. Culture evolves and adapts as new members are born into or join the group, and as the surrounding social and physical environments change. For example, as first-generation immigrants enter a new country, they generally closely follow the cultural patterns of their native lands. As their children grow, the youth maintain some of the family cultural patterns but begin to incorporate some of the new culture (Figure 2–2 🔴).

🔴 **Figure 2–2** Preschoolers from various cultural backgrounds play together. How can nurses partner with families to assist children to understand and respect cultural differences?

■ *Culture is integrated into life and uses symbols.* Culture is integrated through social institutions such as schools, houses of worship, friendships, families, and occupations. This provides a variety of opportunities for learning about one's culture. The sense of integration may be disrupted or harder to maintain if individuals move frequently and as cultures intertwine with each other. Symbols are an important way that many cultures communicate with each other and with the outside world. Language, dress, music, tools, and nonverbal gestures are symbols a culture uses to display and transmit the culture.

Race refers to a group of people who share biologic similarities such as skin color, bone structure, and genetic traits. Examples of races include white (sometimes called Caucasian or European American), black (sometimes called African American in the United States), Hispanic, Natives (such as Native Americans, Alaskan Native, Hawaiian Native, and First Nation people of Canada), and Asian.

Ethnicity describes a "cultural group's sense of identification associated with the group's common social and cultural heritage" (Spector, 2013, p. 357). Examples of ethnic groups include Hmong, Jews, and Irish Americans. Even the mainstream or majority of groups usually identify with an ethnic group. Some beliefs and practices are common among certain ethnic groups, but it is important to avoid **stereotyping** individuals, that is, assuming that all members of a group have the same characteristics. The nurse should assess the woman or child and family to see which characteristics common to a group are possessed by the patient rather than assume that because individuals identify themselves as a specific ethnicity they must practice certain customs.

Acculturation refers to the process of modifying one's culture to fit within the new or dominant culture. **Assimilation** is related to acculturation and is described as adopting and incorporating traits of the new culture within one's practice (Spector, 2013). Acculturation frequently occurs when people leave their country of origin and immigrate to a new country. Often acculturation is associated with improved health status and health behaviors, especially if the immigration is associated with improved socioeconomic status, which leads to better nutrition and access to health care. This is frequently true for people who immigrate to the United States from a developing country. On the other hand, health sometimes declines with acculturation. For example, obesity is a problem that is growing rapidly within the United States and particularly among immigrant populations.

Family Roles and Structure

A family's organization and the roles played by individual family members are largely dependent on cultural influence. The family structure defines acceptable roles and behavior of family members. For example, culture may determine who has authority (head of household) and is the primary decision maker for other members of the family. Additionally, the role of decision maker may change according to specific decisions. In some cultures, decisions regarding the family's health care are primarily the responsibility of the female, while other decisions are male dominated. Family dominance patterns may be *patriarchal,* as

● Figure 2–3 Many cultures value the input of grandparents and other elders in the family or group. In this multigenerational family, the grandmother's guidance is highly valued and significantly influences the family's childrearing practices.

may be seen in Appalachian cultures; *matriarchal,* as may be seen in African American cultures; or more *egalitarian* (equal), as may be seen in European American cultures. Nurses need to be alert to the roles and functions in families since teaching may need to be directed to those responsible for decision making in order to promote health for all family members.

Culture also defines gender roles, the role of the elderly, and the role of the extended family. For example, Native Americans may consult tribal elders (considered part of the extended family) before agreeing to medical care for a pregnant woman or for a child. In some cultures, major decisions for the family, including a child's health care, include input from grandparents and other extended family members (Figure 2–3 ●). Grandparents may even assume responsibility for care of the children in the family. In these cases, nurses must direct teaching for health promotion and demonstration for treatment procedures to the grandparent.

Family goals are also determined by cultural values and practices, as are family member roles and childbearing and childrearing practices and beliefs.

Teaching Highlights Including Grandparents and Cultural Health Practices in the Teaching Plan

When you care for a family in which the grandparents play a key role in decision making, be sure that they are present if you are teaching something that is important for the family to understand and act on if necessary. This might include, for example, signs of illness in the newborn that need immediate follow-up.

If a specific cultural health practice is important to the family and will not cause harm, such as prayer, chanting, or specific foods, respect the family's beliefs and develop a teaching plan that includes those practices. Respecting a family's values improves the likelihood that the newly recommended healthcare actions will be accepted.

Health Beliefs, Approaches, and Practices

Three views of health described by Andrews and Boyle (2012) are magico-religious, scientific, and holistic. In reality, many people ascribe to a view that combines more than one of these belief systems, but it is helpful to examine them separately.

In the *magico-religious belief paradigm,* health and illness are determined by supernatural forces such as God, gods, magic, spirits, or fate. A miscarriage, for example, or the illness of a pregnant woman or of a child may be perceived as a punishment for actions. Children of preschool age and early school age usually have this view of illness; some adults also believe that higher or supernatural powers determine health and illness. It is wise to ask both children and their families what they think caused an illness or how they believe they can stay well. People who believe in this paradigm may gain comfort from prayer, healing rituals, and faith healing. Young children who, because of their developmental level, believe that they have caused their own illness can be expressly told that it was not something they did that caused the illness. This may help decrease their feelings of guilt.

The *scientific or biomedical health paradigm* assumes that physiology explains all illness and life itself (Andrews & Boyle, 2012). Biochemical reactions and the genomic code are used to explain all health states. Illness is always caused by viruses, bacteria, or damage to the body in this framework. This approach is often called "Western medicine." Families who hold this view expect a traditional Western medical intervention, such as medication, treatment, or surgery, to treat the specific health problem. Within this belief system, it is very difficult to understand certain health conditions. Families may struggle to "explain" an illness by wondering if the child was exposed to something harmful during fetal life or exposed to something in the environment. A reason for the condition is needed to understand it.

Most physicians, nurses, and other healthcare professionals adhere primarily to the biomedical or scientific theories to explain and treat illnesses. However, certain therapies such as Therapeutic Touch, biofeedback, and other nontraditional methods that are more common in a holistic health paradigm are gaining popularity within these professions. For the family with this belief system, health professionals sometimes need to emphasize that certain conditions have no known cause, and should suggest treatments other than traditional Western medicine if other approaches may be helpful.

Balance and harmony of the body and nature are important concepts in the *holistic health belief.* It is believed that illness results when the natural balance or harmony is disturbed. Infections and other illnesses gain entry into the body when it is not in balance. This health belief is most common in North American Indian and Asian cultures (Andrews & Boyle, 2012). Increasingly the ideas of holism are being integrated into Western health care and combined with other approaches. An example of integration of approaches is use of a medication or radiation for illness in combination with adequate rest and a diet that is designed to increase immune function.

An associated holistic health belief is the hot and cold theory of disease, which subscribes to the thought that illnesses and diseases are a result of disruption in the hot and cold balance of the body. Therefore, consuming foods of the opposite variety can cure or prevent specific hot and cold illnesses. Hot and cold therapies related to healing are practiced in some African American, Asian, Latino, Arab, Muslim, and Caribbean cultures (Andrews & Boyle, 2012); see Table 2–2.

Healthcare Practitioners

The family seeking care for the child may choose one or a combination of magico-religious, holistic, or biomedical healthcare providers. The use of *folk healers* varies according to the culture. Though the healer's role and position in the community differ among cultures, healers do share commonalities. Healers speak the language of the cultural group, use common methods of communication for the culture, and live in the same community.

Mexican Americans may seek healing by a *curandero* (male healer) or *curandera* (female healer), a holistic healer who deals with physical, psychologic, and social problems (Spector, 2013). The curandero's holistic treatment may include use of herbs, laying on of hands, massaging the afflicted area, cleansing the body with herbs, preparing an amulet to be worn, burning a

Table 2–2	Hot and Cold Conditions and Foods		
Hot Conditions	**Cold Foods Used to Treat Hot Conditions**	**Cold Conditions**	**Hot Foods Used to Treat Cold Conditions**
Diarrhea	Barley water	Cancer	Beef
Fever	Chicken	Earaches	Cheese
Constipation	Dairy products	Headaches	Eggs
Infection	Raisins	Musculoskeletal conditions	Grains (other than barley)
Kidney problems	Fish	Pneumonia	Liquor
Liver conditions	Cucumber	Menstrual cramps	Pork
Sore throats	Fresh fruits	Malaria	Onions
Stomach ulcers	Fresh vegetables	Arthritis	Spicy foods
	Goat meat	Rhinitis	Chocolate
		Colic	Warm water with honey

Source: Data from Purnell, L. D. (2009). *Guide to culturally competent health care.* Philadelphia, PA: F. A. Davis; Purnell, L. D. (2013). *Transcultural health care: A culturally competent approach* (4th ed.). Philadelphia, PA: F. A. Davis; Spector, R. E. (2013). *Cultural diversity in health and illness* (8th ed.). Upper Saddle River, NJ: Pearson.

candle with a specific prayer printed on the candle jar, or calling the spirit of a saint to bless the individual. Essential to the curandero/a and the family is the faith the family has in his or her abilities. Families may combine *curanderismo* (Hispanic medical system) with a Western approach for some conditions. For example, a child with seizures may be given medications for the disorder obtained from Western care and may be fed a tea that the healer believes will treat the condition.

Puerto Ricans may use an ***espiritistas***, a healer who communicates with spirits for the physical and emotional development of the patient (Purnell, 2009). Mexican Americans may use this type of healer when the ailment is thought to be caused by witchcraft. However, use of an *espiritistas* is frowned on in some Hispanic cultures. A *sobador* is an individual who uses massage and manipulation to treat patients with joint and muscle problems, and is another type of healer who might be used by Mexican Americans (Zoucha & Zamarripa, 2013).

African Americans often combine Western and traditional beliefs about illness. Some believe in spirits as causes of illness and may use powders, oils, and ceremonies to maintain health.

Native Americans may seek healing from a **shaman**, "a woman or man who enters an altered state of consciousness, at will, to contact and utilize another type of reality to acquire knowledge and power and to help other people" (Fontaine, 2011, p. 355). Because Native Americans generally believe in the balance of nature and a state of harmony, they seek advice to identify what they have done to disrupt their body harmony. The healer will then prescribe the required treatment for restoration of balance and harmony. Teas, other herbal products, sweats, smudges, meditation, and other approaches are common. Returning to one's family, home, and roots may produce a sense of balance.

Impact of Religion and Spirituality

The terms *religion* and *spirituality* mean different things to different people. Many people view religion, which is sometimes termed *faith-based belief*, as an organized system that shares a common set of beliefs and practices about the significance, cause, and purpose of life and the universe. Religion is usually centered on the belief in or worshipping of a supernatural being or Supreme Being (such as God or Allah). **Spirituality** refers to the individual's experience and own interpretation of his or her relationship with a Supreme Being. Children are spiritual beings and generally express their spirituality through behavior such as imaginative play, art, dance, and song (Mueller, 2010). Prayer, one of the most common expressions of religious faith, is a frequently used therapy in which many children and families engage (Grossoehme, VanDyke, Jacobson, et al., 2010; Lambert, Fincham, & Graham, 2011).

A family's religious beliefs, affiliation, and practices can deeply influence their experiences and attitudes toward health care, childbearing, and childrearing. Members of certain religious groups such as Christian Scientists may attempt to avoid all medical interventions, whereas others such as Jehovah's Witnesses may refuse specific interventions, such as blood transfusions. Roman Catholics may refuse contraception. In most cases,

families gain comfort from acknowledgment of and respect for their religious beliefs and practices in the healthcare setting. However, the agnostic (one who has doubts about the existence of a transcendent being) or the atheist (one who believes that there is no higher power) may be offended if care providers assume that references to God or to a higher power will be comforting.

A religious or spiritual history is often completed when a woman is admitted to a clinic or labor setting or when a child is admitted to the hospital. The assessment can include questions about current spiritual beliefs and practices and preferences for religious rituals. Whenever possible the nurse should attempt to accommodate religious rituals and practices requested by the family.

Considering the diversity of religious beliefs, it is not unusual for nurses to encounter childbearing families whose beliefs conflict with their own. This is not problematic as long as the nurse avoids attempts to influence the family's decision making. For example, a nurse who does not believe in baptism should avoid revealing this to a Catholic seeking baptism for her stillborn infant. Nurses should also examine their religious beliefs related to genetic screening procedures, use of assisted reproductive technology to achieve pregnancy, abortion, use of technology to support life in a severely compromised newborn or a terminally ill child, and even less dramatic issues such as methods of contraception, circumcision, infant feeding, and disciplinary practices for children.

Although spirituality and faith-based belief are generally positive in supporting families to maintain and restore health, at times they can have potentially negative effects for children. Certain groups may blame individuals for their own illnesses, and children may develop guilt as a result. Abuse may result from parental religious beliefs about corporal punishment and discipline. If lifesaving treatments are denied by a religious group, courts may intervene to ensure care for the child.

Although adherence to a religious tradition is predominant in the United States, it should not be assumed that all individuals believe in or practice organized religion. The nurse should always ask the family if they follow a faith tradition and if they would like a leader from that faith to visit when in the hospital (Figure 2–4 ●). Adolescents may follow different faith traditions than their parents and should be asked the question individually.

Collaboration between the healthcare team and family is essential to providing care congruent with the child's and family's expectations. Although spirituality is important for many families, it is often overlooked as a healing strategy. Illness and injury may cause the family to turn to spiritual guidance as a method of understanding and coping. Assessment of the family's and child's spiritual needs is an important aspect of nursing care (Mueller, 2010). The nurse must respect the family's view and avoid being judgmental about their beliefs. Partnering with the child and family to incorporate their traditional practices and beliefs with prescribed therapies will help to ensure the delivery of safe and effective care for the child.

In many institutions, nurses can ask to be reassigned to a different patient if their religious beliefs are in conflict because of health care being provided or refused by the patient and family.

● **Figure 2–4** Today very few communities are limited to one culture. The children in this multicultural choir are representative of the changes in demographics of many Western countries. Even though they may differ in cultural background, a common thread is found in their religious preference.
Source: Myrleen Ferguson/PhotoEdit

However, if other personnel are not available, it is the nurse's responsibility to provide sensitive, appropriate, and nonjudgmental care to that patient.

Childbearing Practices

Children are generally valued all over the world, not only for the joy they bring, but also because they ensure continuation of the family and cultural values. This valuing of children may manifest itself in different ways. Families in the United States and many Western countries commonly have only one or two children out of a desire to provide the children with the best home and education they can afford and to spend as much free time with them as possible. In contrast, in many cultures throughout the world, it is common to have as many children as possible.

In some cultures a woman who gives birth achieves a higher status, especially if the child is male. This is especially true in the traditional Chinese culture and in some Middle Eastern cultures (Bulte, Heerink, & Zhang, 2011). Similarly, in the western United States, people of the Mormon faith view motherhood as the most important aspect of a woman's life, comparable with the male role of priesthood (Mendelkow, 2009). In Mexican American society and among many other Latino groups, having children is evidence of the male's virility and is a sign of manliness or *machismo*, a desired trait.

Culture may also influence attitudes and beliefs about contraception. For example, many Muslims from the Middle East may use birth control but do not believe in sterilization because it is a permanent method (Sueyoshi & Ohtsuka, 2010). Other Muslims might not practice contraception because children are highly valued and it is believed that the traditional role of women is to bear children. In Chinese society, on the other hand, where government policy limits the number of children a couple can have, contraception is common.

Health values and beliefs are also important in understanding reactions and behavior. Certain behaviors can be expected if a culture views pregnancy as a sickness, whereas other behaviors

can be expected if the culture views pregnancy as a natural occurrence. For example, because Native Americans, African Americans, and Mexican Americans generally view pregnancy as a natural and desirable condition, prenatal care may not be a priority. In other cultures, pregnancy may be seen as a time of increased vulnerability. In Orthodox Judaism, for example, it is a man's responsibility to procreate, but it is a woman's right, not her obligation, to do so. This is because, according to Orthodox Jewish law, the health of the mother, both physically and mentally, is of primary concern, and she should never be obliged to do something that threatens her life.

Individuals of many cultures take certain protective precautions based on their beliefs. For example, many Southeast Asian women fear that they will have a complicated labor and birth if they sit in a doorway or on a step. Thus they tend to avoid areas near doors in waiting rooms and examining rooms. In the Mexican American culture, the belief is common that *mal aire,* or bad air, may enter the body and cause harm. Preventive measures, such as keeping the windows closed or covering the head, are used. Some Latinos may place a raisin on the cord stump of a newborn to prevent drafts from entering their bodies.

A **taboo** is a behavior or thing that is to be avoided. Many cultures, including those found in the United States, have taboos centered on the unborn baby or newborn that are meant to ensure that the baby will survive. For example, it is common among Muslims to avoid naming the baby until after birth; similarly many Orthodox Jewish women wait to set up the nursery until after the baby is born.

In developing countries, mortality rates among infants and young children are extremely high; thus certain traditions focus on protecting the baby from evil spirits. For example, many Muslim parents will pin an amulet such as a blue stone or a verse from the Qur'an to the newborn's clothing as protection. Following birth, it is common for a male family member to whisper prayers in the newborn baby's ear to declare faith and protect the baby (Guthrie, Butler, & Elliott, 2010).

Childrearing Practices

In some families children are expected to take on responsibilities early and may be expected to take on tasks such as management of their own chronic disease and nutritional intake. In other families, children are given long periods to grow up and are not expected to manage healthcare needs. Directing teaching to a child with diabetes in the latter family type may not be appropriate. Nurses often provide information and ask about developmental milestones for children; however, there may be variations in family goals and it is not unusual for children to accomplish various tasks at younger or older ages. For example, it is commonly expected that children are weaned by 1 year of age and toilet trained at about 2 years of age, but this is not always the case. The nurse should ask about the norms in the family and whether the child is developing according to the parents' expectations. As long as the child is progressing in motor, language, and social tasks, some variation is expected due to cultural norms.

Table 2–3	Childrearing Practices of Selected Cultures
Culture	**Childrearing Practices**
African American	Grandmothers play an important role in the care of children. Children are expected to demonstrate respectfulness, conformity to rules, obedience, and good behavior. Extended family is very important.
Amish	The family contains, on average, seven children. Childrearing is regarded as the highest priority for parents. Grandparents often provide care to children. Children are expected to continue with the Amish tradition. Children are expected to follow the rules as prescribed by the church district.
Appalachian	Large families are common. Strict parenting practices and physical punishment are common. Grandparents frequently provide care to children.
Arab American	The father is typically the disciplinarian. The child's character is considered a reflection of the family's influence. Children are expected to respect their elders and to have good behavior. Adolescents are expected to do well in their studies. Discipline may include physical punishment and shaming.
Chinese American	The family may lavish resources on child. Children typically depend on family for all needs and may not be expected to earn their own money as adolescents. Male children are often more valued than female children. Children may be taught to avoid displaying their emotions/feelings. Children are expected to assist parents in the home (chores). High educational achievement is expected.
Mexican American	Children are closely protected and are not encouraged to leave the home. Extended family members frequently live close by. Children are expected to demonstrate respect for parents and elderly family members. Discipline may include physical punishment. Education is a priority.
Navajo Indian	Large families are important. Infants may be kept in a cradleboard to protect them. Grandmothers are important decision makers in the family. Children are allowed to make decisions about their care.

Source: Data from Purnell, L. D. (2013). *Transcultural health care: A culturally competent approach* (4th ed.). Philadelphia, PA: F. A. Davis; Purnell, L. D. (2009). *Guide to culturally competent health care* (2nd ed.). Philadelphia, PA: F. A. Davis.

Views about alternative lifestyles such as sexual orientation and single parenting are also established by the family's values and beliefs. Understanding such values assists the nurse in providing sensitive care. Examples of childrearing practices common to particular cultures are listed in Table 2–3. Realize that the practices listed are common in these cultures, but not necessarily practiced by all members of that culture.

CULTURE AND NURSING CARE

Healthcare providers are often unaware of the cultural characteristics they themselves demonstrate. Without cultural awareness, caregivers tend to project their own cultural responses onto foreign-born patients; patients from different socioeconomic, religious, or educational groups; or patients from different regions of the country. This projection leads care providers to assume that the patients are demonstrating a specific behavior for the same reason that they themselves would. Moreover, healthcare providers often fail to realize that medicine has its own culture, which has been dominated historically by traditional middle-class values and beliefs.

Ethnocentrism is the conviction that the values and beliefs of one's own cultural group are the best or only acceptable ones. It is characterized by an inability to understand the beliefs and worldview of another culture. To a certain extent, everyone is guilty of ethnocentrism, at least some of the time. Thus, the nurse who values stoicism during labor may be uncomfortable with the more vocal response of some Latin American women. Another nurse may be disconcerted by a Southeast Asian woman who believes that pain is something to be endured rather than alleviated and who is intent on maintaining self-control in labor.

Developing Cultural Competence
Culture Shock

The experience that people have in attempting to understand or adapt to a culture that is fundamentally different from their own culture is known as *culture shock*. The person may experience feelings of discomfort, powerlessness, anxiety, and disorientation. Immigrants to the United States may experience culture shock when differences or conflicts arise between their own values, beliefs, and customs and the ways of their new surroundings. The nurse should assess childbearing women, children, and their families who have recently immigrated for indications of culture shock. Referring the family to counseling or support from representatives of the family's culture, such as a translator or community group, may be helpful.

Healthcare providers sometimes believe that if members of other cultures do not share Western values and beliefs, they should adopt them. For example, a nurse who believes strongly in equality of the sexes may find it difficult to remain silent if a woman from a Middle Eastern culture defers to her husband in decision making. It is important to remember that pressure to defy cultural values and beliefs can be stressful and anxiety provoking for these women.

To address issues of cultural diversity in the provision of health care, emphasis is being placed on developing **cultural competence**—that is, the ability to understand and effectively respond to the needs of individuals and families from different cultural backgrounds. "Cultural competence is a complex combination of knowledge, attitudes, and skills" (Spector, 2013, p. 356). It involves identifying and integrating the family's health beliefs, practices, and cultural and linguistic needs into patient care (NIH, 2012).

Culturally Influenced Responses

The nurse can begin developing cultural competence by becoming knowledgeable about the cultural differences and practices of various groups. Nurses who are knowledgeable about differences and who take them into account in planning and providing nursing care will be far more effective caregivers than those who do not.

Biologic Differences

Genetic and physical differences occur among cultural groups and can lead to disparity in needs and care. Differences include blood type, body build, skin color, drug metabolism, and susceptibility to certain diseases. Other disparities occur because of fundamental differences between genders, ages, and races. For example, male children are more likely to manifest pyloric stenosis and attention deficit disorder, whereas female children more often have congenital hip dysplasia and systemic lupus erythematosus. Age provides another biologic variation, as infants are more likely to manifest the cancer neuroblastoma, whereas adolescents have a higher incidence of Hodgkin disease. Race is also connected with certain disease processes. Sickle cell disease occurs predominantly in African Americans. African Americans also have a higher incidence of hypertension. American Indians have the highest incidence of diabetes by percentage of population in the United States. However, type 1 diabetes is more common in Caucasians, while type 2 diabetes has a higher incidence in Hispanics and American Indians. Thalassemia, another type of anemia, is most common in Mediterranean people. Lactose intolerance is common in Mexican Americans, African Americans, American Indians, and Asians (Giger, 2013).

Nurses need to understand other genetic characteristics in order to perform culturally competent nursing assessments and interventions. Differences in skin color and tone may make cyanosis, pallor, and jaundice difficult to recognize and describe. Mongolian spots are darkened skin on the lower back and buttocks of some babies with dark skin tones. Variations in texture of hair require different approaches to hygiene among various racial groups.

Communication Patterns

Communication is the method by which members of cultural groups share information and preserve their beliefs, values, norms, and practices. To ensure effective care, it is essential for families to be able to communicate with nurses and other healthcare providers. This becomes an issue when the family does not speak the language of the health professionals. In such cases it is best if the healthcare facility provides translators. Children are most likely to speak both the language of the parents and the healthcare providers and may appear to be likely interpreters. However, it is recommended that children never be used to interpret in healthcare situations due to the confidentiality needs of both parent and child. Additionally, if children are used as interpreters, it can create an imbalance in power that could adversely affect parental authority. Signs, posted literature, and brochures should also be available in the languages of the children and families served. Even when children speak the language of the healthcare providers, written material must be provided at a level that the family can read and understand.

Language can also affect health literacy skills because a large number of instructions are given in writing, including prescriptions and directions on medication bottles, signs hanging in health facilities, consent forms for procedures and surgery, insurance forms, directions for techniques or procedures, future appointment dates, and health promotion materials. Nurses need to verify what the patient and family can read and whether alternative ways of providing the information are needed. For example, nurses could verbally give the information and provide paper and pencil so that the family can take notes in their own language. Translation services should be available in all healthcare settings.

Variations in communication among cultures are reflected in their word meaning, voice inflection and quality, and verbal styles. Culture not only influences the manner in which feelings are expressed, but also which verbal and nonverbal expressions of communication are considered appropriate. An individual's willingness to discuss certain topics or to express or conceal certain thoughts and feelings is also influenced by cultural norms. Some groups may be expected to remain quiet when experiencing pain, while other cultures may loudly and dramatically express pain.

Use of first names and surnames varies among cultural groups, so nurses should not make assumptions, because the use of a person's first name may be considered disrespectful. Address family members respectfully, usually using terms such as Mr., Mrs., and Ms. If the person has a title such as doctor, judge, or senator, it should be used. The nurse should ask what the person prefers to be called and record this in the health record for future reference. In some cultures such as Korean, Cambodian, and Filipino, the first name used is actually the family name. Asking for the "family name" rather than the "last name" may clarify this practice.

Nonverbal Communication.   Nonverbal communication refers to body language such as posture, gestures, facial expressions, eye contact, and touch, as well as the use of silence. The nurse's use of nonverbal communication may hinder or help communication. Gestures and body language may be misunderstood or misinterpreted. Eye contact has different meanings among cultures. European Americans, for example, value eye contact with communication and interpret this as a sign of sincerity and interest. In other cultures, such as Asian and Native American, sustained eye contact may be considered rude or disrespectful. Some African Americans may misinterpret direct eye contact as aggressive behavior (Purnell, 2009).

Silence is considered a sign of respect in some cultures. Among those groups, offering an immediate response to a question may be viewed as being disrespectful since an instant reply could indicate that no thought was given to the matter. Nurses should watch for patterns in various cultures and alter their approach to be more congruent. For example, many nurses commonly nod and say "yes" or "oh, I see" when a patient is speaking. This may seem disruptive to some cultures. If the listener is silent and does not use such patterns of agreement, the nurse should alter his or her response to match more closely the acceptable method of communication for the family.

Touch.   The appropriateness of touch varies with each culture. For example, an Asian may consider touching an unfamiliar person of the opposite gender to be inappropriate, whereas touch between men and women may be viewed as appropriate by another culture. Adults commonly feel that it is acceptable to touch children of all ages, but this may not be accurate. It is best to look for responses from the family to touch and progress accordingly.

Space.   An individual's sense of personal space also differs by culture. Space refers to the physical distance and relationships between the individual and other persons and objects in the environment. Cultures may have specific spatial preferences, such as personal distance and social distance. Some cultures tend to prefer close contact with less space since they use touch as a form of communication. The nurse should be alert for how close a childbearing woman or a child comes to other individuals and try to maintain this space during interactions. Nursing procedures often cause the space barrier to be broken. Nurses need to touch patients to take vital signs, administer injections, change dressings, and the like. This does not mean that close touch is appropriate at all times. It is essential to tell all patients before touching them for procedures so they understand what is happening.

Time Orientation

Cultures have specific values and meanings regarding time orientation. Cultural groups may place emphasis on the events of the past, those events that occur in the present, or those events that will occur in the future. Children reflect the time orientation of their families and the cultures in which they live. Time is also influenced by development so that young children sometimes do not understand the use of clocks, the importance ascribed to being "on time," or other time orientations.

Cultures that are oriented predominantly to the past may want to begin healthcare encounters with lengthy descriptions of past healthcare treatments, family history of diseases, or individual past experiences with health. There may be little interest in learning methods of adapting to or maintaining a new plan of care.

For cultures that are oriented predominantly to the present, little consideration may be given to either the past or the future. For example, adolescents commonly focus on the present, and may not engage in preventive health practices for long-term health. Therefore, short-term goals often provide more incentive to adolescents.

Cultures that are oriented predominantly to the future, such as European American, may not focus on what is important at the present time. For example, the family focusing on the future may focus on the dreams they had for a child's education or sports performance and have trouble setting present goals for treatment of a disease such as juvenile arthritis. One commonly hears that it was a big adjustment to learn to "take one day at a time." Not living up to the family's expectation for their future success may be difficult for a child who has developed an illness that has a chronic course.

Time also refers to punctuality about schedules and appointments. In the United States, the predominant culture respects being on time and considers time valuable and not to be wasted. Other cultures may not emphasize a concern for time. This may be manifested by a family's inability to follow timed medication schedules or treatments or to show up as scheduled for an appointment. In these cases it is not intended as a sign of disrespect.

Nutrition

Nutritional practices begin even before birth as many cultural groups have beliefs that determine foods that are healthy to eat or should be avoided during pregnancy. Nutritional habits and patterns vary among cultures and are related to both religious practices and health beliefs. Certain cultures and religions have restrictions on or prescriptions about specific foods and preparation methods. Ritualistic behaviors involving eating and drinking, for example on special occasions and holidays, are observed by most cultures. Many religions recommend fasts during specific holy seasons, such as Lent for Roman Catholics, Yom Kippur for Jews, and Ramadan for Muslims; however, in most cases, small children, pregnant women, the elderly, and sick individuals are not required to fast.

Additionally, some cultures value large size or may associate a healthy child with being "large." Other cultures value slimness and look down on individuals who are obese. Both of these views influence family eating patterns and expectations for the child; the child's self-esteem can therefore be influenced. The U.S. culture honors being slim in the media but reinforces eating and large size by the availability of fast food and positive image of large sports stars such as some football players, which can result in confusion about health and body image.

Nutrition may also be essential to the culture's practices for health promotion and care during illness. Health problems associated with specific cultures that may require dietary changes are also identified. Nutrition can be closely related to environmental situations, and families with few resources may not be able to obtain or eat cultural foods due to access or financial issues. Nutrition plays a powerful role in maintaining health, so resources for nutritious and desired foods may be needed.

NURSING MANAGEMENT

The focus of nursing care is assessment of cultural influences on the patient's health. The nurse providing culturally competent care to the woman or child and family considers all facets of their culture. Identification of cultural influences as well as cultural barriers will enable the nurse to provide culturally competent nursing care and management. See *Evidence-Based Practice: Investigating Culture and Healthcare Barriers.*

Nursing Assessment

Assessment of the woman or child and family includes determining the family's cultural healthcare beliefs and practices. Questions may include:

- Who in the family must be consulted before decisions are made about a person's care?

- Does the patient, or do the parents of a child, see primarily in the present or do they have a futuristic time orientation?

- What type of health provider is most appropriate for (or preferred by) the woman, the child, or the family?

- Does the family have beliefs or traditions that may affect the plan of care?

Several cultural assessment tools are available to assist the nurse in gathering this information. These tools are becoming increasingly common at healthcare agencies as providers act in response to the expectation of culturally competent care. The nurse who respects cultural diversity is an asset to the childbearing and childrearing family as they adjust to their new role. Establishing a trusting relationship enables the nurse to assist the family in meeting educational needs.

The use of North American Nursing Diagnosis Association (NANDA) nursing diagnoses to describe situations specifically related to culture may in itself be culturally biased because the foci of these diagnoses are based on Western cultural beliefs. Diagnoses such as *Communication: Verbal, Impaired* or *Knowledge, Deficient* should not be used solely because a person does not speak English. Is someone who speaks a different language "impaired" in communication?

Specific nursing diagnoses are dependent on the reason the family seeks contact with healthcare professionals, ranging from a pregnancy to a child's health promotion and health maintenance (e.g., immunizations) to the care of a child with a chronic or terminal illness. Examples include the following (NANDA-I © 2012):

- *Therapeutic Regimen Management: Family, Ineffective,* related to mistrust of healthcare personnel

- *Fear* related to separation from support system in stressful situation such as hospitalization

- *Spiritual Distress* related to discrepancy between spiritual beliefs and prescribed treatment

- *Family Processes, Interrupted,* related to a shift in family roles due to illness

The planning and implementation of nursing care for the culturally diverse family depend specifically on the findings of the previous assessments. Nurses need to partner with the family to establish a safe, effective, and desirable plan of care. Nurses can ensure access to an interpreter if needed and evaluate whether the match with a particular interpreter is appropriate for the child and family.

Recognizing the influence of culture on one's beliefs, values, and healthcare practices is essential for the nurse to deliver culturally competent care. Nurses demonstrate appropriate strategies for delivering culturally sensitive care when they develop techniques in assessing the influence of culture on the pregnant woman or the child and family and incorporate that information into an individualized plan of care.

Culturally competent nurses find effective ways to partner with the family to assist them in determining how they can incorporate prescribed therapies with their healthcare practices. Ensure that the woman herself or the child and family understand the problem or illness, treatment, and health promotion activities. Apply culturally sensitive techniques when dispelling any cultural myths.

Nurses can also collaborate with a multidisciplinary team, including social workers and language specialists, to assist the family in receiving assistance with barriers to care such as transportation, financial issues, remote access, and others.

COMPLEMENTARY AND ALTERNATIVE THERAPIES AND THE FAMILY

Through most of the 20th century in the United States, it was rare for European American childbearing families to consult anyone except their obstetrician for advice about their pregnancy, birth, and postpartum period. Similarly, most childrearing families closely followed the advice of their pediatrician about all aspects of child care. Though such patients are still encountered today, nurses are more likely to care for families who integrate other types of practitioners and therapies with traditional Western medicine.

Although the terms *complementary* and *alternative* are often used interchangeably, they have different meanings and applications. A **complementary therapy** may be defined as any procedure or product that is used as an adjunct to conventional medical treatment (National Center for Complementary and Alternative Medicine [NCCAM], 2011). Although complementary therapies were absent from clinics and hospitals until the past few decades, therapies such as acupuncture, acupressure, and massage therapy are now often used with conventional medical care, and many health insurance plans cover at least a portion of the cost of such therapies.

In contrast, an **alternative therapy** is usually considered a substance or procedure that is used in place of conventional medicine (NCCAM, 2011). It usually has not undergone rigorous scientific testing in this country, although it might have been thoroughly tested in other countries. Alternative therapies are not usually available in conventional clinics and hospitals, and their costs are not typically covered under most health insurance policies. An example of an alternative therapy is the use of herbal medicines instead of biomedicines for the treatment of a child's health condition. In other words, the child would not receive traditional Western medical care for the condition, such as surgery, radiation, prescribed medications, or other medical interventions.

The dramatic increase in complementary and alternative therapies that began in the final decade of the 20th century was probably the result of a combination of several factors:

- Increased consumer awareness of the limitations of conventional Western medicine
- Increased international travel
- Increased media attention
- Advent of the Internet

Evidence-Based Practice   Investigating Culture and Healthcare Barriers

Clinical Question

What barriers to providing accessible health care exist among ethnically diverse families with children?

The Evidence

Ferayorni, Sinha, and McDonald (2011) examined demographic characteristics, socioeconomic status, access to care, perceived barriers to care, compliance with follow-up care, and unmet health needs in foreign-born children who visited a pediatric emergency department. Parents of 385 children were interviewed during a visit to the emergency department and over the telephone 1 week after the visit. Twenty-three percent of these children did not have health insurance. Compared to children with health insurance, those who did not have coverage were less likely to have a regular healthcare provider and a regular place for health and dental care. Parents of 31% of uninsured children cited a perceived barrier to care. Barriers reported most often were language, lack of insurance and inability to pay, and transportation. Parents of 26 children reported unmet healthcare needs, with a slightly higher prevalence among uninsured children as opposed to insured children. Dental care was the most commonly reported unmet healthcare need. Uninsured children who were foreign born were primarily Spanish speaking, poorer, and had poor access to health care. This population was also more likely to use the emergency department for its healthcare needs.

Baker, Dang, Ly, et al. (2010) examined barriers to immunizations for Hmong children in California. Responses from 417 parents were analyzed to determine what factors contributed to perceived barriers. Parents of Hmong children who used traditional Hmong health care, such as herbalists and shamans, and were of lower socioeconomic status had higher perceived barriers to immunizations.

Schneiderman, McDaniel, Xie, et al. (2010) examined the perceptions of 237 parents at a child welfare pediatric medical clinic related to healthcare access barriers and pediatric healthcare use. Difficulty understanding the explanations given by physicians was identified as the greatest healthcare access barrier and could impact compliance with recommended health care among this population.

Best Practice

Socioeconomic status is a theme in all of these studies. These families may not have health insurance, a regular healthcare provider, or adequate transportation. Nurses need to refer families to sources for healthcare services and then follow up to be sure the families were able to access care. Referrals to community health centers and instructions for transportation to the health setting are important for many families. A need for understandable information is another theme among most groups. Explaining why an immunization is needed as well as providing information about the child's condition are important nursing roles. Interpreters may be needed to provide this information. Referring the family to others from the same ethnic or racial group and assisting them in navigating complex systems such as school and social services may also be necessary. Cultural differences and practices were also cited as a barrier to health care. It is essential that healthcare providers become familiar with other cultures and be accepting of practices that are safe for the child. By being open to practices of other cultures, healthcare providers will find families more willing to share openly about how they treat their children. This may lead to an opportunity for education related to unsafe practices.

Clinical Reasoning

What is the process that immigrant families in your state or province must follow to secure health care for their children? How would you help to guide someone through this process? What cultural groups are common in your community? Do you speak their language? If not, what measures should you take to ensure that they understand the teaching offered in clinical settings? What type of support groups will be helpful for families when they have a child with special healthcare needs?

In this century, it seems clear that Western health care will see an ever-increasing integration between conventional medicine and complementary therapies. Some obvious examples of this new integration in perinatal settings include the acceptance of certain herbal teas for antepartum discomforts; the use of massage, Reiki, or Therapeutic Touch during the first stage of labor; music during childbirth; and the increased emphasis on skin-to-skin mother-to-baby bonding in the immediate postpartum period.

Further evidence of this increased integration is the establishment in 1992 of the Office of Alternative Medicine (OAM) at the National Institutes of Health. The OAM was mandated by Congress to promote research into complementary and alternative therapies and dissemination of information to consumers. In 1998 the OAM was incorporated into a new National Center for Complementary and Alternative Medicine (NCCAM) with an expanded mission and increased funding. Many studies of complementary and alternative therapies are currently under way at NCCAM.

Benefits and Risks

Complementary and alternative therapies have many benefits for women and children. Many complementary and alternative therapies emphasize prevention and wellness, and place a higher value on holistic healing than on physical cure.

SAFETY ALERT!

Complementary and alternative therapies must be assessed for safety, including positive and negative benefits, cost, efficacy, and clinical usefulness. The use of herbs and natural products raises many issues, of which these are just a few: standards of products, misleading claims, and safety related to megadoses of some products.

Determine the family's use of complementary and/or alternative therapies such as the type of remedies and healthcare practices used. Also determine the side effects, risks, and other implications to the child receiving this type of therapy. Work with the family to ensure safe practices with the use of complementary and/or alternative therapies.

Types of Complementary and Alternative Therapies

Numerous forms of complementary and alternative therapies are available. Only a few of the most commonly used approaches are presented here.

Homeopathy

Homeopathy is a healing approach in which a person is treated with small doses of medicines that would cause illness when given to someone who is healthy. Traditional Western (or allopathic) medicine generally gives medicine or treatments that suppress symptoms. Analgesics for pain or antibiotics for infection are examples of such treatments. In homeopathy, the symptoms are viewed as the body's method of healing, and small doses of medications are given to enhance the symptoms.

For example, medications are chosen to promote fever and inflammation since they are thought to be healing forces (Fontaine, 2011; Spector, 2013).

Naturopathy

Naturopathy is a form of medicine that utilizes the healing forces of nature and is commonly referred to as natural medicine. It is more precisely defined as a healing system that combines safe and effective traditional means of preventing and treating human disease with the most current advances in modern medicine (American Association of Naturopathic Physicians [AANP], 2011). Many naturopathic physicians are eclectic, employing a variety of therapies in their practice. These might include clinical nutrition, botanical medicine, homeopathy, natural childbirth, traditional Chinese medicine, hydrotherapy, naturopathic manipulative therapy, pharmacology, minor surgery, and counseling for lifestyle modifications (AANP, 2011).

Traditional Chinese Medicine

Traditional Chinese medicine (TCM) developed more than 3,000 years ago in the Chinese culture and then gradually spread with modifications to other Asian countries. The underlying focus of TCM is prevention, although diagnosis and treatment of disease also play an important role.

TCM seeks to ensure the balance of energy, which is called *chi* or *qi* (pronounced "chee"). Chi is the invisible flow of energy in the body that maintains health and energy and enables the body to carry out its physiologic functions. Chi flows along certain pathways or meridians.

Another important concept in TCM is that of *yin* and *yang*, opposing internal and external forces that, together, represent the whole.

TCM includes the following therapeutic techniques:

- *Acupuncture* uses very fine (hairlike) stainless steel needles to stimulate specific acupuncture points, depending on the patient's medical assessment and condition.

- *Acupressure* (Chinese massage) uses pressure from the fingers and thumbs to stimulate pressure points.

- *Herbal therapy* is an important part of TCM, but it is sometimes difficult to locate a skilled herbalist because there are relatively few in the United States and other English-speaking countries.

- *Qi gong* (pronounced "chee-goong") is a self-discipline that involves the use of breathing, meditation, self-massage, and movement. Typically practiced daily, the movements are nontiring and are designed to stimulate the flow of chi.

- *T'ai chi* (pronounced "ty chee") is a form of martial art. It originally focused on physical fitness and self-defense, but it is currently used to improve health as well (Fontaine, 2011).

- *Moxibustion* involves the application of heat from a small piece of burning herb called *moxa (Artemisia vulgaris)*. The moxa stick is typically burned at the lateral side of the little toe. In TCM moxibustion has many uses. For example, studies from China demonstrate good success when moxibustion is used to help turn a fetus who is breech to a vertex presentation (van den Berg, Kaandorp, Bosch, et al., 2010).

Mind-Based Therapies

Biofeedback is a method used to help individuals learn to control their physiologic responses based on the concept that the mind controls the body. An individual is hooked up to a system of highly sensitive instruments that relay information about the body back to that person. Currently biofeedback has more than 150 applications for disease prevention and the restoration of health. The effectiveness of biofeedback has been proven in countless studies, and it is now considered a conventional therapy more than a complementary one.

Hypnosis, whether guided by a trained hypnotherapist or induced through self-hypnosis, is a state of great mental and physical relaxation during which a person is very open to suggestions. In this state the individual is able to modify body responses. Pregnant women who receive hypnosis before childbirth have reported shorter, less painful labors and births.

Visualization is a complementary therapy in which a person goes into a relaxed state and focuses on or "visualizes" soothing or positive scenes such as a beach or a mountain glade. Visualization helps reduce stress and encourage relaxation.

Guided imagery is a state of intense, focused concentration used to create compelling mental images. It is sometimes considered a form of hypnosis. Guided imagery is useful in imagining a desired effect such as weight loss or in mentally rehearsing a new procedure or activity.

Chiropractic

Chiropractic, the third largest independent health profession in the United States (behind medicine and dentistry), is based on concepts of manipulation to address health problems that are thought to be the result of abnormal nerve transmissions (subluxation) caused by misalignment of the spine. In the United States doctors of chiropractic perform more than 90% of all spinal manipulations (American Chiropractic Association, 2011). Chiropractors also stress the importance of proper nutrition and regular exercise to good health. Chiropractic is widely available, and popular demand has earned it a higher level of insurance coverage than most other alternative therapies.

Massage Therapy

Massage has been used for centuries as a form of therapy. *Massage therapy* involves manipulation of the soft tissues of the body to reduce stress and tension, increase circulation, diminish pain, and promote a sense of well-being. Different techniques have been developed, including Swedish massage, shiatsu massage, Rolfing, and trigger point massage. Most forms use techniques such as pressing, kneading, gliding, circular motion, tapping, and vibrational strokes.

Certain massage therapists specialize in massage for women during pregnancy. Massage is often helpful as women adapt to the discomforts of their changing bodies. Certified nurse-midwives often use perineal massage prior to labor to stretch the muscles of the perineum around the vaginal opening and thereby prevent tearing of the tissues during childbirth. During labor, massage of the back and buttocks by the nurse, labor coach, or doula can help the woman relax and may help decrease her discomfort.

Infant massage is also growing in popularity in the United States, and many parents have learned to massage their infants and young children (Figure 2–5 ●). Massage also plays a role in therapy for children with a variety of conditions, including eczema.

● **Figure 2–5** Infant massage.

Herbal Therapies

Herbal therapy or herbal medicine has been used since ancient times to treat illnesses and ailments. Well-known herbal remedies include ginger, rosemary, ginseng, ginkgo, chamomile, oil of evening primrose, *Echinacea*, garlic, lemon balm, and black cohosh.

Herbs are categorized as dietary supplements and are controlled by the Dietary Supplement Health Education Act. They do not require approval by the Food and Drug Administration (FDA) as do prescription and over-the-counter medications; however, the FDA does have the authority to pull a product off the market if it is proven to be dangerous (Cranwell-Bruce, 2008; Fontaine, 2011). Consequently, most of what is known about herbs comes from Germany where they have been studied for some time (Fontaine, 2011).

SAFETY ALERT!

The use of herbs during pregnancy is an especially important consideration for nurses working with childbearing families. Pregnant and lactating women interested in using herbs are best advised to consult with their healthcare provider before taking any herbs, even as teas. Lists identifying common herbs that women are advised to avoid or use with caution during pregnancy and lactation are available. Certain herbs may be harmful to children with some conditions (e.g., renal disorders), or they may interact with prescribed medication, and should not be used.

In cases when the family's cultural practice is placing the child in a hazardous situation, civil courts may intervene to provide care for the child, for example, by mandating a life-preserving chemotherapy procedure for a child even when the family is opposed to treatment. Support families in their beliefs and healthcare practices, but remain alert for any care that could be harmful for the child and report it promptly.

Therapeutic Touch

Therapeutic Touch is grounded in the belief that people are a system of energy with a self-healing potential. The Therapeutic Touch practitioner, often a nurse, can unite his or her energy

Video   Infant Massage

field with that of the patient's, directing it in a specific way to promote well-being and healing. Healing is promoted when the body's energies are in balance. By passing their hands over the patient, without touching the patient, healers can identify energy imbalances. Proponents of Therapeutic Touch believe that a strong desire to help the recipient is essential, as is a conscious use of the self to act as a link between the universal life energy and the other person (Fontaine, 2011).

Like many other conventional and complementary therapies, Therapeutic Touch should be applied cautiously to pregnant women, newborns, and children by trained providers (Figure 2–6 ●).

Other Types of Complementary and Alternative Therapies

This discussion only touched on some of the most common forms of complementary and alternative therapies. Other examples include Ayurveda (the traditional medicine of India), meditation, craniosacral therapy, reflexology, hydrotherapy, hatha yoga, regular physical exercise, aromatherapy, color and light therapy, music and sound therapies, magnetic therapy, and Reiki, to name a few. Readers interested in these therapies are referred to specialty texts.

● **Figure 2–6** During pregnancy, Therapeutic Touch is often helpful in easing pain and reducing anxiety.

Source: dean bertoncelj/Shutterstock

Nursing Care of the Family Using Complementary Therapies

Some form of complementary and alternative medicine (CAM) is currently being used by 36% of adults in the United States. When prayer for health reasons and megavitamin therapy are added to the definition, the number increases to 62%. Women use CAM more often than men do, as do people with higher educational levels and people who have been hospitalized within the past year. By race, when megavitamin therapy and prayer are included in the definition, blacks are the greatest users of CAM. When those elements are excluded, Asians are the greatest users, followed by whites (Fontaine, 2011).

The reality that families may use CAM and not reveal it raises some concern. Certain CAM modalities such as biofeedback, acupuncture, aromatherapy, and massage are not likely to cause adverse effects. However, the possibility exists that there might be interactions between herbal therapies and other medications prescribed by the care provider (Cranwell-Bruce, 2008; Fontaine, 2011). Complications may also develop from the use of vitamin supplements.

The use of CAM in the care of children must be addressed because of the limited research with this age group and developmental variations that may influence efficacy and safety. While many CAM therapies may have been proven effective in adults, they may have little effect on children, or even be harmful.

Nurses who create a climate of respect and openness tend to be more effective in gathering information about a family's use of complementary or alternative therapies. The nurse should use a nonjudgmental approach in assessing pregnant women and families for the use of CAM. Identify the expected outcome of the herbal or dietary supplement. Ask specifically about the use of herbs and other supplements, as the pregnant woman, parent, or child may not think to include them in their list of medications.

Nurses should use complementary modalities that are in the scope of their nursing practice and the nursing practice act in their state. Their use should also be supported by evidence-based research (Fontaine, 2011). Nurses working with a pregnant woman might use acupressure wristbands for the treatment of nausea. Other therapies nurses often employ include progressive relaxation, exercise and movement, Therapeutic Touch, visualization and guided imagery, prayer, meditation, music therapy, massage, storytelling, aromatherapy, and journaling.

Nurses who use complementary modalities should document their use within the context of nursing practice. This is most effective when the modality is identified as an intervention to address a specific nursing diagnosis or identified patient need. Thus, music therapy might be used for a laboring woman or a child to help address the identified nursing diagnosis of ***Pain, Acute*** (NANDA-I © 2012).

Clinical Tip

A recent study examined the frequency of CAM use in general pediatrics as compared to specialty pediatrics. Children with specific conditions such as epilepsy, cancer, and sickle cell disease were more likely to use CAM than those with acute illnesses or injury. This difference is perhaps related to recurring symptoms that are more likely to occur in children with chronic illnesses. Use of CAM in a child, however, was most directly related to whether or not CAM was used by the child's parents. Assessment of the child should include questions related to the use of CAM so that any concerns or questions related to its use can be addressed (Post-White, Fitzgerald, Hageness, et al., 2009).

Nurses have a role in conducting and supporting research on CAM. Because of the variety of CAM therapies in use, research is needed in a host of areas. The results of research on CAM can be found in professional journals and at the National Institutes of Health website. As the evidence supporting the use of certain interventions grows, nurses and other healthcare providers are incorporating the results as part of their evidence-based practice.

Critical Concept Review

LEARNING OUTCOME 2.1: Compare the characteristics of different types of families.

1. Nuclear families consist of a mother, father, and children.
2. Dual-career/dual-earner families make up the majority of contemporary families in the United States.
3. Childless families are a growing trend in American culture.
4. Extended family members can play an active role in family life, decision making, and family roles.
5. Extended kin network families share a social support network, chores, goods, and services.
6. Single-parent families account for almost a third of all U.S. families.
7. The blended or reconstituted nuclear family has become increasingly common due to high rates of divorce and remarriage and consists of two parents with biologic children from a previous marriage or relationship who marry or cohabitate.
8. In a binuclear family, the biologic children are members of two nuclear households, with co-parenting by the father and the mother.
9. A nonmarital heterosexual cohabiting family is often chosen for financial reasons or for companionship.
10. Gay and lesbian families have children who show no significant differences from children raised in more traditional families.

LEARNING OUTCOME 2.2: Identify the stages of a family life cycle.

1. Stage I: Beginning families
2. Stage II: Childbearing families
3. Stage III: Families with preschool children
4. Stage IV: Families with school-age children
5. Stage V: Families with teenagers
6. Stage VI: Families launching young adults
7. Stage VII: Middle-aged parents
8. Stage VIII: Retirement and old age

LEARNING OUTCOME 2.3: Identify prevalent cultural norms related to childbearing and childrearing.

Childbearing and childrearing are influenced by the following cultural norms:

1. Status of the family unit:
   - Pregnancy may elevate the status of both the man and the woman depending on the culture.
   - The role of extended family in the care of the child varies depending on the culture.
2. Contraception:
   - Culture may prohibit the use of contraception or may determine the type used.
3. View of pregnancy:
   - May be seen as an honor.
   - May be viewed as a sickness.
   - May determine the responsibilities of the mother or father.
4. Existence of taboos.
5. Discipline.

LEARNING OUTCOME 2.4: Summarize the importance of cultural competency in providing nursing care.

The nurse who provides culturally competent care:

1. Recognizes the importance of the childbearing family's value system.
2. Acknowledges that differences occur among people.
3. Seeks to respect and respond to ethnic diversity in a way that leads to mutually desirable outcomes.

LEARNING OUTCOME 2.5: Discuss the use of a cultural assessment tool as a means of providing culturally sensitive care.

A cultural assessment tool provides information of health practices based on:

1. Patient beliefs
2. Patient values
3. Patient customs

LEARNING OUTCOME 2.6: Identify key considerations in providing spiritually sensitive care.

To provide spiritually sensitive care, the nurse should:

1. Determine the current spiritual and religious beliefs and practices that will affect the mother and baby.
2. Accommodate these practices where possible.
3. Examine one's own spiritual or religious beliefs to be more aware and able to provide nonjudgmental care.

LEARNING OUTCOME 2.7: Differentiate between complementary and alternative therapies.

1. A complementary therapy is an adjunct to conventional medical treatment that has been through rigorous scientific testing, which shows that it has some reliability.
2. An alternative therapy is usually considered a substance or procedure that has not undergone rigorous scientific testing in this country, although it might have been thoroughly tested in other countries.

LEARNING OUTCOME 2.8: Determine the benefits and risks of complementary and alternative therapies.

1. CAM therapies have several benefits. Many of them emphasize prevention and wellness, place a higher value on holistic healing than on physical cure, are noninvasive, and have few side effects. In addition, many are more affordable and available than conventional therapies.
2. Risks of CAM therapies include lack of standardization, lack of regulation and research substantiating safety and effectiveness, inadequate training and certification of some healers, and financial and health risks of unproven methods.

LEARNING OUTCOME 2.9: Summarize complementary therapies appropriate for the nurse to use with childbearing and childrearing families.

Nurses may choose to use the following CAM therapies:

1. Guided imagery
2. Acupressure
3. Prayer
4. Music therapy
5. Massage
6. Storytelling
7. Exercise and movement
8. Meditation
9. Aromatherapy
10. Journaling
11. Progressive relaxation

Clinical Reasoning in Action

While working in an inner-city clinic for adolescents, you meet a new patient, a 14-year-old Latina girl named Juanita. Her parents accompany her to the clinic. None of them speak English. Through an interpreter, Juanita tells you that she recently moved here with her parents. They have brought her here today because she has a sore throat. The curandero they took her to see prescribed the herbal remedy Echinacea, but her throat is still sore. The rapid test you perform for strep throat is positive and the nurse practitioner prescribes an antibiotic.

1. According to the national standards for culturally and linguistically appropriate services in health care set by the government, what are examples of important standards of care you as the nurse can provide in the care of this adolescent?
2. How can you, as the nurse, take steps to achieve cultural competence?
3. How would you, as the nurse, be able to address some of the disparities that can exist when this patient comes to the clinic?
4. What are some examples of common food preferences in the Latino-American culture?

See www.nursing.pearsonhighered.com for possible responses.

References

American Association of Naturopathic Physicians (AANP). (2011). *What is naturopathic medicine?* Retrieved from http://naturopathic.org/content.asp?contentid=59

American Chiropractic Association. (2011). *Spinal manipulation.* Retrieved from http://www.acatoday.org

Andrews, M. M., & Boyle, J. S. (2012). *Transcultural concepts in nursing care* (6th ed.). Philadelphia, PA: Lippincott Williams & Wilkins.

Baker, D. L., Dang, M. T., Ly, M. Y., & Diaz, R. (2010). Perception of barriers to immunization among parents of Hmong origin in California. *American Journal of Public Health, 100*(5), 839–845.

Balch, P. A. (2010). *Prescription for nutritional healing* (5th ed.). New York, NY: Avery Trade.

Bulte, E., Heerink, N., & Zhang, X. (2011). China's one-child policy and "the mystery of missing women": Ethnic minorities and male-biased sex ratios. *Oxford Bulletin of Economics and Statistics, 73*(1), 21–39.

Chamberlain, J., Miller, M. K., & Bornstein, B. H. (2008). The rights and responsibilities of gay and lesbian parents: Legal developments, psychological research, and policy implications. *Social Issues and Policy Review, 2*(1), 103–126.

Cranwell-Bruce, L. (2008). Herb-drug interactions. *MEDSURG Nursing, 17*(1), 52–54.

Duvall, E. M. (1977). *Marriage and family development* (5th ed.). New York, NY: Harper & Row.

Duvall, E. M., & Miller, B. L. (1985). *Marriage and family development* (6th ed.). New York, NY: Harper & Row.

Ferayorni, A., Sinha, M., & McDonald, F. W. (2011). Health issues among foreign born uninsured children visiting an inner city pediatric emergency department. *Journal of Immigrant and Minority Health, 13*(3), 434–444.

Fontaine, K. L. (2011). *Complementary and alternative therapies for nursing practice* (3rd ed.). Upper Saddle River, NJ: Pearson.

Friedman, M. M., Bowden, V. R., & Jones, E. G. (2003). *Family nursing: Research, theory, and practice* (5th ed.). Upper Saddle River, NJ: Prentice Hall.

Gedaly-Duff, V., Nielsen, A., Heims, M. L., & Pate, M. D. (2010). Family child health nursing. In J. R. Kaakinen, V. Gedaly-Duff, D. P. Coehlo, & S. M. H. Hanson (Eds.), *Family health care nursing: Theory, practice, and research* (4th ed., pp. 332–378). Philadelphia, PA: F. A. Davis.

Giger, J. N. (2013). *Transcultural nursing: Assessment & intervention* (6th ed.). St. Louis, MO: Elsevier Mosby.

Grossoehme, D. H., VanDyke, R., Jacobson, C. J., Cotton, S., Ragsdale, J. R., & Seid, M. (2010). Written prayers in a pediatric hospital: Linguistic analysis. *Psychology of Religion and Spirituality, 2*(4), 227–233.

Guthrie, J., Butler, W. J., & Elliott, R. L. (2010). A Muslim woman and childbirth. *Journal of the Medical Association of Georgia, 99*(2), 28–29.

Lambert, N. M., Fincham, F. D., & Graham, S. M. (2011). Understanding the layperson's perception of prayer: A prototype analysis of prayer. *Psychology of Religion and Spirituality, 3*(1), 55–65.

Mendelkow, J. L. (2009). The cult of true motherhood: A narrative. *All Graduate Theses and Dissertations. Paper 383.* Retrieved from http://digitalcommons.usu.edu/etd/383

Mueller, C. R. (2010). Spirituality in children: Understanding and developing interventions. *Pediatric Nursing, 36*(4), 197–203, 208.

National Center for Complementary and Alternative Medicine (NCCAM). (2011). *What is CAM?* Retrieved from http://nccam.nih.gov/health/whatiscam

National Institutes of Health. (2012). *Cultural competency.* Retrieved from http://www.nih.gov/clearcommunication/culturalcompetency.htm

Post-White, J., Fitzgerald, M., Hageness, S., & Sencer, S. F. (2009). Complementary and alternative medicine use in children with cancer and general and specialty pediatrics. *Journal of Pediatric Oncology Nursing, 26*(1), 7–15.

Purnell, L. D. (2009). *Guide to culturally competent health care* (2nd ed.). Philadelphia, PA: F. A. Davis.

Purnell, L. D. (2013). *Transcultural health care: A culturally competent approach* (4th ed.). Philadelphia, PA: F. A. Davis.

Schneiderman, J. U., McDaniel, D. D., Xie, B., Cabassa, L. J., & Suh, J. (2010). Child welfare caregivers of differing English-language use: Perceptions of pediatric health care access barriers. *Journal of Ethnic & Cultural Diversity in Social Work, 19,* 18–33.

Spector, R. E. (2013). *Cultural diversity in health and illness* (8th ed.). Upper Saddle River, NJ: Pearson.

Sueyoshi, S., & Ohtsuka, R. (2010). Significant effects of Fatwa-based perception on contraceptive practice among Muslim women in south Jordan under the early stage of fertility transition. *Biodemography and Social Biology, 56*(1), 67–79. doi:10.1080/19485561003709263

U.S. Census Bureau. (2012). *Definition: Household and family.* Retrieved from https://ask.census.gov

van den Berg, I., Kaandorp, G. C., Bosch, J. L., Duvekot, J. J., Arends, L. R., & Hunink, M. G. (2010). Cost-effectiveness of breech version by acupuncture-type interventions on BL 67, including moxibustion, for women with a breech fetus at 33 weeks gestation: A modeling approach. *Complementary Therapies in Medicine, 18*(2), 67–77.

Zoucha, R., & Zamarripa, C. A. (2013). People of Mexican heritage. In L. D. Purnell, *Transcultural health care: A culturally competent approach* (4th ed., pp. 374–390). Philadelphia, PA: F. A. Davis.

Reproductive Anatomy and Physiology

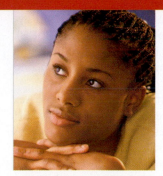

I am amazed by how little many of our students know about anatomy, physiology, and reproduction. As nurses, we must use every opportunity we have to teach young people about their bodies and those of their partners. Information is the key to helping keep them safe and well! —University Health Clinic Nurse

LEARNING OUTCOMES

3.1 Identify the structures and functions of the female reproductive system.

3.2 Explain the significance of specific female reproductive structures during pregnancy and childbirth.

3.3 Summarize the actions of the hormones that affect reproductive functioning.

3.4 Identify the two phases of the ovarian cycle and the changes that occur in each phase.

3.5 Describe the phases of the uterine (menstrual) cycle, their dominant hormones, and the changes that occur in each phase.

3.6 Identify the structures and functions of the male reproductive system.

Understanding childbearing requires more than understanding sexual intercourse, or the process by which the female and male sex cells unite. The nurse must also become familiar with the structures and functions that make childbearing possible and the phenomena that initiate it. This chapter presents the anatomic and physiologic aspects of the female and male reproductive systems.

The female and male reproductive organs are *homologous;* that is, they are fundamentally similar in structure and function. The primary functions of both female and male reproductive systems are to produce sex cells and transport them to locations where their union can occur. The sex cells, called *gametes,* are produced by specialized organs called *gonads.* A series of ducts and glands within both male and female reproductive systems contributes to the production and transport of the gametes.

PHYSIOLOGY OF ONSET OF PUBERTY

The term *puberty* refers to the developmental period between childhood and attainment of adult sexual characteristics and functioning. The age at onset and progress of puberty vary widely, physical changes overlap, and the sequence of events can vary from person to person. (For a detailed discussion of physical changes associated with puberty, see Chapter 34 🔗.)

Puberty is initiated by the maturation of the hypothalamic-pituitary-gonad complex (the *gonadostat*) and input from the central nervous system. The process, which begins during fetal life, is sequential and complex.

The central nervous system releases a neurotransmitter that stimulates the hypothalamus to synthesize and release **gonadotropin-releasing hormone (GnRH).** GnRH is transmitted to the anterior pituitary, where it causes the synthesis and secretion of the gonadotropins **follicle-stimulating hormone (FSH)** and **luteinizing hormone (LH)** (Figure 3–1 ●).

Although the gonads do produce small amounts of *androgens* (male sex hormones) and *estrogens* (female sex hormones) before the onset of puberty, FSH and LH stimulate increased secretion of these hormones. Androgens and estrogens influence the development of secondary sex characteristics. FSH and LH stimulate the processes of spermatogenesis and maturation of ova. The external and internal female reproductive organs develop and mature in response to estrogen and progesterone. Other hormones are involved in the onset of puberty. Abnormally high or low levels of adrenocorticotropic hormone (ACTH), thyroid hormone, or growth hormone (GH) can disrupt the onset of normal puberty (see Chapter 54 🔗 for a detailed discussion).

FEMALE REPRODUCTIVE SYSTEM

The female reproductive system consists of the external and internal genitals and the accessory organs of the breasts. Because of its importance to childbearing, the bony pelvis is also discussed in this chapter.

External Genitals

The appearance of the external genitalia varies greatly among women. Heredity, age, race, and the number of children a woman has borne influence the size, color, and shape of her external organs. The female external genitals, also referred to as the *vulva,* include the following structures (Figure 3–2 ●):

- Mons pubis
- Labia majora
- Labia minora
- Clitoris

● **Figure 3–1** Physiologic changes leading to onset of puberty. *A,* In females, and *B,* in males. Solid lines illustrate stimulation of hormone production, and broken lines illustrate inhibition. Through a neurotransmitter the central nervous system stimulates the hypothalamus, which in turn produces a gonadotropin-releasing factor that causes the anterior pituitary to produce gonadotropins (follicle-stimulating hormone, FSH; or luteinizing hormone, LH). These hormones stimulate specific structures in the gonads to secrete steroid hormones (estrogen, progesterone, or testosterone). The rise in pituitary hormone production increases hypothalamus activity. Elevated steroid hormone levels stimulate the central nervous system and pituitary gland to inhibit hormone production.

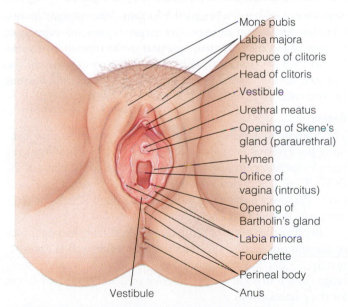

● **Figure 3–2** Female external genitals, longitudinal view.

- Urethral meatus and opening of the paraurethral (Skene's) glands
- Vaginal vestibule (vaginal orifice, vulvovaginal [Bartholin] glands, hymen, and fossa navicularis)
- Perineal body

Although they are not true parts of the female reproductive system, the urethral meatus and perineal body are considered here because of their proximity and relationship to the vulva. The vulva has a generous supply of blood and nerves. As a woman ages, estrogen secretions decrease, causing the vulvar organs to atrophy.

Mons Pubis

The *mons pubis* is a softly rounded mound of subcutaneous fatty tissue beginning at the lowest portion of the anterior abdominal wall (see Figure 3–2). The mons pubis is covered with pubic hair, typically with the hairline forming a transverse line across the lower abdomen. The hair is short and varies from sparse and fine in Asian women to heavy, coarse, and curly in women of African descent. The mons pubis protects the symphysis pubis, especially during coitus.

Labia Majora

The *labia majora* are longitudinal, raised folds of pigmented skin, one on either side of the vulvar cleft. Their chief function is to protect the structures lying between them. The labia majora are covered by hair follicles and sebaceous glands, with underlying adipose and muscle tissue. The inner surface of the labia majora in women who have not had children is moist and looks like mucous membrane, whereas after many births it is more skinlike. With each pregnancy, the labia majora may become less prominent.

Because of the extensive venous network in the labia majora, varicosities may occur during pregnancy, and obstetric or sexual trauma may cause hematomas. The labia majora share an extensive lymphatic supply with the other structures of the vulva, which can facilitate the spread of cancer in the female

Animation | *Female Reproductive System*

reproductive organs. Because of the nerves supplying the labia majora (from the first lumbar and third sacral segment of the spinal cord), certain regional anesthesia blocks will affect them and cause numbness.

Labia Minora

The *labia minora* are soft folds of skin within the labia majora that converge near the anus, forming the *fourchette*. Each labium minus has the appearance of shiny mucous membrane, moist and devoid of hair follicles. The labia minora are rich in sebaceous glands, which lubricate and waterproof the vulvar skin and provide bactericidal secretions. Because the sebaceous glands do not open into hair follicles but open directly onto the surface of the skin, sebaceous cysts commonly occur in this area. The labia minora are composed of erectile tissue and involuntary muscle tissue. Vulvovaginitis in this area is irritating because the labia minora have many tactile nerve endings. The labia minora increase in size at puberty and decrease after menopause because of changes in estrogen levels.

Clitoris

The *clitoris,* located between the labia minora, is about 5 to 6 mm long and 6 to 8 mm across. Its tissue is essentially erectile. The glans of the clitoris is partly covered by a fold of skin called the *prepuce,* or clitoral hood. This area resembles an opening to an orifice and may be confused with the urethral meatus. Accidental attempts to insert a catheter in this area produce extreme discomfort. The clitoris has rich blood and nerve supplies and is the primary erogenous organ of women. It secretes *smegma,* which along with other vulval secretions has a unique odor that may be sexually stimulating to the male.

Urethral Meatus and Paraurethral Glands

The *urethral meatus* is located 1 to 2.5 cm beneath the clitoris in the midline of the vestibule; it often appears as a puckered, slit-like opening. At times the meatus is difficult to visualize because of the presence of blind dimples, small mucosal folds, or wide variations in location.

The paraurethral glands, or *Skene's glands,* open into the posterior wall of the urethra close to its opening (see Figure 3–2). Their secretions lubricate the vaginal opening, facilitating sexual intercourse.

Vaginal Vestibule

The vaginal vestibule is a boat-shaped depression enclosed by the labia majora and minora, which is visible when they are separated (see Figure 3–2). The vestibule contains the vaginal opening, or *introitus,* which is the border between the external and internal genitals.

The *hymen* is a thin, elastic collar or semicollar of tissue that surrounds the vaginal opening. The appearance changes during the woman's lifetime. At birth, the hymen is essentially avascular. For thousands of years, some societies have perpetuated the belief that the hymen covers the vaginal opening and thus an intact hymen is a sign of virginity. However, modern studies of female genital anatomy have revealed that the hymen surrounds rather than entirely covers the vaginal opening, and can be torn not only through sexual intercourse but also through strenuous physical activity, masturbation, menstruation, or the use of tampons, thus dispelling old beliefs. For discussion of the nurse's role in discussing these topics, see Chapter 5 🔴.

The *vulvovaginal (Bartholin's) glands' duct openings* lie under the constrictor muscle of the vagina. These glands secrete a clear, thick, alkaline mucus that enhances the viability and motility of the sperm deposited in the vaginal vestibule. These gland ducts can harbor *Neisseria gonorrhoeae* and other bacteria, which can cause pus formation and abscesses in the Bartholin's glands.

The vestibular area is innervated predominantly by the perineal nerve from the sacral plexus. The area is not sensitive to touch generally; however, the hymen contains numerous free nerve endings as receptors to pain.

Perineal Body

The *perineal body* is a wedge-shaped mass of fibromuscular tissue found between the lower part of the vagina and the anus (see Figure 3–2). The superficial area between the anus and the vagina is referred to as the *perineum.*

The muscles that meet at the perineal body are the external sphincter ani, both levator ani (the superficial and deep transverse perineal), and the bulbocavernosus. These muscles mingle with elastic fibers and connective tissue in an arrangement that allows a remarkable amount of stretching. During the last part of labor, the perineal body thins out until it is just a few centimeters thick. This tissue is often the site of lacerations or episiotomy during childbirth (see Chapter 22 🔴).

Female Internal Reproductive Organs

The female internal reproductive organs—the vagina, uterus, fallopian tubes, and ovaries—are target organs for estrogenic hormones and they play a unique part in the reproductive cycle (Figure 3–3 🔴). Certain internal reproductive organs can be palpated during vaginal examination and assessed with various instruments.

Vagina

The **vagina** is a muscular and membranous tube that connects the external genitals with the uterus. It extends from the vulva to the uterus in a position nearly parallel to the plane of the pelvic brim. The vagina is often called the *birth canal* because it forms the lower part of the pelvic axis through which the fetus must pass during birth.

Because the cervix of the uterus projects into the upper part of the anterior wall of the vagina, the anterior wall is approximately 2.5 cm shorter than the posterior wall. Measurements range from 6 to 8 cm for the anterior wall and from 7 to 10 cm for the posterior wall.

In the upper part of the vagina, which is called the vaginal vault, there is a recess or hollow around the cervix. This area is called the *vaginal fornix.* Since the walls of the vaginal vault are very thin, various structures can be palpated through them, including the uterus, a distended bladder, the ovaries, the appendix, the cecum, the colon, and the ureters. The upper fourth of the vagina is separated from the rectum by the pouch of Douglas (sometimes referred to as the cul-de-sac of Douglas). This deep pouch or recess is posterior to the cervix.

When a woman lies on her back after intercourse, the space in the fornix permits the pooling of semen. The collection of a

Suspensory ligament
Fallopian tube
Fimbriae
Ovary
Fundus of uterus
Round ligament
Urinary bladder
Symphysis pubis
Mons pubis
Urethra
Clitoris
Labium minus
Labium majus

Sacrum
Perimetrium
Pouch of Douglas
Posterior fornix
Cervix
Anterior fornix
Rectum
Vagina
Urogenital diaphragm
Anus
Bartholin's gland
Perineal body

● **Figure 3–3** Female internal reproductive organs.

large number of sperm near the cervix at or near the time of ovulation increases the chances of pregnancy.

The walls of the vagina are covered with ridges, or rugae, crisscrossing each other. These rugae allow the vaginal tissues to stretch enough for the fetus to pass through during childbirth as well as stretch during coitus.

During a woman's reproductive life, an acidic vaginal environment is normal (pH 4–5). Secretion from the vaginal epithelium provides a moist environment. The acidic environment is maintained by a symbiotic relationship between lactic acid–producing bacilli (Döderlein bacillus or lactobacillus) and the vaginal epithelial cells. These cells contain glycogen, which is broken down by the bacilli into lactic acid. The amount of glycogen is regulated by the ovarian hormones. Any interruption of this process can destroy the normal self-cleaning action of the vagina. Such interruption may be caused by antibiotic therapy, douching, frequent intercourse, or use of vaginal sprays or deodorants. (For further discussion, see Chapter 5 ✐.) The acidic vaginal environment is normal only during the mature reproductive years and in the first days of life, when maternal hormones are operating in the infant. A relatively neutral pH of 7.5 is normal from infancy until puberty and after menopause.

Each third of the vagina is supplied by a distinct vascular pattern (Figure 3–4 ●). Although one would expect venous drainage going to the heart and lungs, anastomoses of the veins are present and make it possible for a pelvic embolism or carcinoma to bypass the heart and lungs and lodge in the brain, spine, or other remote part of the body.

Vaginal lymphatic fluids drain into the external and internal iliac nodes, the hypogastric nodes, and the inguinal glands. The posterior wall drains into nodes lying in the rectovaginal septum. Any vaginal infection follows these routes.

The pudendal nerve supplies what relatively little somatic innervation there is to the lower third of the vagina. Thus sensation during sexual excitement and coitus is reduced in this area, as is vaginal pain during the second stage of labor.

The vagina has three functions:

- To serve as the passage for sperm and for the fetus during birth

- To provide passage for the menstrual products from the uterine cavity to the outside of the body

- To protect against trauma from sexual intercourse and infection of the uterus, ovaries, and pelvis from pathogenic organisms

A

Uterus

The **uterus** is a hollow, muscular, thick-walled organ shaped like an upside-down pear (Figure 3–5 ●). It lies in the center of the pelvic cavity between the base of the bladder and the rectum and above the vagina. It is level with or slightly below the brim of the pelvis, with the external opening of the cervix (external os) at about the level of the ischial spines. The uterus of the mature woman is 7 to 8 cm long and 4 to 5 cm at its widest point and weighs 30 to 40 g (Heitmann, 2013).

About a fourth of women exposed to diethylstilbestrol (DES) in utero have structural variations of the cervix, uterus, and vagina (Khachikyan & Stratton, 2013). These women have increased incidence of miscarriage, ectopic pregnancy, cervical incompetency, and preterm births.

The body of the uterus can move freely forward or backward. Only the cervix is anchored laterally. Thus the position of the uterus can vary, depending on a woman's posture and musculature, number of children borne, bladder and rectal fullness, and even normal respiratory patterns. Generally, the uterus bends forward, forming a sharp angle with the vagina. If there is a bend in the area of the isthmus of the uterus and from there the cervix points downward, the uterus is said to be anteverted or anteflexed. Four pairs of ligaments (i.e., the cardinal, uterosacral, round, and broad) support the uterus. Single anterior and posterior ligaments also support the uterus.

The uterus is divided into two major parts: the upper triangular portion called the **corpus**, or uterine body; and the lower cylindric portion called the cervix. The corpus comprises the upper two thirds of the uterus and is composed mainly of a smooth muscle layer (myometrium). The lower third is the cervix, or neck. The rounded uppermost portion of the corpus that extends above the points of attachment of the fallopian tubes is called the **fundus**. The elongated portion of the uterus where the fallopian tubes enter is called the **cornua**.

The *isthmus* is that portion of the uterus between the internal cervical os and the endometrial cavity. The isthmus is about 6 mm above the uterine opening of the cervix (the internal os),

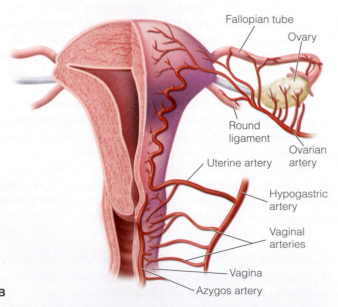

B

● **Figure 3–4** Blood supply to internal reproductive organs. *A,* Pelvic blood supply. *B,* Blood supply to vagina, ovaries, uterus, and fallopian tube.

● **Figure 3–5** Structures of the uterus.

and it is in this area that the uterine lining changes into the mucous membrane of the cervix; it joins the corpus to the cervix. The isthmus takes on importance in pregnancy because it becomes the lower uterine segment. At birth, this thin lower segment, situated behind the bladder, is the site for lower-segment cesarean births (see Chapter 23 ⊘).

The blood and lymphatic supplies to the uterus are extensive. Innervation of the uterus is entirely by the autonomic nervous system. Even without an intact nerve supply, the uterus can contract adequately for birth; for example, hemiplegic women have adequate uterine contractions.

Pain of uterine contractions is carried to the central nervous system by the 11th and 12th thoracic nerve roots. Pain from the cervix and upper vagina passes through the ilioinguinal and pudendal nerves. The motor fibers to the uterus arise from the 7th and 8th thoracic vertebrae. Because the sensory and motor levels are separate, epidural anesthesia can be used during labor and birth.

The function of the uterus is to provide a safe environment for fetal development. The uterine lining is cyclically prepared by steroid hormones for implantation of the embryo, a process known as **nidation**. Once the embryo is implanted, the developing fetus is protected until it is expelled.

Both the uterine body and the cervix are changed permanently by pregnancy. The body never returns to its prepregnant size, and the external os changes from a circular opening of about 3 mm to a transverse slit with irregular edges.

Uterine Corpus.

The uterine corpus is made up of three layers. The outermost layer is the *serosal layer,* or **perimetrium**, which is composed of peritoneum. The middle layer is the *muscular uterine layer,* or **myometrium**. This muscular uterine layer is continuous with the muscle layers of the fallopian tubes and the vagina. This characteristic helps these organs present a unified reaction to various stimuli—ovulation, orgasm, or the deposit of sperm in the vagina. These muscle fibers also extend into the ovarian, round, and cardinal ligaments and minimally into the uterosacral ligaments, which helps explain the vague but disturbing pelvic "aches and pains" reported by many pregnant women.

The myometrium has three distinct layers of uterine (smooth) involuntary muscles (Figure 3–6 ●). The outer layer, found mainly over the fundus, is made up of longitudinal muscles that cause the descent of the fetus, which places pressure on the cervical fibers leading to cervical effacement and delivery of the fetus. The thick middle layer is made up of interlacing muscle fibers in figure-eight patterns, which assist the longitudinal fibers in expelling the fetus. These muscle fibers also surround large blood vessels, and their contraction produces a hemostatic action (a tourniquet-like action on blood vessels to stop bleeding) after birth. The inner muscle layer consists of circular fibers that form sphincters at the fallopian tube attachment sites and at the internal os. The internal os sphincter inhibits the expulsion of the uterine contents during pregnancy but relaxes in labor as cervical dilatation occurs. An incompetent cervical os can be caused by a torn, weak, or absent sphincter at the internal os. The sphincters at the fallopian tubes prevent menstrual blood from flowing backward into the fallopian tubes from the uterus.

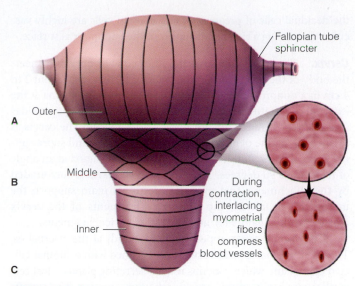

● **Figure 3–6** Myometrium uterine muscle layer placement and function. *A,* Outer layer (longitudinal muscles) is suited to expelling fetus. *B,* Middle layer (interlacing muscle fibers in figure-eight pattern) surrounds and constricts blood vessels to stop bleeding. *C,* Inner layer (circular muscle fibers form sphincters at fallopian tubes and internal os) prevents backflow of menstrual blood into fallopian tubes and stretches during labor as cervical dilatation occurs.

Although each layer of muscle has been discussed as having a unique function, it must be remembered that the uterine musculature works as a whole. The uterine contractions of labor are responsible for the dilatation of the cervix and provide the major force for the passage of the fetus through the pelvis and vaginal canal at birth.

The *mucosal layer,* or **endometrium**, of the uterine corpus is the innermost layer. This single layer consists of columnar epithelium, glands, and stroma. From menarche (first menstruation) to menopause, the endometrium undergoes monthly degeneration and renewal in the absence of pregnancy. As it responds to the governing hormonal cycle and prostaglandin influence as well, the endometrium varies in thickness from 0.5 to 5 mm.

The glands of the endometrium produce a thin, watery, alkaline secretion that keeps the uterine cavity moist. This endometrial milk not only helps sperm travel to the fallopian tubes but also nourishes the developing embryo before it implants in the endometrium (see Chapter 4 ⊘).

The blood supply to the endometrium is unique. In the myometrium, the radial arteries branch off from the arcuate arteries at right angles. Once inside the endometrium, they become the basal arteries supplying the zona basalis (a layer of the endometrium) and ultimately become the coiled arteries supplying the zona functionalis (also part of the endometrium). The basal arteries are not sensitive to cyclic hormonal control; hence, the zona basalis portion remains intact and is the site of new endometrial tissue generation. The coiled arteries are extremely sensitive to hormonal control. Their response is alternate relaxation and constriction during the ischemic, or terminal, phase of the menstrual cycle. These differing responses allow part of the endometrium to remain intact while other endometrial tissue is shed during menstruation.

When pregnancy occurs and the endometrium is not shed, the reticular stromal cells surrounding the endometrial glands become the decidual cells of pregnancy. The stromal cells are highly vascular, channeling a rich blood supply to the endometrial surface.

Cervix. The narrow neck of the uterus is the **cervix**. It meets the body of the uterus at the internal os and descends about 2 to 4 cm in a nonpregnant woman to connect with the vagina at the external os (Heitmann, 2013) (see Figure 3–3). Thus it provides a protective entrance for the body of the uterus. The cervix is divided by its line of attachment into the vaginal and supravaginal areas. The *vaginal cervix* projects into the vagina at an angle of from 45 to 90 degrees. The *supravaginal cervix* is surrounded by the attachments that give the uterus its main support: the uterosacral ligaments, the transverse ligaments of the cervix (Mackenrodt's ligaments), and the pubocervical ligaments.

The vaginal cervix appears pink and ends at the external os. The cervical canal appears rosy red and is lined with columnar ciliated epithelium, which contains mucus-secreting glands. Most cervical cancer begins at this *squamocolumnar* junction. The specific location of the junction varies with age and number of pregnancies. Elasticity is the chief characteristic of the cervix. Its ability to stretch results from both the high fibrous and collagenous content of the supportive tissues and the vast number of folds in the cervical lining.

The cervical mucus has three functions:

- To lubricate the vaginal canal
- To act as a bacteriostatic agent
- To provide an alkaline environment to shelter deposited sperm from the acidic vaginal secretions

At ovulation, cervical mucus is clearer, thinner, more profuse, and more alkaline than at other times.

Uterine Ligaments

The uterine ligaments support and stabilize the various reproductive organs. The ligaments shown in Figure 3–7 ● are described as follows:

1. The **broad ligament** keeps the uterus centrally placed and provides stability within the pelvic cavity. It is a double layer that is continuous with the abdominal peritoneum. The broad ligament covers the uterus anteriorly and posteriorly and extends outward from the uterus to enfold the fallopian tubes. The round and ovarian ligaments are at the upper border of the broad ligament. At its lower border, it forms the cardinal ligaments. Between the folds of the broad ligament are connective tissue, involuntary muscle, blood and lymph vessels, and nerves.

2. The **round ligaments** help the broad ligament keep the uterus in place. The round ligaments arise from the sides of the uterus near the fallopian tube insertions. They extend outward between the folds of the broad ligament, passing through the inguinal ring and canals and eventually fusing with the connective tissue of the labia majora. Made up of longitudinal muscle, the round ligaments enlarge during pregnancy. During labor the round ligaments steady the uterus, pulling downward and forward so that the presenting part of the fetus is moved into the cervix.

3. The **ovarian ligaments** anchor the lower pole of the ovary to the cornua of the uterus. They are surrounded by muscle fibers that allow the ligaments to contract. This contractile ability influences the position of the ovary to some extent, thus helping the fimbriae of the fallopian tubes to "catch" the ovum as it is released each month.

4. The **cardinal ligaments** are the chief uterine supports and suspend the uterus from the side walls of the true pelvis. These ligaments, also known as Mackenrodt's or transverse cervical ligaments, arise from the sides of the pelvic walls and attach to the cervix in the upper vagina. These ligaments prevent uterine prolapse and also support the upper vagina.

5. The **infundibulopelvic ligament** suspends and supports the ovaries. Arising from the outer third of the broad ligament, the infundibulopelvic ligament contains the ovarian vessels and nerves.

6. The **uterosacral ligaments** provide support for the uterus and cervix at the level of the ischial spines. Arising on each

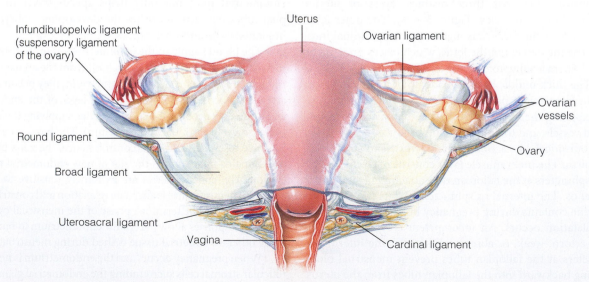

● **Figure 3–7** Uterine ligaments.

side of the pelvis from the posterior wall of the uterus, the uterosacral ligaments sweep back around the rectum and insert on the sides of the first and second sacral vertebrae. The uterosacral ligaments contain smooth muscle fibers, connective tissue, blood and lymph vessels, and nerves. They also contain sensory nerve fibers that contribute to dysmenorrhea (painful menstruation) (see Chapter 5 🔗).

Fallopian Tubes

The two **fallopian tubes**, also known as the *oviducts* or *uterine tubes,* arise from each side of the uterus and reach almost to the sides of the pelvis, where they turn toward the ovaries (Figure 3–8 ●). Each tube is approximately 8 to 13.5 cm long. A short section of each fallopian tube is inside the uterus; its opening into the uterus is only 1 mm in diameter. The fallopian tubes link the peritoneal cavity with the uterus and vagina. This linkage increases a woman's biologic vulnerability to disease processes in the pelvis.

Each fallopian tube may be divided into three parts: the *isthmus,* the *ampulla,* and the *fimbria (ends of the infundibulum).* The fallopian tube **isthmus** is straight and narrow, with a thick muscular wall and an opening (lumen) 2 to 3 mm in diameter. It is the site of tubal ligation, a surgical procedure to prevent pregnancy (see Chapter 5 🔗).

Next to the isthmus is the curved **ampulla**, which comprises the outer third of the tube. Fertilization of the secondary oocyte by a spermatozoon usually occurs here. The ampulla ends at the **fimbria**, which is a funnel-like enlargement with many fingerlike projections (fimbriae) reaching out to the ovary. The longest of these, the fimbria ovarica, is attached to the ovary to increase the chances of intercepting the ovum as it is released.

The wall of the fallopian tube consists of four layers: peritoneal (serous), subserous (adventitial), muscular, and mucous tissues. The peritoneum covers the tubes. The subserous layer contains the blood and nerve supply, and the muscular layer is responsible for the peristaltic movement of the tube. The mucosal layer, immediately next to the muscular layer, is composed of ciliated and nonciliated cells, with the number of ciliated cells more abundant at the fimbria. Nonciliated cells secrete a protein-rich, serous fluid that nourishes the ovum. The constantly moving tubal cilia propel the ovum toward the uterus. Because the ovum is a large cell, this ciliary action is needed to assist the tube's muscular layer peristalsis. Any malformation or malfunction of the tubes or cilia can result in infertility, ectopic pregnancy, or even sterility.

A well-functioning tubal transport system involves active fimbriae close to the ovary, peristalsis of the tube created by the muscular layer, ciliated currents beating toward the uterus, and the proximal contraction and distal relaxation of the tube caused by different types of prostaglandins.

A rich blood and lymphatic supply serves each fallopian tube. Thus the tubes have an unusual ability to recover from an inflammatory process (see Figure 3–4). The fallopian tubes have three functions:

■ To provide transport for the ovum from the ovary to the uterus (transport time through the fallopian tubes varies from 3 to 4 days)

■ To provide a site for fertilization

■ To serve as a warm, moist, nourishing environment for the ovum or zygote (fertilized egg) (See Chapter 4 🔗 for further discussion.)

Ovaries

The *ovaries* are two almond-shaped structures just below the pelvic brim. One ovary is located on each side of the pelvic cavity. Their size varies among women and with the stage of the menstrual cycle. Each ovary weighs approximately 6 to 10 g and is 1.5 to 3 cm wide, 2 to 5 cm long, and 1 to 1.5 cm thick. The ovaries of girls are small, but they become larger after puberty and then decrease in size following menopause. They also change in appearance from a dull white, smooth-surfaced organ to a pitted gray organ as the woman ages. The pitting appearance on their surface is the result of scarring after ovulation. The ovaries

● **Figure 3–8** Fallopian tubes and ovaries.

are maintained in their position by the broad, ovarian, and infundibulopelvic ligaments. It is rare for both ovaries to be at the same level in the pelvic cavity.

There is no peritoneal covering for the ovaries. Although this lack of covering assists the mature ovum to erupt, it also allows easier spread of malignant cells from cancer of the ovaries. A single layer of cuboidal epithelial cells, called the germinal epithelium, covers the ovaries. The ovaries are composed of three layers: the tunica albuginea, the cortex, and the medulla. The *tunica albuginea* is dense and dull white and serves as a protective layer. The *cortex* is the main functional part because it contains ova, graafian follicles, corpora lutea, the degenerated corpora lutea (corpora albicantia), and degenerated follicles. The *medulla* is completely surrounded by the cortex and contains the nerves and the blood and lymphatic vessels.

The ovaries are the primary source of two important hormones: estrogen and progesterone. *Estrogens* are associated with those characteristics contributing to femaleness, including breast alveolar lobule growth and duct development. The ovaries secrete large amounts of estrogen, while the adrenal cortex (extraglandular sites) produces minute amounts of estrogen in nonpregnant women, and the fat cells produce a secondary estrogen.

Progesterone is often called the *hormone of pregnancy* because it inhibits uterine contractions and relaxes smooth muscle to cause vasodilation, allowing pregnancy to be maintained. The interplay between the ovarian hormones and other hormones such as follicle-stimulating hormone (FSH) and luteinizing hormone (LH) is responsible for the cyclic changes that allow pregnancy to occur. The hormonal and physical changes that occur during the female reproductive cycle are discussed in depth later in this chapter. Between the ages of 45 and 55, a woman's ovaries secrete decreasing amounts of estrogen. Eventually, ovulatory activity ceases and menopause occurs.

Bony Pelvis

The female bony pelvis has two unique functions:

- To support and protect the pelvic contents
- To form the relatively fixed axis of the birth passage

Because the pelvis is so important to childbearing, its structure must be understood clearly.

Bony Structure

The pelvis is made up of four bones: two innominate bones, the sacrum, and the coccyx (or tailbone). The pelvis resembles a bowl or basin; its sides are the innominate bones, and its back is the sacrum and coccyx. Lined with fibrocartilage and held tightly together by pelvic ligaments (Figure 3–9 ●), the four bones join at the symphysis pubis, the two sacroiliac joints, and the sacrococcygeal joints.

The *innominate bones,* also known as the hip bones, are made up of three separate bones: the ilium, ischium, and pubis. These bones fuse to form a circular cavity, the *acetabulum,* which articulates with the femur.

The *ilium* is the broad, upper prominence of the hip. The iliac crest is the margin of the ilium. The ischial spines, the foremost projections nearest the groin, are the site of attachment for ligaments and muscles.

The *ischium,* the strongest bone, is under the ilium and below the acetabulum. The L-shaped ischium ends in a marked protuberance, the ischial tuberosity, on which the weight of a seated body rests. The **ischial spines** arise near the junction of the ilium and ischium and jut into the pelvic cavity. The shortest diameter of the pelvic cavity is between the ischial spines. The ischial spines serve as reference points during labor to evaluate the descent of the fetal head into the birth canal (see Chapter 17 🔗 and Figure 17–8 🔗 on page 359).

● Figure 3–9 Pelvic bones with supporting pelvic ligaments.

The **pubis** forms the slightly bowed front portion of the innominate bone. Extending medially from the acetabulum to the midpoint of the bony pelvis, each pubis meets the other to form a joint called the *symphysis pubis*. The triangular space below this junction is known as the pubic arch. The fetal head passes under this arch during birth. The symphysis pubis is formed by heavy fibrocartilage and the superior and inferior pubic ligaments. The mobility of the inferior ligament increases during a first pregnancy and to a greater extent in subsequent pregnancies.

The sacroiliac joints also have a degree of mobility that increases near the end of pregnancy as the result of an upward, gliding movement. The pelvic outlet may be increased by 1.5 to 2 cm in the squatting, sitting, and dorsal lithotomy positions. Relaxation of the pelvic joints is induced by the hormones of pregnancy.

The *sacrum* is a wedge-shaped bone formed by the fusion of five vertebrae. The anterior upper portion of the sacrum has a projection into the pelvic cavity known as the **sacral promontory**. This projection is another obstetric guide in determining pelvic measurements. (For a discussion of pelvic measurements, see Chapter 10 🔗.)

The small triangular bone last on the vertebral column is the coccyx. It articulates with the sacrum at the sacrococcygeal joint. The coccyx usually moves backward during labor to provide more room for the fetus.

Pelvic Floor

The muscular floor of the bony pelvis is designed to overcome the force of gravity exerted on the pelvic organs. It acts as a supportive structure to the irregularly shaped pelvic outlet, thereby providing stability for surrounding structures.

Deep fascia, the levator ani, and coccygeal muscles form the part of the pelvic floor known as the **pelvic diaphragm**. The components of the pelvic diaphragm function as a whole, yet they are able to move over one another. This feature provides an exceptional capacity for relaxation during birth and return to prepregnancy condition following birth. Above the pelvic diaphragm is the pelvic cavity; below and behind it is the perineum. The sacrum is located posteriorly.

The levator ani muscle makes up the major portion of the pelvic diaphragm and consists of four muscles: the iliococcygeus, pubococcygeus, puborectalis, and pubovaginalis. The iliococcygeal muscle, a thin muscular sheet underlying the sacrospinous ligament, helps the levator ani support the pelvic organs. Muscles of the pelvic floor are shown in Figure 3–10 ● and discussed in Table 3–1.

Pelvic Division

The **pelvic cavity** is divided into the false pelvis and the true pelvis (Figure 3–11*A* ●). The **false pelvis**, the portion above the pelvic brim, or linea terminalis, serves to support the weight of the enlarged pregnant uterus and direct the presenting fetal part into the true pelvis below.

The **true pelvis** is the portion that lies below the pelvic brim. The bony circumference of the true pelvis is made up of the sacrum, coccyx, and innominate bones and represents the bony limits of the birth canal. The relationship between the true pelvis and the fetal head is of paramount importance: The size and shape of the true pelvis must be adequate for normal fetal passage during labor and at birth. The true pelvis consists of three parts: the inlet, the pelvic cavity, and the outlet (Figure 3–11*B* ●). Each part has distinct measurements that aid in evaluating the adequacy of

Animation | 3-D Female Pelvis

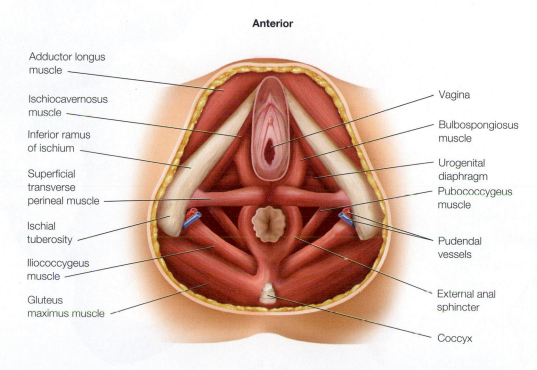

Anterior

Adductor longus muscle

Ischiocavernosus muscle

Inferior ramus of ischium

Superficial transverse perineal muscle

Ischial tuberosity

Iliococcygeus muscle

Gluteus maximus muscle

Vagina

Bulbospongiosus muscle

Urogenital diaphragm

Pubococcygeus muscle

Pudendal vessels

External anal sphincter

Coccyx

Posterior

● **Figure 3–10** Muscles of the pelvic floor. (The puborectalis, pubovaginalis, and coccygeal muscles cannot be seen from this view.)

Table 3–1	Muscles of the Pelvic Floor			
Muscle	Origin	Insertion	Innervation	Action
Levator ani	Pubis, lateral pelvic wall, and ischial spine	Blends with organs in pelvic cavity	Inferior rectal, second, and third sacral nerves, plus anterior rami of third and fourth sacral nerves	Supports pelvic viscera; helps form pelvic diaphragm
Iliococcygeus	Pelvic surface of ischial spine and pelvic fascia	Central point of perineum, coccygeal raphe, and coccyx		Assists in supporting abdominal and pelvic viscera
Pubococcygeus	Pubis and pelvic fascia	Coccyx		Forms part of levator ani and pelvic diaphragm
Puborectalis	Pubis	Blends with rectum; meets similar fibers from opposite side		Forms sling for rectum, just posterior to it; raises anus
Pubovaginalis	Pubis	Blends into vagina		Supports vagina
Coccygeus	Ischial spine and sacrospinous ligament	Lateral border of lower sacrum and upper coccyx	Third and fourth sacral nerves	Supports pelvic viscera; helps form pelvic diaphragm; flexes and abducts coccyx

● **Figure 3–11** Female pelvis. *A,* False pelvis is a shallow cavity above the inlet; true pelvis is the deeper portion of the cavity below the inlet. *B,* True pelvis consists of inlet, cavity (midpelvis), and outlet.

the pelvis for childbirth. Measurement techniques are discussed in Chapter 10 🔗. The effects of inadequate or abnormal pelvic diameters on labor and birth are considered in Chapter 17 🔗.

The **pelvic inlet** is the upper border of the true pelvis and is typically rounded in the female. The size and shape of the pelvic inlet are determined by assessing three anteroposterior diameters. The **diagonal conjugate** extends from the subpubic angle to the middle of the sacral promontory and is typically 12.5 cm. The diagonal conjugate can be measured manually during a pelvic examination. The **obstetric conjugate** extends from the middle of the sacral promontory to an area approximately 1 cm below the pubic crest. Its length is estimated by subtracting 1.5 cm from the length of the diagonal conjugate (Figure 3–12 ●). The fetus passes through the obstetric conjugate, and the size of this diameter determines whether the fetus can move down into the birth canal in order for engagement to occur. The true (anatomic) conjugate, or **conjugate vera**, extends from the middle of the sacral promontory to the middle of the pubic crest (superior surface of the symphysis). One additional measurement, the transverse diameter, helps determine the shape of the inlet. The **transverse diameter** is the largest diameter of the inlet and is measured by using the linea terminalis as the point of reference.

The *pelvic cavity* (canal) is a curved canal with a longer posterior than anterior wall. A change in the lumbar curve can increase or decrease the tilt of the pelvis and can influence the progress of labor because the fetus has to adjust itself to this curved path as well as to the different diameters of the true pelvis (see Figure 3–11*B*).

The **pelvic outlet** is at the lower border of the true pelvis. The size of the pelvic outlet can be determined by assessing the outlet *transverse diameter*. The anteroposterior diameter of the pelvic outlet increases during birth as the presenting part pushes the coccyx posteriorly at the mobile sacrococcygeal joint. Decreased mobility, a large head, and/or a forceful birth can

cause the coccyx to break. As the infant's head emerges, the long diameter of the head (occipital frontal) parallels the long diameter of the outlet (anteroposterior).

The transverse diameter *(bi-ischial or intertuberous)* extends from the inner surface of one ischial tuberosity to the other. In the pelvic outlet, the transverse diameter is the shortest diameter and becomes even shorter if the woman has a narrowed pubic arch. The pubic arch is of great importance because the fetus must pass under it during birth. If it is narrow, the baby's head may be pushed backward toward the coccyx, making extension of the head difficult. This situation, known as outlet dystocia, may require the use of forceps or a cesarean birth. The shoulders of a large baby may also become wedged under the pubic arch, making birth more difficult (see Chapter 23 🔗). The clinical assessment of each of these obstetric diameters is discussed further in Chapter 10 🔗.

Pelvic Types

The Caldwell–Moloy classification of pelves is widely used to differentiate bony pelvic types (Caldwell & Moloy, 1933). The four basic types are *gynecoid, android, anthropoid,* and *platypelloid* (see Figure 17–1 🔗 on page 355). However, variations in the female pelvis are so great that classic types are not usual. Each type has a characteristic shape, and each shape has implications for labor and birth, which are discussed in detail in Chapter 22 🔗.

Breasts

The *breasts,* or *mammary glands,* considered accessories of the reproductive system, are specialized sebaceous glands (Figure 3–13 ●). They are conical and symmetrically placed on the sides of the chest. The pectoral and anterior serratus muscles underlie each breast. Suspending the breasts are fibrous tissues, called *Cooper's ligaments,* which extend from the deep fascia in the chest outward to just under the skin covering the breast. Frequently, the left breast is larger than

● **Figure 3–12** Pelvic planes: coronal section and diameters of the bony pelvis.

- **Figure 3–13** Anatomy of the breast.

Labels on figure:
- Pectoralis minor muscle
- First rib
- Skin
- Pectoralis major muscle
- Fascia of pectoralis muscles
- Intercostal muscle
- Alveoli (glandular tissue)
- Ductule
- Connective tissue stroma
- Areola
- Nipple
- Opening of lactiferous sinus
- Nipple pores
- Ampulla
- Lactiferous duct
- Suspensory ligaments of Cooper
- Adipose tissue
- Sixth rib

the right. In different racial groups breasts develop at slightly different levels in the pectoral region of the chest.

In the center of each mature breast is the *nipple*, a protrusion about 0.5 to 1.3 cm in diameter. The nipple is composed mainly of erectile tissue, which becomes more rigid and prominent during the menstrual cycle, sexual excitement, pregnancy, and lactation. The nipple is surrounded by the heavily pigmented **areola**, which is 2.5 to 10 cm in diameter. Both the nipple and the areola are roughened by small papillae called *tubercles of Montgomery*. As an infant suckles, these tubercles secrete a fatty substance that helps lubricate and protect the nipple (Karam, 2013).

The breasts are composed of glandular, fibrous, and adipose tissue. The glandular tissue consists of acini, or alveoli, which are arranged in a series of 15 to 24 lobes separated from each other by adipose and fibrous tissue. Each lobe is made up of several lobules that are made up of many grapelike clusters of alveoli clustered around tiny ducts. The lining of these ducts secretes the various components of milk. The ducts from several lobules share common openings, called nipple pores, and open on the surface of the nipple. The smooth muscle of the nipple causes erection of the nipple on contraction (Karam, 2013).

The biologic function of the breasts is to:

- Provide nourishment and protective maternal antibodies to infants through the lactation process.
- Be a source of pleasurable sexual sensation.

THE FEMALE REPRODUCTIVE CYCLE

The **female reproductive cycle (FRC)** is composed of the ovarian cycle, during which ovulation occurs, and the uterine (menstrual) cycle, during which menstruation occurs. These two cycles take place simultaneously (Figure 3–14 ●).

Effects of Female Hormones

After menarche, a woman undergoes a cyclic pattern of ovulation and menstruation for a period of 30 to 40 years. Menstruation is an orderly process under neurohormonal control. Each month multiple oocytes mature, with one rupturing from the ovary, and entering the fallopian tube. The ovary, vagina, uterus, and fallopian tubes are major target organs for female hormones.

The ovaries produce mature gametes and secrete hormones. Ovarian hormones include estrogen, progesterone, and testosterone. The ovary is sensitive to follicle-stimulating hormone (FSH) and luteinizing hormone (LH). The uterus is sensitive to estrogen and progesterone. The relative proportion of these hormones to each other controls the events of both ovarian and menstrual cycles.

Estrogens

The ovaries secrete large amounts of estrogen, while the adrenal cortex (extraglandular sites) produces minute amounts of estrogens in nonpregnant women, and the fat cells produce a secondary estrogen. Estrogens are hormones that are associated with characteristics contributing to "femaleness." The major estrogenic effects are primarily the result of three classical estrogens: estrone, β-estradiol, and estriol. The major estrogen is β-estradiol.

Estrogens control the development of the female secondary sex characteristics: breast development (including breast alveolar lobule growth and duct development), growth of body hair, widening of the hips, and deposits of tissue (fat) in the buttocks and mons pubis. Estrogens also assist in the maturation of the ovarian follicles and cause the endometrial mucosa to proliferate following menstruation. The amount of estrogens is greatest during the proliferative (follicular or estrogenic) phase of the menstrual cycle. Estrogens also cause the uterus to increase in size and weight because of increased glycogen, amino acids, electrolytes, and water. Blood supply is expanded as well. Under the influence of estrogens, myometrial contractility increases in both the uterus and the fallopian tubes, and uterine sensitivity to oxytocin increases. Estrogens inhibit FSH production and stimulate LH production.

Estrogens have effects on many hormones and other carrier proteins, such as contributing to the increased amount of protein-bound iodine in pregnant women and women who use oral contraceptives containing estrogen. Estrogens may also increase libidinal feelings in humans. They decrease the excitability of the hypothalamus, which may cause an increase in sexual desire.

Progesterone

Progesterone is secreted by the corpus luteum and is found in greatest amounts during the secretory (luteal or progestational) phase of the menstrual cycle. Progesterone is often called the *hormone of pregnancy* because its effects on the uterus allow pregnancy to be maintained. Under the influence of progesterone:

- Vaginal epithelium proliferates.
- Cervix secretes thick, viscous mucus.
- Breast glandular tissue increases in size and complexity.
- Breasts prepare for lactation.
- Temperature rise of about 0.3°C to 0.6°C (0.5°F to 1.0°F) accompanies ovulation and persists throughout the secretory phase of the menstrual cycle.

● **Figure 3–14** Female reproductive cycle: interrelationships of hormones with the four phases of the uterine cycle and the two phases of the ovarian cycle in an ideal 28-day cycle.

Prostaglandins

Prostaglandins (PGs) are oxygenated fatty acids that are produced by the cells of the endometrium and are also classified as hormones. Prostaglandins have varied action in the body. The two primary types of prostaglandins are group E and F. Generally PGE relaxes smooth muscles and is a potent vasodilator; PGF is a potent vasoconstrictor and increases the contractility of muscles and arteries. Although the primary actions of PGE and PGF seem antagonistic, their basic regulatory functions in cells are achieved through an intricate pattern of reciprocal events.

Prostaglandin production increases during follicular maturation, is dependent on gonadotropins, and seems to be critical to follicular rupture. Extrusion of the ovum, resulting from follicular swelling and increased contractility of the smooth muscle in the theca externa layer of the mature follicle, is thought to be caused in part by PGF$_{2\alpha}$. Significant amounts of PGs are found in and around the follicle at the time of ovulation.

Neurohormonal Basis of the Female Reproductive Cycle

The female reproductive cycle is controlled by complex interactions between the nervous and endocrine systems and their target tissues.

The hypothalamus secretes *gonadotropin-releasing hormone (GnRH)* to the pituitary gland in response to signals received from the central nervous system. This releasing hormone is often called both luteinizing hormone-releasing hormone (LHRH) and follicle-stimulating hormone-releasing hormone (FSHRH) (Blackburn, 2013). In response to GnRH, the anterior pituitary secretes the gonadotropic hormones *follicle-stimulating hormone (FSH)* and *luteinizing hormone (LH)*.

FSH is primarily responsible for the maturation of the ovarian follicle. As the follicle matures, it secretes increasing amounts of estrogen, which enhance the development of the follicle (Alford & Nurudeen, 2013). (This estrogen is also responsible for the rebuilding/proliferation phase of the endometrium after it is shed during menstruation.)

Final maturation of the follicle cannot come about without the action of LH. The anterior pituitary's production of LH increases six- to tenfold as the follicle matures. The peak production of LH can precede ovulation by as much as 12 to 24 hours (Blackburn, 2013). LH is also responsible for "luteinizing" the increase in production of progesterone by the granulosa cells of the follicle. As a result, estrogen production is reduced and progesterone secretion continues. Thus estrogen levels fall a day before ovulation; tiny amounts of inhibin and progesterone are in evidence (Blackburn, 2013). **Ovulation** takes place following the very rapid growth of the follicle, as the sustained high level of estrogen diminishes and progesterone secretion begins.

The ruptured follicle undergoes rapid change, complete luteinization is accomplished, and the mass of cells becomes the *corpus luteum*. The lutein cells secrete large amounts of progesterone with smaller amounts of estradiol. (Concurrently, the excessive amounts of progesterone are responsible for the secretory phase of the uterine cycle.) On day 7 or 8 following ovulation, the corpus luteum begins to involute, losing its secretory function. The production of both progesterone and estrogen is severely diminished. The anterior pituitary responds with increasingly large amounts of FSH; a few days later LH production begins. As a result, new follicles become responsive to another ovarian cycle and begin maturing.

Ovarian Cycle

The ovarian cycle has two phases: the *follicular phase* (days 1–14) and the *luteal phase* (days 15–28 in a 28-day cycle). Figure 3–15 ● depicts the changes that the follicle undergoes during the ovarian cycle. In women whose menstrual cycles vary, usually only the length of the follicular phase varies, because the luteal phase is of fixed length. During the follicular phase, the immature follicle matures as a result of FSH. Within the follicle, the oocyte grows.

Animation | Ovulation

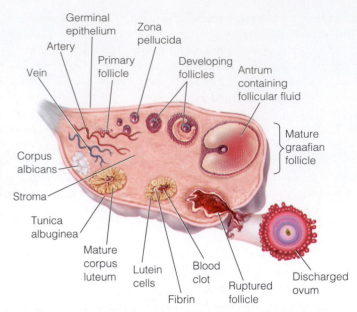

● **Figure 3–15** Various stages of development of the ovarian follicles.

A mature **graafian follicle** appears on about the 14th day under dual control of FSH and LH. It is a large structure, measuring about 5 to 10 mm. The mature follicle produces increasing amounts of estrogen. In the mature graafian follicle, the cells surrounding the fluid-filled antral cavity are granulosa cells. The mass of granulosa cells surrounding the oocyte and follicular fluid is called the *cumulus oophorus*. In the fully mature graafian follicle, the zona pellucida, a thick elastic capsule, develops around the oocyte. Just before ovulation, the mature oocyte completes its first meiotic division (see Chapter 4 ● for a description of meiosis). As a result of this division, two cells are formed: a small cell, called a *polar body*, and a larger cell, called the *secondary oocyte*. The secondary oocyte matures into the ovum (see Figure 4–1 ● on page 64).

As the graafian follicle matures and enlarges, it comes close to the surface of the ovary. The ovary surface forms a blister-like protrusion 10 to 15 mm in diameter, and the follicle walls become thin. The secondary oocyte, polar body, and follicular fluid are pushed out. The ovum is discharged near the fimbria of the fallopian tube and is pulled into the tube to begin its journey toward the uterus.

In some women, ovulation is accompanied by midcycle pain known as *mittelschmerz*. This pain may be caused by a local peritoneal reaction to the expelling of the follicular contents. Vaginal discharge may increase during ovulation, and a small amount of blood (midcycle spotting) may be discharged as well.

The body temperature increases about 0.3°C to 0.6°C (0.5°F to 1.0°F) 24 to 48 hours after the time of ovulation. It remains elevated until the day before menstruation begins. There may be an accompanying sharp basal body temperature drop before the increase. These temperature changes are useful clinically to determine the approximate time ovulation occurs (Blackburn, 2013).

Generally the ovum takes several minutes to travel through the ruptured follicle to the fallopian tube opening. The contractions of the tube's smooth muscle and its ciliary action propel the ovum through the tube. The ovum remains in the ampulla, where, if it is fertilized, cleavage can begin. The ovum is thought to be fertile for only 6 to 24 hours. It reaches the uterus 72 to 96 hours after its release from the ovary.

The luteal phase begins when the ovum leaves its follicle. Under the influence of LH, the corpus luteum develops from the ruptured follicle. Within 2 or 3 days, the corpus luteum becomes yellowish and spherical and increases in vascularity. If the ovum is fertilized and implants in the endometrium, the fertilized egg begins to secrete **human chorionic gonadotropin (hCG)**, which is needed to maintain the corpus luteum. If fertilization does not occur, within about a week after ovulation the corpus luteum begins to degenerate, eventually becoming a connective tissue scar called the *corpus albicans*. With degeneration comes a decrease in estrogen and progesterone. This allows for an increase in LH and FSH, which triggers the hypothalamus.

Uterine (Menstrual) Cycle

Menstruation is cyclic uterine bleeding in response to cyclic hormonal changes. Menstruation occurs when the ovum is not fertilized and begins about 14 days after ovulation (in an ideal 28-day cycle) in the absence of pregnancy. The menstrual discharge, also referred to as the *menses,* or *menstrual flow,* is composed of blood mixed with fluid, cervical and vaginal secretions, bacteria, mucus, leukocytes, and other cellular debris. The menstrual discharge is dark red and has a distinctive odor.

Menstrual parameters vary greatly among individuals. Generally, menstruation occurs every 29 days, but varies from 21 to 35 days. Some women normally have longer cycles, which can skew standard calculations of the estimated date of birth (EDB) when they become pregnant. Emotional and physical factors such as illness, excessive fatigue, stress or anxiety, and vigorous exercise programs can alter the cycle interval. Certain environmental factors such as temperature and altitude may also affect the cycle. The duration of menses is from 2 to 8 days, with the blood loss averaging 25 to 60 mL, and the loss of iron averaging 0.5 to 1 mg daily.

The uterine (menstrual) cycle has four phases: menstrual, proliferative, secretory, and ischemic (see Figure 3–14). Menstruation occurs during the *menstrual phase.* Some endometrial areas are shed, although others remain. Some of the remaining tips of the endometrial glands begin to regenerate. The endometrium is in a resting state following menstruation. Estrogen levels are low, and the endometrium is 1 to 2 mm deep. During this part of the cycle, the cervical mucosa is scanty, viscous, and opaque.

The *proliferative phase* begins when the endometrial glands enlarge, becoming twisted and longer in response to increasing amounts of estrogen. The blood vessels become prominent and dilated, and the endometrium increases in thickness six- to eightfold. This gradual process reaches its peak just before ovulation. The cervical mucosa becomes thin, clear, watery, and more alkaline, making the mucosa more favorable to spermatozoa. As ovulation nears, the cervical mucosa shows increased elasticity, called *spinnbarkeit.* At ovulation, the mucus will stretch more than 5 cm. The cervical mucosa pH increases from below 7.0 to 7.5 at the time of ovulation. On microscopic examination, the mucosa shows a characteristic ferning pattern (see Figure 7–3B 🔗 on page 138). This fern pattern is a useful aid in assessing ovulation time.

The *secretory phase* follows ovulation. The endometrium, under estrogenic influence, undergoes slight cellular growth.

Progesterone, however, causes such marked swelling and growth that the epithelium is warped into folds. The glandular epithelial cells begin to fill with cellular debris, become twisted, and dilate. The glands secrete small quantities of endometrial fluid in preparation for a fertilized ovum. The vascularity of the entire uterus increases greatly, providing a nourishing bed for implantation. If implantation occurs, the endometrium, under the influence of progesterone, continues to develop and become even thicker (see Chapter 4 🔗 for a discussion of implantation).

If fertilization does not occur, the *ischemic phase* begins. The corpus luteum begins to degenerate, and as a result both estrogen and progesterone levels fall. Areas of necrosis appear under the epithelial lining. Extensive vascular changes also occur. Small blood vessels rupture, and the spiral arteries constrict and retract, causing a deficiency of blood in the endometrium, which becomes pale. This ischemic phase is characterized by the escape of blood into the stromal cells of the uterus. The menstrual flow begins, thus beginning the menstrual cycle again. After menstruation the basal layer remains, so that the tips of the glands can regenerate the new functional endometrial layer. For further discussion, see Table 3–2.

MALE REPRODUCTIVE SYSTEM

The primary reproductive functions of the male genitals are to produce and transport sex cells (sperm) through and eventually out of the male genital tract and into the female genital tract. The external and internal genitals of the male reproductive system are shown in Figure 3–16 ●.

External Genitals

The two external reproductive organs are the penis and scrotum.

Penis

The *penis* is an elongated, cylindrical structure consisting of a body, called the *shaft,* and a cone-shaped end, called the *glans.* The penis lies in front of the scrotum. The shaft of the penis is made up of three longitudinal columns of erectile tissue: the paired *corpora cavernosa* and the *corpus spongiosum.* These columns are covered by dense fibrous connective tissue and then enclosed by elastic tissue. The penis is covered by a thin outer layer of skin.

The corpus spongiosum contains the urethra and becomes the glans at the distal end of the penis. The urethra widens within the glans and ends in a slitlike opening, located in the tip of the glans, called the *urethral meatus.* A circular fold of skin arises just behind the glans and covers it. Known as the *prepuce,* or *foreskin,* it may be removed by the surgical procedure of circumcision (see Chapter 26 🔗 for a discussion of circumcision). If the corpus spongiosum does not surround the urethra completely, the urethral meatus may occur on the ventral aspect of the penile shaft (hypospadias) or on the dorsal aspect (epispadias).

The penis is innervated by the pudendal nerve. Sexual stimulation causes the penis to elongate, thicken, and stiffen, a process called *erection.* The penis becomes erect when its blood vessels become engorged, a consequence of parasympathetic nerve stimulation. If sexual stimulation is intense enough, the

Table 3–2	Summary of Female Reproductive Cycle		
Cycle	Phase	Days	Events
Ovarian Cycle	Follicular phase	Days 1–14	Primordial follicle matures under influence of FSH and LH up to the time of ovulation.
	Luteal phase	Days 15–28	Ovum leaves follicle; corpus luteum develops under LH influence and produces high levels of progesterone and low levels of estrogen.
Uterine (Menstrual) Cycle	Menstrual phase	Days 1–6	Estrogen levels are low. Cervical mucus is scant, viscous, and opaque. Endometrium is shed.
	Proliferative phase	Days 7–14	Endometrium and myometrium thickness increases. Estrogen peaks just before ovulation. Cervical mucus at ovulation: Is clear, thin, watery, alkaline Is more favorable to sperm; shows ferning pattern on microscopic exam Has spinnbarkeit greater than 5 cm Just before ovulation, body temperature may drop slightly, then at ovulation basal body temperature increases 0.3°C to 0.6°C (0.5°F to 1.0°F). Mittelschmerz and/or midcycle spotting may occur.
	Secretory phase	Days 15–26	Estrogen drops sharply, and progesterone dominates. Vascularity of entire uterus increases. Tissue glycogen increases, and the uterus is made ready for implantation.
	Ischemic phase	Days 27–28	Both estrogen and progesterone levels drop. Spiral arteries undergo vasoconstriction. Endometrium becomes pale, blood vessels rupture. Blood escapes into uterine stromal cells, gets ready to be shed.

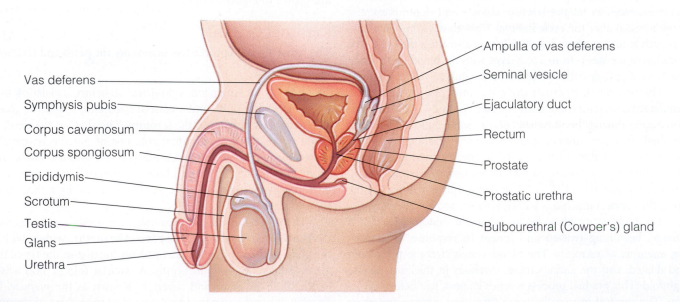

● **Figure 3–16** Male reproductive system, sagittal view.

forceful and sudden expulsion of semen occurs through the rhythmic contractions of the penile muscles. This phenomenon is called *ejaculation.*

The penis serves both the urinary and the reproductive systems. Urine is expelled through the urethral meatus. The reproductive function of the penis is to deposit sperm in the vagina so that fertilization of the ovum can occur.

Scrotum

The *scrotum* is a pouchlike structure that hangs in front of the anus and behind the penis. Composed of skin and the *dartos* muscle, the scrotum shows increased pigmentation and scattered hairs. The sebaceous glands open directly onto the scrotal surface; their secretion has a distinctive odor. Contraction of the dartos and cremasteric muscles shortens the scrotum and draws it closer to the body, thus wrinkling its outer surface. The degree of wrinkling is greatest in young men and at cold temperatures and is least in older men and at warm temperatures.

Inside the scrotum are two lateral compartments. Each compartment contains a testis with its related structures. Because the left spermatic cord grows longer, the left testis and its scrotal sac hang lower than the right. A ridge (raphe) on the external scrotal surface marks the position of the medial septum and continues anteriorly on the urethral surface of the penis, disappearing in the perineal area.

The function of the scrotum is to protect the testes and the sperm by maintaining a temperature lower than that of the body. Spermatogenesis cannot occur if the testes fail to descend and thus remain at body temperature. Because it is sensitive to touch, pressure, temperature, and pain, the scrotum defends against potential harm to the testes.

Male Internal Reproductive Organs

The male internal reproductive organs include the gonads (testes or testicles), a system of ducts (epididymides, vas deferens, ejaculatory duct, and urethra), and accessory glands (seminal vesicles, prostate gland, bulbourethral glands, and urethral glands) (Table 3–3).

Testes

The *testes* are a pair of oval, compound glandular organs contained in the scrotum. In the sexually mature male, they are the site of spermatozoa (male gamete) production and the secretion of several male sex hormones.

Each testis is 4 to 6 cm long, 2 to 3 cm wide, and 3 to 4 cm thick and weighs about 10 to 15 g. Each is covered by an outer serous membrane and an inner capsule that is tough, white, and fibrous. The connective tissue sends projections inward to form septa, dividing the testis into 250 to 400 lobules. Each lobule contains one to three tightly packed, convoluted *seminiferous tubules* containing sperm cells in all stages of development.

The seminiferous tubules are surrounded by loose connective tissue that houses abundant blood and lymph vessels and *interstitial (Leydig's) cells.* The interstitial cells produce testosterone, the primary male sex hormone. The tubules also contain Sertoli's cells, which nourish and protect the spermatocytes (phase between spermatids and spermatozoa). The seminiferous tubules come together to form 20 to 30 straight tubules, which in turn form an anastomotic network of thin-walled spaces, the *rete testis.* The rete testis forms 10 to 15 efferent ducts that empty into the duct of the epididymis.

Most of the cells lining the seminiferous tubules undergo *spermatogenesis,* a process of maturation in which spermatocytes become spermatozoa. (Chapter 4 ● further discusses the process of spermatogenesis.) Sperm production varies among and within the tubules, with cells in different areas of the same tubule undergoing different stages of spermatogenesis. The sperm are eventually released from the tubules into the epididymis, where they mature further.

Like the female reproductive cycle, the process of spermatogenesis and other functions of the testes are the result of complex neural and hormonal controls. The hypothalamus secretes releasing factors that stimulate the anterior pituitary to release the gonadotropins—FSH and LH. These hormones cause the testes to produce testosterone, which maintains spermatogenesis, increases sperm production by the seminiferous tubules, and stimulates production of seminal fluid.

Table 3–3	Summary of Male Reproductive Organ Functions	
Organ	**Structure**	**Function**
Testes	Seminiferous tubules	Contain sperm cells in various stages of development and undergoing meiosis.
	Sertoli's cells	Nourish and protect spermatocytes (phase between spermatids and spermatozoa—see Chapter 4 ●).
	Interstitial (Leydig's) cells	Provide the main source of testosterone.
Ducts	Epididymides	Provide an area for maturation of sperm and a reservoir for mature spermatozoa.
	The vas deferens	Connects the epididymis with the prostate gland, then connects with ducts from the seminal vesicle to become an ejaculatory duct.
	Ejaculatory ducts	Provide a passageway for semen and seminal fluid into the urethra.
Accessory glands	Seminal vesicles	Secrete yellowish fluid rich in fructose, prostaglandins, and fibrinogen. This provides nutrition that increases motility and fertilizing ability of sperm. Prostaglandins also aid fertilization by making the cervical mucus more receptive to sperm.
	The prostate gland	Secretes thin, alkaline fluid containing calcium, citric acid, and other substances. Alkalinity counteracts acidity of ductus and seminal vesicle secretions.
	Bulbourethral (Cowper's) glands	Secrete alkaline, viscous fluid into semen, aiding in neutralization of acidic vaginal secretions.
	Urethral (Littré's) glands	Add secretions to those of the bulbourethral glands.

Testosterone is the most prevalent and potent of the testicular hormones. It is also responsible for the development of secondary male characteristics and certain behavioral patterns. The effects of testosterone include structural and functional development of the male genital tract, emission and ejaculation of seminal fluid, distribution of body hair, promotion of growth and strength of long bones, increased muscle mass, and enlargement of the vocal cords. The action of testosterone on the central nervous system is thought to produce aggressiveness and sexual drive. The action of testosterone is constant, not cyclic like that of the female hormones. Its production is not limited to a certain number of years, but it is thought to decrease with age.

The testes have two primary functions:

- To serve as the site of spermatogenesis
- To produce testosterone

Epididymis

The *epididymis* (plural, *epididymides*) is a duct about 5.6 m long, although it is convoluted into a compact structure about 3.75 cm long. An epididymis lies behind each testis. It arises from the top of the testis, courses downward, and then passes upward, where it becomes the vas deferens.

The epididymis provides a reservoir for maturing spermatozoa. When discharged from the seminiferous tubules into the epididymis, the sperm are immotile and incapable of fertilizing an ovum. The spermatozoa usually remain in the epididymis for 2 to 10 days but can be stored in the body for up to 42 days. As the sperm move along the tortuous course of the epididymis they become both motile and fertile.

Vas Deferens and Ejaculatory Ducts

The *vas deferens,* also known as the *ductus deferens,* is about 40 cm long and connects the epididymis with the prostate. One vas deferens arises from the posterior border of each testis. It joins the spermatic cord and weaves over and between several pelvic structures until it meets the vas deferens from the opposite side. Each vas deferens terminus expands to form the *terminal ampulla.* It then unites with the seminal vesicle duct (a gland) to form the ejaculatory duct, which enters the prostate gland and ends in the prostatic urethra. The ejaculatory ducts serve as passageways for semen and fluid secreted by the seminal vesicles. The main function of the vas deferens is to rapidly squeeze the sperm from their storage sites (the epididymis and distal part of the vas deferens) into the urethra.

Men who choose to take total responsibility for birth control may elect to have a vasectomy. In this procedure, the scrotal portion of the vas deferens is surgically incised or cauterized. Although sperm continues to be produced for the next several years, they can no longer reach the outside of the body. Eventually, the sperm deteriorate and are reabsorbed.

Urethra

The *male urethra* is the passageway for both urine and semen. The urethra begins in the bladder and passes through the prostate gland, where it is called the *prostatic urethra.* The urethra emerges from the prostate gland to become the *membranous*

urethra. It terminates in the penis, where it is called the *penile urethra.* In the penile urethra, goblet secretory cells are present, and smooth muscle is replaced by erectile tissue.

Accessory Glands

The male accessory glands secrete a unique and essential component of the total seminal fluid in an ordered sequence.

The *seminal vesicles* are two glands composed of many lobes. Each vesicle is about 7.5 cm long. They are situated between the bladder and the rectum, immediately above the base of the prostate. The epithelium lining the seminal vesicles secretes an alkaline, viscous, clear fluid rich in high-energy fructose, prostaglandins, fibrinogen, and amino acids. During ejaculation, this fluid mixes with the sperm in the ejaculatory ducts. This fluid helps provide an environment favorable to sperm motility and metabolism.

The *prostate gland* encircles the upper part of the urethra and lies below the neck of the bladder. Made up of several lobes, it measures about 4 cm in diameter and weighs 20 to 30 g. The prostate is made up of both glandular and muscular tissue. It secretes a thin, milky, alkaline fluid containing high levels of zinc, calcium, citric acid, and acid phosphatase. This fluid protects the sperm from the acidic environment of the vagina and the male urethra, which would otherwise be spermicidal.

The *bulbourethral (Cowper's) glands* are a pair of small, round structures on either side of the membranous urethra. The glands secrete a clear, thick, alkaline fluid rich in mucoproteins that becomes part of the semen. This secretion also lubricates the penile urethra during sexual excitement and neutralizes the acid in the male urethra and the vagina, thereby enhancing sperm motility.

● **Figure 3–17** Schematic representation of a mature spermatozoon.

The *urethral (Littré's) glands* are tiny mucus-secreting glands found throughout the membranous lining of the penile urethra. Their secretions add to those of the bulbourethral glands.

Semen

The male ejaculate, *semen* or *seminal fluid,* is made up of spermatozoa and the secretions of all the accessory glands. The seminal fluid transports viable and motile sperm to the female reproductive tract. Effective transportation of sperm requires adequate nutrients, an adequate pH (about 7.5), a specific concentration of sperm to fluid, and an optimal osmolarity.

A spermatozoon is made up of a head and a tail (Figure 3–17 ●). The head's main components are the acrosome and nucleus. The head carries the male's haploid number of chromosomes (23), and it is the part that enters the ovum at fertilization (see Chapter 4 ✪). The tail, or *flagellum,* is specialized for motility. The tail is divided into the middle and end piece.

Sperm may be stored in the epididymis and distal vas deferens for up to 42 days, depending primarily on the frequency of ejaculations. The average volume of ejaculate following abstinence for several days is 2 to 5 mL but may vary from 1 to 10 mL. Repeated ejaculation results in decreased volume. Once ejaculated, sperm can live only 2 or 3 days in the female genital tract.

Critical Concept Review

LEARNING OUTCOME 3.1: Identify the structures and functions of the female reproductive system.

1. Ovaries:
   - Produce female gametes and female sex hormones.
2. Fallopian tubes:
   - Capture the ovum.
   - Allow transport of the ovum to the uterus.
3. Uterus:
   - Implantation site for the fertilized ovum.

4. Cervix:
   - Connection between the vagina and the uterus.
   - Protective portal for the body of the uterus.
5. Vagina:
   - Passageway from the external genitals to the uterus.
   - Provides for discharge of menstrual products out of the body.

LEARNING OUTCOME 3.2: Explain the significance of specific female reproductive structures during pregnancy and child birth.

1. Ischial spines:
   - Serve as a reference point during labor to evaluate the descent of the fetal head.
2. Pubic arch (symphysis pubis):
   - Fetal head passes under this arch during birth.
3. False pelvis:
   - Serves to support the weight of the enlarged pregnant uterus and direct the presenting fetal part into the true pelvis.

4. True pelvis:
   - Shape and size must be adequate for normal fetal passage.
   - Fetus must change its position to move through the diameter of the true pelvis.
5. Pelvic cavity:
   - Can influence the length of labor.

LEARNING OUTCOME 3.3: Summarize the actions of the hormones that affect reproductive functioning.

1. Estrogen:
   - Controls development of female secondary sex characteristics.
   - Assists in the maturation of the ovarian follicles.
   - Causes endometrial mucosa to proliferate following menstruation.
   - Causes uterus to increase in size and weight.
   - Increases myometrial contractility in both the uterus and fallopian tubes.
   - Increases uterine sensitivity to oxytocin.
   - Inhibits FSH production.
   - Stimulates LH production.

2. Progesterone:
   - Decreases uterine motility and contractility.
   - Causes uterine endometrium to increase its supply of glycogen, arterial blood, secretory glands, amino acids, and water.
   - Vaginal epithelium proliferates.
   - Cervix secretes thick, viscous mucus.
   - Increases breast glandular tissue, both in size and in complexity.
   - Prepares breasts for lactation.
3. Prostaglandins:
   - Necessary for follicular rupture.

LEARNING OUTCOME 3.4: Identify the two phases of the ovarian cycle and the changes that occur in each phase.

1. Follicular phase:
   - Primordial follicle matures under the influence of FSH and LH until ovulation occurs.

2. Luteal phase:
   - Ovum leaves the follicle.
   - Corpus luteum develops under the influence of LH.
   - Corpus luteum produces high levels of progesterone and low levels of estrogen.

LEARNING OUTCOME 3.5: Describe the phases of the uterine (menstrual) cycle, their dominant hormones, and the changes that occur in each phase.

1. Menstrual phase:
   - Shedding of the endometrial lining.
   - Low estrogen levels.
2. Proliferative phase:
   - Enlargement of the endometrial glands under influence of estrogen.
   - Changes in cervical mucus; peak at ovulation.
   - Increasing estrogen levels.
3. Secretory phase:
   - Follows ovulation.
   - Influenced primarily by progesterone.
   - Increase in vascularity of the uterus to make ready for possible implantation.
4. Ischemic phase:
   - Decreasing levels of estrogen and progesterone.
   - Degeneration of the corpus luteum.
   - Constriction of the spiral arteries.
   - Escape of blood into the stromal cells of the endometrium.

LEARNING OUTCOME 3.6: Identify the structures and functions of the male reproductive system.

1. Penis:
   - Deposits sperm in the vagina so fertilization of the ovum can occur.
   - Reproductive organ of intercourse.
2. Scrotum:
   - Protects the testes and sperm by maintaining a temperature lower than the body.
3. Testes:
   - Serve as a site for spermatogenesis.
   - Produce testosterone.
   - Produce male gametes and male sex hormones.
4. Epididymis:
   - Provides a reservoir for maturing spermatozoa.
5. Vas deferens:
   - Rapidly squeeze the sperm from their storage sites into the urethra.
6. Ejaculatory duct:
   - Passageway for semen and fluid secreted by the seminal vesicles.
   - In conjunction with epididymis and vas deferens, transports spermatozoa outside the body.
7. Urethra:
   - Passageway for both urine and semen.
8. Accessory glands:
   - Produce secretions necessary for sperm nutrition, survival, and transport.
9. Seminal fluid:
   - Provides environment favorable to sperm mobility and metabolism.
   - Transports viable and mobile sperm to the female reproductive tract.

Clinical Reasoning in Action

You are working in the OB/GYN clinic when Sally Smith, a 17-year-old teenager, comes in complaining of irregular menses. She believes her periods are really "messed up" and interfering with her active schedule. She wants them to be more regular and asks you for birth control. She tells you that she is a member of the swimming team and is a senior in high school. She says she is planning to start community college next year to obtain an associate degree in computer technology. You assess Sally's history as follows: menarche began at age 12; periods occur every 28 to 32 days. She usually experiences cramping in the first 2 days and the flow lasts 4 to 5 days. She uses an average of 4 to 5 tampons a day during her period. She has never been hospitalized, has no prior medical problems, and is up to date on her immunizations except for meningitis.

1. Based on your knowledge of menstruation, how would you describe Sally's menstrual cycle?
2. What is your primary goal in discussing Sally's menstrual cycle with her?
3. What information would you give Sally relating to her menstrual cycle?
4. What important request does Sally have?
5. Sally expresses problems dealing with the cramping she experiences with the first 2 days of her menses. What would you suggest to Sally to cope with the discomfort?

See www.nursing.pearsonhighered.com for possible responses.

References

Alford, C., & Nurudeen, S. (2013). Physiology of reproduction in women. In A. H. DeCherney, L. Nathan, N. Lauffer, & A. S. Roman (Eds.), *Current diagnosis and treatment: Obstetrics & gynecology* (10th ed.). Boston, MA: McGraw-Hill.

Blackburn, S. T. (2013). *Maternal, fetal, & neonatal physiology: A clinical perspective* (4th ed.). St. Louis, MO: Saunders.

Caldwell, W. E., & Moloy, H. C. (1933). Anatomical variations in the female pelvis and their effect on labor with a suggested classification [Historical article]. *American Journal of Obstetrics and Gynecology, 26,* 479–505.

Heitmann, R. J. (2013). Anatomy of the female reproductive system. In A. H. DeCherney, L. Nathan, N. Lauffer, & A. S. Roman (Eds.), *Current diagnosis and treatment: Obstetrics & gynecology* (10th ed.). Boston, MA: McGraw-Hill.

Karam, A. (2013). The breast. In A. H. DeCherney, L. Nathan, N. Lauffer, & A. S. Roman (Eds.), *Current diagnosis and treatment: Obstetrics & gynecology* (10th ed.). Boston, MA: McGraw-Hill.

Khachikyan, I., & Stratton, P. (2013). Benign disorders of the uterine cervix. In A. H. DeCherney, L. Nathan, N. Lauffer, & A. S. Roman (Eds.), *Current diagnosis and treatment: Obstetrics & gynecology* (10th ed.). Boston, MA: McGraw-Hill.

Conception and Fetal Development

Peter Bowater/Science Source

My friends tease me when I say this, but I know the moment my son was conceived. My husband and I had both been so busy at work, but finally we planned a getaway weekend. It was wonderful. We got back some of the magic as we took long walks and talked. Until that weekend, whenever we discussed having children it was always "maybe someday."

On the second night, we decided to skip the diaphragm for the first time. Our lovemaking seemed so special and magical—a true reflection of the emotional closeness we had recaptured. We are convinced that Michael is the result of that night together. —Michelle, 29

LEARNING OUTCOMES

4.1 Differentiate between meiotic cellular division and mitotic cellular division.

4.2 Compare the processes by which ova and sperm are produced.

4.3 Describe the components of the process of fertilization as to how each may impact fertilization.

4.4 Summarize the processes that occur during the cellular multiplication and differentiation stages of intrauterine development and their effects on the structures that form.

4.5 Describe the development, structure, and functions of the placenta and umbilical cord during intrauterine life (embryonic and fetal development).

4.6 Compare the factors and processes by which fraternal (dizygotic) and identical (monozygotic) twins are formed.

4.7 Summarize the significant changes in growth and development of the fetus at 4, 6, 12, 16, 20, 24, 28, 36, and 40 weeks' gestation.

4.8 Identify the factors that influence congenital malformations of the various organ systems.

The human genome contains *genes*, which are units of genetic information. Genes are encoded in the DNA that makes up the chromosomes in the nucleus of each cell. These chromosomes, which determine the structure and function of organ systems and traits, are of the same biochemical substances. How then does each person become unique? The answer lies in the physiologic mechanisms of heredity, the processes of cellular division, and the environmental factors that influence our development from the moment we are conceived. This chapter explores the processes involved in conception and fetal development—the basis of human uniqueness.

CELLULAR DIVISION

Each human begins life as a single cell called a fertilized ovum, or **zygote**. This single cell reproduces itself, and in turn each resulting cell also reproduces itself in a continuing process. The new cells are similar to the cells from which they came. Cells are reproduced by either mitosis or meiosis, two different but related processes.

Mitosis

Mitosis results in the production of diploid body (somatic) cells, which are exact copies of the original cell. During mitosis, the cell undergoes several changes, ending in cell division. As the last phase of cell division nears completion, a furrow develops in the cell cytoplasm, which divides it into two daughter cells, each with its own nucleus. Daughter cells have the same **diploid number of chromosomes** (46) and same genetic makeup as the cell from which they came. After a cell with 46 chromosomes goes through mitosis, the result is two identical cells, each with 46 chromosomes. Mitosis makes growth and development possible, and in mature individuals it is the process by which our body cells continue to divide and replace themselves.

Meiosis

Meiosis is a special type of cell division by which diploid cells in the testes and ovaries give rise to gametes (sperm and ova). These cells are different from somatic (body) cells because they contain only half of the parent cell—23 chromosomes—the **haploid number of chromosomes**.

Meiosis consists of two successive cell divisions. In the first division, the chromosomes replicate. Next, a pairing takes place between homologous chromosomes (Sadler, 2012). Instead of separating immediately, as in mitosis, the chromosomes become closely intertwined. At each point of contact, there is a physical exchange of genetic material between the chromatids (the arms of the chromosomes). New combinations are provided by the newly formed chromosomes; these combinations account for the wide variation of traits in people (e.g., hair or eye color). The chromosome pairs then separate, and the members of the pair move to opposite sides of the cell. (In contrast, during mitosis, the chromatids of each chromosome separate and move to opposite poles.) The cell divides, forming two daughter cells, each with 23 double-structured chromosomes—the same amount of deoxyribonucleic acid (DNA) as a normal somatic cell. In the second division, the chromatids of each chromosome separate and move to opposite poles of each of the daughter cells. Cell division occurs, resulting in the formation of four cells, each containing 23 single chromosomes (the haploid number of chromosomes). These daughter cells contain only half the DNA of a normal somatic cell (Sadler, 2012) (Table 4–1).

Chromosomal mutations may occur during the second meiotic division, for example, if two of the chromatids do not move apart rapidly enough when the cell divides. The still-paired chromatids are carried into one of the daughter cells and eventually form an extra chromosome. Another type of chromosomal mutation can occur if chromosomes break during meiosis. The effects of the chromosomal mutations of nondisjunction and translocation are described in Chapter 7 🔗.

Table 4–1	Comparison of Meiosis and Mitosis		
Process	**Purpose**	**Cell Division**	**Number of Daughter Cells**
Meiosis	Produce reproductive cells (gametes). Reduction of chromosome number by half (from diploid [46] to haploid [23]), so that when fertilization occurs the normal diploid number is restored. Introduces genetic variability.	Two-stage reduction.	Four daughter cells, each containing one half the number of chromosomes as the mother cell, or 23 chromosomes. Nonidentical to original cell.
Mitosis	Produce cells for growth and tissue repair. Cell division characteristic of all somatic cells.	One-stage cell division.	Two daughter cells identical to the mother cell, each with the diploid number (46 chromosomes).

GAMETOGENESIS

Meiosis occurs during **gametogenesis**, the process by which germ cells, or **gametes** *(ovum and sperm),* are produced. These cells contain only half the genetic material of a typical body cell. Each gamete must have only the haploid number (23) of chromosomes so that when the female gamete (egg or ovum) and the male gamete (sperm or spermatozoon) unite to form the *zygote* (fertilized ovum), the normal human diploid number of chromosomes (46) is reestablished.

Oogenesis

Oogenesis is the process that produces the female gamete, called an ovum (egg). As discussed in Chapter 3 🕮, the ovaries begin to develop early in the fetal life of the female. All the ova that the female will produce in her lifetime are present at birth. The ovary gives rise to oogonial cells, which develop into oocytes. Meiosis (cell replication by division) begins in all oocytes before the female fetus is born but stops before the first division is complete and remains in this arrested phase until puberty. During puberty, the mature primary oocyte proceeds (by oogenesis) through the first meiotic division in the graafian follicle of the ovary.

The first meiotic division produces two cells of unequal size with different amounts of cytoplasm but with the same number of chromosomes. These two cells are the *secondary oocyte* and a minute *polar body.* Both the secondary oocyte and the polar body contain 22 double-structured autosomal chromosomes and one double-structured sex chromosome (X).

At the time of ovulation, a second meiotic division begins immediately and proceeds as the oocyte moves down the fallopian tube. Division is again not equal, and the secondary oocyte moves into the metaphase stage of cell division, where its meiotic division is arrested until and unless the oocyte is fertilized.

When the secondary oocyte completes the second meiotic division after fertilization, the result is a mature ovum with the haploid number of chromosomes and virtually all the cytoplasm. In addition, the second polar body (also haploid) forms at this time. The first polar body has now also divided, producing two additional polar bodies. Thus, at the completion of meiosis, four haploid cells have been produced: the three polar bodies, which eventually disintegrate, and one ovum (Sadler, 2012) (Figure 4–1 ●).

Spermatogenesis

During puberty, the germinal epithelium in the seminiferous tubules of the testes begins the process of spermatogenesis, which produces the male gamete (sperm). The diploid spermatogonium replicates before it enters the first meiotic division, during which it is called the *primary spermatocyte.* During this first meiotic division, the spermatogonium replicates and forms two cells called *secondary spermatocytes,* each of which contains 22 double-structured autosomal chromosomes and either a double-structured X sex chromosome or a double-structured Y sex chromosome. During the second meiotic division, they divide to form four spermatids, each with the haploid number of chromosomes. The spermatids undergo a series of changes during which they lose most of their cytoplasm and become sperm (spermatozoa) (see Figure 4–1*B*). The nucleus becomes compacted into the head of the sperm, which is covered by a cap called an *acrosome* that is, in turn, covered by a plasma membrane. A long tail is produced from one of the centrioles.

THE PROCESS OF FERTILIZATION

Fertilization is the process by which a sperm fuses with an ovum to form a new diploid cell, or zygote. The zygote begins life as a single cell with a complete set of genetic material, 23 chromosomes from the mother's ovum and 23 chromosomes from the father's sperm, for a total of 46 chromosomes. The following events lead to fertilization.

Preparation for Fertilization

The mature ovum and spermatozoa have only a brief time to unite. Ova are considered fertile for about 12 to 24 hours after ovulation. Sperm can survive in the female reproductive tract for 48 to 72 hours, but are believed to be healthy and highly fertile for only about 24 hours.

The ovum's cell membrane is surrounded by two layers of tissue. The layer closest to the cell membrane is called the *zona pellucida.* It is a clear, noncellular layer whose thickness influences the fertilization rate. Surrounding the zona pellucida is a ring of elongated cells, called the *corona radiata* because they radiate from the ovum like the gaseous corona around the sun. These cells are held together by hyaluronic acid. The ovum has no inherent power of movement. During ovulation, high estrogen levels increase peristalsis within the fallopian tubes, which

● **Figure 4–1** Result of gametogenesis. Gametogenesis involves meiosis within the ovary and testis. *A,* During meiosis each oogonium produces a single haploid ovum once some cytoplasm moves into the polar bodies. *B,* Each spermatogonium produces four haploid spermatozoa.

helps move the ovum through the tube toward the uterus. The high estrogen levels also cause a thinning of the cervical mucus, facilitating movement of the sperm through the cervix, into the uterus, and up the fallopian tube.

The process of fertilization takes place in the ampulla (outer third) of the fallopian tube. In a single ejaculation, the male deposits approximately 200 to 500 million spermatozoa into the vagina, of which only hundreds of sperm actually reach the ampulla (Sadler, 2012). Fructose in the semen, secreted by the seminal vesicles, is the energy source for the sperm. The spermatozoa propel themselves up the female tract by the flagellar movement of their tails. Transit time from the cervix into the fallopian tube can be as short as 5 minutes but usually takes an average of 2 to 7 hours after ejaculation (Sadler, 2012). Prostaglandins in the semen may increase uterine smooth muscle contractions, which help transport the sperm. The fallopian tubes have a dual ciliary action that facilitates movement of the ovum toward the uterus and movement of the sperm from the uterus toward the ovary.

The sperm must undergo two processes before fertilization can occur: capacitation and the acrosomal reaction. **Capacitation** is the removal of the plasma membrane overlying the spermatozoa's acrosomal area and the loss of seminal plasma proteins. If the glycoprotein coat is not removed, the sperm will not be able to fertilize the ovum (Sadler, 2012). Capacitation occurs in the female reproductive tract (aided by uterine enzymes) and is thought to take about 7 hours. Sperm that undergo capacitation now take on three characteristics: (1) the ability to undergo the acrosomal reaction, (2) the ability to bind to the zona pellucida, and (3) the acquisition of hypermotility.

The **acrosomal reaction** follows capacitation, whereby the acrosomes of the sperm surrounding the ovum release their enzymes (hyaluronidase, a protease called acrosin, and trypsin-like substances) and thus break down the hyaluronic acid in the ovum's corona radiata (Sadler, 2012). Hundreds of acrosomes must rupture before enough hyaluronic acid is cleared for a single sperm to penetrate the ovum's zona pellucida successfully.

At the moment of penetration by a fertilizing sperm, the zona pellucida undergoes a reaction that prevents additional sperm from entering a single ovum (Figure 4–2 ●). This is known as the *block to polyspermy.* This cellular change is mediated by release of materials from the cortical granules, organelles found just below the ovum's surface, and is called the *cortical reaction.*

The Moment of Fertilization

After the sperm enters the ovum, a chemical signal prompts the secondary oocyte to complete the second meiotic division, forming the nucleus of the ovum and ejecting the second

● **Figure 4–2** Sperm penetration of an ovum. *A,* The sequential steps of oocyte penetration by a sperm are depicted moving from top to bottom. *B,* Scanning electron micrograph of a human sperm surrounding a human ovum (750X). The smaller spherical cells are granulosa cells of the corona radiata.

Source: B, © Phillips D/Photo Researchers/Getty Images.

polar body. Then the nuclei of the ovum and sperm swell and approach each other. The true moment of fertilization occurs as the nuclei unite. Their individual nuclear membranes disappear, and their chromosomes pair up to produce the diploid zygote. Because each nucleus contains a haploid number of chromosomes (23), this union restores the diploid number (46). The zygote contains a new combination of genetic material that results in an individual different from either parent and from anyone else.

The sex of the zygote is determined at the moment of fertilization. The two chromosomes (the sex chromosomes) of the 23rd pair—either XX or XY—determine the sex of an individual. The X chromosome is larger and bears more genes than the Y chromosome. Females have two X chromosomes, and males have an X and a Y chromosome. The mature ovum produced by oogenesis can have only one type of sex chromosome—an X. Spermatogenesis produces two sperm with an X chromosome and two sperm with a Y chromosome. When each gamete contributes an

X chromosome, the resulting zygote is female. When the ovum contributes an X and the sperm contributes a Y chromosome, the resulting zygote is male. As discussed in more detail in Chapter 5 🔗, certain traits are termed *sex linked* because they are controlled by the genes on the X sex chromosome. Two examples of sex-linked traits are color blindness and hemophilia.

PREEMBRYONIC DEVELOPMENT

The first 14 days of development, starting the day the ovum is fertilized (conception), are called the *preembryonic stage,* or the *stage of the ovum.* Development after fertilization can be divided into two phases: cellular multiplication and cellular differentiation. These phases are characterized by rapid cellular multiplication, and differentiation and establishment of the primary germ layers and embryonic membranes. Synchronized development of both the endometrium and embryo is a prerequisite for implantation to succeed (Moore, Persaud, & Torchia, 2013). These phases and the process of implantation (nidation), which occurs between them, are discussed next.

Cellular Multiplication

Cellular multiplication begins as the zygote moves through the fallopian tube toward the cavity of the uterus. This transport takes 3 days or more and is accomplished mainly by a very weak fluid current in the fallopian tube resulting from the beating action of the ciliated epithelium that lines the tube.

The zygote now enters a period of rapid mitotic divisions called **cleavage**, during which it divides into two cells, four cells, eight cells, and so on. These cells, called *blastomeres,* are so small that the developing cell mass is only slightly larger than the original zygote. The blastomeres are held together by the zona pellucida, which is under the corona radiata. The blastomeres eventually form a solid ball of 12 to 16 cells called the **morula**.

As the morula enters the uterus, two things happen: The intracellular fluid in the morula increases, and a central cavity forms within the cell mass. Inside this cavity is an inner solid mass of cells called the **blastocyst**. The outer layer of cells that surrounds the cavity and replaces the zona pellucida is the **trophoblast**. Eventually, the trophoblast develops into one of the two embryonic membranes, the chorion. The blastocyst develops into a double layer of cells called the *embryonic disk,* from which the embryo and the amnion (embryonic membrane) will develop. Figure 4–3 ● shows the journey of the fertilized ovum to its destination in the uterus.

Early pregnancy factor (EPF), an immunosuppressant protein, is secreted by the trophoblastic cells. This factor appears in the maternal serum within 24 to 48 hours after fertilization and forms the basis of a pregnancy test during the first 10 days of development (Moore et al., 2013).

● **Figure 4–3** Changes in fertilized ovum from conception to implantation. During ovulation, the ovum leaves the ovary and enters the fallopian tube. Fertilization generally occurs in the outer third of the fallopian tube.

Implantation (Nidation)

While floating in the uterine cavity, the blastocyst is nourished by the uterine glands, which secrete a mixture of lipids, mucopolysaccharides, and glycogen. The trophoblast attaches itself to the surface of the endometrium for further nourishment. The most frequent site of attachment is the upper part of the posterior uterine wall. Between days 7 and 10 after fertilization, the zona pellucida disappears and the blastocyst implants itself by burrowing into the uterine lining and penetrating down toward the maternal capillaries until it is completely covered (Moore et al., 2013). The lining of the uterus thickens below the implanted blastocyst, and the cells of the trophoblast grow down into the thickened lining, forming processes that are called *chorionic villi*.

Under the influence of progesterone, the endometrium increases in thickness and vascularity in preparation for implantation and nutrition of the ovum. After implantation, the endometrium is called the decidua. The portion of the decidua that covers the blastocyst is called the **decidua capsularis**, the portion directly under the implanted blastocyst is the **decidua basalis**, and the portion that lines the rest of the uterine cavity is the **decidua vera (parietalis)**. The maternal part of the placenta develops from the decidua basalis, which contains large numbers of blood vessels (see magnified inset in Figure 4–3). The chorionic villi (discussed shortly) in contact with the decidua basalis will form the fetal portion of the placenta.

Cellular Differentiation

Primary Germ Layers

About the 10th to 14th day after conception, the homogeneous mass of blastocyst cells differentiates into the primary germ layers (Figure 4–4 ●). These three layers, the **ectoderm**, **mesoderm**, and **endoderm**, are formed at the same time as the embryonic membranes. All tissues, organs, and organ systems will develop from these primary germ cell layers (Table 4–2). For example, differentiation of the endoderm results in the formation of epithelium lining the respiratory and digestive tracts (Figure 4–5 ●).

Embryonic Membranes

The **embryonic membranes** begin to form at the time of implantation (Figure 4–6 ●). These membranes protect and support the embryo as it grows and develops inside the uterus. The first and outermost membrane to form is the **chorion**. This thick membrane develops from the trophoblast, and has many fingerlike projections called chorionic villi on its surface. These chorionic villi can be used for early genetic testing of the embryo at 8 to 11 weeks' gestation by chorionic villus sampling (CVS) (see Chapter 14 ●). As the pregnancy progresses, the chorionic villi begin to degenerate, except for those just under the embryo, which grow and branch into depressions in the uterine wall, forming the fetal portion of the placenta. By the fourth month of pregnancy, the surface of the chorion is smooth except at the place of attachment to the uterine wall.

The second membrane to form, the amnion, originates from the ectoderm, a primary germ layer, during the early stages of embryonic development. The **amnion** is a thin protective membrane that contains amniotic fluid. The space between the membrane and the embryo is the *amniotic cavity*. This cavity surrounds the embryo and yolk sac, except where the developing embryo (germ-layer disk) attaches to the trophoblast via the umbilical cord. As the embryo grows, the amnion expands until it comes into contact with the chorion. These two slightly adherent membranes form the fluid-filled amniotic sac, also called the **bag of waters (BOW)**, which protects the floating embryo.

Animation Cell Division

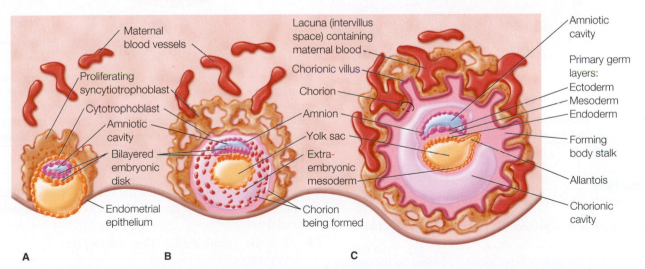

Maternal blood vessels — Proliferating syncytiotrophoblast — Cytotrophoblast — Amniotic cavity — Bilayered embryonic disk — Endometrial epithelium

Lacuna (intervillus space) containing maternal blood — Chorionic villus — Chorion — Amnion — Yolk sac — Extra-embryonic mesoderm — Chorion being formed

Amniotic cavity — Primary germ layers: Ectoderm, Mesoderm, Endoderm — Forming body stalk — Allantois — Chorionic cavity

A   **B**   **C**

● **Figure 4–4** Formation of primary germ layers. *A,* Implantation of a 7½-day blastocyst in which the cells of the embryonic disk are separated from the amnion by a fluid-filled space. The erosion of the endometrium by the syncytiotrophoblast is ongoing. *B,* Implantation is completed by day 9, and extraembryonic mesoderm is beginning to form a discrete layer beneath the cytotrophoblast. *C,* By day 16 the embryo shows all three germ layers, a yolk sac, and an allantois (an outpouching of the yolk sac that forms the structural basis of the body stalk, or umbilical cord). The cytotrophoblast and associated mesoderm have become the chorion, and chorionic villi are developing.

Table 4–2	**Derivation of Body Structures from Primary Cell Layers**	
Ectoderm	**Mesoderm**	**Endoderm**
Epidermis	Dermis	Respiratory tract epithelium
Sweat glands	Wall of digestive tract	Epithelium (except nasal), including pharynx, tongue, tonsils, thyroid, parathyroid, thymus, tympanic cavity
Sebaceous glands	Kidneys and ureter (suprarenal cortex)	
Nails	Reproductive organs (gonads, genital ducts)	
Hair follicles	Connective tissue (cartilage, bone, joint cavities)	Lining of digestive tract
Lens of eye	Skeleton	Primary tissue of liver and pancreas
Sensory epithelium of internal and external ear, nasal cavity, sinuses, mouth, anal canal	Muscles (all types)	Urethra and associated glands
	Cardiovascular system (heart, arteries, veins, blood, bone marrow)	Urinary bladder (except trigone)
Central and peripheral nervous systems		Vagina (parts)
Nasal cavity	Pleura	
Oral glands and tooth enamel	Lymphatic tissue and cells	
Pituitary gland	Spleen	
Mammary glands		

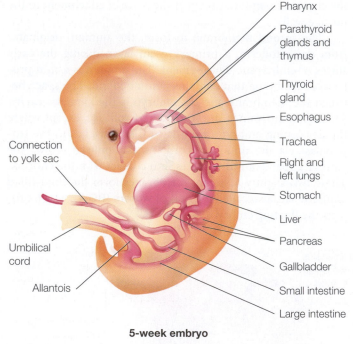

Pharynx
Parathyroid glands and thymus
Thyroid gland
Esophagus
Trachea
Right and left lungs
Stomach
Liver
Pancreas
Gallbladder
Small intestine
Large intestine

Connection to yolk sac
Umbilical cord
Allantois

5-week embryo

● **Figure 4–5** Differentiation of endoderm. Endoderm differentiates to form the epithelial lining of the digestive and respiratory tracts and associated glands.

Decidua basalis
Maternal blood
Chorionic villus
Umbilical blood vessels in umbilical cord
Amnion
Amniotic cavity
Yolk sac
Extraembryonic coelom
Chorion
Decidua capsularis

● **Figure 4–6** Early development of primary embryonic membranes. At 4½ weeks, the decidua capsularis (placental portion enclosing the embryo on the uterine surface) and decidua basalis (placental portion encompassing the elaborate chorionic villi and maternal endometrium) are well formed. The chorionic villi lie in blood-filled intervillous spaces within the endometrium. The amnion and yolk sac are well developed.

Amniotic Fluid

The *primary functions* of **amniotic fluid** are to:

■ Act as a cushion to protect the embryo against mechanical injury

■ Help control the embryo's temperature (relies on the mother to release heat)

■ Permit symmetrical external growth and development of the embryo

■ Prevent adherence of the embryo-fetus to the amnion (decreases chance of amniotic band syndrome) to allow freedom of movement so that the embryo-fetus can change position (flexion and extension), thus aiding in musculoskeletal development

■ Allow the umbilical cord to be relatively free of compression

■ Act as an extension of fetal extracellular space (hydropic infants have increased amniotic fluid)

■ Act as a wedge during labor

■ Provide fluid for analysis to determine fetal health and maturity

Amniotic fluid is slightly alkaline and contains albumin, uric acid, creatinine, lecithin, sphingomyelin, bilirubin, vernix, leukocytes, epithelial cells, enzymes, and fine hair called **lanugo**. The amount of amniotic fluid at 10 weeks is about 30 mL, and it increases to 190 mL at 16 weeks. After 28 weeks, the amniotic fluid volume changes little until 39 weeks, after which it decreases dramatically (Blackburn, 2013). The average volume ranges from 700 to 800 mL in the third trimester. As the pregnancy continues, the fetus influences the volume of amniotic fluid by swallowing the fluid and by excreting lung fluid and urine into the amniotic fluid.

Abnormal variations in amniotic fluid volume are *oligohydramnios* (less than 400 mL of amniotic fluid) and *hydramnios* (more than 2000 mL or amniotic fluid index greater than 97.5 percentile for the corresponding gestational age). Hydramnios is also called *polyhydramnios*. See Chapter 22 for an in-depth discussion of alterations in amniotic fluid volume during childbirth.

Yolk Sac

In humans, the yolk sac is small and functions early in embryonic life. It develops as a second cavity in the blastocyst on about day 8 or 9 after conception. It forms primitive red blood cells during the first 6 weeks of development, until the embryo's liver takes over the process. As the embryo develops, the yolk sac is incorporated into the umbilical cord, where it can be seen as a degenerated structure after birth.

Umbilical Cord

As the placenta is developing, the **umbilical cord** is also being formed from the amnion. The *body stalk,* which attaches the embryo to the yolk sac, contains blood vessels that extend into the chorionic villi. The body stalk fuses with the embryonic portion of the placenta to provide a circulatory pathway from the chorionic villi to the embryo. As the body stalk elongates to become the umbilical cord, the vessels in the cord decrease to one large vein and two smaller arteries. About 1% of umbilical cords have only two vessels, an artery and a vein; this condition may be associated with congenital malformations primarily of the renal, gastrointestinal, and cardiovascular systems. A specialized connective tissue known as **Wharton's jelly** surrounds the blood vessels in the umbilical cord. This tissue, plus the high blood volume pulsating through the vessels, prevents compression of the umbilical cord in utero. The umbilical cord has no sensory or motor innervation, so cutting the cord after birth is not painful. At term (38 to 42 weeks' gestation), the average cord is 2 cm (0.8 in.) across and about 55 cm (22 in.) long. The cord can attach itself to the placenta in various sites. Central insertion into the placenta is considered normal. (See Chapter 22 for a discussion of the various attachment sites.)

Umbilical cords appear twisted or spiraled, which is most likely caused by fetal movement. A true knot in the umbilical cord rarely occurs; if it does, the cord will be longer than usual. More common are so-called "false knots," caused by the folding of cord vessels. A *nuchal cord* is said to exist when the umbilical cord encircles the fetal neck.

TWINS

Twins normally occur in approximately 33.2 in 1000 live births in the United States (Society of Maternal-Fetal Medicine (SMFM), Moise & Argon, 2013). This increase is attributed to delayed childbearing and the use of artificial reproductive treatments.

Twins may be either fraternal or identical (Figure 4–7 ●). If twins are fraternal (nonidentical), they are dizygotic, which means they arise from two separate ova fertilized by two separate spermatozoa. There are two placentas, two chorions, and two amnions; however, the placentas sometimes fuse and look as if they are one. Despite their birth relationship, fraternal twins are no more similar to each other than they would be to siblings born singly. They may be of the same or different sex.

Dizygotic twinning increases with maternal age up to about age 35 and then decreases abruptly. The chance of dizygotic twins increases with parity, in conceptions that occur in the first 3 months of marriage, and also with coital frequency. The chance of dizygotic twinning decreases during periods of malnutrition and during winter and spring for women living in the Northern Hemisphere. Studies indicate that dizygotic twins occur in certain families, perhaps because of genotype (genetic constitution) of the mother that results in elevated serum gonadotropin levels leading to double ovulation (Moore et al., 2013). Fraternal (dizygotic) twins have been reported to occur more often among black women than among white women and more often among white women than among women of Asian origin (Moore et al., 2013). Among all groups, as parity (having given birth to a viable infant) increases, so does the chance for multiple births.

Identical, or monozygotic, twins develop from a single fertilized ovum. They are of the same sex and have the same phenotype (appearance). Identical twins usually have a common placenta. Monozygosity is not affected by environment, race, physical characteristics, or fertility.

Monozygotic twins originate from division of the fertilized ovum at different stages of early development, after the zygote consists of thousands of cells. Complete separation of the cellular mass into two parts is necessary for twin formation. The number of amnions and chorions present depends on the timing of the division:

1. If division occurs within 4 days of fertilization (before the inner cell mass and chorion have formed), two embryos, two amnions, and two chorions will develop. This dichorionic–diamniotic situation occurs about 25% of the time, and there may be two distinct placentas or a single fused placenta.

2. If division occurs about 4 to 8 days after fertilization (when the inner cell mass has formed and the chorion cells have differentiated but those of the amnion have not), two embryos develop with separate amnion sacs. These sacs will eventually be covered by a common chorion; thus there will be a monochorionic–diamniotic placenta (see Figure 4–7*B*).

3. If the amnion has already developed, approximately 8 to 12 days after fertilization, division results in two embryos with a common amnion sac and a common chorion (a monochorionic–monoamniotic placenta). This type rarely occurs (Society of Maternal-Fetal Medicine (SMFM), Moise & Argon, 2013).

Two ova
Sperm
Two blastocysts
Two amnions
Two chorions

One ovum
Sperm
One blastocyst
Inner cell mass splits in two
Two amnions
One chorion

A

B

● **Figure 4–7** *A,* Formation of fraternal twins. (Note separate placentas.) *B,* Formation of identical twins.

Monozygotic twinning is considered a random event and occurs in approximately 3 to 4 per 1000 live births (Blackburn, 2013). The survival rate of monozygotic twins as a group is 10% lower than that of dizygotic twins, and congenital anomalies are more prevalent. Both twins may have the same malformation.

DEVELOPMENT AND FUNCTIONS OF THE PLACENTA

The **placenta** is the means of metabolic and nutrient exchange between the embryonic and maternal circulations. Placental development and circulation do not begin until the third week of embryonic development. The placenta develops at the site where the embryo attaches to the uterine wall. Expansion of the placenta continues until about 20 weeks, when it covers approximately one half of the internal surface of the uterus. After 20 weeks' gestation, the placenta becomes thicker but not wider. At 40 weeks' gestation, the placenta is about 15 to 20 cm (5.9 to 7.9 in.) in diameter and 2.5 to 3.0 cm (1.0 to 1.2 in.) in thickness. At that time, it weighs about 400 to 600 g (14 to 21 oz).

The placenta has two parts: the maternal and fetal portions. The maternal portion consists of the decidua basalis and its circulation. Its surface is red and fleshlike (often called *Dirty Duncan*). The fetal portion consists of the chorionic villi and

their circulation. The fetal surface of the placenta is covered by the amnion, which gives it a shiny, gray appearance (often called *Shiny Schultz*) (Figures 4–8 ● and 4–9 ●).

Development of the placenta begins with the chorionic villi. The trophoblastic cells of the chorionic villi form spaces in the tissue of the decidua basalis. These spaces fill with maternal blood, and the chorionic villi grow into them. As the chorionic villi differentiate, two trophoblastic layers appear: an outer layer, called the *syncytium* (consisting of syncytiotrophoblasts), and an inner layer, known as the *cytotrophoblast* (see Figure 4–4). The cytotrophoblast thins out and disappears about the fifth month, leaving only a single layer of syncytium covering the chorionic villi. The syncytium is in direct contact with the maternal blood in the intervillous spaces. It is the functional layer of the placenta and secretes the placental hormones of pregnancy.

A third, inner layer of connective mesoderm develops in the chorionic villi, forming *anchoring villi*. These anchoring villi eventually form the *septa* (partitions) of the placenta. The septa divide the mature placenta into 15 to 20 segments called **cotyledons** (subdivisions of the placenta made up of anchoring villi and decidual tissue). In each cotyledon, the *branching villi* form a highly complex vascular system that allows compartmentalization of the uteroplacental circulation. The exchange of gases and nutrients takes place across these vascular systems.

Animation | Placenta Formation

● **Figure 4–8** Maternal side of placenta.
Source: Courtesy of M. London.

● **Figure 4–9** Fetal side of placenta.
Source: Courtesy of M. London.

Exchange of substances across the placenta is minimal during the first 3 to 5 months of development because the villous membrane is initially too thick, which limits its permeability. As the villous membrane thins, placental permeability increases until about the last month of pregnancy, when permeability begins to decrease as the placenta ages. In the fully developed placenta, fetal blood in the villi and maternal blood in the intervillous spaces are separated by three to four thin layers of tissue.

Placental Circulation

The completion of the maternal–placental–embryonic circulation occurs about 17 days after conception, when the embryonic heart begins functioning (Moore et al., 2013). By the end of the fourth week, embryonic blood is circulating between the embryo and the chorionic villi. The placenta has begun to function as a means of metabolic exchange between embryo and mother. By 14 weeks, the placenta is a discrete organ. It has grown in

thickness as a result of growth in the length and size of the chorionic villi and accompanying expansion of the intervillous space.

In the fully developed placenta's umbilical cord, fetal blood flows through the two umbilical arteries to the capillaries of the villi, and oxygen-enriched blood flows back through the umbilical vein into the fetus (Figure 4–10 ●). Late in pregnancy, a soft blowing sound (*funic souffle*) can be heard over the area of the umbilical cord. The sound is synchronous with the fetal heartbeat and fetal blood flow through the umbilical arteries.

Maternal blood, rich in oxygen and nutrients, spurts from the arcuate artery to the radial artery to the spiral uterine arteries and then spurts into the intervillous spaces. These spurts are produced by the maternal blood pressure. The spurt of blood is directed toward the chorionic plate, and as the blood loses pressure, it becomes lateral (spreads out). Fresh blood enters continuously and exerts pressure on the contents of the intervillous spaces, pushing blood toward the exits in the basal plate. The blood then drains through the uterine and other pelvic veins. A *uterine souffle,* timed precisely with the mother's pulse, is also heard just above the mother's symphysis pubis during the last months of pregnancy. This souffle is caused by the augmented blood flow entering the dilated uterine arteries.

Braxton Hicks contractions are intermittent painless uterine contractions that may occur every 10 to 20 minutes and occur more frequently near the end of pregnancy (see Chapter 17 ✪). These contractions are believed to facilitate placental circulation by enhancing the movement of blood from the center of the cotyledon through the intervillous space. Placental blood flow is enhanced when the woman is lying on her side because venous return from the lower extremities is not compromised (Blackburn, 2013).

Placental Functions

Placental exchange functions occur only in those fetal vessels that are in intimate contact with the covering syncytial membrane. The syncytium villi have brush borders containing many microvilli, which greatly increase the exchange rate between maternal and fetal circulation (Blackburn, 2013; Sadler, 2012).

The placental functions, many of which begin soon after implantation, include fetal respiration, nutrition, and excretion. To carry out these functions, the placenta is involved in metabolic and transfer activities. In addition, it has endocrine functions and special immunologic properties; see discussion later in this section.

Metabolic Activities

The placenta performs several essential metabolic activities. The placenta:

- Continuously produces glycogen, cholesterol, and fatty acids for fetal use and hormone production

- Produces numerous enzymes required for fetoplacental transfer, including sulfatase, which enhances excretion of fetal estrogen precursors, and insulinase, which increases the barrier to insulin

- Breaks down certain substances such as epinephrine and histamine (Blackburn, 2013)

- Stores glycogen and iron

Umbilical arteries

Umbilical vein

Chorion

Amnion

Umbilical cord

Maternal vein

Myometrium

Maternal artery

Fetal arteriole

Fetal venule

Maternal blood pools within intervillus space

Fetal portion of placenta (chorion)

Maternal portion of placenta (decidua basalis)

● **Figure 4–10** Vascular arrangement of the placenta. Arrows indicate the direction of blood flow. Maternal blood flows through the uterine arteries to the intervillous spaces of the placenta and returns through the uterine veins to maternal circulation. Fetal blood flows through the umbilical arteries into the villous capillaries of the placenta and returns through the umbilical vein to the fetal circulation.

Transport Function

The placental membranes actively control the transfer of a wide range of substances by a variety of transport mechanisms, such as the following:

■ *Simple diffusion* moves substances from an area of higher concentration to an area of lower concentration. Substances that move across the placenta by simple diffusion include water, oxygen, carbon dioxide, electrolytes (sodium and chloride), anesthetic gases, and drugs. Insulin, steroid hormones originating from the adrenals, and thyroid hormones cross the placenta. However, this happens at a very slow rate. Unfortunately, many substances of abuse, such as cocaine and heroin, cross the placenta via simple diffusion. The rate of oxygen transfer across the placental membrane is greater than that allowed by simple diffusion, indicating that oxygen is also transferred by some type of facilitated diffusion transport.

■ *Facilitated transport* involves a carrier system to move molecules from an area of greater concentration to an area of lower concentration. Molecules such as glucose, galactose, and some oxygen are transported by this method. The glucose level in the fetal blood ordinarily is approximately 20% to 30% lower than the glucose level in the maternal blood, because the fetus is metabolizing glucose rapidly. This in turn causes rapid transport of additional glucose from the maternal blood into the fetal blood.

■ *Active transport* can work against a concentration gradient and allows molecules to move from areas of lower concentration to areas of higher concentration. Amino acids, calcium, iron, iodine, water-soluble vitamins, and glucose are transferred across the placenta in this way. The measured amino acid content of fetal blood is greater than that of maternal blood, and calcium and inorganic phosphate occur in greater concentration in fetal blood than in maternal blood (Blackburn, 2013).

Other modes of transfer also exist. *Pinocytosis* is important for transferring large molecules such as albumin and gamma globulin. Materials are engulfed by amoeba-like cells, forming plasma droplets. *Hydrostatic* and *osmotic pressures* allow the bulk flow of water and some solutes. Fetal red blood cells pass into the maternal circulation through breaks in the capillaries and placental membrane, particularly during labor and birth. Certain cells, such as maternal leukocytes, and microorganisms, such as viruses (e.g., the human immunodeficiency virus [HIV], which causes acquired immunodeficiency syndrome [AIDS]), rubella, cytomegalovirus, polio, and the bacterium *Treponema pallidum* (which causes syphilis), can also cross the placental membrane under their own power (Moore et al., 2013). Some bacteria and protozoa infect the placenta by causing lesions and then entering the fetal blood system.

Reduction of the placental surface area, as with abruptio placentae (partial or complete premature separation of an abnormally implanted placenta), decreases the area that is functional for exchange. Placental diffusion distance also affects exchange. In conditions such as diabetes and placental infection, edema of the villi increases the diffusion distance, thus increasing the distance the substance has to be transferred.

Blood flow alteration changes the transfer rate of substances. Decreased blood flow in the intervillous space is seen in labor and with certain maternal diseases such as hypertension. Mild fetal hypoxia increases the umbilical blood flow, but severe hypoxia results in decreased blood flow.

As the maternal blood picks up fetal waste products and carbon dioxide, it drains back into the maternal circulation through the veins in the basal plate. Fetal blood is hypoxic by comparison; it therefore attracts oxygen from the mother's blood. Affinity for oxygen increases as the fetal blood gives up its carbon dioxide, which also decreases its acidity.

Endocrine Functions

The placenta produces hormones that are vital to the survival of the fetus. These include human chorionic gonadotropin (hCG), human placental lactogen (hPL), and two steroid hormones, estrogen and progesterone.

The hormone hCG is similar to luteinizing hormone (LH) and prevents the normal involution of the corpus luteum at the end of the menstrual cycle. If the corpus luteum stops functioning before the 11th week of pregnancy, spontaneous abortion occurs. The hCG also causes the corpus luteum to secrete increased amounts of estrogen and progesterone.

After the 11th week, the placenta produces enough progesterone and estrogen to maintain pregnancy. In the male fetus, hCG also exerts an interstitial cell-stimulating effect on the testes, resulting in the production of testosterone. This small secretion of testosterone during embryonic development is the factor that causes male sex organs to grow. Human chorionic gonadotropin may play a role in the trophoblast's immunologic capabilities (its ability to keep the mother's system from rejecting the placenta and embryo). This hormone is used as a basis for pregnancy tests (see Chapter 9 🕮).

Human chorionic gonadotropin is present in maternal blood serum 8 to 10 days after fertilization, just as soon as implantation has occurred, and is detectable in maternal urine at the time of missed menses. After reaching its maximum level at 50 to 70 days' gestation, hCG begins to decrease as placental hormone production increases.

Progesterone is an essential hormone for pregnancy. It increases the secretions of the fallopian tubes and uterus to provide appropriate nutritive matter for the developing morula and blastocyst. It also appears to aid in ovum transport through the fallopian tube. Progesterone causes decidual cells to develop in the uterine endometrium, and it must be present in high levels for implantation to occur. Progesterone also decreases the contractility of the uterus, thus preventing uterine contractions from causing spontaneous abortion.

Before stimulation by hCG, the corpus luteum's production of progesterone reaches a peak about 7 to 10 days after ovulation. Implantation occurs at about the same time as this peak. At 16 days after ovulation, progesterone reaches a level between 25 and 50 mg per day and continues to rise slowly in subsequent weeks. After 11 weeks, the placenta (specifically, the syncytiotrophoblast) takes over the production of progesterone and secretes it in tremendous quantities, reaching levels of more than 250 mg per day late in pregnancy.

By 7 weeks, the placenta produces more than 50% of the estrogens in the maternal circulation. *Estrogens* serve mainly a proliferative function, causing enlargement of the uterus, breasts, and breast glandular tissue. Estrogens also have a significant role in increasing vascularity and vasodilation, particularly in the villous capillaries toward the end of pregnancy. Placental estrogens increase markedly toward the end of pregnancy, to as much as 30 times the daily production in the middle of a normal monthly menstrual cycle. The primary estrogen secreted by the placenta *(estriol)* is different from the estrogen secreted by the ovaries *(estradiol)*. The placenta cannot synthesize estriol by itself. Essential precursors such as dehydroepiandrosterone sulfate (DHEA-S) are provided by the fetal adrenal glands, are processed by fetal liver, and are transported to the placenta for the final conversion to estrone, estradiol, and estriol (Blackburn, 2013).

The hormone human placental lactogen (hPL), also referred to as human chorionic somatomammotropin (hCS), is similar to human pituitary growth hormone in that hPL stimulates certain changes in the mother's metabolic processes. These changes ensure that more protein, glucose, and minerals are available for the fetus. Secretion of hPL can be detected by about 4 weeks after conception.

Immunologic Properties

The placenta and embryo are transplants of living tissue within the same species and are therefore considered *homografts*. Unlike other homografts, the placenta and embryo appear exempt from immunologic reaction by the host. Most recent data suggest that the placental hormones (progesterone and hCG) suppress cellular immunity during pregnancy. One theory suggests that chorionic villi syncytiotrophoblastic tissue is immunologically inert. The chorionic villi may lack major histocompatibility (MHC) antigens and thus do not evoke rejection responses. They do, however, protect against antibody formation. Extravillous trophoblast (EVT) cells, which invade the uterine deciduas, have human leukocyte antigen (HLA-G), which is not readily recognized by sensitized T lymphocytes and natural killer cells (Blackburn, 2013).

DEVELOPMENT OF THE FETAL CIRCULATORY SYSTEM

The circulatory system of the fetus has several unique features that, by maintaining the blood flow to the placenta, provide the fetus with oxygen and nutrients while removing carbon dioxide and other waste products.

Most of the blood supply bypasses the fetal lungs because they do not carry out respiratory gas exchange. The placenta assumes the function of the fetal lungs by supplying oxygen and allowing the fetus to excrete carbon dioxide into the maternal bloodstream. Figure 4–11 ● shows the fetal circulatory system. The blood from the placenta flows through the umbilical vein, which enters the abdominal wall of the fetus at the site that, after birth, is the umbilicus (belly button). As umbilical venous blood approaches the liver, a small portion of the blood enters the liver sinusoids, mixes with blood from the portal circulation, and then enters the inferior vena cava via hepatic veins. Most of the

● **Figure 4–11** Fetal circulation. Blood leaves the placenta and enters the fetus through the umbilical vein. After circulating through the fetus, the blood returns to the placenta through the umbilical arteries. The ductus venosus, the foramen ovale, and the ductus arteriosus allow the blood to bypass the fetal liver and lungs.

umbilical vein's blood flows through the **ductus venosus** directly into the fetal inferior vena cava, bypassing the liver. This blood then enters the right atrium, passes through the **foramen ovale** into the left atrium, and pours into the left ventricle, which pumps blood into the aorta. Some blood returning from the head and upper extremities by way of the superior vena cava is emptied into the right atrium and passes through the tricuspid valve into the right ventricle. This blood is pumped into the pulmonary artery, and a small amount passes to the lungs for nourishment only. The larger portion of blood passes from the pulmonary artery through the **ductus arteriosus** into the descending aorta, bypassing the lungs. Finally, blood returns to the placenta through the two umbilical arteries, and the process is repeated.

The fetus obtains oxygen via diffusion from the maternal circulation because of the gradient difference of Po_2 of 50 mm Hg in maternal blood in the placenta to 30 mm Hg Po_2 in the fetus. At term the fetus receives oxygen from the mother's circulation at a rate of 20 to 30 mL per minute (Sadler, 2012). Fetal hemoglobin facilitates obtaining oxygen from the maternal circulation, because it carries as much as 20% to 30% more oxygen than adult hemoglobin.

Fetal circulation delivers the highest available oxygen concentration to the head, neck, brain, and heart (coronary circulation) and a lesser amount of oxygenated blood to the abdominal organs and the lower body. This circulatory pattern leads to cephalocaudal (head-to-tail) development in the fetus.

EMBRYONIC AND FETAL DEVELOPMENT

Pregnancy is calculated to last an *average* of 10 lunar months: 40 weeks, or 280 days. This period of 280 days is calculated from the onset of the last normal menstrual period to the time of birth. Many obstetric units in the United States and Australia use a combination of menstrual dates and ultrasonographic dates to perform this calculation. Estimated date of birth (EDB), sometimes referred to as the *estimated date of delivery (EDD)*, is usually calculated by this method. Most fetuses are born within 10 to 14 days of the calculated date of birth. The postconception age (fertilization age) of the fetus is calculated to be *about* 2 weeks less, or 266 days (38 weeks) or 9.5 calendar months. The latter measurement is more accurate because it measures time from the fertilization of the ovum, or conception.

The basic events of organ development in the embryo and fetus are outlined in Table 4–3. The time periods in the table are **postconception age periods**. During the period from fertilization to the end of the embryonic period (8 weeks), age is often expressed in days but can be given in weeks. During the fetal period (9th week until birth), age is given in weeks (Moore et al., 2013). The National Institute for Health and Clinical Excellence (NICE) (2008) guidelines state that the crown-to-rump (C–R) length should be used to determine gestational age and if the C–R length is greater than 84 mm, the head circumference (HC) should be used instead. The foldout poster inserted in this text also summarizes fetal development.

In review, human development follows three stages. The preembryonic stage, as discussed earlier in the chapter, consists of the first 14 days of development after the ovum is fertilized; then the embryonic stage covers the period from day 15 until approximately the end of the eighth week postconception, and the fetal stage extends from the end of the eighth week until birth.

Embryonic Stage

The stage of the **embryo** starts on day 15 (the beginning of the third week after conception) and continues until approximately the eighth week, or until the embryo reaches a crown-to-rump (C–R) length of 3 cm (1.2 in.). This length is usually reached about 56 days after fertilization (the end of the eighth gestational week). During the embryonic stage, tissues differentiate into essential organs, and the main external features develop. The embryo is the most vulnerable to *teratogens* during this period. These are discussed in more depth later in the chapter.

Three Weeks

In the third week, the embryonic disk becomes elongated and pear shaped, with a broad cephalic end and a narrow caudal end. The ectoderm has formed a long cylindrical tube for brain and spinal cord development. The gastrointestinal tract, created from the endoderm, appears as another tubelike structure communicating with the yolk sac. The most advanced organ is the heart. At 3 weeks, a single tubular heart forms just outside the body cavity of the embryo.

Four to Five Weeks

During days 21 to 32, *somites* (a series of mesodermal blocks) form on either side of the embryo's midline. The vertebrae that form the spinal column will develop from these somites. Before 28 days, arm and leg buds are not visible, but the tail bud is present. The pharyngeal arches—which will form the lower jaw, hyoid bone, and larynx—develop at this time. The pharyngeal pouches appear now; these pouches will form the eustachian tube and cavity of the middle ear, the tonsils, and the parathyroid and thymus glands. The primordia of the ear and eye are also present. By the end of 28 days, the tubular heart is beating at a regular rhythm and pushing its own primitive blood cells through the main blood vessels.

During the fifth week, the optic cups and lens vessels of the eye form and the nasal pits develop. Partitioning in the heart occurs with the dividing of the atrium. The embryo has a marked C-shaped body, accentuated by the rudimentary tail and the large head folded over a protuberant trunk (Figure 4–12 ●). By day 35, the arm and leg buds are well developed, with paddle-shaped hand and foot plates. The heart, circulatory system, and brain show the most advanced development. The brain has differentiated into five areas, and 10 pairs of cranial nerves are recognizable.

Six Weeks

At 6 weeks the head structures are more highly developed and the trunk is straighter than in earlier stages. The upper and lower jaws are recognizable, and the external nares are well formed. The trachea has developed, and its caudal end is bifurcated for beginning lung formation. The upper lip has formed, and the palate is developing. The ears are developing rapidly. The arms

● **Figure 4–12** The embryo at 5 weeks. The embryo has a C-shaped body and a rudimentary tail.

Source: Omikron Omikron/Getty Images

Table 4–3   Timeline of Organ System Development in the Embryo and Fetus

AGE: 2 TO 3 WEEKS

Length: 2 mm C–R (crown to rump)
Nervous system: Groove forms along middle back as cells thicken; neural tube forms from closure of neural groove.
Cardiovascular system: Beginning of blood circulation; tubular heart begins to form during third week.
Gastrointestinal system: Liver begins to function.

Genitourinary system: Formation of kidneys beginning.
Respiratory system: Nasal pits forming.
Endocrine system: Thyroid tissue appears.
Eyes: Optic cup and lens pit have formed; pigment in eyes.
Ears: Auditory pit is now enclosed structure.

AGE: 4 WEEKS

Length: 4 to 6 mm C–R
Weight: 0.4 g
Nervous system: Anterior portion of neural tube closes to form brain; closure of posterior end forms spinal cord.
Musculoskeletal system: Noticeable limb buds.

Cardiovascular system: Tubular heartbeats at 28 days, and primitive red blood cells circulate through fetus and chorionic villi.
Gastrointestinal system: Mouth: formation of oral cavity; primitive jaws present; esophagotracheal septum begins division of esophagus and trachea.
Digestive tract: stomach forms; esophagus and intestine become tubular; ducts of pancreas and liver forming.

AGE: 5 WEEKS

Length: 8 mm C–R
Weight: Only 0.5% of total body weight is fat (to 20 weeks).
Nervous system: Brain has differentiated and cranial nerves are present.

Musculoskeletal system: Developing muscles have innervation.
Cardiovascular system: Atrial division has occurred.

AGE: 6 WEEKS

Length: 12 mm C–R
Musculoskeletal system: Bone rudiments present; primitive skeletal shape forming; muscle mass begins to develop; ossification of skull and jaws begins.
Cardiovascular system: Chambers present in heart; groups of blood cells can be identified.

Gastrointestinal system: Oral and nasal cavities and upper lip formed; liver begins to form red blood cells.
Respiratory system: Trachea, bronchi, and lung buds present.
Ears: Formation of external, middle, and inner ear continues.
Sexual development: Embryonic sex glands appear.

AGE: 7 WEEKS

Length: 18 mm C–R
Cardiovascular system: Fetal heartbeats can be detected.
Gastrointestinal system: Mouth: tongue separates; palate folds.
Digestive tract: stomach attains final form.
Genitourinary system: Separation of bladder and urethra from rectum.

Respiratory system: Diaphragm separates abdominal and thoracic cavities.
Eyes: Optic nerve formed; eyelids appear, thickening of lens.
Sexual development: Differentiation of sex glands into ovaries and testes begins.

AGE: 8 WEEKS

Length: 2.5 to 3 cm C–R
Weight: 2 g
Musculoskeletal system: Digits formed; further differentiation of cells in primitive skeleton; cartilaginous bones show first signs of ossification; development of muscles in trunk, limbs, and head; some movement of fetus now possible.
Cardiovascular system: Development of heart essentially complete; fetal circulation follows two circuits—four extraembryonic and two intraembryonic. Heartbeat can be heard with Doppler at 8 to 12 weeks.

Gastrointestinal system: Mouth: completion of lip fusion. Digestive tract: rotation in midgut; anal membrane has perforated.
Ears: External, middle, and inner ear assuming final forms.
Sexual development: Male and female external genitals appear similar until end of ninth week.

AGE: 10 WEEKS

Length: 5 to 6 cm C–R
Weight: 14 g
Nervous system: Neurons appear at caudal end of spinal cord; basic ...isions of brain present.
...skeletal system: Fingers and toes begin nail growth.
...al system: Mouth: separation of lips from jaw; fusion of
...ng intestines enclosed in abdomen.

Genitourinary system: Bladder sac formed.
Endocrine system: Islets of Langerhans differentiated.
Eyes: Eyelids fused closed; development of lacrimal duct.
Sexual development: Males: production of testosterone and physical characteristics between 8 and 12 weeks.

...-H
...utlining of miniature bones (12 to
...s established throughout fetal body;
...s in viscera.
...completion of palate. Digestive tract:
...bile secretion begins; liver is major

Respiratory system: Lungs acquire definitive shape.
Skin: Pink and delicate.
Endocrine system: Hormonal secretion from thyroid; insulin present in pancreas.
Immunologic system: Appearance of lymphoid tissue in fetal thymus gland.

Table 4–3   Timeline of Organ System Development in the Embryo and Fetus—*continued*

AGE: 16 WEEKS

Length: 13.5 cm C–R; 15 cm C–H (crown to heel)
Weight: 200 g
Musculoskeletal system: Teeth beginning to form hard tissue that will become central incisors.
Gastrointestinal system: Mouth: differentiation of hard and soft palate.
Digestive tract: Development of gastric and intestinal glands; intestines begin to collect meconium.

Genitourinary system: Kidneys assume typical shape and organization.
Skin: Appearance of scalp hair; lanugo present on body; transparent skin with visible blood vessels; sweat glands developing.
Eyes, ears, and nose: Formed.
Sexual development: Sex determination possible.

AGE: 18 WEEKS

Musculoskeletal system: Teeth beginning to form hard tissue (enamel and dentine) that will become lateral incisors.

Cardiovascular system: Fetal heart tones audible with fetoscope at 16 to 20 weeks.

AGE: 20 WEEKS

Length: 19 cm C–R; 25 cm C–H
Weight: 435 g (6% of total body weight is fat).
Nervous system: Myelination of spinal cord begins.
Musculoskeletal system: Teeth beginning to form hard tissue that will become canines and first molars. Lower limbs are of final relative proportions.
Gastrointestinal system: Fetus actively sucks and swallows amniotic fluid; peristaltic movements begin.

Skin: Lanugo covers entire body; brown fat begins to form; vernix caseosa begins to form.
Immunologic system: Detectable levels of fetal antibodies (IgG type).
Blood formation: Iron is stored and bone marrow is increasingly important.

AGE: 24 WEEKS

Length: 23 cm C–R; 28 cm C–H
Weight: 780 g
Nervous system: Brain looks like mature brain.
Musculoskeletal system: Teeth are beginning to form hard tissue that will become the second molars.

Respiratory system: Respiratory movements may occur (24 to 40 weeks). Nostrils reopen. Alveoli appear in lungs and begin production of surfactant; gas exchange possible.
Skin: Reddish and wrinkled, vernix caseosa present.
Immunologic system: IgG levels reach maternal levels.

AGE: 28 WEEKS

Length: 27 cm C–R; 35 cm C–H
Weight: 1200 to 1250 g
Nervous system: Begins regulation of some body functions.
Skin: Adipose tissue accumulates rapidly; nails appear; eyebrows and eyelashes present.

Eyes: Eyelids open (26 to 29 weeks).
Sexual development: Males: testes descend into inguinal canal and upper scrotum.

AGE: 32 WEEKS

Length: 31 cm C–R; 38–43 cm C–H
Weight: 2000 g
Nervous system: More reflexes present.

AGE: 36 WEEKS

Length: 35 cm C–R; 42 to 48 cm C–H
Weight: 2500 to 2750 g
Musculoskeletal system: Distal femoral ossification centers present.
Skin: Pale; body rounded, lanugo disappearing, hair fuzzy or woolly; few sole creases; sebaceous glands active and helping to produce vernix caseosa (36 to 40 weeks).

Ears: Earlobes soft with little cartilage.
Sexual development: Males: scrotum small and few rugae present; descent of testes into upper scrotum to stay (36 to 40 weeks). Females: labia majora and minora equally prominent.

AGE: 38 TO 40 WEEKS

Length: 40 cm C–R; 48 to 52 cm C–H
Weight: 3200+ g (16% of total body weight is fat).
Respiratory system: At 38 weeks, lecithin–sphingomyelin (L/S) ratio approaches 2:1 (indicates decreased risk of respiratory distress from inadequate surfactant production if born now).

Skin: Smooth and pink; vernix present in skin folds; moderate to profuse silky hair; lanugo on shoulders and upper back; nails extend over tips or digits; creases cover sole.
Ears: Earlobes firmer because of increased cartilage.
Sexual development: Males: rugous scrotum. Females: labia majora well developed and minora small or completely covered.

Note: Age refers to postfertilization or postconception age.

Source: Data from Moore, K. L., Persaud, T. V. N., & Torchia, M. G. (2013). *The developing human: Clinical oriented embryology* (9th ed.). Philadelphia, PA: Saunders/Elsevier; Sadler, T. W. (2012). *Langman's medical embryology* (12th ed.). Philadelphia, PA: Lippincott Williams & Wilkins.

have begun to extend ventrally across the chest, and both arms and legs have digits, although they may still be webbed. There is a slight elbow bend in the arms, which are more advanced in development than the legs. Beginning at this stage, the prominent tail will recede. The heart now has most of its definitive characteristics, and fetal circulation begins to be established. The liver starts to produce blood cells.

Seven Weeks

At 7 weeks the head of the embryo is rounded and nearly erect (Figure 4–13 ●). The eyes have shifted and are closer together, and the eyelids are beginning to form. The palate is near completion, and the tongue is developing in the formed mouth. The gastrointestinal and genitourinary tracts undergo significant changes during the seventh week. Before this time the rectal and urogenital passages formed one tube that ended in a blind pouch; they now separate into two tubular structures. The intestines enter the extraembryonic coelom in the area of the umbilical cord (called umbilical herniation) (Moore et al., 2013). The beginnings of all essential external and internal structures are present.

Eight Weeks

At 8 weeks the embryo is approximately 3 cm (1.2 in.) C–R length and clearly resembles a human being. Facial features continue to develop. The eyelids begin to fuse. Auricles of the external ears begin to assume their final shape, but they are still set low (Moore et al., 2013). External genitals appear, but the embryo's sex is not clearly identifiable. The rectal passage opens with the perforation of the anal membrane. The circulatory system through the umbilical cord is well established. Long bones are beginning to form, and the large muscles are now capable of contracting.

Fetal Stage

By the end of the eighth week, the embryo is sufficiently developed to be called a **fetus**. Every organ system and external structure that will be found in the full-term newborn is present.

The remainder of gestation is devoted to refining structures and perfecting function.

Nine to Twelve Weeks

By the end of the ninth week the fetus reaches a C–R length of 5 cm (2 in.) and weighs about 14 g (0.5 oz). The head is large and comprises almost half of the fetus's entire size (Figure 4–14 ●). At 12 weeks, the fetus reaches 8 cm (3.2 in.) C–R length and weighs about 45 g (1.6 oz). The face is well formed, with the nose protruding, the chin small and receding, and the ear acquiring a more adult shape. The eyelids close at about the 10th week and will not reopen until about the 26- to 29-week period. Some movement of the lips suggestive of the sucking reflex has been observed at 3 months. Tooth buds now appear for all 20 of the child's first teeth (baby teeth). The limbs are long and slender, with well-formed digits. The fetus can curl the fingers toward the palm and begins to make a tiny fist. The legs are still shorter and less developed than the arms. The urogenital tract completes its development, well-differentiated genitals appear, and the kidneys begin to produce urine. Red blood cells are produced primarily by the liver. Spontaneous movements of the fetus now occur. Fetal heart rates can be ascertained by electronic devices between 8 and 12 weeks. The rate is 120 to 160 beats per minute.

Thirteen to Sixteen Weeks

This is a period of rapid growth. At 13 weeks, the fetus weighs 55 to 60 g (1.9 to 2.1 oz) and is about 9 cm (3.6 in.) in C–R length. Lanugo, or fine hair, begins to develop, especially on the head. The skin is so transparent that blood vessels are clearly visible beneath it. More muscle tissue and body skeleton have developed and hold the fetus more erect (Figure 4–15 ●). Active movements are present; the fetus stretches and exercises its arms and legs. It makes sucking motions, swallows amniotic fluid, and produces meconium in the intestinal tract. Bronchial tubes are branching out in the primitive lungs, and sweat glands are developing. The liver and pancreas now begin producing their appropriate secretions. By the beginning of week 16, skeletal ossification is clearly identifiable.

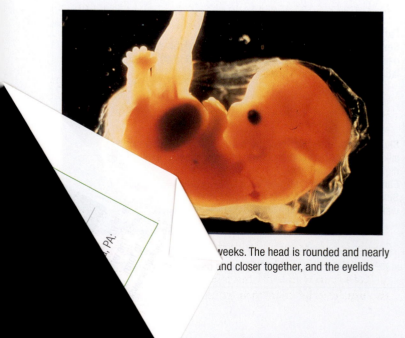

weeks. The head is rounded and nearly ...nd closer together, and the eyelids

● **Figure 4–14** The fetus at 9 weeks. Every organ system and external structure is present.

Source: © Vincent Zuber/Custom Medical Stock

● **Figure 4–15** The fetus at 14 weeks. During this period of rapid growth the skin is so transparent that blood vessels are visible beneath it. More muscle tissue and body skeleton have developed, and they hold the fetus more erect.

Source: NMSB/Custom Medical Stock

● **Figure 4–16** The fetus at 20 weeks. The fetus now weighs 435 to 465 g (15.2 to 16.3 oz) and measures about 19 cm (7.5 in.). Subcutaneous deposits of brown fat make the skin a little less transparent. "Woolly" hair may cover the head, and nails have developed on the fingers and toes.

Source: James Stevenson/Science Source

Twenty Weeks

The fetus doubles its C–R length and now measures 19 cm (8 in.) long. Fetal weight is between 435 and 465 g (15.2 and 16.3 oz). Lanugo covers the entire body and is especially prominent on the shoulders. Subcutaneous deposits of brown fat, which has a rich blood supply, make the skin less transparent. Brown fat is found chiefly at the root of the neck, posterior to the sternum, and in the perirenal area. Nipples now appear over the mammary glands. The head may be covered with fine, "woolly" hair, and the eyebrows and eyelashes are beginning to form. Nails are present on both fingers and toes. Muscles are well developed, and the fetus is active (Figure 4–16 ●). The mother feels fetal movement, known as *quickening*. The fetal heartbeat is audible through a fetoscope. Quickening and fetal heartbeat can help in validating the EDB.

Twenty-Four Weeks

The fetus at 24 weeks reaches a C–R of 23 cm (9.2 in.) or crown-to-heel (C–H) length of 28 cm (11.2 in.). It weighs about 780 g (1 lb, 10 oz). The hair on the head is growing long, and eyebrows and eyelashes have formed. The eye is structurally complete and will soon open. The fetus has a reflex hand grip (grasp reflex) and, by the end of 6 months, a startle reflex. Skin covering the body is reddish and wrinkled, with little subcutaneous fat. Skin on the hands and feet have thickened, with skin ridges on the palms and soles forming distinct foot- and fingerprints. The skin over the entire body is covered with **vernix caseosa**, a protective cheeselike, fatty substance secreted by the sebaceous glands. The alveoli in the lungs are just beginning to form.

Twenty-Five to Twenty-Eight Weeks

At about 25 weeks the fetal skin is still red, wrinkled, and covered with vernix caseosa. The brain is developing rapidly, and the nervous system is complete enough to provide some degree of regulation of body functions. The eyelids, under neural control, open and close. The fetus has nails on both fingers and toes. In the male fetus, the testes begin to descend into the scrotal sac. Even though the lungs are still physiologically immature, they are sufficiently developed to provide gas exchange. A fetus born at this time will require immediate and prolonged intensive care to survive and then to decrease the risk of major handicap. The fetus at 28 weeks is about 27 cm (10.8 in.) C–R or 35 to 38 cm (14 to 15 in.) C–H and weighs 1200 to 1250 g (2 lb, 10.5 oz to 2 lb, 12 oz).

Twenty-Nine to Thirty-Two Weeks

At 30 weeks the pupillary light reflex is present (Moore et al., 2013). The fetus is gaining weight from an increase in body muscle and fat and weighs about 2000 g (4 lb, 6.5 oz), with a C–R length of 31 cm (12.4 in.) or C–H length of about 38 to 43 cm (15 to 17 in.), by 32 weeks of age. The CNS has matured enough to direct rhythmic breathing movements and partially control body temperature; however, the lungs are not yet fully mature. Bones are fully developed but soft and flexible. The fetus begins storing iron, calcium, and phosphorus. In males the testicles may be located in the scrotal sac but are often still high in the inguinal canals.

Thirty-Five to Thirty-Six Weeks

The fetus begins to get plump, and less wrinkled skin covers the deposits of subcutaneous fat. Lanugo begins to disappear, and the nails reach the edge of the fingertips. By 35 weeks of age, the fetus has a firm grasp and exhibits spontaneous orientation to light. By 36 weeks of age the weight is usually 2500 to 2750 g (5 lb, 12 oz to 6 lb, 11.5 oz), and the C–H length of the fetus is about 42 to 48 cm (17 to 19 in.) or C–R 35 cm (14 in.). An infant born at this time has a good chance of surviving but may require special care, especially if there is intrauterine growth restriction.

Thirty-Eight to Forty Weeks

The fetus is considered full term at 38 weeks and up to 40 weeks conception. The C–H length varies from 48 to 52 cm (19 in.) C–R of 40 cm (16 in.), with males usually longer than females. They also usually weigh more than females. The weight

3000 to 3600 g (6 lb, 10 oz to 7 lb, 15 oz) and varies in different ethnic groups. The skin is pink and has a smooth, polished look. The only lanugo left is on the upper arms and shoulders. The hair on the head is no longer woolly but is coarse and about 1 in. long. Vernix caseosa is present, with heavier deposits remaining in the creases and folds of the skin. The body and extremities are plump, with good skin turgor, and the fingernails extend beyond the fingertips. The chest is prominent but still a little smaller than the head, and mammary glands protrude in both sexes. In males, the testes are in the scrotum or palpable in the inguinal canals.

As the fetus enlarges, amniotic fluid diminishes to about an average of 400 mL, and the fetal body mass fills the uterine cavity (Blackburn, 2013). The fetus assumes what is called its *position of comfort,* or lie. The head is generally pointed downward, following the shape of the uterus (and possibly because the head is heavier than the feet). The extremities, and often the head, are well flexed. After 5 months, patterns in feeding, sleeping, and activity become established, so at term the fetus has its own body rhythms and individual style of response. See Table 4–4 for important developmental milestones. For a detailed discussion of each body system's transition to and their functioning in the newborn, see Chapter 24 🌐.

FACTORS INFLUENCING EMBRYONIC AND FETAL DEVELOPMENT

Factors that may affect embryonic development include the quality of the sperm or ovum from which the zygote was formed, the genetic code established at fertilization, and the adequacy of the intrauterine environment. If the environment is unsuitable before cellular differentiation occurs, all the cells of the zygote are affected. The cells may die, which causes spontaneous abortion, or growth may be slowed, depending on the severity of the situation. When differentiation is complete and the fetal membranes have formed, an injurious agent has the greatest effect on those cells undergoing the most rapid growth. Thus the time of injury is critical in the development of anomalies.

Because organs are formed primarily during embryonic development, the growing organism is considered most vulnerable to hazardous agents during the first months of pregnancy. Any agent (e.g., drug, virus, or radiation) that can cause abnormal structures to develop in an embryo is called a **teratogen**. It is important to remember that the effects of teratogens depend on the (1) fetal genotype and maternal genome, (2) stage of development when exposure occurs, and (3) dose and duration of exposure of the agent. Potential teratogens can cause malformations as early as 3 weeks postconception of the heart, limbs, eyes, and central nervous systems (Moore et al., 2013). Chapter 11 🌐 discusses specific teratogenic agents on the developing fetus.

The maternal environment is also important during embryonic and fetal development. Maternal nutrition affects brain and neural tube development. The period of rapid brain growth and myelination begins with the fifth lunar month and continues into adulthood (Blackburn, 2013). Long-chain fatty acids are considered to be the most important for growth. A subtle type of damage to the outer layer of the brain, possibly leading to decreased IQ, can be caused by nutritional deficiency at this

Table 4–4	Fetal Development: What Parents Want to Know
4 weeks:	The fetal heart begins to beat.
8 weeks:	All body organs are formed.
8 to 12 weeks:	Fetal heart rate can be heard by ultrasound Doppler device.
16 weeks:	Baby's sex can be seen. Although thin, the fetus looks like a baby.
20 weeks:	Heartbeat can be heard with fetoscope. Mother feels movement (quickening). Baby develops a regular schedule of sleeping, sucking, and kicking. Hands can grasp. Baby assumes a favorite position in utero. Vernix (lanolinlike covering) protects the body, and lanugo (fine hair) keeps oil on skin. Head hair, eyebrows, and eyelashes present.
24 weeks:	Weighs 780 g (1 lb, 10 oz). Activity is increasing. Fetal respiratory movements begin. Baby makes sucking movements.
28 weeks:	Eyes open and close. Baby can breathe at this time. Surfactant needed for breathing at birth is formed. Baby is two thirds its final length.
32 weeks:	Baby has fingernails and toenails. Subcutaneous fat is being laid down. Baby appears less red and wrinkled.
38+ weeks:	Baby fills total uterus. Baby gets antibodies from mother.

stage. Studies in Tunisia showed that babies of mothers who were pregnant during the observance of Ramadan (the ninth month of the Islamic calendar) and practiced the required strict fasting for 29 to 30 days had reduced birth weight, head circumference, ponderal index, and placental weight (Alwasel, Harrath, Aljarallah, et al., 2013). Similar results were found in studies of pregnant women fasting during Ramadan in Saudi Arabia.

SAFETY ALERT!
Vitamins and folic acid supplements taken before conception can reduce the incidence of neural tube defects. A goal of *Healthy People 2020* is to increase the proportion of women of childbearing potential with daily intake of at least 400 mcg of folic acid from fortified foods or dietary supplementation to 26.2% from the current level of 23.8% (U.S. Department of Health and Human Services, 2011).

Poor maternal nutrition may also predispose babies who were small or disproportionate at birth to the development of adult coronary heart disease, hypertension, and diabetes (Moore et al., 2013). Maternal nutrition is discussed in depth in Chapter 12 🔗.

Another prenatal influence on the intrauterine environment is maternal hyperthermia associated with sauna or hot tub use. Studies of the effects of maternal hyperthermia during the first trimester have raised concern about possible central nervous system defects and failure of neural tube closure. Cigarette smoking during pregnancy is a well-established cause of intrauterine growth restriction (IUGR) (Moore et al., 2013). Maternal substance abuse also affects the intrauterine environment and is discussed in Chapters 15 🔗 and 31 🔗.

Critical Concept Review

LEARNING OUTCOME 4.1: Differentiate between meiotic cellular division and mitotic cellular division.

- Mitosis produces cells that cause growth in the body. Results in daughter cells that are an exact copy of the parent cell. They contain a full diploid set (46) of chromosomes.

- Meiosis produces cells called gametes that are necessary for reproduction of the species. Results in cells that contain only one half (haploid or 23) of the chromosomes of the parent cell.

LEARNING OUTCOME 4.2: Compare the processes by which ova and sperm are produced.

- Ova are present in the female ovary at birth but are dormant until puberty. Meiosis initially produces via oogenesis two haploid cells (secondary oocyte and a minute polar body) that are released at ovulation. At the end of meiosis in the female, there are four haploid cells: the three polar bodies and one ovum.

- Sperm are produced in the seminiferous tubules of the testes beginning at puberty.

- Meiosis in the male creates four haploid sperm able to fertilize the ovum. Two sperm carry the Y chromosome and two sperm contain the X chromosome.

LEARNING OUTCOME 4.3: Describe the components of the process of fertilization as to how each may impact fertilization.

1. Preparation is the first component of fertilization:
   - Ovum released into fallopian tube—viable for 24 hr.
   - Sperm deposited into vagina—viable for 48 to 72 hr (highly fertile for 24 hr).
   - Sperm must undergo capacitation and acrosomal reaction.
   - Sperm penetration causes a chemical reaction that blocks more sperm penetration.

2. Moment of fertilization is the second component of fertilization:
   - It occurs in the ampulla (outer third) of the fallopian tube.
   - Sperm enters the ovum. The nuclei of the ovum and sperm swell, unite, and become a diploid zygote.

LEARNING OUTCOME 4.4: Summarize the processes that occur during the cellular multiplication and differentiation stages of intrauterine development and their effects on the structures that form.

1. Cellular multiplication:
   - Rapid mitotic division (cleavage).
   - Blastomeres grow to morula (solid ball of 12 to 16 cells).
   - Morula divides into a solid mass (blastocyst) surrounded by an outer layer of cells (trophoblast).
   - Implantation occurs in 7 to 10 days.

2. Cellular differentiation:
   - At 10 to 14 days of age, blastocyst differentiates into three primary germ layers (ectoderm, mesoderm, and endoderm) from which all tissues, organs, and organ systems develop.
   - Amniotic fluid is created when the amnion and chorion grow, connect, form the amniotic sac, and produce fluid.

- Embryonic membranes form at implantation and include the chorion and the amnion.
- Amniotic fluid cushions the fetus against mechanical injury, controls the embryo's temperature, allows symmetrical growth, permits freedom of movement, and prevents adherence to the amnion.
- Yolk sac develops as part of the blastocyst and produces primitive red blood cells. It is soon incorporated into the umbilical cord.
- After implantation, the endometrium is called the decidua. Decidua capsularis is the portion that covers the blastocyst. Decidua basalis is the portion that is directly under the blastocyst. The decidua vera (parietalis) is the portion that lines the rest of the uterine cavity.

LEARNING OUTCOME 4.5: Describe the development, structure, and functions of the placenta and umbilical cord during intrauterine life (embryonic and fetal development).

1. Umbilical cord:
   - Develops from amnion. Contains two arteries and one vein and is surrounded by Wharton's jelly, which protects the vessels.
   - Function is to provide a circulatory pathway to the embryo.

2. Placenta:
   - Develops at the site of embryonic attachment to the uterus and is composed of two parts, the maternal side and the fetal side. The placenta is made up of 15 to 20 segments called cotyledons.
   - Provides endocrine (production of hPL, hCG, estrogen, and progesterone), metabolic, and immunologic functions to the fetus. It acts as the fetus's respiratory organ, is an organ of excretion, and aids in the exchange of nutrients.

LEARNING OUTCOME 4.6: Compare the factors and processes by which fraternal (dizygotic) and identical (monozygotic) twins are formed.

1. Fraternal twins:
   - Develop from two separate ova fertilized by two separate sperm.
   - Two placentas.

2. Identical twins:
   - Develop from a single fertilized egg. Both fetuses are the same sex with the same characteristics.
   - Single placenta.

LEARNING OUTCOME 4.7: Summarize the significant changes in growth and development of the fetus at 4, 6, 12, 16, 20, 24, 28, 36, and 40 weeks' gestation.

- 4 weeks: 4 to 6 mm C–R, brain formed from anterior neural tube, limb buds seen, heart begins to beat.
- 6 weeks: 12 mm C–R, primitive skeletal shape, chambers in heart, respiratory system begins to form, ear formation begins.
- 12 weeks: 8 cm C–R, ossification of skeleton begins, liver produces red cells, palate complete in mouth, skin pink, thyroid hormone present, and insulin present in pancreas.
- 16 weeks: 13.5 cm C–R, teeth begin to form, meconium begins to collect in intestines, kidneys assume shape, hair present on scalp. Sex can be determined.

- 20 weeks: 19 cm C–R, myelination of spinal cord begins. Suck and swallow begins, lanugo covers body, vernix begins to form.
- 24 weeks: 23 cm C–R, respiratory movement and surfactant production begins, brain appears mature.
- 28 weeks: 27 cm C–R, nervous system begins regulation of some functions, adipose tissue accumulates rapidly. Nails, eyebrows, and eyelids are present. Eyes open and close.
- 36 weeks: 35 cm C–R, earlobes soft with little cartilage, few sole creases.
- 40 weeks: 40 cm C–R, adequate surfactant, vernix in skin folds and lanugo on shoulders, earlobes firm, and sex apparent.

LEARNING OUTCOME 4.8: Identify the factors that influence congenital malformations of the various organ systems.

- Embryo is most vulnerable to teratogenesis during the first 8 weeks of cell differentiation and organ system development.

- Effects of teratogens depend on the (1) maternal and fetal genotype, (2) stage of development when exposure occurs, and (3) dose and duration of exposure of the agent.

Clinical Reasoning in Action

You are working at the local clinic when Frances, a 28-year-old G2 P1001 at 11 weeks' gestation, comes into the office. Frances tells you that early in the first trimester, her husband experienced a flulike syndrome and that he was later diagnosed with cytomegalovirus (CMV) pneumonia. She tells you that his physician found an enlarged supraclavicular lymph node and an ulcer on one tonsil. Laboratory testing revealed elevated liver enzymes. Further testing led to the discovery of positive cytomegalovirus (CMV) IgM levels. She has come today with symptoms including night sweats, persistent sore throat, joint pain, headache, vomiting, and fatigue. You obtain vital signs of temperature 99°F, pulse 90, respirations 14, BP 110/70. Her physical exam is normal; no lymphadenopathy is present. Her weight gain is 2 lb even with nausea and some vomiting. She is worried that her husband's illness could be related to her current symptoms.

1. How would you respond to Frances's concern?
2. Frances asks you if her baby is formed. How would you discuss the three stages of development?
3. Frances asks when her baby is most vulnerable for developing abnormalities in growth or structure. How would you answer?
4. Frances asks what stage her baby is in. What would you tell her?
5. Develop a concept map that correlates CMV and Frances' signs and symptoms and possible risk factors for her baby.

See www.nursing.pearsonhighered.com for possible responses and an interactive template for a concept map.

References

Alwasel, S. H., Harrath, A., Aljarallah, J. S., Abotalib, Z., Osmond, C., Al Omar, S. Y., Khaled, I., & Barker, D. J. P. (2013). Intergenerational effects of in utero exposure to Ramadan in Tunisia. *American Journal of Human Biology.* Retrieved from http://onlinelibrary.wiley.com/doi/10.1002/ajhb.22374/full doi:10.1002/ajhb.22374

Blackburn, S. T. (2013). *Maternal, fetal, & neonatal physiology: A clinical perspective* (4th ed.). St. Louis, MO: Saunders/Elsevier.

Moore, K. L., Persaud, T. V. N., & Torchia, M. G. (2013). *The developing human: Clinical oriented embryology* (9th ed.). Philadelphia, PA: Saunders/Elsevier.

National Institute for Health and Clinical Excellence (NICE) (2008). Antenatal care: routine care for the healthy pregnant woman. Retrieved from http://www.nice.org.uk/CG62

Sadler, T. W. (2012). *Langman's medical embryology* (11th ed.). Philadelphia, PA: Lippincott Williams & Wilkins.

Society of Maternal-Fetal Medicine (SMFM); Moise, K. J., & Argon, P. S. (2013). The importance of determining chorionicity in twin gestations. *Contemporary OB/GYN,* February 3, 2013, 35–43.

U.S. Department of Health and Human Services. (2011). *Healthy People 2020 topics & objectives.* Retrieved from http://www.healthypeople.gov/2020/topicsobjectives2020/default.aspx

CHAPTER

5

Health Promotion for Women

Steve Smith/Taxi/Getty Images

I am 64 now, an early baby boomer. I am astonished at the changes that have occurred in women's health care in my lifetime. I remember that my mom was shocked when our family doctor taught me to do a breast exam when I turned 18. What a farsighted man. Information on sexually transmitted infections was not as generally available. AIDS was beyond our imagination. Contraceptive options were more limited although the pill was gaining in popularity. Menopause seemed like the end of life—menopausal women were old. Today more and more of us women are becoming savvy healthcare consumers. We have more information, we have treatment options, we decide our own care. I think this is the most exciting change of all! —Alice

LEARNING OUTCOMES

5.1 Describe accurate information to be provided to girls and women so that they can implement effective self-care measures for dealing with menstruation.

5.2 Contrast the signs, symptoms, and nursing management of women with dysmenorrhea and those with premenstrual syndrome.

5.3 Compare the advantages, disadvantages, and effectiveness of the various methods of contraception available today.

5.4 Identify basic gynecologic screening procedures indicated for well women.

5.5 Examine the physical and psychologic aspects and clinical treatment options of menopause when caring for menopausal women.

5.6 Discuss the nurse's role in screening and caring for women who have experienced domestic violence or rape.

A woman's healthcare needs change throughout her lifetime. As a young girl, she needs health teaching about menstruation, sexuality, and personal responsibility. As a teen she needs information about reproductive choices and safe sexual activity. During this time she should also be introduced to the importance of healthcare practices such as breast self-examination and regular Pap smears. The mature woman may need to be reminded of these self-care issues and prepared for the physical changes that accompany childbirth and aging. By educating women about their bodies, their healthcare choices, and their right to be knowledgeable consumers, nurses can help women assume responsibility for the health care they receive. This chapter provides information about selected aspects of women's health care with an emphasis on conditions typically addressed in a community-based setting.

NURSING CARE IN THE COMMUNITY

Women's health refers to a holistic view of women and their health-related needs within the context of their everyday lives. It is based on the awareness that a woman's physical, mental, and spiritual status are interdependent and affect her state of health or illness. The woman's view of her situation, her assessment of her needs, her values, and her beliefs are valid and important factors to be incorporated into any healthcare intervention.

Nurses can work with women to provide health teaching and information about self-care practices in schools, during routine examinations in a clinic or office, at senior centers, at meetings of volunteer organizations, through classes offered by local agencies or schools, or in the home. Nurses oriented to community-based care are especially effective in recognizing the autonomy of each individual and in dealing with patients holistically. This holistic approach is important in addressing not only physical problems but also major health issues such as violence against women, which may go undetected unless care providers are alert for signs of it.

The Nurse's Role in Addressing Issues of Sexuality

Because sexuality and its reproductive implications are such intrinsic and emotion-laden parts of life, people have many concerns, problems, and questions about sex roles, behaviors, education, inhibitions, morality, and related areas such as family planning. The reproductive implications of sexual intercourse must also be considered. Some people desire pregnancy; others wish to avoid it. Health factors are another consideration. The increase in the incidence of sexually transmitted infections, especially HIV/AIDS and herpes, has caused many people to modify their sexual practices and activities. Women frequently ask questions or voice concerns about these issues to the nurse in a clinic or ambulatory setting. Thus, the nurse may need to assume the role of counselor or educator on sexual and reproductive matters.

Nurses who assume this role must recognize their own feelings, values, and attitudes about sexuality so they can be more sensitive when they encounter the values and beliefs of others. Nurses need to have accurate, up-to-date information about anatomy and physiology and about topics related to sexuality, sexual practices, and common gynecologic problems. In addition, when a woman is accompanied by her partner, it is important that the nurse be sensitive to the dynamics of the relationship and communication patterns between the two.

Taking a Sexual History

Nurses are often responsible for taking a woman's initial history, including her gynecologic and sexual history. For the interview to be its most useful, the nurse must have effective communication skills and should conduct the interview in a quiet, private place free of distractions. It is important to phrase questions in a sensitive and nonjudgmental manner and to assure the woman of strict confidentiality.

Opening the discussion with a brief explanation of the purpose of such questions is often helpful. For example, the nurse might say, "As your nurse, I'm interested in all aspects of your well-being. Often women have concerns or questions about sexual matters, especially as their life situations change. I will be asking you some questions about your sexual history as part of your general health history." This explanation helps women understand the nature of this part of their history and encourages more open, honest answers.

It may be helpful to use direct eye contact as much as possible unless the nurse knows it is culturally unacceptable to the woman. The nurse should do little, if any, writing during the interview, especially if the woman seems ill at ease or is discussing very personal issues. Beginning with general questions such as "What brings you here today?" before progressing to more sensitive topics will provide an opportunity for the woman to develop trust with the nurse. Open-ended questions are often useful in eliciting information. For example, "What, if anything, would you change about your sex life?" will elicit more information than "Are you happy with your sex life now?" The nurse needs to clarify terminology and proceed from easier topics to those that are more difficult to discuss.

Throughout the interview the nurse should be alert to body language and nonverbal cues. It is important that the nurse not assume that the patient is heterosexual. Some women are open about lesbian relationships or transgender surgery; others are more reserved until they develop a sense of trust in their caregivers.

After completing the sexual history, the nurse assesses the information obtained. If there is a problem that requires further medical tests and assessments, the nurse refers the woman to a nurse practitioner, certified nurse-midwife, physician, or counselor as necessary. In many instances the nurse alone will be able to develop a nursing diagnosis and then plan and implement therapy. The nurse must be realistic in making assessments and planning interventions. It requires insight and skill to recognize when a woman's problem requires interventions that are beyond a nurse's preparation and ability. In such situations it is essential that the nurse make appropriate referrals.

MENSTRUATION

Girls today begin to learn about puberty and menstruation at a young age. Unfortunately, the source of their "education" is sometimes their peers or the media; thus, the information is often incomplete, inaccurate, and sensationalized. Nurses who work with young girls and adolescents recognize this and are working hard to provide accurate health teaching and to correct misinformation about *menarche* (the onset of menses) and the menstrual cycle.

Cultural, religious, and personal attitudes about menstruation are part of the menstrual experience. Currently in the Western world, there are few customs associated with menstruation. Sexual intercourse during menses is a common practice and is not generally contraindicated. For most couples the decision is one of personal preference. (The physiology of menstruation is discussed in Chapter 3 🔗.)

Counseling the Premenstrual Girl About Menarche

Many young women find it embarrassing to discuss menstruation. However, the most critical factor in successful adaptation to menarche is the adolescent's level of preparedness. Information should be given to premenstrual girls over time rather than all at once. This allows them to absorb information and develop questions.

The following basic information is helpful for girls and young women:

- *Cycle length.* Cycle length is determined from the first day of one menses to the first day of the next menses. Initially a female's cycle length may be irregular. Once established, it is about 29 days, although it may vary from 21 to 35 days. Cycle length frequently varies by a day or two from one cycle to the next, although greater normal variations may also occur.
- *Amount of flow.* The average flow is approximately 25 to 60 mL per period. Usually women characterize the amount of flow in terms of the number of pads or tampons used. Flow is often heavier at first and lighter toward the end of the period.
- *Length of menses.* Menses usually lasts from 3 to 7 days, although this may vary.

The nurse should make it clear that variations in age at menarche, length of cycle, and duration of menses are normal, because girls may worry if their experiences vary from those of their peers. It also is helpful to acknowledge the negative aspects of menstruation (messiness, cramping, embarrassment) while stressing its positive role as a symbol of maturity and womanhood.

Educational Topics

Pads and Tampons

Since early times women have made pads and tampons from cloth or rags, which required washing but were reusable. Commercial tampons were introduced in the 1930s.

Today, adhesive-stripped, disposable minipads and maxipads and tampons are readily available. However, the deodorants and increased absorbency that manufacturers have added to both pads and tampons may prove harmful. The chemical used to deodorize can create irritation of the vulva and inner aspects of the vagina. This irritation may cause an external rash or internal sores from trauma to the tender mucosal lining of the vagina.

Interest is also growing in the use of eco-friendly menstrual products, including reusable menstrual pads made of washable cotton, menstrual cups, and menstrual sponges. These products are becoming more readily available at pharmacies and major discount stores.

The use of superabsorbent tampons has been linked to the development of toxic shock syndrome (TSS). (For more information about TSS, see Chapter 6 🔗.) Women can prevent problems by using tampons with the minimum absorbency necessary to control menstrual flow, changing them every 3 to 6 hours, and avoiding using them for vaginal discharge or light bleeding.

Because *Staphylococcus aureus*, the causative organism of TSS, is frequently found on the hands, a woman should wash her hands before inserting a fresh tampon and should avoid touching the tip of the tampon when unwrapping it or before insertion.

Clinical Tip

If you work with teens and preteens, keep a variety of pads and tampons on hand so that you can help these young girls become familiar with the options available for dealing with menstruation. You can also put colored water in a small glass and insert a tampon to show a girl how much fluid a tampon absorbs. Girls often think that they lose far more blood with a period than they actually do.

In the absence of a heavy menstrual flow, tampons absorb moisture, leaving the vaginal walls dry and subject to injury. The absorbency of regular tampons varies. If the tampon is hard to pull out or shreds when removed, or if the vagina becomes dry, the tampon is probably too absorbent.

A woman may want to use tampons only during the day and switch to pads at night to avoid vaginal irritation. If a woman experiences vaginal irritation, itching, or soreness or notices an unusual odor while using tampons, she should stop using them and be evaluated for infection. The choice of sanitary protection—whether pads or tampons—must meet the individual's needs and feel comfortable. Cultural factors may play a role in this decision and should be considered.

Vaginal Spray, Douching, and Cleansing
Vaginal sprays are unnecessary and can cause infections, itching (pruritus), burning, vaginal discharge, rashes, and other problems. If a woman chooses to use a spray, she needs to know that these sprays are for external use only, should be used infrequently, and should never be applied to irritated or itching skin.

Douching as a hygiene practice is unnecessary because the vagina cleanses itself. Douching washes away the natural mucus and upsets the vaginal flora, which can make the vagina more susceptible to infection. Perfumed douches can cause allergic reactions. Propelling water up the vagina may force bacteria and germs from the vagina into the uterus. Women should avoid douching during menstruation because the cervix is dilated to permit the downward flow of menstrual fluids from the uterine lining. Douching is also contraindicated during pregnancy.

The secretions that bathe the vagina are odor-free while they are in the vagina; odor develops only when they mingle with perspiration and are exposed to the air. Keeping one's skin clean and free of bacteria with plain soap and water is the most effective method of controlling odor. Bathing is as important during menses as at any other time. A long, leisurely soak in a warm tub promotes menstrual blood flow and relieves cramps by relaxing the muscles.

Keeping the vulva fresh throughout the day means keeping it dry and clean. A woman can ensure adequate ventilation by wearing cotton panties and clothes loose enough to permit the vaginal area to "breathe." After using the toilet, a woman should always wipe herself from front to back and, if necessary, follow up with a moistened paper towel or a premoistened wipe. If an unusual odor persists despite these efforts, a visit to one's

Developing Cultural Competence
Use of Tampons

In certain religious or cultural groups, unmarried women are expected to avoid the use of tampons. This is more common among those groups that highly value a girl's virginity and fear that tampon use will break the hymen. Thus it is wise to ask the girl (or her mother if the girl is uncertain) about the issue.

healthcare provider is indicated. Certain conditions such as vaginitis produce a foul-smelling discharge that women often describe as having a "fishy" odor.

Associated Menstrual Conditions
New self-explanatory terminology has been developed to define a variety of menstrual irregularities. These include *abnormal uterine bleeding (AUB), heavy menstrual bleeding (HMB), heavy and prolonged menstrual bleeding (HPMB), intermenstrual bleeding (IMB),* and *postmenopausal bleeding (PMB).* The following terminology is still used to define various menstrual irregularities but an International Review Panel has recommended that they be phased out: *hypomenorrhea* (abnormally short duration of menses), *hypermenorrhea* (abnormally long duration), *menorrhagia* (excessive flow), *metrorrhagia* (bleeding between periods), *oligomenorrhea* (infrequent menses), and *polymenorrhea* (too frequent menses) (Garza-Cavazos & Loret de Mola, 2012).

Amenorrhea
Amenorrhea, the absence of menses, is classified as primary or secondary. Primary amenorrhea (menstruation has not been established by 16 years of age or within 4 years of breast development) necessitates a thorough assessment to determine its cause. Possible causes include congenital obstructions; Turner syndrome; congenital absence of the uterus, ovaries, or vagina; testicular feminization (external genitals appear female but uterus and ovaries are absent and testes are present); chronic anovulation related to polycystic ovarian syndrome, thyroid, or adrenal disorders; or absence or imbalance of hormones. Treatment depends on the causative factors. Some causes are not correctable.

Secondary amenorrhea, or the cessation of regular menses, is caused most frequently by pregnancy. Additional causes include lactation, hormonal imbalances, poor nutrition (anorexia nervosa, obesity, and fad dieting), ovarian lesions, strenuous exercise (associated with long-distance runners, dancers, and other athletes with low body fat ratios), debilitating systemic diseases, stress of high intensity or long duration, stressful life events, a change in season or climate, use of oral contraceptives, use of the phenothiazine and chlorpromazine group of tranquilizers, and syndromes such as Cushing and Sheehan.

The causative factors dictate treatment. The nurse can explain that once the underlying condition has been corrected—for example, when sufficient body weight is gained—menses will resume. Athletes and women who participate in strenuous exercise routines may be advised to increase their caloric intake or reduce their exercise levels for a month or two to see whether a normal cycle ensues. If it does not, medical referral is indicated.

Dysmenorrhea

Dysmenorrhea, or painful menstruation, occurs at, or a day before, the onset of menstruation and disappears by the end of menses. Dysmenorrhea is classified as primary or secondary.

Primary dysmenorrhea is defined as cramps without underlying disease. Prostaglandins F_2 and $F_{2\alpha}$, which are produced by the uterus in higher concentrations during menses, are the primary cause. They increase uterine contractility and decrease uterine artery blood flow, causing ischemia. The end result is the painful sensation of cramps. Dysmenorrhea typically disappears after a first pregnancy and does not occur if cycles are anovulatory. Treatment of primary dysmenorrhea includes combined oral contraceptives, which inhibit ovulation; nonsteroidal anti-inflammatory drugs (NSAIDs) (such as ibuprofen, aspirin, and naproxen), which act as prostaglandin inhibitors; and self-care measures such as regular exercise, rest, application of heat, and good nutrition (Figure 5–1 ●). Research indicates that acupuncture may also provide relief (Smith, Zhu, He, et al., 2011). Some nutritionists suggest that vitamins B and E help relieve the discomforts associated with menstruation. Vitamin B_6 may help relieve the premenstrual bloating and irritability some women experience. Vitamin E, a mild prostaglandin inhibitor, may help decrease menstrual discomfort. Avoiding salt can decrease discomfort from fluid retention. Biofeedback has also been used with some success.

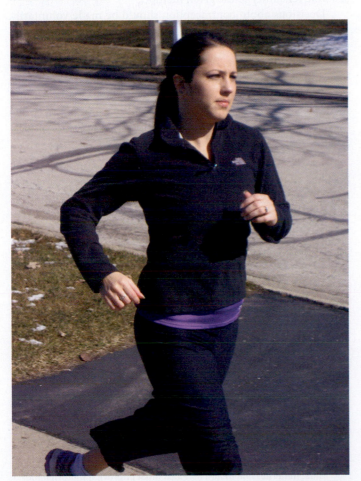

● **Figure 5–1** Regular exercise is an important part of therapy for dysmenorrhea.

Secondary dysmenorrhea is associated with pathology of the reproductive tract and usually appears after menstruation has been established. Conditions that most frequently cause secondary dysmenorrhea include endometriosis; residual pelvic inflammatory disease; cervical stenosis, uterine fibroids, ovarian cysts, benign or malignant tumors of the pelvis or abdomen; and the presence of an intrauterine device. Because primary and secondary dysmenorrhea may coexist, accurate differential diagnosis is essential for appropriate treatment.

For women with severe dysmenorrhea, use of continuous oral contraceptive therapy, which does not allow ovulation or menstruation to occur, may be of benefit. Hysterectomy may be the treatment of choice if there are anatomic disorders and childbearing is not desired.

Premenstrual Syndrome

Premenstrual syndrome (PMS) refers to a symptom complex associated with the luteal phase of the menstrual cycle (2 weeks prior to the onset of menses). The symptoms must, by definition, occur between ovulation and the onset of menses. They repeat at the same stage of each menstrual cycle and include some or all of the following:

- *Psychologic:* irritability, lethargy, depression, low morale, anxiety, sleep disorders, crying spells
- *Neurologic:* classic migraine, vertigo, syncope
- *Respiratory:* rhinitis, hoarseness, and occasionally asthma
- *Gastrointestinal:* nausea, vomiting, constipation, abdominal bloating, craving for sweets
- *Urinary:* retention, oliguria
- *Dermatologic:* acne
- *Mammary:* swelling and tenderness

Most women experience only some of these symptoms. The symptoms usually are most pronounced 2 or 3 days before the onset of menstruation and subside as menstrual flow begins, with or without treatment.

Evidence suggests that progesterone and estradiol levels are involved in PMS in some way. Central nervous system–mediated interactions between neurohormones and sex steroids may also account for the occurrence of PMS. Risk factors include a family history of PMS, emotional stress, a history of depression or other psychiatric disorders, poor nutritional habits, and increased alcohol, salt, and caffeine use (Raines, 2010). Women who are obese are also at increased risk for PMS (Bertone-Johnson, Hankinson, Willett, et al., 2010).

Premenstrual dysphoric disorder (PMDD) is a diagnosis that may be applied to a small subgroup of women with PMS whose symptoms are primarily mood related and severe. Women with PMDD may benefit from selective serotonin reuptake inhibitors (SSRIs) such as fluoxetine hydrochloride (Prozac), sertraline hydrochloride (Zoloft), and paroxetine CR (Paxil CR) or from the use of an oral contraceptive called YAZ (Shulman, 2010).

Nursing Management. Counseling for PMS may include advising the woman to restrict her intake of foods containing methylxanthines such as chocolate, cola, and coffee; restrict her intake of alcohol, nicotine, red meat, and foods containing salt

Evidence-Based Practice   PMS and B-Complex Vitamins

Clinical Question
Are B-complex vitamins effective in preventing the symptoms of premenstrual syndrome (PMS)?

The Evidence
The Harvard School of Public Health conducted a case/control study of more than 1000 women over 10 years to determine the relationship between B-complex vitamins and premenstrual syndrome. This longitudinal, comparative study is classified as Level I evidence of effectiveness. This study was part of the Nurses' Health Study II, a 30-year, highly respected cohort study that has yielded valuable information about women's health issues during the past decade. Intake of thiamine and riboflavin from food sources were each inversely associated with PMS. Women who had the highest intake of naturally occurring thiamine had a 35% lower risk of developing PMS than did those women whose intake was low. Risk was reduced most dramatically

among those women whose symptoms were psychologic, rather than physical. However, no significant associations were found when the B-complex vitamins were taken as supplements, rather than in food-based, naturally occurring forms (Chocano-Bedoya et al., 2011).

Best Practice
Treatment with B-complex vitamins is effective for those women whose primary premenstrual symptoms are psychologic, such as anxiety and depression. Intake of B vitamins—particularly thiamine and riboflavin—from food-based sources is most effective. Other types of vitamin supplements are not effective as a treatment for PMS.

Clinical Reasoning
What foods provide the most naturally occurring thiamine and riboflavin? How can women incorporate these foods into their diets prior to the start of their PMS symptoms?

---

and sugar; increase her intake of complex carbohydrates and protein; and increase the frequency of meals. For women whose primary symptoms are psychologic, supplementation with B-complex vitamins, especially B$_6$, may decrease anxiety and depression. Vitamin E supplements may help reduce breast tenderness. Supplementation with 1200 mg calcium daily may help relieve certain physical and psychologic symptoms. Magnesium supplements may help reduce fluid retention and bloating. See *Complementary Care: Herbal Remedies for PMS.*

A program of aerobic exercise such as fast walking, jogging, and aerobic dancing is generally beneficial. In addition to vitamin supplements, pharmacologic treatments for PMS include diuretics and prostaglandin inhibitors.

Women with PMS may find it helpful to have an empathetic relationship with a healthcare professional to whom she feels free to voice concerns. Encourage the woman to keep a diary to help identify life events associated with PMS. Self-care groups and self-help literature both help women feel they have control over their bodies.

CONTRACEPTION

The decision to use a method of contraception may be made individually by a woman (or, in the case of vasectomy, by a man) or jointly by a couple. The decision may be motivated by a desire

to avoid pregnancy, to gain control over the number of children conceived, or to determine the spacing of future children. In choosing a specific method, consistency of use outweighs the absolute reliability of the given method.

Decisions about contraception should be made voluntarily, with full knowledge of available choices, advantages, disadvantages, effectiveness, side effects, contraindications, and long-term effects. Many outside factors influence this choice, including cultural practices, religious beliefs, attitudes and personal preferences, cost, effectiveness, misinformation, practicality of method, and self-esteem. Different methods of contraception may be appropriate at different times for individuals or couples.

Fertility Awareness–Based Methods

Fertility awareness–based (FAB) methods, also known as *natural family planning,* are based on an understanding of the changes that occur throughout a woman's ovulatory cycle. FAB methods take into account the limited life span of sperm

---

Complementary Care   Herbal Remedies for PMS

Although the research evidence is weak, some women find that herbal remedies such as vitex or chasteberry and evening primrose oil reduce the effects of PMS (National Center for Complementary and Alternative Medicine [NCCAM], 2010a, 2010b). Underlying health conditions may contraindicate the use of herbal or vitamin supplements, however, and must be considered when recommending them.

Developing Cultural Competence
Contraceptive Use

- One in 26 women of reproductive age in Africa dies from a maternal cause, as compared to one in 9400 in Europe (Population Reference Bureau, 2010).
- In more developed countries worldwide, 60% of women of childbearing age use modern methods of contraception; in the least developed countries only 23% of women do so. This number drops to 17% in sub-Saharan Africa (Population Reference Bureau, 2010).
- Most of the causes of maternal mortality are treatable or preventable with adequate health care including contraceptive services. Thus, maternal healthcare services must improve if maternal mortality and morbidity are to be reduced.

in cervical mucus and the upper genital tract (3 to 5 days) and the ovum (12 to 24 hours) in the female reproductive tract (Hatcher, Trussell, Nelson, et al., 2011). Maximum fertility for the woman occurs approximately 5 days before ovulation and decreases rapidly the day after. Therefore, the couple must abstain from intercourse, or use a barrier method, during the fertile days (Hatcher et al., 2011). In conjunction with FAB methods, women may choose to improve identification of their fertile days by use of an over-the-counter ovulation prediction kit (e.g., OvuKIT). They may also use a temperature computer (e.g., Bioself 2000) or a hormone computer (e.g., Persona) to help predict fertile days.

Fertility awareness–based methods are free, safe, and acceptable to many whose religious beliefs prohibit other methods. They provide an increased awareness of the body, involve no artificial substances or devices, encourage a couple to communicate about sexual activity and family planning, and are useful in helping a couple plan a pregnancy.

However, these methods require extensive initial counseling to be used effectively. They may interfere with sexual spontaneity; they require extensive maintenance of records for several cycles before beginning to use them; they may be difficult or impossible for women with irregular cycles to use; and, although theoretically they should be very reliable, in practice they may not be as reliable in preventing pregnancy as other methods.

The *basal body temperature (BBT)* method to detect ovulation requires that a woman take her BBT every morning upon awakening (before any activity) and record the readings on a temperature graph. To do this she uses a BBT thermometer, which shows tenths of a degree rather than the two tenths shown on standard thermometers. She may also use tympanic thermometry (an "ear thermometer"). After 3 to 4 months of recording temperatures, a woman with regular cycles should be able to predict when ovulation will occur. The method is based on the fact that the temperature sometimes drops just before ovulation and almost always rises and remains elevated for several days after. The temperature rise occurs in response to the increased progesterone levels that occur in the second half of the cycle. Figure 7–2B 🔗 on page 137 shows a sample BBT chart of an ovulating woman. To avoid conception, the couple abstains from intercourse on the day of the temperature rise and for 3 days after. Because the temperature rise does not occur until after ovulation, a woman who had intercourse just before the rise is at risk of pregnancy. To decrease this risk, some couples abstain from intercourse for several days before the anticipated time of ovulation and then for 3 days after.

The *ovulation method,* sometimes called the *cervical mucus method* or the *Billings method,* involves the assessment of cervical mucus changes that occur during the menstrual cycle. The amount and character of cervical mucus change because of the influence of estrogen and progesterone. At the time of ovulation, the mucus (estrogen-dominant mucus) is clearer, more stretchable (a quality called *spinnbarkeit*), and more permeable to sperm. It also shows a characteristic fern pattern when placed on a glass slide and allowed to dry (see Figure 7–3 🔗 on page 138). During the luteal phase, the cervical mucus is thick and sticky (progesterone-dominant mucus) and forms a network that traps sperm, making their passage more difficult.

To use the cervical mucus method, the woman abstains from intercourse for the first menstrual cycle. Each day she assesses her cervical mucus for amount, feeling of slipperiness or wetness, color, clearness, and spinnbarkeit, as she becomes familiar with varying characteristics.

The peak day of wetness and clear, stretchable mucus is assumed to be the time of ovulation. To use this method correctly, the woman should abstain from intercourse from the time she first notices that the mucus is becoming clear, more elastic, and slippery until 4 days after the last wet mucus (ovulation) day. Because this method evaluates the effects of hormonal changes, it can be used by women with irregular cycles.

The *symptothermal method* consists of various assessments made and recorded by the couple. These include information regarding cycle days, coitus, cervical mucus changes, and secondary signs such as increased libido, abdominal bloating, *mittelschmerz* (midcycle abdominal pain), and BBT. Through the various assessments, the couple learns to recognize signs that indicate ovulation. This combined approach tends to improve the effectiveness of fertility awareness as a method of birth control.

Situational Contraceptives

Abstinence can be considered a method of contraception, and, partly because of changing values and the increased risk of infection with intercourse, it is gaining increased acceptance.

Coitus interruptus, or *withdrawal*, is one of the oldest and least reliable methods of contraception. This method requires that the male withdraw from the female's vagina when he feels that ejaculation is impending. He then ejaculates away from the external genitalia of the woman. Failure tends to occur for two reasons: (1) This method demands great self-control on the part of the man, who must withdraw just as he feels the urge for deeper penetration with impending orgasm, and (2) some pre-ejaculatory fluid, which can contain sperm, may escape from the penis during the excitement phase prior to ejaculation. The fact that the quantity of sperm in this pre-ejaculatory fluid is increased after a recent ejaculation is especially significant for couples who engage in repeated episodes of intercourse within a short period of time. Couples who use this method should be aware of postcoital contraceptive options in case the man fails to withdraw in time.

Douching after intercourse is an ineffective method of contraception and is not recommended. It may actually facilitate conception by pushing sperm farther up the birth canal.

Spermicides

The **spermicide** approved for use in the United States, nonoxynol-9 (N-9), is available as a cream, jelly, foam, vaginal film, and suppository. Spermicide is inserted into the vagina before intercourse. It destroys sperm by disrupting the cell membrane. Spermicides that effervesce in a moist environment offer more rapid protection, and coitus may take place immediately after they are inserted. Suppositories may require up to 30 minutes to dissolve and do not offer protection until they do so. The woman should be instructed to insert these spermicide preparations high in the vagina and maintain a supine position.

N-9 is minimally effective when used alone, but its effectiveness increases in conjunction with a barrier method of contraception such as a diaphragm, FemCap, contraceptive sponge, or male or female condom. The major advantages of spermicides are their wide availability and low toxicity. Skin irritation and allergic reactions to spermicides are the primary disadvantages. N-9 does not offer protection against infection from the human immunodeficiency virus, which causes HIV/AIDS, or against any other sexually transmitted infection. Moreover, N-9 may actually increase a woman's risk of HIV infection because it irritates vaginal tissue, making them more susceptible to invasion by organisms (U.S. Food and Drug Administration [FDA], 2009b).

Barrier Methods of Contraception

Barrier methods of contraception prevent the transport of sperm to the ovum, immobilize sperm, or are lethal against sperm.

Male and Female Condoms

The male **condom** offers a viable means of contraception when used consistently and properly (Figure 5–2 ●). Acceptance has been increasing as a growing number of men are assuming responsibility for regulation of fertility. The condom is applied to the erect penis, rolled from the tip to the base of the shaft, before vulvar or vaginal contact. A small space must be left at the end of the condom to allow for collection of the ejaculate, so that the condom will not break at the time of ejaculation. If the condom or vagina is dry, a water-soluble lubricant such as K-Y jelly or Astroglide should be used to prevent irritation and possible condom breakage.

Couples should be careful when removing the condom after intercourse. For optimal effectiveness the man should withdraw his penis from the woman's vagina while it is still erect and hold the condom rim to prevent spillage. If after ejaculation the penis becomes flaccid while still in the vagina, the man should hold onto the edge of the condom while withdrawing to avoid spilling semen and to prevent the condom from slipping off.

The effectiveness of male condoms is determined by their use. The condom is small, disposable, and inexpensive; it has no side effects, requires no medical examination, and offers visual evidence of effectiveness. Most condoms are made of latex, although polyurethane and silicone rubber condoms are available for individuals allergic to latex. All condoms, except natural "skin" condoms, made from lamb's intestines, offer protection against both pregnancy and sexually transmitted infections (STIs). Breakage, displacement, perineal or vaginal irritation, and dulled sensation are possible disadvantages. Condoms deteriorate in hot conditions, making them susceptible to breaking. Thus, men should avoid placing them in their car glove box or in their wallets in a rear pant's pocket.

The male condom is becoming increasingly popular because of the protection it offers from infections. For women, an STI increases the risk of pelvic inflammatory disease (PID) and resultant infertility. Many women are beginning to insist that sexual partners use condoms, and many women carry condoms with them.

The *female condom* (Figure 5–3 ●) is a thin sheath with a flexible ring at each end. The inner ring, at the closed end of the

A

B

● **Figure 5–2** The male condom. *A,* Unrolled condom with reservoir tip. *B,* Correct use of a condom.

condom, serves as the means of insertion and fits over the cervix like a diaphragm. The second ring remains outside the vagina and covers a portion of the woman's perineum. It also covers the base of the man's penis during intercourse. Available over the counter and designed for one-time use, the condom may be inserted up to 8 hours before intercourse. The inner sheath is prelubricated but does not contain spermicide and is not designed to be used with a male condom. Because it also covers a

● **Figure 5–3** Application of the female condom. *A,* The condom. To insert: *B,* Remove condom and applicator from wrapper by pulling up on the ring. *C,* Insert condom slowly by gently pushing the applicator toward the small of the back. *D,* When properly inserted, the outer ring should rest on the folds of skin around the vaginal opening, and the inner ring (closed end) should fit loosely against the cervix.

portion of the vulva, it probably provides better protection than other methods against some pathogens. Two female condoms are available: the Reality Female condom, made of polyurethane (see Figure 5–3), and the FC2, which is made of synthetic latex. The FC2 is less expensive and quieter than its predecessor.

Diaphragm and Cervical Cap
The **diaphragm** (Figure 5–4 ●) is used with spermicidal cream or jelly and offers a good level of protection from conception. The woman must be fitted with a diaphragm and instructed in its use by trained personnel. The diaphragm should be rechecked for correct size after each childbirth and whenever a woman has gained or lost 10 or more pounds.

The diaphragm must be inserted before intercourse, with approximately 1 teaspoon (or 1.5 inches from the tube) of spermicidal jelly placed around its rim and in the cup. This chemical barrier supplements the mechanical barrier of the diaphragm. The diaphragm is inserted through the vagina and covers the cervix. The last step in insertion is to push the edge of the diaphragm under the symphysis pubis, which may result in a "popping" sensation. When fitted properly and correctly in place, the diaphragm should not cause discomfort to the woman or her partner. Correct placement of the diaphragm can be checked by touching the cervix with a fingertip through the cup. The cervix feels like a small, firm, rounded structure and has a consistency similar to that of the tip of the nose. The center of the diaphragm

A

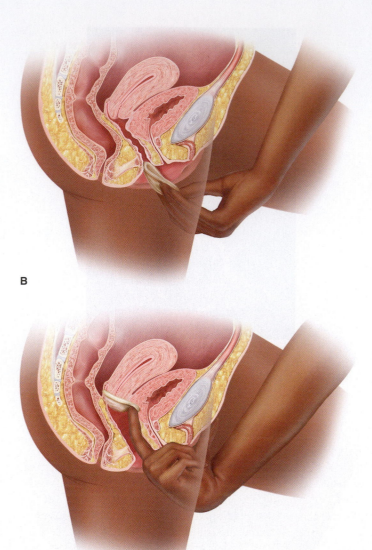

B

C

● **Figure 5–4** Inserting the diaphragm. *A,* Apply jelly to the rim and center of the diaphragm. *B,* Insert the diaphragm. *C,* Push the rim of the diaphragm under the symphysis pubis. Then check placement of the diaphragm. Cervix should be felt through the diaphragm.

should be over the cervix. If more than 6 hours elapse between insertion of the diaphragm and intercourse, additional spermicidal cream or jelly should be used. It is necessary to leave the diaphragm in place for at least 6 hours after coitus. The diaphragm should then be removed, cleaned with mild soap and water, and allowed to air dry before it is stored in its case. If intercourse is desired again within the 6 hours, another type of contraception must be used or additional spermicidal jelly placed in the vagina with an applicator, taking care not to disturb the placement of the diaphragm. Periodically the diaphragm should be held up to the light and inspected for tears or holes.

Some couples feel that the use of a diaphragm interferes with the spontaneity of intercourse. The nurse can suggest that the partner insert the diaphragm as part of foreplay. The woman can then easily verify the placement herself.

Diaphragms are an excellent contraceptive method for women who are lactating, who cannot or do not wish to use the pill (oral contraceptives), who are smokers over age 35, or who wish to avoid the increased risk of PID associated with intrauterine devices. A silicone diaphragm is available for women with latex allergies.

Women who object to manipulating their genitals to insert the diaphragm, check its placement, and remove it may find this method unsatisfactory. It is not recommended for women with a history of urinary tract infection, because pressure from the diaphragm on the urethra may interfere with complete bladder emptying and lead to recurrent urinary tract infections.

SAFETY ALERT!
Women with a history of toxic shock syndrome should not use diaphragms or any of the barrier methods because they are left in place for prolonged periods. For the same reason, the diaphragm should not be used during a menstrual period or if a woman has abnormal vaginal discharge.

The Prentiff Cavity Rim **cervical cap** or *FemCap* is a latex, cup-shaped device, used with spermicidal cream or jelly, that fits snugly over the cervix and is held in place by suction. Advantages, disadvantages, and contraindications are similar to those associated with the diaphragm. The cap is no longer available in the United States.

Lea's shield is a reusable, silicone, one-size-fits-all barrier method that completely covers the cervix and is used with spermicide. It is similar to the cervical cap but contains a centrally located valve that permits the passage of cervical secretions and air. It is held in place by the vaginal walls. It is available by prescription in the United States.

Vaginal Sponge

The *Today vaginal sponge,* available without a prescription, is a pillow-shaped, soft, absorbent synthetic sponge containing spermicide. It is made with a concave or cupped area on one side that fits over the cervix and has a loop for easy removal. The sponge is moistened thoroughly with water before insertion to activate the spermicide and then inserted into the vagina with the cupped side against the cervix (Figure 5–5 ●). It should be left in place for 6 hours following intercourse and may be worn for up to 24 hours, then removed and discarded.

The sponge has the following advantages: professional fitting is not required, it may be used for multiple acts of coitus for up to 24 hours, one size fits all, and it acts as both a barrier and a spermicide. Problems associated with the sponge include difficulty removing it and irritation or allergic reactions. Some women report a problem because the sponge absorbs vaginal secretions, contributing to vaginal dryness. The sponge is more effective for women who have never given birth. Overall, it is slightly less effective than a diaphragm.

Intrauterine Devices

The **intrauterine device (IUD)** is a safe, effective, long-acting, reversible contraceptive that is designed to be inserted into the uterus by a qualified healthcare provider and left in place for an extended period, providing continuous contraceptive protection. Two IUDs are currently available in the United States. The Copper T380A (ParaGard) is nonhormonal, highly effective, and can be left in place for up to 10 years. The levonorgestrel-releasing intrauterine system (LNG-IUS) (Mirena) is a small, T-shaped frame with a reservoir that releases levonorgestrel gradually (Figure 5–6 ●). It is comparable in effectiveness to the Copper T, and may be left in place for up to 5 years. After 3 months of use of the LNG-IUS, bleeding and length of menstrual cycles are reduced, and some women experience amenorrhea, which they welcome once they are advised that the absence of menses is safe and not an indication of pregnancy.

The exact mechanism of the IUD is not clearly understood. Traditionally the IUD was believed to act by preventing the implantation of a fertilized ovum. Thus the IUD was considered an abortifacient (abortion-causing) method. This belief is not accurate. Both IUDs truly are contraceptive. The copper IUD is known to have local inflammatory effects on the endometrium and to impair sperm from functioning properly. The Mirena IUD may alter the endometrium. It also produces thick cervical mucus that is "hostile" or unfriendly to sperm and may inhibit sperm survival.

Advantages of the IUD include high rate of effectiveness, continuous contraceptive protection, no coitus-related activity, and relative inexpensiveness over time. Possible adverse reactions to the IUD include discomfort to the wearer, increased bleeding during menses, PID, perforation of the uterus, intermenstrual bleeding, dysmenorrhea, and expulsion of the device.

There are few women for whom either IUD is contraindicated. The American College of Obstetricians and Gynecologists (ACOG) (2012a) states that the IUD is a safe, reliable choice for adolescents. It is a very effective contraceptive (pregnancy rate of less than 1% per year) and has the highest rates of satisfaction and continuation of all reversible contraceptives. A current pregnancy or current STI or pelvic infection would be contraindications. If a woman has multiple sexual partners, she should be cautioned to use a condom in addition to her IUD. Because the Mirena causes thick cervical mucus, it may have a protective effect against PID (Hatcher et al., 2011).

The IUD is inserted into the uterus with its string or tail protruding through the cervix into the vagina. It may be inserted at any time during a woman's cycle providing she is not pregnant or

Animation | Oral Contraception

● **Figure 5–5** Application of the contraceptive sponge. The contraceptive sponge is moistened well with water and inserted into the vagina with the concave portion positioned over the cervix.

● **Figure 5–6** The Mirena intrauterine system. This contraceptive device releases levonorgestrel gradually and may be left in place for up to 5 years.
Source: © BOUCHARLAT/age fotostock.

during the 4- to 6-week postpartum check. After insertion, the clinician instructs the woman to check for the presence of the string once a week for the first month and then after each menses. She is told that she may have some cramping or bleeding intermittently for 2 to 6 weeks and that her first few menses may be irregular. Follow-up examination is suggested 4 to 8 weeks after insertion.

Women with IUDs should contact their healthcare providers if they are exposed to an STI or if they develop the following warning signs: late period, abnormal spotting or bleeding, pain with intercourse, abdominal pain, abnormal discharge, signs of infection (fever, chills, and malaise), or missing string. If the woman becomes pregnant with an IUD in place, the device should be removed as soon as possible to prevent infection.

Hormonal Contraception

Hormonal contraceptives are available in a variety of forms. They may be progestin-only hormones, most often using a synthetic form of progesterone called progestin, or a combination of estrogen and a progestin.

Combined Estrogen-Progestin Approaches

Combined hormonal approaches work by inhibiting the release of an ovum, by creating an atrophic endometrium, and by maintaining thick cervical mucus that slows sperm transport and inhibits the process that allows sperm to penetrate the ovum.

Combined Oral Contraceptives. Combined oral contraceptives (COCs), also called *birth control pills,* are typically a combination of the hormones estrogen and progesterone. COCs are safe, highly effective, and rapidly reversible. Many COCs are available. The pill is taken daily for 21 days, typically beginning on the Sunday after the first day of the menstrual cycle, although the woman can also start on day 1 of her menstrual cycle. In most cases menses occurs 1 to 4 days after the last pill is taken. Seven days after taking her last pill, the woman restarts the pill. Thus the woman always begins the pill on the same day. Some companies offer a 28-day pack with seven "blank" pills so that the woman never stops taking a pill. The pill should be taken at approximately the same time each day—usually upon arising or before retiring in the evening.

Research suggests that traditional 21/7 approaches may need to be modified. With today's low-dose COCs, the 7 hormone-free days may result in failure to completely suppress ovarian function, resulting in the development of an ovarian follicle and possible ovulation. Consequently, many of the newer COCs with very low estrogen levels (20 mcg) now provide 24/4 formulations (Hatcher et al., 2011). In addition, there is growing interest in extended oral contraceptives. Seasonale and Seasonique are the first FDA-approved extended-cycle COCs. They both are 91-day regimens in which a woman takes an active pill daily for 84 consecutive days followed by 7 days of inactive tablets during which the woman has a period. Thus a woman has only four periods a year. Extended use reduces the side effects of COCs such as bloating, headache, breast tenderness, and cramping.

Although they are highly effective when taken correctly, COCs may produce a variety of side effects, which may be either progesterone or estrogen related (Table 5–1). The use of low-dose (35 mcg or less estrogen) preparations has reduced many

Table 5–1	Side Effects Associated with Oral Contraceptives
Estrogen Effects	**Progestin Effects**
Alterations in lipid metabolism	Acne, oily skin
Breast tenderness, engorgement; increased breast size	Breast tenderness; increased breast size
Cerebrovascular accident	Decreased libido
Changes in carbohydrate metabolism	Decreased high-density lipoprotein (HDL) cholesterol levels
Chloasma (Melasma)	Depression
Fluid retention; cyclic weight gain	Fatigue
Headache	Hirsutism
Hepatic adenomas	Increased appetite; weight gain
Hypertension	Increased low-density lipoprotein (LDL) cholesterol levels
Leukorrhea, cervical erosion, ectopia	Oligomenorrhea, amenorrhea
Nausea	Pruritus
Nervousness, irritability	Sebaceous cysts
Telangiectasia	
Thromboembolic complications—thrombophlebitis, pulmonary embolism	

of the side effects. The newer 20-mcg pills have even fewer side effects, but they may result in less contraceptive effectiveness.

Contraindications to the use of COCs include pregnancy, previous history of thrombophlebitis or thromboembolic disease, acute or chronic liver disease of cholestatic type with abnormal function, presence of estrogen-dependent carcinomas, undiagnosed uterine bleeding, heavy smoking, gallbladder disease, hypertension, diabetes, and hyperlipidemia. In addition, women with the following relative contraindications who use COCs need to be monitored frequently: migraine headaches, epilepsy, depression, oligomenorrhea, and amenorrhea. Women who choose this method of contraception should be fully advised of its potential side effects.

COCs also have some important noncontraceptive benefits. Many women experience relief of uncomfortable menstrual symptoms. Cramps are lessened, flow is decreased, and cycle regularity is increased. Mittelschmerz is eliminated. More important, there is a reduction in the incidence of ovarian cancer, endometrial cancer, colorectal cancer, menstrual migraines, and iron deficiency anemia. In addition, hormonal contraceptives can be effective in improving bone mineral density and in treating acne or hirsutism, pelvic pain due to endometriosis, and bleeding due to leiomyomas (ACOG, 2010). In addition, COCs are considered a good solution to the physiologic problems some women experience during the perimenopause (such as hot flashes). For nonsmoking women over age 40 years, a COC that contains less than 30 mcg of ethinyl estradiol is recommended. COCs are not recommended for women over age 50 (Gardner, 2011).

Because of the increased risk of myocardial infarction (heart attack), women over age 35 who smoke should not take COCs.

Other Combined Hormonal Methods. Hormones can now be administered transdermally using a *contraceptive skin patch* called Ortho Evra. The patch is roughly the size of a silver dollar, but square. The woman applies it weekly for 3 weeks to one of four sites: her abdomen, buttocks, upper outer arm, or trunk (excluding the breasts). During the fourth week, no patch is worn and menses occurs. The patch is highly effective in women who weigh less than 198 lb. The patch is as safe and reliable as a COC and has a better rate of compliance. Product labeling specifies that there is a greater risk of venous thromboembolism (VTE) for women using the patch versus those taking COCs. The U.S. Food and Drug Administration (FDA) (2009a) considers the patch a safe method of contraception for women not at risk of a VTE.

NuvaRing vaginal contraceptive ring (manufactured by Merck), another form of low-dose, sustained-release hormonal contraceptive, is a flexible soft ring that the woman inserts into her vagina (Figure 5–7 ●). The ring is left in place for 3 weeks and then removed for 1 week to allow for withdrawal bleeding. One size fits virtually all women. The ring is highly effective and has minimal side effects. The ring can be worn during intercourse and is comfortable for both the woman and her partner.

Progestin Contraceptives

The progestin-only pill, also called the *minipill,* is another oral contraceptive. It is used primarily by nursing mothers, because it does not interfere with breast milk production. It is also used by women who have a contraindication to the estrogen component of the combination preparation, such as history of thrombophlebitis or hypertension, but are strongly motivated to use this form of contraception. The major problems with progesterone-only pills are amenorrhea or irregular bleeding patterns.

Implanon, a long-acting, progestin-only, reversible contraceptive, is a single-capsule implant inserted subdermally in the woman's upper arm. It is impregnated with etonogestrel, a progestin, and is effective for 3 years. It acts by preventing ovulation. Implanon also stimulates the production of thick cervical mucus, which inhibits sperm penetration. Implanon provides effective continuous contraception removed from the act of coitus. Possible side effects include spotting, irregular bleeding or amenorrhea, an increased incidence of ovarian cysts, weight gain, headaches, fluid retention, acne, hair loss, mood changes, and depression. A minor surgical procedure is required to insert and remove the implant.

Depot-medroxyprogesterone acetate (DMPA) (**Depo-Provera**), another long-acting progestin administered by injection, provides highly effective contraception for 3 months after administration, with subsequent injections every 10 to 14 weeks. It is available in two dosings: DMPA-IM 150 mg for intramuscular use or DMPA-SC 104 mg for subcutaneous use.

DMPA, which acts primarily by suppressing ovulation, is safe, convenient, private, and relatively inexpensive. It also separates birth control from the act of coitus. It can be given to nursing mothers because it contains no estrogen. Side effects include menstrual irregularities, headache, weight gain, breast tenderness, and depression. Return of fertility may be delayed for an average of 9 months.

DMPA is associated with bone demineralization, especially during the first 2 years of use. The rate of calcium loss slows after this time, and bone loss is reversible after discontinuation of DMPA. All women should exercise daily and take 1200 mg of calcium with vitamin D.

Postcoital Emergency Contraception

Postcoital **emergency contraception (EC)** is indicated when a woman is worried about pregnancy because of unprotected intercourse or possible contraceptive failure (e.g., broken condom, slipped diaphragm, missed COCs, or too long a time between DMPA injections).

Plan B, a progestin-only approach (levonorgestrel), is the most commonly used EC. Originally it was given in two 0.75-mg doses—the first as soon after intercourse as possible (but not longer than 72 hours) and a second dose 12 hours later. Studies suggest that a single 1.5-mg dose (Plan B One-Step™) may be as effective. Next Choice™ is a two-pill generic form of Plan B. Both are available over the counter, without prescription, to any woman 15 years or older. A new FDA-approved EC, ulipristal acetate (ella™), is available by prescription only. Ella is a selective progesterone receptor modulator, which can be taken up to 5 days after unprotected intercourse, thus providing two additional days for use (Fine, 2011).

Placement of the copper IUD within 5 days after unprotected intercourse may reduce pregnancy risk by as much as 99% (Hatcher et al., 2011).

● **Figure 5–7** The NuvaRing vaginal contraceptive ring.
Source: © N. Aubrier/age fotostock/Getty Images.

Operative Sterilization

Operative **sterilization** refers to surgical procedures that permanently prevent pregnancy. Before sterilization is performed on either partner, the physician provides a thorough explanation of the procedure to both. Each needs to understand that sterilization is not a decision to be taken lightly or entered into when psychologic stresses, such as separation or divorce, exist. Even though both male and female procedures are theoretically reversible, the permanency of the procedure should be stressed and understood.

Male sterilization is achieved through a relatively minor procedure called a **vasectomy**. This procedure involves surgically severing the vas deferens in both sides of the scrotum. Following vasectomy it takes about 4 to 6 weeks and 6 to 36 ejaculations to clear the remaining sperm from the vas deferens. During that period the couple is advised to use another method of birth control and to bring in two or three semen samples for a sperm count. The man is rechecked at 6 and 12 months to ensure that fertility has not been restored by recanalization. Side effects of a vasectomy include pain, infection, hematoma, sperm granulomas, and spontaneous reanastomosis (reconnecting).

Female sterilization is most frequently accomplished by **tubal ligation**. The tubes are located through a small subumbilical incision or by minilaparotomy techniques and are clipped, ligated, electrocoagulated, banded, or plugged. Tubal ligation may be done at any time. However, the postpartum period is an ideal time to perform a tubal ligation because the tubes are somewhat enlarged and easily located.

Complications of female sterilization procedures include coagulation burns on the bowel, bowel perforation, pain, infection, hemorrhage, and adverse anesthesia effects. Reversal of a tubal ligation depends on the type of procedure performed.

The *Essure* method of permanent sterilization requires no surgical incision and yields no scar. Under hysteroscopy, a stainless steel microinsert is placed into the proximal section of each fallopian tube. Within 3 months, these microinserts create a benign tissue response that occludes the fallopian tubes. Three months after placement, tubal occlusion is confirmed by hysterosalpingogram.

Male Contraception

The vasectomy and the condom, discussed previously, are currently the only forms of male contraception available in the United States. Hormonal contraception for men has yet to be developed, although studies are under way.

Nursing Management

In most cases the nurse who provides information and guidance about contraceptive methods works with the female partner, because most contraceptive methods are female oriented. Because men can purchase condoms without seeing a healthcare provider, counseling and interaction with a nurse are required only with vasectomy. As a nurse, you can play an important role in helping a woman choose a method of contraception acceptable to her and to her partner.

In addition to completing a history and assessing for any contraindications to specific methods, spend time with a woman

Table 5–2	Factors to Consider When Choosing a Method of Contraception
Effectiveness of method in preventing pregnancy	Lifestyle:
Safety of the method:	How frequently does patient have intercourse?
Are there inherent risks?	Does she have multiple partners?
Does it offer protection against STIs or other conditions?	Does she have ready access to medical care in the event of complications?
Patient's age and future childbearing plans	Is cost a factor?
Any contraindications in patient's health history	Partner's support and willingness to cooperate
Religious or moral factors influencing choice	Personal motivation to use method
Personal preferences, biases	

learning about her lifestyle, personal attitudes about particular contraceptive methods, religious beliefs, personal biases, and plans for future childbearing before helping the woman select a particular contraceptive method. Once the method is chosen, help the woman learn to use it effectively. Table 5–2 summarizes factors to consider when choosing an appropriate method of contraception.

Also review any possible side effects and warning signs related to the method chosen and counsel the woman about what action to take if she suspects she is pregnant. In many cases the nurse is involved in telephone counseling of women who call with questions and concerns about contraception. Thus, it is vital to be knowledgeable about this topic and have resources available to find answers to less common questions.

Clinical Reasoning Choosing a Method of Contraception

Monique Hermann, age 37, was divorced 3 years ago. Her only son, now 19, is away at college. Recently, with some trepidation, Monique began dating, and she is now enjoying an active social life. She is being seen today for advice about contraception, which had not been an issue during her marriage because her husband had had a vasectomy. She reports that she is a little nervous about becoming sexually active because until this point her husband had been her only sexual partner. She is very attracted to two different men but does not prefer one over the other at this point. She states that she wants a reliable method that would permit her to have intercourse at any time without having to take action beforehand because she thinks that would be embarrassing for her. Similarly she is not interested in the patch, which is visible. She is not willing to consider a tubal ligation. She is a nonsmoker who drinks occasionally. She has no known contraindications to any available methods. Which methods of contraception might be appropriate for Monique?

See www.nursing.pearsonhighered.com for possible responses.

Weblink   Women's Health Websites

Teaching Highlights   Using a Method of Contraception

- Discuss factors a woman should consider when choosing a method of contraception (see Table 5–2). Note that different methods may be appropriate at different times in a woman's life.
- Review the woman's reasons for choosing a particular method and confirm the absence of any contraindications to specific methods.
- Give a step-by-step description of the correct procedure for using the method chosen. Provide opportunities for questions.
- If a technique is to be learned, such as charting BBT or inserting a diaphragm, demonstrate and then have the woman do a return demonstration as appropriate. (*Note:* If certain aspects are beyond your level of expertise, such as fitting a diaphragm, review the content about its use and confirm that the woman understands what she is to do.)
- Provide information on what the woman should do if unusual circumstances arise (for example, she misses a pill or forgets a morning temperature). These can be presented in a written handout as well.
- Stress warning signs that may require immediate action by the woman and explain why these signs indicate a risk. (These should also be covered in the handout.)
- Arrange to talk with the woman again soon, either by phone or at a return visit, to see if she has any questions or has encountered any problems.

Teaching Highlights: Using a Method of Contraception provides guidelines for helping women use a method of contraception effectively.

Clinical Interruption of Pregnancy

Although abortion was legalized in the United States in 1973, controversy over moral and legal issues continues. Many people are opposed to abortion for religious, ethical, or personal reasons. Others feel that access to a safe, legal abortion is every woman's right. A number of physical and psychosocial factors influence a woman's decision to seek an abortion. Some situations may involve lack of knowledge about contraceptive options, contraceptive failure, rape, or incest. Medical abortion provides an effective alternative to surgical abortion for many women with an unintended pregnancy. Mifepristone (Mifeprex), originally called RU-486, may be used to induce a medical abortion during the first 7 weeks of pregnancy (up to 49 days following conception). Mifepristone blocks the action of progesterone, thereby altering the endometrium. After the length of the woman's gestation is confirmed, she takes a dose of mifepristone. Between 1 and 3 days later (depending on gestation), she returns to her caregiver and takes a dose of the prostaglandin misoprostol, which induces contractions that expel the embryo/fetus. About 14 days after taking the misoprostol, the woman is seen a third time to confirm that the abortion was successful. Some clinicians support the use of a slightly modified dosage regimen through 63 days' gestation (ACOG, 2009).

Surgical abortion in the first trimester is technically easier and safer than abortion in the second trimester. It may be performed by dilation and curettage (D&C), minisuction, or vacuum curettage. Second-trimester abortion may be done using dilation and evacuation (D&E), hypertonic saline, systemic prostaglandins, and intrauterine prostaglandins.

Prior to an elective abortion, women often experience clinically significant anxiety and/or depression. Research suggests that following first-trimester elective abortion, whether medical or surgical, women tend to experience significant improvements in psychologic outcomes. Depression and anxiety are reduced and quality of life improves significantly (Crandell, 2012).

Nursing Management

The nurse needs to recognize that the decision to have an abortion is a major one with psychologic implications for the woman and her partner, if he is involved. In caring for a woman who decides to have an abortion, it is important to do the following:

- Provide information about the methods of abortion and associated risks.
- Counsel the woman about available alternatives to abortion and their implications.
- Encourage the woman to talk about feelings related to her decision to end her pregnancy.
- Provide support before, during, and after the procedure.
- Monitor vital signs, intake, and output.
- Provide for physical comfort and privacy throughout the procedure.
- Teach about self-care, the importance of the postabortion checkup, and contraception review.

HEALTH PROMOTION FOR WOMEN

Healthcare providers and consumers alike are becoming increasingly aware of the importance of activities that promote health and prevent illness, including lifestyle choices. In addition, the value of regular screenings to detect any health problems early cannot be overemphasized. Health screening recommendations vary by age. General screening and immunization guidelines for women can be found on this text's website.

This section focuses on some of the most commonly used screening procedures: breast self-examination and breast examination by a trained healthcare provider, mammography, Pap smear, and pelvic examination.

Breast Examination

Like the uterus, the breast undergoes regular cyclic changes in response to hormonal stimulation. Each month, in rhythm with the cycle of ovulation, the breasts become engorged with fluid in anticipation of pregnancy, and the woman may experience sensations of tenderness, lumpiness, or pain. If conception does not occur, the accumulated fluid drains away via the lymphatic network. *Mastodynia* or *mastalgia* (premenstrual swelling and tenderness of the breasts) is common. It usually lasts for 3 to 4 days before the onset of menses, but the symptoms may persist throughout the month.

After menopause, adipose breast tissue atrophies and is replaced by connective tissue. Elasticity is lost, and the breasts may droop and become pendulous. The recurring breast engorgement associated with ovulation ceases. If estrogen replacement therapy is used to counteract other symptoms of menopause, breast engorgement may resume.

Monthly **breast self-examination (BSE)** is a good method for detecting breast masses early. Women at high risk for breast cancer are especially encouraged to be attentive to the importance of early detection through routine BSE.

The value of BSE, however, has been under continual scrutiny. The U.S. Preventive Services Task Force made a recommendation in November 2009 against teaching women breast self-examination based on studies they reviewed that suggested that BSE did not reduce breast cancer mortality but resulted in additional imaging procedures and biopsies. The American College of Obstetricians and Gynecologists stresses *breast self-awareness,* the need for a woman to be aware of how her breasts normally look and feel. ACOG (2012b) identifies breast self-examination as one way for a woman to develop self-awareness. The American Cancer Society (ACS) (2011a) recommends BSE be presented to the patient as an option. Women who choose to do BSE should have their technique reviewed during the annual examination.

Therefore, in light of the conflicting recommendations, in the course of a routine physical examination, or during an initial visit to the caregiver, women are generally taught the BSE technique. The effectiveness of BSE is determined by the woman's ability to perform the procedure correctly. See *Teaching Highlights: Breast Self-Examination.*

Clinical breast examination (CBE) by a trained healthcare provider, such as a physician, nurse practitioner, or nurse-midwife, is an essential element of a routine gynecologic examination and is generally performed annually. Experience in differentiating among benign, suspicious, and worrisome breast changes lets the caregiver reassure the woman if the findings are normal or move forward with additional diagnostic procedures or referral if the findings are suspicious or worrisome.

Mammography

A **mammogram** is a soft-tissue x-ray of the breast without the injection of a contrast medium. It can detect lesions in the breast before they can be felt and has gained wide acceptance as a screening tool. Currently the American Cancer Society (2011b) recommends that all women age 40 and over have an annual mammogram and CBE. ACOG (2012b) concurs with ACS recommendations.

If a woman has a history of breast cancer in a close relative (i.e., mother, sister) and the cancer was diagnosed before the relative was age 40, many clinicians advocate that the patient begin mammograms 10 years before the age of her close relative's diagnosis. However, the ACS now recommends annual mammogram and MRI beginning at age 30 in women who are at a high risk for breast cancer due to gene mutations, and/or a strong family history of breast cancer, or who had radiation to the chest between the ages of 10 and 30 years because they often develop breast cancer at a younger age (ACS, 2011b).

Pap Smear and Pelvic Examination

The Papanicolaou test (*Pap smear*) is a form of cervical cytology testing used to detect cellular abnormalities by examining a sample containing cells from the cervix and the endocervical canal. Traditionally the test has been done by preparing a Pap smear slide. A newer test, the liquid-based medium Pap smear, is now available. In this test, no slide is prepared. Instead the cervical cells, gathered in the same way as for the Pap smear, are transferred directly to a vial of preservative fluid, thereby preserving the entire specimen. The specimen is sent to a laboratory where a special processor prepares the slide. This test has become the method of choice for cervical cancer screening. Liquid-based Pap smear preparations allow for removal of debris from the sample, such as blood and mucus, thereby increasing accuracy. Additionally, these preparations allow for human papillomavirus (HPV) screening and for some STI infection screening. Pap smear findings are reported using the Bethesda system (see Table 6–1 🥚 on page 123).

In 2012 new guidelines for cervical cancer screening were issued by the U.S. Preventive Services Task Force, the American Cancer Society, and other groups. These guidelines are found in Table 5–3. It is important to recognize that these recommendations are population-based guidelines reflecting statistical analysis. As such, they are not appropriate for all women. Each woman needs to consult her caregiver about the best approach to screening based on her risk factors, history, preexisting conditions, and signs and symptoms.

Table 5–3	Screening for Cervical Cancer
Population	**Test and Frequency**
Women under age 21	No screening
Women ages 21 to 29	Screening with cytology alone every 3 years (*Note:* Co-testing for HPV is not recommended for this group because of the high prevalence of HPV.)
Women ages 30 to 65	Preferred approach: screen with cytology and HPV testing every 5 years Acceptable approach: test with cytology alone every 3 years
Women over age 65 who have had adequate prior screening and are not at high risk	Do not screen
Women who have undergone hysterectomy and have no history of high-grade precancer or cervical cancer	Do not screen

Source: U.S. Preventive Services Task Force. (2012). *Screening for cervical cancer.* Retrieved from http://www.uspreventiveservicestaskforce.org/uspstf11/cervcancer/cervcancerrs.htm

Teaching Highlights   Breast Self-Examination

Describe and demonstrate the correct procedure for BSE.

Inspection

The woman should inspect her breasts by standing or sitting in front of a mirror. She should inspect them in three positions: both arms relaxed at her sides, both arms raised straight over her head, and both hands placed on her hips while she leans forward. Instruct her to note the following:

- *Size and symmetry of the breasts, and their shape, contours, and direction.* Have her check for redness or inflammation, rashes, ulceration, or nipple discharge. A blue hue with a marked venous pattern that is focal or unilateral may indicate an area of increased blood supply due to tumor. Symmetric venous patterns are normal.
- *Thickening or edema.* Skin edema is seen as thickened skin with enlarged pores ("orange peel"). It may indicate blocked lymph drainage due to tumor.
- *Surface of the skin.* Skin dimpling, puckering, or retraction when the hands are pressed together in front of the chest or against the hips suggests malignancy.

- *The nipples.* Note any deviation, flattening, broadening, or recent inversion.

Palpation

The woman should be instructed to palpate her breasts as follows:

- Lie down. Put one hand behind your head. With the other hand, fingers flattened, gently feel your breast. Press lightly (Figure 5–8A ●).
- Still lying down, check each breast as shown in Figure 5–8B ●. Follow the arrows shown in the image, moving in an up and down pattern, feeling gently for a lump or thickening. Remember to feel all parts of each breast, including the "tail" of tissue near the armpit. Repeat the process on the second breast.
- Now repeat the same process on each breast while sitting up, with your hand still behind your head (Figure 5–8C ●).
- Squeeze the nipple between your thumb and forefinger. Look for any discharge—clear, bloody, or milky.

Determine whether the patient has any questions about her findings during this examination. If she has questions, palpate the area and attempt to identify whether it is normal.

With one hand behind your head, flatten your fingers and press lightly on your breast, feeling gently for a lump or thickening.

A

Repeat the same procedure sitting up with your hand still behind your head.

C

B

Check each breast in an up-and-down pattern, feeling all parts of the breast.

● **Figure 5–8** Procedure for breast self-examination.

Clinical Tip

Whenever you teach about pelvic examination and cervical cytology testing, be sure the woman understands that she should not douche for at least 24 hours beforehand. Douching can interfere with the accuracy of the Pap smear. Occasionally a caregiver will specifically request that a woman use a douche before a Pap smear; douching should be done only in this circumstance.

The *pelvic examination* lets the healthcare provider assess a woman's vagina, uterus, ovaries, and lower abdominal area. It is often performed after the Pap smear but may also be performed without a Pap for diagnostic purposes. Women sometimes perceive the pelvic examination as uncomfortable and embarrassing and may delay having yearly gynecologic examinations. This avoidance may pose a threat to life and health.

To make the pelvic examination less threatening and thus improve health-seeking behavior, caregivers can offer the woman a mirror to watch the procedure, point out anatomic parts to her, and position and drape her to allow eye-to-eye contact with the practitioner. Caregivers can encourage the woman to participate by asking questions and giving feedback.

Nurse practitioners, CNMs, and physicians all perform pelvic examinations. Nurses assist the practitioner and the woman during the examination. See *Skill 2–2: Assisting with a Pelvic Examination* in the *Clinical Skills Manual* SKILLS .

MENOPAUSE

Menopause, defined as the absence of menses for a full year, is a time of transition for a woman, marking the end of her reproductive abilities. *Climacteric,* or *change of life* (often used synonymously with menopause), refers to the psychologic and physical alterations that occur around the time of menopause. Today the median age at menopause is 50 to 53 years, and the average life span of a woman in the United States is over 80 years. Thus the average woman will live one third of her life after menopause.

A woman's psychologic adaptation to menopause and the climacteric is multifactorial. She is influenced by her own expectations and knowledge, physical well-being, family views, marital stability, and sociocultural expectations. While some women still accept the negative emotional connotations society once attached to menopause, that has changed dramatically. Today, women in this age group are generally active, engaged, and fit. They simply view menopause as a new stage of life and a time of personal growth and fulfillment.

Perimenopause is the term applied to the time before menopause when ovarian function wanes and hormonal deficiencies begin to produce symptoms. Symptoms of perimenopause may be nonexistent or bothersome. They may include PMS, hot flashes, irregular periods, insomnia, decreased libido, vaginal dryness, and mood changes. Contraception remains a concern during perimenopause. Combined oral contraceptives (the pill, patches, and vaginal rings) are popular among healthy nonsmokers because many women also benefit from the noncontraceptive effects, including regulation of menses, relief of symptoms of estrogen deficiency, and a decreased risk of endometrial and ovarian cancers.

Other contraceptive options for perimenopausal women include sterilization, IUDs, progestin-only methods, and barrier methods such as male and female condoms, diaphragm, cervical cap, and spermicides.

The physical characteristics of menopause are linked to the shift from a cyclic to a noncyclic hormonal pattern. The age at onset may be influenced by nutritional, cultural, or genetic factors. The onset of menopause occurs when estrogen levels become so low that menstruation stops.

Generally, ovulation ceases 1 to 2 years before menopause, but individual variations exist. Atrophy of the ovaries occurs gradually. Follicle-stimulating hormone (FSH) levels rise, and less estrogen is produced. Menopausal symptoms include atrophic changes in the vagina, vulva, and urethra and in the trigonal area of the bladder.

Many menopausal women experience a vasomotor disturbance commonly known as *hot flashes,* a feeling of heat arising from the chest and spreading to the neck and face. The hot flashes are often accompanied by sweating and sleep disturbances. These episodes may occur as often as 20 to 30 times a day and generally last 3 to 5 minutes. Some women also experience dizzy spells, palpitations, and weakness. Many women find their own most effective ways to deal with the hot flashes. Some report that using a fan or drinking a cool liquid helps relieve distress; others seek relief through hormone therapy. In addition, many women use complementary therapies (see later discussion).

The uterine lining (endometrium) and uterine muscle layer (myometrium) atrophy, as do the cervical glands. The uterine cavity constricts. The fallopian tubes and ovaries atrophy extensively. The vaginal mucosa becomes smooth and thin, and the rugae disappear, leading to loss of elasticity. As a result, intercourse can be painful, but this problem may be overcome by using lubricating gel. Dryness of the mucous membrane can lead to burning and itching. The vaginal pH level increases as the number of Döderlein's bacilli decreases.

Vulvar atrophy occurs late, and the pubic hair thins, turns gray or white, and may ultimately disappear. The labia shrink and lose their heightened pigmentation. Pelvic fascia and muscles atrophy, resulting in decreased pelvic support. The breasts become pendulous and decrease in size and firmness.

Sexual functioning generally declines with age although more than 75% of the middle-aged women in the Study of Women's Health Across the Nation (SWAN) cited sex as being moderately to extremely important. Contributing factors to the decline in both interest and occurrence of sexual activity are widespread. Pain during intercourse due to lack of lubrication and thinning vaginal walls is a common cause. Other factors may include a lack of partners, stress in current relationships, psychosocial factors, and a decline in general health. A positive attitude about aging and menopause as well as the overall good health of the women in the study had a highly positive effect on sexual activity and satisfaction (Avis, Brockwell, Randolph, et al., 2009).

Long-range physical changes may include **osteoporosis**, a decrease in the bony skeletal mass. This change is thought to be associated with lowered estrogen levels, lack of physical exercise, inadequate vitamin D, and a chronic low intake of calcium. Moreover, the estrogen deprivation that occurs in menopausal women may significantly increase their risk of coronary heart disease. Loss of protein from the skin and supportive tissues causes wrinkling. Postmenopausal women frequently gain weight, which may be due to excessive caloric intake or to lower caloric need with the same level of intake.

Clinical Therapy

Menopausal **hormone therapy (HT)** refers to the administration of specific hormones, usually estrogen alone (ET) or a combination estrogen-progestogen (EPT), to alleviate menopausal symptoms. ET is used for women who have had a hysterectomy, whereas EPT is used for women with an intact uterus. When estrogen is given alone, it can produce endometrial hyperplasia and increase the risk of endometrial cancer. Thus, in women who still have a uterus, estrogen is opposed by giving a progestin, often Provera, continuously or sequentially.

In 2002 the advisability of hormone replacement therapy (HRT) was called into question because of the results of the Women's Health Initiative (WHI) study, which suggested that the risks of HRT outweigh the benefits, especially for long-term use, because of the slightly increased risk of breast cancer, thromboembolic disease, and stroke (Writing Group for the Women's Health Initiative Investigations, 2002).

The North American Menopause Society (NAMS) (2012b), a nonprofit scientific organization, currently recommends that hormone therapy should be considered when there are clear indications that the potential benefits outweigh the risks and there are no contraindications to its use. Extended use of HT may be an option for women who are at high risk of osteoporotic fracture when alternative therapies are not appropriate or cause adverse effects. Proven risks of HT use include increased risk of venous thrombosis and breast cancer. The recommended duration of use is shorter for EPT (3 to 5 years) because of the increased risk of breast cancer than for ET alone.

HT can be prescribed in a number of ways, including orally; transdermally (patch); intramuscularly; topically as a gel, lotion, or vaginal cream; or through a vaginal ring. It is given in a continuous manner via daily administration of both estrogen and progestogen, or as a cyclic or sequential therapy, with estrogen use daily and a progestogen added on a set sequence. Combination estrogen-progestogen preparations are also available.

Postmenopausal women experiencing decreased libido may experience improved sexual desire, responsiveness, and frequency when testosterone is added to their HT. Options for providing testosterone in doses low enough for women are still limited. Estratest, a combined estrogen-androgen pill, is used by some women. Custom-compounded testosterone preparations are available by prescription and work is under way on low-dose testosterone patches.

Before starting HT, a woman should undergo a thorough history; a physical examination, including Pap smear; measurement of cholesterol, lipid, and liver enzyme levels; and a baseline mammogram. An initial endometrial biopsy is indicated for women with an increased risk of endometrial cancer; biopsy is also indicated if excessive, unexpected, or prolonged vaginal bleeding occurs. Women taking estrogen should be advised to stop immediately if they develop headaches, visual changes, signs of thrombophlebitis, or chest pain.

Complementary and Alternative Therapies

For women who do not wish to take HT or who have medical contraindications to it, a variety of approaches have been proposed as alternative or complementary treatment or preventive measures for the discomforts of the perimenopausal and postmenopausal years. Research suggests that mind-body practices such as yoga, t'ai chi, and meditation are helpful in reducing many of the common symptoms of menopause for some women; acupuncture may also help reduce the severity of symptoms (NCCAM, 2012). Women may also seek relief through diet and nutrition, specifically a high-fiber, low-fat diet with supplements of calcium and vitamins D, E, and B complex. *Phytoestrogens* (plant substances with estrogen properties), found in a number of plant foods, may be helpful.

Soy, an isoflavone, has had inconsistent results in studies in reducing hot flashes. There is some question that daily intake of soy may reduce slightly the levels of LDL or bad cholesterol. Ongoing studies are needed to examine the effects of soy on women's arteries and bones after menopause (NAMS, 2011). Research does suggest that isoflavones are effective in reducing symptoms of insomnia in postmenopausal women (Hachul, Brandão, D'Almeida, et al., 2011).

Natural products (botanicals) are gaining popularity for symptom relief but it is important to remind women that *natural* does not always signify safe. See *Complementary Care: Use of Botanicals for Symptom Relief.*

DHEA is a dietary supplement that is changed in the body to the hormones estrogen and testosterone. It has been suggested that DHEA might have anti-aging effects and might help in improving decreased sexual arousal, mood, cognition, and bone density, although the results of randomized controlled trials and observational studies conflict (Sood, Shuster, Smith, et al., 2011).

Weight-bearing exercises such as walking, jogging, tennis, and low-impact aerobics help increase bone mass and decrease the risk of osteoporosis. Exercise also improves cholesterol profiles and contributes to overall health. Pelvic floor, or Kegel, exercises can help maintain vaginal muscle tone and increase blood circulation to the perineal area. Vaginal lubricants and adequate foreplay can be helpful in maintaining a satisfactory sexual experience. Stress management and relaxation techniques such as biofeedback, meditation, yoga, visualization, and massage may provide a sense of well-being.

Complementary Care Use of Botanicals for Symptom Relief

The following botanicals are often mentioned for treating menopausal symptoms but results are mixed (NCCAM, 2012):

- Black cohosh has received attention for its possible effectiveness but preliminary research suggests that it is no more effective than a placebo in relieving symptoms. In rare cases it has been associated with liver inflammation.
- Red clover is sometimes used to reduce hot flashes but research has failed to demonstrate its effectiveness.
- Ginseng may help relieve mood symptoms and sleep disturbances but has not been effective in treating hot flashes.
- Kava has not been shown to relieve hot flashes but it may decrease anxiety. Like black cohosh, it has been associated with liver disease.

Prevention and Treatment of Osteoporosis

Osteoporosis is more common in women who are middle-aged or older. In fact, one out of every two women over age 50 in the United States will have an osteoporosis-related fracture in her lifetime (Gallagher & Levine, 2011). Table 5–4 identifies risk factors associated with osteoporosis.

Bone mineral density (BMD) testing is useful in identifying individuals who are at risk for osteoporosis. The National Osteoporosis Foundation (NOF) (2010) recommends BMD testing for the following:

- Women age 65 or older and men 70 years and older
- Menopausal and postmenopausal women under age 65 and men ages 50 to 69 with one or more risk factors
- Adults over age 50 who have had a fracture

Prevention of osteoporosis is a primary goal of care. Peri- and postmenopausal women are advised to have a daily calcium intake of 1200 mg (NAMS, 2012a). Most women require supplements to achieve this level. Vitamin D supplements (800 to 1000 International Units per day) may also be indicated for those at risk of deficiency (Gallagher & Levine, 2011). Women are also advised to participate regularly in exercise, to consume only modest quantities of alcohol and caffeine, and to stop smoking. Alcohol and smoking have a negative effect on the rate of bone resorption. Women's height should be measured at each visit, because a loss of height is often an early sign that vertebrae are being compressed because of reduced bone mass. The effectiveness of estrogen in preventing osteoporosis is well documented. However, because of the increased risks associated with long-term use of hormone replacement therapy, other pharmacologic agents are being used more frequently to prevent and treat osteoporosis. These include the following:

- *Bisphosphonates* are calcium regulators that act by inhibiting bone resorption and increasing bone mass. Alendronate (Fosamax) and risedronate (Actonel) are commonly prescribed. Zoledronic acid (Zometa) is administered IV once a year and seems to achieve the same results in treating osteoporosis as other bisphosphonates taken daily or weekly without the troublesome gastrointestinal side effects.
- *Selective estrogen receptor modulators (SERMs)* such as raloxifene (Evista) preserve the beneficial effects of estrogen, including its protection against osteoporosis, but do not stimulate uterine or breast tissue.
- Salmon *calcitonin* is a calcium regulator that may inhibit bone loss. Administered as a nasal spray, its value is less clear than that of the other medications listed.
- *Parathyroid hormone*, taken daily as a subcutaneous injection, activates bone formation, which results in substantial increases in bone density.

Women who are taking medication for osteoporosis should have BMD testing 2 years after beginning therapy and every 2 years thereafter (NOF, 2010).

Nursing Management.   Most menopausal women deal well with this developmental phase of life, although some women may need counseling to adjust successfully. Nurses and other health professionals can help menopausal women achieve high-level functioning at this time in life. Of major importance is the nurse's ability to understand and provide support for the woman's views and feelings. Use an empathetic approach in counseling, health teaching, and when providing physical care.

Explore the question of the woman's comfort during sexual intercourse. In counseling, it may be appropriate to say, "After menopause many women notice that their vagina seems drier and intercourse can be uncomfortable. Have you noticed any changes?" This gives the woman information and may open discussion. Then go on to explain that dryness and shrinking of the vagina can be addressed by use of a water-soluble jelly. Use of estrogen, orally or in vaginal creams, may also be indicated. Increased frequency of intercourse will maintain some elasticity in the vagina. When assessing the menopausal woman, address the question of sexual activity openly but tactfully, because the woman may have been socialized to be reticent about discussing sex.

The crucial need of women in the menopausal period of life is for adequate information about the changes taking place in their bodies and their lives. Supplying that information provides both a challenge and an opportunity for nurses.

VIOLENCE AGAINST WOMEN

Violence against women is a major health concern in society today. Violence affects women of all ages, races, ethnic backgrounds, socioeconomic levels, educational levels, and walks of life. Two of the most common forms of violence are domestic violence and rape. Often people not only accept these forms of violence but also shift the blame for the violence to the women themselves by asking questions such as "How did she make him so mad?" "Why does she stay?" "What was she doing out so late?" and "Why did she dress that way?" Violence against women is also a major health concern. In addition to causing injuries, associated physical and mental health outcomes, and fatalities, violence costs the healthcare system millions of dollars annually. In response to this epidemic, healthcare providers are becoming more knowledgeable

Table 5–4	Risk Factors for Osteoporosis

- Middle-age and elderly women
- European American or Asian ethnic origin
- Small-boned and thin body type
- Low body weight (less than 127 pounds)
- Family history of osteoporosis
- Lack of regular weight-bearing exercise
- Nulliparity
- Early onset of menopause
- Consistently low intake of calcium
- Cigarette smoking
- Moderate to heavy alcohol intake
- Use of certain medications such as anticonvulsants, corticosteroids, or lithium

about actions they should take to identify women at risk, implement preventive measures, and provide effective care.

Domestic Violence

Domestic violence is defined as a pattern of coercive behavior and methods used to exert power and control by one individual over another in an adult domestic or intimate relationship. It is also termed **intimate partner violence** or *relationship violence*. This section focuses on domestic violence experienced by women in heterosexual relationships, although gay and lesbian individuals do experience domestic violence in their relationships as well.

Although the incidence has decreased significantly in the past decade, domestic violence is still staggeringly common in the United States, where one in four women has experienced physical violence by an intimate partner (Black, Basile, Breiding, et al., 2011). Worldwide, the prevalence of physical or sexual violence by a partner tends to be in the 30% to 60% range; however, that varies considerably, ranging, for example, from 15% in urban Japan to 71% in rural areas of Ethiopia (UN Women, 2011).

The woman may be married to her abuser, or she may be living with, dating, or divorced from him. Domestic violence takes many forms, including verbal attacks, insults, intimidation, threats, emotional abuse, social isolation, economic deprivation, intellectual derision, ridicule, stalking, and physical attacks and injury. Physical battering includes slapping, kicking, shoving, punching, forms of torture, attacks with objects or weapons, and sexual assault. Women who are physically abused can also suffer psychologic and emotional abuse.

Cycle of Violence

In an effort to explain the experience of battered women, Walker (1984) developed the theory of the *cycle of violence*. Battering takes place in a cyclic fashion through three phases:

1. In the *tension-building phase*, the batterer demonstrates power and control. This phase is characterized by anger, arguing, blaming the woman for external problems, and possibly minor battering incidents. The woman may blame herself and believe she can prevent the escalation of the batterer's anger by her own actions.

2. The *acute battering incident* is typically triggered by some external event or internal state of the batterer. It is an episode of acute violence distinguished by lack of control, lack of predictability, and major destructiveness. The cycle of violence can be interrupted before the acute battering incident if proper interventions take place.

3. The *tranquil, loving phase* is sometimes termed the honeymoon period. This phase may be characterized by extremely kind and loving behavior on the part of the batterer as he tries to make up with the woman, or it may simply be manifested as an absence of tension and violence. Without intervention this phase will end and the cycle of violence will continue. Over time the violence increases in severity and frequency.

Characteristics of Battered Women

Battered women often hold traditional views of sex roles. Many were raised to be submissive, passive, and dependent and to seek approval from male figures. Some battered women were exposed to violence between their parents, whereas others first experienced it from their partners. Many battered women do not work outside the home. As part of the manipulation of batterers, they are isolated from family and friends and totally dependent on their partners for their financial and emotional needs.

Women with physically abusive partners nearly always experience psychologic abuse as well and have been told repeatedly by their batterers that the family's problems are all their fault. Many believe their batterers' insults and accusations. As these women become more isolated, they find it harder to judge who is right. Eventually they fully believe in their inadequacy, and their low self-esteem reinforces their belief that they deserve to be beaten. Battered women often feel a pervasive sense of guilt, fear, and depression. Their sense of hopelessness and helplessness reduces their problem-solving ability. Battered women may also experience a lack of support from family, friends, and their religious community.

Characteristics of Batterers

Batterers come from all backgrounds. They often have feelings of insecurity, socioeconomic inferiority, powerlessness, and helplessness that conflict with their assumptions of male supremacy. Emotionally immature and aggressive men have a tendency to express these overwhelming feelings of inadequacy through violence. Many batterers feel undeserving of their partners, yet they blame and punish the very women they value.

Battered women often describe their husbands or partners as lacking respect toward women in general, having come from homes where they witnessed abuse of their mothers or were themselves abused as children, and having a hidden rage that erupts occasionally. Batterers accept traditional macho values, yet when they are not angry or aggressive, they appear childlike, dependent, seductive, manipulative, and in need of nurturing. They may be well respected in the community. This dual personality of batterers reflects the conflict between their belief that they must live up to their macho image and their feelings of inadequacy in the role of husband or provider. Combined with low frustration tolerance and poor impulse control, their pervasive sense of powerlessness leads them to strike out at life's inequities by abusing women.

Nursing Management. Nurses often come in contact with abused women but fail to recognize them, especially if their bruises are not visible. Women at high risk for battering often have a history of alcohol or drug abuse, child abuse, or abuse in the previous or present relationship. Other possible signs of abuse include expressions of helplessness and powerlessness; low self-esteem revealed by the woman's dress, appearance, and the way she relates to healthcare providers; signs of depression evidenced by fatigue, hopelessness, and somatic problems such as headache, insomnia, chest pain, back pain, or pelvic pain; and possible suicide attempts. In addition, the abused woman may have a history of missed or frequently changed appointments, perhaps because she had signs of abuse that kept her from coming in or because her partner prevented it.

Because female partner abuse is so prevalent, many caregivers now advocate *universal screening of all female patients at every health encounter*. Screening should be done privately, with only the caregiver and patient present, in a safe and quiet place. Specific language leads to higher disclosure rates. Possible screening questions include the following:

1. During the past year, have you been slapped, kicked, hit, choked, or hurt physically by someone?

2. Has your partner or anyone else ever forced you to have sex?

3. Are you afraid of an ex-partner or anyone at home?

During the screening, assure the woman that her privacy will be respected (Figure 5–9 ●). It is essential to remain nonjudgmental. Create a warm, caring climate conducive to sharing, and demonstrate a willingness to talk about violence. A battered woman may interpret your willingness to discuss violence as permission for her to discuss it as well.

It is important to consider cultural and religious factors that may impact a woman's willingness to disclose abuse. See *Developing Cultural Competence: Supporting Immigrant Women Who Suffer Abuse.*

When a woman seeks care for an injury, be alert to the following cues of abuse:

- Hesitation in providing detailed information about the injury and how it occurred

- Inappropriate affect for the situation

- Delayed reporting of symptoms

- Pattern of injury consistent with abuse, including multiple injury sites involving bruises, abrasions, and contusions to the head (eyes and back of the neck), throat, chest, abdomen, or genitals

- Inappropriate explanation for the injuries

- Lack of eye contact

- Signs of increased anxiety in the presence of the possible batterer, who frequently does much of the talking

When a battered woman comes in for treatment, she needs to feel safe physically and secure in talking about her injuries and problems. If a man is with her, ask or tell him to remain in the waiting room while the woman is examined. A battered woman

● **Figure 5–9** Screening for domestic violence should be done privately.
Source: Courtesy of Al Dodge.

Developing Cultural Competence
Supporting Immigrant Women Who Suffer Abuse

Immigrant women who experience intimate partner violence (IPV) may be reluctant to report it for fear of deportation. Nurses need to be aware that the "U" nonimmigrant visa permits immigrants who have been victims of IPV or other crimes to remain in the United States legally if it is justified on humanitarian grounds, is in the public interest, or ensures family unity (ACOG, 2012a).

also needs to regain a sense of predictability by knowing what to expect and how she can interact. Provide sufficient information about what to expect in terms the woman can understand.

In providing care, let the woman work through her story, problems, and situation at her own pace. Reassure the woman that she is believed and that her feelings are reasonable and normal. Anticipate the woman's ambivalence (due to her fear and possible love-hate relationship with her batterer), but also respect the woman's capacity to change and grow when she is ready. Thus any assessment should include information about a woman's strengths and support systems. The woman may need help identifying specific problems and developing realistic ideas for reducing or eliminating those problems. In all interactions, stress that no one should be abused and that the abuse is not the woman's fault.

Nursing Care in the Community

Inform any woman suspected of being in an abusive situation of the services available in the community. A battered woman may need the following:

- Medical treatment for injuries

- Temporary shelter to provide a safe environment for her and her children

- Counseling to raise her self-esteem and help her understand the dynamics of violence

- Legal assistance for protection from or prosecution of the batterer

- Financial assistance to obtain shelter, food, and clothing

- Job training or employment counseling

If the woman returns to an abusive situation, encourage her to develop an exit plan for herself and her children, if any. As part of the plan, she should pack a change of clothing for herself and her children, including toiletries and an extra set of car and house keys. She should store these items away from the house with a friend or relative and ask a neighbor to call the police if violence begins. In planning she should be aware that her abuser may monitor mail, telephone, and Internet communication. If possible she should have money, identification papers (driver's license, Social Security card, and birth certificates for herself and her children), checkbook, savings account information, other financial information (such as mortgage papers, automobile papers, and pay stubs), court papers or orders, and information about the children to help her enroll them in school. She should also plan where she will go, regardless of the time of day. Ensure that the woman has a planned escape route and emergency telephone numbers she can call, including local police, a phone hotline, and a women's shelter if one is available in the community.

Working with battered women is challenging, and many healthcare providers feel frustrated and impotent when the women repeatedly return to their abusive situations. Nurses must realize that they cannot rescue battered women; battered women must decide on their own how to handle their situations. Effective nurses provide battered women with information that empowers them in decision making and supports their decisions, knowing that incremental assistance over the years may be the only alternative until the battered women are ready to explore other options.

Sexual Assault and Rape

Broadly, **sexual assault** is involuntary sexual contact with another person. **Rape** is forced sexual intercourse as a result of physical force or psychologic coercion. Forced sexual intercourse refers to vaginal, oral, or anal penetration by a body part or by an object.

Research indicates that nearly one in five women (18.3%) in the United States has been the victim of an attempted or completed sexual assault or rape at some time in her life. Of these women, 40.8% have been raped by an acquaintance and over half (51.1%) report being raped by an intimate partner (Black et al., 2011).

Sexual violence often occurs early in life. Almost 80% of female victims of completed rape experience their first rape before age 25; over two fifths (42.2%) occur before age 18 (Black et al., 2011). No woman of any age, cultural or ethnic background, or socioeconomic status is immune, but statistics indicate that young, unmarried women; women who are unemployed or have low family income; and students have the highest incidence of sexual assault or attempted assault.

Why do men rape? Of the many theories put forth, none provides a completely satisfactory explanation. So few assailants are actually caught and convicted that a clear characteristic of the assailant has not been developed. However, rapists tend to be emotionally weak and insecure and may have difficulty maintaining interpersonal relationships. Many assailants also have trouble dealing with the stresses of daily life. Such men may become angry and overcome by feelings of powerlessness. They then commit a sexual assault as an expression of power or anger.

Acquaintance rape, which occurs when the assailant is someone with whom the victim has had previous nonviolent interaction, is the most common form of rape. One type of acquaintance rape, **date rape**, which occurs between a dating couple, is an increasing problem on high school and college campuses. In some cases an assailant uses alcohol or other drugs to sedate his intended victim. One drug, flunitrazepam (Rohypnol), has gained notoriety as a date rape drug. Gamma hydroxybutyrate (GHB), ketamine, MDMA (Ecstasy), clonazepam, and scopolamine have also been identified as date rape drugs that are used to incapacitate a woman. More recently, prescription drugs have been used in combination with alcohol to facilitate many sexual assaults. Because these drugs frequently produce amnesia, the woman may be unable to remember details of her assault, thereby making prosecution more difficult.

Responses to Sexual Assault

Sexual assault is a *situational crisis*. It is a traumatic event that the survivor cannot be prepared to handle because it is unforeseen. Following an assault the victim generally experiences a cluster of symptoms, described by Burgess and Holmstrom (1979) as the *rape trauma syndrome,* that last far beyond the rape itself. These

Table 5–5	Phases of Recovery Following Sexual Assault
Phase	**Response**
Acute phase (disorganization)	Fear, shock, disbelief, desire for revenge, anger, anxiety, guilt, denial, embarrassment, humiliation, helplessness, dependence, self-blame, wide variety of physical reactions, lost or distorted coping mechanisms
Outward adjustment phase (denial)	Survivor appears outwardly composed, denying and repressing feelings (e.g., she returns to work, buys a weapon); refuses to discuss the assault; denies need for counseling
Reorganization	Survivor makes many life adjustments, such as moving to a new residence or changing her phone number; uses emotional distancing; may engage in risky sexual behaviors; may experience sexual dysfunction, phobias, flashbacks, sleep disorders, nightmares, anxiety; has a strong urge to talk about or resolve feelings; may seek counseling or remain silent
Integration and recovery	Time of resolution; survivor begins to feel safe and be comfortable trusting others; places blame on assailant; may become an advocate for others

phases are described in Table 5–5. Although the phases of response are listed individually, they often overlap, and individual responses and their duration may vary. A fourth phase—integration and recovery—has also been suggested (Holmes, 1998).

Research suggests that survivors of sexual assault may exhibit high levels of posttraumatic stress disorder, the same disorder that developed in many of the veterans of the Vietnam War. Posttraumatic stress disorder is marked by varying degrees of intensity. Assault victims with this disorder often require lengthy, intensive therapy to regain a sense of trust and feeling of personal control.

Nursing Management. Survivors of sexual assault often enter the healthcare system by way of the emergency department. Thus, the emergency department nurse is often the first person to counsel them. Because the values, attitudes, and beliefs of the caregiver necessarily affect the competence and focus of the care, it is essential that you clearly understand your feelings about sexual assault and assault survivors and resolve any conflicts that may exist. In many communities a specially trained sexual assault nurse examiner (SANE) coordinates the care of survivors of sexual assault, gathers necessary forensic evidence, and is then available as an expert witness when assailants are tried for the crime.

The first priority in caring for a survivor of a sexual assault is to create a safe, secure environment. Gather admission information in a quiet, private room. Reassure the woman that she is safe and not alone. Assess the survivor's appearance, demeanor, and ways of communicating for the purpose of planning care. Initially the woman is evaluated to determine the need for emergency care. Obtaining a careful, detailed history is essential. After the woman has received any necessary emergency care, complete a forensic chart and kit.

Give the woman a thorough explanation of the procedures to be carried out and have her sign a consent form for the forensic examination and collection of materials. Sexual assault kits contain all the necessary supplies for collecting and labeling evidence. The woman's clothing should be collected and bagged, swabs of stains and secretions taken, hair samples and any fingernail scrapings collected, blood samples drawn, tissue swabs obtained, and photographs taken of any injuries. Vaginal and rectal examinations are performed, along with a complete physical examination for trauma. The woman is offered prophylactic treatment for sexually transmitted infections. If the assailant's HIV status is not known, the woman may be offered postexposure prophylaxis with HIV antiviral medications. In such cases, consultation with an HIV specialist is advised. Question the woman about her menstrual cycle and contraceptive practices. If she could become pregnant as a result of the rape, she should be offered postcoital contraceptive therapy.

Throughout the experience you act as the sexual assault survivor's advocate, providing support without usurping decision making. You need not agree with all the survivor's decisions but should respect and defend her right to make them.

The family members and friends on whom the survivor calls also need nursing care. The reactions of the family will depend on the values to which they ascribe. Many families or mates blame the survivor for the assault and feel angry with her for not having been more careful. They may also incorrectly view the assault as a sexual act rather than an act of violence. They may feel personally wronged and see the survivor as devalued or unclean. Their reactions may compound the survivor's crisis. By spending some time with family members before their first interaction with the

---

Health Promotion   Counseling After Sexual Assault

Sexual assault counseling, provided by qualified nurses or other counselors, is a valuable tool in helping the survivor come to terms with her assault and its impact on her life. In counseling, the woman is encouraged to explore and identify her feelings and determine appropriate actions to resolve her problems and concerns. The counselor must avoid reinforcing the prevalent myth that the assault was somehow the woman's fault. The fault lies with the assailant. The counselor also plays an important role in emphasizing that the loss of control the woman experienced during the rape was temporary and that the woman can regain a feeling of control over life.

---

survivor, you can perhaps reduce their anxiety and absorb some of their frustrations, sparing the woman further trauma.

Prosecution of the Assailant

Legally, sexual assault is considered a crime against the state, and prosecution of the assailant is a community responsibility. The survivor, however, must begin the process by reporting the assault and pressing charges against her assailant. In the past, the police and the judicial system were notoriously insensitive in dealing with survivors. However, many communities now have classes designed to help officers work effectively with sexual assault survivors or have special teams to carry out this important task.

Many women who have sought to use the judicial process have had such a traumatic experience that they refer to it as a second assault. The woman may be asked repeatedly to describe the experience in intimate detail, and her reputation and testimony may be attacked by the defense attorney. In addition, publicity may intensify her feelings of humiliation, and, if her assailant is released on bail or found not guilty, she may fear retaliation.

The nurse acting as a counselor needs to be aware of the judicial sequence to anticipate rising tension and frustration in the survivor and her support system. The woman needs consistent, effective support at this crucial time.

Clinical Tip

Strive to listen nonjudgmentally. Impartial listening can often make the difference in a victim's readiness to disclose the full details of the assault and can also assist her in the recovery process.

Critical Concept Review

LEARNING OUTCOME 5.1: Describe accurate information to be provided to girls and women so that they can implement effective self-care measures for dealing with menstruation.

For effective self-care the woman may need information about:
1. Choice of sanitary protection:
   - Pads
   - Tampons
2. Use of vaginal sprays.
3. Douching practices.
4. Comfort measures:
   - Proper nutrition
   - Exercise
   - Use of heat and massage

LEARNING OUTCOME 5.2: Contrast the signs, symptoms, and nursing management of women with dysmenorrhea and those with premenstrual syndrome.

1. Dysmenorrhea:
   - Begins at onset of menstruation and disappears by the end of menstruation.
   - Treated with oral contraceptives, NSAIDs, or prostaglandin inhibitors.
   - Self-care measures include improved nutrition, exercise, heat application, and extra rest.
2. Premenstrual syndrome:
   - Symptoms are associated with the luteal phase (2 weeks prior to onset of menses).
   - Pronounced symptoms begin 2–3 days before onset of menstruation and subside as menstruation starts.
   - Symptoms disappear with or without treatment.
   - Treatment includes the use of progesterone agonists and prostaglandin inhibitors.
   - Self-care measures include use of vitamin B and E supplements, calcium, avoidance of sodium and caffeine, and increased aerobic exercise.

LEARNING OUTCOME 5.3: Compare the advantages, disadvantages, and effectiveness of the various methods of contraception available today.

1. Fertility awareness methods:
   - Advantages: Natural and noninvasive.
   - Disadvantages: Requires extensive initial counseling for effectiveness. Requires couple to practice abstinence during parts of each month.
   - Effectiveness: In practice, it may be less reliable than other methods.
2. Barrier contraceptives:
   - Advantages: Easy to use with no side effects. Condoms prevent spread of most venereal diseases.
   - Disadvantages: Some types must be fitted by a nurse practitioner or physician. Must be placed prior to intercourse. Must be used with spermicides.
   - Effectiveness: Excellent when used correctly.
3. Spermicides:
   - Advantages: Inexpensive and easy to obtain.
   - Disadvantages: Must be applied prior to intercourse. Considered "messy" by many people.
   - Effectiveness: Minimally effective when used alone.
4. Intrauterine devices:
   - Advantages: Effective for up to 5 years (Mirena) or 10 years (ParaGard) without removal.

- Disadvantages: May cause cramping and bleeding for first 3–6 months. Woman must check for proper placement after each menses. Does not protect from STIs. May predispose woman to PID.
- Effectiveness: Very effective while in place.
5. Hormonal contraceptives:
   - Advantages: Menstrual symptoms are lessened. Menstruation is very predictable.
   - Disadvantages: May increase chance of blood clots. Should not be used by anyone who smokes, has a heart condition, or has previous history of thromboembolic disease. Does not protect from STIs.
   - Effectiveness: Highly effective when used correctly.
6. Sterilization:
   - Advantages: Permanent form of birth control. No additional costs once procedure is completed.
   - Disadvantages: Considered nonreversible. Requires general anesthesia for the woman and local anesthesia for the man. Vasectomy does not produce immediate sterility; semen sample must be clear before other form of contraception is stopped. Does not protect against STIs.
   - Effectiveness: Considered completely effective.

LEARNING OUTCOME 5.4: Identify basic gynecologic screening procedures indicated for well women.

1. Breast examination (yearly).
2. Mammography: Recommended every 1–2 years after age 40 and annually for women age 50 or older.
3. Pap smear and pelvic examination (yearly).

LEARNING OUTCOME 5.5: Examine the physical and psychologic aspects and clinical treatment options of menopause when caring for menopausal women.

1. Physical aspects of menopause:
   - Ovulation ceases 1–2 years prior to menopause.
   - Gradual atrophy of ovaries.
   - FSH levels rise.
   - Less estrogen is produced.
   - Atrophic changes of vagina, vulva, urethra, and bladder.
   - Vasomotor disturbances such as "hot flashes."
   - Atrophy of uterine endometrium and myometrium, and fallopian tubes.
   - Constriction of uterine cavity.
   - Vaginal tissue becomes smooth, thins, and loses elasticity.

- Thinning of pubic hair.
- Decreased pelvic support.
- Decrease in breast firmness.
- Possible development of osteoporosis.
- Increased risk of coronary heart disease.
2. Psychologic aspects of menopause:
   - Possible helpless feelings at physical changes.
   - Fatigue from lack of sleep due to hot flashes.
   - Decreased libido.
   - Possible increase in enjoyment of sexual intercourse due to lack of worry about pregnancy.

LEARNING OUTCOME 5.6: Discuss the nurse's role in screening and caring for women who have experienced domestic violence or rape.

The nurse's role includes the following:
1. Create a safe, secure environment.
2. Obtain a careful, detailed history.
3. Complete a forensic chart and kit.
4. Explain all procedures.
5. Act as the survivor's advocate.

Clinical Reasoning in Action

You are working at a local clinic when Joy Lang, age 20, presents for her first pelvic exam. You obtain the following GYN history: menarche age 12, menstrual cycle 28–30 days lasting 4–5 days, heavy one day, then lighter. She tells you that she needs to use superabsorbent tampons on the first day of her period and then she switches to a regular absorbency tampon for the remaining days. She confirms that she changes the tampon every 6 to 8 hours, never leaving it in overnight. She denies premenstrual syndrome, dysmenorrhea, or medical problems and says that she is not taking any medication on a regular schedule. She tells you that she recently got married, but would like to wait before getting pregnant. She'd like to discuss birth control methods. Joy tells you that doctors make her nervous and she admits to being anxious about her first pelvic exam.

1. What steps would you take to reduce Joy's anxiety relating to the pelvic exam?
2. What position is best to relax Joy's abdominal muscles for the pelvic exam?
3. What precaution should be taken when obtaining a Pap smear?
4. Explain the purpose of the Pap smear.
5. What factors do you include in a discussion of the type of birth control that Joy could practice?

See www.nursing.pearsonhighered.com for possible responses.

References

American Cancer Society (ACS). (2011a). *Breast aware-ness and self-exam*. Retrieved from http://www .cancer.org/Cancer/BreastCancer/MoreInformation/ BreastCancerEarlyDetection/breast-cancer-early-detection-acs-recs-bse?docSelected=breast-cancer-early-detection-ref

American Cancer Society (ACS). (2011b). *Breast cancer: Early detection*. Retrieved from http://www.cancer .org/acs/groups/cid/documents/webcontent/ 003165-pdf.pdf

American College of Obstetricians and Gynecologists (ACOG). (2009). *Medical management of abortion* (ACOG Practice Bulletin No. 67). Washington, DC: Author.

American College of Obstetricians and Gynecologists (ACOG). (2010). *Noncontraceptive uses of hormonal contraceptives* (ACOG Practice Bulletin No. 110). Washington, DC: Author.

American College of Obstetricians and Gynecologists (ACOG). (2012a). *Adolescents and long-acting reversible contraception: Implants and intrauterine devices* (ACOG Committee Opinion 539). Washington, DC: Author.

American College of Obstetricians and Gynecologists (ACOG). (2012b). *Screening for breast problems*. Retrieved from http://www.acog.org/~/media/ For%20Patients/FAQ178.pdf?dmc=1&ts= 20120526T1508258847

Avis, N., Brockwell, S., Randolph, J., Shen, S., Cain, V., Ory, M., & Greendale, G. (2009). *Longitudinal changes in sexual functioning as women transition through menopause: Results from the Study of Women's Health Across the Nation*. Retrieved from http:// www.medscape.com/viewarticle/703258

Bertone-Johnson, E. R., Hankinson, S. E., Willett, W. C., Johnson, S. R., & Manson, J. E. (2010). Adiposity and the development of premenstrual syndrome. *Journal of Women's Health, 19*(11), 1955–1962.

Black, M. C., Basile, K. C., Breiding, M. J., Smith, S. G., Walters, M. L., Merrick, M. T., . . . Stevens, M. R. (2011). *The National Intimate Partner and Sexual Violence Survey, 2010 summary report*. Retrieved from http://www.cdc.gov/ViolencePrevention/pdf/ NISVS_Executive_Summary-a.pdf

Burgess, A. W., & Holmstrom, L. L. (1979). *Rape: Crisis and recovery*. Englewood Cliffs, NJ: Prentice-Hall.

Chocano-Bedoya, P., Manson, J., Hankinson, S., Wilett, W., Johnson, S., Chasan-Taber, L., . . . Bertone-Johnson, E. R. (2011). Dietary B vitamin intake and incident premenstrual syndrome. *American Journal of Clinical Nutrition, 93*(5), 1080–1086.

Crandell, L. (2012). Psychological outcomes of medical versus surgical elective first trimester abortion. *Nursing for Women's Health, 16*(4), 296–307.

Fine, P. M. (2011). A new option for emergency contraception. *The Female Patient, 36*(2), 41–44.

Gallagher, J. C., & Levine, J. P. (2011). Preventing osteoporosis in symptomatic postmenopausal women. *Menopause: The Journal of the North American Menopause Society, 18*(1), 109–118.

Gardner, A. (2011). Contraception for older women. *InnovAiT, 4*(3), 139–143.

Garza-Cavazos, A., & Loret de Mola, J. R. (2012). Abnormal uterine bleeding: New definitions and contemporary terminology. *The Female Patient, 37*(7), 27–36.

Hachul, H., Brandão, L. C., D'Almeida, V., Bittencourt, L. R. A., Baracat, E. C., & Tufik, S. (2011). Isoflavones decrease insomnia in postmenopause. *Menopause: The Journal of the North American Menopause Society, 18*(2), 178–184.

Hatcher, R. A., Trussell, J., Nelson, A., Cates, W., Kowal, D., & Policar, M. S. (2011). *Contraceptive technology* (20th ed.). New York, NY: Ardent Media.

Holmes, M. M. (1998). The clinical management of rape in adolescents. *Contemporary OB/GYN, 43*(5), 62–78.

National Center for Complementary and Alternative Medicine (NCCAM). (2010a). *Herbs at a glance: Chasteberry*. Retrieved from http://nccam.nih.gov/ health/chasteberry

National Center for Complementary and Alternative Medicine (NCCAM). (2010b). *Herbs at a glance: Evening primrose oil*. Retrieved from http://nccam.nih.gov/ health/eveningprimrose

National Center for Complementary and Alternative Medicine (NCCAM). (2012). *Get the facts: Menopausal symptoms and complementary health practices*. Retrieved from http://nccam.nih.gov/health/ menopause/menopausesymptoms#hed2

National Osteoporosis Foundation (NOF). (2010). *Clinician's guide to prevention and treatment of osteoporosis*. Retrieved from http://www.nof.org/sites/ default/files/pdfs/NOF_ClinicianGuide2009_v7.pdf

North American Menopause Society (NAMS). (2011). NAMS 2011 isoflavones report. *Menopause: The Journal of the North American Menopause Society, 18*(7), 732–753.

North American Menopause Society (NAMS). (2012a). *FRAX®: A tool for estimating your fracture risk*. Retrieved from http://www.menopause.org/

for-women/menopauseflashes/frax-sup-sup-a-tool-for-estimating-your-fracture-risk

North American Menopause Society (NAMS). (2012b). The 2012 hormone therapy position statement of the North American Menopause Society. *Menopause, 19*(3), 257–271.

Population Reference Bureau. (2010). *2010 world population data sheet*. Retrieved from http://www.prb.org/ pdf10/10wpds_eng.pdf

Raines, K. (2010). Diagnosing premenstrual syndrome. *Journal for Nurse Practitioners, 6*(3), 224–225.

Shulman, L. P. (2010). Gynecological management of premenstrual symptoms. *Current Pain and Headache Report, 14*, 367–375.

Smith, C. A., Zhu, X., He, L., & Song, J. (2011). Acupuncture for dysmenorrhea. *Cochrane Database of Systematic Reviews*. ISSN: 1469493X CINAHL AN: 2011468788

Sood, R., Shuster, L., Smith, R., Vincent, A., & Jatoi, A. (2011). Counseling postmenopausal women about bioidentical hormones: Ten discussion points for practicing physicians. *Journal of the American Board of Family Medicine, 24*(2), 202–210.

UN Women. (2011). *Violence against women*. Retrieved from http://www.unifem.org/gender_issues/ violence_against_women

U.S. Food and Drug Administration. (2009a). *FDA approves update to label on birth control patch*. Retrieved from http://www.fda.gov/NewsEvents/Newsroom/ PressAnnouncements/2008/ucm116842.htm

U.S. Food and Drug Administration (FDA). (2009b). *Nonoxynol 9 (N9) OTC contraceptive choices*. Retrieved from http://www.fda.gov/Safety/MedWatch/Safety-Information/SafetyAlertsforHumanMedicalProducts/ ucm152690.htm

U.S. Preventive Services Task Force. (2009). *Screening for breast cancer*. Retrieved from http://www.ahrq .gov/clinic/uspstf/uspsbrca.htm

Walker, L. (1984). *The battered woman syndrome*. New York, NY: Springer.

Writing Group for the Women's Health Initiative Investigations. (2002). Risks and benefits of estrogen plus progestin in healthy postmenopausal women: Principal results from the Women's Health Initiative randomized controlled trial. *Journal of the American Medical Association, 288*, 321–333.

Common Gynecologic Problems

Don Klumpp/Getty Images

I was 58 when I learned that I had human papillomavirus infection. My first reaction was denial. I had been a virgin when I married and always thought I had the world's best marriage. When I confronted my husband of 30 years, I learned that he had been unfaithful to me with three different women over the course of our marriage. At first I was ready to walk away. But my husband begged for a second chance, we saw a counselor for almost 6 months, and eventually rebuilt our life together. Many women would call me a fool but I know that, for me, it was important to save something I had committed to—for better or for worse— and to practice the forgiveness so many preach but fail to follow. —Leonora

LEARNING OUTCOMES

6.1   Contrast the contributing factors, signs and symptoms, treatment options, and nursing care management of women with common benign breast disorders.

6.2   Explain the signs and symptoms, medical therapy, and implications for fertility of endometriosis.

6.3   Discuss the signs and symptoms, treatment options, and health implications of polycystic ovarian syndrome (PCOS).

6.4   Summarize the risk factors, treatment options, and nursing interventions for women with toxic shock syndrome.

6.5   Compare the causes, signs and symptoms, treatment options, and nursing care for women with vulvovaginal candidiasis versus bacterial vaginosis.

6.6   Compare the common sexually transmitted infections with regard to their etiology, treatment options, nursing care, and methods of prevention.

6.7   Summarize the pathology, signs and symptoms, treatment, nursing care, and implications for future fertility of pelvic inflammatory disease (PID).

6.8   Identify the implications of an abnormal finding during a pelvic examination in the provision of nursing care.

6.9   Contrast the causes, signs and symptoms, treatment options, and nursing care for women with cystitis versus pyelonephritis.

The contemporary woman is likely to encounter various major or minor gynecologic or urinary problems during her lifetime. Some may be minor and easily treated, others may be more serious. This chapter provides information about a variety of gynecologic conditions, with an emphasis on problems commonly addressed in community-based settings.

CARE OF THE WOMAN WITH A BENIGN DISORDER OF THE BREAST

This section deals with the most common breast disorders women encounter. For information on breast cancer, consult a medical-surgical nursing textbook.

Fibrocystic Breast Changes

Fibrocystic breast changes, also known as *benign breast disease (BBD)*, is the most common of the benign breast disorders. It is most prevalent in women 20 to 50 years of age. *Fibrosis* is a thickening of the normal breast tissue. Cyst formation that may accompany fibrosis is considered a later change in the condition. The exact etiology of fibrocystic breast changes is unclear. Generally fibrocystic changes are not a risk factor for breast cancer. In some rare cases, if the change is proliferative and results in hyperplasia or buildup of the cells of the breast ducts, atypia may occur (Lee, 2009).

The woman often reports pain, tenderness, and swelling that occur cyclically and are most pronounced just before menses. Physical examination may reveal only mild signs of irregularity, or the breasts may feel dense, with areas of irregularity and nodularity. Women often refer to this irregularity as "lumpiness." Some women may also have expressible nipple discharge. Although unilateral discharge and serosanguineous discharge are the most worrisome findings, all breast discharge should be investigated further.

If the woman has a large, fluid-filled cyst, she may experience a localized painful area as the capsule containing the accumulated fluid distends coincident with her cycle. However, if small cysts form, the woman may experience not a solitary tender lump but a diffuse tenderness. A cyst may often be differentiated from a malignancy because a cyst is more mobile (easily moved with palpation) and tender and is not associated with skin retraction (pulling) in the surrounding tissue.

Mammography, sonography, magnetic resonance imaging (MRI), palpation, and fine-needle aspiration are used to confirm fibrocystic breast changes. Often, fine-needle aspiration is the treatment as well, affording relief from the tenderness or pain. Treatment of palpable cysts is conservative; invasive procedures such as biopsy are used only if the diagnosis is questionable.

Women with mild symptoms may benefit from restricting sodium intake and taking a mild diuretic during the week before the onset of menses. This counteracts fluid retention, relieves pressure in the breast, and helps decrease the pain. In other cases a mild analgesic is necessary. In severe cases the hormone inhibitor danazol is often helpful because it suppresses follicle-stimulating hormone (FSH) and luteinizing hormone (LH), resulting in anovulation. However, it can cause undesirable side effects including masculinization. Women who do not respond to other treatment approaches may be given a trial of bromocriptine, a prolactin inhibitor.

Some researchers suggest that methylxanthines (found in caffeine products, such as coffee, tea, colas, and chocolate, and in some medications) may contribute to the development of fibrocystic breast changes and that limiting intake of these substances will help decrease fibrocystic changes.

Other Benign Breast Disorders

Fibroadenoma is a common benign tumor seen in women in their teens and early twenties. It has not been significantly associated with breast cancer. Fibroadenomas are freely movable, solid tumors that are well defined, sharply delineated, and rounded, with a rubbery texture.

Ultrasound is the best method for imaging women under age 35 with a palpable mass because of the density of their breast tissue. Most women can be observed and followed every 6 months with ultrasound for 2 years then once yearly thereafter. Some clinicians may prefer surgical excision to prove that it is benign (Lee, 2009).

The term for nipple discharge not associated with lactation (production of milk for breastfeeding) is **galactorrhea**. Nonclinically significant nipple discharge occurs in women who have fibrocystic changes in the breast, who are using contraceptives, or who are on hormone therapy (Azavedo, 2009). Certain medications that are used to treat psychiatric disorders have a side effect of galactorrhea. The most common types of nipple discharge occur in both breasts, are secreted from several ducts, and vary in color from white to brown. The likelihood of malignancy increases with the presence of a spontaneous discharge arising from a single duct in one breast that is watery or bloody in nature and warrants further investigation.

Intraductal papillomas, most often occurring during the menopausal years, are tumors growing in the terminal portion of a duct or, sometimes, throughout the duct system within a section of the breast. They are typically benign but have the potential to become malignant. Although relatively uncommon, they are the most frequent cause of nipple discharge in women who are not pregnant or lactating.

The majority of papillomas present as solitary nodules. These small, ball-like lesions may be detected on mammography but often are nonpalpable. A papilloma is often frightening to the woman, because her primary symptom is a discharge from the nipple that may be serosanguineous or brownish green due to old blood. The location of the papilloma within the duct system and its pattern of growth determine whether nipple discharge will be present. Papillomas are typically benign but they are generally excised to rule out the possibility of cancer.

Duct ectasia (comedomastitis), an inflammation of the ducts behind the nipple, commonly occurs during or near the onset of menopause and is not associated with malignancy. The condition typically occurs in women who have borne and breastfed children. It is characterized by a thick, sticky nipple discharge and by burning pain, pruritus, and inflammation. Nipple retraction may also be noted, especially in postmenopausal women. Treatment is conservative, with drug therapy aimed at symptomatic relief. The major central ducts of the breast occasionally have to be excised.

NURSING MANAGEMENT *For the Woman with a Breast Disorder*

Nursing Assessment and Diagnosis

During the period of diagnosis of any breast disorder, the woman may be anxious about a possible change in body image or a diagnosis of cancer. Use therapeutic communication to assess the significance the woman places on her breasts, her current emotional status, coping mechanisms used during periods of stress, knowledge and beliefs about cancer, and other variables that may influence her coping and adjustment.

Nursing diagnoses that may apply to a woman with a benign disorder of the breast include the following (NANDA-I © 2012):

- *Knowledge, Readiness for Enhanced,* about diagnostic procedures for breast disorders related to an expressed desire to understand procedures
- *Anxiety* related to threat to body image

Planning and Implementation

During the prediagnosis period, clarify misconceptions and encourage the woman to express her anxiety. Once a diagnosis is made, ensure that the woman understands her condition, its association to breast malignancy, and the treatment options. Also point out that frequent professional breast examinations and regular mammograms help detect any abnormalities. Although recommendations about the importance of monthly breast self-examination (BSE) have been modified (see Chapter 5 🔗; also see Skill 2–2: Teaching Breast Self-Examination in the *Clinical Skills Manual* SKILLS), most professionals agree that women should be familiar with their own breasts so that they are able to note changes should they occur.

Evaluation

Expected outcomes of nursing care include the following:

- The woman is able to discuss her fears, concerns, and questions during the period of diagnosis.
- The diagnosis is made quickly and accurately, and treatment is initiated if indicated.

CARE OF THE WOMAN WITH ENDOMETRIOSIS

Endometriosis, a condition characterized by the presence of endometrial tissue outside the endometrial cavity, occurs in about 10% of reproductive-age women (Schindler, 2011). Endometriosis has been found almost everywhere in the body, including the vagina, lungs, cervix, central nervous system, and gastrointestinal tract. The most common location, however, is the pelvic cavity. This tissue responds to the hormonal changes of the menstrual cycle and bleeds in a cyclic fashion. The bleeding results in inflammation, scarring of the peritoneum, and formation of adhesions.

Endometriosis may occur at any age after puberty, but it is most common in women between ages 20 and 45. The exact cause of endometriosis is unknown. Leading theories include retrograde menstrual flow and inflammation of the endometrium, hereditary tendency, and a possible immunologic defect.

The most common symptom of endometriosis is pelvic pain, which is often dull or cramping. Usually the pain is related to menstruation itself and is often thought to be dysmenorrhea by the affected woman. However, the pain of dysmenorrhea usually begins right before menses starts and lasts for a day or two, decreasing as prostaglandin levels decrease (American College of Obstetricians and Gynecologists [ACOG], 2012). **Dyspareunia** (painful intercourse) and abnormal uterine bleeding are other common signs. The condition is often diagnosed when the woman seeks evaluation for infertility. Bimanual examination may reveal a fixed, tender, retroverted uterus and palpable nodules in the cul-de-sac. Diagnosis is confirmed by laparoscopy.

Treatment may be medical, surgical, or a combination of the two. In women with minimal disease and symptoms, treatment includes observation, analgesics, and nonsteroidal anti-inflammatory drugs (NSAIDs). If the woman does not currently desire pregnancy, she may be started on a combined oral contraceptive (COC), often in combination with an NSAID. The COC creates a pseudopregnancy state with decreased menstrual bleeding and may be used for long-term treatment (Schindler, 2011). If the COC does not relieve symptoms, therapy with medroxyprogesterone acetate (MPA), danazol, or a gonadotropin-releasing hormone (GnRH) agonist may be indicated.

MPA causes endometrial tissue to atrophy, thereby decreasing symptoms. It is administered intramuscularly every 3 months, and the effectiveness of treatment is evaluated every 3 to 6 months. Side effects include weight gain, bloating, acne, headaches, emotional lability, and irregular bleeding.

Danazol is a testosterone derivative that suppresses ovulation and causes amenorrhea. It is intended for short-term therapy. Because of adverse effects on lipid metabolism and significant side effects such as weight gain, hirsutism, acne, oily skin, vaginal dryness, hot flushes, reduced libido, voice changes, clitoral enlargement, and decreased breast size, many clinicians have moved away from danazol to other treatment options.

GnRH agonists such as nafarelin acetate (given as a metered nasal spray twice daily) and leuprolide acetate (Lupron) (given once a month as an intramuscular injection) are gaining popularity because many women tolerate them better than danazol, and their results in treating endometriosis are comparable. GnRH agonists suppress the menstrual cycle through estrogen antagonism. This may result in the hypoestrogen side effects of hot flashes, vaginal dryness, decreased libido, pain in muscles and joints, and loss of bone density. Consequently, the use of GnRH agonists should be limited to 6 months (Schindler, 2011).

In more advanced cases, surgery may be done to remove endometrial implants and break up adhesions. If severe dyspareunia or dysmenorrhea are symptoms, the surgeon may perform a presacral neurectomy. In advanced cases in which childbearing is not an issue, treatment may be a hysterectomy (removal of the uterus) with bilateral salpingo-oophorectomy (removal of the fallopian tubes and ovaries).

NURSING MANAGEMENT *For the Woman with Endometriosis*

Nursing Assessment and Diagnosis

The nurse needs to know the symptoms of endometriosis and elicit an accurate history. If a woman is being treated for endometriosis, assess the woman's understanding of the condition, its implications, and the treatment alternatives.

Nursing diagnoses that may apply to a woman with endometriosis include the following (NANDA-I © 2012):

- *Pain, Acute,* related to peritoneal irritation secondary to endometriosis
- *Family Processes, Dysfunctional,* related to depression secondary to infertility

Planning and Implementation

Be available to explain the condition, its symptoms, treatment alternatives, and prognosis. Help the woman evaluate treatment options and make appropriate choices. If the woman begins taking medication, review the dosage, schedule, possible side effects, and any warning signs. A woman with endometriosis is often advised not to delay pregnancy because of the increased risk of infertility. The woman may wish to discuss the implications of this decision on her life choices, relationship with her partner, and personal preferences. Be a nonjudgmental listener and help the woman consider her options.

Evaluation

Expected outcomes of nursing care include the following:

- The woman is able to discuss her condition, its implications for fertility, and her treatment options.
- After considering the alternatives, the woman chooses appropriate treatment options.

CARE OF THE WOMAN WITH POLYCYSTIC OVARIAN SYNDROME

Polycystic ovarian syndrome (PCOS) is a complex endocrine disorder of ovarian dysfunction that is evidenced by menstrual dysfunction, signs of androgen excess (typically hirsutism, acne), and infertility.

The most common clinical signs and symptoms of PCOS include:

- *Menstrual dysfunction.* Irregular menses, ranging from total absence of periods (amenorrhea) to intermittent or infrequent periods (oligomenorrhea), are the hallmarks of PCOS. Anovulation is usually a chronic problem with PCOS and may present as a history of menstrual irregularities.
- *Hyperandrogenism.* Women with PCOS consistently have elevated serum androgen levels. These elevated androgen levels often lead to clinical manifestations such as hirsutism (excessive hair growth), acne, deepening voice, and increased muscle mass.
- *Obesity.* About half of women with PCOS are clinically obese (Smith & Taylor, 2011). The obesity is generally of the android type, with an increased hip-to-waist ratio.
- *Hyperinsulinemia.* Women with PCOS may be insulin resistant. This insulin resistance, characterized by the failure of insulin to enter the cells appropriately, places these women at increased risk for impaired glucose tolerance and type 2 diabetes mellitus (Smith & Taylor, 2011).
- *Infertility.* The majority of women who have been diagnosed with PCOS struggle with some degree of infertility related to anovulation. (See Chapter 7 🔗.)

Clinical Therapy

If a woman presents with complaints of hirsutism, menstrual irregularities, acne, difficulty conceiving, and unexplained weight gain, several other disorders must be ruled out. Important disorders to

Evidence-Based Practice   Dietary Modifications for PCOS

Clinical Question

What dietary modifications are effective in treating the symptoms of polycystic ovary syndrome (PCOS)?

The Evidence

Several randomized controlled trials have contributed evidence to support the effectiveness of dietary changes in treating the symptoms of PCOS. Multiple trials compared a balanced diet with a low-glycemic-index diet, a high-protein diet, and a diet rich in calcium and vitamin D. A second randomized trial focused on increasing protein consumption while decreasing carbohydrates as compared to a balanced diet. A Cochrane systematic review evaluated six studies using any diet change in combination with overall lifestyle modification. Randomized control trials and systematic reviews provide the strongest, Level I evidence for effectiveness. The low-glycemic-index diet as well as the high-protein diet helped women with PCOS lose weight and improve their body mass index (Marsh et al., 2010). The low-glycemic-index diet seemed to have the most impact on insulin sensitivity and improving menstrual cycles, particularly when combined with

metformin use. The high-protein diet produced decreases in blood glucose, while simultaneously decreasing waist circumference (Sorensen et al., 2012). Eating a calcium- and vitamin D-rich diet contributed to weight loss, menstrual regularity, and improvement in some of the androgenic symptoms (Firouzabadi et al., 2012). The Cochrane systematic review demonstrated that both types of diets result in changes in anthropometric measures such as weight and BMI (Moran, Hutchison, Norman, et al., 2011). None of the diets had an effect on other physical manifestations of PCOS, such as hirsutism, acne, or clinical reproductive outcomes.

Best Practice

A diet high in protein with a low glycemic index may help women with PCOS lose weight, improve menstrual irregularities, and enhance glucose metabolism.

Clinical Reasoning

What foods are high in protein and have a low glycemic index? How can the nurse encourage compliance with this type of diet change?

---

consider include hyperthyroidism or hypothyroidism, congenital adrenal hyperplasia, Cushing's syndrome, hyperprolactinemia, and androgen-producing tumors. The diagnostic process is fourfold: history, physical examination, laboratory studies, and imaging.

Once PCOS is diagnosed, the goals for treatment include decreasing the effects of hyperandrogenism (hirsutism, acne, etc.), restoring reproductive functioning for women desiring pregnancy, protecting the endometrium (increased risk for uterine cancer), and reducing long-term risks, specifically type 2 diabetes and cardiovascular disease.

If pregnancy is not an immediate goal, menstrual irregularities can be treated with a combined oral contraceptive (COC) or cyclic progesterone. COCs help to regulate menstrual cycles; provide a balance between estrogen and progesterone, thereby protecting the endometrium and decreasing the risk of uterine cancer; and may improve acne by inhibiting ovarian androgen production (Guzick & Hoeger, 2009). If pregnancy is an immediate goal, then another option is the use of medications that improve insulin sensitivity and use.

Antiandrogens such as spironolactone (Aldactone) may be used to decrease symptoms of androgen excess. Metformin (Glucophage) improves tissue sensitivity to insulin, inhibits glucose production in the liver, and improves glucose uptake by fat and muscle cells. It improves ovarian function, reduces the degree of hyperandrogenism, restores normal ovulation in women with PCOS, and is associated with an improved ability to lose weight. In addition, lifestyle changes are important. Modifications should include weight loss, regular exercise, balanced diet, and smoking cessation.

If initial approaches to helping a woman with PCOS become pregnant fail, assisted reproductive technology (ART) may be recommended using in vitro fertilization, intrauterine insemination, or intracytoplasmic sperm injection. This may be combined with gonadotropin therapy (McFarland, 2012).

Long term, PCOS may increase a woman's risk for developing type 2 diabetes, hypertension, cardiovascular disease, endometrial cancer, breast cancer, and ovarian cancer. Additionally, the woman with PCOS may struggle with significant emotional responses to this chronic disorder. She will likely face issues related to body image, infertility, problematic menses, and depression.

Nursing Management

The nurse plays a vital role in the identification of PCOS and its evaluation, management, and follow-up. The signs of PCOS, especially hirsutism, negatively impact women's feelings of femininity, and they may feel physically inferior and lack self-confidence (Weiss & Bulmer, 2011). Nurses can help women recognize these feelings and find ways to develop a more positive body image. The nurse also has an important role in providing accurate information, education, and counseling for a woman diagnosed with PCOS. Finally, because the woman with PCOS is at risk for developing long-term complications, the nurse can play a key role in follow-up and continuity of care throughout the life of a woman facing this challenging disorder.

CARE OF THE WOMAN WITH TOXIC SHOCK SYNDROME

Toxic shock syndrome (TSS) is primarily a disease of women at or near menses or during the postpartum period. The causative organism is a toxin released by a strain of *Staphylococcus aureus*. The use of superabsorbent tampons was once related to an increased incidence of TSS. That incidence has declined. Occluding the cervical os with a contraceptive device such as a diaphragm or cervical cap during menses may also increase the risk of TSS.

Activity | Case Study: Toxic Shock Syndrome

Early diagnosis and treatment are important in preventing death. For a diagnosis of TSS to be made, certain criteria must be met, including fever (often greater than 38.9°C [102°F]), hypotension (systolic BP less than 90 mm Hg), rash, and multisystem involvement (Silversides, Lappin, & Ferguson, 2010). The fever and a rash on the trunk present initially followed by desquamation of the skin, especially the palms and soles, which usually occurs 1 to 2 weeks after the onset of symptoms; hypotension; and dizziness. Systemic symptoms often include vomiting, diarrhea, severe myalgia, and inflamed mucous membranes (oropharyngeal, conjunctival, or vaginal). Disorders of the central nervous system, including alterations in consciousness, disorientation, and coma, may also occur. Laboratory findings reveal elevated blood urea nitrogen (BUN), creatinine, aspartate aminotransferase (AST), alanine aminotransferase (ALT), and total bilirubin levels, whereas platelets are often less than 100,000/mm^3.

Women with TSS are gravely ill. They are hospitalized and given antibiotics and supportive therapy, including oxygen, and intravenous fluids to maintain blood pressure. Severe cases may require renal dialysis, administration of vasopressors, and intubation.

Nursing Management

Nurses play a major role in helping educate women about preventing the development of TSS. It is crucial that women understand the importance of avoiding prolonged use of tampons. Women who choose to continue using tampons may reduce their risk of TSS by alternating them with pads and avoiding overnight use of tampons. Women should avoid the use of tampons for 6 to 8 weeks after childbirth. Women who use diaphragms or cervical caps should not leave them in place for prolonged periods and should not use them during the postpartum period or when they are menstruating. Also, help make women aware of the signs and symptoms of TSS so that they will seek treatment promptly if symptoms occur.

CARE OF THE WOMAN WITH A VAGINAL INFECTION

Vaginitis is one of the most common reasons why women seek gynecologic care. Symptoms of vaginitis or vulvovaginitis may include increased vaginal discharge, vulvar irritation, pruritus, foul odor, dyspareunia (painful sexual intercourse), bleeding with intercourse, and pain when urine touches irritated vulvar tissue. It may be caused directly by an infection or it may result from an alteration of normal flora, as in the case of bacterial vaginosis or *Candida albicans*.

Bacterial Vaginosis

Bacterial vaginosis (BV) is more prevalent among sexually active women, but it is not considered a sexually transmitted infection. BV is an alteration of normal vaginal bacterial flora that results in the loss of hydrogen peroxide–producing lactobacilli, which are normally the main vaginal flora. With the loss of this natural defense, bacteria such as *Gardnerella vaginalis*, mycoplasmas,

● **Figure 6–1** Clue cells characteristically seen in bacterial vaginosis. Unlike normal epithelial cells, which appear translucent and have a clear border, clue cells are desquamated epithelial cells with bacteria adhering to them. The presence of the bacteria makes the cell appear to be speckled with black dots. The borders are also obscured because of the bacteria.
Source: Courtesy of Centers for Disease Control and Prevention.

and anaerobes overgrow in large numbers, causing vaginitis. The cause of this overgrowth is not clear, although tissue trauma from douching, frequent sexual intercourse without condom use, and an upset in normal vaginal flora are predisposing factors. BV during pregnancy may be a factor in premature rupture of the membranes and preterm birth.

The infected woman often notices an excessive amount of thin, watery, white or gray vaginal discharge with a foul odor described as "fishy." The characteristic "clue" cell is seen on a wet-mount preparation (Figure 6–1 ●). The addition of 10% potassium hydroxide (KOH) solution to the vaginal secretions, called a "whiff" test, releases a strong, fishy odor. The vaginal pH is usually greater than 4.5.

The symptomatic woman, whether nonpregnant or pregnant, is generally treated with metronidazole (Flagyl) orally or as a vaginal cream. (See *Drug Guide: Metronidazole [Flagyl].*) Alternately, tinidazole orally or clindamycin (Cleocin) orally or as vaginal cream may be used (Centers for Disease Control and Prevention [CDC], 2010). Women should avoid intercourse or use condoms during the treatment period.

SAFETY ALERT!

Alcohol should be avoided when taking either metronidazole or tinidazole. When combined with alcohol, both metronidazole and tinidazole can produce effects similar to that of alcohol and Antabuse—abdominal pain, flushing, and tremors. The CDC (2010) recommends abstaining from alcohol for 24 hours after completing metronidazole and 72 hours after completing tinidazole.

Vulvovaginal Candidiasis

Vulvovaginal candidiasis (VVC), also called moniliasis or yeast infection, is one of the most common forms of vaginitis that women experience. Recurrences are frequent for some women.

Drug Guide Metronidazole (Flagyl)

Overview of Action

Metronidazole is an antiprotozoal and antibacterial agent. It possesses direct trichomonacidal and amebicidal activity against *Trichomonas vaginalis* and *Entamoeba histolytica*. Metronidazole is active in vitro against most obligate anaerobes but does not appear to possess any clinically relevant activity against facultative anaerobes or obligate aerobes. It is used in the treatment of various infections caused by organisms that are sensitive to this drug. It is used predominantly to treat the following infections in women: *T. vaginalis*, bacterial vaginosis, endometritis, endomyometritis, tubo-ovarian abscess, and postsurgical vaginal cuff infection.

Route, Dosage, Frequency

Trichomoniasis—Nonpregnant women: 1-day treatment: 2 g orally in a single dose; alternately 500 mg orally twice a day for 7 consecutive days; pregnant women: 2 g orally in a single dose (CDC, 2010). Amebiasis—Adults: 750 mg orally three times a day for 5–10 days; children: 35–50 mg/kg/24 hours orally divided into 3 doses for 10 days. Bacterial vaginosis—Nonpregnant woman: 500 mg orally twice a day for 7 consecutive days or one full applicator of metronidazole gel 0.75% intravaginally, once daily for 5 days; pregnant women: 500 mg orally twice a day for 7 consecutive days or 250 mg orally three times a day for 7 days (CDC, 2010).

Contraindications

Blood dyscrasias
Breastfeeding women (drug secreted in breast milk)
Impaired kidney or liver function
Active CNS disease

Side Effects

Convulsive seizures
Weakness
Peripheral neuropathy
Insomnia
Nausea/vomiting
Cystitis
Headache
Reversible neutropenia and thrombocytopenia
Anorexia
Diarrhea
Flattening of the T wave on electrocardiogram (ECG)
Epigastric distress
Polyuria
Abdominal cramping
Incontinence
Constipation
Pelvic pressure
Metallic taste in mouth
Proliferation of *Candida* in the vagina and mouth
Dizziness
Vertigo
Joint pains
Uncoordination
Decreased libido
Ataxia
Dryness in the mouth, vulva, and vagina
Confusion
Irritability
Dyspareunia
Depression

Nursing Considerations

- Inform the woman about potential side effects.
- Stress the importance of contraceptive compliance during course of treatment.
- Obtain baseline renal and liver function tests as ordered.
- Teach the woman about the signs, symptoms, and treatment of vulvovaginal candidiasis.
- Counsel the woman to avoid alcoholic beverages while taking the medication.
- If the woman is taking oral contraceptives, a backup nonhormonal contraceptive method is recommended during treatment.
- Teach the woman to monitor the signs and symptoms of her infection.
- Encourage cooperation with the entire course of treatment.

Candida albicans is the fungal species responsible for most vaginal yeast infections. Factors that contribute to VVC are the use of COCs, immunosuppressants, and antibiotics, which destroy normal bacteria that usually keep the yeast cells in check. Other factors are frequent douching, pregnancy, and diabetes mellitus.

The woman with VVC often complains of thick, curdy vaginal discharge, severe itching, dysuria, and dyspareunia. A male sexual partner may experience a rash or excoriation of the skin of the penis and possibly pruritus. The male may be symptomatic and the female asymptomatic.

On physical examination the woman's labia may be swollen and excoriated if pruritus has been severe. A speculum examination reveals thick, white, tenacious cheeselike patches adhering to the vaginal mucosa. Diagnosis is confirmed by microscopic examination of the vaginal discharge; hyphae and spores are usually seen on a wet-mount preparation (Figure 6–2 ●).

Medical treatment of VVC includes intravaginal butoconazole, miconazole, tioconazole, or clotrimazole cream or vaginal suppositories, which are available over the counter (OTC). Terconazole cream or suppositories or nystatin vaginal tablets are available by prescription (CDC, 2010). Single-dose and short-course (3 days) approaches are effective for 80% to 90% of women with uncomplicated VVC. Women who continue to have symptoms after using an OTC preparation and women who have a recurrence of symptoms within 2 months should be evaluated during an office visit because inappropriate use of OTC preparations can lead to a delay in treatment (CDC, 2010).

Treatment of the male partner is generally not necessary unless candidal balanitis (inflammation of the glans penis) is

● **Figure 6–2** The hyphae and spores of *Candida albicans*. This is the fungus that is responsible for vulvovaginal candidiasis.

Source: Courtesy of Centers for Disease Control and Prevention.

Clinical Tip

To distinguish among the common types of vaginitis and their treatments, it is useful to remember the following:

Vulvovaginal Candidiasis (moniliasis)
- Cause: *Candida albicans*
- Appearance of discharge: Thick, curdy, like cottage cheese
- Diagnostic test: Slide of vaginal discharge (treated with potassium hydroxide) shows characteristic hyphae and spores
- Treatment: Azole vaginal cream or suppositories

Bacterial Vaginosis (*Gardnerella vaginalis* vaginitis)
- Cause: *Gardnerella vaginalis*
- Appearance of discharge: Gray, milky
- Diagnostic test: Slide of vaginal discharge shows characteristic "clue" cells
- Treatment: Metronidazole or tinidazole

Trichomoniasis
- Cause: *Trichomonas vaginalis*
- Appearance of discharge: Greenish white and frothy
- Diagnostic test: Saline slide of vaginal discharge shows motile flagellated organisms
- Treatment: Metronidazole

present. Then treatment with a topical antifungal medication is indicated (CDC, 2010).

If a woman experiences recurrent VVC (four or more symptomatic episodes in 1 year), she should be tested for an elevated blood glucose level to determine whether a diabetic or prediabetic condition is present. Women at high risk for sexually transmitted infections should also be tested for HIV. Recurrent infection is then treated with an intensive regimen of oral and local agents for 7 to 14 days followed by maintenance antifungal therapy. Pregnant women with VVC are treated only with topical azole preparations applied for 7 days (CDC, 2010). Infection at the time of birth may cause *thrush* (a mouth infection) in the newborn.

NURSING MANAGEMENT *For the Woman with Vulvovaginal Candidiasis*

Nursing Assessment and Diagnosis

The nurse should suspect VVC if a woman complains of intense vulvar itching and a curdy, white discharge. Because pregnant women with diabetes mellitus are especially susceptible to this infection, be alert for symptoms in these women. In some areas, nurses are trained to do speculum examinations and wet-mount preparations and can confirm the diagnosis themselves. In most cases, however, the nurse who suspects a vaginal infection reports it to the woman's healthcare provider.

Nursing diagnoses that might apply to the woman with VVC include the following (NANDA-I © 2012):

- *Skin Integrity, Risk for Impaired,* related to scratching secondary to discomfort of the infection
- *Knowledge, Readiness for Enhanced,* regarding information about yeast infection related to an expressed desire to learn about ways of preventing VVC

Planning and Implementation

If the woman is experiencing discomfort because of pruritus, recommend gentle bathing of the vulva with a weak sodium bicarbonate solution. If a topical treatment is being used, the woman will need to bathe the area before applying the medication.

Also discuss with the woman the factors that contribute to the development of VVC and suggest ways to prevent recurrences, such as wearing cotton underwear and avoiding vaginal powders or sprays that may irritate the vulva. Stress the importance of completing the course of medication even during menses. Some women report that the addition of yogurt to the diet or the use of activated culture of plain yogurt as a vaginal douche helps prevent recurrence by maintaining high levels of lactobacilli. For the same reason, some clinicians recommend that women who are taking antibiotics consume yogurt or probiotics supplements (containing acidophilus and other helpful bacteria) simultaneously.

Evaluation

Expected outcomes of nursing care include the following:

- The woman's symptoms are relieved, and the infection is cured.
- The woman is able to identify self-care measures to prevent further episodes of VVC.

CARE OF THE INDIVIDUAL WITH A SEXUALLY TRANSMITTED INFECTION

The occurrence of **sexually transmitted infections (STIs)**, or *sexually transmitted diseases (STDs),* has increased during the past few decades. In fact, vaginitis and STIs are the most common reasons for outpatient, community-based treatment of women.

Children and adolescents can also become infected with sexually transmitted organisms through sexual experimentation, sexual play, molestation, and sexual abuse. Among adolescents

Activity | Care Plan: Gynecologic Infection

and young adults the incidence of STIs is significant. Although young people ages 15 to 24 account for approximately one fourth of the sexually experienced population in the United States, they acquire almost half of all new STIs (CDC, 2011b).

Results from the CDC's *Youth Risk Behavior Surveillance—United States, 2009,* reveal that 46.0% of high school students had engaged in sexual intercourse and 38.9% of sexually active adolescents had not used a condom at last sexual intercourse (Eaton, Kann, Kinchen, et al., 2010). Adolescents are considered an at-risk population because of their inexperience and lack of knowledge about STIs. They may disregard the importance of using barrier protection, may have multiple sexual partners, may have sex frequently, and often do not seek medical treatment until symptoms are well advanced.

Frequently diagnosed STIs include chlamydia, genital herpes (herpes simplex type 2), gonorrhea, genital warts (human papilloma virus), trichomoniasis, and syphilis. For more detailed information on the specific signs, symptoms, and treatment of males with STIs, consult a medical-surgical nursing textbook.

Trichomoniasis

Trichomoniasis is an infection caused by *Trichomonas vaginalis,* a microscopic motile protozoan that thrives in an alkaline environment. Almost all infections are acquired through sexual intimacy. Transmission by shared bath facilities, wet towels, or wet swimsuits, though possible, is unlikely.

In females, symptoms of trichomoniasis include a yellow-green, frothy, odorous discharge frequently accompanied by inflammation of the vagina and cervix, dysuria, and dyspareunia. Visualization of *T. vaginalis* under the microscope on a wet-mount preparation of vaginal discharge confirms the diagnosis (Figure 6–3 ●). Two other tests with greater sensitivity than the wet-mount preparation are also available and are performed on vaginal secretions: the OSOM Trichomonas Rapid Test (results available in 10 minutes) and the Affirm VPIII (results available in 45 minutes) (CDC, 2010).

Treatment for trichomoniasis is metronidazole (Flagyl) administered in a single 2-g dose or tinidazole, which is also administered in a single 2-g dose. Sex partners should be treated as well (CDC, 2010). Partners should avoid intercourse until both are cured.

● **Figure 6–3** Microscopic appearance of *Trichomonas vaginalis.*
Source: Courtesy of Centers for Disease Control and Prevention.

Pregnant women with trichomoniasis may be at increased risk for premature rupture of the membranes, preterm birth, and a low-birth-weight newborn. Pregnant women who are symptomatic should be treated with a single 2-g dose of metronidazole (CDC, 2010).

Chlamydial Infection

Chlamydial infection, caused by *Chlamydia trachomatis,* is the most commonly reported STI in the United States (CDC, 2010). A strain of chlamydia is responsible for trachoma, the world's leading cause of preventable blindness.

In males, chlamydia is a major cause of nongonococcal urethritis (NGU). In females it can cause infections similar to those that occur with gonorrhea. Pelvic inflammatory disease, infertility, and ectopic pregnancy are associated with chlamydia. The newborn of a woman with untreated chlamydia is at risk of developing ophthalmia neonatorum, which responds to erythromycin ophthalmic ointment prophylaxis at birth. The newborn may also develop chlamydia pneumonia.

In females, symptoms of chlamydia include a thin or purulent discharge, burning and frequency of urination, and lower abdominal pain. Women, however, are often asymptomatic. Diagnosis is often made after treatment of a male partner for NGU or in a symptomatic woman with a negative gonorrhea culture. Of the laboratory tests available to diagnose chlamydia,

Video ⎸ Acyclovir

Developing Cultural Competence
Racial Disparity in STIs

Racial disparities exist in all STIs, with the highest rates found among African Americans. In 2010, African Americans accounted for 69% of reported gonorrhea cases and almost half the cases of syphilis (47.4%) (CDC, 2011b). Though less marked, disparities also exist among Hispanics. These disparities may result, in part, because people from minority populations are more likely to seek care in public health clinics, which report STIs more accurately than private providers do. However, socioeconomic barriers to high-quality health care and to STI prevention and treatment play a role. It is essential that these barriers be addressed if such disparities are to be eliminated.

Clinical Reasoning Sexually Transmitted Infections

Ella Matlosz is a 21-year-old, single woman, never pregnant, who comes to the office complaining of excessive, odorous vaginal discharge. She uses an IUD for contraception and has several sex partners. She states that she douches with a medicated douche after intercourse.

What should you tell Ella about feminine hygiene? What would you tell Ella about the relationship between contraceptives and sexually transmitted infections?

See www.nursing.pearsonhighered.com for possible responses.

nucleic acid amplification testing (NAAT) is the most sensitive. Other tests for diagnosis include culture, direct immunofluorescence, enzyme immunoassay (EIA), and nucleic acid hybridization tests (CDC, 2010). The recommended treatment is a single 1-g dose of azithromycin orally or doxycycline orally twice daily for 7 days. Sexual partners should be treated, and couples should abstain from intercourse for 7 days (CDC, 2010). Doxycycline is contraindicated in pregnancy. The CDC (2010) recommends that pregnant women be treated with azithromycin or amoxicillin.

Gonorrhea

Gonorrhea is an infection caused by the bacteria *Neisseria gonorrhoeae*. If a nonpregnant female contracts the disease, she is at risk of developing pelvic inflammatory disease. If a woman becomes infected after the third month of pregnancy, the mucous plug in the cervix will prevent the infection from ascending, and it will remain localized in the urethra, cervix, and Bartholin's glands until the membranes rupture. Then it can spread upward. A newborn exposed to a gonococcal-infected birth canal is at risk of developing ophthalmia neonatorum. To prevent this infection, all newborns should receive eye prophylaxis at birth, generally with erythromycin ophthalmic ointment.

Often girls and women with gonorrhea are asymptomatic. Thus it is routine to screen for this infection using a cervical culture during the initial prenatal examination. For women at high risk, the culture may be repeated during the last month of pregnancy. Cultures of the urethra, throat, and rectum may also be required for diagnosis, depending on the body orifices used for intercourse.

In females the most common symptoms of gonorrheal infection include a purulent, greenish yellow vaginal discharge, dysuria, and urinary frequency. Some women also develop inflammation and swelling of the vulva. The cervix may appear swollen and eroded and may secrete a foul-smelling discharge in which gonococci are present. In males, urethritis, or inflammation of the urethra, is the cardinal symptom. This is marked by burning during urination and the presence of discharge from the urethra.

The preferred treatment for nonpregnant women consists of antibiotic therapy with ceftriaxone intramuscularly or, if that is not an option, with cefixime orally. This treatment is combined with azithromycin or doxycycline orally to address the risk of co-infection with chlamydia because gonorrhea and chlamydia often occur together (CDC, 2010). Additional treatment may be required if the cultures remain positive 7 to 14 days after completion of treatment. All sexual partners must also be treated or the woman may become reinfected.

Pregnant women should be treated with ceftriaxone intramuscularly or cefixime orally plus azithromycin or amoxicillin to prevent co-infection. Doxycycline is contraindicated during pregnancy (CDC, 2010).

Females should be informed of the need for reculture to verify cure and the need for abstinence or condom use until cure is confirmed. Both sexual partners should be treated if either has a positive test for gonorrhea.

Herpes Genitalis

Herpes infections are caused by the herpes simplex virus (HSV). Two types of herpes infections can occur: HSV-1 (the cold sore), which can cause genital herpes through oral-genital contact, and HSV-2, which is usually associated with genital infections. The clinical symptoms and treatment of both types are the same. At least 50 million people in the United States have been diagnosed with genital HSV-2 infection—*herpes genitalis* (Akhter, Beckmann, & Gorelick, 2009).

The primary episode of herpes genitalis is characterized by the development of single or multiple blisterlike vesicles. In males these usually occur on the penis or anal area. In females the vesicles occur in the genital area and sometimes affect the vaginal walls, cervix, urethra, and anus. The vesicles may appear within a few hours to 20 days after exposure and rupture spontaneously to form painful, open, ulcerated lesions. Inflammation and pain secondary to the presence of herpes lesions can cause difficult urination and urinary retention. Inguinal lymph node enlargement may be present. Flulike symptoms and genital pruritus or tingling also may be noticed. Primary episodes usually last the longest and are the most severe. Lesions heal spontaneously in 2 to 4 weeks.

After the lesions heal, the virus enters a dormant phase, residing in the nerve ganglia of the affected area. Some individuals never have a recurrence, whereas others have regular recurrences. Recurrences are usually less severe than the initial episode and seem to be triggered by emotional stress, menstruation, ovulation, pregnancy, frequent or vigorous intercourse, poor health status or a generally run-down physical condition, tight clothing, or overheating. Diagnosis is most often made on the basis of the clinical appearance of the lesions, culture of the lesions, polymerase chain reaction (PCR) identification, and HSV-specific glycoprotein G2 and glycoprotein G1 assays (CDC, 2010).

No known cure for herpes exists. The recommended treatment of the first clinical episode of genital herpes is oral acyclovir, valacyclovir, or famciclovir. These same medications, in somewhat different dosages, are also recommended for recurrent herpes infection and for daily suppression therapy for people who have frequent recurrences. Because there is more documented information on the use of acyclovir during pregnancy, it may be administered orally to pregnant women with first-episode genital herpes or severe recurrent herpes. Its use in the third trimester may reduce the frequency of cesarean births by decreasing the incidence of recurrences at term (CDC, 2009).

Keeping the genital area clean and dry, wearing loose clothing, and wearing cotton underwear or none at all help promote healing. If herpes is present in the genital tract of a woman during childbirth, it can have a devastating effect on the newborn. Women with herpetic lesions when labor begins should give birth by cesarean to prevent neonatal herpes. Note that cesarean birth does not completely prevent the risk of neonatal transmission (CDC, 2010). See Chapter 16 🔗 for more information.

Syphilis

Syphilis is a chronic STI caused by the spirochete *Treponema pallidum*. Syphilis is divided into early and late stages. During the early stage (primary), a chancre appears at the site where the

T. pallidum organism entered the body. Symptoms include slight fever, loss of weight, and malaise. The chancre persists for about 4 weeks and then disappears. In 6 weeks to 6 months, secondary symptoms appear. Skin eruptions called condylomata lata, which resemble wartlike plaques and are highly infectious, may appear on the vulva. Other secondary symptoms are acute arthritis, enlargement of the liver and spleen, nontender enlarged lymph nodes, iritis, and a chronic sore throat with hoarseness.

Syphilis may also be transmitted transplacentally. When infected in utero, the newborn exhibits secondary-stage symptoms of syphilis. Transplacentally transmitted syphilis may cause intrauterine growth restriction, preterm birth, and stillbirth. As a result of the disease's impact on the fetus in utero, serologic testing of every pregnant woman is recommended; some state laws require it. Testing is done at the initial prenatal screening and may be repeated in the third trimester. Blood studies in early pregnancy may be negative if the woman has only recently contracted the infection.

Diagnosis of syphilis is made by dark-field examination for spirochetes. Blood tests such as the Venereal Disease Research Laboratory (VDRL) test, the rapid plasma reagin (RPR) test, or the more specific fluorescent treponemal antibody absorption (FTA-ABS) test are commonly done.

For nonpregnant and pregnant women with syphilis of less than a year's duration (early latent syphilis), the CDC (2010) recommends 2.4 million units of benzathine penicillin G administered intramuscularly in a single dose. If syphilis is of long (more than a year) duration, 2.4 million units of benzathine penicillin G is given intramuscularly once a week for 3 weeks. For nonpregnant women allergic to penicillin, doxycycline or tetracycline can be given. The pregnant woman who is allergic to penicillin should be desensitized to penicillin and then treated with it (CDC, 2010). Maternal serologic testing may remain positive for 8 months, and the newborn may have a positive test for 3 months.

Condylomata Acuminata (Venereal Warts)

The infection **condylomata acuminata**, also called *venereal warts,* is a common sexually transmitted condition caused by the human papillomavirus (HPV). Transmission can occur through vaginal, oral, or anal sex. The infection has received considerable attention because HPV is almost always the cause of cervical cancer.

Over 100 HPV subtypes have been identified. Of these, about 40 can infect the genital tract (CDC, 2010). HPV types 6 and 11 account for most visible genital warts, whereas high-risk HPV types such as 16 and 18 cause most of the cervical cancer (CDC, 2010).

Often an individual seeks medical care after noticing a single or multiple soft, grayish pink, cauliflower-like lesions on the penis or in the genital area (Figure 6–4 ●). The moist, warm environment of the genital area is conducive to the growth of the warts, which may be present on the vulva, vagina, cervix, and anus. The incubation period following exposure is 3 weeks to 3 years.

Because condylomata sometimes resemble other lesions and malignant transformation is possible, all atypical, pigmented, and persistent warts should be biopsied and treatment should be instituted promptly. The CDC (2010) does not specify

● **Figure 6–4** Condylomata acuminata on the vulva.
Source: Courtesy of Centers for Disease Control and Prevention.

a treatment of choice for genital warts but recommends that treatment be determined based on patient preference, available resources, and experience of the healthcare provider. Patient-applied therapies include podofilox solution or gel, imiquimod cream, or sinecatechin ointment.

SAFETY ALERT!

If a patient-applied therapy is prescribed, the patient must understand exactly how to apply the medication and must be able to identify and reach all the warts. These regimens have specific directions for application, frequency, and length of use, which the nurse should review carefully. Both imiquimod and sinecatechin ointment must be washed off after specified time periods.

Provider-administered therapies include cryotherapy with liquid nitrogen; trichloroacetic acid (TCA); bichloroacetic acid (BCA); intralesional interferon surgical removal by tangential scissor excision, shave excision, curettage, or electrocautery; or laser surgery (CDC, 2010). Imiquimod, podophyllin, and podofilox are not used during pregnancy because they are thought to be teratogenic and in large doses have been associated with fetal death.

Two HPV vaccines are now available against herpes simplex virus (HSV) types 16 and 18, which cause 70% of cervical cancers. Gardasil, the first vaccine to receive FDA approval, is a quadrivalent vaccine and also provides protection against types 6 and 11, which cause 90% of genital warts. The second vaccine, Cervarix, is bivalent, only offering protection against HSV types 16 and 18. Either vaccine is recommended for girls ages 11 to 12 (preferably before they are sexually active) and for 13- to 26-year-old females who did not receive or complete the 3-dose vaccine series. The CDC (2011a) now recommends that the 3-dose HPV vaccine be routinely given to boys ages 11 to 12 to protect against HPV and also help provide indirect protection of women by reducing HPV transmission.

Women who have received the vaccine should receive regular Pap smears as recommended. Sex partners are probably infected but do not require treatment unless large lesions are present. The use of male or female condoms may reduce the risk of transmitting the virus to an uninfected partner.

Acquired Immunodeficiency Syndrome

Acquired immunodeficiency syndrome (AIDS) is a serious, often fatal disorder caused by the human immunodeficiency virus (HIV). Medical-surgical texts more fully describe care of people with HIV/AIDS. However, because HIV/AIDS has profound implications for the pregnant woman's fetus, AIDS is discussed in more detail in Chapter 15 .

NURSING MANAGEMENT *For the Individual with a Sexually Transmitted Infection*

Nursing Assessment and Diagnosis

Nurses need to become adept at taking a thorough history and identifying people at risk for STIs. Risk factors include multiple sexual partners, a partner's involvement with other partners, high-risk sexual behaviors such as intercourse without barrier contraception or anal intercourse, partners with high-risk behaviors, treatment with antibiotics while taking oral contraceptives, and young age at onset of sexual activity. Be alert for signs and symptoms of STIs and be familiar with diagnostic procedures if an STI is suspected.

> ### ◯ Clinical Tip
>
> ■ When a child younger than 10 years of age is found to have gonorrhea or another STI, consider the possibility of sexual abuse.
> ■ Whenever anorectal symptoms are found in a child, suspect molestation.

When children or adolescents have a possible STI, the nurse usually encounters them and their families in the emergency department, outpatient clinic, or nursing unit. Because adolescents are often afraid of the consequences of reporting symptoms, it is important to develop good assessment skills, particularly when asking questions about sexual activity, partners, and the possibility of abuse. When a child or adolescent is diagnosed with one STI, it is important to screen for others because these diseases may coexist. Adolescents who are symptomatic may postpone care because of their discomfort with examinations and cultures. Routine screening of sexually active adolescents is recommended because many have subclinical infections or are asymptomatic.

Although each STI has certain distinctive characteristics, the following complaints warrant further investigation: presence of a sore or lesion on the penis or vulva, increased vaginal discharge, malodorous vaginal discharge, urethral discharge (males), burning with urination, dyspareunia, bleeding after intercourse, and pelvic pain. In many instances a woman is asymptomatic but may report symptoms in her partner, especially painful urination or urethral discharge. It is often helpful to ask the woman whether her partner is experiencing any symptoms.

Nursing diagnoses that may apply when an STI is diagnosed include the following (NANDA-I © 2012):

■ *Family Processes*, *Interrupted,* related to the effects of a diagnosis of STI on the couple's relationship

■ *Knowledge, Readiness for Enhanced,* about preventing STIs related to an expressed desire to prevent infection

Planning and Implementation

Some STIs such as trichomoniasis or chlamydia may cause a woman concern but, once diagnosed, are rather easily treated. Other STIs may be simple to treat medically but may carry a stigma and be emotionally difficult to accept. Stress prevention with all patients and encourage them to require partners, especially new partners, to use condoms. While condoms offer protection from many STIs, they do not protect against infections like herpes and HPV, which are transmitted by direct skin-to-skin contact (Fantasia, Fontenot, Sutherland, et al., 2011). It is important to emphasize that, to be effective, condoms must remain in place during each and every act of intercourse. See *Teaching Highlights: Preventing STIs and Their Consequences.*

Refer the child with signs of an STI for evaluation of sexual assault by a facility or healthcare provider specializing in collecting evidence and providing specialized care. Similarly refer any adolescent who has been sexually assaulted to a sexual assault nurse examiner or other healthcare provider who can collect evidence and coordinate medical treatment and mental health support.

As a nurse, you can be especially helpful in encouraging a patient to explore feelings about the diagnosis. People may, for example, experience anger or feel betrayed by a partner, they may feel guilt or see their diagnosis as a form of punishment, or they may feel concern about the long-term implications for future childbearing or ongoing intimate relationships. Opportunities to discuss personal feelings in a nonjudgmental environment can be very helpful. Offer suggestions about support groups, if indicated, and assist the person in planning for future sexual activity.

Evaluation

Expected outcomes of nursing care include the following:

■ The infection is identified and cured, if possible; if not, supportive therapy is provided.

■ The individual and partner can describe the infection, its method of transmission, its implications, and the therapy.

■ The person copes successfully with the impact of the diagnosis on self-concept.

Teaching Highlights Preventing STIs and Their Consequences

The risk of contracting an STI increases with the number of sexual partners. Because of the extended time between infection with HIV and evidence of infection, intercourse with an individual exposes a female or male to all the other sexual partners of that individual for the past 5 or more years. In light of this risk, it is important to take the following actions:

- Plan ahead and develop strategies to refuse sex (especially important for adolescents who may be less confident about saying "no" to casual sexual encounters). Abstinence is the best method of preventing STIs.
- Limit the number of sexual contacts and practice mutual monogamy with an uninfected partner.
- The condom is the best contraceptive method currently available (other than abstinence) for protection from STIs. Use one for every act of vaginal or anal intercourse. Other contraceptives such as the diaphragm, cervical cap, and spermicides also offer some protection against STIs.
- Plan strategies for negotiating condom use with a partner. Do not assume that a sexually experienced partner knows how to practice safe sex.
- Reduce high-risk behaviors. Use of recreational drugs and alcohol can increase sexual risk taking.
- Refrain from oral sex if your partner has active sores in the mouth, on the genitals, or around the anus.
- Refrain from sexual interaction when signs and symptoms of an STI are present.
- Seek care as soon as you notice symptoms and make sure your partner gets treatment if indicated. Absence of symptoms or disappearance of symptoms does not mean that treatment is unnecessary if you suspect an STI. Take all prescribed medications completely.
- The presence of a genital infection may lead to an abnormal Pap smear. Women with certain infections should have more frequent Pap smears according to a schedule recommended by their caregiver. Ask your healthcare provider if you need more frequent Pap tests.

Health Promotion
Information for the Woman with an STI

In a supportive, nonjudgmental way, provide the woman who has an STI with information about the infection, methods of transmission, implications for pregnancy or future fertility, and the importance of thorough treatment. If treatment of her partner is indicated, help her understand that it is necessary to prevent a cycle of reinfection. She should also understand the need to abstain from sexual activity, if necessary, during treatment.

The organisms most frequently identified with PID are *Chlamydia trachomatis* and *Neisseria gonorrhoeae* although not all cases of chlamydia or gonorrhea develop into PID. Symptoms of PID include bilateral sharp, cramping pain in the lower quadrants, fever, chills, purulent vaginal discharge, irregular bleeding, malaise, nausea, and vomiting. However, it is also possible to be asymptomatic and have normal laboratory values.

Diagnosis is based on examination, cultures for gonorrhea and chlamydia, a complete blood count (CBC) with differential, and a rapid plasma reagin (RPR) or Venereal Disease Research Laboratory (VDRL) test to check for syphilis. The woman may have an elevated C-reactive protein and an elevated sedimentation rate. Physical examination usually reveals direct abdominal tenderness with palpation, adnexal tenderness, and cervical and uterine tenderness with movement (chandelier sign). A palpable mass is evaluated with ultrasound. Laparoscopy may confirm the diagnosis and enable the examiner to obtain cultures from the fimbriated ends of the fallopian tubes.

Oral outpatient therapy is comparable to inpatient intravenous therapy in women with PID of mild to moderate severity (CDC, 2010). The decision to hospitalize is based on clinical judgment. Inpatient treatment includes intravenous fluids, pain medications, and intravenous antibiotics—often either cefoxitin or cefotetan, plus doxycycline or clindamycin plus gentamicin. Outpatient oral therapy usually includes ceftriaxone plus doxycycline with or without metronidazole (Holland-Hall, 2012). Other antibiotic combinations may also be used. In addition, supportive therapy is often indicated for severe symptoms. The sexual partner should be treated. If the woman has an IUD, it is generally removed 24 to 48 hours after antibiotic therapy is started.

CARE OF THE WOMAN WITH PELVIC INFLAMMATORY DISEASE

Pelvic inflammatory disease (PID) is a clinical syndrome of inflammatory disorders of the upper female genital tract that includes any combination of endometritis, salpingitis (tubal infection), tubo-ovarian abscess, pelvic abscess, and pelvic peritonitis (CDC, 2010). The disease is more common in sexually active women younger than age 25. Other risk factors include multiple sexual partners, a history of PID, recent insertion of an intrauterine device, and regular douching. Perhaps the greatest problem of PID is postinfection tubal damage, which is closely associated with infertility.

NURSING MANAGEMENT *For the Woman with Pelvic Inflammatory Disease*

Nursing Assessment and Diagnosis

Be alert to factors in a woman's history that put her at risk for PID. Question the woman who has an IUD about possible symptoms, such as aching pain in the lower abdomen, foul-smelling discharge, malaise, and the like. The woman who is acutely ill will have obvious symptoms, but a low-grade infection is more difficult to detect.

Nursing diagnoses that may apply to a woman with PID include the following (NANDA-I © 2012):

- *Pain, Acute,* related to peritoneal irritation
- *Knowledge, Deficient,* related to a lack of information about the possible effects of PID on fertility

Planning and Implementation

The nurse plays a vital role in helping to prevent or detect PID. Accordingly, spend time discussing risk factors related to this infection. The woman who uses an IUD for contraception and has multiple sexual partners needs to understand clearly the risk she faces. Discuss signs and symptoms of PID and stress the importance of early detection.

Counsel the woman who develops PID on the importance of completing her antibiotic treatment and of returning for follow-up evaluation. She should also understand the possibility of decreased fertility following the infection.

Evaluation

Expected outcomes of nursing care include the following:

- The woman describes her condition, her therapy, and the possible long-term implications of PID on her fertility.
- The woman completes her course of therapy and the PID is cured.

CARE OF THE WOMAN WITH AN ABNORMAL FINDING DURING PELVIC EXAMINATION

Abnormal Pap Smear Results

As discussed in Chapter 5 🌎, a Papanicolaou (Pap) smear is a cervical cytology test done to screen for the presence of cellular anomalies. Although the Pap smear is useful in detecting a variety of abnormalities, it has had its greatest impact on the detection of cervical cancer. The *Bethesda system* (Table 6–1) has become the most widely used system in the United States for reporting Pap smear results. Early detection of abnormalities allows changes to be treated before cells reach the precancerous or cancerous stage. Notification of an abnormal Pap smear usually causes anxiety for a woman, so it is important that she be told in a caring way. The woman needs accurate, complete information about the meaning of the results and the next steps to be taken. She should also be given time to ask questions and express her concerns.

Colposcopy, the direct, detailed visualization and examination of the cervix, has become a common second step in many cases of abnormal Pap smears. The examination, done in an office or clinic, permits more detailed visualization of the cervix in bright light, using a high-magnification microscope. The cervix can be visualized directly and again following application of acetic acid. The acetic acid causes abnormal epithelium to assume a characteristic white appearance. The colposcope can also be used to obtain a directed biopsy.

Ovarian Masses

Ovarian masses may be palpated during the pelvic examination. Between 70% and 80% of ovarian masses are benign. More than 50% are functional cysts (cysts that develop from ovarian follicles, from the corpus luteum, or from the theca luteum), occurring most commonly in women 20 to 40 years of age. Functional cysts are rare in women who take oral contraceptives. Ovarian cysts usually represent physiologic variations in the menstrual cycle. Dermoid cysts (cystic teratomas) and endometriomas, or "chocolate cysts," are common types of ovarian masses. No relationship exists between ovarian masses and ovarian cancer. However, ovarian cancer is the most fatal of all cancers in women because it is difficult to diagnose and often has spread throughout the pelvis before it is detected. Refer to medical-surgical nursing texts for an in-depth discussion of ovarian cancer.

Many women with a benign ovarian mass are asymptomatic; the mass may be noted on a routine pelvic examination. Others experience a sensation of fullness or cramping in the lower abdomen (often unilateral), dyspareunia, irregular bleeding, or delayed menstruation. Diagnosis is made on the basis of a palpable mass with or without tenderness and other related symptoms. Radiography or ultrasonography may be used to assist in the diagnosis.

The woman is often kept under observation for a month or two because most cysts resolve on their own and are harmless. Oral contraceptives may be prescribed for 1 to 2 months to suppress ovarian function. If this regimen is effective, a repeat pelvic examination should be normal. If the mass is still present after 60 days of observation and oral contraceptive therapy, a diagnostic laparoscopy or laparotomy may be considered. Tubal or ovarian lesions, ectopic pregnancy, cancer, infection, or appendicitis also must be ruled out before a diagnosis can be confirmed.

Surgery is not always necessary but is considered if the mass is larger than 6 to 7 cm in circumference; if the woman is over 40 years of age with an adnexal mass, a persistent mass, or continuous pain; or if the woman is taking oral contraceptives. Surgical exploration is also indicated when a palpable mass is found in an infant, a young girl, or a postmenopausal woman.

Women may need clear explanations about why the initial therapy is observation. A discussion of the origin and resolution of ovarian cysts may clarify this treatment plan. If a surgical treatment removes or impairs the function of one ovary, the woman needs to be assured that the remaining ovary can be expected to take over ovarian functioning and that pregnancy is still possible if desired.

Uterine Abnormalities

Fibroid tumors, or *leiomyomas,* are among the most common benign disease entities in women and are the most common reason for gynecologic surgery. Between 20% and 50% of reproductive age women develop leiomyomas (Matthews & Hurst, 2010). The potential for cancer is minimal. Leiomyomas are more common in women of African heritage.

Most uterine fibroid tumors are asymptomatic and require no treatment. Treatment is indicated when fibroids cause symptoms such as lower abdominal pain, fullness or pressure,

Table 6–1	The Bethesda System for Classifying Pap Smears

Specimen Type

Indicate conventional smear (Pap smear) vs. liquid based vs. other

Specimen Adequacy

Satisfactory for evaluation *(describe presence or absence of endocervical/transformation zone component and any other quality indicators, e.g., partially obscuring blood inflammation, etc.)*
Unsatisfactory for evaluation . . . *(specify reason)*
Specimen rejected/not processed *(specify reason)*
Specimen processed and examined, but unsatisfactory for evaluation of epithelial abnormality because of *(specify reason)*

General Categorization (optional)

Negative for intraepithelial lesion or malignancy.
Epithelial cell abnormality. See Interpretation/Result *(specify squamous or glandular as appropriate).*
Other: See Interpretation/Result *(e.g., endometrial cells in a woman ≥40 years of age).*

Automated Review

If case examined by automated device, specify device and result.

Ancillary Testing

Provide a brief description of the test methods and report the result so that it is easily understood by the clinician.

Interpretation/Result

Negative for intraepithelial lesion or malignancy (when there is no cellular evidence of neoplasia, state this in the General Categorization above and/or in the Interpretation/Result section of the report, whether or not there are organisms or other nonneoplastic findings)
  ORGANISMS:
    Trichomonas vaginalis
    Fungal organisms morphologically consistent with *Candida* spp.
    Shift in flora suggestive of bacterial vaginosis
    Bacteria morphologically consistent with *Actinomyces* spp.
    Cellular changes associated with herpes simplex virus
  OTHER NONNEOPLASTIC FINDINGS *(Optional to report list not inclusive)*
  Reactive cellular changes associated with
  —inflammation (includes typical repair)
  —radiation
  —intrauterine contraceptive device (IUD)
  Glandular cells status post-hysterectomy
  Atrophy

Other

Endometrial cells (in a woman ≥40 years of age) (Specify if negative for squamous intraepithelial lesion)
Epithelial cell abnormalities
SQUAMOUS CELL
  Atypical squamous cells
    —of undetermined significance (ASC-US)
    —cannot exclude HSIL (ASC-H)
  Low-grade squamous intraepithelial lesion (LSIL)
    —encompassing HPV/mild dysplasia/CIN-1
  High-grade squamous intraepithelial lesion (HSIL)
    —encompassing moderate and severe dysplasia CIS/CIN-2
      and CIN-3
    —with features suspicious for invasion *(if invasion is suspected)*
  Squamous cell carcinoma
GLANDULAR CELL
  Atypical
    —endocervical cells *(NOS or specify in comments)*
    —endometrial cells *(NOS or specify in comments)*
    —glandular cells *(NOS or specify in comments)*
  Atypical
    —endocervical cells, favor neoplastic
    —glandular cells, favor neoplastic
  Endocervical adenocarcinoma in situ
  Adenocarcinoma
    —endocervical
    —endometrial
    —extrauterine
    —not otherwise specified (NOS)
Other malignant neoplasms (specify)

Educational Notes and Suggestions (optional)

Suggestions should be concise and consistent with clinical follow-up guidelines published by professional organizations (references to relevant publications may be included).

Source: Courtesy of National Cancer Institute.

menorrhagia, metrorrhagia, or increased dysmenorrhea. Ultrasonography revealing masses or nodules can assist and confirm the diagnosis. Leiomyoma is also considered a possible diagnosis when masses or nodules involving the uterus are palpated on a pelvic examination.

The majority of these masses require no treatment and will shrink after menopause. Close observation for symptoms or an increase in size of the uterus or the masses is the only management most women need.

If a woman is troubled by symptoms, or pelvic examination reveals that the mass is increasing in size, interventions are recommended. Gonadotropin-releasing hormone (GnRH) analogs such as Lupron are used off-label to reduce the size and subsequent bleeding due to these tumors. Once discontinued, however, growth of the fibroid can reoccur. Treatment with GnRH analogs may be used before surgery to reduce the size of the fibroid and decrease complications. *Myomectomy* (surgical removal of the fibroid) is used most often if the woman wishes to maintain her ability to have a child. However, fibroids may regrow after myomectomy. *Hysterectomy* is often used to treat fibroids when the primary symptom is heavy menstrual bleeding. *Uterine artery embolization (UAE)* has become a viable alternative for the woman who wishes to avoid surgery and retain her uterus (Moss, Cooper, Khaund, et al., 2011). Small particles are injected through a catheter placed in the umbilical artery. These particles block the blood supply to the fibroid, leading to shrinkage and symptom relief. If symptoms recur, hysterectomy may be necessary.

Endometrial cancer, most commonly a disease of postmenopausal women, has a high rate of cure if detected early. The hallmark sign is vaginal bleeding in postmenopausal women not treated with hormone replacement therapy. Endometrial biopsy, transvaginal ultrasound, and post-hysterectomy pathologic examination of the uterus are used in the diagnosis. The treatment is total abdominal hysterectomy (TAH) and bilateral salpingo-oophorectomy (BSO). Radiation therapy may also be indicated, depending on the stage of the cancer.

Nursing Management

Pelvic examinations and Pap smears are not done by nurses except those with special training. In most cases, nursing assessment is directed toward an evaluation of the woman's understanding of the findings and their implications and her psychosocial response.

The woman needs accurate information on etiology, symptomatology, and treatment options. Encourage her to report symptoms and keep appointments for follow-up examination and evaluation. The woman needs realistic reassurance if her condition is benign; she may require counseling and effective emotional support if a malignancy is likely. If the management plan includes surgery, she may need the nurse's support in obtaining a second opinion and making her decision about treatment.

CARE OF THE WOMAN WITH A URINARY TRACT INFECTION

A **urinary tract infection (UTI)**, defined as significant bacteriuria in the presence of symptoms, is one of the most common problems women experience. Estimates indicate that more than 60% of women will experience a UTI in their lifetime (Minkin, 2011). Bacteria usually enter the body by way of the urethra. The organisms are capable of migrating against the downward flow of urine. The shortness of the female urethra facilitates the passage of bacteria into the bladder. Other conditions associated with bacterial entry are relative incompetence of the urinary sphincter, frequent enuresis (bed-wetting) before adolescence, and urinary catheterization. Wiping from back to front after urination may transfer bacteria from the anorectal area to the urethra. Voluntarily suppressing the desire to urinate is a predisposing factor. Retention overdistends the bladder and can lead to an infection. Sexual activity is a strong risk factor for UTI, especially in younger women. General poor health or lowered resistance to infection can increase a woman's susceptibility to UTI.

Asymptomatic bacteriuria (ASB) (bacteria in the urine actively multiplying without accompanying clinical symptoms) is a condition that becomes especially significant if the woman is pregnant because, if untreated, ASB can lead to pyelonephritis in the pregnant woman and low birth weight in the newborn (Lumbiganon, Laopaiboon, & Thinkhamrop, 2010). ASB is almost always caused by a single organism, typically *Escherichia coli*. A woman who has had a UTI is susceptible to recurrent infection. If a pregnant woman develops an acute UTI, especially with a high temperature, amniotic fluid infection may develop and retard the growth of the placenta.

Lower Urinary Tract Infection

Because UTIs are ascending, it is important to recognize and diagnose a lower UTI early to avoid the sequelae associated with an upper UTI. *Cystitis*, or inflammation of the bladder, usually occurs secondary to an ascending infection. *E. coli* is present in the majority of cases. Other common causative organisms include *Klebsiella pneumonia, Proteus mirabilis, Enterococcus* species, and *Staphylococcus saprophyticus*.

When cystitis develops, the initial symptom is often dysuria, specifically at the end of urination. Urgency and frequency also occur. Cystitis is usually accompanied by a low-grade fever (38.3°C [101°F] or lower), and hematuria is occasionally seen. Urine specimens usually contain an abnormal number of leukocytes and bacteria. Diagnosis is made with a urine culture.

Treatment depends on the causative organism. Nitrofurantoin has reemerged as an effective first-line therapy and is given twice daily for 5 days. A 3-day, twice daily course of oral trimethoprim-sulfamethoxazole (TMP-SMZ) is recommended as a viable alternative if local resistance to it is low. Fluoroquinolones (FQ) such as ciprofloxacin, levofloxacin, gatifloxacin, or norfloxacin should be reserved for treatment failures and for women with suspected upper UTI infection (Schultz & Edson, 2011).

Upper Urinary Tract Infection (Pyelonephritis)

Pyelonephritis (inflammatory disease of the kidneys) is less common but more serious than cystitis and is often preceded by lower UTI. It is more common during the latter part of pregnancy or early postpartum and poses a serious threat to maternal and fetal well-being. Women with symptoms of pyelonephritis during pregnancy have an increased risk of preterm birth and of intrauterine growth restriction.

Acute pyelonephritis has a sudden onset, with chills, high temperature of 39.6°C to 40.6°C (103°F to 105°F), and flank pain (either unilateral or bilateral). The right side is almost always involved if the woman is pregnant, because the large bulk of intestines to the left pushes the uterus to the right, putting pressure on the right ureter and kidney. Nausea, vomiting, and general malaise may ensue. With accompanying cystitis, the woman may experience frequency, urgency, and burning with urination.

Edema of the renal parenchyma or ureteritis with blockage and swelling of the ureter may lead to temporary suppression of urinary output. This is accompanied by severe colicky (spastic, intense) pain, vomiting, dehydration, and ileus of the large bowel. Women with acute pyelonephritis generally have increased diastolic blood pressure, positive fluorescent antibody titer (FA test), low creatinine clearance, significant bacteremia in urine culture, pyuria, and presence of white blood cell casts.

Many women can be treated as outpatients or given IV fluids and one IV dose of antibiotics, then discharged on oral medications. Fluoroquinolones are the first-line treatment in communities where FQ resistance is low, specifically ciprofloxacin, extended-release ciprofloxacin, or levofloxacin. If local FQ resistance is high, an initial dose of ceftriaxone or gentamicin is given followed by an oral FQ regimen (Colgan, Williams, & Johnson, 2011).

A woman who is severely ill or has complications may require hospitalization. She is started on intravenous antibiotics. Therapy also includes IV hydration, urinary analgesics such as Pyridium, pain management, and medications to manage fever. In the case of obstructive pyelonephritis, a blood culture is necessary. The woman is kept on bed rest. After the sensitivity report is received, the antibiotic is changed as necessary. If signs of urinary obstruction occur or continue, the ureter may be catheterized to establish adequate drainage.

With appropriate drug therapy, the woman's temperature should return to normal. The pain subsides and the urine shows no bacteria within 2 to 3 days. Follow-up urinary cultures are needed to determine that the infection has been eliminated completely.

NURSING MANAGEMENT *For the Woman with a Urinary Tract Infection*

Nursing Assessment and Diagnosis

During a woman's visit, obtain a sexual and medical history to identify whether she is at risk for UTI. A clean-catch urine specimen is evaluated for evidence of asymptomatic bacteriuria (ASB).

Nursing diagnoses that may apply to a woman with an upper UTI include the following (NANDA-I © 2012):

- *Pain, Acute,* related to dysuria, systemic discomforts, or renal pain secondary to UTI
- *Fear* related to the possible long-term effects of the disease

Planning and Implementation

Give the woman information to help her recognize the signs of UTI. Also discuss hygiene practices, the advantages of wearing cotton underwear, and the need to void frequently to prevent urinary stasis. Stress the importance of maintaining a good fluid intake. UTIs usually respond quickly to treatment, but follow-up clinical evaluation and urine cultures are important. See *Teaching Highlights: Preventing Cystitis.*

Evaluation

Expected outcomes of nursing care include the following:

- The woman completes her prescribed course of antibiotic therapy.
- The woman's infection is cured.
- The woman incorporates preventive self-care measures into her daily regimen.

PELVIC RELAXATION

A **cystocele** is the downward displacement of the bladder, which appears as a bulge in the anterior vaginal wall. Genetic predisposition, childbearing, obesity, and increased age are factors that may contribute to cystocele. Symptoms of stress urinary incontinence (SUI) are most common, including loss of urine

---

Teaching Highlights Preventing Cystitis

Following is information for women about ways to avoid cystitis:

- If you use a diaphragm for contraception, try changing methods or using another size of diaphragm.
- Avoid bladder irritants such as alcohol, caffeine products, and carbonated beverages.
- Increase fluid intake, especially water, to a minimum of six to eight glasses per day.
- Make regular urination a habit; avoid long waits.
- Practice good genital hygiene, including wiping from front to back after urination and bowel movements.
- Be aware that vigorous or frequent sexual activity may contribute to the development of urinary tract infections.
- Urinate before and after intercourse to empty the bladder and cleanse the urethra.
- Complete medication regimens even if symptoms decrease.
- Do not use medication left over from previous infections.
- Drink cranberry juice to acidify the urine. This has been found to relieve symptoms in some cases.

---

with coughing, sneezing, laughing, or sudden exertion. Vaginal fullness, a bulging out of the vaginal wall, or a dragging sensation may also be noticeable.

If pelvic relaxation is mild, Kegel exercises help restore tone. The exercises involve contraction and relaxation of the pubococcygeal muscle (see the *Perineal Exercises* section in Chapter 11 🔗 for more information). Women have found these exercises helpful before and after childbirth in maintaining vaginal muscle tone. Estrogen may improve the condition of vaginal mucous membranes, especially in menopausal women.

Duloxetine, a balanced serotonin and norepinephrine reuptake inhibitor used to treat major depressive disorders and the pain of fibromyalgia or diabetic neuropathy, is the only medication shown to help decrease SUI. Although approved for the treatment of SUI in the European Union, it is not approved for that purpose in the United States, and its administration would be an off-label use (Elliott & Sokol, 2011). Vaginal pessaries or rings may be used if surgery is undesirable or impossible or until surgery can be scheduled. Surgery may be considered for cystoceles considered moderate to severe.

The nurse can instruct the woman in the use of Kegel exercises. Information on causes and contributing factors and discussion of possible alternative therapies greatly help the woman.

A **rectocele** may develop when the posterior vaginal wall is weakened. The anterior wall of the rectum can then sag forward, ballooning into the vagina, pushing the weakened posterior wall of the vagina in front of it. When the woman strains to have a bowel movement, a pocket of rectum develops that traps stool, and constipation results. To defecate, a woman with a rectocele may find it necessary to press the tissue between the vagina and rectum, which elevates the rectocele.

Diagnosis is based on history and physical examination. Decisions about treatment are based on the size of the rectocele, the presence and severity of symptoms, and the woman's individual situation, including her overall health. Surgery is often indicated.

Uterine prolapse occurs when the uterus protrudes downward (drops) into the upper vagina, pulling the vagina with it. The extent of the prolapse is determined by the location of the cervix in the vagina. In severe cases the uterus may prolapse below the vaginal introitus. The woman may report a "dragging" sensation in her groin and a backache over the sacrum, which is caused by pulling on the uterosacral ligaments. Typically these symptoms are relieved when the woman lies down. As with cystocele, conservative treatment includes the use of topical or systemic estrogen and vaginal pessaries. Surgery for uterine prolapse often involves hysterectomy and repair of the prolapsed vaginal walls.

CARE OF THE WOMAN REQUIRING A HYSTERECTOMY

Hysterectomy is the surgical removal of the uterus. In the United States, it is the most common nonpregnancy-related surgical procedure that women undergo. Removal of the uterus through a surgical incision is called a *total abdominal hysterectomy (TAH),* and removal of both fallopian tubes and ovaries is called a *bilateral salpingo-oophorectomy (BSO).* When both procedures are performed at the same time it is called a TAH-BSO. When the uterus is removed through the vagina, it is termed a *total vaginal hysterectomy (TVH).*

A laparoscopic-assisted vaginal hysterectomy (LAVH) may also be used. In this technique, the surgeon inserts the laparoscope through an incision near the umbilicus and uses it to assist with visualization and dissection to facilitate vaginal removal of the uterus. The benefit is that the surgeon can achieve results similar to those of a TAH without a large abdominal incision.

Abdominal hysterectomy is the usual treatment for several conditions, including cancer of the cervix, endometrium, or ovary; large fibroids; severe endometriosis; chronic PID; and adenomyosis. TAH is preferred when cancer is expected because it permits easier exploration of the abdomen. It is also helpful when large uterine masses are present.

Vaginal hysterectomy is generally done for pelvic relaxation, abnormal uterine bleeding, or small fibroids. Advantages of vaginal hysterectomy include earlier ambulation, less postoperative pain, less anesthesia and operative time, less blood loss, no visible scar, and a shorter hospital stay. The major disadvantage is the increased risk of trauma to the bladder.

NURSING CARE MANAGEMENT *For the Woman Requiring a Hysterectomy*

Nursing Assessment and Diagnosis

Preoperatively the nurse needs to identify the woman's physiologic and psychologic needs as she approaches surgery. Additionally it is important to evaluate her learning needs in relation to the surgery and its implications postoperatively. In assessing the woman, consider her age, her culture and educational level, the attitudes of her partner and family, her preoperative status, and whether the hysterectomy is being performed because of a cancer diagnosis. The significance of her reproductive health to her self-image is also a consideration.

Nursing diagnoses that may apply to a woman having a hysterectomy include the following (NANDA-I © 2012):

- ■ *Knowledge, Deficient,* related to a lack of information about preoperative routines, postoperative activities, and expected postoperative changes
- ■ *Fear* related to the risk of possible surgical complications

Planning and Implementation

Preoperative teaching should include information about the procedure, expected preparation, type of anesthesia to be used, possible risks and complications, postoperative care routines, and expected recovery time (Figure 6–5 ●).

Routine postoperative care includes monitoring of physiologic and emotional responses and implementation of nursing interventions to ensure physical well-being and comfort. The woman should be aware of possible complications and when to follow up with her surgeon. Follow up with the woman regarding any psychosocial implications discussed preoperatively, such as support at home and potential for sadness or depression related to perception of changed sexuality or self-image.

Evaluation

Expected outcomes of nursing care include the following:

- ■ The woman can discuss the reasons for her hysterectomy and the type of procedure performed, the alternatives, and aspects of self-care following surgery.
- ■ The woman has an uneventful recovery without complications.
- ■ The woman participates in decision making about her care.
- ■ The woman can identify available resources if she has physical or emotional concerns in the postoperative period.

● **Figure 6–5** The nurse provides information for the woman during preoperative teaching.

Critical Concept Review

LEARNING OUTCOME 6.1: Contrast the contributing factors, signs and symptoms, treatment options, and nursing care management of women with common benign breast disorders.

1. Fibrocystic breast changes:
   - May be caused by an imbalance in progesterone and estrogen.
   - Breasts have increased tenderness and swelling before beginning of menses.
   - Sodium and caffeine restriction may help.
2. Fibroadenoma:
   - Freely movable solid benign tumor.
   - Asymptomatic and nontender.
   - Surgically removed if malignancy is suspected.

3. Intraductal papilloma:
   - Tumor within the ductal system of the breast.
   - Potentially malignant.
   - Most frequent cause of nipple discharge.
   - Must be surgically removed.
4. Duct ectasia (comedomastitis):
   - Inflammation of duct behind the nipple.
   - Occurs during or near menopause.
   - Treatment is symptom relief or surgical removal.

LEARNING OUTCOME 6.2: Explain the signs and symptoms, medical therapy, and implications for fertility of endometriosis.

1. Signs and symptoms:
   - Pelvic pain
   - Dyspareunia
   - Abnormal uterine bleeding
2. Treatment:
   - Surgical removal of visible endometrial tissue.
   - Oral contraceptives.
   - Hormonal therapy.
   - Surgical removal of uterus and ovaries in severe cases if childbearing is not an issue.
3. Implications for fertility:
   - Pregnancy must be delayed until oral contraceptive or hormonal therapy is over, due to suppression of the menstrual cycle.

LEARNING OUTCOME 6.3: Discuss the signs and symptoms, treatment options, and health implications of polycystic ovarian syndrome (PCOS).

1. Signs and symptoms:
   - Menstrual dysfunction, most often anovulation
   - Signs of androgen excess including hirsutism, acne, deepening voice, increased muscle mass
   - Obesity
   - Hyperinsulinemia
   - Infertility
2. Treatment options:
   - If pregnancy not an immediate issue, combined oral contraceptives
   - If pregnancy desired, antiandrogens (spironolactone), metformin to inhibit glucose production and improve ovarian function
   - Lifestyle changes including weight loss, regular exercise, balanced diet, no smoking
3. Health implications:
   - Increased risk for type 2 diabetes, hypertension, cardiovascular disease, and certain cancers

LEARNING OUTCOME 6.4: Summarize the risk factors, treatment options, and nursing interventions for women with toxic shock syndrome.

1. Risk factors:
   - Use of superabsorbent tampons
   - Use of cervical cap or diaphragm during menses
2. Treatment options:
   - IV fluids for hydration
   - Broad-spectrum antibiotics
3. Nursing interventions:
   - Instruct women about proper use of superabsorbent tampons, cervical caps, and diaphragms.
   - Instruct women not to use tampons for first 6–8 weeks after childbirth.

LEARNING OUTCOME 6.5: Compare the causes, signs and symptoms, treatment options, and nursing care for women with vulvovaginal candidiasis versus bacterial vaginosis.

1. Vulvovaginal candidiasis:
   - Most common form of vaginitis.
   - Related to use of oral contraceptives, immunosuppressants, and antibiotics.
   - Thick, curdy, white vaginal discharge.
   - Severe itching, dysuria, and dyspareunia.
   - Treated topically or systemically with antifungal drugs.
2. Bacterial vaginosis:
   - Caused by an alteration in normal vaginal bacterial flora.
   - Most common cause of vaginal discharge or odor.
   - Thin vaginal discharge with a "fishy" smell.
   - Treated with metronidazole (Flagyl).

LEARNING OUTCOME 6.6: Compare the common sexually transmitted infections with regard to their etiology, treatment options, nursing care, and methods of prevention.

1. Trichomoniasis:
   - Yellow-green, frothy, odorous discharge.
   - Causes vaginal itching.
   - Both partners are treated with metronidazole (Flagyl).
2. Chlamydial infection:
   - May cause disease in newborn.
   - Often asymptomatic.
   - Both partners are treated with doxycycline or azithromycin.

3. Gonorrhea:
   - May cause pelvic inflammatory disease.
   - Often asymptomatic.
   - Purulent, green-yellow discharge, dysuria, and urinary frequency.
   - Both partners are treated with antibiotics.
4. Herpes genitalis:
   - Cannot be cured.
   - Recurrences may be triggered by physical or emotional stress.
   - Treatment with antiviral medication may decrease length of outbreak.
   - May cause fatal fetal infection if herpes lesion is present in genital tract during childbirth.
5. Syphilis:
   - Testing for disease is required during pregnancy.
   - Treated with penicillin.
6. Human papillomavirus (HPV)/condylomata acuminata:
   - Genital warts.
   - Certain forms of HPV have been linked to cervical cancer.
   - Treatment is removal of warts by chemical or surgical means.

7. Acquired immunodeficiency syndrome (AIDS):
   - Fatal disorder caused by the human immunodeficiency virus (HIV).
   - Has profound implications for the fetus if infected woman is pregnant.
8. The nurse must provide the woman with information about:
   - The infection
   - Methods of transmission of the infection
   - Implications of the infection on present pregnancy, future fertility, and general health
   - Importance of completion of treatment
   - Treatment of both partners
   - Need for abstinence until treatment is completed

LEARNING OUTCOME 6.7: Summarize the pathology, signs and symptoms, treatment, nursing care, and implications for future fertility of pelvic inflammatory disease (PID).

1. Pathology:
   - Often caused by chlamydia or gonorrhea.
   - Infection may cause scarring of fallopian tubes, preventing union of sperm and ova.
2. Signs and symptoms:
   - Chills and fever
   - Purulent vaginal discharge
   - Irregular vaginal bleeding
   - Nausea and vomiting
3. Treatment:
   - Antibiotics (IV or PO)
   - Treatment of sexual partner

LEARNING OUTCOME 6.8: Identify the implications of an abnormal finding during a pelvic examination in the provision of nursing care.

1. Abnormal Pap smear results:
   - May indicate abnormal cervical cells or cervical malignancy.
2. Ovarian masses:
   - May indicate cysts or malignancy.
   - Cysts are often observed closely unless they cause symptoms.
3. Uterine abnormalities:
   - Fibroid tumors are most common.
   - May be observed or removed depending on symptoms of woman.

LEARNING OUTCOME 6.9: Contrast the causes, signs and symptoms, treatment options, and nursing care for women with cystitis versus pyelonephritis.

1. Cystitis:
   - Infection of lower urinary tract.
   - Often causes dysuria, urgency, and frequency.
   - Treated with PO antibiotics.
2. Pyelonephritis:
   - Infection of upper urinary tract.
   - May be preceded by lower urinary tract infection.
   - Sudden onset of chills, high temperature, and flank pain.
   - May also have dysuria, urgency, and frequency.
   - More serious than cystitis.
   - Treated with IV or PO antibiotics.

Clinical Reasoning in Action

Linda Knoll, 35 years old, presents to you at the GYN clinic for her annual physical and pelvic exam. You obtain the following menstrual history: LMP 8 days ago. Periods occur every 29 days and last 5 days. She tells you that she uses super-absorbent tampons during the first 2 days of her period and then changes to regular absorbency tampons for the duration, and that she currently has an IUD in place for contraception. She tells you that her husband has been complaining for the past few months that she seems irritable, tense, and moody near "that time of the month." Linda admits that she doesn't feel well before her period and describes having low pelvic discomfort, breast tenderness, "bloating," and some constipation. She seems to cry easily 2 to 3 days before her period. She has noticed this pattern over the last 4 or 5 months. You recognize these symptoms as related to premenstrual syndrome (PMS). Linda asks you if these changes are due to female hormones.

1. How would you answer Linda's question concerning female hormones?
2. After reviewing Linda's diet with her, what would you recommend to help?
3. Linda has an IUD in place. What other type of contraceptive might help reduce the symptoms of PMS?
4. What other activities can you suggest to help Linda reduce PMS symptoms?
5. What should you tell Linda about using tampons during heavy menstrual flow?

See www.nursing.pearsonhighered.com for possible responses.

References

Akhter, S., Beckmann, K., & Gorelick, M. (2009). Update on sexually transmitted infections, 2008. *Pediatric Emergency Care, 25*(9), 608–618.

American College of Obstetricians and Gynecologists (ACOG). (2012). *FAQ: Dysmenorrhea.* Retrieved from http://www.acog.org/~/media/For%20Patients/faq046.pdf?dmc=1&ts=20121227T1451215783

Azavedo, E. (2009). Breast, nipple discharge evaluation. *E-Medicine Radiology.* Retrieved from http://www.emedicine.medscape.com/article/347305

Centers for Disease Control and Prevention (CDC). (2009). *Trends in reportable sexually transmitted diseases in the United States, 2007: National surveillance data for chlamydia, gonorrhea, and syphilis.* Retrieved from http://www.cdc.gov

Centers for Disease Control and Prevention (CDC). (2010). Sexually transmitted diseases treatment guidelines, 2010. *Mortality and Morbidity Weekly Report, 59*(RR-12), 1–114.

Centers for Disease Control and Prevention (CDC). (2011a). *ACIP recommends all 11–12 year old males get vaccinated against HPV.* Retrieved from http://www.cdc.gov/media/releases/2011/t1025_hpv_12yroldvaccine.html

Centers for Disease Control and Prevention (CDC). (2011b). *Sexually transmitted disease surveillance 2010.* Atlanta, GA: U.S. Department of Health and Human Services.

Colgan, R., Williams, M., & Johnson, J. R. (2011). Diagnosis and treatment of acute pyelonephritis in women. *American Family Physician, 84*(5), 519–526.

Eaton, D. K., Kann, L., Kinchen, S., Shanklin, S., Ross, J., Hawkins, J., . . . Wechsler, H. (2010). Youth risk behavior surveillance—United States, 2009. *Morbidity and Mortality Weekly Report, 59*(SS-5), 1–148.

Elliott, C. S., & Sokol, E. R. (2011). New techniques for treating stress urinary incontinence. *Contemporary OB/GYN, 56*(1), 28–38.

Fantasia, H. C., Fontenot, H. B., Sutherland, M., & Harris, A. L. (2011). Sexually transmitted infections in women: An overview. *Nursing for Women's Health, 15*(1), 46–57.

Firouzabadi, R., Aflatoonian, A., Modarresi, S., Sekhavat, L., & Taheri, S. (2012). Therapeutic effects of calcium and vitamin D supplementation in women with PCOS. *Complementary Therapies in Clinical Practice, 18,* 85–88.

Guzick, D., & Hoeger, K. (2009). *Clinical updates in women's health care. Polycystic ovary syndrome* (Vol. VIII, No. 1). Washington, DC: American College of Obstetricians and Gynecologists.

Holland-Hall, C. (2012). Pelvic inflammatory disease. *The Female Patient, 37*(5), 23–29.

Lee, E. (2009). Evidence-based management of benign breast diseases. *American Journal for Nurse Practitioners, 13*(7/8), 22–31.

Lumbiganon, P., Laopaiboon, M., & Thinkhamrop, J. (2010). Screening and treating asymptomatic bacteriuria in pregnancy. *Current Opinion in Obstetrics and Gynecology, 22,* 95–99.

Marsh, K., Steinbeck, K., Atkinson, F., Petoca, P., & Brand-Miller, J. (2010). Effect of a low glycemic index compared with a conventional healthy diet on polycystic ovary syndrome. *American Journal of Clinical Nutrition, 92*(1), 83–92.

Matthews, M. L., & Hurst, B. S. (2010). Fibroids and assisted reproduction. *The Female Patient, 35*(10), 18–25.

McFarland, C. (2012). Treating polycystic ovary syndrome and infertility. *American Journal of Maternal/Child Nursing, 37*(2), 116–121.

Minkin, M. J. (2011). Urinary tract infection 101: Diagnosis and therapy. *The Female Patient, 36*(10), 14–18.

Moran, L., Hutchison, S., Norman, R., & Teeded, H. (2011). Lifestyle changes in women with polycystic ovary syndrome. *Cochrane Database of Systematic Reviews.* NLM ID: 100909747.

Moss, J. G., Cooper, K. G., Khaund, A., Murray, L. S., Murray, G. D., Wu, O., . . . Lumsden, M. A. (2011). Randomized comparison of uterine artery embolization (UAE) with surgical treatment in patients with symptomatic uterine fibroids (REST trial): 5-year results. *BJOG: International Journal of Obstetrics & Gynaecology, 118,* 936–944.

Schindler, A. E. (2011). Dienogest in long-term treatment of endometriosis. *International Journal of Women's Health, 3,* 175–184.

Schultz, H. J., & Edson, R. S. (2011). Cystitis treatment in women, circa 2011: New role for an old drug. *Mayo Clinic Proceedings, 86*(6), 477–479.

Silversides, J. A., Lappin, E., & Ferguson, A. J. (2010). Staphylococcal toxic shock syndrome: Mechanisms and management. *Current Infectious Disease Reports, 12*(5), 392–400.

Smith, J. W., & Taylor, J. S. (2011). Polycystic ovarian syndrome: Evidence-based strategies for managing symptoms and preventing long-term sequelae. *Nursing for Women's Health, 15*(5), 403–410.

Sorensen, L., Soe, M., Halkier, K., Stigsby, B., & Astrup, A. (2012). Effects of increased dietary protein to carbohydrate ratios in women with polycystic ovary syndrome. *American Journal of Clinical Nutrition, 95*(1), 39–48.

Weiss, T. R., & Bulmer, S. M. (2011). Young women's experiences living with polycystic ovary syndrome. *Journal of Obstetric, Gynecologic & Neonatal Nursing, 40*(6), 709–718.

Families with Special Reproductive Concerns

As we sat in the in vitro clinic waiting room, I felt great apprehension. For 4 years we had been unable to conceive. I'd been through two surgeries, dozens of blood tests, and hormone drugs that made me irrational and emotional. It was difficult at times—I blamed myself, felt out of control, and had surprisingly painful reactions to seeing mothers with babies. We were on the brink of the most expensive infertility treatment—the last resort for most infertile couples. Was this the right thing to do? —Samantha, 38

Walter Hodges/Getty Images

LEARNING OUTCOMES

7.1 Compare the essential components of fertility with the possible causes of infertility.

7.2 Describe the elements of the preliminary investigation of infertility and the nurse's role in supporting/teaching patients during this phase.

7.3 Summarize the indications for the tests and associated treatments, including assisted reproductive technologies, that are done in an infertility workup.

7.4 Relate the physiologic and psychologic effects of infertility on a couple to the nursing management of the couple.

7.5 Describe the nurse's role as counselor, educator, and advocate for couples during infertility evaluation and treatment.

7.6 Identify couples who may benefit from preconceptual chromosomal analysis and prenatal testing when providing care to couples with special reproductive concerns.

7.7 Identify the characteristics of autosomal dominant, autosomal recessive, and X-linked (sex-linked) recessive disorders.

7.8 Compare prenatal and postnatal diagnostic procedures used to determine the presence of genetic disorders.

7.9 Examine the emotional impact on a couple undergoing genetic testing or coping with the birth of a baby with a genetic disorder, and explain the nurse's role in supporting the family undergoing genetic counseling.

Most couples who want children are able to conceive them with little difficulty. Pregnancy and childbirth usually take their normal course, and a healthy baby is born without problems. But some less fortunate couples are unable to fulfill their dream of having the desired baby because of infertility or genetic problems.

This chapter explores two particularly troubling reproductive problems facing some couples: the inability to conceive and the risk of bearing babies with genetic abnormalities.

INFERTILITY

Infertility, a lack of conception despite unprotected sexual intercourse for at least 12 months (American Society for Reproductive Medicine [ASRM], 2012d), has a profound emotional, psychologic, and economic impact on affected couples and society. The term *sterility* is applied when there is an absolute factor preventing reproduction. **Subfertility** is used to describe a couple who has difficulty conceiving because both partners have reduced fertility. The term *second infertility* is applied to couples who have been unable to conceive after one or more successful pregnancies or who cannot sustain a pregnancy.

In the United States approximately 15% of couples in their reproductive years are infertile (ASRM, 2012e). Public perception is that the incidence of infertility is increasing, but in fact there has been no significant change in the proportion of infertile couples in the United States. What has changed is the composition of the infertile population, which has increased in the age group 25 to 44 because of delayed childbearing and the entry of the baby boom cohort into this age range in Western society (Fritz & Speroff, 2011). The perception that infertility is on the rise may be related to the following factors (Fritz & Speroff, 2011):

- The increase in assisted reproductive techniques, which has increased the prognosis for many infertile couples
- The increase in availability and use of infertility services
- The increase in insurance coverage of more socioeconomic groups for diagnosis of and treatment for infertility
- The increased number of childless women over age 35 seeking medical attention for infertility

Essential Components of Fertility

Understanding the elements essential for normal fertility can help the nurse identify the many factors that may cause infertility. The components necessary for normal fertility are correlated with possible causes of deviation in Table 7–1. In couples who suffer infertility, about one third of infertility cases are a result of a male factor, one third are the result of a female factor, and one-third are the result of a problem with both partners, or unexplained infertility (ASRM, 2012c). Professional intervention can help approximately 65% of infertile couples achieve pregnancy.

Young couples with no history that is suggestive of reproductive disorders should be referred for infertility evaluation if they have been unable to conceive after at least 1 year of attempting to achieve pregnancy. An earlier workup is indicated in couples with positive history for fertility-lowering disease or advancing maternal age. If the woman is over age 35, it may be appropriate to refer the couple after only 6 months of unprotected intercourse without conception or earlier if clinically indicated (Matthews, 2011). The most important determinant of a couples' fertility is the age of the woman.

Table 7–1	Possible Causes of Infertility

Necessary Norms	Deviations from Normal
Female	
Favorable cervical mucus	Cervicitis, cervical stenosis, use of coital lubricants, antisperm antibodies (immunologic response)
Clear passage between cervix and tubes	Myomas, adhesions, adenomyosis, polyps, endometritis, cervical stenosis, endometriosis, congenital anomalies (e.g., septate uterus, diethylstilbestrol [DES] exposure)
Patent tubes with normal motility	Pelvic inflammatory disease, peritubal adhesions, endometriosis, intrauterine device (IUD), salpingitis (e.g., chlamydia, recurrent sexually transmitted infections [STIs]), neoplasm, ectopic pregnancy, tubal ligation
Ovulation and release of ova	Primary ovarian failure, polycystic ovarian disease, hypothyroidism, pituitary tumor, lactation, periovarian adhesions, endometriosis, premature ovarian failure, hyperprolactinemia, Turner syndrome
No obstruction between ovary and tubes	Adhesions, endometriosis, pelvic inflammatory disease
Endometrial preparation	Anovulation, luteal phase defect, malformation, uterine infection, Asherman syndrome
Male	
Normal semen analysis	Abnormalities of sperm or semen, polyspermia, congenital defect in testicular development, mumps after adolescence, cryptorchidism, infections, gonadal exposure to x-rays, chemotherapy, smoking, alcohol abuse, malnutrition, chronic or acute metabolic disease, medications (e.g., morphine, aspirin [ASA], ibuprofen), cocaine, marijuana use, constrictive underclothing, heat
Unobstructed genital tract	Infections, tumors, congenital anomalies, vasectomy, strictures, trauma, varicocele
Normal genital tract secretions	Infections, autoimmunity to semen, tumors
Ejaculate deposited at the cervix	Premature ejaculation, impotence, hypospadias, retrograde ejaculation (e.g., as can occur with diabetes), neurologic cord lesions, obesity (inhibiting adequate penetration)

Health Promotion *Healthy People 2020* Infertility Objectives

The *Healthy People 2020* objectives for infertile parents are as follows:

- Reduce the proportion of women ages 18 to 44 years who have impaired fecundity (i.e., a physical barrier preventing pregnancy or carrying a pregnancy to term).
- Reduce the proportion of men ages 18 to 44 years who have impaired fecundity

Initial Investigation: Physical and Psychosocial Issues

The easiest and least intrusive infertility testing approach is used first. Extensive testing for infertility is avoided until data confirm that the timing of intercourse and length of coital exposure have been adequate. The nurse provides information about the most fertile times to have intercourse during the menstrual cycle. Teaching the couple the signs and timing of ovulation, the most effective times for intercourse within the cycle, and other fertility awareness behaviors may solve the problem (see *Teaching Highlights: Suggestions for Improving Fertility*). Primary assessment, including a comprehensive history (with a discussion of genetic conditions) and physical examination for any obvious causes of infertility, is done before a costly, time-consuming, and emotionally trying investigation is initiated.

The initial infertility evaluation offers nurses a unique opportunity to initiate preconception counseling, thereby helping infertile couples maximize their chances of delivering a healthy baby. The use of prenatal vitamins is often one of the earliest recommendations made to women planning to conceive. Studies show that folic acid supplementation of at least 400 micrograms (0.4 mg/day) taken 1 to 3 months preconceptually and continued through the first trimester greatly reduces the incidence of neural tube defects such as anencephaly and spina bifida. Preconception is the optimal time to review the importance of rubella and varicella immunity and the risk of congenital anomalies associated with exposure. It also provides the opportunity to address risks associated with alcohol, tobacco, and medication use. Women may warrant a change in medications or stricter management of chronic illnesses.

Teaching Highlights Suggestions for Improving Fertility

- Avoid douching and artificial lubricants (gels, oils, saliva) that can alter sperm motility. Prevent alteration of pH of vagina and introduction of spermicidal agents.
- Promote retention of sperm. The male superior position with female remaining recumbent for at least 20 to 30 minutes after intercourse maximizes the number of sperm reaching the cervix.
- Avoid leakage of sperm. Elevate the woman's hips with a pillow after intercourse for 20 to 30 minutes to allow liquefaction of seminal fluid and motility of the sperm toward the egg. Avoid getting up to urinate or shower for 1 hour after intercourse.
- Maximize the potential for fertilization. Instruct the couple that it is optimal if sexual intercourse occurs every other day during the fertile period. Because each woman's menstrual cycle varies in

length, the fertile period can extend from cycle day (CD) 7 through CD 17. Note CD 1 is considered the first day of actual menstrual flow.
- Avoid emphasizing conception during sexual encounters to decrease anxiety and potential sexual dysfunction.
- Maintain adequate nutrition and reduce stress. Stress reduction techniques and good nutritional habits increase sperm production.
- Explore other methods to increase fertility awareness, such as home assessment of cervical mucus and basal body temperature (BBT) recordings, and use of a home ovulation predictor kit (tests luteinizing hormone (LH) surge to time intercourse).
- Consider incorporating culturally appropriate methods to enhance fertility.

The basic investigation depends on the couple's history and usually includes assessment of ovarian function, cervical mucus adequacy and receptivity to sperm, sperm adequacy, tubal patency, and the general condition of the pelvic organs.

The mutual desire to have children is a cornerstone of many marriages. A fertility problem is a deeply personal, emotion-laden area in a couple's life. The self-esteem of one or both partners may be threatened if the inability to conceive is perceived as a lack of virility or femininity. It is never easy to discuss one's sexual activity, especially when potentially irreversible problems with fertility exist. The nurse can provide comfort to couples by offering a sympathetic ear, a nonjudgmental approach, and appropriate information and instructions throughout the diagnostic and therapeutic process (McGrath, Samra, Zukowsky, et al., 2010). Because counseling includes discussion of very personal matters, nurses who are comfortable with their own sexuality are able to establish rapport and elicit relevant information from couples with fertility problems.

The first interview should involve both partners and include a comprehensive history and physical examination. Table 7–2 lists the items in a complete infertility physical workup and laboratory evaluation for both partners. Because about one third of cases of infertility are related to a male factor, a semen analysis should be one of the first diagnostic tests done before moving on to more invasive diagnostic procedures involving the woman. Figure 7–1 ● outlines the couple's history and physical exam data, diagnostic tests usually performed, and healthcare interventions used in cases of infertility.

Assessment of the Woman's Fertility

After a thorough history and physical examination, both partners may undergo tests to identify causes of infertility. A thorough female evaluation includes assessment of the hypothalamic-pituitary axis in terms of ovulatory function, as well as structure and function of the cervix, uterus, fallopian

tubes, and ovaries. See Chapter 3 ● for an in-depth discussion of the fertility cycle.

Evaluation of Ovulatory Factors

Ovulation problems account for approximately 20% of couples' infertility.

Basal Body Temperature Recording. One basic test of ovulatory function is the **basal body temperature (BBT)** recording, which aids in identifying follicular and luteal phase abnormalities. At the initial visit, the nurse instructs the woman in the technique of recording BBT on a special form. The woman is instructed to begin a new chart on the first day of every monthly cycle. The temperature can be taken with an oral or rectal thermometer that is calibrated by tenths of a degree, making slight temperature changes readily apparent. A special BBT thermometer may be used to measure temperatures only between 35.6°C and 37.8°C (96°F and 100°F) (Fritz & Speroff, 2011). In addition to the traditional or digital thermometers, tympanic thermometry, which provides a reading in only a few seconds, may also be a valid method.

The woman records daily variations on a temperature graph. The temperature graph shows a typical biphasic pattern during ovulatory cycles, whereas in anovulatory cycles it remains monophasic. The woman uses the readings on the temperature graph to detect ovulation and timing of intercourse (see Figure 7–2 ●).

Basal temperature for females in the preovulatory (follicular) phase is usually below 36.7°C (98°F). As ovulation approaches, production of estrogen increases and at its peak may cause a slight drop, then a rise, in the basal temperature. The slight drop in temperature before ovulation is often difficult to capture on the BBT chart. After ovulation, there is a surge of luteinizing hormone (LH), which stimulates production of progesterone. Because progesterone is thermogenic (produces heat), it causes a 0.3°C to 0.6°C (0.5°F to 1.0°F) sustained rise in basal temperature during the second half of the menstrual cycle (luteal phase).

Table 7–2	Initial Infertility Physical Workup and Laboratory Evaluations

Screening	Female	Male
Physical Examination	Assessment of height, weight, blood pressure, temperature, and general health status Endocrine evaluation of thyroid for exophthalmos, lid lag, tremor, or palpable gland Optic fundi evaluation for presence of increased intracranial pressure, especially in oligomenorrheal or amenorrheal women (possible pituitary tumor) Reproductive features (including breast and external genital area) Physical ability to tolerate pregnancy	General health (assessment of height, weight, blood pressure) Endocrine evaluation (e.g., presence of gynecomastia) Visual fields evaluation for bitemporal hemianopia (blindness in one half of the visual field) Abnormal hair patterns
Laboratory Examination (*Note:* Adequate reproductive hormones must be present.)	Complete blood count Sedimentation rate, if indicated Serology Urinalysis Rh factor and blood grouping Rubella IgG Follicle-stimulating hormone (FSH) level regardless of age and regularity of menstrual cycles If indicated depending on age and regularity of menstrual cycles: thyroid-stimulating hormone (TSH), prolactin levels (PRL), glucose tolerance test, hormonal assays including estradiol (E_2), luteinizing hormone (LH), midluteal progesterone (MLP), dehydroepiandrosterone (DHEA), androstenedione, testosterone, 17 alpha-hydroxyprogesterone (17–OHP).	Complete blood count Sedimentation rate, if indicated Serology Urinalysis Rh factor and blood grouping Semen analysis If indicated, testicular biopsy, buccal smear (to determine number of Barr bodies) Hormonal assays, FSH, LH, prolactin
Gender-Specific Examinations	**Pelvic Examination** Papanicolaou (PAP) smear Culture for gonorrhea if indicated and possibly chlamydia or mycoplasma culture (opinions vary) Signs of vaginal infections (see Chapter 6 🩸) Shape of escutcheon (e.g., does pubic hair distribution resemble that of a male?) Size of clitoris (enlargement caused by endocrine disorders) Evaluation of cervix: old lacerations, tears, erosion, polyps, condition and shape of os, signs of infections, cervical mucus (evaluate for estrogen effect of spinnbarkeit and cervical ferning) **Rectovaginal Examination** Presence of retroflexed or retroverted uterus Presence of rectouterine pouch masses Presence of possible endometriosis **Bimanual Examination** Size, shape, position, and motility of uterus Presence of congenital anomalies Evaluation for endometriosis Evaluation of adnexa: ovarian size, cysts, fixations, or tumors	**Urologic Examination** Presence or absence of phimosis (narrowing of the preputial orifice) Location of urethral meatus Size and consistency of each testis, vas deferens, and epididymis Presence of varicocele (enlargement of spermatic cord veins above testicles) **Rectal Examination** Size and consistency of prostate, with microscopic evaluation of prostate fluid for signs of infection Size and consistency of seminal vesicles

Immediately before or coincident with the onset of menses, the temperature again falls below 36.7°C (98°F). These changes in the basal temperature create the typical biphasic pattern. Figure 7–2B shows a biphasic ovulatory BBT chart. Temperature elevation does not predict the day of ovulation, but it does provide supportive evidence of ovulation about a day after it has occurred.

Although there are other, more reliable methods to detect ovulatory function, BBT offers couples a low-tech, noninvasive, and inexpensive option. Based on serial BBT charts, the clinician might recommend sexual intercourse *every other day* beginning 3 to 4 days before and continuing for 2 to 3 days after the expected time of ovulation. See *Teaching Highlights: Methods of Determining Ovulation.*

Hormonal Assessments of Ovulatory Function.   Hormonal assessments of ovulatory function fall into the following categories.

1. *Gonadotropin levels (FSH, LH).* Baseline hormonal assessment of FSH and LH provides valuable information about normal ovulatory function. Measured on cycle day (CD) 3,

● **Figure 7–1** Flowchart for management of the infertile couple.

FSH is the single most valuable test of ovarian reserve (number of remaining oocytes or follicles in the ovary) and function. FSH should always be measured, particularly in women over age 35, to predict the potential for successful treatment with ovulation-induction treatment cycles (ASRM, 2012f). LH levels may be measured early in the cycle to rule out androgen excess disorders, which disrupt normal follicular development and oocyte maturation. Daily sampling of LH at midcycle can detect the LH surge. The day of the LH surge is believed to be the day of maximum fertility. Ovulation occurs 14 to 26 hours after the onset of the LH surge. Urine LH ovulation prediction and serum LH assay (predictor) kits are available for home use to better time postcoital testing, insemination, and intercourse (ASRM, 2012f).

2. *Progesterone assays.* Progesterone levels furnish the best evidence of ovulation and corpus luteum function. Serum levels begin to rise with the LH surge and peak about 8 days later. A level of 3 ng/mL 3 days after the LH surge confirms ovulation (ASRM, 2012e).

Hormonal assessment may also be conducted for prolactin, thyroid-stimulating hormone, and androgen (testosterone, dehydroepiandrosterone [DHEA], and androstenedione) levels.

Endometrial Biopsy. **Endometrial biopsy (EMB)** provides information about the effects of progesterone produced by the corpus luteum after ovulation and endometrial receptivity. EMB is reliable for determining the presence of ovulation. Histologic evidence of secretory endometrium detected by endometrial biopsy shows ovulation and corpus luteum

● **Figure 7–2** *A,* Monophasic, anovulatory basal body temperature (BBT) chart. *B,* Biphasic BBT chart illustrating probable time of ovulation, the different types of testing, and the time in the cycle that each would be performed.

formation. However, it is not effective for diagnosing luteal phase deficiency (ASRM, 2012e).

Transvaginal Ultrasound. **Transvaginal ultrasound** is the method of choice for follicular monitoring of women undergoing induction cycles, for timing ovulation for insemination and intercourse, for retrieving oocytes for in vitro fertilization (IVF), and for monitoring early pregnancy.

Evaluation of Cervical Factors

The mucous cells of the endocervix consist predominantly of water. As ovulation approaches, the ovary increases its secretion of estrogen and produces changes in the cervical mucus. The amount of mucus increases tenfold, and the water content rises significantly. At ovulation, mucus elasticity (**spinnbarkeit**) increases to at least 5 cm in length and viscosity decreases. Excellent spinnbarkeit exists when the mucus can be stretched 8 to 10 cm

or longer. Mucous elasticity is determined by using two glass slides (Figure 7–3A) or by grasping some mucus at the external os (see *Teaching Highlights: Methods of Determining Ovulation*).

The **ferning capacity** (crystallization) (Figure 7–3B) of the cervical mucus also increases as ovulation approaches. Ferning is caused by decreased levels of salt and water interacting with the glycoproteins in the mucus during the ovulatory period and is thus an indirect indication of estrogen production. To test for ferning, mucus is obtained from the cervical os, spread on a glass slide, allowed to air dry, and examined under the microscope. Within 24 to 48 hours postovulation, rising levels of progesterone markedly decrease the quantity of cervical mucus and increase its viscosity and cellularity. The resulting absence of spinnbarkeit and ferning capacity decreases sperm survival.

Teaching Highlights Methods of Determining Ovulation

Basal Body Temperature Method

The basal body temperature (BBT) method relies on assessing the woman's temperature pattern.

Describe the expected findings with an ovulatory (biphasic) cycle and stress the need to monitor BBT for 3 to 4 months to establish a pattern. BBT can be used to time intercourse if pregnancy is desired or as a method of natural family planning. Describe the timing of intercourse to achieve or avoid pregnancy.

Procedure for Measuring BBT

- Using a BBT thermometer, the woman chooses one site (oral, vaginal, or rectal), which she uses consistently.
- The woman takes her temperature every day before arising and before starting any activity, including smoking. Any activity can produce an increase in body temperature.
  Note: Read and follow manufacturers' instructions for each type of BBT thermometer in regard to the amount of time needed for an accurate reading.
- The result is then recorded immediately on a BBT chart, and the temperature dots for each day are connected to form a graph.
- The woman then shakes the thermometer down and cleans it in preparation for use the next day.

Explain that certain situations can disturb body temperature such as large alcohol intake, sleeplessness, fever, warm climate, jet lag, shift work, the use of an electric blanket, or use of heated waterbed.

Cervical Mucus Method

Explain that cervical mucus changes throughout a woman's menstrual cycle and that the quality of the mucus can be used to predict ovulation (see Figure 7–3 ●).

Procedure for Assessing Cervical Mucus Changes

- Every day when she uses the bathroom the woman checks her vagina, either by dabbing the vaginal opening with toilet paper or by putting a finger in the opening.
- She notes the wetness (presence of mucus), collects some mucus, determines its color and consistency, and records her findings on a chart. For discussion of mucus characteristics, see page 137.
- She washes her hands before and after the procedure.

LH Predictor Kit Method

Explain that LH kits are a good predictor of ovulation for a woman with a history of regular menstrual cycles.

Procedure for Using an LH Predictor Kit

- Determine the length of the woman's menstrual cycle. Use a calendar to determine the cycle day on which the woman will initiate testing.
- The testing must occur at the same time daily. The morning is recommended, because the LH concentration is highest on wakening.
- Begin testing with the first morning urine void and examine the test strips for color changes that indicate if ovulation has occurred or is close to occurring.

Mittelschmerz

Explain that mittelschmerz (midcycle pain) located in the lower pelvis is a common symptom of ovulation. Encourage the woman to document this occurrence (or its absence) on her BBT chart.

A

B

● **Figure 7–3** *A,* Spinnbarkeit (elasticity). *B,* Ferning pattern.

● **Figure 7–4** Sperm passage through cervical mucus. *A*, Appearance at the time of ovulation with channels favoring efficient sperm penetration and migration upward. *B*, Unfavorable mazelike configuration found at other times during the menstrual cycle.

To be receptive to sperm, cervical mucus must be thin, clear, watery, profuse, alkaline, and acellular. As shown in Figure 7–4 ●, the mazelike microscopic mucoid strands align in a parallel manner to allow for easy sperm passage. The mucus is termed *inhospitable* if these changes do not occur.

Cervical mucus inhospitable to sperm survival can have several causes, some of which are treatable. For example, estrogen secretion may be inadequate for development of receptive mucus. Cone biopsy, electrocautery, or cryosurgery of the cervix may remove large numbers of mucus-producing glands, creating a "dry cervix" that decreases sperm survival. Treatment with clomiphene citrate may have harmful effects on cervical mucus because of its antiestrogenic properties. Therapy with supplemental estrogen for approximately 6 days before expected ovulation encourages the formation of suitable spinnbarkeit. However, intrauterine insemination (IUI) is more often the most appropriate therapy to overcome these obstacles. When mucosal hostility to sperm is because of cervical infection, antimicrobial therapy may be effective.

The cervix can also be the site of secretory immunologic reactions in which antisperm antibodies are produced, causing agglutination or immobilization of sperm. The most widely used serum–sperm bioassay to detect specific classes of antibodies in serum and seminal fluid is immunobead testing (IBT) (Fritz & Speroff, 2011). IBT is considered clinically significant when 50% of the sperm are coated with immunobeads. The treatment for antisperm antibodies may include IUI of the man's washed sperm to bypass the cervical factor.

The **postcoital test (PCT)**, also called the **Huhner test**, is performed 1 or 2 days before the expected date of ovulation as determined by previous BBT charts, the length of prior cycles, or a urinary LH kit. Its use is controversial and it has limited use in infertility workups because it reliably assesses the presence of sperm only after intercourse (ASRM, 2012e).

Evaluation of Uterine Structures and Tubal Patency

Uterine abnormalities are a relatively uncommon cause of infertility but should be considered. A few tests offer the ability to evaluate the uterine cavity and tubal patency simultaneously. These tests are usually done after BBT evaluation, semen analysis, and other less invasive tests. Tubal patency and uterine structure are usually evaluated by hysterosalpingography or laparoscopy.

Other invasive tests used to evaluate only the uterine cavity are hysteroscopy and sonohysterography. Hysteroscopy may be performed earlier in the evaluation if the woman's history suggests the potential for adhesive disease or uterine abnormalities.

Hysterosalpingography. Hysterosalpingography (HSG), or *hysterogram,* involves the instillation of a radiopaque substance into the uterine cavity. In addition, the oil-based dye and injection pressure used in HSG may have a therapeutic effect. This effect may be caused by the flushing of debris, breaking of adhesions, or induction of peristalsis by the instillation.

The HSG should be performed in the follicular phase of the cycle to avoid interrupting an early pregnancy. This timing also avoids the lush secretory changes in the endometrium that occur after ovulation, which may prevent the passage of the dye through the tubes and present a false picture of obstruction of the entry point of the fallopian tube into the uterus.

HSG causes moderate discomfort. The pain is referred from the peritoneum (which is irritated by the subdiaphragmatic collection of gas) to the shoulder. The cramping may be decreased if the radiopaque dye is warmed to body temperature before instillation. Women can take an over-the-counter (OTC) prostaglandin synthesis inhibitor (such as ibuprofen) 30 minutes before the procedure to decrease the pain, cramping, and discomfort. HSG can also cause recurrence of pelvic inflammatory disease, so prophylactic antibiotics are recommended to prevent infection that could be triggered by the procedure (ASRM, 2012f).

Hysteroscopy and Laparoscopy. *Hysteroscopy* is the definitive method for both diagnosis and treatment of intrauterine pathology (ASRM, 2012b). Hysteroscopy allows the physician to further evaluate any areas of suspicion within the uterine cavity or fallopian tubes revealed by the HSG. It can be done in conjunction with a laparoscopy or independently in the office and does not require general anesthesia. A fiber-optic instrument called a hysteroscope is placed into the uterus for further evaluation of polyps, fibroids, or structural variations. The newest generation hyperscope allows for minor operative procedures to be performed in the office setting.

Laparoscopy enables direct visualization of the pelvic organs to evaluate endometriosis and pelvic adhesions. It is used only if there is strong clinical suspicion of these conditions or before considering more aggressive treatments with higher risks and/or costs (ASRM, 2012f). In routine preanesthesia instructions, the woman is told that she may have some discomfort from organ displacement and shoulder and chest pain caused by gas in the abdomen as a result of distending the peritoneal cavity with carbon dioxide gas in order to better visualize the pelvic organs. She should be informed that she can resume normal activities as tolerated after 24 hours. Using postoperative pain medication and assuming a supine position may help relieve discomfort caused by any remaining gas.

Assessment of the Man's Fertility

Male infertility can be caused by numerous factors, some of which can be identified and are reversible, such as ductal obstruction and varicocele. Varicocele, which is an abnormal dilation of scrotal veins, is present in 10% to 15% of the normal population and accounts for approximately 30% of male

Teaching Highlights Obtaining a Sperm Specimen

- To obtain accurate results, the specimen is collected after 3 days of abstinence, usually by masturbation, to avoid contamination or loss of any ejaculate.
- If the man has difficulty producing sperm by masturbation, special medical-grade condoms are available to collect the sperm during intercourse.
- Regular latex and nonlatex condoms should not be used because they contain agents that impair the motility of sperm, which can result in sperm loss in the condom.
- Lubricants should not be used (most are spermicidal) unless approved by the andrology laboratory.
- If the specimen is obtained at home, it needs to be brought to the lab within 1 hour and kept at body temperature so as not to impair motility.
- Seasonal and incidental variability may be seen in count and motility in successive semen analyses from the same individual. A repeat semen analysis may be required to assess the man's fertility potential adequately; a minimum of two separate analyses is recommended for confirmation.
- In cases in which a known testicular insult has occurred (infection, high fevers, or surgery), a repeat analysis may not be done for at least 2.5 months to allow for new sperm maturation.

Table 7–3 Normal Semen Analysis

Factor	Value
Volume	≥ 1.5 mL
pH	7.2–7.8
Sperm concentration	$\geq 15 \times 10^6$/mL
Total sperm count	$\geq 39 \times 10^6$
Progressive motility	$\geq 32\%$
Total motility	$\geq 40\%$
Normal morphology (strict criteria)	$\geq 4\%$
Vitality	$\geq 58\%$

Source: Cooper, T., Noonan, E., von Eckardstein, S., et al. (2010). World Health Organization reference values for human semen characteristics. *Human Reproduction Update, 16*(3), 231–245.

infertility (Fritz & Speroff, 2011). Other identifiable conditions are not reversible, such as bilateral testicular atrophy secondary to viral orchitis and *congenital bilateral absence of the vas deferens (CBAVD)*. Idiopathic male factor infertility occurs when the etiology of an abnormal semen analysis is not identifiable.

If a male infertility factor is present, it is usually defined by the findings of an abnormal semen analysis. A semen analysis of sperm quality, quantity, and motility is the single most important diagnostic study of the man. It should be done early in the couple's evaluation, before invasive testing of the woman. See *Teaching Highlights: Obtaining a Sperm Specimen.*

Sperm analysis provides information about sperm motility and morphology and a determination of the absolute number of spermatozoa present (Table 7–3). Although low numbers and motility may indicate compromised fertility, other parameters, such as morphology, motion patterns, and progression, are important prognostic indicators. The quality of sperm decreases with increasing paternal age and may result in chromosomal damage. For example, fathers older than 40 years may be at an increased risk for offspring with chromosome abnormalities or new gene mutations.

Genetic factors may affect male fertility. Men with oligospermia (semen with a low concentration of sperm) and nonobstructive azoospermia (impaired or nonexistent sperm production) have an increased risk for chromosome abnormalities and Y chromosome deletions (ASRM, 2012e). Men with obstructive azoospermia, such as CBAVD, have an up to 80% risk for cystic fibrosis genetic mutations (ASRM, 2012e).

Spermatozoa have been shown to possess intrinsic antigens that can provoke male immunologic infertility. Any disruption in the blood-testes barrier, such as vasectomy reversals, or genital trauma, such as testicular torsion, can lead to the

production of antisperm antibodies (ASAs) (ASRM, 2012e). Treatment for antisperm antibodies is directed toward preventing the formation of antibodies or arresting the underlying mechanism that compromises sperm function. The treatment of choice for clinically significant antisperm antibodies is intracytoplasmic sperm injection (ICSI) in conjunction with IVF. If the man's history indicates, he may be referred to a urologist for further testing.

Methods of Infertility Management

Methods of managing infertility include pharmacologic agents, therapeutic insemination, in vitro fertilization, and other assisted reproductive techniques. In addition, many couples choose adoption as their preferred response to infertility.

Pharmacologic Agents

This section provides a brief overview of the drugs commonly used for ovarian stimulation in the follicular phase, control of midcycle release, and support of the luteal phase. The pharmacologic treatment chosen depends on the specific cause of infertility.

Clomiphene Citrate. If a woman has normal ovaries, a normal prolactin level, and an intact pituitary gland, *clomiphene citrate* (Clomid or Serophene) is often used as a first-line therapy to induce ovulation. This medication induces ovulation in 80% of women by actions at both the hypothalamic and ovarian levels; 40% of these women will become pregnant. Clomiphene citrate works by stimulating the hypothalamus to secrete more gonadotropin-releasing hormone (GnRH). This increases the secretion of LH and FSH, which stimulates follicle growth and facilitates the release of ova (Fritz & Speroff, 2011).

For the first course the woman usually takes 50 mg/day orally for 5 days from cycle day (CD) 3 to day 7 or CD 5 to day 9. In nonresponders, the dose may be increased to 100 mg/day to a maximum of 250 mg/day, although doses in excess of 100 mg/day are not approved by the FDA (Wilson, Shannon, & Shields, 2013). The woman may need to take estrogen simultaneously if a decrease in cervical mucus occurs.

The woman is informed that if ovulation occurs, it is expected 5 to 9 days after the last dose. The nurse determines if the couple has been advised to have sexual intercourse every other day for 1 week, beginning 5 days after the last day of medication. Upon a negative pregnancy test, another trial of clomiphene can be initiated. After the first treatment cycle, a pelvic ultrasound should be done to rule out ovarian enlargement, ovarian cysts, or hyperstimulation. Ovarian enlargement and abdominal discomfort (bloating) may result from follicular growth and formation of multiple corpora lutea. Persistence of ovarian cysts is a contraindication for further treatment regimens. Other side effects include hot flashes, abdominal distention, bloating, breast discomfort, nausea and vomiting, vision problems (such as visual spots), headache, and dryness or loss of hair (Casper, 2011). Supplemental low-dose estrogen may be given to ensure appropriate quality and quantity of cervical mucus, or IUI may be employed to overcome this obstacle. Women can assess the presence of ovulation and possible response to clomiphene therapy by doing BBT and urinary LH tests. The woman should be knowledgeable about side effects and call her healthcare provider if they occur. When visual disturbances (flashes, blurring, or spots) occur, bright lighting should be avoided. This side effect disappears within a few days or weeks after discontinuation of therapy. The occurrence of hot flashes may be because of the antiestrogenic properties of clomiphene citrate. The woman can obtain some relief by increasing intake of fluids and using fans.

Fecundability (the ability to become pregnant) declines with advancing age as described earlier; therefore, prolonged treatment with clomiphene is unjustified in women in their later reproductive years. Clomiphene treatment should generally be limited to the minimum effective dose and to no more than six ovulatory cycles. Failure to conceive after clomiphene induction is an indication to expand the diagnostic evaluation or to change the overall treatment plan if evaluation is complete.

Insulin Sensitizing Agents.
Insulin resistance and hyperinsulinemia are common features of polycystic ovarian syndrome (PCOS) and a contributing cause of chronic anovulation. Anovulatory women with PCOS are hyperinsulinemic and subsequently are more resistant to clomiphene treatment. The best initial treatment for anovulatory women who are obese is weight loss. Recently, studies have shown that oral hypoglycemic agents (e.g., metformin and rosiglitazone) can induce ovulation in women with PCOS. Clinical trials are under way to determine the appropriateness of oral hypoglycemic agents with and without clomiphene in the infertility setting.

Gonadotropins.
Therapy using *human menopausal gonadotropins (hMGs)* is indicated as a first line of therapy for anovulatory infertile women with low to normal levels of gonadotropins (FSH and LH). It is a second line of therapy in women who fail to ovulate or conceive with clomiphene citrate therapy and in women undergoing controlled ovarian stimulation with assisted reproduction.

Recently, recombinant gonadotropins (rFSH and rLH) have been produced, giving rise to more consistent preparations. Recombinant FSH is homogenous and free of contaminants by proteins. Luveris, a recombinant form of LH, is used concomitantly with recombinant FSH in women with profound LH deficiency. It is thought that the use of recombinant gonadotropins will eventually become the preferred preparation and that the use of urinary preparations will be phased out.

Gonadotropin therapy requires close observation by means of serum estradiol levels and ultrasound. Monitoring of follicle development is necessary to minimize the risk of multiple fetuses and to avoid ovarian hyperstimulation syndrome. The daily dose of medication given is titrated based on serum estradiol and ultrasound findings. Then once follicle maturation has occurred, hCG may be administered by intramuscular or subcutaneous injection to induce final follicular maturation and stimulate ovulation. The couple is advised to have intercourse 24 to 36 hours after hCG administration and for the next 2 days. Women who elect to undergo ovarian stimulation with gonadotropins have usually passed through all other forms of management without conceiving. Strong emotional support and thorough education are needed because of the numerous office visits and injections. Often the male partner is instructed, with return demonstration, to administer the daily injections.

Bromocriptine.
High prolactin levels may impair the glandular production of FSH and LH or block their action on the ovaries. When hyperprolactinemia accompanies anovulation, the infertility may be treated with bromocriptine (Parlodel). This medication acts directly on the prolactin-secreting cells in the anterior pituitary. It inhibits the pituitary's secretion of prolactin, thus preventing suppression of the pulsatile secretion of FSH and LH. This restores normal menstrual cycles and induces ovulation by allowing FSH and LH production. If treatment is successful, the tests of ovulatory function will indicate that ovulation is occurring with a normal luteal phase. Bromocriptine should be discontinued if pregnancy is suspected or at the anticipated time of ovulation because of its possible teratogenic effects. Other side effects include nausea, diarrhea, dizziness, headache, and fatigue, which can be attributed to the dopaminergic action of bromocriptine. To minimize side effects for women who are extremely sensitive, treatment may be initiated with a dose of 1.25 mg, slowly building tolerance toward the usual dose of 2.5 mg bid. An intravaginal preparation may also be used to decrease the occurrence of side effects.

Other Pharmacologic Agents

Pharmacologic treatments for endometriosis-related infertility involve use of danazol (Danocrine), oral contraceptives or oral medroxyprogesterone acetate, and gonadotropin-releasing hormone (GnRH) agonists. The management and care of endometriosis are discussed further in Chapter 6 🔗. Treatment of luteal phase defects may include the use of progesterone to augment luteal phase progesterone levels. Ovulation-induction agents, such as clomiphene citrate or menotropins, may be used to augment proliferative phase FSH production in the developing follicle, because women with luteal phase defects have been found to have decreased FSH production in the proliferative phase. It is also common to use progesterone supplementation in conjunction with these ovulation-induction agents for luteal phase support, thereby increasing endometrial receptivity for embryonic implantation. Occasionally hCG therapy may be used in the luteal phase to stimulate corpus luteum production of progesterone.

Evidence-Based Practice Herbal Treatments for Infertility

Clinical Question

What herbal and/or dietary supplements are helpful as treatments for infertility?

The Evidence

Several systematic reviews have focused on herbal therapies and/or dietary supplements as methods to enhance fertility. Two systematic reviews studied the evidence for the use of Chinese herbal medicine. One study reviewed multiple randomized trials, cohort studies, and case series comparing Chinese herbal medicine to medical treatment alone; these studies involved more than 1,800 women. A second study compared treatment with clomiphene citrate and the same treatment supplemented with Chinese herbal medicine. This study of 14 randomized controlled trials involved 1,316 women.

The use of Chinese herbal medicine with or without medical treatments for infertility demonstrated improved pregnancy rates (Ried & Stuart, 2011; See, McCulloch, Smikle, et al., 2011). Women in these studies also reported improved menstrual cycles while using the herbal medicines. Assessment of the quality of the menstrual cycle is integral to the use of Chinese herbal medicine, so a higher level of sensitivity to existing cycles may be an element of its effectiveness.

Best Practice

Women who may be considering herbal or other supplements as a means to enhance fertility can be counseled that Chinese herbal medicines are safe and may be effective in improving the chance of a pregnancy. A thorough baseline assessment of the quality of menstrual cycles is a key part of any infertility assessment process.

Clinical Reasoning

What are the elements of an assessment of menstrual cycles? Which women may be candidates for herbal or other supplement therapies for infertility?

Complementary Care Common Treatments for Infertility

Couples experiencing infertility may seek alternative treatments. Some common treatments include acupuncture and herbs.

Acupuncture

Acupuncture is used in traditional Chinese medicine (TCM), and has become a popular complementary treatment. Acupuncture involves inserting sterile needles into specific points on the body to control the flow of *chi*, or life energy. Acupuncture treatment focuses on the regulation of uterine and ovarian blood flow through supraspinal pathways. Several clinical studies have shown acupuncture to be effective in treating infertility in both men and women by inhibiting uterine motility during embryo transfer and improving the endometrial environment for embryo implantation (Bennington, 2010). Acupuncture in conjunction with embryo transfer improves the rate of pregnancy and live birth in women undergoing in vitro fertilization.

Herbal Treatments

Herbs frequently recommended to treat infertility include ginseng and astragalus. Herbalists cite the healing and hormone-balancing effects of these herbs. Ginseng has historically been used in TCM to enhance male virility and fertility. Several studies also cite ginseng, as well as astragalus, in enhancing in vitro sperm motility (Skidmore-Roth, 2010).

The nurse should be alert for signs that the couple is pursuing complementary therapies out of desperation. A sensitive, nonjudgmental approach will go a long way toward comforting a couple and assuring them that many complementary therapies used are helpful and not harmful.

Therapeutic Insemination

Therapeutic insemination has replaced the previously used term *artificial insemination* and involves the depositing of semen at the cervical os or in the uterus by mechanical means. *Therapeutic husband insemination (THI)* is the current term for use of the husband's semen, and *therapeutic donor insemination (TDI)* is the current term for use of donor semen.

THI is generally indicated for such seminal deficiencies as oligospermia (low sperm count), asthenospermia (decreased motility), and teratospermia (low percentage, abnormal morphology); for anatomic defects accompanied by inadequate deposition of semen such as hypospadia (a congenital abnormal male urethral opening on the underside of the penis); and for ejaculatory dysfunction (such as retrograde ejaculation). THI is also indicated in cases of unexplained infertility and some cases of female factor infertility, such as scant or inhospitable mucus, persistent cervicitis, or cervical stenosis. In some cases, IUI would be indicated to bypass the cervical factor. Seminal fluid contains high levels of prostaglandins, which can cause nausea, severe cramps, abdominal pain, and diarrhea when absorbed by the uterine lining. Therefore, sperm preparation for IUI involves washing sperm from the seminal plasma. IUI, with or without ovulation-induction therapy, is an option for many couples before more aggressive treatments such as in vitro fertilization are employed.

The couple undergoing genetic counseling may consider assisted reproduction techniques, such as therapeutic donor insemination. This alternative is appropriate in several instances; for example, if the man has an autosomal dominant disease, TDI would decrease to zero the risk of having an affected child (if the sperm donor is not at risk) because the child would not inherit any genes from the affected parent. If the man is affected with a male sex-linked disorder and does not wish to continue the gene in the family (all his daughters will be carriers), TDI would be an alternative to terminating all pregnancies with a female fetus. If the man is a carrier for a balanced translocation and if termination of pregnancy is against family ethics, TDI is an appropriate alternative. If both parents are carriers of an autosomal recessive disorder, TDI lowers the risk to a very low level or to zero if a carrier test is available. Finally, TDI may be appropriate if the family is at high risk for a multifactorial disorder or in cases of azoospermia (absence of sperm), severe oligospermia, or asthenospermia.

In the past several years, indications for donor insemination have expanded to include single women or lesbians who want to become pregnant. Some states have specified the parental rights of single women and donors, but most are silent on this issue.

TDI has become more complicated and expensive in the past decade because of the need for strict screening and processing procedures to prevent transmission of a genetic defect or sexually transmitted infection to the offspring or recipient. Guidelines have been established and updated by the American Society for Reproductive Medicine (2011) that include mandatory medical (genetic) and infectious disease screening of both donor and recipient, the need for informed consent from all parties, the need to limit the number of pregnancies per donor, and the need for accurate means of record keeping. Finally, because of the risk of transmitting infectious diseases, donated sperm must be frozen and quarantined for 6 months from the time of acquisition, and the donor must be retested before sperm can be released for use.

Numerous factors need to be evaluated before TDI is performed. Has every possible effort been made to diagnose and treat the cause of the male infertility? Do tests indicate normal fertility and sperm–ovum transport in the woman? Has the couple had an opportunity to discuss this option with an infertility counselor to explore the issues of secrecy, disclosure, and potential feelings of loss the couple (particularly the male partner) may feel about not having a genetic child? Are there any religious constraints? After making the decision, the couple should allow themselves time to further assess their concerns and explore their feelings individually and together to ensure that this option is acceptable to both.

In Vitro Fertilization

In vitro fertilization (IVF) is selectively used in cases when infertility has resulted from tubal factors, mucous abnormalities, male infertility, unexplained infertility, male and female immunologic infertility, and cervical factors. In IVF a woman's eggs are collected from her ovaries, fertilized in the laboratory, and placed into her uterus after normal embryo development has begun. If the procedure is successful, the embryo continues to develop in the uterus, and pregnancy proceeds naturally.

The potential for a successful pregnancy with IVF is maximized when three to four embryos (rather than one) are placed into the uterus. For this reason, fertility drugs are used to induce ovulation before the process. Follicular development and oocyte maturity are monitored frequently with ultrasound and hormonal assays. Monitoring usually begins around cycle day 5, and medications are titrated according to individual response. When follicles appear mature, hCG is given to stimulate final egg maturation and control the induction of ovulation. Egg retrieval is performed approximately 35 hours later, before ovulation occurs.

In the majority of cases, egg retrieval is performed by a transvaginal approach under ultrasound guidance (Figure 7–5 ●). It is an outpatient procedure performed with intravenous sedation and a cervical block for anesthesia. Many follicles can be aspirated with only one puncture, and the procedure generally lasts no more than 30 minutes. Once the eggs are fertilized and progress to the embryo stage, the embryos are placed in the uterus. This occurs 1 to 2 days after conception. After the procedure, the woman is advised to engage in only minimal activity for 12 to 24 hours, and

---

Developing Cultural Competence
Infertility Treatments

The acceptance of infertility treatments varies widely around the world. Some belief systems do not allow various treatments, because using a treatment is considered interfering with God's design or because the treatment itself is seen as tainted or sinful. For example, fertility practices in Arab cultures are influenced by traditional Arab Bedouin values that support tribal dominance and beliefs that "God decides family sizes." In Arab cultures, procreation is the purpose of marriage.

If a couple is infertile, the approved methods for treating infertility are limited to use of therapeutic insemination using the husband's sperm and in vitro fertilization involving fertilization of the wife's ovum by the husband's sperm because of lineage concerns (ASRM, 2012a). Sterility in a woman can lead to rejection and divorce. Also with the use of ICSI, male-initiated divorce is becoming more common for aging wives of infertile husbands. Infertile women are encouraged by their own families and their husbands' families to suggest a second wife (ASRM, 2012a). Infertility in Jordanian men is denied so that the man will not be viewed as an incomplete person (ASRM, 2012a). Contemporary Islamic religious opinion forbids any kind of egg, embryo, or semen donation, as well as surrogacy.

In Jewish cultures, infertile couples are to try all possible means to have children, including egg and sperm donation. However, Orthodox Jewish opinion is virtually unanimous in prohibiting therapeutic insemination when the semen donor is a Jewish man other than the woman's husband, because it may constitute adultery. If the infertility is because of a male factor, therapeutic insemination with sperm from a non-Jewish sperm donor is acceptable because "Jewishness" is conferred through the matriline. IVF and embryo transfer (ET) are also acceptable artificial insemination methods because they do not involve putting sperm into another's wife (Schenker, 2010).

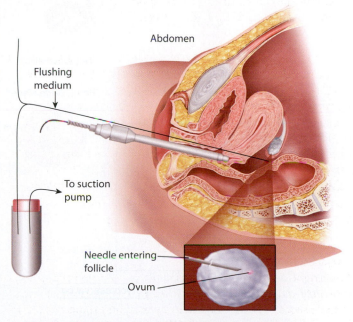

● **Figure 7–5** Transvaginal ultrasound-guided oocyte retrieval.

progesterone supplementation is prescribed. The progesterone supplementation is given to promote implantation and support the early pregnancy; therefore, she will not have a period even if she is not pregnant (the pregnancy is usually determined by transvaginal ultrasound).

Sperm used to fertilize the eggs in vitro can be obtained naturally or via microsurgical epididymal sperm aspiration (MESA) or testicular sperm aspiration (TESA). These are procedures that address severe male factor infertility. MESA and TESA involve the retrieval of sperm from the gonadal tissue of men who have azoospermia or an ejaculatory disorder (Figure 7–6 ●). Percutaneous epididymal sperm aspiration (PESA) and TESA are replacing MESA as the preferred techniques for retrieval of sperm because they are not surgical procedures. ICSI is a microscopic procedure to inject a single sperm into the outer layer of an ovum so that fertilization will occur (ASRM, 2011).

Success with IVF depends on many factors, but especially the woman's age and the specific indication. Women have a good chance of achieving pregnancy with an average of three cycles of IVF. Many couples find the emotional, physical, and financial costs of going beyond three cycles too great. Costs vary by treatment and by region of the country (ASRM, 2012e). Clinical birth rates reported by the Society for Assisted Reproductive Technology (SART) were 50% per egg donation for women regardless of age or indication in the United States

(ASRM, 2011). The increase in maternal and neonatal morbidity is associated with IVF because the rates of multiple fetuses remain an issue.

Other Assisted Reproductive Techniques

Other assisted reproductive techniques include procedures for transfer of gametes, zygotes, or embryos; cryopreservation of embryos; IVF using donor oocytes; assisted hatching (AH); and use of a gestational carrier.

Gamete intrafallopian transfer (GIFT) involves the retrieval of oocytes by laparoscopy; immediate placement of the oocytes in a catheter with washed, motile sperm; and placement of the gametes into the fimbriated end of the fallopian tube. Fertilization occurs in the fallopian tube as with normal conception (in vivo) rather than in the laboratory (in vitro). The fertilized egg then travels through the fallopian tube to the uterus for implantation as in normal reproduction. GIFT may be more acceptable than other procedures such as ZIFT to adherents of some religions (Roman Catholic Church), because fertilization does not occur outside the woman's body.

From the GIFT technology evolved procedures such as **zygote intrafallopian transfer (ZIFT)** and **tubal embryo transfer (TET)**. In these procedures eggs are retrieved and incubated with the man's sperm. However, the eggs are transferred back to the woman's body at a much earlier stage of cell division than in

● **Figure 7–6** Assisted reproductive techniques.

IVF and, as in GIFT, are placed in the fallopian tube or tubes and not the uterus. In TET the placement is done at the embryo stage. These procedures allow fertilization to be documented, which is not possible with GIFT, and the pregnancy rate is theoretically increased when the fertilized ovum is placed in the fallopian tube.

A micromanipulation procedure called *assisted embryo hatching (AH)* has proved to be an effective adjunct therapy in IVF. In vitro fertilization using a *gestational carrier* allows infertile women who are genetically sound but unable to carry a pregnancy to exercise the option of having their own biologic child. Other technologies involve oocyte donation (women donate ovum to another woman) and cryopreservation of the embryo (embryos are frozen and then thawed at a later date) (Michalakis, DeCherney, & Penzias, 2013).

Preimplantation Genetic Diagnosis

Recent advances in micromanipulation allow a single cell to be removed from the embryo for genetic study. Couples at risk for having a detectable single-gene or chromosomal anomaly may wish to undergo such preimplantation genetic testing, called *blastomere analysis* or, more recently, *preimplantation genetic diagnosis (PGD)*. PGD is a term used when one or both genetic parents carry a gene mutation or balanced chromosome rearrangement and testing is performed to determine whether that mutation or unbalanced chromosomal complement has been passed to the oocyte or embryo (Laliota, 2011). *Preimplantation genetic screening (PGS)* is a term used when the genetic parents are known or presumed to have normal chromosomes, and their embryos are screened for aneuploidy with the purpose of increasing the likelihood of a viable pregnancy with normal chromosomes (Laliota, 2011). The single cell is obtained from an eight-cell embryo by a process known as blastomere biopsy. The genetic content of the cell is examined using comparative genome hybridization (CGH) (Laliota, 2011). The cell's deoxyribonucleic acid (DNA) is amplified and labeled with fluorochrome. CGH requires several days to do. Biopsied embryos are examined so that embryos affected with a particular genetic disease or chromosome abnormality are not placed in the mother. Both PGD and PGS can produce false-positive and false-negative results. Prenatal diagnostic testing to confirm the results is strongly encouraged (Laliota, 2011).

The diagnosis of genetic disorders before implantation provides couples with the option of foregoing the attempt to establish a pregnancy and thereby avoiding a difficult decision about terminating an affected pregnancy (Kalfoglou, Kammersell, Philpott, et al., 2013). This technology also raises several ethical issues, including the following:

■ Identification of couples at risk. There is a need for criteria that identify couples at risk for diseases that constitute significant hardship and suffering so that "wrongful birth" cases can be avoided.

■ Availability of and access to centers providing PGD. Should society provide access for those at risk for genetic transfer of disease but without the financial resources to pay for the services?

■ Analysis of blastomeres for sex chromosome testing when a genetic disorder carried on the sex chromosomes is

suspected. In X-linked diseases, the only way to prevent the disorder is to select against the blastomere with the Y chromosome.

■ Identification of late-onset diseases. The Human Genome Project has aided in the identification of genetic markers for late-onset disease. Couples may wish to choose to implant blastomeres that do not carry these markers.

■ Effect on the offspring as a result of removing cells from the embryo.

■ Selection for nonmedical reasons and potential concern of eugenics "designer babies".

Sperm Sorting. Sperm sorting is a technology designed to separate sperm that primarily produce females or those that primarily produce males. Sorted sperm enriched with male- or female-producing sperm is then used for IUI or IVF. The accuracy depends on the laboratory that performs the sorting and the technology it uses. Study data indicate that 9 out of 10 patients sorting for a girl will conceive a female. Approximately 3 out of 4 patients who sort for a boy will conceive a male. This technology is used to increase the likelihood of having a child of a particular gender in couples at risk for an X-linked genetic disorder or for couples interested in family balancing (gender selection when a couple has two or more children of the same gender) (Kalfoglou et al., 2013).

Adoption

Infertile couples consider various alternatives for resolving their infertility, and adoption is one option that may be considered at several points during the treatment process. As couples begin to consider adoption, important aspects of this exploration are the gathering of information from magazines, books, informational websites, and organizations such as the National Adoption Information Clearinghouse; attending adoption support groups and conferences; and meeting with adoptive parents to discuss their experiences with adoption.

The adoption of a healthy American infant can be difficult and frustrating, often involving long waiting periods, continual setbacks, and high costs. Thus many couples seek international adoption or consider adopting older children, children with handicaps, or children of mixed parentage, because the adoption process in such cases may be quicker and more children are available. Nurses in the community can assist couples considering adoption by providing information on community resources for adoption and support through the adoption process. Couples need support if they remain childless, either by choice or circumstance. Informational books, websites such as Childless by Choice, and support groups such as San Francisco RESOLVE's "living without children" are available for couples who remain childless by choice or circumstance.

Pregnancy After Infertility

The feeling of being infertile does not necessarily disappear with pregnancy. Although there may be initial ecstasy, couples may face a whole new arena of fear and anxiety, and the parents-to-be often do not know where they "fit in." They may feel a great sense of isolation because those who have had no trouble conceiving cannot relate to the physical and emotional pain they endured to achieve the pregnancy. Contact with their past support system of other infertile couples may vanish when peers learn the couple has resolved their infertility. Although the desperation to become pregnant may have superseded the couple's ability to acknowledge their concerns about undergoing various treatments or procedures, questions about the repeated cycle of fertility drugs or the achievement of pregnancy through IVF technology or cryopreservation may now arise. The expectant couple may be very concerned about the potential of these treatments to adversely affect the fetus (McGrath et al., 2010). Couples may need reassurance throughout the pregnancy to allay these anxieties. The nurse can assist couples who conceive after infertility by acknowledging their past experiences of infertility treatment; validating their fears and anxieties as they face childbirth classes, birth, and parenting issues; and providing support and education about what to anticipate physically and emotionally throughout the pregnancy. The nurse can also counsel couples that infertility because of nonstructural causes may correct itself following a successful pregnancy and birth; therefore, postchildbirth contraception counseling may be warranted. These interventions will go a long way toward normalizing the experience for the couple.

Recurrent Pregnancy Loss

Recurrent pregnancy loss (RPL) is a disease distinct from infertility. It is defined by two or more failed pregnancies (ASRM, 2012d). Estimates suggest that RPL occurs in 1% to 5% of fertile couples attempting pregnancy (Marquard, Westphal, Milki, et al., 2010). There are several etiologies, including maternal medical complications, chromosome abnormalities and other genetic conditions, autoimmune disorders, and thrombotic causes. However, in up to 50% of couples with RPL, an etiology will not be identified (ASRM, 2012d).

Maternal medical complications associated with RPL include luteal phase defects or progesterone deficiency and congenital uterine abnormalities. Autoimmune disorders such as antiphospholipid antibody syndrome, alloimmune factors, and blood group isoimmunization have been associated with RPL. Chromosome abnormalities (primarily autosomal trisomies) such as recurrent aneuploidy and parental chromosome abnormalities are associated with RPL. One partner will have a balanced chromosome rearrangement in 3% to 5% of couples with RPL. Single-gene disorders such as alpha-thalassemia major, some metabolic diseases, and some X-linked dominant disorders that are lethal in utero in males can account for RPL. Hereditary thrombophilias, such as factor V Leiden, prothrombin gene, protein C or S deficiency, and antithrombin III deficiency are known to predispose individuals to pregnancy complications including RPL (ASRM, 2012d).

Nursing Management of the Infertile Couple

Infertility therapy taxes a couple's financial, physical, and emotional resources. Treatment can be costly, and insurance coverage is limited. Years of effort and numerous evaluations and examinations may take place before conception occurs, if it occurs at all. In a society that values children and considers them to be the natural result of marriage, infertile couples face a myriad of tensions and discrimination.

Clinic nurses need to be constantly aware of the emotional needs of the couple confronting infertility evaluation and treatment. Often an intact marriage will become stressed with intrusive infertility procedures and treatments. Constant attention to temperature charts and instructions about their sex life from a person outside the relationship naturally affects the spontaneity of a couple's interactions. Tests and treatments may heighten feelings of frustration or anger between partners. The need to share this intimate area of a relationship, especially when one or the other is identified as "the cause" of infertility, may precipitate feelings of guilt or shame. Infertility often becomes a central focus for role identity, especially for women (McGrath et al., 2010).

The couple may experience feelings of loss of control, feelings of reduced competency and defectiveness, loss of status and ambiguity as a couple, a sense of social stigma, stress on the marital and sexual relationship, and a strained relationship with healthcare providers. The nurse's roles can be summarized as those of counselor, educator, and advocate.

Tasks of the infertile couple and appropriate nursing interventions are summarized in Table 7–4. Throughout the evaluation process nurses play a key role in lessening the stress these couples must endure by providing resources and accurate information about what is entailed in treatment and what physical, emotional, and financial demands they can anticipate throughout the process (Van den Broeck, Emery, Wischmann, et al., 2010).

The nurse's ability to assess and respond to emotional and educational needs is essential to give infertile couples a sense of control and help them negotiate the treatment process. It is important to use a nursing framework that recognizes the multidimensional needs of the infertile individual or couple within physical, social, psychologic, spiritual, and environmental contexts.

Infertility may be perceived as a loss by one or both partners. Affected individuals have described this as a loss of their relationship with spouse, family, or friends; their health; their status or prestige; their self-esteem and self-confidence; their security; and the potential child. Any one of these losses may lead to depression, but in many cases the crisis of infertility evokes feelings

Table 7–4	Tasks of the Infertile Couple
Tasks	**Nursing Interventions**
Recognize how infertility affects their lives and express feelings (may be negative toward self or mate)	Supportive: Help to understand and facilitate free expression of feelings
Grieve the loss of potential offspring	Help to recognize feelings
Evaluate reasons for wanting a child	Help to understand motives
Decide about management	Identify alternatives; facilitate partner communication

Source: Sawatzky, M. (1981). Tasks of the infertile couple. *Journal of Obstetric, Gynecologic, and Neonatal Nursing, 10,* 132.

Care Plan: Infertile Couple

Activity

similar to those associated with all these losses (McGrath et al., 2010). Each couple passes through several stages of feelings: surprise, denial, anger, isolation, guilt, grief, and resolution. The impact of these feelings on the couple and how fast they move into resolution, if ever, may depend on the cause and on the duration of treatment. Each partner may progress through the stages at different rates (McGrath et al., 2010). Nonjudgmental acceptance and a professional, caring attitude on the nurse's part can go far in dissipating the negative emotions the couple may experience while going through these stages.

This is also a time when the nurse may assess the couple's relationship: Are both partners able and willing to communicate verbally and share feelings? Are the partners mutually supportive? The answers to such questions may help the nurse to identify areas of strength and weakness and to construct an appropriate plan of care.

Referral to mental health professionals is helpful when the emotional issues become too disruptive in the couple's relationship or life. The couple should be aware of infertility support and education organizations such as RESOLVE (National Infertility Association), which may help meet some of their needs and validate their feelings. Finally, individual or group counseling with other infertile couples can help the couple resolve feelings brought about by their own difficult situation.

GENETIC DISORDERS

Even when conception has been achieved, families can have special reproductive concerns. The desired and expected outcome of any pregnancy is the birth of a healthy, "perfect" baby. Parents experience grief, fear, and anger when they discover that their baby has been born with a defect or a genetic disease. Such an abnormality may be evident at birth or may not appear for some time. The baby may have inherited a disorder from one parent or both, creating guilt and strife within the family.

Regardless of the type or scope of the problem, parents will have many questions: "What did I do?" "What caused it?" "How do I cope with it?" "Will it happen again?" The nurse must anticipate the couple's questions and concerns and guide, direct, and support the family. To do so, the nurse must have a basic knowledge of genetics and genetic counseling. Professional nurses can help expedite this process if they understand the principles involved and can direct the family to the appropriate resources.

Chromosomes and Chromosomal Analysis

All hereditary material is carried on tightly coiled strands of DNA known as **chromosomes**. The chromosomes carry the *genes,* the smallest units of inheritance, as discussed in greater detail in Chapter 4 🔗. The Human Genome Project has made remarkable advances toward determining the exact DNA sequence of human genes and the precise genes that are associated with certain abnormalities such as fragile X syndrome and cystic fibrosis, as discussed in greater detail later in the chapter (National Human Genome Research Institute, 2011).

All *somatic (body) cells* have 23 pairs of homologous chromosomes (a matched pair of chromosomes, one inherited from each parent) (see Chapter 4 🔗). Twenty-two of the pairs are **autosomes**

● **Figure 7–7** Normal female karyotype.

Source: Courtesy of Susan Olson, PhD, The Oregon Health & Science University Cytogenics Laboratory.

(nonsex chromosomes), and one pair is made up of the sex chromosomes, X and Y. A normal female has a 46, XX chromosome constitution, the normal male, 46, XY (Figures 7–7 ● and 7–8 ●).

The **karyotype**, or pictorial analysis of these chromosomes, is usually obtained from specially treated and stained peripheral blood lymphocytes. Placental tissue taken from a site near the insertion of the cord and deep enough to include chorion can also be sent for karyotyping of the fetus.

Chromosome abnormalities can occur in either the autosomes or the sex chromosomes and can be divided into two categories: abnormalities of number and abnormalities of structure. Even small alterations in chromosomes can cause problems, especially those associated with delayed growth and development. Some of these abnormalities can be passed on to other offspring. Thus in some cases chromosomal analysis is appropriate even if clinical manifestations are mild.

Abnormalities of Chromosomal Number

Abnormalities of chromosomal number are most commonly seen as trisomies, monosomies, and mosaicism. In all three cases, the abnormality is most often caused by *nondisjunction,* a failure of paired chromosomes to separate during cell division. If nondisjunction occurs in either the sperm or the egg before fertilization, the resulting zygote (fertilized egg) will have an abnormal chromosome makeup in all of the cells (trisomy or monosomy). If nondisjunction occurs after fertilization, the developing zygote will have cells with two or more different chromosome makeups, evolving into two or more different cell lines (mosaicism).

● **Figure 7–8** Normal male karyotype.

Source: Courtesy of Susan Olson, PhD, The Oregon Health & Science University Cytogenics Laboratory.

Video | What Is a Gene?

Trisomies are the product of the union of a normal gamete (egg or sperm) with a gamete that contains an extra chromosome. The resulting individual will have 47 chromosomes and be trisomic (have three copies of the same chromosome) for whichever chromosome is extra (Table 7–5). Down syndrome (formerly called *mongolism*) is the most common trisomy seen in children (Figure 7–9 ●). The presence of the extra chromosome 21 produces distinctive clinical features (Figure 7–10 ●). Although children born with Down syndrome have a variety of physical ailments, advances in medical science have extended their life expectancy.

Two other common trisomies are trisomy 18 and trisomy 13 (refer to Table 7–5 and Figures 7–11 ● and 7–12 ●). The prognosis for both trisomies 13 and 18 is extremely poor. Most children (70%) die within the first 3 months of life secondary to complications related to respiratory and cardiac abnormalities. However, 10% survive the first year of life; therefore, the family needs to plan for the possibility of long-term care of a severely affected infant and for family support.

Monosomies occur when a normal gamete unites with a gamete that is missing a chromosome. In this case, the individual

Table 7–5	Chromosomal Syndromes
Altered Chromosome: 21	**Characteristics**
Genetic defect: trisomy 21 (Down syndrome) (secondary nondisjunction or 14/21 unbalanced translocation) Incidence: average 1 in 700 live births, incidence variable with age of woman (Figures 7–9 and 7–10)	CNS: intellectual disability; hypotonia at birth Head: flattened occiput; depressed nasal bridge; mongoloid slant of eyes; epicanthal folds; white specking of the iris (Brushfield spots); protrusion of the tongue; high, arched palate; low-set ears Hands: broad, short fingers; abnormalities of finger and foot; dermal ridge patterns (dermatoglyphics); transverse palmar crease (simian line) Other: congenital heart disease
Altered Chromosome: 18	**Characteristics**
Genetic defect: trisomy 18 Incidence: 1 in 3,000 live births (Figure 7–11*B*)	CNS: intellectual disability; severe hypotonia Head: prominent occiput; low-set ears; corneal opacities; ptosis (drooping eyelids) Hands: third and fourth fingers overlapped by second and fifth fingers; abnormal dermatoglyphics; syndactyly (webbing of fingers) Other: congenital heart defects; renal abnormalities; single umbilical artery; gastrointestinal tract abnormalities; rocker-bottom feet; cryptorchidism; various malformations of other organs
Altered Chromosome: 13	**Characteristics**
Genetic defect: trisomy 13 Incidence: 1 in 5,000 live births	CNS: intellectual disability; severe hypotonia; seizures Head: microcephaly; microphthalmia, and/or coloboma (keyhole-shaped pupil); malformed ears; aplasia of external auditory canal; micrognathia (abnormally small lower jaw); cleft lip and palate Hands: polydactyly (extra digits); abnormal posturing of fingers; abnormal dermatoglyphics Other: congenital heart defects; hemangiomas; gastrointestinal tract defects; various malformations of other organs
Altered Chromosome: 5P	**Characteristics**
Genetic defect: deletion of short arm of chromosome 5 (*cri du chat*, or cat-cry syndrome) Incidence: 1 in 20,000 live births	CNS: severe intellectual disability; a catlike cry in infancy Head: microcephaly; hypertelorism (widely spaced eyes); epicanthal folds; low-set ears Other: failure to thrive; various organ malformations
Altered Chromosome: X (sex chromosome)	**Characteristics**
Genetic defect: only one X chromosome or partially missing second X chromosome in female (Turner syndrome) Incidence: 1 in 300 to 7,000 live female births (see Figure 7–13)	CNS: no intellectual impairment; some perceptual difficulties Head: low hairline; webbed neck Trunk: short stature; cubitus valgus (increased carrying angle of arm); excessive nevi (congenital discoloration of skin because of pigmentation); broad, shieldlike chest with widely spaced nipples; puffy feet; no toenails Other: fibrous streaks in ovaries; underdeveloped secondary sex characteristics; primary amenorrhea; usually infertile; renal anomalies; coarctation of the aorta
Altered Chromosome: XXY (sex chromosome)	**Characteristics**
Genetic defect: extra X chromosome in male (Klinefelter syndrome) Incidence: 1 in 1,000 live male births	CNS: mild intellectual disability Trunk: occasional gynecomastia (abnormally large male breasts); eunuchoid body proportions (lack of male muscular and sexual development) Other: small, soft testes; underdeveloped secondary sex characteristics; usually sterile

● **Figure 7–9** Karyotype of a female who has trisomy 21, Down syndrome. Note the extra 21 chromosome.

Source: Courtesy of Susan Olson, PhD, The Oregon Health & Science University Cytogenics Laboratory.

● **Figure 7–10** A boy with Down syndrome.

Source: Joni Hofmann/Fotolia.

B

● **Figure 7–11** *A,* Karyotype of a male who has trisomy 18. *B,* Infant girl with trisomy 18.

Source: Courtesy of Susan Olson, PhD, The Oregon Health & Science University Cytogenics Laboratory.

● **Figure 7–12** Karyotype of male with trisomy 13.

Source: Courtesy of Susan Olson, PhD, The Oregon Health & Science University Cytogenics Laboratory.

has only 45 chromosomes and is said to be monosomic. Monosomy of an entire autosomal chromosome is incompatible with life.

Mosaicism occurs after fertilization and results in an individual who has two different cell lines, each with a different chromosomal number. Mosaicism tends to be more common in the sex chromosomes than in the autosomes; when it occurs in the autosomes, it is most common in Down syndrome.

Abnormalities of Chromosome Structure

Abnormalities of chromosome structure involve only parts of the chromosome and occur in two forms: translocation and deletions or duplications. Most (>95%) children born with Down syndrome have trisomy 21, whereas some (<5%) have an abnormal rearrangement of chromosomal material known as a *translocation.* Clinically the two types of Down syndrome are indistinguishable; the only way to distinguish them is to do a chromosome analysis.

The translocation occurs when the carrier parent has 45 chromosomes, usually with one chromosome fused to another. For example, a common translocation is one in which a particle of chromosome 14 breaks and fuses to chromosome 21. The parent has one normal 14, one normal 21, and one 14/21 chromosome. Because all the chromosomal material is present and functioning normally, the parent is clinically normal. This individual is known as a *balanced translocation carrier.* When a person who

is a balanced translocation carrier has a child with a partner who has a structurally normal chromosome constitution, the child can have a normal number of chromosomes, be a carrier, or have an extra chromosome 21. Such a child has an *unbalanced translocation* and has Down syndrome.

Structure abnormality is also caused by *duplications* or *deletions* of chromosomal material. Any portion of a chromosome may be lost or added, generally leading to some adverse effect. Depending on how much chromosomal material is involved, the clinical effects may be mild or severe. Many types of duplications and deletions have been described, such as the deletion of the short arm of chromosome 5 (*cri du chat,* or cat-cry syndrome) or the deletion of the long arm of chromosome 18 (Edwards syndrome). Table 7–5 lists other chromosomal syndromes.

Sex Chromosome Abnormalities

To better understand abnormalities of the sex chromosomes, the nurse should know that in a female, at an early embryonic stage, one of the two normal X chromosomes becomes inactive. The inactive X chromosome forms a dark staining area known as the *Barr body*. The normal female has one Barr body, because one of her two X chromosomes has been inactivated. The typical male has no Barr bodies because he has only one X chromosome.

The most common sex chromosome abnormalities are Turner syndrome in females (45, X with no Barr bodies present; see Figure 7–13 ●) and Klinefelter syndrome in males (47, XXY with one Barr body present). See Table 7–5 for clinical descriptions of these abnormalities.

The mosaic form of the X chromosome is associated with daughters of women who took the drug diethylstilbestrol (DES) during pregnancy. The fertility of women with the mosaic form of the XO chromosome may not be impaired; however, there is a higher percentage of uterine malformation and hormonal difficulty associated with it and therefore a high degree of miscarriage.

There is a concern that children born as a result of ICSI might be at increased risk for chromosomal and other major congenital anomalies, cancer, or infertility, because intracytoplasmic sperm

injection (ICSI) may override natural safeguards that serve to prevent fertilization. Therefore, it is strongly recommended that karyotyping and Y chromosome deletion analysis be offered to all men with severe male factor infertility who are candidates for IVF and ICSI (ASRM, 2011).

Modes of Inheritance

Many inherited diseases are produced by an abnormality in a single gene or pair of genes. In such instances, the chromosomes are grossly normal. The defect is at the gene level. Some of these gene defects can be detected by technologies such as DNA and other biochemical assays. The two major categories of inheritance are **Mendelian (single-gene) inheritance** and **non-Mendelian (multifactorial) inheritance**. Each single-gene trait is determined by a pair of genes working together. These genes are responsible for the observable expression of the traits (e.g., brown eyes, dark skin), referred to as the **phenotype**. The total genetic makeup of an individual is referred to as the **genotype** (pattern of the genes on the chromosomes).

One of the genes for a trait is inherited from the mother, the other from the father. An individual who has two identical genes at a given locus is considered to be *homozygous* for that trait. Individuals are considered to be *heterozygous* for a particular trait when they have two different alleles (alternate forms of the same gene) at a given locus on a pair of homologous chromosomes.

The best known modes of single-gene inheritance are autosomal dominant, autosomal recessive, and X-linked (sex-linked).

Autosomal Dominant Inheritance

A person is said to have an autosomal dominant inherited disorder if the disease trait is heterozygous—that is, the abnormal gene overshadows the normal gene of the pair to produce the trait. It is essential to remember that in autosomal dominant inheritance the following occurs:

- An affected individual generally has an affected parent. Thus the family **pedigree** (graphic representation of a family tree) usually shows multiple generations with the disorder.

- Affected individuals have a 50% chance of passing on the abnormal gene to each of their children (Figure 7–14 ●).

- Males and females are equally affected, and a father can pass the abnormal gene on to his son. This is an important principle when distinguishing autosomal dominant disorders from X-linked disorders.

- Autosomal dominant inherited disorders have varying degrees of presentation. This is an important factor when counseling families concerning autosomal dominant disorders. Although a parent may have a mild form of the disease, the child may have a more severe form.

Autosomal dominant conditions such as phocomelia (a developmental anomaly characterized by the absence of the upper portion of the limbs) can have minimal expression in a parent but severe effects in a child. Other common autosomal dominant inherited disorders are Huntington disease, myotonic dystrophy, and fragile X syndrome (an X-linked disorder).

A

B

● **Figure 7–13** *A,* Karyotype of a female with Turner syndrome. *B,* Toddler girl with Turner syndrome.

Source: A, Courtesy of Susan Olson, PhD, The Oregon Health & Science University Cytogenics Laboratory. *B,* Courtesy of the Turner Syndrome Society U.S.A.

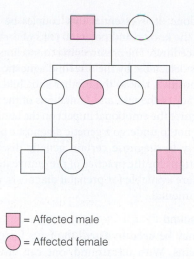

☐ = Affected male

◯ = Affected female

● **Figure 7–14** Autosomal dominant pedigree. One parent is affected. Statistically 50% of offspring will be affected regardless of sex.

Autosomal Recessive Inheritance

In an autosomal recessive inherited disorder, the individual must have two abnormal genes to be affected. A *carrier* is an individual who is heterozygous for the abnormal gene and clinically normal. It is not until two individuals mate and pass on the same abnormal gene that affected children may appear. It is essential to remember that in autosomal recessive inheritance the following occurs:

- An affected individual may have clinically normal parents, but both parents are carriers of the abnormal gene (Figure 7–15 ●).

- In the case where both parents are carriers, there is a 25% chance that the abnormal gene will be passed on to any of their offspring. Each pregnancy has a 25% chance of resulting in an affected child.

- If a child of two carrier parents is clinically normal, there is a 50% chance that the child is a carrier of the gene.

- Both males and females are equally affected.

- There is an increased history of consanguineous matings (mating of close relatives).

Some common autosomal recessive inherited disorders are cystic fibrosis, phenylketonuria (PKU), galactosemia, sickle cell disease, Tay-Sachs disease, and most metabolic disorders.

X-Linked Recessive Inheritance

X-linked (or sex-linked) disorders are those for which the abnormal gene is carried on the X chromosome. Thus an X-linked disorder is manifested in a male who carries the abnormal gene on his only X chromosome and is considered hemizygous for the condition. His mother is considered to be a carrier when the normal gene on one X chromosome overshadows the abnormal gene on the other X chromosome. It is essential to remember that in X-linked recessive inheritance the following occurs:

- There is no male-to-male transmission. Affected males are related through the female line (see Figure 7–16 ●).

- There is a 50% chance that a carrier mother will pass the abnormal gene to each of her sons, who will thus be affected.

- There is a 50% chance that a carrier mother will pass the normal gene to each of her sons, who will thus be unaffected.

- There is a 50% chance that a carrier mother will pass the abnormal gene to each of her daughters, who become carriers.

- Fathers affected with an X-linked disorder cannot pass the disorder to their sons, but all their daughters become carriers of the disorder.

Common X-linked recessive disorders are hemophilia, Duchenne muscular dystrophy, and color blindness. Fragile X syndrome is an X-linked recessive disorder that exhibits anticipation. This condition is the most common form of inherited intellectual disability (mental retardation) second only to Down syndrome. It is caused by an increased number of CGG trinucleotide repeats in the *FMR1* gene, located at a "fragile site" on the long arm of the X chromosome. The normal number of CGG repeats is up to 60. Individuals with a repeat number ranging between 60 and 200

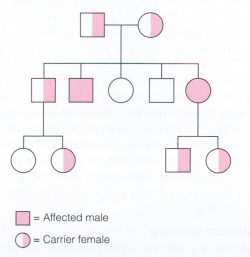

☐ = Affected male

◐ = Carrier female

● **Figure 7–15** Autosomal recessive pedigree. Both parents are carriers. Statistically 25% of offspring are affected regardless of sex.

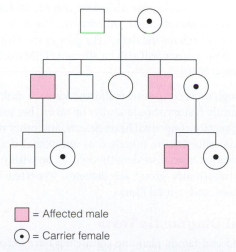

☐ = Affected male

⊙ = Carrier female

● **Figure 7–16** X-linked recessive pedigree. The mother is the carrier. Statistically 50% of male offspring are affected, and 50% of female offspring are carriers.

have a *premutation* allele, meaning the copy number can increase during maternal (but not paternal) meiosis. If the CGG repeat number increases to over 200, the individual (particularly hemizygous males) can have fragile X syndrome. Approximately one third of females with over 200 CGG repeats will be affected with fragile X syndrome, one third will have mild developmental or learning disabilities, and one third will have no symptoms at all.

X-Linked Dominant Inheritance

X-linked dominant disorders are extremely rare, the most common being vitamin D–resistant rickets. When X-linked dominance does occur, the pattern is similar to that of X-linked recessive inheritance except that heterozygous females are affected. It is essential to remember that in X-linked dominant inheritance there is no male-to-male transmission. Affected fathers will have affected daughters; however, because they pass only the Y chromosome to male offspring, any sons will not be affected.

Multifactorial Inheritance

Many common congenital malformations such as cleft palate, heart defects, spina bifida, dislocated hips, clubfoot, and pyloric stenosis are caused by an interaction of many genes and environmental factors. They are, therefore, multifactorial in origin. It is essential to remember that in multifactorial inheritance the following occurs:

- The malformations may vary from mild to severe. For example, spina bifida may range in severity from mild (spina bifida occulta) to more severe (myelomeningocele). The more severe the defect, the greater the number of genes present for that defect.

- There is often a sex bias. For example, pyloric stenosis is more common in males, whereas cleft palate is more common in females. When a member of the less commonly affected sex shows the condition, a greater number of genes must usually be present to cause the defect.

- Not only is increased risk greatest among closest relatives and decreases with distance of relationship, but the risk is increased when multiple family members are affected.

- In contrast to single-gene disorders, there is an additive effect in multifactorial inheritance. The more family members who have the defect, the greater the risk that the next pregnancy will also be affected (DiMaio, Fox, & Mahoney, 2010).

Although most congenital malformations are multifactorial, a careful family history should always be taken, because cleft lip and palate, certain congenital heart defects, and other malformations occasionally can be inherited as autosomal dominant or recessive traits. Other disorders thought to be within the multifactorial inheritance group are diabetes, hypertension, some heart diseases, and mental illness.

Prenatal Diagnostic Tests

Parent-child and family planning counseling have become a major responsibility of professional nurses. To be effective counselors, nurses must have the most up-to-date information about prenatal diagnosis. Appropriate counseling should occur before prenatal

screening is done. It is essential that couples be completely informed about the known and potential risks of each of the genetic diagnostic procedures. The prescreening counseling should include the conditions detectable by the screen, diagnostic test available if the screen is positive, risk to the mother and child of the test performed, accuracy of the test, and limitations of the test. The nurse needs to recognize the emotional impact on the family of a decision to undergo or not to undergo a genetic diagnostic procedure.

The ability to diagnose certain genetic diseases has enormous implications for the practice of preventive health care. Several methods are available for prenatal diagnosis, although some are still experimental.

Genetic Ultrasound

Ultrasound may be used to assess the fetus for genetic or congenital problems. With ultrasound, one can visualize the fetal head for abnormalities in size, shape, and structure. (For a detailed discussion of ultrasound technology, see Chapter 14 .) Craniospinal defects (anencephalus, microcephaly, hydrocephalus), thoracic malformations (diaphragmatic hernia), gastrointestinal malformations (omphalocele, gastroschisis), renal malformations (dysplasia or obstruction), and skeletal malformations (caudal regression, conjoined twins) are just some of the disorders that have been diagnosed in utero by ultrasound. Screening by ultrasound for congenital anomalies is best done at 16 to 20 weeks, when fetal structures have developed completely. With the addition of a fetal nuchal translucency measurement at 10 to 14 weeks, there is high correlation with fetal chromosome abnormalities (Gilbert, 2011). The nuchal translucency is a fluid-filled space at the back of the fetal neck. An increased amount of fluid is associated with an increased risk for chromosome abnormalities, birth defects, genetic syndromes, and poor pregnancy outcome—the larger the nuchal translucency, the higher the risk for abnormalities. There is no information documenting harm to the fetus or long-term effects with exposure to ultrasound. However, there is no guarantee of complete safety; therefore, the practitioner and the parents must evaluate the risks against the benefits on an individual basis.

Screening and invasive diagnostic testing for chromosome abnormalities should be available to all women who present for prenatal care before 20 weeks of pregnancy regardless of maternal age. Women should be counseled regarding the differences between screening and invasive diagnostic testing. Screening tests, such as the nuchal translucency ultrasound and maternal serum screening, are designed to gather information about the risk that the pregnancy could have chromosome abnormalities or open spina bifida. If the risk is increased above a specific cutoff, the woman is offered invasive prenatal diagnosis. These diagnostic techniques, such as amniocentesis and chorionic villus sampling (CVS), obtain cells from the pregnancy to rule out or diagnose a chromosome abnormality or certain genetic disorders. They are associated with a small risk of pregnancy complications, including miscarriage.

Maternal Serum Screening

Measuring specific hormones and proteins in the maternal serum during the first and/or second trimester can determine the risk for Down syndrome, trisomy 18, or open spina bifida. In the first trimester, the nuchal translucency measurement is often added to improve the detection rate for Down syndrome and trisomy 18. Detection and false-positive rates differ depending on the type of screening test that is performed and may also differ depending on the laboratory that performs the screening.

Genetic Amniocentesis

A major method of prenatal diagnosis is genetic amniocentesis (Figure 7–17 ●). The procedure is described in Chapter 14 🔗. The risk for pregnancy complications, including infection and miscarriage, are thought to be less than 0.5%. The indications for genetic amniocentesis include the following:

1. *Maternal age 35 or older.* Women ages 35 or older are at greater risk for having children with chromosomal abnormalities. Chromosomal abnormalities because of maternal age include trisomy 21, trisomy 13, trisomy 18, XXX, or XXY. The risk of having a live-born infant with a chromosome problem is 1 in 192 for a 35-year-old woman; the risk for trisomy 21 is 1 in 385. At age 44, the risks are 1 in 20 and 1 in 37, respectively (Harper, 2010).

2. *Previous child born with a chromosomal abnormality.* Young couples who have had a child with a trisomy 21, 18, or 13 have an approximately 1% to 2% risk of a future child having a chromosomal abnormality.

3. *Parent carrying a chromosomal abnormality (balanced translocation).* A woman who carries a balanced 14/21 translocation has a risk of approximately 10% to 15% that her children will be affected with the unbalanced translocation of Down syndrome; if the father is the carrier, there is a 2% to 5% risk.

4. *Mother carrying an X-linked disease.* In families in which the woman is a known or possible carrier of an X-linked disorder such as hemophilia A or B or Duchenne muscular dystrophy, the risk of an affected male fetus is 50%. Now DNA testing may make it possible to identify affected males from nonaffected males in some disorders.

5. *Parents carrying an inborn error of metabolism that can be diagnosed in utero.* Inborn error of metabolism disorders are detectable in utero by DNA analysis or biochemical testing, and include Fabry disease, galactosemia, Gaucher

A Amniocentesis

B Chorionic villus sampling

Human karyotype

● **Figure 7–17** *A,* Genetic amniocentesis. This method used for prenatal diagnosis is done at 15 to 21 weeks' gestation. *B,* Chorionic villus sampling is done at 10 to 13 weeks, and the cells are cultured and karyotyped. Results take 7 to 14 days.

disease, homocystinuria, Hunter syndrome, Hurler syndrome, Krabbe disease, Lesch-Nyhan disease, maple syrup urine disease, metachromatic leukodystrophy, methylmalonic aciduria, Niemann-Pick disease, Pompe disease, and Tay-Sachs disease.

6. *Both parents carrying an autosomal recessive disease.* When both parents are carriers of an autosomal recessive disease, there is a 25% risk for *each pregnancy* that the fetus will be affected. Autosomal recessive diseases identified by amniocentesis are hemoglobinopathies such as sickle cell disease, thalassemia, and cystic fibrosis.

7. *Family history of neural tube defects.* Genetic amniocentesis is available to couples who have had a child with neural tube defects or who have a family history of these conditions, which include anencephaly, spina bifida, and myelomeningocele. Neural tube defects are usually multifactorial traits.

Percutaneous Umbilical Blood Sampling and Chorionic Villus Sampling

Percutaneous umbilical blood sampling (PUBS) is a technique used for obtaining blood that allows for rapid chromosome diagnosis, genetic studies, or transfusion for Rh isoimmunization or hydrops fetalis. *Chorionic villus sampling (CVS)* is used in selected regional centers, and its diagnostic capability is similar to that of amniocentesis. Its advantage is that diagnostic information is available at 10 to 13 weeks' gestation. The risk for pregnancy complications, including infection and pregnancy loss, is estimated to be around 1%. For further discussion of these techniques, see Chapter 14 ⊘.

Noninvasive Prenatal Diagnosis

In the near future, noninvasive methods of prenatal diagnosis for chromosome abnormalities or genetic disorders will be available by obtaining maternal blood as early as 8 weeks of pregnancy. Fetal ribonucleic acid (RNA) and/or DNA can be isolated in the maternal serum to test for specific disorders. This technology is currently used for fetal Rh determination in women who are Rh negative. Commercial biotechnology companies plan to introduce this testing, particularly for the diagnosis of chromosomal trisomies such as Down syndrome. Preliminary data estimate that the accuracy of the test is >99%.

Nursing Management

Nurses are on the front line of patient care and need to be competent in genetic- and genomic-related health care, know how to find reliable genetic information, and know where to refer patients and families for further genetic information and counseling (Consensus Panel on Genetic/Genomic Nursing Competencies, 2009). In both prospective and retrospective genetic counseling, timely nursing intervention is a crucial factor. During annual exam and other clinical appointments, the nurse should interview all women of childbearing age to determine any family history or other risk factors for genetic disorders. If the woman is planning to conceive, genetic counseling should be encouraged before discontinuation of contraception.

Nursing Implications of Prenatal Diagnostic Testing

It is imperative that counseling precede any procedure for prenatal diagnosis. Many questions and points must be considered if the family is to reach a satisfactory decision. See *Health Promotion: Couples Who May Benefit from Prenatal Diagnosis*.

Every pregnancy has a 3% to 4% risk of resulting in an infant with a birth defect. When an abnormality is detected or suspected before birth, an attempt is made to determine the diagnosis by assessing the family health history (via the pedigree) and the pregnancy history and by evaluating the fetal anomaly or anomalies via ultrasound. After experts on a specific disorder have been consulted, healthcare professionals can then present the parents with options. Treatment of prenatally diagnosed disorders may begin during the pregnancy, thus possibly preventing irreversible damage. In light of the philosophy of preventive health care, information that can be obtained prenatally should be made available to all couples who are expecting a baby or who are contemplating pregnancy.

With the advent of diagnostic techniques such as amniocentesis, at-risk couples who would not otherwise have a first child or additional children can decide to conceive. Following prenatal diagnosis, a couple can decide not to have a child with a genetic disease. For many couples, prenatal diagnosis is not a solution because they choose not to prevent the genetic disease by aborting the fetus. The decision about whether to use prenatal diagnosis can only be made by the family. Even when termination is not an option, prenatal diagnosis can give parents an opportunity to

---

Health Promotion   Couples Who May Benefit from Prenatal Diagnosis

- Women ages 35 or older at time of birth
- Couples with a balanced translocation (chromosomal abnormality)
- Family history of known or suspected Mendelian genetic disorder (e.g., cystic fibrosis, hemophilia A and B, Duchenne muscular dystrophy)
- Couples with a previous child with chromosomal abnormality
- Couples in which either partner or a previous child is affected with, or in which both partners are carriers for, a diagnosable metabolic disorder
- Family history of birth defects and/or intellectual disability (e.g., neural tube defects, congenital heart disease, cleft lip and/or palate)

- Ethnic groups at increased risk for specific disorders (see *Developing Cultural Competence: Genetic Screening Recommendations for Various Ethnic and Age Groups* on page 157)
- Couples with history of two or more first-trimester spontaneous abortions
- Women with an abnormal maternal serum alpha-fetoprotein (MSAFP or AFP) test
- Women with a teratogenic risk secondary to an exposure or maternal health condition (e.g., diabetes)

Clinical Tip

- Remember that prenatal screening and diagnosis are optional parts of routine prenatal care.
- Present options to patients using a nondirective manner. *Nondirective counseling* is a technique designed to allow patients to talk about their problems or emotional difficulties and reach the decision that is best for themselves or their families with a minimum of direction from the person serving as their counselor.
- Give patients accurate, up-to-date information about the various prenatal screening and diagnostic testing options, but remain impartial and do not recommend any specific course of action.
- Be aware of the language you use when discussing these options with patients. For example, in discussing prenatal screening for Down syndrome, terms such as *handicapped* or *retarded* should be replaced with *disabled* and/or *developmentally/cognitively/intellectually disabled*. Use the words *risk for*, or consider using the terms *chance of* or *possibility of*.

prepare for the birth of a child with special needs, contact the families of children with similar problems, or access support services before the birth.

Postnatal Diagnosis

The nurse has a key role in preventing recurrence. The perinatal nursing team frequently has the first contact with the family who has an affected newborn. One cannot expect a couple who has just learned that their child has a birth defect or Down syndrome to take in any information concerning future risks. However, the couple should never be "put off" from genetic counseling for so long that they conceive another affected child because of lack of information. The nurse can inform the parents that before they attempt to have another child, genetic counseling is available.

Questions concerning genetic disorders (cause, treatment, and prognosis) are most often first discussed in the newborn nursery or during the infant's first few months of life. When a child is born with anomalies, has a stormy newborn period, or does not progress as expected, a genetic evaluation may be warranted. An accurate diagnosis and an optimal treatment plan incorporate the following:

- Complete detailed history to determine whether the problem is prenatal (congenital), postnatal, or familial in origin
- Thorough physical and dermatoglyphic examination by a trained clinical geneticist.
- Laboratory analysis, which includes chromosome analysis; enzyme assay for inborn errors of metabolism; DNA studies (both direct and by linkage); and antibody titers for infectious teratogens, such as toxoplasmosis, rubella, cytomegalovirus, and herpes virus (TORCH syndrome) (see Chapter 16 🔗).

To make an accurate diagnosis, the geneticist consults with other specialists and reviews the current literature, evaluating all the available information before arriving at a diagnosis and plan of action.

The Human Genome Project has significant implications for the identification and management of inherited disorders. Once genes are identified, it will be possible to detect their presence in carriers and provide better genetic counseling. However, concerns have been voiced about ethical considerations with genetic research. What guidelines are needed to protect children and families so that genetic testing does not lead to discrimination in future employment or health insurance? Who should be tested for genetic diseases, and who should have access to the results? Because children cannot yet give informed consent for genetic testing (see Chapter 1 🔗 for discussion of informed consent), it is recommended that children and adolescents should have genetic testing only when medical treatment can help if the disease is identified, or when another family member might benefit from the knowledge for their own health and the child will not be harmed by testing (American Academy of Pediatrics, Committee on Genetics, 2000, reaffirmed 2009). Whenever genetic testing is performed, counseling about the results must be available.

Genetic Counseling

Genetic counseling is a communication process in which a genetic counselor, physician, or specially trained and certified nurse helps a family or individuals understand and adapt to the medical, psychologic, and familial implications of genetic contributions to disease (National Society of Genetic Counselors, 2005, reaffirmed 2011).

Referral

Genetic counseling referral is advised for any of the following categories:

- *Congenital abnormalities.* These include *developmental/cognitive/intellectual disabilities.* Any couple who has a child or a relative with a congenital malformation may be at increased risk and should be so informed. If a developmental/cognitive/intellectual disability of unidentified cause has occurred in a family, there may be an increased risk of recurrence. In some cases, the genetic counselor will identify the cause of a malformation as a teratogen (for more information about teratogens, see Chapter 11 🔗). The family should be aware of teratogenic substances so they can avoid exposure during any subsequent pregnancy.

- *Familial disorders.* Families should be told that certain diseases may have a genetic component and that the risk of their occurrence in a particular family may be higher than that in the general population. Such disorders as diabetes, heart disease, cancer, and mental illness fall into this category.

- *Known inherited diseases.* Families may know that a disease is inherited but not know the mechanism or the specific risk for them. An important point to remember is that family members who are not at risk for passing on a disorder should be as well informed as family members who are at risk.

- *Metabolic disorders.* Any families at risk for having a child with a metabolic disorder or biochemical defect should be referred for genetic counseling. Because most inborn errors of metabolism are autosomal recessively inherited, a family may not be identified as being at risk until the birth of an affected child.

Weblink | Human Genome Project

■ *Chromosomal abnormalities.* As discussed previously, any couple who has had a child with a chromosomal abnormality may be at increased risk of having another child similarly affected. This group includes families in which there is concern about a possible translocation.

After a couple has been referred to the genetics clinic, they are sent a form requesting information on the health status of various family members. This information assists the genetic counselor in creating the family's pedigree.

The pedigree and history facilitate identification of other family members who might also be at risk for the same disorder (Figure 7–18 ●). The couple being counseled may wish to notify relatives at risk so that they, too, can begin genetic counseling. When done correctly, the family history and pedigree can be powerful tools for determining a family's risk.

Initial Session

During the initial session, the counselor gathers additional information about the pregnancy, the affected child's growth and development, and the family's understanding of the problem. The counselor also elicits information concerning ethnic background and family origin. Many genetic disorders are more common among certain ethnic groups or in particular geographic areas. (See *Developing Cultural Competence:*

Developing Cultural Competence
Consanguineous Marriages

In the United States, marriage between related individuals is generally taboo. In Western medicine, there is a concern that a child conceived by people who are related by blood may have an increased risk for birth defects. This has not, however, been supported by recent research unless the relationship is closer than first cousins. In many other cultures, marriage of first cousins and others who are related by blood is acceptable and even common. Egypt has a high rate of consanguineous (blood relationship) marriages. Reasons for consanguineous marriage include: "increase family links," "they knew each other and everything would be clear before marriage," "customs and traditions," and "less cost." The most common type of consanguineous marriage in Egypt is between first cousins.

Genetic Screening Recommendations for Various Ethnic and Age Groups.)

Generally the child undergoes a physical examination. Other family members may also be examined. If laboratory tests such as chromosomal analyses, metabolic studies, or viral titers are indicated, they are performed at this time. The genetic counselor may then give the parents some preliminary information based on the data at hand.

Follow-Up Counseling

After all the data have been carefully examined and analyzed, the couple returns for a follow-up visit. At this time, the genetic counselor gives the parents all the information available, including:

■ Medical facts

■ Diagnosis

■ Probable course of the disorder and any available management

■ Inheritance pattern for this particular family

■ Risk of recurrence and the options or alternatives for dealing with recurrence

The remainder of the counseling session is spent discussing the course of action that seems appropriate to the family in view of the risk and family goals. For couples who desire to become parents or who want a subsequent child, options include prenatal diagnosis, early detection and treatment, preimplantation genetic diagnosis or other assisted reproductive therapies, delayed childbearing until prenatal diagnosis is available or a disease can be detected and treated early to prevent irreversible damage, or in some cases, adoption. When the parents have completed the counseling sessions, the counselor sends them and their certified nurse-midwife or physician a letter detailing the contents of the sessions. The parents keep this document for reference.

The family may return to the genetic counselor a number of times to ask questions and express concerns, especially if the couple is considering having more children, or if siblings want information about their affected brother or sister. It is most desirable for the nurse working with the family to attend many or

● **Figure 7–18** Screening pedigree. Arrow indicates the nearest family member affected with the disorder being investigated. Numbers refer to the ages or birth dates of family members.

Developing Cultural Competence
Genetic Screening Recommendations for Various Ethnic and Age Groups

Background of Population at Risk	Disorder	Screening Test	Definitive Test
Ashkenazi Jewish, French-Canadian, Cajun	Tay-Sachs disease	Decreased serum hexosaminidase-A or DNA mutation analysis	Chorionic villus sampling (CVS) or amniocentesis for hexosaminidase-A assay or DNA mutation analysis
Ashkenazi Jewish	Cystic fibrosis, Canavan disease, familial dysautonomia, several other disorders	DNA mutation analysis	CVS or amniocentesis for DNA mutation analysis
African; Hispanic from Caribbean, Central America, or South America; Arab, Egyptian; Asian Indian	Sickle cell disease	Presence of sickle cell hemoglobin; confirmatory hemoglobin electrophoresis	CVS or amniocentesis for DNA mutation analysis
Greek, Italian	Beta-thalassemia	Mean corpuscular volume less than 80% confirmatory hemoglobin electrophoresis	CVS or amniocentesis for DNA mutation analysis
Southeast Asian (Vietnamese, Laotian, Cambodian), Filipino	Alpha-thalassemia	Mean corpuscular volume less than 80%; confirmatory hemoglobin electrophoresis	CVS or amniocentesis for DNA mutation analysis or gene deletion studies
Women over age 35 (all ethnic groups)	Chromosomal trisomies	Prenatal serum and/or ultrasound screening	CVS or amniocentesis for cytogenetic analysis
Women of any age (all ethnic groups; particularly suggested for women from British Isles, Ireland)	Neural tube defects and selected other anomalies	Maternal serum alpha-fetoprotein (MSAFP)	Amniocentesis for amniotic fluid alpha-fetoprotein (AFP) and acetyl-cholinesterase assays
Caucasian (northern European, Celtic population), Ashkenazi Jewish	Cystic fibrosis	DNA mutation analysis of the cystic fibrosis transmembrane regulation (CFTR) gene	CVS or amniocentesis for DNA mutation analysis

all of these counseling sessions. Because the nurse has already established a rapport with the couple, she or he can act as a liaison between the family and the genetic counselor. Hearing directly what the genetic counselor says helps the nurse clarify the issues for the family, which in turn helps them formulate questions. Many genetic centers have found the public health nurse to be the ideal health professional to provide such follow-up care. Nurses must be careful not to assume a diagnosis, determine carrier status or recurrence risks, or provide genetic counseling without adequate information and training. Inadequate, inappropriate, or inaccurate information may be misleading or harmful. Healthcare professionals need to learn the appropriate referral systems and options for care in their region.

After genetic counseling, the nurse with the appropriate knowledge of genetics is in an ideal position to help couples review what has been discussed during the counseling sessions and to answer any additional questions they might have. As families return to daily living, the nurse can provide helpful information on the day-to-day aspects of caring for a child, answer questions as they arise, support parents in their decisions, and refer families to other health and community agencies. Nursing care of children with various genetic issues is discussed in Part 7, *Caring for Children with Alterations in Health Status*, of this text.

 Clinical Tip

Nursing responsibilities in genetic counseling include:

- Identifying families at risk for genetic problems
- Determining how the genetic problem is perceived and what information is desired before proceeding
- Assisting families in acquiring accurate information about the specific problem
- Acting as a liaison between the family and genetic counselor
- Assisting the family in understanding and dealing with information received
- Providing information on support groups
- Aiding families in coping with this crisis
- Providing information about known genetic factors
- Assuring continuity of nursing care to the family

Critical Concept Review

LEARNING OUTCOME 7.1: Compare the essential components of fertility with the possible causes of infertility.

1. Female:
   - Cervical mucus must be favorable.
   - Fallopian tubes must be patent.
   - Ovaries must produce and release ova in a regular, cyclic fashion.
   - Endometrium must be prepared for implantation of the blastocyst.
   - Adequate reproductive hormones must be present.

2. Male:
   - Testes must produce adequate numbers of sperm.
   - Genital tract must be unobstructed.
   - Genital tract secretions must be normal.
   - Ejaculated sperm must reach cervix.

LEARNING OUTCOME 7.2: Describe the elements of the preliminary investigation of infertility and the nurse's role in supporting/teaching patients during this phase.

1. Information about most fertile times for intercourse.
2. Explanation of basic infertility workup.
3. Basic assessments:
   - Ovarian function.
   - Cervical mucus adequacy.
   - Receptivity to sperm.
   - Sperm adequacy.
   - Tubal patency.
   - General condition of pelvic organs.
   - Semen analysis.
4. Complete physical examination of both partners.

5. Laboratory examination:
   - CBC.
   - UA.
   - Hormonal assays.
6. Nurse's role:
   - Provide information about most fertile times to have intercourse.
   - Explain the basic infertility workup.
   - Provide comfort to couples by using a nonjudgmental approach and information and instruction throughout the diagnostic and therapeutic process.

LEARNING OUTCOME 7.3: Summarize the indications for the tests and associated treatments, including assisted reproductive technologies, that are done in an infertility workup.

1. If lack of ovarian function is suspected:
   - Basal body temperature recording.
   - Hormonal assessments.
   - Endometrial biopsy.
   - Transvaginal ultrasound.
2. If cervical problems are suspected:
   - Ferning capacity of cervical mucus.
   - Postcoital test.
3. If tubal or uterine problems are suspected:
   - Hysterosalpingography.
   - Hysteroscopy.
   - Laparoscopy.

4. If male's fertility is suspected:
   - Semen analysis.
   - Screening for antisperm antibodies.
5. Pharmacologic intervention is prescribed if ovarian or endometrial function is abnormal.
6. Therapeutic insemination is indicated for low or abnormal sperm counts or structural defects in the male reproductive tract.
7. In vitro fertilization (IVF) is used when infertility has resulted from tubal factors, mucus abnormalities, male infertility, female immunologic infertility, and cervical factors.

LEARNING OUTCOME 7.4: Relate the physiologic and psychologic effects of infertility on a couple to the nursing management of the couple.

1. Development of lack of spontaneity of sexual intercourse.
2. Feelings of loss of control.
3. Feelings of reduced competency.
4. Loss of status and ambiguity as a couple.

5. Sense of social stigma.
6. Stress on marital and sexual relationship.
7. Strained relationship with healthcare providers.

LEARNING OUTCOME 7.5: Describe the nurse's role as counselor, educator, and advocate for couples during infertility evaluation and treatment.

1. Support the couple and help them to understand and facilitate the free expressions of feelings.
2. Help the couple to recognize feelings.

3. Help the couple to understand motives.
4. Help the couple identify alternatives, and facilitate partner communication.

LEARNING OUTCOME 7.6: Identify couples who may benefit from preconceptual chromosomal analysis and prenatal testing when providing care to couples with special reproductive concerns.

1. Women who are of advanced maternal age.
2. Family history of a chromosomal disorder, birth defects, or mental retardation.
3. Previous child with chromosomal disorder.

4. Ethnic group with history of chromosomal disorders.
5. Couples with a history of two or more first-trimester spontaneous abortions.
6. Women with an abnormal serum alpha-fetoprotein test.

LEARNING OUTCOME 7.7: Identify the characteristics of autosomal dominant, autosomal recessive, and X-linked (sex-linked) recessive disorders.

1. Autosomal dominant disorder:
   - An affected parent has a 50% chance of having an affected child with each pregnancy.
2. Autosomal recessive disorders:
   - Both parents must be carriers.
   - Each offspring has a 25% chance of having the disease and a 50% chance of being a carrier.
3. X-linked recessive disorders:
   - No male-to-male transmission.
   - Effects limited to males.
   - 50% chance a carrier mother will pass abnormal gene to her son.
   - 50% chance the daughter of a carrier mother will be a carrier.
   - 100% chance that daughter of an affected father will be a carrier.

LEARNING OUTCOME 7.8: Compare prenatal and postnatal diagnostic procedures used to determine the presence of genetic disorders.

1. Prenatal diagnostic tests:
   - Invasive procedure performed on mother, though it may affect the fetus.
   - Genetic ultrasound.
   - Serum alpha-fetoprotein tests.
   - Genetic amniocentesis.
   - Chorionic villus sampling.
   - Percutaneous umbilical blood sampling.
2. Postnatal diagnostic tests:
   - Physical examination and laboratory analysis is performed on the newborn.

LEARNING OUTCOME 7.9: Examine the emotional impact on a couple undergoing genetic testing or coping with the birth of a baby with a genetic disorder, and explain the nurse's role in supporting the family undergoing genetic counseling.

1. Emotional impact:
   - Concern for infant's survival and possible lifelong difficulties.
   - Fear of results of testing.
   - Blame for infant's disorder.
2. The nurse's role:
   - Help families to acquire adequate information and understand this information.
   - Act as a liaison between family and genetic counselor.
   - Provide information about support groups.
   - Provide continuity of care to the family.

Clinical Reasoning in Action

Marie Neives, age 19, presents while you are working at a Planned Parenthood Clinic. She is there for a GYN exam and tells you that she is sexually active with her boyfriend but doesn't want to become pregnant. Because she lives at home with her parents, she does not want to use "the pill" because her mother might find out. Marie tells you she has a family history of sickle cell disease and is concerned that she will pass the disease on. Marie asks you for information concerning fertility awareness. You obtain a menstrual history as follows: menarche age 12, cycle every 28 days for 5 days, dysmenorrhea the first 2 days with moderate flow. She has had one sexual partner. She states her boyfriend doesn't like to use condoms and that she has been lucky so far in not getting pregnant. You assist the nurse practitioner with a physical and pelvic exam. The results show that Marie is essentially healthy. The nurse practitioner asks you to review with Marie the basal body temperature (BBT) method of fertility awareness.

1. Explore with Marie "natural family planning." How would you explain this to her?
2. Briefly explain why the basal body temperature (BBT) method can predict ovulation.
3. How would you describe to Marie the procedure for obtaining BBT?
4. After figuring out her menstruation cycle, to avoid conception when would you tell Marie to abstain from unprotected intercourse?
5. Develop a concept map for a woman who has genetic issues to help her understand her conceptive choices.

See www.nursing.pearsonhighered.com for possible responses and an interactive template for a concept map.

References

American Academy of Pediatrics, Committee on Genetics. (2000, reaffirmed 2009). Molecular genetic testing in pediatric practice: A subject review. *Pediatrics, 106,* 1494–1497. doi:10.1542/peds106.6.1494

American Society for Reproductive Medicine (ASRM). (2011). *Assisted reproductive technologies: A guide for parents.* Retrieved from http://www.asrm.org/patientbooklets

American Society for Reproductive Medicine (ASRM). (2012a). Adversities of being infertile: The experience of Jordanian women. *Fertility and Sterility, 98*(2), 444–449. doi:10.1016/j.fertnstert.2012.04.036

American Society for Reproductive Medicine (ASRM). (2012b). Diagnostic evaluation of the infertile female: A committee opinion. *Fertility and Sterility, 98*(2), 302–307. doi:10.1016/j.fertnstert.2012.05.032

American Society for Reproductive Medicine (ASRM). (2012c). Diagnostic evaluation of the infertile male: A committee opinion. *Fertility and Sterility, 98*(2), 294–301. doi:10.1016/j.fertnstert.2012.05.033

American Society for Reproductive Medicine (ASRM). (2012d). Evaluation and treatment of recurrent pregnancy loss: A committee opinion. *Fertility and Sterility, 98*(5),1103–1111. doi:10.1016/j.fertnstert.2012.06.048

American Society for Reproductive Medicine (ASRM). (2012e). *Frequently asked questions about infertility.* Retrieved from http://www.asrm.org/awards/index.aspx?id=3012

American Society for Reproductive Medicine (ASRM). (2012f). *Infertility: An overview.* Retrieved from http://www.asrm.org/patientbooklets

Bennington, L. K. (2010). Can complementary/alternative medicine be used to treat infertility? *American Journal of Maternal/Child Nursing, 35*(3), 140–149.

Casper, R. E. (2011). Physiologic basis of ovulation induction. In E. Seli (Ed.), *Infertility* (pp. 102–113). West Sussex, UK: Wiley-Blackwell.

Consensus Panel on Genetic/Genomic Nursing Competencies. (2009). *Essentials of genetic and genomic nursing: competencies, curricula guidelines, and outcome indicators* (2nd ed.). Silver Spring, MD: American Nurses Association.

DiMaio, M. S., Fox, J. E., & Mahoney, M. J. (2010). *Prenatal diagnosis: Cases & clinical challenges*. West Sussex, UK: Wiley-Blackwell.

Fritz, M. A., & Speroff L. (2011). *Clinical gynecologic endocrinology and infertility* (8th ed.). Philadelphia, PA: Lippincott Williams & Wilkins.

Gilbert, E. S. (2011). *Manual of high risk pregnancy & delivery* (5th ed.). St. Louis, MO: Mosby Elsevier.

Harper, P. S. (2010). *Practical genetic counseling* (7th ed.) London, UK: Hodder Arnold.

Kalfoglou, A., Kammersell, M., Philpott, S., & Dahl, E. (2013). Ethical arguments for and against sperm sorting for non-medical sex selection: a review. *Reproductive Biomedicine Online, 26*(3), 231–239. doi:10.1016/j.rbmo.2012.11.007

Laliota, M. D. (2011). Preimplantation genetic diagnosis. In E. Seli (Ed.), *Infertility* (pp. 155–163). West Sussex, UK: Wiley-Blackwell.

Marquard, K., Westphal, L. M., Milki, A. A., & Lathi, R. B. (2010). Etiology of recent pregnancy loss in women over the age of 35 years. *Fertility and Sterility, 94*(4), 1473–1477.

Matthews, M. L. (2011). Evaluation of the infertile couple. In E. Seli (Ed.), *Infertility* (pp. 8–17). West Sussex, UK: Wiley-Blackwell.

McGrath, J. M., Samra, H. A., Zukowsky, K., & Baker, B. (2010). Parenting after infertility: Issues for families and infants. *American Journal of Maternal/Child Nursing, 35*(3), 156–165.

Michalakis, K. G., DeCherney, A. H., & Penzias, A. S. (2013). Assisted reproductive technologies: In vitro fertilization & related techniques. In A. H. DeCherney, L. Nathan, N. Laufer, & A. S. Roman (Eds.), *Current diagnosis & treatment: Obstetrics & gynecology* (11th ed., pp. 920–947). New York, NY: McGraw-Hill.

National Human Genome Research Institute. (2011). *Frequently asked questions about genetic disorders.* Retrieved from http://www.genome.gov/19016930

National Society of Genetic Counselors. (2005, reaffirmed 2011). *Genetic counseling as a profession.* Retrieved from http://www.nsgc.org/about/definition/cfm

Ried, K., & Stuart, K. (2011). Efficacy of traditional Chinese herbal medicine in the management of female infertility: A systematic review. *Complementary Therapies in Medicine, 19*(6), 319–331.

Schenker, J. G. (2010). *Infertility evaluation and treatment according to Jewish law.* Retrieved from http://www.obgyn.net/women/women.asp?page=/eago/art13

See, C., McCulloch, M., Smikle, C., & Gao, J. (2011). Chinese herbal medicine and clomiphene citrate for anovulation: A meta-analysis of randomized controlled trials. *Alternative and Complementary Medicine, 17*(5), 397–405.

Skidmore-Roth, L. (2010). *Mosby's handbook of herbs & natural supplements* (4th ed.). St. Louis, MO: Mosby Elsevier.

Van den Broeck, U., Emery, M., Wischmann, T., & Thorn, P. (2010). Patient education and counseling. *Patient Education and Counseling, 422*–428. doi:10.1016j.pec.2010.10.009

Wilson, B. A., Shannon, M. T., & Shields, K. M. (2013). *Prentice Hall nurse's drug guide—2013.* Upper Saddle River, NJ: Pearson Education.

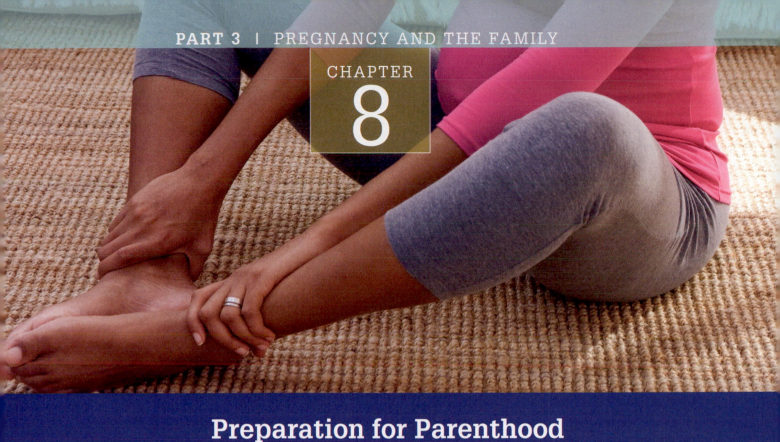

CHAPTER
8

Preparation for Parenthood

We took our childbirth education classes with seven other couples. Our instructor, who was a nurse, was great—warm and funny but very knowledgeable. After we all had given birth, she had everyone over to her house for a "reunion." We lined the babies up together on the sofa and took a picture. They leaned against each other, topsy-turvy. It was hilarious. My son is now 23 but I still love that picture of him. What memories it triggers of such a very special time! —Trish, 47

Kevin Peterson/Getty Images

LEARNING OUTCOMES

8.1   Determine the most appropriate nursing care for couples during preconception to help ensure their best possible health state.

8.2   Identify ways to assist expectant parents in making the best decisions possible about issues related to pregnancy, labor, and birth.

8.3   Summarize the goals and content of the various types of antepartum education programs when providing nursing care for expectant couples and their families.

8.4   Compare methods of childbirth preparation and the nursing interventions for each.

8.5   Explore ways in which the nurse conveys respect for patient individuality in preparing for childbirth.

As pregnancy progresses, expectant parents begin to look forward to their birth experience and the challenges of parenthood. This is a time for plans and decisions. Where will the birth be? Whom do they wish to be present? How will they prepare themselves for this experience?

Today's professional nurse can assist a pregnant woman or expectant couple, if the partner is involved, to make the choices that are part of pregnancy and birth (Figure 8–1 ●). For first-time parents, the decisions may seem numerous and complicated, and the nurse has a unique opportunity to help them establish a pattern of decision making that will serve them well in their years as parents.

PRECONCEPTION COUNSELING

One of the first questions a couple should ask themselves is whether they wish to have children. This decision involves consideration of each person's goals, expectations of the relationship, and desire to be a parent. Sometimes one person wishes to have a child, but the other does not. In such situations, an open discussion is essential to reach a mutually acceptable decision.

Couples who wish to have children need to decide about the timing of pregnancy. When do they believe it would be best to become parents? For couples who have religious beliefs that do not support contraception or who feel that fertility planning is unnatural, planning the timing of the pregnancy is unacceptable and irrelevant. These couples can still take steps to ensure that they are in the best possible physical and mental health when pregnancy occurs.

Preconception Health Measures

The nurse begins by teaching the couple about known or suspected health risks. The nurse advises the woman who smokes to cease smoking if possible or to limit her cigarette intake to less than half a pack per day. The National Cancer Institute (NCI) and the American College of Obstetricians and Gynecologists (ACOG) have advocated for the use of the "five A's" model, which includes (ACOG, 2011):

1. Ask about tobacco use.

2. Advise to quit.

3. Assess willingness to make a quit attempt.

4. Assist in quit attempt.

5. Arrange follow-up.

● **Figure 8–1** The nurse helps prepare couples for their roles as parents.

Smoking interventions offer an effective tool to decrease smoking use among pregnant women and are associated with better fetal outcomes. Because of the hazards of secondhand smoke, it is helpful for the woman to avoid environments where secondhand smoke is common and to ask her partner to refrain from smoking around her.

Although the effects of caffeine on pregnancy are less clearly understood, the woman is advised to avoid or limit her intake of caffeine. ACOG has issued an opinion stating that consuming less than 200 mg per day (approximately 12 oz of coffee) does not appear to increase the risk of adverse fetal outcomes such as prematurity, intrauterine growth restriction, and spontaneous abortion (ACOG, 2010).

Prenatal exposure to alcohol is a leading preventable cause of developmental disabilities and birth defects, therefore caregivers should screen for alcohol use and advise total abstinence for women who are planning a pregnancy and those who are not using an effective method of birth control. Alcohol consumption during pregnancy has been linked to numerous adverse fetal effects including the following (Cheng, Kettinger, Kelechi, et al., 2011):

- Growth deficiencies
- Facial deformities
- Central nervous system impairment
- Behavioral disorders
- Impaired intellectual development
- Spontaneous abortion
- Low-birth-weight infants
- Stillbirth

Likewise, social drugs and street drugs pose a real threat to the fetus and should not be used when planning a pregnancy or during pregnancy (Cheng et al., 2011).

A woman who uses any prescription or over-the-counter medications needs to discuss the implications of their use with her healthcare provider. It is best to avoid using any medication if possible. Because of the possible teratogenic effects of environmental hazards, the nurse urges the couple contemplating pregnancy to determine whether they are exposed to any environmental hazards at work or in their community.

With an increase in the number of women traveling globally for professional or personal reasons, providing healthcare education on disease prevention is often warranted. Women should be assessed during the preconception stage for varicella, rubella, hepatitis B, and HIV. In addition, if global travel is expected, appropriate vaccinations should be obtained prior to attempting pregnancy. Some vaccines require the woman to wait 28 days prior to attempting pregnancy. There are multiple vaccinations that can be given during pregnancy; however, others are contraindicated and should not be administered, so it is important to obtain these prior to pregnancy if travel out of the country is anticipated in the next calendar year (Centers for Disease Control and Prevention [CDC], 2012b). Table 8–1 lists vaccination recommendations from the CDC.

Physical Examination

It is wise for both partners to have a physical examination to identify any health problems so that they can be corrected if possible. These problems might include medical conditions such as high blood pressure, diabetes, or obesity; problems that threaten fertility, such as certain sexually transmitted infections; or conditions that keep the individual from achieving optimal health, such as anemia or colitis. If the family history indicates previous genetic disorders, or if the couple is planning pregnancy when the woman is over age 35, the healthcare provider may suggest that the couple consider genetic counseling. Some ethnic groups have higher incidences of certain genetic conditions, therefore testing should be offered when risks are identified. For example,

 Evidence-Based Practice   Preconception Health Behaviors

Clinical Question
What are the conditions under which women practice preconception health behaviors?

The Evidence
A systematic review and two large cohort studies focused on the prevalence of preconception health behaviors among men and women. The systematic review determined the characteristics of this population and the prevalence of preconception health. One cohort study included 2,736 subjects from a large, multistate survey; the other was a statewide study that described the preconception predictors of optimal birth outcome. Systematic reviews and large cohort studies form the strongest level of evidence, Level 1. The majority of both men and women were unaware they had ever had information about preconception health from their primary care provider (Mitchell, Levis, & Prue, 2012). Women reported seeking out information more frequently than men. Increased educational achievement

was associated with a higher rate of preconception planning. Lower education attainment and young age were associated with fewer preconception behavioral changes (Delissaint & Kisako, 2011). The characteristics of preconception health that were most strongly associated with birth weight and fetal growth were obesity and nutrition (Weisman, Misra, Hillemeier, et al., 2011).

Best Practice
There is a need to educate young people regarding the importance and benefits of practicing preconception health planning. Teaching about preconception health behaviors should be provided to both men and women and should focus on achieving optimal health before pregnancy.

Clinical Reasoning
What are the most important changes a woman can make in preparation for conception? How would you design a teaching plan for both men and women?

Table 8–1	Vaccinations During Pregnancy

Vaccine Type	Considered Safe in Pregnancy	Contraindicated	Special Recommendation
Hepatitis A			The risk associated with vaccination should be weighed against the risk for hepatitis A in pregnant women who may be at high risk for exposure to hepatitis A.
Hepatitis B	X		Prenatal serologic pregnancy screening recommended.
Human papillomavirus (HPV)		X	Quadrivalent HPV vaccine is not recommended for use in pregnancy. Adverse fetal outcomes have not been reported when administered.
Influenza (inactivated)	X		
Influenza (LAIV)*		X	
Measles*		X	
Meningococcal (MCV4)			Safety during pregnancy has not been established.
Mumps*		X	
Pneumococcal		X	Not advised in pregnancy.
Polio (IPV)			Theoretical risk exists.
Rubella*		X	Prenatal serologic pregnancy screening recommended.
Tetanus-diphtheria (Td)	X		
Tetanus-diphtheria-pertussis (Tdap)	X		Tdap is recommended for all pregnant women regardless of previous vaccination or disease history. Optional timing for Tdap administration is between 27 and 36 weeks of gestation although Tdap may be given at any time during pregnancy.
Varicella*		X	
Anthrax			Pregnant women should be vaccinated against anthrax only if the potential benefits of vaccination outweigh the potential risks to the fetus. No studies on safety exist.
BCG*		X	
Japanese encephalitis (JE)			Vaccine should not be routinely administered in pregnancy. Pregnant women who must travel to an area where risk of JE is high should be vaccinated when the theoretical risks of immunization are outweighed by the risk of infection to the mother and developing fetus.
Meningococcal (MPSV4)	X		Pregnancy should not preclude (polysaccharide) vaccination.
Rabies	X		
Typhoid (parenteral and oral*)		X	No information on use in pregnant women is available so the vaccine is not recommended.
Vaccinia* (smallpox)		X	Vaccinia vaccine should not be administered to pregnant women for routine nonemergency indications. It should, however, be administered if definite exposure occurred.
Yellow fever*		X	Since vaccine safety has not been established, vaccine should be administered only if travel to an endemic area is unavoidable and if an increased risk for exposure exists.
Zoster		X	

*Live viruses.

Source: Adapted from Centers for Disease Control and Prevention (CDC). (2012b). *Guidelines for vaccinating pregnant women.* Retrieved from http://www.cdc.gov/vaccines/pubs/downloads/b_preg_guide.pdf

Complementary Care Ayurveda and Preconception Lifestyle

One form of complementary care that nurses may encounter is ayurveda. Ayurveda is an ancient system of natural and medical healing that originated in India. It encompasses a wide range of modalities, including the use of diet, herbs, massage, exercise, music therapy, aromatherapy, meditation, and yoga. Ayurvedic practitioners believe that these modalities should be practiced not only during pregnancy, but also prior to conception for optimal maternal and fetal health.

Ayurvedic practitioners recommend that both the mother and the father take part in a healthy lifestyle prior to conception. Some of the preconception lifestyle recommendations include:

- Avoid stress and overwork.
- Avoid alcohol, tobacco, and drugs.
- Avoid meat and dairy products, and eat primarily a vegetarian diet. (*Note:* Pregnant women who follow this diet may need supplementation with calcium and other vitamins. They will also need to ensure a sufficient intake of complete protein, as discussed in Chapter 12 .)
- Strive for a positive emotional relationship between the man and woman.

individuals of African descent have a higher incidence of sickle cell disease, therefore, serology testing should be offered to anyone of African or African American descent. (See *Genetic Disorders* section in Chapter 7 .) In addition to the history and physical examination, the woman may have a variety of laboratory tests. (See *Assessment Guide: Initial Prenatal Assessment* on pages 205–206 in Chapter 10 .) The woman is advised to have a dental examination and any necessary dental work done prior to conception to avoid exposure to x-rays and the risk of infection while she is pregnant.

Nutrition

Prior to conception it is advisable for the woman to be at an average weight for her body build and height. The woman is advised to follow a nutritious diet that contains ample quantities of all the essential nutrients. Some nutritionists advocate emphasizing the following nutrients: calcium, protein, iron, B-complex vitamins, vitamin C, and magnesium. Folic acid supplementation before conception is recommended to decrease the risk of neural tube defects. Intake of certain vitamins in megadoses can cause severe fetal problems and should be avoided.

Health Promotion Healthy People 2020 Goals for Pregnancy

All women are advised to follow a nutritious diet that contains ample quantities of all the essential nutrients to ensure healthy nutrition and weight gain patterns during pregnancy. *Healthy People 2020* goals for pregnancy include increasing the proportion of mothers who achieve a recommended weight gain during their pregnancies (U.S. Department of Health and Human Services [USDHHS], 2012).

With the epidemic proportions of obesity in the United States, more and more women are having bariatric surgical interventions. Women with a history of bariatric surgical intervention should be advised to avoid pregnancy for the next 12 to 24 months while rapid weight loss is occurring. In addition, if postsurgical complications are going to arise, they are likely to occur during this time period (ACOG, 2009a). Women who have had bariatric surgery have fewer complications when they do become pregnant compared to women with obesity, and they show a reduced incidence of gestational diabetes, preeclampsia, and fetal macrosomia (Lesko & Peaceman, 2012). For women with a previous history of eating disorders, nutritional consultation is warranted (Davidson, 2012). See Chapter 12 for further discussion of nutrition.

Exercise

A woman is advised to continue her present pattern of exercise or to establish a regular exercise plan beginning at least 3 months before she attempts to become pregnant. During pregnancy at least 30 minutes of moderate exercise daily for at least 5 days per week or most days is recommended. An exercise routine that she enjoys and maintains will provide the best results. Exercise that includes some aerobic conditioning and some general muscle toning improves the woman's circulation and general health. Once an exercise program is well established, the woman is generally encouraged to continue it during pregnancy. Contact sports, downhill skiing, and scuba diving are contraindicated in pregnancy. Other sports with high potential for falling, such as horseback riding, gymnastics, and water skiing, should also be avoided (ACOG, 2009b). Warning signs that warrant discontinuation of physical activity and notification of the provider include (March of Dimes, 2012):

- Vaginal bleeding
- Chest pain
- Headache
- Shortness of breath prior to beginning exercise
- Muscle weakness
- Calf swelling
- Preterm labor
- Amniotic fluid leakage
- Absence of fetal movement
- Decreased fetal movement

Contraception

A woman who uses hormonal contraception, such as combined oral contraceptives, the NuvaRing, or Depo-Provera, is advised to stop using the hormonal birth control method and have at least one normal menstrual period before attempting to conceive. This waiting period allows the natural hormonal cycle to return and facilitates dating the subsequent pregnancy. A woman using an intrauterine device is advised to have it removed and to wait 1 month before attempting to conceive. During the waiting period, she can use barrier methods of contraception (condom, diaphragm, or cervical cap with spermicide).

Conception

Conception is a personal and emotional experience. Even if a couple is prepared, they may feel some ambivalence. Ambivalence is a normal response, especially if the pregnancy is unintended, but they may need reassurance that the feeling will pass. Although couples in the United States have access to more contraceptive choices than those in developing countries, approximately 51% of the pregnancies that occur in the United States are unintended (CDC, 2012c). *Healthy People 2020* goals include increasing the proportion of pregnancies that are intended to 56% up from current levels of 51% (USDHHS, 2012).

A couple planning a pregnancy may get so caught up in preparation and in their efforts to "do things right" that they lose sight of the pleasure they derive from each other and their lives together and cease to value the joy of spontaneity in their relationship. It is often helpful for the healthcare provider to remind an overly zealous couple to take pleasure in the present moment.

Healthcare providers can assist the couple to achieve conception by identifying the woman's most fertile period. The nurse can also educate the woman about possible signs of ovulation (presence of ovulatory mucus, changes in the woman's temperature, and the presence of mittelschmerz [ovulation-related pain]). See Chapter 3 🔗 for information about ovulation. Women over the age of 35 should be referred for evaluation after 6 months of not conceiving. For women with known fertility issues, such as endometriosis, a history of pelvic inflammatory disease (PID), or known reproductive tract abnormalities, immediate referral is warranted. These factors are discussed in Chapter 7 🔗.

CHILDBEARING DECISIONS

Once the couple has conceived, they should begin exploring their options for a healthcare provider and birth setting, as well as labor support and sibling preparation, if appropriate. Some women may want to minimize medical interventions, whereas others may desire different childbirth education programs to assist them with specific goals for their birth experience. These decisions are influenced by a variety of factors.

Healthcare Provider

One of the first decisions facing expectant parents is the selection of a healthcare provider. The nurse assists them by explaining the various options and outlining what can be expected from each. Expectant parents should have a thorough understanding of the differences of educational preparation, skill level, general philosophy, and characteristics of practice of certified nurse-midwives, obstetricians, family practice physicians, certified professional midwives, and direct entry (lay) midwives. The nurse can encourage expectant parents to investigate the care provider's credentials, education and training, philosophy of childbirth, fee schedule or insurance plans accepted, availability

to new patients, and on-call coverage issues. Many practitioners in the United States are selected based on insurance coverage issues and enrollment in public assistance programs. Women should be encouraged to check their programs' participation with certain healthcare providers regarding the inclusion of pregnancy care. They can often get this information by telephoning the provider's office. The nurse can help the expectant parents develop a list of questions for their first visit to a care provider to help determine compatibility. These questions might include the following:

- Who is in practice with you, or who covers for you when you are unavailable?

- How do your partners' philosophies compare with yours?

- How do you feel about my partner, other support person, or other children coming to the prenatal visits?

- What are your feelings about _____ (fill in special desires for the birth event, such as different positions assumed during labor, episiotomy, induction of labor, other people present during the birth, breastfeeding immediately after the birth, no separation of infant and parents following birth, and so on)?

- If a cesarean birth is necessary, could my partner be present?

- Are you familiar with _____ (fill in complementary or alternative forms of health care that may be used if applicable)? How will this practice affect my plan of care?

- What type of insurance plans do you accept? Do you care for women on public assistance, such as Medicaid? Are payment options available for out-of-pocket expenses or if self-pay arrangements are needed?

Expectant parents also need to consider the qualities they want in a care provider for the newborn. They may want to visit several before the birth to select someone who will meet their needs and those of their child.

Pregnant women and couples will make many more choices. Some are explored in Table 8–2. A method that has helped many couples make these choices is a **birth preference plan**. By writing down preferences, prospective parents identify aspects of the childbearing experience that are most important to them

---

Developing Cultural Competence
Birth Choices

Sometimes nurses make the mistake of assuming that a pregnant woman will make the same decisions about the birth experience as the nurse would have. However, the choices a woman and her family make are influenced by many factors, including ethnic background, culture, and religious beliefs. These factors may profoundly influence decisions such as care provider (male or female), birth setting, labor support person(s), use of medications for analgesia, position during birth, saving the placenta, dietary practices immediately postpartum, and a host of other issues. There is no one right way to give birth.

Table 8–2	Advantages and Disadvantages of Some Consumer Decisions During Pregnancy, Labor, and Birth	

Issue	Advantages	Disadvantages
Breastfeeding	■ Economic savings related to savings on formula and healthcare costs ■ Decreased incidence of asthma, SIDS, and childhood obesity ■ Decreased incidence of infant otitis media, vomiting, and diarrhea, hospitalizations during the first year of life, and allergies ■ Easier to digest than formula ■ Immediately after birth, promotes uterine contractions and decreases incidence of postpartum hemorrhage ■ Promotes maternal-infant attachment ■ Reduces incidence of maternal breast and ovarian cancers ■ Provides passive immunity during breastfeeding duration by transmission of maternal antibodies that help protect babies from infections and illnesses, such as diarrhea, ear infections, and pneumonia	■ Although rare, transmission of maternal infection, such as HIV, to newborn can occur ■ Irregular ovulation and menses can cause false sense of security and nonuse of combined hormonal contraceptives ■ Increased nutritional requirement in mother ■ Limitation of birth control options in the postpartum period ■ Women who are modest may feel uncomfortable breastfeeding in public

Ambulation during labor	■ Comfort for laboring woman
	■ May assist in labor progression by (if appropriate):
	  ■ Stimulating contractions
	  ■ Allowing gravity to help descent of fetus
	  ■ Giving sense of independence and control
		■ Cord prolapse possible with ruptured membranes unless engagement has occurred
		■ Inability to continually monitor fetal heart rate (FHR) if medically indicated if telemetry unit is not available (Intermittent monitoring can be used for low-risk women.)

Electronic fetal monitoring	■ Helps evaluate fetal well-being ■ Helps identify nonreassuring fetal status ■ Useful in diagnostic testing ■ Helps evaluate labor progress	■ Intrauterine perforation (with internal uterine pressure device) ■ Infection (with internal monitoring) ■ Decreases personal interaction with mother because of attention paid to the machine ■ Mother is unable to ambulate or change her position freely
Whirlpool (jet hydrotherapy)	■ Increased relaxation ■ Decreased anxiety ■ Stimulation of labor ■ Provides pain relief ■ Slight decrease in blood pressure ■ Increased diuresis ■ Decreased incidence of vacuum- and forceps-assisted births ■ Increased pain threshold ■ Higher satisfaction with birth ■ Decreased use of pain medication	■ May slow contractions if used before active labor is established ■ Possible risk of infection if membranes are ruptured ■ Slight increase in maternal temperature and pulse in tub ■ Hypothermia
Analgesia	■ Maternal relaxation facilitates labor	■ All drugs reach the fetus in varying degrees and with varying effects ■ May cause changes in FHR variability
Episiotomy	May assist in facilitating immediate birth when non-reassuring status is present by providing an immediate intervention to correct nonreassuring FHR status	■ Increased pain after birth and for 1 to 3 months following birth ■ Dyspareunia ■ Infection ■ Increased frequency of third- and fourth-degree lacerations ■ Increased bleeding from episiotomy site

Birth Preference Plan

Choice	Choice
Care provider:	Position during birth:
Certified nurse-midwife	On side
Obstetrician	Hands and knees
Family physician	Kneeling
Direct entry midwife	Squatting
Birth setting:	Birthing chair
Hospital:	Birthing bed
Birthing room	Other:
Delivery room	Family present (siblings)
Birth center	Filming of birth (videotaping)
Home	Photography of birth
Support during labor and birth:	Use of LeBoyer Method
Partner present	Episiotomy
Doula present	No sterile drapes
During labor:	Partner to cut umbilical cord
Ambulate as desired	Hold baby immediately after birth
Shower if desired	Breastfeed immediately after birth
Wear own clothes	No separation after birth
Use hot tub	Save the placenta
Use own rocking chair	Collect cord blood for banking
Have perineal prep	Newborn care:
Have enema	Eye treatment for the baby
Membranes:	Vitamin K injection
Rupture naturally	Heptovac injection
Amniotomy if needed	Breastfeeding
Labor stimulation if needed	Formula feeding
Medication:	Pacifier use
Identify type desired	Glucose water
Fluids or ice as desired	Circumcision
Music during labor and birth	Postpartum care:
Massage	Short stay
Therapeutic touch	48-hour stay after vaginal birth
Healing touch	Home visits after discharge
	Home doula
	Other:

● **Figure 8–2** Birth preference plan. The columns list the various choices that a couple may consider during their childbirth experience. Once the couple has considered each of the choices, they can circle the items they desire.

(Figure 8–2 ●). Used as a tool for communication among the expectant parents, the healthcare provider, and the healthcare professionals at the birth setting, the written plan identifies options that are available. Nurses should be aware that a birth plan form may include options that are not available in their particular area or institution. Such options should be identified for the couple so they do not consider them.

Although many birth experiences are very close to the desired experience, at times expectations cannot be met. This may be because of the unavailability of some choices in the community, limitations set by insurance providers, or unexpected problems during pregnancy or birth. It is important for the nurse to help expectant parents keep sight of what is realistic for their situation while also acting as an advocate for them. In some circumstances, couples may request choices that are not available either by that care provider or that birth setting. In these circumstances, couples may wish to select a different care provider or birthing site.

Birth Setting

The nurse can help expectant parents choose a birth setting by suggesting they tour facilities and talk with nurses there and talk with friends or acquaintances who are recent parents. However,

it is important to note that the birth setting may be largely determined by the choice of the care provider. Special homelike labor–delivery–recovery–postpartum (LDRP) rooms in hospitals are becoming very popular.

SAFETY ALERT!

It is important for the woman to question her provider about backup physician availability, the closest hospital should an emergency arise, and emergency procedures that are in place for the practice.

The majority of women in the United States give birth in hospital settings; however, of the 1.2% of babies born outside of hospitals, 67% were born in homes and 28% were born in freestanding birth centers (Martin, Hamilton, Ventura, et al., 2012). Women who opt for less traditional birth settings should be carefully screened. Women with medical risk factors, including those who have had a previous cesarean birth, are not candidates for alternative birth settings.

Women desiring a nonhospital birth experience should obtain recommendations from healthcare providers or other parents who have utilized these services in the past and had positive birth experiences. Questions that expectant parents may ask of new parents include the following:

- What kind of care and support did you receive during labor?
- If the setting has both labor and birthing rooms, was a birthing room available when you wanted it?
- Were you encouraged to be mobile during labor or to do what you wanted to do (walk, sit in a rocking chair, sit in a whirlpool bath, stand in a shower, and so on)? If not, were there reasonable circumstances that prevented you from doing so?
- Were you encouraged to be actively involved in your plan of care and kept well informed of progress or proposed changes?
- Was your labor partner or support person treated well?
- Were your birth preferences respected? Did you share them with the facility before the birth? If something did not work, why do you think there were problems?
- During labor, did the nurse offer or suggest a variety of comfort measures?
- How were medications handled during labor? Were you comfortable with this arrangement?
- Were siblings welcomed in the birth setting? After the birth?
- Was the nursing staff helpful after the baby was born? Did you receive self-care and infant care information?
- Did you have a choice about what information was provided?

 Clinical Tip

Call the birthing facilities in your community and inquire about what options and choices are available for childbearing women at each facility.

Labor Support

Another important choice the expectant family faces is how active a support role the father or partner wants to take during labor and birth. Fathers often play a key role in the support of mothers during labor, birth, and the postpartum period. Although many partners are comfortable acting as the primary physical and emotional support for the laboring woman, some partners are not. One study examined the maternal response to the presence of the father during the labor and birth and found that women who had the father present had "significantly lower pain, anxiety and stress perception than those of the control group" (D'Aliesio, Vellone, Amato, et al., 2009, p. 5). Women with the father present reported being "less irritable, agitated, worried, felt more efficient, self-confident and able to relax" (D'Aliesio et al., 2009, p. 5).

In lieu of the partner, other options for labor support include asking a friend or family member to attend the birth and help with comfort needs, contacting a local childbirth advocate group for a volunteer referral, or hiring a specialized childbirth support person, known as a **doula**.

The doula attends to the needs of the childbearing family and acts as an advocate for them. Specially trained to assist with births and provide support to new parents and family members, the doula is an adjunct to the healthcare team. Doulas do not perform clinical tasks but they have a role in providing labor support, offering support and encouragement, building a good team relationship, helping the laboring woman cover gaps in her care, and encouraging good communication among the woman and her family and caregivers. The presence of doulas at the bedside has been associated with a reduced cesarean section rate and higher patient satisfaction rates (Emeis, Jacobson-Dunlop, Guise, et al., 2011). In a managed care environment in which nursing staff are often stretched thinly, a doula can be an asset to the nurse by attending to the many comfort needs of the laboring mother and her family. In some military hospitals, doulas are provided free of charge to women whose husbands are deployed overseas.

Sibling Participation in the Birth

Some expectant parents may wish to have their other children present at the birth. Children who will attend a birth can be prepared through books, audiovisual materials, use of models, discussion, and sibling classes. Nurses can assist parents with sibling preparation by helping them understand the stresses a child may experience. For example, the child may become frightened if the laboring mom is irritable and visibly showing discomfort, feel left out when there is a new child to love, or feel disappointed if, for example, a brother is born when a sister was expected.

During the birth it is important that a sibling have his or her own support person whose sole responsibility is tending to the child's needs. The support person needs to be familiar to the child; warm, sensitive, and flexible; knowledgeable about the birth process; and comfortable with sexuality and birth. This person must be prepared to interpret what is happening for the child and to intervene when necessary. For example, the support person needs to be prepared to remove the child from the birthing room at the child's request or if the situation warrants that action.

Siblings should be allowed to relate to the birth in whatever manner they choose, as long as it is not disruptive. They should understand that they can stay or leave the room as they choose. They should also feel free to ask questions and express feelings.

Only a few studies have examined the reactions of children witnessing the births of their siblings, but some research suggest that boys and preschool-age children may need additional support and could be fearful of viewing their mothers in distress or verbalizing pain (Okubo, Sankai, Yanagisawa, et al., 2008). Discussing childbirth pain in advance can decrease children's anxiety.

CLASSES FOR FAMILY MEMBERS DURING PREGNANCY

Prenatal education programs provide important opportunities to share information about pregnancy and childbirth and to enhance the parents' decision-making skills (Figure 8–3 ●). The content of each class is generally directed by the overall goals of the program. The nurse who knows the types of prenatal programs available in the community can direct expectant parents to programs that meet their special needs and learning goals.

Developing Cultural Competence
Childbirth Attendance

Women from Hispanic cultures typically want their partner with them during labor. These women like both emotional and physical support, such as verbal reassurance, hand-holding, or assistance with ambulation. The woman may also want female relatives present during the labor and birth to provide additional support.

On the other hand, in most Middle Eastern cultures, childbirth is exclusively attended by the laboring woman's female relatives and friends. It is customary for the expectant father to be excluded from the birthing area or delivery room.

● **Figure 8–3** In a group setting with a nurse-instructor, expectant parents share information about pregnancy and childbirth.
Source: Purestock/Alamy

From the expectant parents' point of view, class content is best presented in chronology with the pregnancy. Thus, prenatal classes are often divided into early and late classes.

Early Classes: First Trimester

Early prenatal classes often include prepregnant women and couples as well as those in early pregnancy. The classes cover the following topics:

- Early gestational changes
- Self-care during pregnancy
- Fetal development and environmental dangers for the fetus
- Sexuality in pregnancy
- Birth settings and types of care providers
- Nutrition, rest, and exercise suggestions
- Relief measures for common discomforts of pregnancy
- Methods for coping with stress
- Psychologic changes in pregnancy for both the woman and her partner
- Information for getting the pregnancy off to a good start
- Availability of prenatal and genetic testing
- Risk factors for preterm labor or other adverse pregnancy-related conditions—how to recognize the symptoms and what to do if they occur

Early classes should also present information about breastfeeding and formula feeding. Breastfeeding has greater nutritional value for the infant along with health-related benefits for the woman. Although 81.9% initiate breastfeeding, only 60% are breastfeeding at 6 months, and 34.1% are doing so at 12 months despite recommendations to continue breastfeeding for 1 year (CDC, 2012a). The majority of women have made their infant feeding decision before the sixth month of pregnancy.

Factors influencing a woman's choice of feeding method include (CDC, 2012a; Kogan, Singh, Dee, et al., 2008):

- Preference of husband (partner)
- Ability to breastfeed independently at hospital discharge
- Influence of family and friends
- Perceptions of professional support
- Society's view of breastfeeding
- Residence in a state with pro-breastfeeding legislation
- Perception of ability to adequately pump breasts at work following leave
- Knowledge about breastfeeding
- Delivery at a "baby-friendly" designated hospital (DeliFraie, Langabeer, Williams, et al., 2011)
- Supportive employment policies in place to facilitate pumping in the workplace
- Use of kangaroo care in very low birth weight (VLBW) infants (Flacking, Ewald, & Wallin, 2011)
- Childcare facilities that allow the mother to feed her child on site

Later Classes: Second and Third Trimesters

The later classes focus on these topics:

- Preparation for birth process
- Birth choices (e.g., position for vaginal birth, possibility of cesarean birth, use of restricted episiotomy, medications, epidural, fetal monitoring, and so forth)
- Cesarean birth: procedures, fear, pain
- Relaxation techniques
- Breathing techniques
- Postpartum self-care
- Infant care and feeding
- Infant stimulation or infant massage
- Newborn safety issues such as how to select an approved car seat and install it correctly
- Sibling preparation and adjustment

SAFETY ALERT!

Because the majority of car seats installed by parents are installed incorrectly, parents should be encouraged to read the directions thoroughly before installing the seat themselves or have it professionally installed or checked by a local group that provides free installation services or car seat inspection clinics. Advise parents of the community resources available for inspecting the installation of car seats. Many police departments and fire stations have car seat inspection clinics that are conducted within the community. Some fire stations have set hours when parents can bring in their car seat and have it installed free of charge. Remind new parents that newborns should be in a rear-facing position until the age of 2 years or until they reach the maximum weight and height for the seat (American Academy of Pediatrics, 2011).

Many childbirth education classes are now provided at local hospitals or medical offices. In these settings, women may be given information that is specific to that facility and a specific provider and may not truly represent evidence-based practice care. For example, in some facilities, trial of labor after cesarean (TOLAC) is not encouraged. This could be interpreted by the pregnant woman as TOLAC being an unrealistic option for care when, in fact, TOLAC is warranted for many women and may result in a shorter recovery period.

Adolescent Parenting Classes

Adolescents have special learning needs during pregnancy. Adolescents usually display strong emotional responses toward an undesired pregnancy. Pregnant teens have higher school dropout rates, increased rates of social punishment, and peer segregation when an unexpected pregnancy occurs. Ambivalence, anxiety, stress, and depression are among the most frequently encountered reactions from young women (Salazar-Pousada, Arroyo, Hidalgo, et al., 2010). Areas of concern for teens include:

- Discomforts of pregnancy
- Healthy diet during pregnancy
- Body image issues

- The birth process, especially coping with pain
- Newborn care
- Health dangers for the baby
- How to recognize when the baby is ill
- How to keep the baby safe from accidents
- How to make the baby feel happy and loved
- How to be a good parent
- Sexuality
- Peer relationships
- Challenges of teen parenting
- Importance of continuation of education after the birth

Breastfeeding Programs

Programs offering information on breastfeeding are increasing. For many years a primary source of information has been **La Leche League**, a nonprofit organization that promotes breastfeeding. Certified lactation educators; clinical lactation consultants; and nurses at birthing centers, hospitals, and health clinics can also provide information.

Online support groups can also be an important resource for new mothers. From these sources, expectant parents can learn:

- Advantages and challenges of breastfeeding
- Techniques and positioning
- Methods of breast pumping and milk storage
- How to involve the father in the feeding process, such as having him bring the baby to the mother for feedings, burp the baby between breasts and/or after feeding, or rock the baby back to sleep
- Ways of successfully breastfeeding and returning to work

Sibling Preparation: Adjustment to a Newborn

The birth of a new sibling is a significant event in a child's life. Positive adjustment can be enhanced by attendance at sibling preparation classes (see Figure 8–4 ●). The classes usually focus on:

- Reducing anxiety in the child
- Providing opportunities for the child to express feelings and concerns

Health Promotion *Healthy People 2020* **Breastfeeding Initiatives**

Healthy People 2020 (USDHHS, 2012) encourages multiple breast-feeding initiatives including:

- Increasing the total number of infants ever breastfed to 81.9%
- Increasing the rate of breastfeeding at 1 year to 34.1%
- Increasing the rate of breastfeeding at 6 months to 60.6%
- Increasing exclusive breastfeeding at 3 months (46.2%) and 6 months (25.5%)
- Increasing the number of worksite-supported lactation programs (38%)

● **Figure 8–4** It is especially important that siblings be well prepared when they are going to be present for the birth. However, all siblings can benefit from information about birth and the new baby ahead of time.

- Encouraging realistic expectations of the newborn
- Teaching the older child to be an active participant in the baby's care by showing how to safely hold the newborn, feed and burp the baby, or even change diapers; this enables the sibling to be an active participant when the new baby arrives

Parents learn strategies to help prepare the child for the birth and to assist the child in coping with a new family member. Suggested strategies aimed at transitioning older children to the arrival of a new sibling include the following (University of Michigan Health System, 2012):

- Tell children about the baby before you tell other friends and extended family members since hearing the news from the parent is preferred.
- Make any major household changes far in advance of the baby's arrival (potty training, changes in room, weaning, child care, etc.).
- Allow children to attend prenatal visits to become an active participant.
- Arrange for siblings to attend a hospital tour or sibling classes.
- Provide realistic expectations for what to expect from Mom after the birth (fatigue, less time to spend with them, reduction in out-of-the-home activities initially).
- Provide realistic expectations about baby's normal behavior (sleeping, crying, eating, bodily functions).
- Reminisce about their births by viewing videos or looking at pictures.
- Visit a friend's or family member's baby or point out new babies in public to your child.
- Allow them to practice with a doll to mimic diapering, feeding, and holding the baby.
- Involve siblings with the preparations whenever possible. After the baby has arrived, ask for their support and help so they feel involved with the baby's care.

● **Figure 8–5** Grandparents play a key role in many childbearing families' lives by taking an active role with grandchildren.

- Bear in mind that 2-year-olds, children very close to their mother, and those with personality characteristics such as jealousy may have more difficulty adjusting than other children.
- Spend focused time with an older child during which someone else cares for newborn.
- Practice reassurance and active listening about the children's feelings and insecurities.
- Have the baby "give" the older child a special gift or allow the children to exchange gifts.
- Clarify expectations and give firm direction that no hitting or hurting is allowed.
- Accept regression and be patient with older children if regression occurs.
- Identify the positives of being the older child and all the things older children can do (playing with friends, watching movies, swinging at the playground).
- Utilize children's literature to teach coping with new babies and common feelings.

Classes for Grandparents

Grandparents are an important source of support and information for prospective and new parents. They are often included in the birthing process. Prenatal programs for grandparents can be a valuable source of information about current beliefs and practices in childbearing. The most useful content may include changes in birthing and parenting practices and helpful tips for being a supportive grandparent. Grandparents who will be integral members of the labor and birth team need information about that role (Figure 8–5 ●).

EDUCATION OF THE FAMILY HAVING CESAREAN BIRTH

Cesarean birth is an alternative method of birth that now accounts for 32.8% of births in the United States (Hamilton, Martin, & Ventura, 2012). Consequently, although the need for a cesarean is not often known in advance, more and more childbirth preparation classes are integrating content on cesarean birth into the curriculum.

Class content should cover what the parents can expect to happen during a cesarean birth, what they might feel, and what choices are available. All pregnant women and couples should be encouraged to discuss with their certified nurse-midwife or physician the progression of events if a cesarean birth becomes necessary.

When expectant parents are anticipating a repeat cesarean birth, they have time to plan and prepare. Many birthing units provide preparation classes for repeat cesarean birth. Parents who have had previous negative experiences need an opportunity to describe what contributed to their feelings. They should be encouraged to identify what they would like to change and to list interventions that would make the experience more positive. Those who have had positive experiences require reassurance that their needs and desires will be met in a similar manner. All parents should be encouraged to air any fears or anxieties.

Often a woman facing a repeat cesarean is concerned about postoperative pain. She needs reassurance that subsequent cesarean births are often less painful than the first. In addition, planned cesarean births involve less fatigue than unplanned procedures because they are not preceded by a long, strenuous labor. Providing this information will help the woman cope more effectively with stressful stimuli, including pain.

PREPARATION FOR PARENTS DESIRING TRIAL OF LABOR AFTER CESAREAN BIRTH

Trial of labor after cesarean birth (TOLAC) was previously termed *vaginal birth after cesarean (VBAC)* and is discussed in detail in Chapter 23 . Parents who have had a cesarean birth and are now anticipating a vaginal birth have unique needs. Because they may have unresolved questions and concerns about the last birth, it is helpful to begin the series of classes with an informational session. The nurse can supply information about the criteria necessary to attempt a trial of labor and identify decisions to be made regarding the birth experience. Some childbirth educators suggest that parents prepare two birth plans: one for vaginal birth and one for cesarean birth. Preparing birth plans seems to give parents some sense of control over the birth experience and tends to increase the positive aspects of the experience.

CHILDBIRTH PREPARATION METHODS

Childbirth preparation classes are usually taught by certified childbirth educators. Various types of childbirth preparation are available. Vital to each method is the educational component, which helps alleviate fear. The classes vary in coverage of subjects related to the maternity cycle, but all teach relaxation and coping techniques, as well as what to expect during labor and birth. Most classes also feature exercises to relax and condition muscles and breathing exercises for use in labor. The greatest differences among the methods lie in the theories of why they work and in the specific comfort techniques and breathing patterns they teach.

Childbirth preparation offers several advantages. It helps a pregnant woman and her support person understand the choices in the birth setting, promotes awareness of available options, and provides tools for them to use during labor and birth. Another advantage is the satisfaction of the parents, for whom childbirth becomes a shared and profound emotional experience. In addition, each method has been shown to shorten labor. All nurses should know how these techniques differ, so that they can support each birth experience effectively. A Cochrane review recently found that women who receive continuous support during labor require less analgesia, have fewer cesarean and instrument births, and experience a shorter period of labor (Hodnett, Gates, Hofmeyr, et al., 2011). This provides additional evidence-based practice guidance regarding the need to provide ongoing support of the woman's partner during the labor and birth process.

Programs for Preparation

Some antepartum classes, specifically oriented to preparation for labor and birth, have a name associated with a theory of pain reduction in childbirth. The most common methods are:

- *Lamaze (psychoprophylactic):* Dissociative relaxation, controlled muscle relaxation, and specified breathing patterns are used to promote birth as a normal process.
- *Kitzinger (sensory-memory):* Women use chest breathing, abdominal breathing, and their sensory memory to help work through the birthing process.
- *Bradley (partner-coached childbirth):* Consists of a 12-week session in which the woman works on controlled breathing and deep abdominopelvic breathing with a focus on achieving natural childbirth.
- *HypnoBirthing:* Breathing and relaxation techniques help prepare the body to work in neuromuscular harmony to make the birth process easier, safer, and more comfortable.

One of the most important components of childbirth education is instilling confidence in a woman's ability to give birth (Hodnett et al., 2011). Many childbirth education specialists and educators embrace contemporary models that focus on the interconnectedness of the body and spirit. After that connection is established and understood by pregnant women, coping strategies, stress reduction, and relaxation techniques can be taught.

Teaching Highlights Internet Resources

Explain to women who are using Internet childbirth education resources that some sites may not use health professionals or experts in the childbirth field and may be written by individuals who lack formal education and training. Advise women to look for resources that are supported by licensed professionals or well-known, credible organizations.

Another prominent organization that provides educational resources and certification for educators is the International Childbirth Education Association (ICEA). This organization does not advocate a particular method of childbirth preparation but rather promotes a philosophy of "freedom of choice based on knowledge of alternatives" (ICEA, 2012). Many expectant parents find this approach consistent with their own desires to experience birth as informed healthcare consumers. ICEA educators often teach a combination of techniques designed to meet individual needs.

Body-Conditioning Exercises

Some body-conditioning exercises, such as the pelvic tilt, pelvic rock, and Kegel exercises, are taught in childbirth preparation classes. Other exercises strengthen the abdominal muscles for the expulsive phase of labor. (See Chapter 11 for a description of some recommended exercises.) Exercises aimed at adducting the legs into an extended McRobert's position, which is performed by flexing the mother's thighs toward her shoulders while she is lying on her back, help enable the woman to stretch her hamstring muscles, a task usually required during the second stage of labor (O'Leary, 2009). Many childbirth methods utilize body-conditioning as a portion of their education program. With the encouragement of daily exercise in pregnancy, women can incorporate exercises into their daily programs that will help build endurance and strength for the labor and birth process.

Relaxation Exercises

Relaxation during labor allows the woman to conserve energy and the uterine muscles to work more efficiently. Most childbirth education methods use a form of relaxation exercise as part of their philosophical basis. Without practice it is difficult to relax the whole body in the midst of intense uterine contractions. Progressive relaxation exercises such as those taught to induce sleep can be helpful during labor. *Teaching Highlights: Touch Relaxation* provides information on one approach.

An additional exercise is *disassociation relaxation*. The woman is taught to become familiar with the sensation of contracting and relaxing the voluntary muscle groups throughout her body. She then learns to contract a specific muscle group and relax the rest of her body. The exercise conditions the woman to relax uninvolved muscles while the uterus contracts, creating an active relaxation pattern.

Breathing Techniques

Breathing techniques are a key element of most childbirth preparation programs. The Bradley method encourages abdominopelvic breathing, whereas the Kitzinger method utilizes chest breathing in collaboration with abdominal relaxation. HypnoBirthing utilizes deep slow breathing as a center component of its philosophy. Breathing exercises help keep the mother and her unborn baby adequately oxygenated, and help the mother relax and focus her attention appropriately. Breathing techniques are best taught during the final trimester of pregnancy. The nurse then supports the mother's use of breathing techniques during labor. Breathing techniques are described in more detail in Chapter 19.

Teaching Highlights Touch Relaxation

The touch relaxation technique often combines patterned abdominal breathing with focused relaxation. It may be used to achieve relaxation of specific body parts or for general body relaxation.

Goals

The woman learns to release tension in the areas that her partner touches. The partner learns to watch his or her partner carefully and becomes attuned to tense, tightened muscles.

Technique

- The partner gently touches the woman's brow.
- The woman uses abdominal breathing. As she breathes in through her nose, her abdomen rises, and as she breathes out through her mouth, her abdomen falls. As each breath is released, she lets all tightness and tension flow out with the breath.
- The partner continues to lightly touch her brow until the woman feels relaxed. The partner may want to provide quiet encouragement such as "You are doing fine, you are releasing the tension in your forehead." After at least five breaths, the partner may touch the woman's shoulders and repeat the pattern described earlier.

- The partner moves on to the arms, chest, abdomen, thighs, and calves. The last aspect is to breathe in, let the whole body relax and go limp, and slowly release the breath. It will be helpful at the end of each labor contraction to let the body go limp and release all tension.
- As the couple practices, it is important for the woman to relax each part of her body. When she is in labor, it will not be possible to go through the whole body; however, the woman can indicate what would be most helpful (e.g., touch her shoulder during each contraction). The partner can also be alert for signs of muscle tension and tightening. As the partner and woman practice touch relaxation, they may want to make the situation more realistic. They could decide that uterine contractions are occurring every 5 minutes and are lasting for 30 seconds. A clock will help the partner keep track of time. The partner can indicate that a contraction is beginning and suggest the woman begin her breathing. To help her focus, the partner may touch her shoulder or hand. In some instances, it is helpful for the partner to breathe along with the woman. Each couple can determine what works best for them.

PREPARATION FOR CHILDBIRTH THAT SUPPORTS INDIVIDUALITY

Childbirth educators stress the value of individuality when providing information to expectant parents. The goal is to encourage women to incorporate their own natural responses into coping with the pain of labor and birth. Self-care activities that may be used include vocalization or "sounding" to relieve tension in pregnancy and labor, massage (light touch) to facilitate relaxation, use of warm water for showers or bathing during labor, visualization (imagery), relaxing music, subdued lighting, and the use of a birthing ball (Figure 8–6 ●).

Additional ways in which the nurse can help the couple during labor and birth include the following:

- Identify the methods of childbirth preparation commonly used in your area and learn the basics of their approaches to relaxation and breathing; practice these methods so that you can support a laboring couple more effectively.

- Encourage expectant mothers and couples to make the birth a personal experience.

- Suggest the couple bring items from home that help create a more personal birthing space, such as warm socks, extra pillows or a favorite blanket, bath powder, lotion, or meaningful photos.

- Encourage the couple to listen to soothing music or watch favorite DVDs to increase personalization of the childbearing experience.

● **Figure 8–6** A birthing ball is just one of many options that a family may choose to promote maternal comfort during labor.

Critical Concept Review

LEARNING OUTCOME 8.1: Determine the most appropriate nursing care for couples during preconception to help ensure their best possible health state.

1. Information is a major nursing responsibility during the preconception period. Preconception counseling is designed to:
   - Teach the patient about environmental and lifestyle hazards that could affect conception and pregnancy.
   - Identify any health problems that could impede a successful pregnancy.
   - Advise the patient about contraception and fertility.

LEARNING OUTCOME 8.2: Identify ways to assist expectant parents in making the best decisions possible about issues related to pregnancy, labor, and birth.

1. Couples are faced with the need to make decisions about issues such as:
   - Choice of a healthcare provider.
   - Birth experience plan.
   - Choice of birth setting.
   - Choice of support person during labor.
   - Choice of who should be present during the birth, such as other family members and siblings.

LEARNING OUTCOME 8.3: Summarize the goals and content of the various types of antepartum education programs when providing nursing care for expectant couples and their families.

1. A broad range of classes are available, including:
   - Description of each stage of pregnancy.
   - Childbirth preparation.
   - Breastfeeding.
   - Sibling preparation.

LEARNING OUTCOME 8.4: Compare methods of childbirth preparation and the nursing interventions for each.

1. There are many different methods to prepare patients for childbirth. They all emphasize measures that help to decrease anxiety and pain. The childbirth methods discussed in this chapter are:
   - Lamaze: uses breathing patterns, controlled muscular relaxation techniques (psychoprophylactic).
   - Bradley: partner-coached childbirth.
   - Kitzinger: sensory-memory techniques.
   - HypnoBirthing: deep relaxation techniques.
2. The nurse should support the approach the family has chosen.

LEARNING OUTCOME 8.5: Explore ways in which the nurse conveys respect for patient individuality in preparing for childbirth.

1. Nurses convey respect during childbirth preparation by:
   - Emphasizing the uniqueness of each birth experience.
   - Providing the patient with tools such as breathing and relaxation to choose the best childbirth methods.

Clinical Reasoning in Action

Terry Dole, a 38-year-old G1 P0000, at 6 weeks' gestation, presents to you at the OB clinic for her first prenatal visit with the certified nurse-midwife (CNM). One of the first decisions facing Terry is the selection of a healthcare provider. The midwife explains the various options available to Terry at the clinic related to the differences in educational preparation, skill level, practice characteristics, and general philosophy of CNMs and obstetricians. Terry tells you that she has been married for 6 years and works as a massage therapist. You obtain the following data: BP 110/70, temperature 97.0°F, pulse 76, respirations 12, weight 140 lb, height 5'7''. The physical and pelvic exams are essentially normal. The CNM asks you to teach Terry about birth plans.

1. Discuss the advantages of a birth plan.
2. Discuss the disadvantages of a birth plan.
3. Explain the role of a doula.
4. What gender differences are there in moving toward parenthood?
5. Develop a concept map based on the scenario that shows key components of Terry's care.

See www.nursing.pearsonhighered.com for possible responses and an interactive template for a concept map.

References

American Academy of Pediatrics (AAP). (2011). *AAP policy statement: Child passenger safety.* Retrieved from http://pediatrics.aappublications.org/content/early/2011/03/21/peds.2011-0213.abstract

American College of Obstetricians and Gynecologists (ACOG). (2009a). *Bariatric surgery and pregnancy* (ACOG Practice Bulletin No. 105). Washington, DC: Author.

American College of Obstetricians and Gynecologists (ACOG). (2009b). *Exercise during pregnancy and the postpartum period* (ACOG Committee Opinion No. 267). Washington, DC: Author.

American College of Obstetricians and Gynecologists (ACOG). (2010). *Moderate caffeine consumption during pregnancy* (ACOG Committee Opinion No. 462). Washington, DC: Author.

American College of Obstetricians & Gynecologists (ACOG). (2011). *Smoking cessation during pregnancy: A clinician's guide to helping pregnant women quit smoking.* Retrieved from http://www.acog.org/departments/healthIssues/scdp/files/scdp.pdf

Centers for Disease Control and Prevention (CDC). (2012a). *CDC Breastfeeding report card.* Retrieved from http://www.cdc.gov/breastfeeding/data/reportcard.htm

Centers for Disease Control and Prevention (CDC). (2012b). *Immunization and pregnancy.* Retrieved from http://www.cdc.gov/vaccines/pubs/downloads/f_preg_chart.pdf

Centers for Disease Control & Prevention (CDC). (2012c). *Unintended pregnancy prevention.* Retrieved from http://www.cdc.gov/reproductivehealth/unintendedpregnancy

Cheng, D., Kettinger, L., Kelechi, U., & Hurt, L. (2011). Alcohol consumption during pregnancy: Prevalence and provider assessment. *Obstetrics & Gynecology, 117*(2, Part 1), 212–217. doi:10.1097/AOG.0b013e3182078569

D'Aliesio, L., Vellone, E., Amato, E., & Alvaro, R. (2009). The positive effects of father's attendance to labour and delivery: A quasi-experimental study. *International Nursing Perspectives, 9*(1), 5–10.

Davidson, M. R. (2012). *A nurse's guide to women's mental health.* New York, NY: Springer.

DeliFraie, J., Langabeer, J., Williams, J., Gong, A., Delgado, R. I., & Gill, S. (2011). Cost comparison of baby friendly and non–baby friendly hospitals in the United States. *Pediatrics, 127*(4), e989–e994. doi:10.1542/peds.2010-1591

Delissaint, D., & Kisako, J. (2011). A systematic review of factors utilized in preconception health behavior research. *Health Education & Behavior, 38*(6), 603–616.

Emeis, C., Jacobson-Dunlop, N., Guise, J. M., & O'Haire, C. (2011). *Doula care for vulnerable populations.* Western Institute of Nursing Conference. Retrieved from http://www.nursinglibrary.org/vhl/handle/10755/157493

Flacking, R., Ewald, U., & Wallin, L. (2011). Positive effect of kangaroo mother care on long-term breastfeeding in very preterm infants. *Journal of Obstetric, Gynecologic, & Neonatal Nursing, 40*, 190–197. doi:10.1111/j.1552-6909.2011.01226.x

Hamilton, B. E., Martin, J. A., & Ventura, S. J. (2012). Births: Preliminary data for 2011. *National Vital Statistics Reports, 61*(5), 1–29.

Hodnett, E. D., Gates, S., Hofmeyr, G. J., Sakala, C., & Weston, J. (2011). Continuous support for women during childbirth. *Cochrane Database of Systematic Reviews,* Issue 2. Art. No.: CD003766. doi:10.1002/14651858.CD003766.pub3

International Childbirth Education Association (ICEA). (2012). *ICEA philosophy statement.* Retrieved from http://www.icea.org

Kogan, M. D., Singh, G. K., Dee, D. L., Belanoff, C., & Grummer-Strawn, L. M. (2008). Multivariate analysis of state variation in breastfeeding rates in the United States. *American Journal of Public Health, 98*(10), 1872–1880. doi:1254074

Lesko, J., & Peaceman, A. (2012). Pregnancy outcomes in women after bariatric surgery compared with obese and morbidly obese controls. *Obstetrics & Gynecology, 119* (3),547–554. doi:10.1097/AOG.0b013e318239060e

March of Dimes. (2012). *Warning signs to stop exercising.* Retrieved from http://www.marchofdimes.com/pnhec/159_637.asp

Martin, J. A., Hamilton, B. E., Ventura, S. J., Osterman, M. J. K., Wilson, E. C., & Matthews, T. J. (2012). Births: Final data for 2010. *National Vital Statistics Reports, 61*(1), 1–100. Retrieved from http://www.cdc.gov/nchs/data/nvsr/nvsr61/nvsr61_01.pdf

Mitchell, E., Levis, D., & Prue, C. (2012). Preconception health: Awareness, planning and communication among a sample of US men and women. *Maternal & Child Health Journal, 16*(1), 31–39.

Okubo, C., Sankai, C., Yanagisawa, H., & Kano, N. (2008). Witnessing the birth of a sibling—Looking at drawings to understand the possible effects on children. *Journal of Japan Academy of Midwifery, 22*(2), 233–248. doi:101125965

O'Leary, J. A. (2009). The McRoberts maneuver. *Shoulder Dystocia and Birth Injury, 2*, 107–117. doi:10.1007/978-1-59745-473-5_8

Salazar-Pousada, D., Arroyo, D., Hidalgo, L., Pérez-López, F. R. & Chedraui, P. (2010). Depressive symptoms and resilience among pregnant adolescents: A case-control study. *Obstetrics and Gynecology International.* Article ID 952493. doi:10.1155/2010/952493

University of Michigan Health System. (2012). *New baby sibling: Helping your older child (or children) adjust.* Retrieved from http://www.med.umich.edu/yourchild/topics/newbaby.htm

U.S. Department of Health and Human Services (USDHHS). (2012). *Implementing* Healthy People. Retrieved from http://www.healthypeople.gov/2020/default.aspx

Weisman, C., Misra, D., Hillemeier, M., Downs, D., Chuang, C., & Camacho, F. (2011). Preconception predictors of birth outcomes: Prospective findings from the Central Pennsylvania Women's Health Study. *Maternal & Child Health, 15*(7), 829–835.

Physical and Psychologic Changes of Pregnancy

Our son and his wife just told us they are pregnant. I am going to be a grand-father! I have tried to be a good father, to give my boy love, to teach him to respect others, to show him what it means to be a real man, someone a family can count on. Guess time will tell if the lessons took—I'm betting they have. —Patrick, 52

Kevin Peterson/Getty Images

LEARNING OUTCOMES

9.1   Identify the anatomic and physiologic changes that occur during pregnancy.

9.2   Assess the subjective (presumptive), objective (probable), and diagnostic (positive) changes of pregnancy in patients.

9.3   Contrast the various types of pregnancy tests.

9.4   Examine the emotional and psychologic changes that commonly occur in a woman, her partner, and her family during pregnancy when providing nursing care.

9.5   Discuss cultural factors that may influence a family's response to pregnancy in the provision of nursing care.

Pregnancy is divided into three trimesters, each approximately a 3-month period. Each trimester brings predictable changes for both the mother and the fetus. How does pregnancy affect the woman physically and psychologically? How does it affect her family, including siblings, partner, and grandparents? This chapter describes these physical and psychologic changes and the responses of the entire family to pregnancy. It also presents the various cultural factors that can affect a pregnant woman's well-being. Subsequent chapters build on this information in describing effective approaches to planning and providing care.

ANATOMY AND PHYSIOLOGY OF PREGNANCY

Reproductive System

Some of the most dramatic changes of pregnancy occur in the reproductive organs.

Uterus

Before pregnancy the uterus is a small, almost solid, pear-shaped organ measuring approximately 7.5 × 5 × 2.5 cm and weighing about 60 g (2 oz). At the end of pregnancy, it measures about 28 × 24 × 21 cm and weighs approximately 1100 g; its capacity has also increased from about 10 mL to 5000 mL (5 L) or more (Cunningham, Leveno, Bloom, et al., 2010). The change is primarily a result of the enlargement (hypertrophy) of the preexisting myometrial cells in response to the stimulating influence of estrogen and the distention caused by the growing fetus. Only a limited increase in cell number (hyperplasia) occurs. The fibrous tissue between the muscle bands increases markedly, which adds to the strength and elasticity of the muscle wall. The enlarging uterus, developing placenta, and growing fetus require additional blood flow to the uterus. By the end of pregnancy, one sixth of the total maternal blood volume is contained within the vascular system of the uterus.

Braxton Hicks contractions, which are irregular, generally painless contractions of the uterus, occur intermittently throughout pregnancy. They may be felt through the abdominal wall beginning about the fourth month of pregnancy. In later months these contractions become uncomfortable and may be confused with true labor contractions.

Cervix

Estrogen stimulates the glandular tissue of the cervix, which increases in cell number and becomes hyperactive. The endocervical glands secrete a thick, sticky mucus that accumulates and forms the mucous plug, which seals the endocervical canal and prevents the ascent of organisms into the uterus. This mucous plug is expelled at the onset of labor or before, when cervical dilatation begins. The hyperactivity of the glandular tissue also increases the normal physiologic mucorrhea, at times resulting in profuse discharge. Increased cervical vascularity also causes both the softening of the cervix (Goodell's sign) and its bluish discoloration (Chadwick's sign).

Ovaries

The ovaries stop producing ova during pregnancy, but the corpus luteum continues to produce hormones until about weeks 6 to 8. It secretes progesterone until about the seventh week of pregnancy, maintaining the endometrium until the placenta assumes the task. The corpus luteum then begins to disintegrate slowly.

Vagina

Estrogen causes a thickening of the vaginal mucosa, a loosening of the connective tissue, and an increase in vaginal secretions (leukorrhea). These secretions are thick, white, and acidic (pH 3.5 to 6.0). The acid pH helps prevent bacterial infection but favors the growth of yeast organisms. Thus, the pregnant woman is more susceptible to *Candida* infection than usual.

The supportive connective tissue of the vagina loosens throughout pregnancy. By the end of pregnancy, the vagina and perineal body are sufficiently relaxed to

Clinical Tip

Beginning early in pregnancy, have the woman feel her uterus periodically so that she becomes familiar with the size and the way it feels. As her pregnancy progresses, she then will be more likely to identify Braxton Hicks contractions and preterm labor, if it occurs.

permit passage of the infant. Because blood flow to the vagina is increased, the vagina may show the same blue-purple color (Chadwick's sign) as the cervix.

Breasts

Estrogen and progesterone cause many changes in the mammary glands. The breasts enlarge and become more nodular as the glands increase in size and number in preparation for lactation. Superficial veins become more prominent, the nipples become more erectile, and the areolae darken. Montgomery's tubercles (sebaceous glands) enlarge, and striae (reddish stretch marks that slowly turn silver after childbirth) may develop.

Colostrum, an antibody-rich yellow secretion, may leak or be expressed from the breasts during the last trimester. Colostrum gradually converts to mature milk during the first few days after childbirth.

Respiratory System

Many respiratory changes occur to meet the increased oxygen requirements of a pregnant woman. The volume of air breathed each minute increases 30% to 40%. In addition, progesterone decreases airway resistance, permitting a 15% to 20% increase in oxygen consumption, as well as increases in carbon dioxide production and in the respiratory functional reserve.

As the uterus enlarges, it presses upward and elevates the diaphragm. The subcostal angle increases, so that the rib cage flares. The anteroposterior diameter increases, and the chest circumference expands by as much as 6 cm; as a result there is no significant loss of intrathoracic volume. Breathing changes from abdominal to thoracic as pregnancy progresses, and descent of the diaphragm on inspiration becomes less possible. Some hyperventilation and difficulty in breathing may occur.

Nasal stuffiness and epistaxis (nosebleeds) may also occur because of estrogen-induced edema, hypersecretion of mucus, and vascular congestion of the nasal mucosa.

Cardiovascular System

Blood volume progressively increases beginning in the first trimester, increases rapidly until about 30 to 34 weeks, and then plateaus until birth at about 40% to 50% above nonpregnant levels. This increase is a result of increases in both erythrocytes and plasma (Gordon, 2012).

During pregnancy, blood flow increases to organ systems with an increased workload. Thus, blood flow increases to the uterus, placenta, and breasts, whereas hepatic and cerebral flow remain unchanged. Cardiac output begins to increase early in pregnancy and peaks at 25 to 30 weeks' gestation at 30% to 50% above prepregnant levels. It generally remains elevated in the third trimester.

The pulse may increase by as many as 10 to 15 beats per minute at term. The blood pressure decreases slightly, reaching its lowest point during the second trimester. It gradually increases to near prepregnant levels by the end of the third trimester. The enlarging uterus puts pressure on pelvic and femoral vessels, interfering with returning blood flow and causing stasis of blood in the lower extremities. This condition may lead to dependent edema and varicosity of the veins in the legs, vulva, and rectum (hemorrhoids) in late pregnancy. This increased blood volume in the lower legs may also make the pregnant woman prone to postural hypotension.

When the pregnant woman lies supine, the enlarging uterus may press on the vena cava, thus reducing blood flow to the right atrium, lowering blood pressure, and causing dizziness, pallor, and clamminess. The enlarging uterus may also press on the aorta and its collateral circulation (Cunningham et al., 2010). This condition is called **supine hypotensive syndrome**. It may also be referred to as *vena caval syndrome* or *aortocaval compression* (Figure 9–1 ●). It can be corrected by having the woman lie on her left side or by placing a pillow or wedge under her right hip.

The total erythrocyte (red blood cell [RBC]) volume increases by about 30% in women who receive iron supplementation but only about 18% without iron supplementation. This increase in erythrocytes is necessary to transport the additional oxygen required during pregnancy. However, the increase in plasma volume during pregnancy averages about 50%. Because the plasma volume increase (50%) is greater than the erythrocyte increase (30%), the hematocrit, which measures the concentration of red blood cells in the plasma, decreases slightly (Gordon, 2012). This decrease is referred to as the **physiologic anemia of pregnancy** (pseudoanemia).

Iron is necessary for hemoglobin formation, and hemoglobin is the oxygen-carrying component of erythrocytes. Thus, the increase in erythrocyte levels results in an increased need for iron by the pregnant woman. Even though the gastrointestinal absorption of iron is moderately increased during pregnancy, it is usually necessary to add supplemental iron to the diet to meet the expanded red blood cell and fetal needs.

● **Figure 9–1** Supine hypotensive syndrome (vena caval syndrome). The gravid uterus compresses the vena cava when the woman is supine. This reduces the blood flow returning to the heart and may cause maternal hypotension.

Leukocyte production increases slightly to a range of 5600 to 12,200/mm³. During labor and early postpartum, these levels may reach 25,000/mm³ or higher (Gordon, 2012). Although the exact cause of the leukocytosis is not known, this increase is a normal finding (Cunningham et al., 2010).

Both fibrin and plasma fibrinogen levels increase during pregnancy. Although the blood-clotting time of the pregnant woman does not differ significantly from that of the nonpregnant woman, clotting factors VII, VIII, IX, and X increase; thus, pregnancy is a somewhat hypercoagulable state. These changes, coupled with venous stasis in late pregnancy, increase the pregnant woman's risk of developing venous thrombosis.

Gastrointestinal System

Nausea and vomiting are common during the first trimester and may result from several factors, including elevated human chorionic gonadotropin (hCG) levels, relaxation of the smooth muscle of the stomach, and changed carbohydrate metabolism (Gordon, 2012). Gum tissue may soften and bleed easily. The secretion of saliva may increase and even become excessive (ptyalism).

Elevated progesterone levels cause smooth muscle relaxation, resulting in delayed gastric emptying and decreased peristalsis. As a result the pregnant woman may complain of bloating and constipation. These symptoms are aggravated as the enlarging uterus displaces the stomach upward and the intestines are moved laterally and posteriorly. The cardiac sphincter also relaxes, and heartburn (pyrosis) may occur because of reflux of acidic secretions into the lower esophagus. Hemorrhoids frequently develop in late pregnancy from constipation and from pressure on vessels below the level of the uterus.

The emptying time of the gallbladder is prolonged during pregnancy as a result of smooth muscle relaxation from progesterone. This, coupled with the elevated levels of cholesterol in the bile, can predispose the woman to gallstone formation.

Urinary Tract

During the first trimester, the enlarging uterus is still a pelvic organ and presses against the bladder, producing urinary frequency. This symptom decreases during the second trimester, when the uterus becomes an abdominal organ and pressure against the bladder lessens. Frequency reappears during the third trimester, when the presenting part descends into the pelvis and again presses on the bladder, reducing bladder capacity, contributing to hyperemia, and irritating the bladder.

The ureters (especially the right ureter) elongate and dilate above the pelvic brim. The glomerular filtration rate rises by as much as 50% beginning in the second trimester and remains elevated until birth. To compensate for this increase, renal tubular reabsorption also increases. However, glycosuria is sometimes seen during pregnancy because of the kidneys' inability to reabsorb all the glucose filtered by the glomeruli. Glycosuria may be normal or may indicate gestational diabetes, so it always warrants further testing.

Skin and Hair

Changes in skin pigmentation commonly occur during pregnancy. They are thought to be stimulated by increased estrogen,

● **Figure 9–2** Linea nigra.
Source: George Dodson/Lightworks Studio/Pearson Education.

progesterone, and α-melanocytic-stimulating hormone levels. Pigmentation of the skin increases primarily in areas that are already hyperpigmented: the areolae, the nipples, the vulva, and the perianal area. The skin in the middle of the abdomen may develop a pigmented line, the **linea nigra**, which usually extends from the pubic area to the umbilicus or higher (Figure 9–2 ●). Facial **chloasma (melasma gravidarum)**, also known as the "mask of pregnancy," a darkening of the skin over the forehead and around the eyes, may develop. Melasma is more prominent in dark-haired women and is aggravated by exposure to the sun. Fortunately, it fades or becomes less prominent soon after childbirth when the hormonal influence of pregnancy subsides. The sweat and sebaceous glands are often hyperactive during pregnancy. **Striae (striae gravidarum** when they result from pregnancy), or stretch marks, may appear on the abdomen, thighs, buttocks, and breasts. They result from reduced connective tissue strength because of elevated adrenal steroid levels.

Vascular spider nevi, small, bright-red elevations of the skin radiating from a central body, may develop on the chest, neck, face, arms, and legs. They may be caused by increased subcutaneous blood flow in response to elevated estrogen levels.

The proportion of hair in the growing phase increases during pregnancy compared with the number of hair follicles in the resting or dormant phase. After birth the number of hair follicles in the resting phase increases sharply, and the woman may notice increased hair shedding beginning 1 to 4 months postpartum. Practically all hair is replaced within 6 to 12 months, however (Cunningham et al., 2010).

Musculoskeletal System

No demonstrable changes occur in the teeth of pregnant women. The dental caries that sometimes accompany pregnancy are

12 weeks   20 weeks   28 weeks   36 weeks   40 weeks

● **Figure 9–3** Postural changes during pregnancy. Note the increasing lordosis of the lumbosacral spine and the increasing curvature of the thoracic area.

probably caused by inadequate oral hygiene and dental care, especially if the woman has problems with bleeding gums or nausea and vomiting.

The joints of the pelvis relax somewhat because of hormonal influences. The result is often a waddling gait. As the pregnant woman's center of gravity gradually changes, the lumbar spinal curve becomes accentuated (lordosis), and her posture changes (Figure 9–3 ●). This posture change compensates for the increased weight of the uterus anteriorly and frequently results in low backache.

Pressure of the enlarging uterus on the abdominal muscles may cause the rectus abdominis muscle to separate, producing **diastasis recti**. If the separation is severe and muscle tone is not regained postpartum, subsequent pregnancies will not have adequate support and the woman's abdomen may appear pendulous.

Central Nervous System

Pregnant women frequently describe decreased attention, concentration, and memory during and shortly after pregnancy, but few studies have explored this phenomenon. One study did find a decline in memory that could not be attributed to depression, anxiety, sleep deprivation, or other physical changes of pregnancy. This memory loss disappeared soon after childbirth (Cunningham et al., 2010).

Metabolism

Most metabolic functions increase during pregnancy because of the increased demands of the growing fetus and its support system. For a detailed discussion of nutrient, vitamin, and mineral metabolism, see Chapter 12 🔗.

Weight Gain

The recommended total weight gain during pregnancy for a woman of normal weight before pregnancy is 11.5 to 16 kg (25 to 35 lb); for women who were overweight before becoming pregnant, the recommended gain is 6.8 to 11.5 kg (15 to 25 lb). Women with obesity are advised to limit weight gain to 5 to 9 kg (11 to 20 lb). Underweight women are advised to gain 12.7 to 18.1 kg (28 to 40 lb) (Institute of Medicine [IOM], 2009). A normal weight woman should gain about 0.5 to 2 kg (1.1 to 4.4 lb) during the first trimester, followed by an average gain of about 0.45 kg (1 lb) per week during the last two trimesters (IOM, 2009).

Water Metabolism

Increased water retention, a basic alteration of pregnancy, is caused by several interrelated factors. The increased level of steroid sex hormones affects sodium and fluid retention. The lowered serum protein also influences fluid balance, as do increased intracapillary pressure and permeability. The extra water is needed for the fetus, the placenta, amniotic fluid, and the mother's increased blood volume, interstitial fluids, and enlarged organs.

Nutrient Metabolism

The fetus makes its greatest protein and fat demands during the second half of pregnancy, doubling in weight during the last 6 to 8 weeks. Protein (contributing nitrogen) must be stored during pregnancy to maintain a constant level within the breast milk and to avoid depletion of maternal tissues. Carbohydrate needs also increase, especially during the second and third trimesters. Fats are more completely absorbed during pregnancy, and the level of free fatty acids increases in response to human placental lactogen (hPL). The levels of lipoproteins and cholesterol also increase. Because of these changes, increased levels of dietary fat or reduced carbohydrate production may lead to ketonuria in the pregnant woman.

Endocrine System

Thyroid

The thyroid gland often enlarges slightly during pregnancy because of increased vascularity and hyperplasia of glandular tissue. Estrogen increases its capacity to bind thyroxine, resulting in an increase in serum protein-bound iodine. The basal metabolic rate increases by as much as 20% to 25% during pregnancy.

Activity | Case Study: Prenatal Education

Evidence-Based Practice Cultural Influences on Perception of Weight Gain During Pregnancy

Clinical Question

What are the cultural influences on perception of weight gain during pregnancy?

The Evidence

A large cohort study and a cross-sectional study investigated the association between cultural and physical traits and beliefs about appropriate gestational weight gain. These large, multisite studies involved 1700 women and form the strongest level of evidence. In addition, a large qualitative study focused on perceptions of weight gain specific to ethnicity. Various personal characteristics affect the perception of "appropriate weight gain" during pregnancy. Body image was associated with gestational weight, but not as clearly as one might think (Mehta, Siega-Riz, & Herring, 2011). Racial background had the greatest influence on the perception of weight gain during pregnancy. Caribbean black and African American women had low perceived risk of gaining too much pregnancy weight; the highest perceived risk for both was gaining too little (Brooten, Youngbult, Golembeski, et al., 2012). These groups also had some of the highest nutritional intake during pregnancy. Specifically, low-income African American women did not

focus on limiting their gestational weight gain and, in fact, were often of the belief that gaining more weight is indicative of a healthy infant (Groth, Morrison-Beedy, & Meng, 2012). White, non-Hispanic women had greater concern for gaining too much weight. Hispanic women did not exhibit a clear preference, although Hispanic women who had acculturated to the United States reported perceptions much like their white counterparts. The majority of Hispanic women could not remember getting specific advice from their provider about weight gain. Women in all racial groups had inadequate intake of protein and several vitamins.

Best Practice

Cultural sensitivity is called for when counseling pregnant women about weight gain. Belief systems affect how women perceive appropriate weight gain during pregnancy. Good teaching materials will take into account the differing beliefs that may affect health behaviors.

Clinical Reasoning

How can the nurse design culturally sensitive materials for teaching pregnant women about appropriate gestational weight gain?

However, within a few weeks after birth, all thyroid function returns to normal limits.

Pituitary

Pregnancy is made possible by the hypothalamic stimulation of the anterior pituitary gland. The anterior pituitary produces follicle-stimulating hormone (FSH), which stimulates ovum growth, and luteinizing hormone (LH), which brings about ovulation. Stimulation of the pituitary also prolongs the ovary's corpus luteal phase. This maintains the endometrium in case conception occurs. Prolactin, another anterior pituitary hormone, is responsible for initial lactation.

The posterior pituitary secretes vasopressin (antidiuretic hormone) and oxytocin. Vasopressin causes vasoconstriction, which results in increased blood pressure; it also helps regulate water balance. Oxytocin promotes uterine contractility and stimulates ejection of milk from the breasts (the letdown reflex) in the postpartum period.

Adrenals

During pregnancy, circulating cortisol, which regulates carbohydrate and protein metabolism, increases in response to increased estrogen levels. Cortisol blood levels return to normal within 1 to 6 weeks postpartum. The adrenals secrete increased levels of aldosterone by the early part of the second trimester. This increase in aldosterone in a normal pregnancy may be the body's protective response to the increased sodium excretion associated with progesterone (Cunningham et al., 2010).

Pancreas

The pregnant woman has increased insulin needs, and the pancreatic islets of Langerhans, which secrete insulin, are stressed to meet this increased demand. Any marginal pancreatic function quickly becomes apparent, and the woman may show signs of

Complementary Care Herbs During Pregnancy

Pharmaceutical companies have not included pregnant women in their studies of drug safety. As a result, very few over-the-counter or prescription drugs can claim to be safe for pregnant women and breastfeeding mothers. The same can be said for herbal medicines. Although many herbs have been researched extensively in Europe and Asia, little clinical research has been done in the United States on the use of herbs during pregnancy.

Nurses would do well to learn about many of the commonly used herbs so that they can provide pregnant women with accurate information. Pregnant or breastfeeding women must be cautious about everything they ingest—foods, liquids, medications, and herbs. If a problem warrants intervention, the woman and her primary healthcare provider should discuss the benefits and risks of all treatments, synthetic and natural.

gestational diabetes mellitus (GDM). (For a discussion of GDM, see Chapter 15 .)

Hormones in Pregnancy

Human Chorionic Gonadotropin

The trophoblast secretes human chorionic gonadotropin (hCG) in early pregnancy. This hormone stimulates progesterone and estrogen production by the corpus luteum to maintain the pregnancy until the placenta is developed sufficiently to assume that function.

Human Placental Lactogen

Also called *human chorionic somatomammotropin*, human placental lactogen (hPL) is produced by the syncytiotrophoblast.

Human placental lactogen is an antagonist of insulin; it increases the amount of circulating free fatty acids for maternal metabolic needs and decreases maternal metabolism of glucose to favor fetal growth.

Estrogen

Secreted originally by the corpus luteum, estrogen is produced primarily by the placenta as early as the seventh week of pregnancy. Estrogen stimulates uterine development to provide a suitable environment for the fetus. It also helps develop the ductal system of the breasts in preparation for lactation.

Progesterone

Also produced initially by the corpus luteum and then by the placenta, progesterone plays the greatest role in maintaining pregnancy. It maintains the endometrium and inhibits spontaneous uterine contractility, thus preventing early spontaneous abortion. Progesterone also helps develop the acini and lobules of the breasts in preparation for lactation.

Relaxin

Relaxin is detectable in the serum of a pregnant woman by the time of the first missed menstrual period. Relaxin inhibits uterine activity, diminishes the strength of uterine contractions, aids in the softening of the cervix, and has the long-term effect of remodeling connective tissue, which is necessary for the uterus to accommodate pregnancy (Cunningham et al., 2010). Its primary source is the corpus luteum, but small amounts are believed to be produced by the placenta and uterine decidua.

Prostaglandins in Pregnancy

Prostaglandins are lipid substances that can arise from most body tissues but occur in high concentrations in the female reproductive tract and are present in the decidua during pregnancy. The exact functions of prostaglandins during pregnancy are still unknown, although it has been proposed that they are responsible for maintaining reduced placental vascular resistance. Decreased prostaglandin levels may contribute to hypertension and preeclampsia. Prostaglandins may also play a role in the complex biochemistry that initiates labor.

SIGNS OF PREGNANCY

Many of the changes women experience during pregnancy are used to diagnose the pregnancy itself. They are called the subjective, or presumptive, changes; the objective, or probable, changes; and the diagnostic, or positive, changes of pregnancy.

Subjective (Presumptive) Changes

The subjective changes of pregnancy are the symptoms the woman experiences and reports. Because they can be caused by other conditions, they cannot be considered proof of pregnancy (Table 9–1). Several subjective signs can be diagnostic clues when other signs and symptoms of pregnancy are also present.

Amenorrhea, or the absence of menses, is the earliest symptom of pregnancy. Missing more than one menstrual period, especially in a woman whose cycle is ordinarily regular, is an especially useful diagnostic clue.

Table 9–1	Differential Diagnosis of Pregnancy—Subjective Changes	
Subjective Changes	**Possible Alternative Causes**
Amenorrhea	*Endocrine factors:* early menopause; lactation; thyroid, pituitary, adrenal, ovarian dysfunction *Metabolic factors:* malnutrition, anemia, climatic changes, diabetes mellitus, degenerative disorders, long-distance running *Psychologic factors:* emotional shock, fear of pregnancy or sexually transmitted infection, intense desire for pregnancy (pseudocyesis), stress Obliteration of endometrial cavity by infection or curettage Systemic disease (acute or chronic), such as tuberculosis or malignancy
Nausea and vomiting	Gastrointestinal disorders Acute infections such as encephalitis Emotional disorders such as pseudocyesis or anorexia nervosa
Urinary frequency	Urinary tract infection Cystocele Pelvic tumors Urethral diverticula Emotional tension
Breast tenderness	Premenstrual tension Chronic cystic mastitis Pseudocyesis Hyperestrogenism
Quickening	Increased peristalsis Flatus ("gas") Abdominal muscle contractions Shifting of abdominal contents

Nausea and vomiting in pregnancy (NVP) occur frequently during the first trimester. It may be mild or may cause considerable distress. Because these symptoms often occur in the early part of the day, they are commonly referred to as **morning sickness**. In reality the symptoms may occur at any time and can range from a mere distaste for food to severe vomiting. Women who experience NVP often have a more favorable pregnancy outcome than those who do not.

Excessive fatigue may be noted within a few weeks after the first missed menstrual period and may persist throughout the first trimester.

Urinary frequency is experienced during the first trimester as the enlarging uterus presses on the bladder.

Changes in the breasts are frequently noted in early pregnancy. These changes include tenderness and tingling sensations, increased pigmentation of the areola and nipple, and changes in Montgomery's glands. The veins also become more visible and form a bluish pattern beneath the skin.

Quickening, or the mother's perception of fetal movement, occurs about 18 to 20 weeks after the last menstrual period in a

Clinical Tip

Some women suggest that it is easiest to imagine the fluttering associated with quickening by letting the outer tips of the eyelashes brush a finger and then imagining that same sensation deep inside the abdomen.

woman pregnant for the first time but may occur as early as 16 weeks in a woman who has been pregnant before. Quickening is a fluttering sensation in the abdomen that gradually increases in intensity and frequency.

Objective (Probable) Changes

An examiner can perceive the objective changes that occur in pregnancy. Because these changes can have other causes, they do not confirm pregnancy (Table 9–2).

Changes in the pelvic organs—the only physical changes detectable during the first 3 months of pregnancy—are caused by increased vascular congestion. These changes are noted on pelvic examination. As noted earlier, there is a softening of the cervix called **Goodell's sign**. **Chadwick's sign** is a bluish, purple, or deep-red discoloration of the mucous membranes of the cervix, vagina, and vulva (some sources consider this a presumptive sign). **Hegar's sign** is a softening of the isthmus of the uterus, the area between the cervix and the body of the uterus (Figure 9–4 ●). **McDonald's sign** is an ease in flexing of the body of the uterus against the cervix.

General enlargement and softening of the body of the uterus can be noted after the eighth week of pregnancy. The fundus of the uterus is palpable just above the symphysis pubis at about 10 to 12 weeks' gestation and at the level of the umbilicus at 20 to 22 weeks' gestation (Figure 9–5 ●).

Enlargement of the abdomen during the childbearing years is usually regarded as evidence of pregnancy, especially if it is continuous and accompanied by amenorrhea.

Braxton Hicks contractions can be palpated most commonly after the 28th week. As the woman approaches the end of pregnancy, these contractions may become uncomfortable. They are often called *false labor.*

Uterine souffle may be heard when the examiner auscultates the abdomen over the uterus. It is a soft, blowing sound that occurs at the same rate as the maternal pulse and is caused by the increased uterine blood flow and blood pulsating through the placenta. It is sometimes confused with the funic souffle, a soft, blowing sound of blood pulsating through the umbilical cord. The funic souffle occurs at the same rate as the fetal heart rate.

Changes in pigmentation of the skin are common in pregnancy. The nipples and areolae may darken, and the linea nigra may develop. Facial melasma (chloasma) may become noticeable, and striae may appear.

The *fetal outline* may be identified by palpation in many pregnant women after 24 weeks' gestation. **Ballottement** is the

Table 9–2	Differential Diagnosis of Pregnancy—Objective Changes
Objective Changes	**Possible Alternative Causes**
Changes in pelvic organs: Goodell's sign Chadwick's sign Hegar's sign Uterine enlargement	Increased vascular congestion Estrogen-progestin oral contraceptives Vulvar, vaginal, cervical hyperemia Excessively soft walls of nonpregnant uterus Uterine tumors
Enlargement of abdomen	Obesity, ascites, pelvic tumors
Braxton Hicks contractions	Hematometra, pedunculated, submucous, and soft myomas
Uterine souffle	Large uterine myomas, large ovarian tumors, or any condition with greatly increased uterine blood flow
Pigmentation of skin: Chloasma (melasma) Linea nigra Nipples/areolae	Estrogen-progestin oral contraceptives Melanocyte hormonal stimulation
Abdominal striae	Obesity, pelvic tumor
Ballottement	Uterine tumors/polyps, ascites
Positive pregnancy test	Increased pituitary gonadotropins at menopause, choriocarcinoma, hydatidiform mole
Palpation for fetal outline	Uterine myomas

● **Figure 9–4** The presence of Hegar's sign, which is a softening of the isthmus of the uterus, can be determined by the examiner during a vaginal examination.

● **Figure 9–5** Approximate height of the fundus at various weeks of pregnancy.

passive fetal movement elicited when the examiner inserts two gloved fingers into the vagina and pushes against the cervix. This action pushes the fetal body up, and, as it falls back, the examiner feels a rebound.

Pregnancy tests detect the presence of hCG in the maternal blood or urine. These are not considered a positive sign of pregnancy because other conditions can cause elevated hCG levels.

Clinical Pregnancy Tests

A variety of assay techniques are available to detect human chorionic gonadotropin (hCG) in either blood or urine during early pregnancy. Most healthcare providers use urine screening tests because the results are immediate, the cost is minimal, the tests are reasonably accurate, and no invasive procedure (blood draw) is required (Levin, Hopkins, & Tiffany, 2011).

Most pregnancy tests available today are based on an approach called *enzyme-linked immunosorbent assay (ELISA)*. ELISA uses a substance that results in a color change after binding. The assay, which can be done on blood or urine, is sensitive,

---

Clinical Reasoning Evaluating Fundal Height

At 33 weeks' gestation, Elena Martinez, G2P1, who is 5 feet 4 inches tall and weighs 144 lb (prepregnancy weight of 120 lb), is examined by her certified nurse-midwife. At that time her fundal height is measured as 33 cm. Because of a vacation trip, she is not seen again by her midwife until 36 weeks' gestation. At that time her fundus measures 35 cm and she weighs 147 lb. Elena asks if there is something wrong with her baby's growth. What is your assessment?

See www.nursing.pearsonhighered.com for possible responses.

---

quick, and can detect hCG levels as early as 7 to 9 days after ovulation and conception, which is 5 days before the first missed period.

Another approach to testing is called a *fluoroimmunoassay (FIA)*. The FIA uses an antibody tagged with a fluorescent label to detect serum hCG. The test, which takes about 2 to 3 hours to perform, is extremely sensitive and is used primarily to identify and follow hCG concentrations.

Over-the-Counter Pregnancy Tests

Home pregnancy tests are available over the counter at a reasonable cost. These ELISA tests, performed on urine, detect even low levels of hCG. Test instructions should be followed carefully. If the results are negative, the woman should repeat the test in 1 week if she has not started her period.

Diagnostic (Positive) Changes

The positive signs of pregnancy are completely objective, cannot be confused with a pathologic state, and offer conclusive proof of pregnancy.

■ *Fetal heartbeat* can be detected with an electronic Doppler device as early as weeks 10 to 12 of pregnancy.

■ *Fetal movement* is actively palpable by a trained examiner after about the 20th week of pregnancy.

■ *Visualization of the fetus by ultrasound examination* confirms a pregnancy. The gestational sac can be observed by 4 to 5 weeks' gestation (2 to 3 weeks after conception). Fetal parts and fetal movement can be seen as early as 8 weeks' gestation. Transvaginal ultrasound has been used to detect a gestational sac as early as 10 days after implantation (Cunningham et al., 2010).

PSYCHOLOGIC RESPONSE OF THE EXPECTANT FAMILY TO PREGNANCY

Pregnancy is a turning point in a family's life, accompanied by stress and anxiety, whether the pregnancy is desired or not. Especially if this is their first child, the expectant couple may be unaware of the physical, emotional, and cognitive changes of pregnancy and may anticipate no problems from such a normal event. Thus, they may be confused and distressed by new feelings and behaviors that are essentially normal.

For beginning families, pregnancy is the transition period from childlessness to parenthood. If the expectant woman is married or has a stable partner, she no longer is only a mate but must also assume the role of mother. Her partner, whether male or female, will become a parent, too. Career goals and mobility may be affected, and the couple's relationship takes on a different meaning to them and their families and community. If the pregnancy results in the birth of a child, the couple enters a new, irreversible stage of their life together. With each subsequent pregnancy, routines and family dynamics are again altered, requiring readjustment and realignment.

If the pregnant woman has no stable partner, she must deal alone with the role changes, fears, and adjustments of pregnancy or seek support from family or friends. She also faces the reality of planning for the future as a single parent. Even if the pregnant woman plans to relinquish her infant, she must still deal with the adjustments of pregnancy. This adjustment can be especially difficult without a good support system.

In most pregnancies, finances are an important consideration. Traditional lore relegates to the father the role of primary breadwinner, and indeed finances are often a very real concern for fathers. In today's society, however, even pregnant women with stable partners recognize the financial impact of a child and may feel concern about financial issues. For the single mother, finances may be a major source of concern.

Decisions about financial matters need to be made at this time. Will the woman work during her pregnancy and return to work after her child is born? If so, who will provide child care? Couples may also need to decide about the division of domestic tasks. Any differences of opinion must be discussed openly and resolved so that the family can meet the needs of its members.

Pregnancy can be viewed as a developmental stage with its own distinct developmental tasks. For a couple it can be a time of support or conflict, depending on the amount of adjustment each is willing to make to maintain the family's equilibrium.

During a first pregnancy, the woman and her partner plan together for the child's arrival, collecting information on how to be parents. At the same time, each continues to participate in some separate activities with friends or family members. The availability of a social support network is an important factor in psychosocial well-being during pregnancy. Most pregnant parents find that their partners are their greatest source of support followed by family and friends (Widarsson, Kerstis, Sundquist, et al., 2012). The broader social network is often a major source of advice for the pregnant woman. However, both sound and unsound information may be conveyed.

During any pregnancy, the expectant parents face significant changes and must deal with major psychosocial adjustments (Table 9–3). Other family members, especially other children of the woman or couple and the grandparents-to-be, must also adjust to the pregnancy.

For some, pregnancy is more than a developmental stage; it is a crisis. *Crisis* can be defined as a disturbance or conflict in which the individual cannot maintain a state of equilibrium. Pregnancy can be considered a *maturational crisis*, as it is a common event in the normal growth and development of the family.

Table 9–3	Parental Reactions to Pregnancy	
First-Trimester	**Second-Trimester**	**Third-Trimester**
Mother's Reactions	**Mother's Reactions**	**Mother's Reactions**
Informs father secretively or openly. Feels ambivalent toward pregnancy, anxious about labor and responsibility of child. Is aware of physical changes, daydreams of possible miscarriage. Develops special feelings for and renewed interest in her own mother, begins to form a personal identity as a mother.	Remains regressive and introspective, projects all preexisting problems with authority figures onto partner, may become angry if she perceives his lack of interest as a sign of weakness in him. Continues to deal with feelings about motherhood; shops for nursery furniture as something concrete to do. May experience anxiety or, alternately, may be very lackadaisical and wait until ninth month to look for furniture and clothes for baby. Feels movement and is aware of fetus and incorporates it into herself. May dream that partner will be killed, telephones him often for reassurance. Experiences more distinct physical changes; sexual desires may increase or decrease.	Experiences more anxiety and tension, with physical awkwardness. Feels much discomfort and insomnia from physical condition. Prepares for birth, assembles layette, picks out names. Dreams often about misplacing baby or not being able to give birth, fears birth of deformed baby. Feels ecstasy and excitement, has spurt of energy during last month.
Father's Reactions	**Father's Reactions**	**Father's Reactions**
Differ according to age, parity, desire for child, economic stability. Acceptance of pregnant woman's attitude or complete rejection and lack of communication. Is aware of his sexual feelings, may develop more or less sexual arousal. Accepts, rejects, or resents mother-in-law. May develop new hobby outside of family as sign of stress.	If he can cope, will give her extra attention she needs; if he cannot cope, will develop a new time-consuming interest outside of home. May develop a creative feeling and a "closeness to nature." May become involved in pregnancy and buy or make furniture. Feels for movement of baby, listens to heartbeat, or remains aloof, with no physical contact. May have fears and fantasies about himself being pregnant, may become uneasy with this feminine aspect in himself. May react negatively if partner is too demanding, may become jealous of physician and of physician's importance to partner and her pregnancy.	Adapts to alternative methods of sexual contact. Becomes concerned over financial responsibility. May show new sense of tenderness and concern, treats partner like doll. Daydreams about child as if older and not newborn, dreams of losing partner. Renewed sexual attraction to partner. Feels he is ultimately responsible for whatever happens.

If the crisis is not resolved, it will result in maladaptive behaviors in one or more family members and possible disintegration of the family. Families that are able to resolve a maturational crisis will return successfully to normal functioning and can even strengthen the bonds in the family relationship.

The Mother

Pregnancy alters body image and also necessitates a reordering of social relationships and changes in roles of family members. The way each woman meets the stresses of pregnancy is influenced by her emotional makeup, her sociologic and cultural background, and her acceptance or rejection of the pregnancy. However, many women manifest similar psychologic and emotional responses during pregnancy, including ambivalence, acceptance, introversion, mood swings, and changes in body image.

A woman's attitude toward her pregnancy can be a significant factor in its outcome. Even if the pregnancy is planned, there is an element of surprise at first. Many women commonly experience feelings of ambivalence during early pregnancy. This ambivalence may be related to feelings that the timing is somehow wrong; worries about the need to modify existing relationships or career plans; fears about assuming a new role; unresolved emotional conflicts with the woman's own mother; and fears about pregnancy, labor, and birth. These feelings may be more pronounced if the pregnancy is unplanned or unwanted. Indirect expressions of ambivalence include complaints about considerable physical discomfort, prolonged or frequent depression, significant dissatisfaction with changing body shape, excessive mood swings, and difficulty accepting the life changes resulting from the pregnancy.

Many pregnancies are unintended, but not all unintended pregnancies are unwanted. A pregnancy can be unintended and wanted at the same time. For some women, an unintended pregnancy has more psychologic and social advantages than disadvantages. It provides purpose and direction to life and allows a woman to test the devotion and love of her partner and family. However, an unintended pregnancy can be a risk factor for depression.

Acceptance of pregnancy is influenced by many factors. Lower acceptance tends to be related to an unplanned pregnancy and greater evidence of fear and conflict. When a pregnancy is well accepted, the woman demonstrates feelings of happiness and pleasure in the pregnancy. She experiences less physical discomfort and shows a high degree of tolerance for the discomforts associated with the third trimester (Lederman & Weis, 2009).

Conflicts about adapting to pregnancy are no more pronounced for older pregnant women (age 35 and over) than for younger ones. Moreover, older pregnant women tend to be less concerned about the normal physical changes of pregnancy and are confident about handling issues that arise during pregnancy and parenting. This difference may result because mature pregnant women have more experience with problem solving.

Pregnancy produces marked changes in a woman's body within a relatively short period. Pregnant women experience changes in body image because of physical alterations and may feel a loss of control over their bodies during pregnancy and later during childbirth. These perceptions are to a certain extent related to personality factors, social network responses, and attitudes toward pregnancy. Although changes in body image are normal, they can be stressful for the woman. Explanation and discussion of the changes may help both the woman and her partner deal with the stress associated with this aspect of pregnancy.

First Trimester

During the first trimester, feelings of disbelief and ambivalence are paramount. The woman's baby does not seem real, and she focuses on herself and her pregnancy. She may experience one or more of the early symptoms of pregnancy, such as breast tenderness or morning sickness, which are unsettling and at times unpleasant.

At this time, the expectant mother begins to exhibit some characteristic behavioral changes. She may become increasingly introspective and passive. She may be emotionally labile, with characteristic mood swings from joy to despair. She may fantasize about a miscarriage and feel guilt because of these fantasies. She may worry that these thoughts will harm the baby in some way.

Second Trimester

During the second trimester, quickening occurs. This perception of fetal movement helps the woman think of her baby as a separate person, and she generally becomes excited about the pregnancy even if earlier she was not. The woman becomes increasingly introspective as she evaluates her life, her plans, and her child's future. This introspection helps the woman prepare for her new mothering role. Emotional lability, which may be unsettling to her partner, persists. In some instances the partner may react by withdrawing. This withdrawal is especially distressing to the woman, because she needs increased love and affection. Once the couple understands that these behaviors are characteristic of pregnancy, they are easier to accept; however, they may be sources of stress to some extent throughout pregnancy.

As pregnancy becomes more noticeable, the woman's body image changes. She may feel great pride, embarrassment, or concern. Generally women feel best during the second trimester, which is a relatively tranquil time.

Third Trimester

In the third trimester, the woman feels pride about her pregnancy and anxiety about labor and birth. Physical discomforts increase, and the woman is eager for the pregnancy to end. She experiences increased fatigue, her body movements are awkward, and her interest in sexual activity may decrease. The woman tends to be concerned about the health and safety of her unborn child and may worry that she will not cope well during childbirth. Toward the end of this period, there is often a surge of energy as the woman prepares a "nest" for the infant. Many women report bursts of energy, during which they vigorously clean and organize their homes.

Psychologic Tasks of the Mother

Rubin (1984) identified four major tasks that the pregnant woman undertakes to maintain her intactness and that of her family and to incorporate her new child into the family system. These tasks form the foundation for a mutually gratifying relationship with her infant:

1. *Ensuring safe passage through pregnancy, labor, and birth.* The pregnant woman feels concern for both her unborn child and herself. She looks for competent maternity care to provide a sense of control. She may seek information from literature, observation of other pregnant women and new

mothers, and discussion with others. She often engages in self-care activities related to diet, exercise, alcohol consumption, and so forth. In the third trimester, she becomes more aware of external threats in the environment—a toy on the stairs, the awkwardness of an escalator—that pose a threat to her well-being. Sleep becomes more difficult and she longs for birth even though it, too, is frightening.

2. *Seeking acceptance of this child by others.* The birth of a child alters a woman's primary support group (her family) and her secondary affiliative groups. The woman slowly and subtly alters her network to meet the needs of her pregnancy. In this adjustment the woman's partner is the most important figure. The partner's support and acceptance help form a maternal identity. If there are other children in the home, the mother also works to ensure their acceptance of the coming child. The woman without a partner looks to others such as a family member or friend for this support.

3. *Seeking commitment and acceptance of herself as mother to the infant (binding-in).* During the first trimester, the child remains a rather abstract concept. With quickening, however, the child begins to become a real person, and the mother begins to develop bonds of attachment. The mother experiences movement of the child within her in an intimate, exclusive way, and bonds of love form. The mother develops a fantasy image of her ideal child. This binding-in process, characterized by its strong emotional component, motivates the pregnant woman to become competent in her role and provides satisfaction for her in the role of mother.

4. *Learning to give of oneself on behalf of one's child.* Childbirth involves many acts of giving. The man "gives" a child to the woman; she in turn "gives" a child to him. Life is given to an infant; a sibling is given to older children of the family. The woman begins to develop a capacity for self-denial and learns to delay immediate personal gratification to meet the needs of another. Baby showers and gifts are acts of giving that increase the mother's self-esteem and help her recognize the separateness and needs of the coming baby.

Accomplishment of these tasks helps the pregnant woman develop her self-concept as mother. The expectant mother who was well nurtured by her own mother may view her as a role model and emulate her; the woman who views her mother as a "poor mother" may worry that she will make similar mistakes. A woman's self-concept as a mother expands with actual experience and continues to grow through subsequent childbearing and childrearing.

The Father

For the expectant father, pregnancy is a psychologically stressful time because he, too, must make the transition from nonparent to parent or from parent of one or more to parent of two or more. Most men handle the transition to fatherhood well, and generally any anxieties they feel resolve over time. Fathers' feelings of anxieties often stem from inadequate preparation and can be addressed by recognizing paternal needs and including fathers more in antepartum education.

Initially, expectant fathers may feel pride in their virility, which pregnancy confirms, but also have many of the same ambivalent feelings as expectant mothers. The extent of ambivalence depends on many factors, including the father's relationship with his partner, his previous experience with pregnancy, his age, his economic stability, and whether the pregnancy was planned.

In adjusting to his role, the expectant father must first deal with the reality of the pregnancy and then gain recognition as a parent from his partner, family, friends, coworkers, and society—and from his baby as well. Preliminary research suggests that fathers who perceive that they have more marital intimacy and support from their partners tend to develop stronger bonds of attachment to their infants after birth (Yu, Hung, Chan, et al., 2012). The expectant mother can help her partner adjust if she has a definite sense of the experience as their pregnancy and their infant, and not her pregnancy and her infant.

The expectant father must establish a fatherhood role, just as the woman develops a motherhood role. Fathers who are most successful at this task generally like children, are excited about the prospect of fatherhood, are eager to nurture a child, and have confidence in their ability to be a parent. They also share the experiences of pregnancy and birth with their partners (Lederman & Weis, 2009). (See Table 9–3.)

First Trimester

After the initial excitement attending the announcement of the pregnancy, an expectant father may begin to feel left out. He may be confused by his partner's mood changes. He might resent the attention she receives and her need to modify their relationship as she experiences fatigue and possibly a decreased interest in sex. He might also be concerned about what kind of father he will be. During this time, his child is a "potential" baby. Fathers often picture interacting with a child of 5 or 6 years, not a newborn. The pregnancy itself may seem unreal until the woman shows more physical signs.

Second Trimester

The father's role in the pregnancy is still vague, but his involvement may increase as he watches and feels fetal movement and listens to the fetal heartbeat during a prenatal visit. For many men, seeing their infant on ultrasound is an important experience in accepting the reality of pregnancy. Like expectant mothers, expectant fathers need to confront and resolve some of their conflicts about the parenting they received. A father needs to sort out which behaviors of his own father he wants to imitate and which he wants to avoid.

The father-to-be's anxiety is lessened if both parents agree on the paternal role the man is to assume. For example, if both see his role as that of breadwinner, the man's stress is low. However, if the man views his role as that of breadwinner and the woman expects him to be actively involved in child care, his stress increases. An open, honest discussion about the expectations the parents have about their roles will help the father-to-be in his transition to fatherhood.

As the woman's appearance begins to change, her partner may have several reactions. Her appearance may decrease his sexual interest, or it may have the opposite effect. Because of the variety of emotions both partners may feel, communication and acceptance remain important.

Third Trimester

If the couple's relationship has grown through effective communication of their concerns and feelings, the third trimester is often a rewarding time. They may attend childbirth classes and make concrete preparations for the arrival of the baby. If the father has developed a detached attitude about the pregnancy, however, it is unlikely he will become a willing participant, even though his role becomes more obvious.

Concerns and fears may recur. The father may worry about hurting the unborn baby during intercourse or become concerned about labor and birth. He may also wonder what kind of parents he and his partner will be.

Couvade

Couvade has traditionally referred to the observance of certain rituals and taboos by the male to signify the transition to fatherhood. This observance affirms his psychosocial and biophysical relationship to the woman and child. More recently the term has been used to describe the unintentional development of physical symptoms such as fatigue, increased appetite, difficulty sleeping, depression, headache, or backache by the partner of a pregnant woman. Men who demonstrate couvade syndrome tend to have a higher degree of paternal role preparation and be involved in more activities related to this preparation.

Siblings

Bringing a new baby home often marks the beginning of sibling rivalry. The siblings view the baby as a threat to the security of their relationships with their parents. Parents who recognize this potential problem early in pregnancy and begin constructive actions can minimize the problem of sibling rivalry.

Preparation of the young child begins several weeks before the anticipated birth. Because they do not have a clear concept of time, young children should not be told too early about the pregnancy. From the toddler's point of view, several weeks is an extremely long time. The mother may let the child feel the baby moving in her uterus, explaining that the uterus is "a special place where babies grow." The child can help the parents put the baby clothes in drawers or prepare the baby's room.

Consistency is important in dealing with young children. They need reassurance that certain people, special things, and familiar places will continue to exist after the new baby arrives. Pregnant women may find it helpful to bring their children on a prenatal visit to the certified nurse-midwife or physician to give them an opportunity to listen to the fetal heartbeat. Such a visit helps make the baby more real to the children.

If siblings are school-age children, pregnancy should be viewed as a family affair. Teaching should be suitable to the child's level of understanding and may be supplemented with appropriate books. Taking part in family discussions, attending sibling preparation classes, feeling fetal movement, and listening to the fetal heartbeat help the school-age child take part in the experience of pregnancy and not feel like an outsider.

Older children or adolescents may appear to have sophisticated knowledge but may have many misconceptions about pregnancy and birth. The parents should make opportunities to discuss their concerns and involve the children in preparations for the new baby.

Sibling preparation is essential, but other factors are equally important. These include the amount of parental attention the new arrival receives, the amount of attention the older child receives after the baby comes home, and parental skill in dealing with regressive or aggressive behavior. See the discussion of sibling preparation in Chapter 8 🔗.

Grandparents

The first relatives told about a pregnancy are usually the grandparents. The expectant grandparents often become increasingly supportive of the couple, even if conflicts previously existed. But it can be difficult for even sensitive grandparents to know how deeply to become involved in the childrearing process.

Because grandparenting can occur over a wide expanse of years, people's response to this role can vary considerably. Younger grandparents leading active lives may not demonstrate as much interest as the young couple would like. In other cases, expectant grandparents may give advice and gifts unsparingly. For grandparents, conflict may be related to the expectant couple's need to feel in control of their lives, or it may stem from events signaling changing roles in the grandparents' own lives (e.g., retirement, financial concerns, menopause, or death of a friend). Some parents of expectant couples may already be grandparents with a developed style of grandparenting. This influences their response to the pregnancy. Clarifying the role of the helping grandparent ensures a comfortable situation for all.

Because childbearing and childrearing practices have changed, family cohesiveness is promoted by effective communication and frank discussion between young couples and interested grandparents about the changes and the reasons for them.

CULTURAL VALUES AND PREGNANCY

Cultures have a universal tendency to create ceremonial rituals or rites around important life events. The rituals and customs of a group are a reflection of the group's values. In many developed countries, such as the United States, Canada, England, and Germany, populations are becoming more and more ethnically diverse as the number of immigrants continues to grow. It is not realistic or appropriate to assume that people who are new to a country or area will automatically abandon their ways and adopt the practices of the dominant culture (Dean, 2010). Consequently the identification of cultural values is useful in planning and providing culturally sensitive care.

Generalization about cultural characteristics or values is difficult because not every individual in a culture may display these characteristics. Just as variations are seen between cultures, variations are also seen within cultures. For example, because of their exposure to the American culture, a third-generation

Activity | Care Plan: Prepare Siblings for New Baby

Developing Cultural Competence Providing Effective Prenatal Care to Families of Different Cultures

Nurses who are interacting with expectant families from a different culture or ethnic group can provide more effective, culturally sensitive nursing care by:

- Critically examining their own cultural beliefs
- Identifying personal biases, attitudes, stereotypes, and prejudices
- Making a conscious commitment to respect the values and beliefs of others
- Using sensitive, current language when describing others' cultures
- Learning the rituals, customs, and practices of the major cultural and ethnic groups with whom they have contact
- Including cultural assessment and assessment of the family's expectations of the healthcare system as a routine part of prenatal nursing care
- Incorporating the family's cultural and spiritual practices into prenatal care as much as possible
- Fostering an attitude of respect for and cooperation with alternative healers and caregivers whenever possible
- Providing for the services of an interpreter if language barriers exist
- Learning the language (or at least several key phrases) of at least one of the cultural groups with whom they interact
- Recognizing that ultimately it is the woman's right to make her own healthcare choices
- Evaluating whether the woman's healthcare beliefs have any potential negative consequences for her health

---

Chinese American family might have very different values and beliefs from those of a Chinese family that has recently immigrated to the United States. For this reason, the nurse needs to supplement a general knowledge of cultural values and practices with a complete assessment of the individual's values and practices. *Developing Cultural Competence: Providing Effective Prenatal Care to Families of Different Cultures* summarizes the key actions a nurse can take to become more culturally aware.

Cultural assessment is an important aspect of prenatal care. The nurse needs to identify the prospective parents'

main beliefs, values, and behaviors about pregnancy and childbearing. This includes information about ethnic background, amount of affiliation with the ethnic group, patterns of decision making, religious preference, language, communication style, and common etiquette practices. The nurse can also explore the woman's (or family's) expectations of the healthcare system. Once this information is gathered, the nurse can then plan and provide care that is appropriate and responsive to family needs. See Chapter 2 🔴 for more detail on these topics.

Critical Concept Review

LEARNING OUTCOME 9.1: Identify the anatomic and physiologic changes that occur during pregnancy.

1. Uterus: Increased amounts of estrogen and growing fetus cause enlargement in size and weight, strength, elasticity, and vascularity.
2. Cervix: Hyperplasia occurs (increase in cell number) due to increased estrogen level. Mucous plug forms to prevent organisms from entering uterus.
3. Vagina: Increased thickness of mucosa, increased vaginal secretions to prevent bacterial infections. Connective tissue relaxes. Caused by increased estrogen level.
4. Breasts: Estrogen and progesterone cause an increase in size and number of mammary glands; nipples more erectile, areolae darken, colostrum produced in last trimester.
5. Respiratory system: Increasing levels of progesterone cause increased volume of air, deceased airway resistance, increased anteroposterior diameter. Thoracic breathing occurs as uterus enlarges.

6. Cardiovascular system: Cardiac output increases, blood volume increases. Increased size of uterus interferes with blood return from lower extremities. Increased level of red cells increases oxygen delivery to cells. Clotting factors increase. Caused by increased level of estrogen and progesterone. The pulse may increase by 10–15 beats near term; BP decreases, reaching its lowest point in second trimester.
7. Gastrointestinal system: Delayed gastric emptying and decreased peristalsis. Caused by increased progesterone levels.
8. Genitourinary system: Glomerular filtration rate and renal tubular reabsorption increase as a result of increased blood volume.
9. Skin and hair: Increased skin pigmentation caused by increased estrogen and progesterone.
10. Musculoskeletal: Relaxation of joints caused by increased estrogen and progesterone.

LEARNING OUTCOME 9.2: Assess the subjective (presumptive), objective (probable), and diagnostic (positive) changes of pregnancy in patients.

1. Subjective (presumptive) changes:
   - Amenorrhea.
   - Nausea and vomiting.
   - Fatigue.
   - Urinary frequency.
   - Breast changes.
   - Quickening.
2. Objective (probable) changes:
   - Goodell's and Chadwick's sign.
   - Hegar's and McDonald's sign.
   - Enlargement of the abdomen.
   - Braxton Hicks contractions.
   - Uterine souffle.
   - Skin pigmentation changes.
   - Pregnancy tests.
3. Diagnostic (positive) changes:
   - Fetal heartbeat.
   - Fetal movement.
   - Visualization of the fetus.

LEARNING OUTCOME 9.3: Contrast the various types of pregnancy tests.

1. Urine tests: Detect hCG during early pregnancy.
2. Serum tests: Also may detect hCG but may detect presence earlier than urine tests.
3. Home (OTC) tests: Urine tests designed to detect hCG.

LEARNING OUTCOME 9.4: Examine the emotional and psychologic changes that commonly occur in a woman, her partner, and her family during pregnancy when providing nursing care.

1. Mother:
   - First trimester: Disbelief and ambivalence.
   - Second trimester: Quickening helps mother to view fetus as separate from herself.
   - Third trimester: Anxiety about labor and birth. Nesting (bursts of energy) occurs.
   - Rubin identified four tasks:
     - Ensuring safe passage through pregnancy, labor, and birth.
     - Seeking acceptance of this child by others.
     - Seeking commitment and acceptance of herself as mother to infant.
     - Learning to give of oneself on behalf of one's child.
2. Father/partner:
   - First trimester: May feel left out. Disbelief.
   - Second trimester: Begins to decide which behaviors of own father he wants to imitate or discard.
   - Third trimester: Anxiety about labor and birth.
3. Family:
   - Siblings' reaction depends on age of siblings, but preparation is essential.
   - Grandparents are usually supportive and excited about the birth.

LEARNING OUTCOME 9.5: Discuss cultural factors that may influence a family's response to pregnancy in the provision of nursing care.

1. Cultural assessment should be done to determine the beliefs, wishes, and traditions of the family. Factors such as religious preference, language, and communication style will affect the family's plans for the pregnancy.

Clinical Reasoning in Action

Twenty-two-year-old Jean Simmons is an aerobics instructor, G1, P0000 in her first trimester of pregnancy. She presents to you at the local clinic complaining of frequent nausea, urinary frequency, and fatigue. You obtain her vital signs: BP 108/60, temperature 97°F, pulse 68, respirations 12, weight 125 lb, height 64 inches. Her urine tests negative for ketones, albumin, leukocytes, and sugar. You note that Jean has lost 3 lb since her last visit. You assist the certified nurse-midwife with a physical exam, the findings of which are essentially normal. Jean says that while she knows it could become an issue, she would like to continue working as an aerobic instructor for as long as she possibly can during the pregnancy. You identify Jean's complaints as normal discomforts of pregnancy, and proceed with prenatal education.

1. What advice would you suggest to cope with the nausea of pregnancy?
2. What advice might you suggest to cope with urinary frequency?
3. What teaching would be important relating to exercise in pregnancy?
4. What symptoms related to exercise should Jean report to her physician?

See www.nursing.pearsonhighered.com for possible responses.

References

Brooten, D., Youngbult, J., Golembeski, S., Magnus, M., & Hannan, J. (2012). Perceived weight gain, risk, and nutrition in pregnancy in five racial groups. *Journal of the American Academy of Nurse Practitioners, 24*(1), 32–42.

Cunningham, F. G., Leveno, K. J., Bloom, S. L., Hauth, J. C., Rouse, D. J., & Spong, C. Y. (2010). *Williams obstetrics* (23rd ed.). New York, NY: McGraw-Hill.

Dean, R. A., K. (2010). Cultural competence: Nursing in a multicultural society. *Nursing for women's health, 14*(1), 51–56.

Gordon, M. C. (2012). Maternal physiology. In S. G. Gabbe, J. R. Niebyl, J. L. Simpson, M. B. Landon, H. L. Galan, E. R. M. Jauniaux, & D. A. Driscoll (Eds.), *Obstetrics:*

Normal and problem pregnancies (6th ed.). Philadelphia, PA: Churchill Livingstone.

Groth, S., Morrison-Beedy, D., & Meng, Y. (2012). How pregnant African American women view pregnancy weight gain. *JOGNN: Journal of Obstetric, Gynecologic & Neonatal Nursing, 41*(6), 798–808.

Institute of Medicine (IOM). (2009). *Weight gain during pregnancy: Reexamining the guidelines.* Washington, DC: National Academies Press.

Lederman, R. P., & Weis, K. (2009). *Psychosocial adaptation to pregnancy* (3rd ed.). New York, NY: Springer.

Levin, L., Hopkins, P., & Tiffany, D. (2011). Experts weigh in on hCG testing. *Medical Laboratory Observer, 43*(2), 22–24.

Mehta, U., Siega-Riz, A., & Herring, A. (2011). Effect of body image in pregnancy weight gain. *Maternal & Child Health Journal, 15*(3), 324–332.

Rubin, R. (1984). *Maternal identity and the maternal experience.* New York, NY: Springer.

Widarsson, M., Kerstis, B., Sundquist, K., Engstrom, G., & Sarkadi, A. (2012). Support needs of expectant mothers and fathers: A qualitative study. *Journal of Perinatal Education, 21*(1), 36–44.

Yu, C. Y., Hung, C. H., Chan, T. F., Yeh, C. H., & Lai, C. Y. (2012). Prenatal predictors for father-infant attachment after childbirth. *Journal of Clinical Nursing, 21*(11/12), 1577–1583.

Pearson Nursing Student Resources Find additional review materials at: nursing.pearsonhighered.com

Antepartum Nursing Assessment

Joe McBride/Getty Images

I'm 16—just got my license—so it was weird telling my friends that my mom is pregnant. I was embarrassed (and a little jealous) at first but now I kind of like the idea of having a baby sister. Mom had an amniocentesis because she is 37, so we know it's a girl. My mom has been great about including me and telling me what is going on. I've gone to a couple of her prenatal appointments so I got to hear the heartbeat and I saw the baby moving on ultrasound. I'm surprised by how interesting I am finding everything. Don't laugh, but I think I might like to be a nurse-midwife someday. —Krista, 16

LEARNING OUTCOMES

10.1   Use information provided on a prenatal history to identify risk factors for the mother and/or fetus.

10.2   Define common obstetric terminology found in the history of maternity patients.

10.3   Identify risk factors related to the father's health that are generally recorded on the prenatal record when assessing risk factors for the mother and/or fetus.

10.4   Evaluate those areas of the initial assessment that reflect the psychosocial and cultural factors related to a woman's pregnancy.

10.5   Predict the normal physiologic changes a nurse would expect to find when performing a physical assessment of a pregnant woman.

10.6   Calculate the estimated date of birth using the common methods.

10.7   Describe the essential measurements that can be determined by clinical pelvimetry.

10.8   Summarize the results of the major screening tests used during the prenatal period in the assessment of the prenatal patient.

10.9   Assess the prenatal patient for any of the danger signs of pregnancy.

10.10   Relate the components of the subsequent prenatal history and assessment to the progress of pregnancy and the nursing care of the prenatal patient.

During the antepartum period, the role of the nurse is determined by academic preparation, clinical expertise, and professional credentials. The RN may complete many areas of prenatal assessment. Advanced practice nurses such as certified nurse-midwives (CNMs) and nurse practitioners are able to perform complete antepartum assessments. This chapter focuses on the prenatal assessments completed initially and at subsequent visits to provide optimum care for the childbearing family.

INITIAL PATIENT HISTORY

The course of a pregnancy depends on a number of factors, including the woman's prepregnancy health, presence of disease states, emotional status, and past health care. A thorough history helps determine the status of a woman's prepregnancy health.

Definition of Terms

The following terms are used in recording the history of maternity patients:

Gestation: the number of weeks of pregnancy since the first day of the last menstrual period

Abortion: birth that occurs before the end of 20 weeks' gestation or the birth of a fetus-newborn who weighs less than 500 g (Cunningham, Leveno, Bloom, et al., 2010). Abortion is abbreviated as ab. An abortion may occur spontaneously or it may be induced by medical or surgical means. If induced, it is often termed a therapeutic abortion.

Term: the normal duration of pregnancy (38 to 42 weeks' gestation). The stand-alone use of this term is now discouraged because it represents such a wide range of time and related risk (Spong, 2013).

    Early term: births occurring between 37 weeks 0 days and 38 weeks 6 days

    Full term: births occurring between 39 weeks 0 days and 40 weeks 6 days

    Late term: births occurring between 41 weeks 0 days through 41 weeks 6 days

Antepartum: time between conception and the onset of labor; describes the period during which a woman is pregnant; used interchangeably with *prenatal*

Intrapartum: time from the onset of true labor until the birth of the infant and placenta

Postpartum: time from the delivery of the placenta and membranes until the woman's body returns to a nonpregnant condition; typically about 6 weeks

Preterm or premature labor: labor that occurs after 20 weeks' but before completion of 37 weeks' gestation (Cunningham et al., 2010)

Postterm labor: labor that occurs after 42 weeks' gestation

Gravida: any pregnancy, regardless of duration, including present pregnancy. Gravida is often abbreviated as G.

Nulligravida: a woman who has never been pregnant

Primigravida: a woman who is pregnant for the first time

Multigravida: a woman who is in her second or any subsequent pregnancy

Para: birth after 20 weeks' gestation regardless of whether the infant is born alive or dead. Para is often abbreviated as P.

Nullipara: a woman who has had no births at more than 20 weeks' gestation

Primipara: a woman who has had one birth at more than 20 weeks' gestation, regardless of whether the infant was born alive or dead

Multipara: a woman who has had two or more births at more than 20 weeks' gestation

Stillbirth: an infant born dead after 20 weeks' gestation

The terms *gravida* and *para* are used in relation to pregnancies, not to the number of fetuses. Thus twins, triplets, and so forth count as one pregnancy and one birth.

The following examples illustrate how these terms are applied in clinical situations:

1. Jean Sanchez has one child born at 38 weeks' gestation and is pregnant for the second time. At her initial prenatal visit, the nurse indicates her obstetric history as "gravida 2 para 1 ab 0." (She might also be identified as a G2P1Ab0.) Jean Sanchez's present pregnancy terminates at 16 weeks' gestation. She is now "gravida 2 para 1 ab 1."

2. Tracy Hopkins is pregnant for the fourth time. At home she has a child who was born at term. Her second pregnancy ended at 10 weeks' gestation. She then gave birth to twins at 35 weeks. One twin died soon after birth. At her ante-partum assessment, the nurse records her obstetric history as "gravida 4 para 2 ab 1."

This approach is confusing, however, because it fails to identify the number of children that a woman might have. To provide comprehensive data, a more detailed approach is used in some settings. Using the detailed system, the first number, gravida, still refers to the number of pregnancies. However, para now is identified by a series of numbers that refer to the number of term infants, preterm infants, aborted fetuses, and living children the woman has (Cunningham et al., 2010). For example, triplets count as one pregnancy but three babies. Using this approach the nurse would have initially described Jean Sanchez (see the first example) as "gravida 2 para 1001" or "G2P1001." Following Jean's spontaneous abortion, she would be "gravida 2 para 1011" or "G2P1011." Tracy Hopkins would be described as "gravida 4 para 1212" or "G4P1212" (Figure 10–1 ●).

A useful acronym for remembering the system is TPAL:

T: number of term infants born (number of infants born at the completion of 37 weeks' gestation or beyond)
P: number of preterm infants born (number of infants born after 20 weeks but before the completion of 37 weeks' gestation)
A: number of pregnancies ending in either spontaneous or therapeutic abortion
L: number of currently living children

 Clinical Tip

In general, it is best to avoid an initial discussion of a woman's gravida and para status in front of her partner. It is possible that the woman had a previous pregnancy that she has not mentioned to her partner, and revealing the information could violate her right to privacy.

Patient Profile

The history is essentially a screening tool to identify factors that may place the mother or fetus at risk during the pregnancy. The following information is obtained for each pregnant woman at the first prenatal assessment:

1. Current pregnancy
   - First day of last normal menstrual period (LMP) (Is she sure of the dates or uncertain? Do her cycles normally occur every 28 days, or do her cycles tend to be longer?)
   - Presence of cramping, bleeding, or spotting since LMP
   - Woman's opinion about the time when conception occurred and when infant is due
   - Woman's attitude toward pregnancy (Is this pregnancy planned? Wanted?)
   - Results of pregnancy tests, if completed
   - Any discomforts since LMP such as nausea, vomiting, urinary frequency, fatigue, or breast tenderness

2. Past pregnancies
   - Number of pregnancies
   - Number of abortions, spontaneous or induced
   - Number of living children
   - History of previous pregnancies, length of pregnancy, length of labor and birth, type of birth (vaginal, forceps- or vacuum-assisted birth, or cesarean), location of birth, type of anesthesia used (if any), woman's perception of the experience, and complications (antepartum, intrapartum, and postpartum)
   - Neonatal status of previous children: Apgar scores, birth weights, general development, complications, and feeding patterns (breast milk, formula, or both). If breastfed, for how long?
   - Loss of a child (miscarriage, elective or medically indicated abortion, stillbirth, neonatal death, relinquishment, or death after the neonatal period). Cause of loss? What was the experience like for her? What coping skills helped? How did her partner, if involved, respond?
   - Blood type and Rh factor (If Rh negative, was Rh immune globulin received after birth/miscarriage/abortion?)
   - Prenatal education classes and resources (books, websites); knowledge about pregnancy, childbirth, and parenting

3. Gynecologic history
   - Date of last Pap smear; result? Any history of abnormal Pap smear; any follow-up therapy completed
   - Previous infections: vaginal, cervical, pelvic inflammatory disease (PID), or sexually transmitted infections
   - Previous surgery (uterine, ovarian)
   - Age at menarche
   - Regularity, frequency, and duration of menstrual flow

Name	Gravida	Term	Preterm	Abortions	Living Children
Jean Sanchez	2	1	0	1	1
Tracy Hopkins	4	1	2	1	2

● **Figure 10–1** The TPAL approach provides detailed information about a woman's pregnancy history.

- History of dysmenorrhea
- History of infertility
- Sexual history
- Contraceptive history (If hormonal method used, did pregnancy occur immediately following cessation of method? If not, how long after? When was contraception last used?)
- Any issues related to infertility or fertility treatments

4. Current medical history
   - Weight (prepregnancy and current), height, body mass index (BMI) (determine recommended weight gain)
   - General health, including nutrition (dietary practices such as vegetarianism; lactose intolerance; food allergies?), regular exercise program (type, frequency, and duration); monthly breast self-examination; eye exam; date of last dental exam
   - Any medications presently being taken (including prescription, nonprescription, homeopathic, or herbal medications) or taken since the onset of pregnancy
   - Previous or present use of alcohol, tobacco, or caffeine (Ask specifically about the amounts of alcohol, cigarettes, and caffeine [specify coffee, tea, colas, or chocolate] consumed each day.)
   - Illicit drug use or abuse (Ask about specific drugs such as cocaine, crack, methamphetamines, and marijuana; planning cessation?)
   - Drug allergies and other allergies (Ask about latex allergies or sensitivities.)
   - Potential teratogenic insults to this pregnancy such as viral infections, medications, x-ray examinations, surgery, or cats in the home (possible source of toxoplasmosis)
   - Presence of chronic disease conditions such as diabetes, hypertension, cardiovascular disease, renal problems, cancer, or thyroid disorder
   - Infections or illnesses since LMP (flu, measles)
   - Record of immunizations (especially rubella); up to date?
   - Presence of any abnormal signs/symptoms

5. Past medical history
   - Childhood diseases
   - Past treatment for any disease condition (Any hospitalizations? Major injuries?)
   - Surgical procedures
   - Presence of bleeding disorders or tendencies (Has she received blood transfusions? Will she accept blood transfusions?)

6. Family medical history
   - Presence of diabetes, cardiovascular disease, cancer, hypertension, hematologic disorders, tuberculosis, thyroid disease
   - Occurrence of multiple births

- History of congenital diseases or deformities
- Occurrence of cesarean births and cause, if known

7. Genetic history (patient, father of the child [FOC], and both families)
   - Birth defects
   - Recurrent pregnancy loss
   - Stillbirth
   - Down syndrome, intellectual disability, developmental delay, chromosomal abnormalities
   - Ethnic background (Mediterranean descent, Jewish, Asian)
   - Genetic disorders (cystic fibrosis, sickle cell disease/trait, muscular dystrophy).

8. Religious, spiritual, and cultural history
   - Does the woman wish to specify a religious preference on her chart? Does she have any spiritual beliefs or practices that might influence her health care or that of her child, such as a prohibition against receiving blood products, dietary considerations, or circumcision rites?
   - What practices are important for her spiritual well-being?
   - Might practices in her culture or that of her partner influence her care or that of her child?

9. Occupational history
   - Occupation
   - Physical demands (Does she stand all day, or are there opportunities to sit and elevate her legs? Any heavy lifting?)
   - Exposure to chemicals or other harmful substances
   - Opportunity for regular meals and breaks for nutritious snacks
   - Provision for maternity or family leave

10. Partner's history
    - Age
    - Significant health problems
    - Previous or present alcohol intake, drug use, or tobacco use
    - Blood type and Rh factor
    - Occupation
    - Educational level; methods by which he or she learns best
    - Thoughts/feelings about the pregnancy

11. Personal history
    - Age
    - Relationship status (Married? Partner involved?)
    - Educational level; methods by which she learns best
    - Race or ethnic group (to identify need for prenatal genetic screening and racially or ethnically related risk factors)

- Housing; stability of living conditions
- Economic level
- Acceptance of pregnancy, whether intended or unintended
- Any history of emotional or physical deprivation or abuse of herself or children or any abuse in her current relationship (Has she been hit, slapped, kicked, or hurt within the past year or since she has been pregnant? Is she afraid of her partner or anyone else? If yes, of whom is she afraid? [*Note:* Ask these questions when the woman is alone.])
- History of emotional/mental health problems (depression in general, postpartum depression, anxiety, bipolar disorder)
- Support systems
- Personal preferences about the birth (expectations of both the woman and her partner, presence of others, and so on). (For more information see Chapter 8 🔗.)
- Plans for care of child following birth; plans for circumcision if the infant is male.
- Feeding preference for the baby (Breast milk or formula?)

Obtaining Data

A questionnaire is often used to obtain information. Some clinics and offices send the form via e-mail or regular mail, or post the form on their website for downloading, so the woman can complete it prior to her first prenatal visit; others prefer that it be done in person. In either case, the woman should complete the questionnaire in a quiet place with a minimum of distractions. The nurse can get further information in an interview, which allows the pregnant woman to clarify her responses to questions and gives the nurse and patient the opportunity to develop rapport.

SAFETY ALERT!

Because some medications may pose a risk to the fetus if taken during pregnancy, it is crucial to develop a list of all the medications the pregnant woman is currently taking as well as those she had been taking before she learned she was pregnant. This list should be given to the patient's primary caregiver. (See discussion of classification system for medications taken during pregnancy in Chapter 11 🔗.)

The expectant father or partner can be encouraged to attend the prenatal examinations. The partner is often able to contribute to the history and may use the opportunity to ask questions or express concerns that are important to him or her.

Risk-Factor Screening

Risk factors are any findings that suggest the pregnancy may have a negative outcome, for either the woman or her unborn child. Screening for risk factors is an important part of the prenatal assessment. Many risk factors can be identified during the initial assessment; others may be detected during subsequent prenatal visits. It is important to identify high-risk pregnancies early so that appropriate interventions can be started promptly. Not all risk factors threaten a pregnancy equally; thus, many agencies use a scoring sheet to determine the degree of risk. Information must be updated throughout pregnancy as necessary. Any pregnancy may begin as low risk and change to high risk because of complications.

Table 10–1 identifies the major risk factors currently recognized. The table also identifies maternal and fetal or newborn implications if the risk is present in the pregnancy.

INITIAL PRENATAL ASSESSMENT

The initial prenatal assessment focuses on the woman holistically by considering physical, cultural, and psychosocial factors that influence her health. The establishment of the nurse-patient relationship is a chance to develop an atmosphere conducive to interviewing, support, and education. Because many women are excited and anxious at the first antepartum visit, the initial psychosocial-cultural assessment is general.

As part of the initial psychosocial-cultural assessment, discuss with the woman any religious or spiritual, cultural, or socioeconomic factors that influence the woman's expectations of the childbearing experience. It is especially helpful to be familiar with common practices of the members of various religious and cultural groups who reside in the community.

After obtaining the history, prepare the woman for the physical examination. The physical examination begins with assessment of vital signs; then the woman's body is examined. The pelvic examination is performed last.

Before the examination the woman should provide a clean urine specimen for screening. When her bladder is empty, the woman is more comfortable during the pelvic examination and the examiner can palpate the pelvic organs more easily. After the woman empties her bladder, the nurse should ask her to disrobe and give her a gown and sheet or some other protective covering.

Increasing numbers of nurses, such as CNMs, nurse practitioners, and other nurses in advanced practice, are educationally prepared to perform complete physical examinations. The nurse who is not an advanced practitioner assesses the woman's vital signs, explains the procedures to allay apprehension, positions her for examination, and assists the examiner as necessary.

Thoroughness and a systematic procedure are the most important considerations when performing the physical portion of an antepartum examination. See *Assessment Guide: Initial Prenatal Assessment*. To promote completeness, the assessment guide is organized in three columns that address the areas to be assessed (and normal findings), the variations or alterations that may be observed, and nursing responses to the data. Certain organs and systems are assessed concurrently with others during the physical portion of the examination.

Table 10–1	Prenatal High-Risk Factors	
Factor	Maternal Implications	Fetal or Neonatal Implications
Social and Personal		
Low income level and/or low educational level	Insufficient antenatal care or late antenatal care ↑ risk preterm birth Poor nutrition ↑ risk preeclampsia	Low birth weight Prematurity Intrauterine growth restriction (IUGR)/small for gestational age (SGA)
Poor diet	Inadequate nutrition ↑ risk preterm birth ↑ risk anemia ↑ risk preeclampsia	Fetal malnutrition IUGR/SGA Prematurity
Living at high altitude	↑ hemoglobin	Prematurity IUGR ↑ hemoglobin (polycythemia)
Multiparity greater than 3	↑ risk antepartum or postpartum hemorrhage	Anemia Fetal death
Weight less than 45.5 kg (100 lb)	Poor nutrition Cephalopelvic disproportion Prolonged labor	IUGR Hypoxia associated with difficult labor and birth
Weight greater than 91 kg (200 lb)	↑ risk hypertension ↑ risk cephalopelvic disproportion ↑ risk diabetes	↓ fetal nutrition ↑ risk macrosomia
Age less than 16 years	Poor nutrition Insufficient antenatal care ↑ risk preeclampsia ↑ risk cephalopelvic disproportion	Low birth weight ↑ fetal demise
Age older than 35	↑ risk preeclampsia ↑ risk cesarean birth	↑ risk congenital anomalies ↑ chromosomal abnormalities
Smoking one pack/day or more	↑ risk hypertension ↑ risk cancer	↓ placental perfusion → ↓ O_2 and nutrients available Low birth weight IUGR/SGA Preterm birth
Use of addictive drugs	↑ risk poor nutrition ↑ risk infection with IV drugs ↑ risk HIV, hepatitis C	↑ risk congenital anomalies ↑ risk low birth weight Neonatal withdrawal Lower serum bilirubin
Excessive alcohol consumption	↑ risk poor nutrition Possible hepatic effects with long-term consumption	↑ risk fetal alcohol syndrome
Preexisting Medical Disorders		
Diabetes mellitus	↑ risk preeclampsia, hypertension Episodes of hypoglycemia and hyperglycemia ↑ risk cesarean birth	Low birth weight Macrosomia Neonatal hypoglycemia ↑ risk congenital anomalies ↑ risk respiratory distress syndrome

Table 10–1	Prenatal High-Risk Factors—continued

Factor	Maternal Implications	Fetal or Neonatal Implications
Preexisting Medical Disorders		
Cardiac disease	Cardiac decompensation Further strain on mother's body ↑ maternal death rate	↑ risk fetal demise ↑ prenatal mortality
Anemia: hemoglobin less than 11 g/dL or less than 32% hematocrit	Iron-deficiency anemia Low energy level Decreased oxygen-carrying capacity	Fetal death Prematurity Low birth weight
Hypertension	↑ vasospasm ↑ risk central nervous system irritability → convulsions ↑ risk cerebrovascular accident ↑ risk renal damage	↓ placental perfusion → low birth weight Preterm birth
Thyroid disorder	↑ infertility	↑ spontaneous abortion
Hypothyroidism	↓ basal metabolic rate, goiter, myxedema ↑ risk miscarriage, preterm labor/birth ↑ risk preeclampsia	↑ risk congenital goiter ↑ risk IUGR/SGA ↑ risk stillbirth
Hyperthyroidism	↓ risk postpartum hemorrhage ↑ risk preeclampsia Danger of thyroid storm	Mental retardation → cretinism ↑ incidence congenital anomalies ↑ incidence preterm birth, IUGR/SGA ↑ risk neonatal hyperthyroidism ↑ tendency to thyrotoxicosis
Renal disease (moderate to severe)	↑ risk renal failure	↑ risk IUGR/SGA ↑ risk preterm birth
Diethylstilbestrol (DES) exposure	↑ infertility, spontaneous abortion ↑ cervical incompetence	↑ risk preterm birth
Obstetric Considerations		
Previous Pregnancy Stillborn	↑ emotional or psychologic distress	↑ risk IUGR/SGA ↑ risk preterm birth
Habitual abortion	↑ emotional or psychologic distress	↑ risk abortion
Cesarean birth	↑ possibility repeat cesarean birth	↑ risk preterm birth ↑ risk respiratory distress
Rh or blood group sensitization		↑ risk erythroblastosis fetalis Hydrops fetalis Icterus gravis Neonatal anemia Kernicterus Hypoglycemia

(continued)

Table 10–1	Prenatal High-Risk Factors—continued	
Factor	Maternal Implications	Fetal or Neonatal Implications
	Obstetric Considerations	
Large baby	↑ risk cesarean birth ↑ risk gestational diabetes	Birth injury Hypoglycemia
Current Pregnancy Rubella (first trimester)		Congenital heart disease Cataracts Nerve deafness Bone lesions Prolonged virus shedding
Toxoplasmosis		Retinochoroiditis Convulsions, coma, microcephaly
Rubella (second trimester)		Hepatitis Thrombocytopenia
Cytomegalovirus		IUGR Encephalopathy
Herpes virus type 2	Severe discomfort Concern about possibility of cesarean birth, fetal infection	Neonatal herpes virus type 2 2% hepatitis with jaundice Neurologic abnormalities
Syphilis	↑ incidence abortion	↑ fetal demise Congenital syphilis
Abruptio placentae and placenta previa	↑ risk hemorrhage Bed rest Extended hospitalization	Fetal or neonatal anemia Intrauterine hemorrhage ↑ fetal demise
Preeclampsia or eclampsia	See hypertension	↑ placental perfusion → low birth weight
Multiple gestation	↑ risk postpartum hemorrhage ↑ risk preterm labor ↑ risk gestational diabetes mellitus ↑ risk placenta previa ↑ risk preeclampsia	↑ risk preterm labor/birth ↑ risk fetal demise ↑ risk fetal demise, IUGR/SGA ↑ risk malpresentation ↑ risk stillbirth
Elevated hematocrit Greater than 41% (white) Greater than 38% (black)	Increased viscosity of blood	Fetal death rate 5 times normal rate
Spontaneous premature rupture of membranes	↑ uterine infection	Preterm birth Fetal demise

Assessment Guide Initial Prenatal Assessment

Physical Assessment/Normal Findings	Alterations and Possible Causes*	Nursing Responses to Data†
Vital Signs		
Blood pressure (BP): Less than or equal to 120/80 mm Hg	High BP (essential hypertension; renal disease; pregestational hypertension, apprehension; preeclampsia if initial assessment not done until after 20 weeks' gestation)	120–139/80–89 is considered prehypertensive. BP greater than 140/90 requires immediate consideration; establish woman's BP; refer to healthcare provider if necessary. Assess woman's knowledge about high BP; counsel on self-care and medical management.
Pulse: 60–100 beats/min; rate may increase 10 beats/min during pregnancy	Increased pulse rate (excitement or anxiety, dehydration, cardiac disorders)	Count for 1 full minute; note irregularities. Evaluate temperature, increase fluids.
Respirations: 12–20 breaths/min (or pulse rate divided by 4); pregnancy may induce a degree of hyperventilation; thoracic breathing predominant	Marked tachypnea or abnormal patterns	Assess for respiratory disease.
Temperature: 36.2°C–37.6°C (97°F–99.6°F)	Elevated temperature (infection)	Assess for infection process or disease state if temperature is elevated; refer to healthcare provider.
Weight		
Depends on body build	Weight less than 45 kg (100 lb) or greater than 91 kg (200 lb); rapid, sudden weight gain (preeclampsia)	Evaluate need for nutritional counseling; obtain information on eating habits, cooking practices, food regularly eaten, food allergies, income limitations, need for food supplements, and pica and other abnormal food habits. Note initial weight to establish baseline for weight gain throughout pregnancy. Determine body mass index (BMI) and recommend amount of weight gain for pregnancy.
Skin		
Color: Consistent with racial background; pink nail beds	Pallor (anemia); bronze, yellow (hepatic disease; other causes of jaundice) Bluish, reddish, mottled; dusky appearance or pallor of palms and nail beds in dark-skinned women (anemia)	The following tests should be performed: complete blood count (CBC), bilirubin level, urinalysis, and blood urea nitrogen (BUN). If abnormal, refer to healthcare provider.
Condition: Absence of edema (slight edema of lower extremities is normal during pregnancy)	Edema (preeclampsia, normal pregnancy changes); rashes, dermatitis (allergic response)	Counsel on relief measures for slight edema. Initiate preeclampsia assessment; refer to healthcare provider.
Lesions: Absence of lesions	Ulceration (varicose veins, decreased circulation)	Further assess circulatory status; refer to healthcare provider if lesion is severe.
Spider nevi common in pregnancy	Petechiae, multiple bruises, ecchymosis (hemorrhagic disorders; abuse) Change in size or color (carcinoma)	Evaluate for bleeding or clotting disorder. Provide opportunities to discuss abuse if suspected. Refer to healthcare provider.
Moles		
Pigmentation: Pigmentation changes of pregnancy include linea nigra, striae gravidarum, melasma		Assure woman that these are normal manifestations of pregnancy and explain the physiologic basis for the changes.
Cafe-au-lait spots	Six or more (Albright syndrome or neurofibromatosis)	Consult with healthcare provider.
Nose		
Character of mucosa: Redder than oral mucosa; in pregnancy nasal mucosa is edematous in response to increased estrogen, resulting in nasal stuffiness (rhinitis of pregnancy) and nosebleeds	Olfactory loss (first cranial nerve deficit)	Counsel woman about possible relief measures for nasal stuffiness and nosebleeds (epistaxis); refer to healthcare provider for olfactory loss.

(continued)

Assessment Guide   Initial Prenatal Assessment—continued

Physical Assessment/Normal Findings	Alterations and Possible Causes*	Nursing Responses to Data†
Mouth		
May note hypertrophy of gingival tissue because of estrogen	Edema, inflammation (infection); pale in color (anemia)	Assess hematocrit for anemia; counsel regarding dental hygiene habits. Refer to healthcare provider or dentist if necessary. Routine dental care appropriate during pregnancy.
Neck		
Nodes: Small, mobile, nontender nodes	Tender, hard, fixed, or prominent nodes (infection, carcinoma)	Examine for local infection; refer to healthcare provider.
Thyroid: Small, smooth, lateral lobes palpable on either side of trachea; slight hyperplasia by third month of pregnancy	Enlargement or nodule tenderness (hyperthyroidism)	Test to perform: thyroid-stimulating hormone (TSH). Listen over thyroid for bruits, which may indicate hyperthyroidism. Question woman about dietary habits (iodine intake). Ascertain history of thyroid problems; refer to healthcare provider.
Chest and Lungs		
Chest: Symmetric, elliptic, smaller anteroposterior (AP) than transverse diameter	Increased AP diameter, funnel chest, pigeon chest (emphysema, asthma, chronic obstructive pulmonary disease [COPD])	Evaluate for emphysema, asthma, COPD.
Ribs: Slope downward from nipple line	More horizontal (COPD) angular bumps rachitic rosary (vitamin C deficiency)	Evaluate for COPD. Evaluate for fractures. Consult healthcare provider. Consult nutritionist.
Inspection and palpation: No retraction or bulging of intercostal spaces (ICS) during inspiration or expiration; symmetric expansion.	ICS retractions with inspirations, bulging with expiration; unequal expansion (respiratory disease)	Do thorough initial assessment. Refer to healthcare provider.
Tactile fremitus	Tachypnea, hyperpnea, Cheyne-Stokes respirations (respiratory disease)	Refer to healthcare provider.
Percussion: Bilateral symmetry in tone	Flatness of percussion, which may be affected by chest wall thickness	Evaluate for pleural effusions, consolidations, or tumor.
Low-pitched resonance of moderate intensity	High diaphragm (atelectasis or paralysis), pleural effusion	Refer to healthcare provider.
Auscultation: Upper lobes: bronchovesicular sounds above sternum and scapulas; equal expiratory and inspiratory phases	Abnormal if heard over any other area of chest	Refer to healthcare provider.
Remainder of chest: vesicular breath sounds heard; inspiratory phase longer (3:1)	Rales, rhonchi, wheezes; pleural friction rub; absence of breath sounds; bronchophony, egophony, whispered pectoriloquy	Refer to healthcare provider.
Breasts		
Supple: Symmetric in size and contour; darker pigmentation of nipple and areola; may have supernumerary nipples, usually 5–6 cm below normal nipple line	"Pigskin" or orange-peel appearance, nipple retractions, swelling, hardness (carcinoma); redness, heat, tenderness, cracked or fissured nipple (infection)	Encourage monthly self-examination; instruct woman how to examine her own breasts.
Axillary nodes nonpalpable or pellet sized	Tenderness, enlargement, hard node (carcinoma); may be visible bump (infection)	Refer to healthcare provider for evaluation of abnormal breast findings. Plan ultrasound/mammogram/MRI of breasts.

Assessment Guide Initial Prenatal Assessment—continued

Physical Assessment/Normal Findings	Alterations and Possible Causes*	Nursing Responses to Data†
Pregnancy changes: 1. Size increase noted primarily in first 20 weeks. 2. Become nodular. 3. Tingling sensation may be felt during first and third trimester; woman may report feeling of heaviness. 4. Pigmentation of nipples and areolae darkens. 5. Superficial veins dilate and become more prominent. 6. Striae seen in multiparas. 7. Tubercles of Montgomery enlarge. 8. Colostrum may be present after 12th week. 9. Secondary areola appears at 20 weeks, characterized by series of washed-out spots surrounding primary areola. 10. Breasts less firm, old striae may be present in multiparas.		Discuss normalcy of changes and their meaning with the woman. Teach and/or institute appropriate relief measures. Encourage use of supportive, well-fitting brassiere.
Heart Normal rate, rhythm, and heart sounds **Pregnancy changes:** 1. Palpitations may occur due to sympathetic nervous system disturbance. 2. Short systolic murmurs that increase in held expiration are normal due to increased volume.	Enlargement, thrills, thrusts, gross irregularity or skipped beats, gallop rhythm or extra sounds (cardiac disease)	Complete an initial assessment. Explain normal pregnancy-induced changes. Refer to healthcare provider if indicated.
Abdomen Normal appearance, skin texture, and hair distribution; liver nonpalpable; abdomen nontender **Pregnancy changes:** 1. Purple striae may be present (or silver striae on a multipara) as well as linea nigra. 2. Diastasis of the rectus muscles is seen late in pregnancy.	Muscle guarding (anxiety, acute tenderness); tenderness, mass (ectopic pregnancy, inflammation, carcinoma)	Assure woman of normalcy of diastasis. Provide initial information about appropriate prenatal and postpartum exercises. Evaluate woman's anxiety level. Refer to healthcare provider if indicated.
3. Size: Flat or rotund abdomen; progressive enlargement of uterus due to pregnancy: *10–12 weeks:* Fundus slightly above symphysis pubis. *16 weeks:* Fundus halfway between symphysis and umbilicus. *20–22 weeks:* Fundus at umbilicus. *28 weeks:* Fundus three finger breadths above umbilicus. *36 weeks:* Fundus just below ensiform cartilage.	Size of uterus inconsistent with length of gestation (intrauterine growth restriction [IUGR], multiple pregnancy, fetal demise, incorrect estimated date of birth (EDB), abnormal amniotic fluid, hydatidiform mole)	Reassess menstrual history regarding pregnancy dating. Evaluate increase in size using McDonald's method. (See Figure 10–3 on page 209.) Use ultrasound to establish diagnosis.
4. Fetal heart rate: 110–160 beats/min may be heard with Doppler at 10–12 weeks' gestation; may be heard with fetoscope at 17–20 weeks.	Failure to hear fetal heartbeat with Doppler (fetal demise, hydatidiform mole)	Refer to healthcare provider. Administer pregnancy tests. Use ultrasound to establish diagnosis.
5. Fetal movement palpable by a trained examiner after the 18th week.	Failure to feel fetal movements after 20 weeks' gestation (fetal demise, hydatidiform mole)	Refer to healthcare provider.
6. Ballottement: During fourth to fifth month, fetus rises and then rebounds to original position when uterus is tapped sharply.	No ballottement (oligohydramnios)	Refer to healthcare provider.

(continued)

Assessment Guide   Initial Prenatal Assessment—continued

Physical Assessment/Normal Findings	Alterations and Possible Causes*	Nursing Responses to Data†
Extremities		
Skin warm, pulses palpable, full range of motion; may be some edema of hands and ankles in late pregnancy; varicose veins may become more pronounced; palmar erythema may be present	Unpalpable or diminished pulses (arterial insufficiency); marked edema (preeclampsia)	Evaluate for other symptoms of heart disease; initiate follow-up if woman mentions that her rings feel tight. Discuss prevention and self-treatment measures for varicose veins; refer to healthcare provider if indicated.
Spine		
Normal spinal curves: Concave cervical, convex thoracic, concave lumbar In pregnancy, lumbar spinal curve may be accentuated	Abnormal spinal curves; flatness, kyphosis, lordosis Backache	Refer to healthcare provider if indicated. May have implications for administration of spinal anesthetics; see Chapter 20 🔴 for relief measures.
Shoulders and iliac crests should be even	Uneven shoulders and iliac crests (scoliosis)	Refer very young women to healthcare provider; discuss back-stretching exercise with older women.
Reflexes		
Normal and symmetric	Hyperactivity, clonus (preeclampsia)	Evaluate for other symptoms of preeclampsia.
Pelvic Area		
External female genitals: Normally formed with female hair distribution; in multiparas, labia majora loose and pigmented; urinary and vaginal orifices visible and appropriately located	Lesions, genital warts, hematomas, varicosities, inflammation of Bartholin's glands; clitoral hypertrophy (masculinization)	Explain pelvic examination procedure. Encourage woman to minimize her discomfort by relaxing her hips. Provide privacy.
Vagina: Pink or dark pink, vaginal discharge odorless, nonirritating; in multiparas, vaginal folds smooth and flattened; may have episiotomy scar	Abnormal discharge associated with vaginal infections	Obtain vaginal smear. Provide understandable verbal and written instructions about treatment for woman and partner, if indicated.
Cervix: Pink color; os closed except in multiparas, in whom os admits fingertip	Eversion, reddish erosion, nabothian or retention cysts, cervical polyp; granular area that bleeds (carcinoma of cervix); lesions (herpes, human papillomavirus [HPV]); presence of string or plastic tip from cervix (intrauterine device [IUD] in uterus)	Provide woman with a hand mirror and identify genital structures for her; encourage her to view her cervix if she wishes. Refer to healthcare provider if indicated. Advise woman of potential serious risks of leaving an IUD in place during pregnancy; refer to healthcare provider for removal.
Pregnancy changes: *1–4 weeks' gestation:* enlargement in anteroposterior diameter *4–6 weeks' gestation:* softening of cervix (Goodell's sign); softening of isthmus of uterus (Hegar's sign); cervix takes on bluish coloring (Chadwick's sign) *8–12 weeks' gestation:* vagina and cervix appear bluish violet in color (Chadwick's sign)	Absence of Goodell's sign (inflammatory conditions, carcinoma)	Refer to healthcare provider.
Uterus: Pear shaped, mobile; smooth surface	Fixed (pelvic inflammatory disease [PID]); nodular surface (fibromas)	Refer to healthcare provider.
Ovaries: Small, walnut shaped, nontender (ovaries and fallopian tubes are located in the adnexal areas)	Pain on movement of cervix (PID); enlarged or nodular ovaries (cyst, tumor, tubal pregnancy, corpus luteum of pregnancy)	Evaluate adnexal areas; refer to healthcare provider.

Assessment Guide Initial Prenatal Assessment—continued

Physical Assessment/Normal Findings	Alterations and Possible Causes*	Nursing Responses to Data†
Pelvic Measurements		
Internal measurements:		
1. Diagonal conjugate at least 11.5 cm (see Figure 10–5 on page 210)	Measurement below normal	Vaginal birth may not be possible if deviations are present.
2. Obstetric conjugate estimated by subtracing 1.5–2 cm from diagonal conjugate	Disproportion of pubic arch	
3. Inclination of sacrum	Abnormal curvature of sacrum	
4. Motility of coccyx; external intertuberosity diameter greater than 8 cm	Fixed or malposition of coccyx	
Anus and Rectum		
No lumps, rashes, excoriation, tenderness; cervix may be felt through rectal wall	Hemorrhoids, rectal prolapse; warts (HPV infection); nodular lesion (carcinoma)	Counsel about appropriate prevention and relief measures; refer to healthcare provider for further evaluation.
Laboratory Evaluation		
Hemoglobin: 12–16 g/dL; women residing in areas of high altitude may have higher levels of hemoglobin	Less than 11 g/dL in the first trimester, less than 10.5 g/dL in the second trimester, and less than 11 g/dL in the third trimester (anemia) (American College of Obstetricians and Gynecologists [ACOG], 2010)	Hemoglobin less than 12 g/dL requires nutritional counseling; less than 11 g/dL requires iron supplementation.
ABO and Rh typing: Normal distribution of blood types	Rh negative	If Rh negative, check for presence of anti-Rh antibodies. Check blood type of father of child; if he is Rh positive, discuss with woman the need for Rh immune globulin administration at 28 weeks, management during the intrapartum period, and possible need for Rh immune globulin after birth. (See discussion in Chapter 16 🔗.)
Complete Blood Count (CBC)		
Hematocrit: 38%–47% physiologic anemia (pseudoanemia) may occur	Marked anemia or blood dyscrasias	Perform CBC and Schilling differential cell count.
Red blood cells (RBC): 4.2–5.4 million/microliter		
White blood cells (WBC): 5000–12,000/microliter	Presence of infection; may be elevated in pregnancy and with labor	Evaluate for other signs of infection.
Differential Neutrophils: 40%–60% Bands: up to 5% Eosinophils: 1%–3% Basophils: up to 1% Lymphocytes: 20%–40% Monocytes: 4%–8%		
First-trimester aneuploidy screening (testing to detect conditions related to abnormal chromosome number): If nuchal translucency (NT) testing is available, offer first-trimester screening for Down syndrome using nuchal translucency and serum markers (PAPP-A and free β-hCG). Normal range. *Integrated screening:* Combines first-trimester aneuploidy screening results with second-trimester quad screen to detect aneuploidy and neural tube defects; may be used in areas in which NT testing is not available. (See discussion in *Assessment Guide: Subsequent Prenatal Assessment.*)	Increased nuchal translucency, elevated β-hCG, and reduced PAPP-A (Down syndrome, trisomy 18, trisomy 13, Turner syndrome)	If findings are positive, genetic counseling and diagnostic testing using chorionic villus sampling (CVS) or second-trimester amniocentesis are offered.

(continued)

Assessment Guide   Initial Prenatal Assessment—continued

Physical Assessment/Normal Findings	Alterations and Possible Causes*	Nursing Responses to Data†
Syphilis tests: Serologic tests for syphilis (STS), complement fixation test, Venereal Disease Research Laboratory (VDRL) test—nonreactive	Positive reaction STS—tests may have 25%–45% incidence of biologic false-positive results; false results may occur in individuals who have acute viral or bacterial infections, hypersensitivity reactions, recent vaccinations, collagen disease, malaria, or tuberculosis	Positive results may be confirmed with the fluorescent treponemal antibody-absorption (FTA-ABS) test; all tests for syphilis give positive results in the secondary stage of the disease; antibiotic tests may cause negative test results. Refer to healthcare provider for treatment.
Gonorrhea culture: Negative	Positive	Refer for treatment.
Urinalysis (u/a): Normal color, specific gravity; pH 4.6–8	Cloudy appearance (infection; pus or tissue) Abnormal color (porphyria, hemoglobinuria, bilirubinemia): alkaline urine (metabolic alkalemia, *Proteus* infection, old specimen)	Repeat u/a; refer to healthcare provider.
Negative for protein, red blood cells, white blood cells, casts	Positive findings (contaminated specimen, UTI, kidney disease)	Repeat u/a; refer to healthcare provider.
Glucose: Negative (small degree of glycosuria may occur in pregnancy)	Glycosuria (low renal threshold for glucose, diabetes mellitus)	Assess blood glucose level; test urine for ketones.
Rubella titer: Hemagglutination-inhibition (HAI) test–1:10 or above indicates woman is immune	HAI titer less than 1:10	Immunization will be given postpartum. Instruct woman whose titers are less than 1:10 to avoid children who have rubella.
Hepatitis B screen: For hepatitis B surface antigen (HBsAg): negative	Positive	If positive, refer to physician. Infants born to women who test positive are given hepatitis B immune globulin soon after birth followed by first dose of hepatitis B vaccine.
HIV screen: Opt-out screening offered to all women; encouraged for those at risk; negative	Positive	Refer to healthcare provider.
Illicit drug screen: Offered to all women; negative	Positive	Refer to healthcare provider.
Sickle cell screen for patients of African or Latino descent: Negative	Positive; test results would include a description of cells	Refer to healthcare provider.
Pap smear: Negative	Test results that show abnormal cells with negative or positive high-risk HPV.	Refer to healthcare provider. Discuss with the woman the meaning of the findings and the importance of follow-up. Plan colposcopy if indicated.

Cultural Assessment	Variations to Consider*	Nursing Responses to Data†
Determine the woman's fluency in written and oral English.	Woman may be fluent in language other than English.	Work with a knowledgeable translator to provide information and answer questions.
Ask the woman how she prefers to be addressed. Nickname?	Some women prefer informality; others prefer to use titles.	Address the woman according to her preference. Maintain formality in introducing oneself if that seems preferred.
Determine customs and practices regarding prenatal care:	Practices are influenced by individual preference, cultural expectations, or religious beliefs.	Honor a woman's practices and provide for specific preferences unless they are contraindicated because of safety.
■ Ask the woman if there are certain practices she expects to follow when she is pregnant. ■ Ask the woman if there are any activities she cannot do while she is pregnant.	Some women believe that they should perform certain acts related to sleep, activity, or clothing. Some women have restrictions or taboos they follow related to work, activity, sexual, environmental, or emotional factors.	Have information printed in the language of different cultural groups that live in the area.
■ Ask the woman whether there are certain foods she is expected to eat or avoid while she is pregnant. Determine whether she has lactose intolerance.	Food is an important cultural factor. Some women may have certain foods they must eat or avoid; many women have lactose intolerance and have difficulty consuming sufficient calcium.	Respect the woman's food preferences, help her plan an adequate prenatal diet within the framework of her preferences, and refer to a dietitian if necessary.

Assessment Guide   Initial Prenatal Assessment—continued

Cultural Assessment	Variations to Consider*	Nursing Responses to Data†
■ Ask the woman whether the gender of her caregiver is of concern. ■ Ask the woman about the degree of involvement in her pregnancy that she expects or wants from her support person, mother, and other significant people. ■ Ask the woman about her sources of support and counseling during pregnancy.	Some women are comfortable only with a female caregiver. A woman may not want her partner involved in the pregnancy. For some the role falls to the woman's mother or a female relative or friend. Some women seek advice from a family member, *curandera*, tribal healer, and so forth.	Arrange for a female caregiver if it is the woman's preference. Respect the woman's preferences about her partner or husband's involvement; avoid imposing personal values or expectations. Respect and honor the woman's sources of support.

Psychologic Status

Excitement and/or apprehension, ambivalence	Marked anxiety (fear of pregnancy diagnosis, fear of medical facility)	Establish lines of communication. Active listening is useful. Establish trusting relationship. Encourage woman to take active part in her care.
	Apathy; display of anger with pregnancy diagnosis	Establish communication and begin counseling. Use active listening techniques.

Educational Needs

May have questions about pregnancy or may need time to adjust to reality of pregnancy		Establish educational, supporting environment that can be expanded throughout pregnancy.

Support System

Can identify at least two or three individuals with whom woman is emotionally intimate (partner, parent, sibling, friend)	Isolated (no telephone, unlisted number); cannot name a neighbor or friend whom she can call on in an emergency; does not perceive parents as part of her support system	Institute support system through community groups. Help woman to develop trusting relationship with healthcare professionals.

Family Functioning

Emotionally supportive Communications adequate Mutually satisfying Cohesiveness in times of trouble	Long-term problems or specific problems related to this pregnancy, potential stressors within the family, pessimistic attitudes, unilateral decision making, unrealistic expectations of this pregnancy or child	Help identify the problems and stressors, encourage communication, and discuss role changes and adaptations. Refer to counseling if indicated.

Economic Status

Source of income is stable and sufficient to meet basic needs of daily living and medical needs	Limited prenatal care; poor physical health; limited use of healthcare system; unstable economic status	Discuss available resources for health maintenance and the birth. Institute appropriate referral for meeting expanding family's needs—food stamps, WIC (a federally funded nutrition program for women, infants, and children), and so forth.

Stability of Living Conditions

Adequate, stable housing for expanding family's needs	Crowded living conditions; questionable supportive environment for newborn	Refer to appropriate community agency. Work with family on self-help ways to improve situation.

*Possible causes of alterations are identified in parentheses.
†This column provides guidelines for further assessment and initial intervention.

Clinical Tip

Gloves are worn for procedures that involve contact with body fluids such as drawing blood for lab work, handling urine specimens, and conducting pelvic examinations. Because of the increased incidence of latex allergies, it is becoming more common for nonlatex gloves to be used. It is important to inquire about latex allergies with any patient before beginning an exam.

Clinical Reasoning   Hot Tub Use in Pregnancy

Karen Blade, a 23-year-old, G1P0, is 10 weeks' pregnant when she sees you for her first prenatal examination. She has been experiencing some mild nausea and fatigue but otherwise is feeling well. She asks you about continuing with her routine exercises (walking 3 miles a day and lifting light weights). She also asks about using the heated pool and a hot tub. What should you tell her?
See www.nursing.pearsonhighered.com for possible responses.

Nursing interventions based on assessment of the normal physical and psychosocial changes of pregnancy, evaluation of the cultural influences associated with pregnancy, and mutually defined patient teaching and counseling needs are discussed further in Chapter 11 🔗.

Determination of Due Date

Childbearing families generally want to know the "due date," or the date around which childbirth will occur. Historically the due date has been called the *estimated date of confinement (EDC)*. However, the concept of confinement is rather negative, and many caregivers avoid it by referring to the due date as the *estimated date of delivery (EDD)*. Childbirth educators often stress that babies are not "delivered" like a package; they are born. In keeping with a view that emphasizes the normality of the process, the authors of this text refer to the due date as the **estimated date of birth (EDB)**.

To calculate the EDB, it is essential to know the first day of the last menstrual period (LMP). However, some women have episodes of irregular bleeding or fail to keep track of menstrual cycles. Thus, other techniques also help to determine how far along a woman is in her pregnancy—that is, at how many weeks' gestation she is. Techniques include evaluating uterine size, determining when quickening occurs (or occurred), using early ultrasound, and auscultating fetal heart rate with a Doppler device or ultrasound. An early ultrasound should be obtained if an accurate LMP is not available to help establish an accurate EDB.

Nägele's Rule

The most common method of determining the EDB is **Nägele's rule**, which uses 280 days as the mean length of pregnancy. To use this method, begin with the first day of the LMP, subtract 3 months, and add 7 days. For example:

First day of LMP	November 21
Subtract 3 months	− 3 months
	August 21
Add 7 days	+ 7 days
EDB	August 28

It is simpler to change the months to numeric terms:

November 21 becomes	11 − 21
Subtract 3 months	− 3
	8 − 21
Add 7 days	+ 7
EDB	8 − 28

Developing Cultural Competence
Using Cultural Information Effectively

Although it is important to avoid stereotyping, race and ethnicity may provide valuable starting information about cultural, behavioral, environmental, and medical factors that might affect a pregnant woman's health. With this general knowledge as a framework, it is essential to ask the woman about specific practices in her culture to determine their meaning for her.

● **Figure 10–2** The EDB wheel can be used to calculate the due date. To use it, place the "last menses began" arrow on the date of the woman's LMP. Then read the EDB at the arrow labeled 40. In this case the LMP is September 8, and the EDB is June 15.

A gestation calculator or wheel lets the caregiver calculate the EDB even more quickly (Figure 10–2 ●).

Nägele's rule may be a fairly accurate determiner of the EDB if the woman has a history of menses every 28 days, remembers her LMP, and was not taking oral contraceptives before becoming pregnant. However, ovulation usually occurs 14 days *before* the onset of the next menses, not 14 days after the previous menses. Consequently, if a woman's cycle is irregular, or more than 28 days long, the time of ovulation may be delayed. If a woman has been using oral contraceptives, ovulation may be delayed several weeks following her last menses. Then, too, a postpartum woman who is breastfeeding may resume ovulating but be amenorrheic for a time, making calculation based on the LMP impossible. Thus Nägele's rule, although helpful, is not foolproof and, in such cases, an ultrasound is done to visualize the gestational sac and obtain measurements of the embryo-fetus to determine EDB.

Uterine Assessment
Physical Examination

When a woman is examined in the first 10 to 12 weeks of her pregnancy and her uterine size is compatible with her menstrual history, uterine size may be the single most important clinical method for dating her pregnancy. In many cases, however, women do not seek maternity care until well into their second trimester, when it becomes much more difficult to evaluate specific uterine size. In obese women it is difficult to determine uterine size early in a pregnancy because the uterus is more difficult to palpate.

Fundal Height

Fundal height may be used as an indicator of uterine size, although this method is less accurate late in pregnancy. A tape measure is

● **Figure 10–3**   A cross-sectional view of fetal position when McDonald's method is used to assess fundal height.

● **Figure 10–4**   This practitioner is using an ultrasonic Doppler device to listen to the fetal heartbeat.

used to measure the distance in centimeters from the top of the symphysis pubis to the top of the uterine fundus (McDonald's method) (Figure 10–3 ●). Fundal height in centimeters correlates well with weeks of gestation between 22 and 34 weeks. Thus, at 26 weeks' gestation, for example, fundal height is probably about 26 cm. If the woman is very tall or very short, fundal height will differ. To be most accurate, fundal height should be measured by the same examiner each time. The woman should have voided within one half hour of the examination and should lie in the same position each time. In the third trimester, variations in fetal weight decrease the accuracy of fundal height measurements.

A lag in progression of measurements of fundal height from month to month and week to week may signal intrauterine growth restriction (IUGR). A sudden increase in fundal height may indicate twins or hydramnios (excessive amount of amniotic fluid).

Assessment of Fetal Development

Quickening

Fetal movements felt by the mother, called quickening, may indicate that the fetus is nearing 20 weeks' gestation. However, quickening may be experienced between 16 and 22 weeks' gestation, so this method is not completely accurate.

Fetal Heartbeat

The ultrasonic Doppler device (Figure 10–4 ●) is the primary tool for assessing fetal heartbeat. It can detect fetal heartbeat, on average, at 8 to 12 weeks' gestation. The normal range for fetal heart tones (FHT) is 110 to 160 beats/min. An ultrasound should be completed if the nurse is unable to auscultate between 10 and 12 weeks because there may be a discrepancy in the EDB, twins, or a missed abortion. In the case of twins or a woman with obesity, it may be later before the fetal heartbeat can be detected.

Ultrasound

In the first trimester, transabdominal ultrasound can detect a gestational sac as early as 4 to 5 weeks after the LMP, fetal heart activity by 6 to 7 weeks, and fetal breathing movements by 10 to 11 weeks of pregnancy. Crown-to-rump measurements can be made to assess fetal age from 4 days until about 12 weeks (until the fetal head can be visualized clearly). Biparietal diameter (BPD) can then be used. BPD measurements can be made by approximately 12 to 13 weeks and are most accurate between 14 and 26 weeks, when rapid growth in the biparietal diameter occurs. (See Chapter 14 🔗 for further discussion of fetal ultrasound scanning.)

ASSESSMENT OF PELVIC ADEQUACY (CLINICAL PELVIMETRY)

The pelvis can be assessed vaginally to determine whether its size is adequate for a vaginal birth. This procedure, clinical pelvimetry, is performed by physicians or by advanced practice nurses such as CNMs or nurse practitioners. For a detailed description of how clinical pelvimetry is done, refer to a nurse-midwifery text. This section provides basic information about the assessment of the inlet and outlet (see Figures 10–5 ● and 10–6 ●), which were described in detail in Chapter 3 🔗.

1. Pelvic inlet (Figure 10–5):
   - **Diagonal conjugate** (the distance from the lower posterior border of the symphysis pubis to the sacral promontory): at least 11.5 cm
   - **Obstetric conjugate** (a measurement approximately 1.5 cm smaller than the diagonal conjugate): 10 cm or more
2. Pelvic outlet (Figures 10–5 and 10–6):
   - Anteroposterior diameter: 9.5 to 11.5 cm
   - Transverse diameter (bi-ischial or intertuberous diameter): 8 to 10 cm

The pelvic cavity (midpelvis) cannot be accurately measured by clinical examination. Examiners estimate its adequacy.

A

B

● **Figure 10–5** Manual measurement of inlet and outlet. *A,* Estimation of the diagonal conjugate, which extends from the lower border of the symphysis pubis to the sacral promontory. *B,* Estimation of the anteroposterior diameter of the outlet, which extends from the lower border of the symphysis pubis to the tip of the sacrum.

Screening Tests

Many screening tests are routinely performed either at the initial prenatal visit or at a specified time during pregnancy. These tests include a Pap smear, a complete blood count, HIV screening, urine culture, rubella titer, ABO and Rh typing, and a hepatitis B screen as well as testing for sexually transmitted infections such as syphilis, chlamydia, and gonorrhea. The urine is screened for abnormal findings initially and at each prenatal visit. Hemoglobin electrophoresis should be performed in women of African, Southeast Asian, and Mediterranean descent to evaluate for sickle cell disease and thalassemias. Prenatal screening for cystic fibrosis has been a routine screening test for all pregnant women for over a decade. To avoid redundant testing, caregivers should determine whether the woman was screened for cystic fibrosis during a previous pregnancy (ACOG, 2011b). A tuberculin test (PPD) should also be completed on women who are considered to be high risk. High-risk populations include women who were not born in the United States or who have a known exposure to tuberculosis, and healthcare workers who care for patients with tuberculosis.

● **Figure 10–6** Use of a closed fist to measure the outlet. Most examiners know the distance between their first and last proximal knuckles. If they do not, they can use a measuring device.

All pregnant women, regardless of age, should be offered screening for fetal chromosome anomalies *(aneuploidy)* including Down syndrome, trisomy 18, trisomy 13, and Turner syndrome. First-trimester screening is available at many centers using ultrasound assessment of the thickness of the fetal nuchal fold (called *nuchal translucency* [NT]) combined with serum screening for free β-hCG and for pregnancy-associated plasma protein A (PAPP-A). Increased NT, elevated free β-hCG, and reduced PAPP-A suggest aneuploidy. Women with these findings are offered genetic counseling and chorionic villus sampling or second-trimester amniocentesis for diagnosis. If these tests are all negative, no further testing is indicated. Instead, during the second trimester, the woman is simply offered a test for maternal serum alpha-fetoprotein to detect the risk of neural tube defects.

The *quadruple screen* (quad screen) is a safe, useful screening test performed on the mother's serum between weeks 15 and 20 of pregnancy. The test is used to detect levels of specific serum markers—alpha-fetoprotein (AFP), human chorionic gonadotropin (hCG), unconjugated estriol (UE), and inhibin-A (a placental hormone). Test results that reveal higher than normal AFP levels might indicate an increased risk of a fetal neural tube defect, a multiple gestation, or a pregnancy that is farther along than believed. Lower than normal AFP could indicate that the woman's child is at risk for Down syndrome or trisomy 18. Higher than normal levels of hCG and inhibin-A and lower than normal UE may also indicate that a woman is at increased risk of having a baby with Down syndrome.

NT evaluation requires a skilled ultrasonographer and specialized training. In areas where NT is not available, first-trimester free β-hCG screening and PAPP-A screening may be combined with second-trimester quad screening in an integrated approach to detection of aneuploidy.

It is important for healthcare professionals to provide parents with factual information about the results of tests that detect chromosomal defects or fetal anomalies including the false-positive and detection rates and the implications of the findings. Parents then need to decide on any course of action based on their own spiritual and cultural beliefs.

Recommendations about screening for gestational diabetes mellitus (GDM) are in flux. ACOG (2011a) continues to recommend that pregnant women have a 50-g 1-hour glucose screen between 24 and 28 weeks' gestation. However, the American Diabetes Association (2011) now recommends that pregnant women at average risk should be screened at 24 to 28 weeks' gestation using a 75-g 2-hour oral glucose tolerance test (OGTT). A consensus conference is currently working to determine the best approach to screening (ACOG, 2011a). Additional testing is indicated if abnormal results are obtained. (For a discussion of GDM, see Chapter 15 🅔.) A hemoglobin or hematocrit is also completed at this time to evaluate for iron-deficiency anemia.

Group B streptococcus (GBS) can cause serious problems for a newborn. Consequently rectal and vaginal swabs of the mother are taken at 35 to 37 weeks' gestation to screen for the infection. Women with GBS in the urine at any time during the pregnancy are considered to be positive and do not need a culture completed. This infection is discussed in more detail in Chapter 16 🅔.

SUBSEQUENT PATIENT HISTORY

At subsequent prenatal visits the nurse continues to gather data about the course of the pregnancy to date and the woman's responses to it. The nurse also asks about:

- Adjustment of the support person and of other children, if any, in the family
- Preparations the family has made for the new baby
- Discomfort, especially the kinds of discomfort that are often seen at specific times during a pregnancy.
- Physical changes that relate directly to the pregnancy, such as fetal movement
- Exposure to contagious illnesses
- Medical treatments and therapies prescribed for nonpregnancy problems since the last visit
- Consumption of prescription or over-the-counter medications or herbal supplements that were not prescribed as part of the woman's prenatal care
- Danger signs of pregnancy (Table 10–2). (*Note:* Many of the danger signs indicate conditions that are potential complications.)

Periodic prenatal examinations offer a chance to assess the childbearing woman's psychologic needs and emotional status.

Table 10–2	Danger Signs in Pregnancy
Danger Sign	**Possible Cause**
Sudden gush of fluid from vagina	Premature rupture of membranes
Vaginal bleeding	Abruptio placentae, placenta previa
	Lesions of cervix or vagina
	"Bloody show"
Abdominal pain	Premature labor, abruptio placentae
Temperature above 38.3°C (101°F) and chills	Infection
Dizziness, blurring of vision, double vision, spots before eyes	Hypertension, preeclampsia
Persistent vomiting	Hyperemesis gravidarum
Severe headache	Hypertension, preeclampsia
Edema of hands, face, legs, and feet	Preeclampsia
Muscular irritability, convulsions	Preeclampsia, eclampsia
Epigastric pain	Preeclampsia, ischemia in major abdominal vessel
Oliguria	Renal impairment, decreased fluid intake
Dysuria	Urinary tract infection
Absence of fetal movement	Maternal medication, obesity, fetal death

The woman should report the following danger signs in pregnancy immediately:

If the woman's partner attends the antepartum visits, they can also be a time to identify the partner's needs and concerns. The woman should have sufficient time to ask questions and air concerns. If a nurse provides the time and demonstrates genuine interest, the woman will be more at ease bringing up questions that she may believe are silly or has been afraid to verbalize.

Be sensitive to religious or spiritual, cultural, and socioeconomic factors that may influence a family's response to pregnancy, as well as to the woman's expectations of the healthcare system. One way to avoid stereotyping patients is simply to ask each woman about her expectations for the antepartum period. Although many women's responses may reflect what are thought to be traditional norms, other women will have decidedly different views or expectations that represent a blending of beliefs or cultures. During the antepartum period, it is also essential to begin assessing the readiness of the woman and her partner (if possible) to assume their responsibilities as parents successfully.

SUBSEQUENT PRENATAL ASSESSMENT

The *Assessment Guide: Subsequent Prenatal Assessment* provides a systematic approach to the regular physical examinations the pregnant woman should undergo for optimal antepartum care and also provides a model for evaluating both the pregnant woman and the expectant father, if he is involved in the pregnancy.

The recommended frequency of antepartum visits in an uncomplicated pregnancy is as follows:

- Every 4 weeks for the first 28 weeks' gestation
- Every 2 weeks until 36 weeks' gestation
- After week 36, every week until childbirth

During the subsequent antepartum assessments, most women demonstrate ongoing psychologic adjustment to pregnancy. However, some women may exhibit signs of possible psychologic problems such as the following:

- Increasing anxiety
- Inability to establish communication
- Inappropriate responses or actions
- Denial of pregnancy
- Inability to cope with stress
- Intense preoccupation with the gender of the baby
- Failure to acknowledge quickening
- Failure to plan and prepare for the baby (e.g., living arrangements, clothing, and feeding methods)
- Indications of substance abuse

If the woman's behavior indicates possible psychologic problems, the nurse can provide ongoing support and counseling and also refer the woman to appropriate professionals.

Clinical Tip

When assessing blood pressure, have the pregnant woman sit up with her arm resting on a table so that her arm is at the level of her heart. Expect a decrease in her blood pressure from baseline during the second trimester because of normal physiologic changes.

Assessment Guide Subsequent Prenatal Assessment

Physical Assessment/Normal Findings	Alterations and Possible Causes*	Nursing Responses to Data†
Vital Signs		
Temperature: 36.2°C–37.6°C (97°F–99.6°F)	Elevated temperature (infection)	Evaluate for signs of infection. Refer to healthcare provider.
Pulse: 60–100 beats/min	Increased pulse rate (anxiety, cardiac disorders)	Note irregularities. Assess for anxiety and stress.
Rate may increase 10 beats/min during pregnancy.		
Respiration: 12–20 breaths/min	Marked tachypnea or abnormal patterns (respiratory disease)	Refer to healthcare provider.
Blood pressure: Less than or equal to 120/80 (falls in second trimester)	BP of 120–139/80–89 is considered prehypertensive. Greater than 140/90 or increase of 30 mm systolic and 15 mm diastolic (preeclampsia)	Assess for edema, proteinuria, and hyperreflexia. Refer to healthcare provider.
		Schedule appointments more frequently.
Weight Gain		
Prepregnant weight based on body mass index (BMI):		
Normal BMI: Total recommended weight gain 11.5–16 kg (25–35 lb)		
First trimester: 1.6–2.3 kg (3.5–5 lb)	Inadequate weight gain (poor nutrition, nausea, IUGR)	Discuss appropriate weight gain.
Second trimester: 5.5–6.8 kg (12–15 lb)	Excessive weight gain (excessive caloric intake, edema, preeclampsia)	Provide nutritional counseling. Assess for presence of edema or anemia. Refer to a dietitian as needed.
Third trimester: 5.5–6.8 kg (12–15 lb)		

Assessment Guide Subsequent Prenatal Assessment—continued

Physical Assessment/Normal Findings	Alterations and Possible Causes*	Nursing Responses to Data†
Edema Small amount of dependent edema, especially in last weeks of pregnancy	Edema in hands, face, legs, and feet (preeclampsia)	Identify any correlation between edema and activities, blood pressure, or proteinuria: Refer to healthcare provider if indicated.
Uterine Size See *Assessment Guide: Initial Prenatal Assessment* on page 203 for normal changes during pregnancy	Unusually rapid growth (multiple gestation, hydatidiform mole, hydramnios, miscalculation of EDB)	Evaluate fetal status. Determine height of fundus (page 208). Use diagnostic ultrasound.
Fetal Heartbeat 110–160 beats/min Funic souffle	Absence of fetal heartbeat after 20 weeks' gestation (maternal obesity, fetal demise)	Evaluate fetal status.
Laboratory Evaluation *Hemoglobin:* 12–16 g/dL Pseudoanemia of pregnancy	Less than 11 g/dL (anemia)	Provide nutritional counseling. Hemoglobin is repeated at 7 months' gestation. Women of Mediterranean heritage need a close check on hemoglobin because of possibility of thalassemia.
Quad marker screen: Blood test performed at 15–20 weeks' gestation. Evaluates four factors: maternal serum alpha-fetoprotein (MSAFP), unconjugated estriol (UE), hCG, and inhibin-A: normal levels	Elevated MSAFP (neural tube defect, underestimated gestational age, multiple gestation); lower than normal MSAFP (Down syndrome, trisomy 18); higher than normal hCG and inhibin-A (Down syndrome); lower than normal UE (Down syndrome)	Offered to all pregnant women. If quad screen is abnormal, further testing such as ultrasound or amniocentesis may be indicated.
Indirect Coombs' test done on Rh negative women: Negative (done at 28 weeks' gestation)	Rh antibodies present (maternal sensitization has occurred)	If Rh negative and unsensitized, Rh immune globulin given (see discussion in Chapter 16 🔗). If Rh antibodies present, Rh immune globulin not given; fetus monitored closely for isoimmune hemolytic disease.
50-g 1-hour glucose screen (done between 24 and 28 weeks' gestation)	Plasma glucose level greater than 140 mg/dL (gestational diabetes mellitus [GDM])	
Urinalysis: See *Assessment Guide: Initial Prenatal Assessment* on page 206 for normal findings	See *Assessment Guide: Initial Prenatal Assessment* on page 206 for deviations	Urinalysis and culture is completed at initial visit and at subsequent visits as indicated. Repeat dipstick test at each visit.
Protein: Negative	Proteinuria, albuminuria (contamination by vaginal discharge, urinary tract infection, preeclampsia)	Obtain dipstick urine sample. Refer to healthcare provider if deviations are present.
Glucose: Negative *Note:* Glycosuria may be present due to physiologic alterations in glomerular filtration rate and renal threshold	Persistent glycosuria (diabetes mellitus)	Refer to healthcare provider.
Screening for Group B streptococcus (GBS): Rectal and vaginal swabs obtained at 35–37 weeks' gestation for all pregnant women.	Positive culture (maternal infection)	Explain maternal and fetal/neonatal risks (see Chapter 16 🔗). Refer to healthcare provider for therapy.

(continued)

Assessment Guide Subsequent Prenatal Assessment—continued

Cultural Assessment	Variations to Consider*	Nursing Responses to Data†
Determine the mother's (and family's) attitudes about the gender of the unborn child.	Some women have no preference about the gender of the child; others do. In many cultures, boys are especially valued as firstborn children.	Provide opportunities to discuss preferences and expectations; avoid a judgmental attitude to the response.
Ask about the woman's expectations of childbirth. Will she want someone with her for the birth? Whom does she choose? What is the role of her partner?	Some women want their partner present for labor and birth; others prefer a female relative or friend. Some women expect to be separated from their partner once labor begins.	Provide information on birth options but accept the woman's decision about who will attend.
Ask about preparations for the baby. Determine what is customary for the woman.	Some women may have a fully prepared nursery; others may not have a separate room for the baby.	Explore reasons for not preparing for the baby. Support the mother's preferences and provide information about possible sources of assistance if the decision is related to a lack of resources.

Expectant Mother

Psychologic status	Increased stress and anxiety	Encourage woman to take an active part in her care.
First trimester: Period of adjustment. Incorporates idea of pregnancy; may feel ambivalent or anxious, especially if she must give up desired role; usually looks for signs of verification of pregnancy, such as increase in abdominal size or fetal movement.	Inability to establish communication; inability to accept pregnancy; inappropriate response or actions; denial of pregnancy; inability to cope	Establish lines of communication. Discuss and provide anticipatory guidance regarding normalcy of feelings and actions. Establish a trusting relationship. Counsel as necessary. Refer to appropriate professional as needed.
Second trimester: Period of radiant health. Baby becomes more real to woman as abdominal size increases and she feels movement; she begins to turn inward, becoming more introspective.		
Third trimester: Period of watchful waiting. Begins to think of baby as separate being; may feel restless, uneasy, and may feel that time of labor will never come; remains self-centered and concentrates on preparing place for baby. Fears for her well-being and that of her baby.		
Educational needs:	Inadequate information	Provide information and counseling.

Self-care measures and knowledge about the following:
  Health promotion
  Breast care
  Hygiene
  Rest
  Exercise
  Nutrition
  Relief measures for common discomforts of pregnancy
  Danger signs in pregnancy (see Table 10–2)		

Sexual activity: Woman knows how pregnancy affects sexual activity	Lack of information about effects of pregnancy and/or alternative positions during sexual intercourse	Provide counseling.
Preparation for parenting: Appropriate preparation	Lack of preparation (denial, failure to adjust to baby, unwanted child)	Counsel. If lack of preparation is due to inadequacy of information, provide information.

Assessment Guide   Subsequent Prenatal Assessment—continued

Cultural Assessment	Variations to Consider*	Nursing Responses to Data†
Preparation for childbirth: Patient aware of the following: 1. Prepared childbirth techniques		If couple chooses particular technique, refer to classes (see Chapter 8 🔗 for description of childbirth preparation techniques).
2. Normal processes and changes during childbirth		Encourage prenatal class attendance. Educate woman during visits based on current physical status. Provide reading list for more specific information.
3. Problems that may occur as a result of drug and alcohol use and of smoking	Continued abuse of drugs and alcohol; denial of possible effect on self and baby	Review danger signs that were presented on initial visit.
Woman has met other physician or nurse-midwife who may be attending her birth in the absence of primary caregiver	Introduction of new individual at birth may increase stress and anxiety for woman and partner	Introduce woman to all members of group practice.
Impending labor: Patient knows signs of impending labor: 1. Uterine contractions that increase in frequency, duration, and intensity 2. Bloody show 3. Expulsion of mucous plug 4. Rupture of membranes	Lack of information	Provide appropriate teaching, stressing importance of seeking appropriate medical assistance.
Expectant Father/Partner *Psychologic status*		
First trimester: May express excitement over confirmation of pregnancy and of his virility; concerns move toward providing for financial needs; energetic; may identify with some discomforts of pregnancy and may even exhibit symptoms (couvade)	Increasing stress and anxiety; inability to establish communication; inability to accept pregnancy diagnosis; withdrawal of support; abandonment of the mother	Encourage partner to come to prenatal visits. Establish line of communication. Establish trusting relationship.
Second trimester: May feel more confident and be less concerned with financial matters; may have concerns about wife's changing size and shape and her increasing introspection		Counsel. Let expectant partner know that it is normal for him to experience these feelings.
Third trimester: May have feelings of rivalry with fetus, especially during sexual activity; may make changes in his physical appearance and exhibit more interest in himself; may become more energetic; fantasizes about child but usually imagines older child; fears mutilation and death of woman and child		Include expectant partner in pregnancy activities as he desires. Provide education, information, and support. Increasing numbers of expectant partners are demonstrating desire to be involved in many or all aspects of prenatal care, education, and preparation.

*Possible causes of alterations are identified in parentheses.
†This column provides guidelines for further assessment and initial intervention.

Critical Concept Review

LEARNING OUTCOME 10.1: Use information provided on a prenatal history to identify risk factors for the mother and/or fetus.

1. To identify all of the risk factors included in Table 10–1, all aspects of a women's history should be reviewed. A detailed prenatal history includes the following:
   - Details of current pregnancy (such as LMP).
   - History of past pregnancies.
   - Gynecologic history (such as last Pap and contraceptive use).
   - Current medical history (such as weight, prescription medications, chronic diseases).
   - Past medical history (past surgeries).
   - Family medical history (cancer or diabetes).
   - Religious, spiritual, and cultural history.
   - Occupational history (physical demands of present job).
   - Partner's history (genetic conditions, blood type).
   - Demographic information about woman (age, educational level, and ethnic background).

LEARNING OUTCOME 10.2: Define common obstetric terminology found in the history of maternity patients.

1. Terms about the number of pregnancies and births: gravida, parity, and TPAL.
2. Terms that denote the phase of pregnancy: ante-, intra-, and postpartum.
3. Terms that denote age and developmental status of fetus at birth: prematurity, postmaturity, and term.

LEARNING OUTCOME 10.3: Identify risk factors related to the father's health that are generally recorded on the prenatal record when assessing risk factors for the mother and/or fetus.

1. Father's health details to be recorded:
   - History of chronic illness in father or immediate family member.
   - Blood type and Rh factor.
   - Present use of alcohol, tobacco, or recreational drugs.
   - Occupation.
   - Age.

LEARNING OUTCOME 10.4: Evaluate those areas of the initial assessment that reflect the psychosocial and cultural factors related to a woman's pregnancy.

1. Determine language preference.
2. Determine how woman should be addressed.
3. Determine food customs and preferences.
4. Determine significant people to woman, and degree of involvement of these persons.
5. Psychologic status.
6. Educational needs.
7. Support system.
8. Family functioning.
9. Economic status.
10. Stability of living conditions.

LEARNING OUTCOME 10.5: Predict the normal physiologic changes a nurse would expect to find when performing a physical assessment of a pregnant woman.

1. Vital signs:
   - Pulse may increase by 10 beats/min.
   - Respiration may be increased, and thoracic breathing predominant.
   - Temperature and blood pressure within normal limits.
2. Weight:
   - Varies, but should be proportional to the gestational age of the fetus.
3. Skin:
   - Linea nigra.
   - Striae gravidarum.
   - Melasma.
   - Spider nevi.
4. Nose:
   - Nasal stuffiness.
5. Mouth:
   - Gingival hypertrophy.
6. Neck:
   - Small, nontender nodes.
   - Slight hyperplasia of thyroid in third trimester.
7. Chest and lungs:
   - Transverse diameter greater than anteroposterior diameter.
8. Breasts:
   - Increasing size.
   - Pigmentation of nipples and areolae.
   - Tubercles of Montgomery enlarge.
   - Colostrum appears in third trimester.
9. Abdomen:
   - Progressive enlargement by Doppler.
   - Fetal heart rate heard by Doppler at approximately 12 weeks' gestation.
10. Extremities:
    - Possible edema late in pregnancy.
11. Spine:
    - Lumbar spinal curve may be accentuated.
12. Pelvic area:
    - Vagina without significant discharge.
    - Cervix closed.
    - Uterus shows progressive growth.
13. Laboratory tests:
    - Physiologic anemia may occur (hematocrit).
    - Small degree of glycosuria may occur.

LEARNING OUTCOME 10.6: Calculate the estimated date of birth using the common methods.

1. Nägele's rule:
   - Date of LMP minus 3 months plus 7 days.
   - Accurate only if woman has 28-day cycles.
2. Physical examination:
   - Uterine size.
3. Fundal height:
   - Measurement should be made from the top of the symphysis pubis to the top of the uterine fundus.
4. Ultrasound:
   - BPD.

LEARNING OUTCOME 10.7: Describe the essential measurements that can be determined by clinical pelvimetry.

1. These measurements are estimates to determine probable adequacy of the pelvis to allow a vaginal birth:
   - Pelvic inlet:
     - Diagonal conjugate: at least 11.5 cm.
     - Obstetric conjugate: 10 cm or more.
   - Pelvic outlet:
     - Anteroposterior diameter: 9.5 to 11.5 cm.
     - Transverse diameter: 8 to 10 cm.

LEARNING OUTCOME 10.8: Summarize the results of the major screening tests used during the prenatal period in the assessment of the prenatal patient.

1. Screening tests are useful in identifying risk factors and potential complications.
   - Basic screening tests such as Pap smear, u/a, complete blood count, hemoglobin, Rubella titer, ABO and Rh typing, a hepatitis B screen, and tests for syphilis and gonorrhea.
   - Urine culture at 12–16 weeks.

   - Other tests that may be indicated or are offered include drug screen, HIV testing, sickle cell screen, cystic fibrosis screen, screening for chromosomal anomalies, and neural tube defects.
   - 50-g 1-hr GTT at 24–28 weeks.
   - Rectal and vaginal swabs for Group B strep at 35 to 37 weeks.

LEARNING OUTCOME 10.9: Assess the prenatal patient for any of the danger signs of pregnancy.

1. The danger signs of pregnancy indicate that potential complications may be developing.
   - Ask patient about the occurrence of any signs.

   - Assess for danger signs at each visit.

LEARNING OUTCOME 10.10: Relate the components of the subsequent prenatal history and assessment to the progress of pregnancy and the nursing care of the prenatal patient.

1. At each visit the woman will be assessed for:
   - Vital signs.
   - Weight gain.
   - Edema.
   - Uterine size.

   - Fetal heartbeat.
   - Urinalysis.
   - Blood tests for alpha-fetoprotein, glucose.
   - Vaginal swab for Group B streptococcus.
   - Expected psychologic stage of pregnancy.

Clinical Reasoning in Action

Wendy Stodard, age 40, G3, P0020, comes to the obstetrician's office where you are working for a prenatal visit. Wendy has experienced two spontaneous abortions followed by a D&C at 14 and 15 weeks' gestation during the previous year. She has a history of *Chlamydia trachomatis* infection 3 years ago, which was treated with azithromycin. She is at 10 weeks' gestation. Wendy tells you that she is afraid of losing this pregnancy as she did previously. She says that she has been experiencing some mild nausea, breast tenderness, and fatigue, which did not occur with her other pregnancies. You assist the obstetrician with an ultrasound. The gestational sac is clearly seen, fetal heartbeat is observed, and crown-to-rump measurements are consistent with gestational age of 10 weeks. The pelvic exam demonstrates a closed cervix, and positive Goodell's, Hegar's, and Chadwick's signs. You discuss with Wendy the signs of a healthy pregnancy.

1. What signs are reassuring with this pregnancy?
2. What symptoms should be reported to the obstetrician immediately?
3. What is the frequency of antepartum visits?
4. Develop a concept map for a woman who has a blood pressure of 130/86 at her first prenatal visit.

See www.nursing.pearsonhighered.com for possible responses and an interactive template for a concept map.

References

American College of Obstetricians and Gynecologists (ACOG). (2010). *Anemia in pregnancy* (ACOG Practice Bulletin No. 95, issued July 2008, reaffirmed 2010). Washington, DC: Author.

American College of Obstetricians and Gynecologists (ACOG). (2011a). *Screening and diagnosis of gestational diabetes mellitus* (ACOG Committee Opinion No. 504). Washington, DC: Author.

American College of Obstetricians and Gynecologists (ACOG). (2011b). *Update on carrier screening for cystic fibrosis* (ACOG Committee Opinion No. 486). Washington, DC: Author.

American Diabetes Association. (2011). Position statement: Standards of medical care in diabetes—2011. *Diabetes Care, 34*(Suppl. 1), S11–S61.

Cunningham, F. G., Leveno, K. J., Bloom, S. L., Hauth, J. C., Rouse, D. J., & Spong, C. Y. (2010). *Williams obstetrics* (23rd ed.). New York, NY: McGraw-Hill.

Spong, C. Y. (2013). Defining "term" pregnancy: Recommendations from the defining "term" pregnancy workgroup. Published online May 3, 2013. doi:10.1001/jama.2013.6235.

CHAPTER
11

The Expectant Family: Needs and Care

Ken Huang/Getty Images

We have what I guess you would call a blended family. I have two college-age sons from my first marriage, and my wife has a 12-year-old boy. She is expecting our first child now. Because she is 38, she had an amniocentesis done and we know that this baby is a girl. How excited we all are! I don't think anything could have done more to unite us as a new family. Now if we can just agree on a name. —Ricardo, 46

LEARNING OUTCOMES

11.1 Describe the most appropriate nursing care to help maintain the well-being of the expectant father and siblings during a family's pregnancy.

11.2 Explain the causes of the common discomforts of pregnancy in each of the three trimesters.

11.3 Summarize appropriate relief measures and interventions to alleviate the common discomforts of pregnancy.

11.4 Describe self-care measures that a pregnant woman can take to maintain and promote her well-being during pregnancy.

11.5 Examine the concerns that an expectant couple might have about sexual activity.

11.6 Discuss the medical risks and special concerns of expectant women older than age 35.

From the moment a woman finds out she is pregnant, she faces a future marked by dramatic changes—changes in her appearance, in her relationships, and in her psychologic state. In coping with these changes, she and her loved ones need to make adjustments in their daily lives.

Nurses caring for pregnant women need an up-to-date understanding of pregnancy to be effective in implementing the nursing process as they plan and provide care. With this in mind, Chapter 9 🕑 provided a database for the nurse by presenting material related to the normal physical, social, cultural, and psychologic changes of pregnancy. Chapter 10 🕑 then used that database to begin discussing nursing care management by focusing on assessment. This chapter further addresses nursing care management as it relates to the needs of the expectant woman and her loved ones.

NURSING CARE DURING THE PRENATAL PERIOD

Nursing Diagnosis During Pregnancy

The nurse may see a pregnant woman only once every 3 to 4 weeks during the first several months of her pregnancy. Therefore, a written care plan or clinical path that incorporates the database, nursing diagnoses, and patient goals is essential to ensure continuity of care.

The nurse can anticipate that, for many women with a low-risk pregnancy, certain nursing diagnoses will be made more frequently than others. The diagnoses will, of course, vary from woman to woman and according to the time in the pregnancy. After formulating an appropriate diagnosis, the nurse and woman establish related goals to guide the nursing plan and interventions.

Planning and Implementation During Pregnancy

Once nursing diagnoses have been identified, the next step is to establish priorities of nursing care. Sometimes priorities of care are based on the most immediate needs or concerns expressed by the woman. For example, during the first trimester, when she is experiencing nausea or is concerned about sexual intimacy with her partner, the woman is not likely to want to hear about labor and birth. At other times, priorities may develop from findings during a prenatal examination. For example, a woman who is showing signs of preeclampsia (a pregnancy complication discussed in Chapter 16 🕑) may feel physically well and find it hard to accept the nurse's emphasis on the need for frequent rest periods. It then becomes the responsibility of medical and nursing professionals to help the woman and her family to understand the significance of a problem and to plan interventions to deal with it.

Health Promotion   Anticipatory Guidance for the Postpartum Period

Throughout the prenatal period, the nurse shares information with the family, both verbally and through written materials. Anticipatory guidance helps the expectant couple identify and discuss issues that could be sources of postpartum stress. Issues to be addressed beforehand may include the sharing of infant and household chores, help in the first few days after childbirth, options for babysitting to allow the mother (and couple) some free time, the mother's return to work after the baby's birth, and sibling rivalry. Couples resolve these issues in different ways, but postpartum adjustment tends to be easier for couples who agree on the issues beforehand than for couples who do not confront and resolve these issues.

Nursing Care in the Community

Prenatal care, especially for women with low-risk pregnancies, is community based, typically in a clinic or a private office. The nurse in a clinic or health maintenance organization may be the only source of continuity for the woman, who may see a different physician or certified nurse-midwife at each visit. The nurse can be extremely effective in working with the expectant family by answering questions; providing complete information about pregnancy, prenatal healthcare activities, and community resources; and supporting the healthcare activities of the woman and her family. Communities often have a wealth of services and educational opportunities available for pregnant women and their families, and the knowledgeable nurse can help expectant mothers to assess and access these services.

Home Care. Home care can be of benefit to any pregnant woman, but it is especially effective in removing barriers for women who have difficulty accessing health care. These barriers may include lack of locally available healthcare facilities, problems with transportation to the facility, or schedule conflicts with available appointment times because of employment hours or family responsibilities.

In-home nursing assessments vary according to the experience and preparation of the nurse and include current history, vital signs, weight, urine screen, physical activity, dietary intake, reflexes, tests of fetal well-being, and cervical examinations, if indicated. Once the assessments are completed, the nurse can determine the level of follow-up home care or telephone contact needed. See Chapter 30 🔗 for further discussion of home care of the childbearing family.

Currently, home care is not routinely used because of the cost, but when home care is available, it is most often used for women with prenatal complications that can be managed without hospitalization if effective nursing assessment and care are provided in the home.

CARE OF THE PREGNANT WOMAN'S FAMILY

The well-being of the pregnant woman is intertwined with the well-being of those to whom she is closest. Thus, the nurse also addresses the needs of the woman's family. Although the expectant father is often involved in the pregnancy, his presence cannot be assumed. If he is not part of the family structure, it is important to assess the woman's support system to determine which significant people in her life will play a major role during this childbearing experience.

Anticipatory guidance of the expectant father, if he is involved in the pregnancy, is a necessary part of any plan of care. He may need information about the anatomic, physiologic, and emotional changes that occur for the expectant mother and father during and after pregnancy; the couple's sexuality and sexual response; and the reactions that he is experiencing. He may wish to express his feelings about the sex of the child, his ability to parent, and other topics.

If it is culturally acceptable to the couple and personally acceptable to the expectant father, refer the couple to expectant parents' classes. These classes provide valuable information about pregnancy and childbirth, using a variety of teaching strategies such as discussion, films, demonstrations with educational

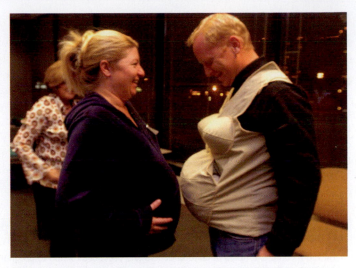

● **Figure 11–1** The Empathy Belly® is a pregnancy simulator that allows men and women to experience some of the symptoms of pregnancy. The "belly," which weighs 33 lb, produces symptoms such as shortness of breath, bladder pressure, shift in the center of gravity with resulting waddling gait, increased lordosis and backache, and fatigue. It also can simulate fetal kicking movements.

Source: ZUMA Press, Inc./Alamy

models, and written handouts. Some classes even give the father the opportunity to get a "feel" for pregnancy by wearing a pregnancy simulator (Figure 11–1 ●). Such classes also offer the couple an opportunity to gain support from other couples.

The nurse assesses the father's intended degree of participation during labor and birth and his knowledge of what to expect. If the couple prefers that his participation be minimal or restricted, support their decision. With this type of consideration and collaboration, the father is less apt to develop feelings of alienation, helplessness, and guilt during the pregnancy. As a result, he is better able to provide physical and emotional support to his partner during labor and birth.

In the plan for prenatal care, the nurse also incorporates a discussion about the negative feelings older children may develop. Parents may be distressed to see an older child regress to "babyish" behavior or become aggressive toward the newborn. Parents who are unprepared for an older child's feelings of anger, jealousy, and rejection may respond inappropriately in their confusion and surprise. The nurse emphasizes that open communication between parents and children (or acting out feelings with a doll if the child is too young to verbalize) helps children master their feelings. Children may feel less neglected and more secure if they know that their parents are willing to help with their anger and aggressiveness.

The nurse also addresses the couple's expectations of the grandparents and encourages the couple to explore ways of dealing with any conflicts that may arise over childrearing approaches. Couples resolve these issues in different ways. However, postpartum adjustment is easiest for couples who acknowledge potential problems and develop strategies to address them beforehand.

CULTURAL CONSIDERATIONS IN PREGNANCY

As discussed in Chapter 2 🖉, actions taken during pregnancy are often determined by cultural beliefs. Table 11–1 presents activities encouraged or forbidden by some specific cultures. The table is not meant to be all-inclusive, nor is it meant to imply that all members of a given culture hold these beliefs. Rather, it offers a few examples of cultural activities that may be important to some women during the prenatal period.

In working with patients of other cultures, health professionals should be open to and respectful of others' beliefs.

Effective nurses recognize that each childbearing family, shaped by culture and life experience, has expectations of both its members and the healthcare system during pregnancy and birth.

Language barriers often pose a challenge in providing effective prenatal nursing care. When possible, it is important to have an interpreter—family member, friend, or staff person—present at prenatal visits so that the nurse can provide basic information about pregnancy and prenatal care. It is essential to have printed material available in the woman's language. (See *Nursing Care Plan: Language Barriers at First Prenatal Visit.*)

Table 11–1	Cultural Beliefs and Practices During Pregnancy

Here are some examples of cultural beliefs and practices related to pregnancy. It is important not to make assumptions about a patient's beliefs, because cultural norms vary greatly within a culture and from generation to generation. The nurse should observe the patient carefully and take the time to ask questions. Patients will benefit greatly from the nurse's increased awareness of their cultural beliefs and practices.

Belief or Practice	Nursing Consideration
Home Remedies	
Pregnant women of Native American background may use herbal remedies. An example is the dandelion, which contains a milky juice in its stem believed to increase breast milk flow in mothers who choose to breastfeed (Spector, 2009). Patients of Chinese descent may drink ginseng tea for faintness after childbirth or as a sedative when mixed with bamboo leaves. Some people of African heritage may use self-medication for pregnancy discomforts—for example, laxatives to prevent or treat constipation (Spector, 2009).	Find out what medications and home remedies your patient is using and counsel your patient regarding overall effects. It is common for individuals to avoid telling healthcare workers about home remedies because the patient may feel their use will be judged unfavorably. Phrase your questions in a sensitive, accepting way.
Nutrition	
Some women of Italian background may believe that it is necessary to satisfy desires for certain foods in order to prevent congenital anomalies. Also, they may believe that they must eat food that they smell, or else the fetus will move "inside," which will result in a miscarriage. Pregnant women of Vietnamese descent are considered to be in a weak, cold state and must correct this by eating and drinking hot foods during the first trimester (Purnell, 2009).	Discuss the woman's beliefs and practices in regard to nutrition during pregnancy. Obtain a diet history from her. Discuss the importance of a well-balanced diet during pregnancy, with consideration of the patient's cultural beliefs and practices.
Alternative Healthcare Providers	
Pregnant women of Mexican background may choose to seek out the care of a *partera* (midwife) for prenatal and intrapartum care. A *partera* speaks their language, shares a similar culture, and can help pregnant women give birth at home or in a birthing center instead of a hospital. Some people in Hispanic American communities may use the *curandero*, the folk healer. *Curanderos* are believed to have been given their healing gifts by God and may prescribe over-the-counter medications (Purnell, 2009).	Discuss the variety of choices of healthcare providers available to the pregnant woman. Contrast the benefits and risks of different settings for prenatal care and birth. Provide reassurance that the goal of health care during pregnancy and birth is a healthy outcome for mother and baby, with respect for the specific cultural beliefs and practices of the patient.
Exercise	
Pregnant women of Korean descent may work hard toward the end of pregnancy to increase the chances of giving birth to a small baby (Purnell, 2009). Some people of European, African, and Mexican descent believe that reaching over the head during pregnancy can harm the baby.	Ask your patient whether there are any activities she is afraid to do because of the pregnancy. Assure her that reaching over her head will not harm the baby and evaluate other activities in terms of their effect on the pregnancy.
Spirituality	
Navajo Indians are aware of the mind–soul connection and may try to follow certain practices to have a healthy pregnancy and birth. Practices could include focusing on peaceful and positive thoughts as well as certain types of prayers and ceremonies. A traditional healer may assist them (Purnell, 2009). Some people of European background may tend to pay more attention to spirituality in their life to alleviate fears and ensure a safe birth.	Encourage the use of support systems and spiritual aids that provide comfort for the mother.

Nursing Care Plan   Language Barriers at First Prenatal Visit

Intervention	Rationale	Expected Outcome

Nursing Diagnosis: *Health Maintenance, Ineffective,* related to alterations in verbal and written communication skills (NANDA-I © 2012)

Intervention	Rationale	Expected Outcome
NIC Priority Intervention: *Effective communication:* Developing and providing prenatal instruction for a non–English-speaking patient.		**NOC Suggested Outcome:** Effective communication occurs. The patient will gain an understanding of basic prenatal information as evidenced by using hand gestures, by pointing to pictures on posters and translated phrases on handouts, and through an interpreter, if one is available.

Goal: Patient will demonstrate understanding of health information received during prenatal visits.

- If no interpreter is available, refer to posters with pictures to explain routine care and procedures during the prenatal examination.

  - Posters put words into verbal images and are helpful in communicating information.

- Provide handouts and brochures about prenatal care in the woman's native language.

  - Translated handouts provide information that the patient can refer to at home. This reinforces information discussed during the visit and helps the family understand what the woman will experience during the pregnancy and at each visit.

- Use teaching models to demonstrate procedures. Teaching models may include plastic pelvis, knitted uterus, fetal model, breast model, birth control devices, ultrasound equipment, and so forth.

  - Visual aids help to communicate information during the examination.

- Schedule an interpreter for subsequent prenatal visits.

  - If a family member cannot translate the health information to the patient, an independent translator is essential to ensure that information is accurately provided. When an interpreter is used (especially a family member), the nurse should be sure that the interpreter is translating information received from the woman and not simply answering the questions for her.

- Refer the woman to prenatal classes taught in her own language, if available.

  - Prenatal classes taught in the woman's language enable her to receive health information that is easily understood, which will provide a better understanding of what she should expect during pregnancy, birth, and postpartum. Prenatal classes may also provide a social outlet for patients.

- Involve other members of the healthcare team in planning and providing care.

  - Cultures vary in language, nonverbal expression, dietary habits, use of time, spatial expectations, and so forth. Use of medication and blood products may also be influenced by cultural beliefs. Social workers who are familiar with the patient's cultural beliefs, for example, may help the patient adjust to different healthcare practices while providing suggestions to ensure prenatal care that is more in line with the woman's cultural beliefs. Dietitians may help the woman plan meals that are aligned with her cultural practices while meeting the nutritional needs of pregnancy.

COMMON DISCOMFORTS OF PREGNANCY

The common discomforts of pregnancy result from physiologic and anatomic changes and are fairly specific to each of the three trimesters. Table 11–2 identifies the common discomforts of pregnancy, their possible causes, and self-care measures that often help relieve the discomfort.

First Trimester

Nausea and Vomiting

Nausea and vomiting of pregnancy (NVP) are early, common symptoms occurring in three fourths of pregnant women (Gregory, Niebyl, & Johnson, 2012). These symptoms appear sometime after the first missed menstrual period and usually cease by the fourth missed menstrual period. Some women develop an aversion to specific foods, many experience nausea when they get up in the morning, and others experience nausea throughout the day or in the evening.

The exact cause of NVP is unknown, but it is thought to be multifactorial. An elevated human chorionic gonadotropin (hCG) level is believed to be a major factor, but relaxation of the smooth muscle of the stomach, changes in carbohydrate metabolism, fatigue, and emotional factors may also play a role.

In addition to common self-care measures (see *Complementary Care: Ginger for Morning Sickness*) and the use of acupressure wristbands (Figure 11–2 ●), some women find pyridoxine (vitamin B_6) or pyridoxine plus doxylamine (Unisom), an over-the-counter antihistamine, helpful in reducing symptoms. Antihistamine H_1-receptor blockers, benzamines, and phenothiazines are considered safe and effective for treating refractory cases.

Clinical Tip

At each prenatal visit, focus your teaching on changes or possible discomforts the woman might encounter during the coming month and the next trimester. If the pregnancy is progressing normally, spend a few minutes describing her baby at this stage of development.

Table 11–2	Self-Care Measures for Common Discomforts of Pregnancy	
Discomfort	**Influencing Factors**	**Self-Care Measures**
First Trimester		
Nausea and vomiting	Increased levels of human chorionic gonadotropin Changes in carbohydrate metabolism Emotional factors Fatigue	Avoid odors or causative factors. Eat dry crackers or toast before arising in morning. Have small but frequent meals. Avoid greasy or highly seasoned foods. Take dry meals with fluids between meals. Drink carbonated beverages.
Urinary frequency	Pressure of uterus on bladder in both first and third trimesters	Void when urge is felt. Increase fluid intake during the day. Decrease fluid intake only in the evening to decrease nocturia.
Fatigue	Specific causative factors unknown May be aggravated by nocturia due to urinary frequency	Plan time for a nap or rest period daily. Go to bed earlier. Seek family support and assistance with responsibilities so that more time is available to rest.
Breast tenderness	Increased levels of estrogen and progesterone	Wear well-fitting, supportive bra.
Increased vaginal discharge	Hyperplasia of vaginal mucosa and increased production of mucus by the endocervical glands due to the increase in estrogen levels	Promote cleanliness by daily bathing. Avoid douching, nylon underpants, and pantyhose; cotton underpants are more absorbent; powder can be used to maintain dryness if not allowed to cake.

(continued)

Table 11–2	Self-Care Measures for Common Discomforts of Pregnancy—continued

Discomfort	Influencing Factors	Self-Care Measures
First Trimester		
Nasal stuffiness and nosebleed (epistaxis)	Elevated estrogen levels	May be unresponsive, but cool air vaporizer may help; avoid use of nasal sprays and decongestants.
Ptyalism (excessive, often bitter salivation)	Specific causative factors unknown	Use astringent mouthwashes, chew gum, or suck hard candy.
Second and Third Trimesters		
Heartburn (pyrosis)	Increased production of progesterone, decreasing gastrointestinal motility and increasing relaxation of cardiac sphincter, displacement of stomach by enlarging uterus, thus regurgitation of acidic gastric contents into the esophagus	Eat small and more frequent meals. Use low-sodium antacids. Avoid overeating, fatty and fried foods, lying down after eating, and sodium bicarbonate.
Ankle edema	Prolonged standing or sitting Increased levels of sodium due to hormonal influences Circulatory congestion of lower extremities Increased capillary permeability Varicose veins	Practice frequent dorsiflexion of feet when prolonged sitting or standing is necessary. Elevate legs when sitting or resting. Avoid tight garters or restrictive bands around legs.
Varicose veins	Venous congestion in the lower veins that increases with pregnancy Hereditary factors (weakening of walls of veins, faulty valves) Increased age and weight gain	Elevate legs frequently. Wear supportive hose. Avoid crossing legs at the knees, standing for long periods, garters, and hosiery with constrictive bands.
Hemorrhoids	Constipation (see following discussion) Increased pressure from gravid uterus on hemorrhoidal veins	Avoid constipation. Apply ice packs, topical ointments, anesthetic agents, warm soaks, or sitz baths; gently reinsert into rectum as necessary.
Constipation	Increased levels of progesterone, which cause general bowel sluggishness Pressure of enlarging uterus on intestine Iron supplements Diet, lack of exercise, and decreased fluids	Increase fluid intake, fiber in the diet, and exercise. Develop regular bowel habits. Use stool softeners as recommended by physician.
Backache	Increased curvature of the lumbosacral vertebrae as the uterus enlarges Increased levels of hormones, which cause softening of cartilage in body joints Fatigue Poor body mechanics	Use proper body mechanics. Practice the pelvic tilt exercise. Avoid uncomfortable working heights, high-heeled shoes, lifting of heavy loads, and fatigue.
Leg cramps	Imbalance of calcium/phosphorus ratio Increased pressure of uterus on nerves Fatigue Poor circulation to lower extremities Pointing the toes	Practice dorsiflexion of feet to stretch affected muscle. Evaluate diet. Apply heat to affected muscles. Rise slowly from resting position.
Faintness	Postural hypotension Sudden change of position causing venous pooling in dependent veins Standing for long periods in warm area Anemia	Avoid prolonged standing in warm or stuffy environments. Evaluate hematocrit and hemoglobin.
Dyspnea	Decreased vital capacity from pressure of enlarging uterus on the diaphragm	Use proper posture when sitting and standing. Sleep propped up with pillows for relief if problem occurs at night.
Flatulence	Decreased gastrointestinal motility leading to delayed emptying time Pressure of growing uterus on large intestine Air swallowing	Avoid gas-forming foods. Chew food thoroughly. Get regular daily exercise. Maintain normal bowel habits.
Carpal tunnel syndrome	Compression of median nerve in carpal tunnel of wrist Aggravated by repetitive hand movements	Avoid aggravating hand movements. Use splint as prescribed. Elevate affected arm.

● **Figure 11–2** Morning sickness relief. Acupressure wristbands are sometimes used to help relieve nausea during early pregnancy.
Source: Patrick Watson/Pearson Education.

The nurse should advise a woman to contact her healthcare provider if she vomits more than once a day or shows signs of dehydration such as dry mouth and concentrated urine. In such cases the physician or certified nurse-midwife might order an antiemetic. However, antiemetics should be avoided if possible during this time because of possible harmful effects on embryo development.

Urinary Frequency

Urinary frequency, a common discomfort of pregnancy, occurs early in pregnancy and again during the third trimester because the enlarging uterus puts pressure on the bladder. Although frequency is considered normal during the first and third trimesters, advise the woman to tell her healthcare provider about signs of bladder infection such as pain, burning with voiding, or blood in the urine. Fluid intake should never be decreased to prevent frequency. The woman needs to maintain an adequate fluid intake—at least 2000 mL (eight to ten 8-oz glasses) per day. Also, encourage her to empty her bladder frequently (about every 2 hours while awake).

Fatigue

Marked fatigue is so common in early pregnancy that it is considered a presumptive sign of pregnancy. It is aggravated if the woman cannot sleep through the night because of urinary frequency. Typically it resolves after the end of the first trimester.

Complementary Care **Ginger for Morning Sickness**

Ginger, long used in traditional Chinese medicine, is becoming increasingly popular for the treatment of NVP, and its safety has been demonstrated (National Center for Complementary and Alternative Medicine [NCCAM], 2012). Ginger is available in a variety of forms, including fresh or dried root, capsules, tea, candy, cookies, crystals, inhaled powdered ginger, and sugared ginger. It has few side effects when taken in small doses (NCCAM, 2012).

Breast Tenderness

Sensitivity of the breasts occurs early and continues throughout the pregnancy. Increased levels of estrogen and progesterone contribute to soreness and tingling of the breasts and increased sensitivity of the nipples.

Increased Vaginal Discharge

Increased whitish vaginal discharge, called **leukorrhea**, is common in pregnancy. It occurs as a result of hyperplasia of the vaginal mucosa and increased mucus production by the endocervical glands. The increased acidity of the secretions encourages the growth of *Candida albicans,* so the woman is more susceptible to monilial vaginitis.

Nasal Stuffiness and Epistaxis

Once pregnancy has progressed somewhat, elevated estrogen levels may produce edema of the nasal mucosa, which results in nasal stuffiness, nasal discharge, and obstruction. *Epistaxis* (nosebleeds) may also result. Cool air vaporizers and normal saline nasal sprays may help, but the problem is often unresponsive to treatment. Women experiencing these problems find it difficult to sleep and may resort to using medicated nasal sprays and decongestants. Such interventions may provide initial relief but can actually increase nasal stuffiness over time.

Ptyalism

Ptyalism is a rare discomfort of pregnancy in which excessive, often bitter saliva is produced. The cause is unknown, and effective treatments are limited.

Second and Third Trimesters

The discomforts discussed in this section usually do not appear until the third trimester in primigravidas but may occur earlier with each succeeding pregnancy.

Heartburn (Pyrosis)

Heartburn is the regurgitation of acidic gastric contents into the esophagus. It creates a burning sensation in the esophagus and sometimes leaves a bad taste in the mouth. Heartburn during pregnancy appears to be primarily a result of the displacement of the stomach by the enlarging uterus. The increased production of progesterone in pregnancy, decreased gastrointestinal motility, and relaxation of the cardiac (esophageal) sphincter also contribute to heartburn.

Liquid forms of low-sodium antacids are often most effective in providing relief. However, many women prefer chewable over-the-counter antacid tablets. The nurse should advise women that antacids containing aluminum may cause constipation, and antacids containing magnesium can cause diarrhea. The nurse should also let women know that they should avoid sodium bicarbonate (baking soda) and Alka-Seltzer because they may lead to electrolyte imbalance.

If maternal heartburn is severe, not relieved by antacids, and accompanied by gastrointestinal reflux, an antisecretory agent (H₂ blocker) such as ranitidine (Zantac), cimetidine (Tagamet), or omeprazole (Losec) may be helpful. To date they have not been linked with an excessive risk of birth defects.

Ankle Edema

Most women experience ankle edema in the last part of pregnancy because of the increasing difficulty of venous return from the lower extremities. Prolonged standing or sitting and warm weather increase the edema. It is also associated with varicose veins. Ankle edema becomes a concern only when accompanied by hypertension or proteinuria or when the edema is not postural in origin.

Varicose Veins

Varicose veins are a result of weakening of the walls of veins or faulty functioning of the valves. Poor circulation in the lower extremities predisposes people to varicose veins in the legs and thighs, as does prolonged standing or sitting. The pregnant uterus puts pressure on the pelvic veins, preventing good venous return, so it may aggravate existing problems or contribute to obvious changes in the veins of the legs (Figure 11–3 ●).

Surgical correction of varicose veins is not generally recommended during pregnancy. The nurse should advise the woman that treatment may be needed after she gives birth because the problem will be aggravated by a succeeding pregnancy.

Although less common, varicosities in the vulva and perineum may also develop. They produce aching and a sense of heaviness. Wearing a foam rubber commercial product that is placed across the perineum and held in place by a sanitary pad type belt can provide support for vulvar varicosities (Cunningham, Leveno, Bloom, et al., 2010). It is important that the pelvic area be elevated to promote venous drainage into the trunk of the body. The woman may best relieve uterine pressure on the pelvic veins by resting on her side. Blocks may also be placed under the foot of her bed to elevate it slightly.

Flatulence

Flatulence results from decreased gastrointestinal motility, leading to delayed emptying, and from pressure on the large intestine by the growing uterus. Air swallowing may also contribute to the problem.

Hemorrhoids

Hemorrhoids are varicosities of the veins in the lower rectum and the anus. During pregnancy the gravid uterus presses on the veins and interferes with venous circulation. In addition, the straining that accompanies constipation is frequently a contributing cause of hemorrhoids.

Some women may not be bothered by hemorrhoids until the second stage of labor, when the hemorrhoids appear as they push. These hemorrhoids usually become asymptomatic a few days after childbirth. Symptoms of hemorrhoids include itching, swelling, pain, and bleeding. Women who have had hemorrhoids before pregnancy will probably experience difficulties with them during pregnancy.

Some women find relief by gently reinserting the hemorrhoid. The woman lies on her side, places some lubricant on her finger, and presses against the hemorrhoids, pushing them inside. She holds them in place for 1 to 2 minutes and then gently withdraws her finger. The anal sphincter should then hold them inside the rectum. The woman will find it especially helpful if she can maintain a side-lying (Sims') position for a time, so this method is best done before bed or prior to a daily rest period.

The woman should contact her healthcare provider if the hemorrhoids become hardened and noticeably tender to touch. Rectal bleeding that is more than spotting following defecation should also be reported.

Constipation

Conditions that predispose the pregnant woman to constipation include general bowel sluggishness caused by increased progesterone and steroid metabolism; displacement of the intestines, which increases with growth of the fetus; and the oral iron supplements most pregnant women need. In severe or preexisting cases of constipation, the woman may need stool softeners, mild laxatives, or suppositories as recommended by her healthcare provider.

Backache

Over 50% of pregnant women experience backache (Kimberly, Niebyl, & Johnson, 2012), due primarily to exaggeration of the lumbosacral curve that occurs as the uterus enlarges and becomes heavier. Maintaining good posture and using proper body mechanics throughout pregnancy can help prevent backache. Advise the pregnant woman to avoid bending over at the waist to

● **Figure 11–3** Relief from varicose veins. Swelling and discomfort from varicosities can be decreased by lying down with the legs and one hip elevated (to avoid compression of the vena cava).

● **Figure 11–4** Body mechanics in pregnancy. When picking up objects from floor level or lifting objects, the pregnant woman must use proper body mechanics.

pick up objects and to bend from the knees instead (Figure 11–4 ●). She should place her feet 12 to 18 inches apart to maintain body balance. If the woman uses work surfaces that require her to bend, advise her to adjust the height of the surfaces.

Leg Cramps

Leg cramps are painful muscle spasms in the gastrocnemius muscles. They occur most often after the woman has gone to bed at night but may occur at other times. Extension of the foot can often cause leg cramps. The nurse should warn the pregnant woman not to extend the foot during childbirth preparation exercises or during rest periods.

Stretching provides immediate relief of the muscle spasm. With the woman lying on her back, another person presses the woman's knee down to straighten her leg while pushing her foot toward her leg (Figure 11–5 ●). The woman may also stand and put her foot flat on the floor. Massage and warm packs can alleviate the discomfort of leg cramps. A diet that includes daily portions of both calcium and phosphorus may help prevent leg cramps.

Faintness

Many pregnant women occasionally feel faint, especially in warm, crowded areas. Faintness is caused by a combination of changes in the blood volume and postural hypotension due to pooling of blood in the dependent veins. Sudden change of position or standing for prolonged periods can also cause this sensation, and the woman may faint.

If a woman begins to feel faint from prolonged standing or from being in a stuffy room, she should sit down and lower

● **Figure 11–5** Leg cramp relief. The expectant father can help relieve the woman's painful leg cramps by flexing her foot and straightening her leg.
Source: Yanik Chauvin/Fotolia

her head between her knees. If this procedure does not help, she should ask someone to help her to an area where she can lie down and get fresh air. The nurse should advise the woman that when getting up from a resting position, it is important to move slowly. Women whose jobs require standing in one place for long periods should march in place regularly to increase venous return from the legs.

Shortness of Breath (Dyspnea)

Shortness of breath occurs as the uterus rises into the abdomen and causes pressure on the diaphragm. This problem worsens in the last trimester because the enlarged uterus presses directly on the diaphragm, decreasing vital capacity. The primigravida experiences considerable relief from shortness of breath in the last few weeks of pregnancy, when **lightening** occurs, and the fetus and uterus move down in the pelvis. Because the multigravida does not usually experience lightening until labor, she tends to feel short of breath throughout the latter part of her pregnancy.

Difficulty Sleeping

Many physical factors in late pregnancy may make sleeping difficult. The enlarged uterus may make it difficult to find a comfortable position for sleep, and an active fetus may aggravate the problem. Other discomforts of pregnancy such as urinary frequency, shortness of breath, and leg cramps may also make it hard to sleep.

Round Ligament Pain

As the uterus enlarges during pregnancy, the round ligaments stretch and hypertrophy as the uterus rises up in the abdomen, causing pain. The woman may feel concern when she first experiences round ligament pain, because it is often intense and causes a "grabbing" sensation in the lower abdomen and inguinal area. The nurse should warn the pregnant woman of this possible discomfort. Once it has been determined that the cause of the pain is not a medical complication such as appendicitis, the woman may find that applying a heating pad to the abdomen brings relief.

Carpal Tunnel Syndrome

Carpal tunnel syndrome, characterized by numbness and tingling of the hand near the thumb, occurs in about 25% to 50%

of pregnant women (Kimberly et al., 2012). It is caused by compression of the median nerve in the carpal tunnel of the wrist. The syndrome is aggravated by repetitive hand movements such as typing and may disappear following childbirth. Fluid retention during pregnancy and high weight gain may aggravate the condition (Gregory et al., 2012). Treatment usually involves splinting and avoiding aggravating movements, but surgery may be needed in severe cases if more conservative approaches are not effective.

PROMOTION OF SELF-CARE DURING PREGNANCY

Fetal Activity Monitoring

Many healthcare providers encourage pregnant women to monitor their unborn child's well-being by regularly assessing fetal activity beginning at 28 weeks' gestation. Vigorous activity generally provides reassurance of fetal well-being, but a marked decrease in activity or cessation of movement may indicate a problem that needs immediate evaluation. Fetal activity is affected by fetal sleep, sound, time of day, blood glucose levels, cigarette smoking, and some illicit drugs such as crack and cocaine. At times a healthy fetus may be minimally active or inactive. See Chapter 14 ❷ for an in-depth discussion of maternal–fetal activity monitoring; also see in Chapter 14, *Teaching Highlights: What to Tell the Pregnant Woman About Assessing Fetal Activity* on ❷ page 279.

Breast Care

Whether the pregnant woman plans to formula-feed or breastfeed her infant, support of the breasts is important to promote comfort, retain breast shape, and prevent back strain, particularly if the breasts become large and pendulous. The sensitivity of the breasts in pregnancy is often relieved by good support.

A well-fitting, supportive brassiere has the following qualities:

- The straps are wide and do not stretch (elastic straps soon lose their tautness with the weight of the breasts and frequent washing).
- The cups hold all breast tissue comfortably.
- The brassiere has tucks or other devices that allow it to expand and accommodate the enlarging chest circumference.
- The brassiere supports the nipple line approximately midway between the elbow and shoulder but is not pulled up in the back by the weight of the breasts.

Cleanliness of the breasts is important, especially as the woman begins producing colostrum. Colostrum that crusts on the nipples can be removed with warm water. The nurse should advise the woman planning to breastfeed not to use soap on her nipples because of its drying effect.

Some women have flat or inverted nipples. True nipple inversion, which is rare, is usually diagnosed during the initial prenatal assessment. Breast shields designed to correct inverted nipples are effective for some women but others gain no benefit from them. For further discussion of inverted nipples, see Chapter 30 ❷.

Clothing

Traditionally maternity clothes have been constructed with fuller lines to allow for the increase in abdominal size that occurs during pregnancy. However, in recent years maternity clothing has changed and now also includes more clothes that are fitted with little attempt to hide the pregnant abdomen. Maternity clothing can be expensive and is worn for a relatively short time, so women can economize by sharing clothes with friends, sewing their own garments, or buying used maternity clothes.

High-heeled shoes tend to aggravate back discomfort by increasing the curvature of the lower back. Women who experience backache or have problems with balance do best to avoid them. Shoes should fit properly and feel comfortable.

Bathing

Hygiene is important because perspiration and mucoid vaginal discharge increase during pregnancy. Keep in mind, however, that cultural norms often influence bathing and cleansing practices. A pregnant woman may choose to cleanse only some portions of her body regularly or may elect to take showers or tub baths. Advise women to be careful in the tub because balance becomes a problem in late pregnancy. Rubber mats and hand grips are important safety devices. Vasodilation due to warm water may cause the woman to feel faint when she gets out of the tub, so she may need assistance, especially during the last trimester.

Employment

In general, women with low-risk pregnancies can continue working until the start of labor if their jobs do not present risks greater than those they encounter in daily life (Kimberly et al., 2012).

Overfatigue, prolonged standing, excessive physical strain, fetotoxic hazards in the environment, and medical or obstetric complications are the major deterrents to certain types of employment during pregnancy. In the second half of pregnancy, women whose occupations involve balance should make adjustments as needed.

Fetotoxic hazards are always a concern to the expectant couple. The pregnant woman (or the woman contemplating pregnancy) who works in industry should contact her company physician or nurse about possible hazards in her work environment and should do her own reading and research on environmental hazards as well. Her partner can also find out how hazards in his workplace might affect his sperm.

Travel

Pregnant women without complications can travel as usual. Pregnant women should avoid travel if they have a history of preterm birth, bleeding, or preeclampsia or if multiple births are anticipated.

Travel by automobile can be tiring, aggravating many of the discomforts of pregnancy. The pregnant woman needs frequent opportunities to get out of the car and walk. (A good pattern is to stop every 2 hours and walk around for about 10 minutes.) She should wear both lap and shoulder belts. The lap belt should fit snugly and be positioned under the abdomen and across the upper thighs; the shoulder strap should rest comfortably between the woman's breasts. Seat belts play an important role in preventing fetal and maternal injury and death (Cunningham et al., 2010). Fetal death in car accidents is sometimes caused by placental separation (abruptio placentae) as a result of uterine distortion. Shoulder belts decrease the risk of traumatic flexion of the woman's body, making placental separation less likely.

As pregnancy progresses, long-distance trips are best taken by plane or train. Before flying the woman should check with her airline to see if they have any travel restrictions because many prohibit flying after 36 weeks' gestation. To avoid the development of phlebitis or blood clots, pregnant women should drink plenty of fluid to avoid dehydration and hemoconcentration. They should also walk about the plane at regular intervals and change position frequently. Air travel is not recommended during pregnancy for women who have obstetric or medical conditions that could require emergency care or that might be exacerbated by flight (American College of Obstetricians and Gynecologists [ACOG], 2009a). Remind near-term women who travel to think about the availability of medical care at the destination.

Activity and Rest

Exercise during pregnancy helps maintain maternal fitness and muscle tone, leads to improved self-image, promotes regular bowel function, improves cardiovascular function, increases energy, improves sleep, relieves tension, helps control weight gain, and is associated with improved postpartum recovery. Fetal benefits include advanced neurobehavioral maturation and improved stress tolerance (Melzer, Schutz, Boulvain, et al., 2010). Normal participation in exercise can continue throughout an uncomplicated pregnancy and, in fact, is encouraged.

The woman can check with her certified nurse-midwife or physician about taking part in strenuous sports. ACOG (2009b) recommends that women avoid activities with a high risk for falling, such as skiing, gymnastics, and horseback riding, and those activities that have a high risk of blunt trauma, such as ice hockey and basketball.

Certain conditions contraindicate exercise. These conditions include rupture of the membranes, preeclampsia, incompetent cervix or cerclage placement, persistent vaginal bleeding, risk factors for preterm labor or a history of preterm labor in the current pregnancy, placenta previa after 26 weeks' gestation, significant heart disease, and restrictive lung disease (ACOG, 2009b).

The following guidelines are helpful in counseling pregnant women about exercise.

- Even mild to moderate exercise is beneficial during pregnancy. Regular exercise—at least 30 minutes of moderate exercise daily or at least most days—is preferred (Kimberly et al., 2012).
- After the first trimester, women should avoid exercising in the supine position. In most pregnant women,

the supine position is associated with decreased cardiac output. Because uterine blood flow is reduced during exercise as blood is shunted from the visceral organs to the muscles, the remaining cardiac output is further decreased. Similarly, women should also avoid standing motionless for prolonged periods (ACOG, 2009b).

- Light muscle strengthening training using lighter weights (or resistance bands) and more repetitions done once or twice per week helps improve overall fitness and does not negatively affect the fetus. Heavy weights should be avoided because they may overload joints that are looser than normal because of the effects of the hormone relaxin (Zavorsky & Longo, 2011). Because decreased oxygen is available for aerobic exercise during pregnancy, women should modify the intensity of their exercise based on their symptoms, should stop when they become fatigued, and should avoid exercising to the point of exhaustion.

- Non–weight-bearing exercises such as swimming and cycling are recommended and provide fitness with comfort. As pregnancy progresses and the center of gravity changes, especially in the third trimester, women should avoid exercises in which the loss of balance could pose a risk to mother or fetus. Similarly, the woman should avoid any type of exercise that has a high potential for physical contact such as basketball, soccer, and ice hockey because it could result in trauma to the woman or her fetus.

- A normal pregnancy requires an additional 300 kcal per day. Women who exercise regularly during pregnancy should be careful to ensure that their diet is adequate. To avoid overheating, especially during the first trimester, pregnant women who exercise should wear clothing that is comfortable and loose, drink plenty of fluids, and avoid the prolonged overheating.

- As a result of the cardiovascular changes of pregnancy, heart rate is not an accurate indicator of the intensity of exercise for pregnant women. If a pregnant, exercising woman is unable to maintain a conversation, then the exercise effort is too high.

The woman should wear a supportive bra and appropriate shoes when exercising. She should also warm up and stretch to help prepare the joints for activity and cool down with a period of mild activity to help restore circulation and avoid pooling of blood. A moderate, rhythmic exercise routine involving large muscle groups such as swimming, cycling, or brisk walking is best. Jogging or running is acceptable for women already conditioned to these activities as long as they avoid exercising at maximum effort and overheating.

During exercise, warning signs include chest pain, calf pain or swelling, decreased or absent fetal movement, dizziness, headache, muscle weakness, dyspnea before exertion, uterine contractions, vaginal bleeding, or fluid loss from the vagina (ACOG, 2009b). The woman should stop exercising if these symptoms occur, and modify her exercise program. If the symptoms persist, the woman should contact her caregiver.

Complementary Care   Yoga During Pregnancy

The following advice is important for women who practice yoga during pregnancy (Fontaine, 2011):

- During pregnancy, some yoga poses or positions are contraindicated. In particular pregnant women should avoid those poses that put pressure on the uterus as well as any extreme stretching positions.
- Because of the changed center of gravity that occurs as pregnancy progresses, women need to be especially careful to maintain balance when doing stretching.
- Pregnant women should avoid stomach-lying for any poses. After 20 weeks' gestation, women should lie on their left side rather than their back for floor positions.
- Pregnant women should immediately stop any pose that is uncomfortable.
- Warning signs that indicate the need to contact the physician or certified nurse-midwife immediately include the following: dizziness, extreme shortness of breath, sudden swelling, vaginal bleeding.

Clinical Reasoning   Counseling About Strenuous Physical Activity

Ana Gonzalez, a 24-year-old, G1P0, is 11 weeks pregnant when she presents for her first prenatal examination. She has been a long-distance runner for 6 years. Because of her low body fat, her menses have always been irregular, and it had not occurred to Ana that she might be pregnant. Ana says she has been told that it is fine to continue any physical activity at which one is proficient and says that she would like to continue running long distances while pregnant. What should you tell Ana about running long distances?

See www.nursing.pearsonhighered.com for possible responses.

During pregnancy, adequate rest is important for both physical and emotional health. Women need more sleep, particularly in the first and last trimesters, when they tire easily. Without enough rest, pregnant women have less resilience. Finding time to rest during the day may be difficult for women who work outside the home or who have small children. The nurse can help the expectant mother examine her daily schedule to develop a realistic plan for short periods of rest and relaxation.

Sleeping becomes more difficult during the last trimester because of the enlarged abdomen, increased frequency of urination, and greater activity of the fetus. Finding a comfortable position becomes difficult. Figure 11–6 shows a position most pregnant women find comfortable. Women can also prepare for sleep with progressive relaxation techniques similar to those taught in prepared childbirth classes.

Exercises to Prepare for Childbirth

Certain exercises help strengthen muscle tone in preparation for birth and promote more rapid restoration of muscle tone after birth. A few of the more common body-conditioning exercises for pregnancy are discussed here.

The **pelvic tilt**, or pelvic rocking, helps maintain pelvic flexibility and prevent or reduce back strain as it helps strengthen abdominal muscles. To do the pelvic tilt in early pregnancy, the pregnant woman lies on her back and puts her feet flat on the floor. This flexes the knees and helps prevent strain or discomfort. She decreases the curvature in her back by pressing her spine toward the floor. With her back pressed to the floor, the woman tightens her abdominal muscles as she tightens and tucks in her buttocks. In the second and third trimesters, the woman can also do the pelvic tilt on her hands and knees (Figure 11–7 •), while sitting in a chair, or while standing with her back against a wall. The woman should maintain the body alignment that results when the pelvic tilt is done correctly as much as possible throughout the day.

Clinical Tip

Doing the pelvic tilt on hands and knees may aggravate back strain. Teach women with a history of minor back problems to do the pelvic tilt only in the standing position.

Abdominal Exercises

A basic exercise to increase abdominal muscle tone is tightening abdominal muscles with each breath. It can be done in any

● **Figure 11–6** Position for relaxation and rest as pregnancy progresses.

A

B

● **Figure 11–7** When the pelvic tilt is done on hands and knees, the starting position is back flat and parallel to the floor, hands below the head, and knees directly below the buttocks. *A,* For the first part of the tilt, head is up, neck is long and separated from the shoulders, buttocks are up, and pelvis is thrust back, allowing the back to drop and release on an inhaled breath. *B,* The next part of the tilt is done on a long exhalation, allowing the pregnant woman to arch her back, drop her head loosely, push away from her hands, and draw in the muscles of her abdomen to strengthen them. Note that in this position the pelvis and buttocks are tucked under, and the buttock muscles are tightened.

Source: Bubbles Photolibrary/Alamy.

position, but it is best learned while lying supine. With knees flexed and feet flat on the floor, the woman expands her abdomen and slowly takes a deep breath. Exhaling slowly, she gradually pulls in her abdominal muscles until they are fully contracted. She relaxes for a few seconds and then repeats the exercise. The pregnant woman should avoid the supine position after the first trimester.

Partial sit-ups strengthen abdominal muscle tone and are done according to individual comfort levels. In early pregnancy, partial sit-ups may be done with the knees flexed and the feet flat on the floor to avoid strain on the lower back. The woman stretches her arms toward her knees as she slowly pulls her head and shoulders off the floor to a comfortable level (if she has poor abdominal muscle tone, she may not be able to pull up very far). She then slowly returns to the starting position, takes a deep breath, and repeats the exercise. To strengthen the oblique abdominal muscles, she repeats the process but stretches the left arm to the side of her right knee, returns to the floor, takes a deep breath, and then reaches with the right arm to the left knee. During the second and third trimesters, these exercises can be done on a large exercise ball.

Women can do these exercises approximately five times in a sequence and repeat the sequence at other times during the day as desired. It is important to do the exercises slowly to prevent muscle strain and overtiring.

Perineal Exercises

Perineal muscle tightening, also called **Kegel exercises**, strengthens the pubococcygeus muscle and increases its elasticity (Figure 11–8 ●). The woman can feel the specific muscle

Pubococcygeus muscle with good tone

Pubococcygeus muscle with poor tone

● **Figure 11–8** Kegel exercises. The woman learns to tighten the pubococcygeus muscle, which improves support to the pelvic organs.

group to be exercised by stopping urination midstream. Doing Kegel exercises while urinating is discouraged, however, because this practice has been associated with urinary stasis and urinary tract infection.

Childbirth educators sometimes use the following technique to teach Kegel exercises. They tell the woman to think of her perineal muscles as an elevator. When she relaxes, the elevator is on the first floor. To do the exercises, she contracts, bringing the elevator to the second, third, and fourth floors. She keeps the elevator on the fourth floor for a few seconds, and then gradually relaxes the area. If the exercise is properly done, the woman does not contract the muscles of the buttocks and thighs. Kegel exercises can be done at almost any time. Some women use ordinary events—for instance, stopping at a red light or talking on the telephone—as a cue to remember to do the exercise.

Inner Thigh Exercises

The nurse can advise the pregnant woman to assume a cross-legged sitting position whenever possible. This "tailor sit" stretches the muscles of the inner thighs in preparation for labor and birth. See Figure 11–9 ●.

Sexual Activity

Because of the physiologic, anatomic, and emotional changes of pregnancy, couples usually have many questions and concerns about sexual activity during pregnancy. Often these questions are about possible injury to the baby or the woman during intercourse and about changes in the desire each partner feels for the other.

In the past, couples were often warned to avoid sexual intercourse during the last 6 to 8 weeks of pregnancy to prevent

complications such as infection or premature rupture of the membranes. However, these fears seem to be unfounded. In a healthy pregnancy, there is no medical reason to limit sexual activity. Intercourse is contraindicated for medical reasons such as threatened miscarriage or risk of preterm labor (Cunningham et al., 2010).

The expectant mother may experience changes in sexual desire and response. Often these changes are related to the various discomforts that occur throughout pregnancy. For instance, during the first trimester, fatigue or nausea and vomiting may decrease sexual desire. During the second trimester, many of these discomforts are lessened and sexual satisfaction increases. During the third trimester, interest in sex may again decrease as the woman becomes more uncomfortable and tired. Shortness of breath, urinary frequency, leg cramps, and decreased mobility may also lessen sexual desire and activity. If they are not already doing so, the couple should consider coital positions other than male superior, such as side-by-side, female superior, and vaginal rear entry.

Sexual activity does not have to include intercourse. Many of the nurturing and sexual needs of the pregnant woman can be satisfied by cuddling, kissing, and being held. The warm, sensual feelings that accompany these activities can be an end in themselves. Her partner, however, may choose to masturbate for satisfaction.

Many factors in pregnancy also affect the sexual desires of men. The man's previous relationship with the partner, acceptance of the pregnancy, attitudes toward the partner's change of appearance, and concern about hurting the expectant mother or baby can all play a role. Some men find it difficult to view their partners as sexually appealing while they are adjusting to the concept of them as mothers. Other men find their partners' pregnancies arousing and experience feelings of increased happiness, intimacy, and closeness.

The expectant couple should be aware of their changing sexual desires, the normality of these changes, and the importance of communicating these changes to each other so that they can make nurturing adaptations. It is important that the couple feel free to express concerns about sexual activity. Use a relaxed manner when responding to questions and giving anticipatory guidance. (See *Teaching Highlights: Sexual Activity During Pregnancy.*)

Dental Care

Proper dental hygiene is important in pregnancy because ensuring a healthy oral environment is essential to overall health. In spite of such discomforts as nausea and vomiting, gum hypertrophy, and heartburn, it is important for pregnant women to maintain regular oral hygiene by brushing at least twice a day and flossing daily. Dental treatment is safe throughout pregnancy; however, the second trimester is considered the most appropriate time for dental treatment because the risk of pregnancy loss tends to be lower and the woman tends to be more comfortable. It is important to encourage the woman to have a dental checkup early in pregnancy. She should inform her dentist that she is pregnant so that she is not exposed to teratogenic substances.

● **Figure 11–9** Tailor sitting. To help prepare her inner thigh muscles for labor and birth, the pregnant woman should assume a cross-legged sitting position whenever possible during the day.

Teaching Highlights Sexual Activity During Pregnancy

In starting a discussion about sexual activity during pregnancy, universal statements that give permission, such as "Many couples experience changes in sexual desire during pregnancy. What kind of changes have you experienced?" are often effective.

In your teaching, explain the following points to the woman and her partner:

- The pregnant woman may experience changes in desire during the course of pregnancy. During the first trimester, discomforts such as nausea, fatigue, and breast tenderness may make intercourse less desirable for many women. In the second trimester, as symptoms decrease, desire may increase. In the third trimester, discomfort and fatigue may lead to decreased desire in the woman.
- Men may notice changes in their level of desire, too. This may be related to feelings about their partner's changing appearance, their belief about the acceptability of sexual activity with a pregnant woman, or concern about hurting the woman or fetus. Some men find the changes of pregnancy erotic; others must adjust to the notion of their partners as mothers.
- The woman may notice that orgasms are much more intense during the last weeks of pregnancy and may be followed by cramping.
- Because of the pressure of the enlarging uterus on the vena cava, the woman should not lie flat on her back for intercourse after about the fourth month. If the couple prefer that position, a pillow should be placed under her right hip to displace the uterus. Alternative positions such as side-by-side, female superior, or vaginal rear entry may become necessary as her uterus enlarges.
- Sexual activities that both partners enjoy are generally acceptable. It is not advisable for couples who favor anal sex to go from anal penetration to vaginal penetration because of the risk of introducing *Escherichia coli* into the vagina.
- Alternative methods of expressing intimacy and affection such as cuddling, holding and stroking each other, and kissing may help maintain the couple's feelings of warmth and closeness. If the man feels desire for further sexual release, his partner may help him masturbate to ejaculation, or he may prefer to masturbate in private.
- Sexual intercourse is contraindicated once the membranes are ruptured or if bleeding is present. Women with a history of preterm labor may be advised to avoid intercourse because the oxytocin that is released with orgasm stimulates uterine contractions and may trigger preterm labor. Because oxytocin is also released with nipple stimulation, fondling the breasts may also be contraindicated in those cases.

Stress the importance of open communication so that the couple feels comfortable expressing their feelings, preferences, and concerns. Deal with any specific questions about the physical and psychologic changes that the couple may have.

Immunizations

Immunizations with attenuated live viruses, such as rubella vaccine, should not be given in pregnancy because of the teratogenic effect of the live viruses on the developing embryo. The most current recommendations on vaccines during pregnancy should be obtained from the Centers for Disease Control and Prevention website; also see Table 8-1, Vaccinations During Pregnancy, on page 164.

Complementary and Alternative Therapies

As discussed in Chapter 2 🔗, many women use complementary and alternative medicine (CAM) such as homeopathy, herbal medicine, acupressure and acupuncture, biofeedback, Therapeutic Touch, massage, and chiropractic as part of a holistic approach to their health care. Thus the nurse should inquire about the use of CAM as part of routine antepartum assessment. Nurses working with pregnant women and childbearing families need to develop a general understanding of the more commonly used therapies to be able to answer basic questions and to provide resources as needed.

It is important for the pregnant woman to understand that herbs are considered dietary supplements and are not regulated as prescription or over-the-counter drugs are through the FDA. In general, it is best to advise pregnant women not to ingest any herbs, except ginger, during the first trimester of pregnancy. The website of the National Center for Complementary and Alternative Medicine is a reliable source of information about herbs, homeopathic remedies, and other alternative options.

CenteringPregnancy®

CenteringPregnancy® is a model of prenatal health care designed to empower women to choose health-promoting behaviors and, as a result, improve prenatal care outcomes (Manant & Dodgson, 2011). CenteringPregnancy® integrates the three major components of care—*health assessment*, *education*, and *support*—into a unified program providing complete prenatal care to women within a group setting. This model replaces the traditional one-on-one visits. Instead, group meetings are held where moms-to-be and their partners receive care and education and form a sense of community with other group members.

Patients begin monthly meetings in small groups at 12 to 16 weeks' gestation and then meet biweekly as their due dates approach. Each group session begins with the expectant mothers taking their own blood pressure, monitoring weight gain, checking urine samples, and recording data on medical charts under their provider's or nurse's guidance. The provider then reviews each group member's information and completes any further assessments that are indicated. After all assessments have been completed, the group members convene in a circle to discuss topics such as nutrition, fetal development, common discomforts of pregnancy and possible remedies, exercise, relaxation, labor and birth procedures, parenting and relationship issues, contraception, and infant care. Both mothers and fathers report an increased investment in the pregnancy and self-care after attending group sessions.

Teratogenic Substances

Substances that adversely affect the normal growth and development of the fetus are called teratogens. Many substances are known or suspected teratogens, including certain medications, psychotropic drugs, and alcohol. The harmful effects of other substances, such as some pesticides or exposure to x-rays in the first trimester of pregnancy, have also been documented. It is essential to provide pregnant women with information about recognized teratogens and environmental risks.

Medications

The use of medications during pregnancy, including prescriptions, over-the-counter drugs, and herbal remedies, is of great concern because maternal drug exposure is thought to account for at least 10% of all birth defects (Yankowitz, 2008). Many pregnant women need medication to treat infections, allergies, or other pathologic processes. In these situations the problem can be complex. Even when a woman is highly motivated to avoid taking any medications, she may have taken potentially teratogenic medications before her pregnancy was confirmed, especially if she has an irregular menstrual cycle.

The fetus is at highest risk for gross abnormalities during the first trimester of pregnancy, when fetal organs are first developing. The classic period of teratogenesis in a woman with a 28-day cycle extends from day 31 after the last menstrual period (17 days after fertilization) to day 71 (57 days after fertilization) (Niebyl & Simpson, 2012). Many factors influence teratogenic effects, including the type of teratogen and the dose, the stage of embryo development, and the genetic sensitivity of the mother and fetus. For example, the commonly prescribed acne medication isotretinoin (Accutane) is associated with a high incidence of spontaneous abortion and congenital malformations if taken early in pregnancy.

To provide information for healthcare providers and patients, the U.S. Food and Drug Administration has developed the following classification system for medications administered during pregnancy:

Category A: Controlled studies in women have demonstrated no associated fetal risk. Few drugs fall into this category.

Category B: Animal studies show no risk, but there are no controlled studies in women; or animal studies indicate a risk, but controlled human studies fail to demonstrate a risk. The penicillins fall into this category.

Category C: Either (1) no adequate animal or human studies are available or (2) animal studies show teratogenic effects, but no controlled studies in women are available. Many drugs fall into this category, which, because of the lack of information, is a problematic one for caregivers. Epinephrine, beta-blockers, and zidovudine (a drug used to decrease perinatal transmission of HIV) fall into this category.

Category D: Evidence of human fetal risk exists, but the benefits of the drug in certain situations are thought to outweigh the risks. Examples of drugs in this category include tetracycline, vincristine, lithium, and hydrochlorothiazide.

Category X: The demonstrated fetal risks clearly outweigh any possible benefit. Examples of drugs in this category include isotretinoin (Accutane), the acne medication, which can cause multiple central nervous system (CNS), facial, and cardiovascular anomalies.

Caregivers do not prescribe teratogenic medications to a pregnant woman. However, if a woman has taken a drug in category D or X, she should be informed of the risks associated with that drug and of her alternatives. A woman who has taken a drug in the safer categories can be reassured (Cunningham et al., 2010).

This system, although useful, has been criticized because the use of letters suggests a risk grading that is not necessarily accurate. More importantly, not all drugs in a category have the same risk level. Currently the FDA has proposed a new labeling system that would eliminate the current categories and require a pregnancy subsection for all medications, even those that are not absorbed systemically. The new label has three main sections: (1) fetal risk summary, (2) clinical considerations, and (3) data (Frederikson, 2011).

Although the first trimester is the critical period for teratogenesis, some medications are known to have a teratogenic effect when taken in the second and third trimesters. For example, tetracycline taken in late pregnancy is commonly associated with staining of teeth in children and has been shown to depress skeletal growth, especially in premature infants. Sulfonamides taken in the last few weeks of pregnancy are known to compete with bilirubin attachment of protein-binding sites, increasing the risk of jaundice in the newborn (Niebyl & Simpson, 2012).

Pregnant women need to avoid all medication—prescribed, homeopathic, or over-the-counter—if possible. If no alternative exists, it is wisest to select a well-known medication rather than a newer drug whose potential teratogenic effects may not be known. When possible, the oral form of a drug should be used, and it should be prescribed in the lowest possible therapeutic dose for the shortest time possible. Caution is the watchword for pregnant women who have been taking medications. The advantage of using a particular medication must outweigh the risks. Any medication with possible teratogenic effects is best avoided.

SAFETY ALERT!

It is essential that pregnant women check with their CNMs or physicians about any herbs or medications they were taking when pregnancy began and about any nonprescription drugs they are thinking of using.

Tobacco

In the United States, smoking during pregnancy is one of the most significant, modifiable causes of poor pregnancy outcomes. It is associated with an increased risk of intrauterine growth restriction, low birth weight, preterm birth, premature rupture of the membranes, perinatal mortality, placenta previa, abruptio placentae, preterm premature rupture of membranes, and ectopic pregnancy (ACOG, 2010b). Research also links maternal smoking, both during pregnancy and afterward, with an increased risk of sudden infant death syndrome (SIDS) (Niebyl & Simpson, 2012). Maternal smoking exposes young children to other risks of secondhand smoke including middle ear infections, acute and chronic respiratory tract illnesses, and behavioral and learning disabilities (L. T. Martin, McNamara, Milot, 2008).

The ingredients in cigarette smoke, such as carbon monoxide, nicotine, lead, and cotinine, are toxic to the fetus and decrease the availability of oxygen to maternal and fetal tissues (Cunningham et al., 2010).

In response to public health education campaigns in the United States, smoking during pregnancy has decreased significantly. In fact, approximately 46% of women who smoke quit during pregnancy. Unfortunately, 60% to 80% of women who

Evidence-Based Practice   Characteristics of Mothers Who Smoke During Pregnancy

Clinical Question

What are the characteristics of mothers who are likely to continue smoking during the prenatal period?

The Evidence

Four large cohort studies involving more than 6000 women focused on the characteristics of mothers who continued to smoke during pregnancy. The large size of the overall samples and the longitudinal nature of the studies make them the strongest evidence for practice. The mother's education and socioeconomic status were inversely related to smoking during pregnancy across all four studies (Homish, Eiden, Leonard, et al., 2012). One of the strongest predictors in all of the studies was whether the mother's partner or spouse continued to smoke during the pregnancy (Page, Padilla, & Hamilton, 2012). One study that focused on mental health issues determined that stressful life events were associated with smoking, but overall mood and depression were not (Gyllstrom, Hellerstedt, & Hennrikus, 2012). Two of the studies identified that the amount of prepregnancy smoking was a predictor of continued smoking during pregnancy (Maxon, Edwards, Ingram, et al., 2012).

The number of previous pregnancies was identified as a predictor in one of the studies. Relapse of smoking after the baby was born was highest in those who did not breastfeed.

Best Practice

Understanding who smokes during pregnancy and what factors influence this behavior is critical to improving the effectiveness of smoking cessation intervention programs. It can also help the nurse identify at-risk mothers so that they can be encouraged to take advantage of supports available for smoking cessation. The woman's partner or spouse should be included in teaching about the importance of both of them ceasing cigarette smoking during the pregnancy.

Clinical Reasoning

How can the nurse involve the spouse or partner in taking action to quit smoking during pregnancy? What assessment questions should be included in the first prenatal assessment to determine if mothers are at risk of continuing to smoke?

quit smoking during their pregnancy resume smoking within a year after birth (ACOG, 2010b). This finding suggests that although women are aware of the potential impact of smoking on the fetus, they may be less knowledgeable about the effects of passive smoke on the baby.

Any decrease in smoking during pregnancy most likely improves fetal outcome, and researchers continue to explore approaches designed to help women quit smoking. Pregnancy may be a difficult time for a woman to stop smoking, but the nurse should encourage her to reduce the number of cigarettes she smokes daily. The perceived need to protect her unborn child may increase her motivation.

Alcohol

Fetuses of women who drink heavily are at increased risk of developing **fetal alcohol syndrome (FAS)** (see Chapter 27 🔗). This syndrome, which is characterized by growth restriction, facial anomalies, and CNS dysfunction of varying severity, is the major cause of mental retardation in the United States (Cunningham et al., 2010).

The effects of moderate drinking during pregnancy are unclear. Research indicates an increased incidence of lowered birth weight and some neurologic effects, such as attention deficit disorder. Evidence suggests that the risk of teratogenic effects increases proportionately with increased average daily intake of alcohol. Although an occasional drink during pregnancy does not carry any known risk, no safe level of drinking during pregnancy has been identified; thus, healthcare providers recommend that pregnant women abstain from all alcohol during pregnancy. In most cases once a woman becomes aware of her pregnancy, she decreases her consumption of alcohol. However, the alcohol consumed after conception and before pregnancy is diagnosed remains a cause for concern. For this reason and for their general well-being, women of childbearing age—and indeed all women—should be counseled to avoid heavy or binge drinking.

Assessment of alcohol intake is a major part of every woman's medical history. The nurse should ask questions in a direct, nonjudgmental manner. All women need to be counseled about the role of alcohol in pregnancy. If heavy consumption is involved, the nurse should refer the pregnant woman immediately to an alcohol treatment program. Counselors in these programs need to know about a woman's pregnancy before drug therapy is suggested, since certain drugs may be harmful to the developing fetus. For example, the drug disulfiram (Antabuse), often used in conjunction with alcohol treatment, is contraindicated during pregnancy because it potentiates the teratogenic effect of alcohol (Wisner, Sit, Alternus, et al., 2012).

Caffeine

Current research reveals no evidence that moderate caffeine intake (less than 200 mg/day) is linked to birth defects, spontaneous abortion, or preterm birth, nor is there any clear evidence of a link between caffeine intake and intrauterine growth restriction (ACOG, 2010a). However, high caffeine intake may be linked to an increased risk of miscarriage (Niebyl & Simpson, 2012). (The average cup of brewed coffee has about 100 mg and a 12-oz can of cola has about 50 mg.). Until more definitive data are available, nurses can advise women about common sources of caffeine, including coffee, tea, colas, and chocolate, and suggest that they limit their caffeine intake to less than 200 mg/day (ACOG, 2010a).

Marijuana

The prevalence of marijuana use raises many concerns about its effect on the fetus, but no teratogenic effects of marijuana use during pregnancy have yet been documented (Niebyl & Simpson, 2012). Research on marijuana use in pregnancy is difficult, however, because it is an illegal drug. Unreliability of reporting, lack of a representative population, inability to determine strength or composition of the marijuana used (including the presence of herbicides), and use of other drugs at the same time all complicate the research being done.

Cocaine

A woman who uses cocaine during pregnancy is at increased risk for acute myocardial infarction, cardiac arrhythmias, ruptured ascending aorta, seizures, cerebrovascular accidents, hyperthermia, bowel ischemia, and sudden death (Cunningham et al., 2010). Cocaine use during pregnancy has been related to spontaneous abortion and abruptio placentae, neonatal irritability or lethargy, poor infant feeding, neonatal seizures (Keegan, Parva, Finnegan, et al., 2010), preterm birth, and low-birthweight and small-for-gestational age (SGA) infants (Gouin, Murphy, & Shah, 2011), as well as SIDS and developmental delays as a toddler (March of Dimes [MOD], 2009). Several congenital anomalies in the newborn have also been linked to maternal cocaine use, including genitourinary anomalies, congenital heart defects, limb reduction defects, and CNS anomalies (Cunningham et al., 2010).

As the number of women of childbearing age using cocaine increases, healthcare providers must be alert to early signs of cocaine use. It is often difficult for a nurse or physician to face the fact that a patient is using cocaine, but ongoing alertness and an open, nonjudgmental approach are important in early detection. Urine screening for cocaine is valuable, but because cocaine is metabolized rapidly, the drug screen is negative within 24 to 48 hours after cocaine use. Thus it is probable that many expectant mothers who use cocaine are not identified.

Evaluation

Throughout the antepartum period, evaluation is an ongoing and essential part of effective nursing care. In evaluating the effectiveness of the interactions, try creative solutions that are logical and carefully thought out. Creative solutions are especially important in dealing with families from other cultures. If a practice is important to a woman and not harmful, the culturally competent nurse will not discourage it.

Be alert for situations that require referral for further evaluation. For example, a woman who has gained 4 lb in a single week does not require counseling about nutrition; she needs further assessment for preeclampsia. The nurse who has a sound knowledge of theory will recognize this need and act immediately.

Throughout the course of pregnancy, certain criteria determine the quality of care. In essence, nursing care has been effective if the following occur:

- The common discomforts of pregnancy are quickly identified and are relieved or lessened effectively.
- The woman is able to discuss the physiologic and psychologic changes of pregnancy.
- The woman uses self-care measures, if needed, during pregnancy.
- The woman avoids substances and situations that pose a risk to her or her child's well-being.
- The woman seeks regular prenatal care.

CARE OF EXPECTANT PARENTS OVER AGE 35

Today an increasing number of women are choosing to have their first baby after age 35. In the United States in 2010, 14.5% of all live births occurred to women age 35 or older (J. A. Martin, Hamilton, Ventura, et al., 2012). Many factors have contributed to this trend, including the following:

- The availability of effective birth control methods
- The expanded roles and career options available for women
- The increased number of women getting advanced education, pursuing careers, and delaying parenthood until they are established professionally
- The increased incidence of later marriage and second marriage
- The high cost of living, which causes some young couples to delay childbearing until they are more secure financially
- The increased number of women in this older reproductive age group due to the baby boom between 1946 and 1964
- The increased availability of specialized fertilization procedures, which may help women previously considered infertile

There are advantages to having a first baby after age 35. Single women or couples who delay childbearing until they are older tend to be well educated and financially secure. Usually their decision to have a baby was deliberately and thoughtfully made (Figure 11–10 ●). Because of their greater life experiences, they

● **Figure 11–10** For many older couples, the decision to have a child may be very rewarding.

Source: Bill Bachmann/PhotoEdit

also are more aware of the realities of having a child and what it means to have a baby at their age. Many of the women have experienced fulfillment in their careers and feel secure enough to take on the added responsibility of a child. Some women are ready to make a change in their lives, wanting to stay home with a new baby. Those who plan to continue working typically can afford good child care.

Medical Risks

In the United States and Canada, the risk of death has declined dramatically during the past 30 years for women of all ages. However, the risk of maternal death is higher for women over age 35 and even higher for women age 40 and older. These women are more likely to have chronic medical conditions that can complicate a pregnancy. Preexisting medical conditions such as hypertension or diabetes probably play a more significant role than age in maternal well-being and the outcome of pregnancy. In addition, the rate of miscarriage, stillbirth, low birth weight, and perinatal morbidity and mortality is significantly higher in pregnant women over age 35 (Franz & Hussein, 2010). These women also have an increased risk for gestational diabetes mellitus, hypertension, placenta previa, and difficult labor (MOD, 2009). The cesarean birth rate is increased in pregnant women over age 35 (Bayrampour & Heaman, 2010). This practice may be related to pregnancy complications as well as to increased concern by the woman and physician about the pregnancy outcome.

The risk of conceiving a child with Down syndrome increases with age, especially over age 35. Consequently, all pregnant women, regardless of age, are offered screening for Down syndrome. Chapter 14 🔗 discusses screening tests in detail. Amniocentesis is routinely offered to all women over age 35 to permit the early detection of several chromosomal abnormalities, including Down syndrome. Genetic testing is not routinely offered to couples in whom there is only advanced paternal age, because there is not enough evidence to determine a paternal age at which to start genetic testing. Advanced paternal age is associated with adverse fetal and neonatal outcomes (Dechanet, Belaisch-Allart, & Hédon, 2010) and with increased risk of autism spectrum disorder (Ben Itzchak, Lahat, & Zachor, 2011).

Special Concerns of Expectant Parents over Age 35

No matter what their age, most expectant parents have concerns about the well-being of the fetus and their ability to parent. Expectant parents over age 35 often have additional concerns about their age, especially the closer they are to age 40. Some couples are concerned about whether they will have enough energy to care for a new baby. Of greater concern is their ability to deal with the needs of the child as they age.

The financial concerns of the older couple are usually different from those of the younger couple. The older couple is generally more financially secure, but when their "baby" is ready for college, the older couple may be close to retirement and might not have the means to provide for their child. The older couple may also be forced to face their own mortality. Certainly the realization of one's mortality is not uncommon in midlife, but older expectant parents may confront the issue earlier as they consider what will happen as their child grows.

Older couples facing pregnancy in a late or second marriage or after therapy for infertility may find themselves somewhat isolated socially. They may feel different because they are often the only couple in their peer group expecting their first baby. In fact, many of their peers are likely to be parents of adolescents or young adults and may be grandparents as well.

Older couples who already have children may respond quite differently to learning that the woman is pregnant, depending on whether the pregnancy was planned or unexpected. Other factors influencing their response include their children's, family's, and friends' attitudes toward the pregnancy; the impact on their lifestyle; and the financial implications of having another child. Sometimes couples who had previously been married to other mates will choose to have a child together. *Blended families* are formed when "her" children, "his" children, and "their" children come together as a new family group.

Healthcare professionals may treat older expectant parents differently than they would a younger couple. They may offer older women more medical procedures, such as amniocentesis and ultrasound, than younger women. They may also discourage an older woman from using a birthing room or birthing center even if she is healthy because her age is considered to put her at risk.

The woman who has delayed pregnancy may be concerned about the limited amount of time that she has to bear children. When pregnancy does not occur as quickly as she had hoped, the older woman may become increasingly anxious as time slips away on her "biological clock." When an older woman becomes pregnant but has a spontaneous abortion, her grief for the loss of her unborn child is exacerbated by anxiety about her ability to conceive again in the time remaining to her.

NURSING MANAGEMENT *For the Pregnant Woman over Age 35*

Nursing Assessment and Diagnosis

In working with a woman in her late 30s or 40s who is pregnant, make the same assessments as are indicated in caring for any woman who is pregnant. Assess physical status, the woman's understanding of pregnancy and its changes, the couple's attitudes about the pregnancy and their expectations of the impact a baby will have on their lives, their health teaching needs, the degree of support the woman has, and her knowledge of infant care.

The nursing diagnoses applicable to pregnant women in general apply to pregnant women over age 35. Examples of other nursing diagnoses that may apply include the following (NANDA-I © 2012):

- *Decisional Conflict* related to unexpected pregnancy
- *Anxiety* (moderate) related to uncertainty about fetal well-being

Planning and Implementation

Once an older couple has made the decision to have a child, respect and support the couple in this decision. As with any patient, discuss risks, identify concerns, and promote strengths. Do not make the woman's age an issue. It is helpful in promoting a sense of well-being to treat the pregnancy as normal unless the woman has specific health risks.

As the pregnancy continues, identify and discuss concerns the woman may have related to her age or to specific health problems. The older woman who has made a conscious decision to become pregnant often has carefully thought through potential problems and may actually have fewer concerns than a younger woman or one with an unplanned pregnancy.

Childbirth education classes are important in promoting adaptation to the event of childbirth for expectant parents of any age. However, older expectant parents often feel uncomfortable in classes in which most of the participants are much younger. Consequently, classes for expectant parents over age 35 are now available in many communities.

Women who are over age 35 and having their first baby tend to be better educated than other healthcare consumers. These patients frequently know the kind of care and services they want and may be assertive in their interactions with the healthcare system. You should not be intimidated by these individuals and should not assume that anticipatory guidance and support are not needed. Instead, support the couple's strengths and be sensitive to their individual needs.

In working with older expectant couples or an older single woman, the nurse should be sensitive to special needs. A particularly difficult issue these couples face is the possibility of bearing an unhealthy child or a child with a genetic disorder. As discussed previously, a quad screening test, also called multiple marker screen, is useful in assessing for Down syndrome. Because of the risk of Down syndrome in these families, amniocentesis is often suggested.

For couples who agree to amniocentesis, the first few months of pregnancy are a difficult time. Amniocentesis cannot be done until week 14 of pregnancy, and the chromosomal studies take roughly 2 weeks to complete. Their fear that the fetus is at risk may delay the successful completion of the psychologic tasks of early pregnancy.

You can support couples who decide to have amniocentesis by providing information and answering questions about the procedure and by providing comfort and emotional support during the amniocentesis. If the results indicate that the fetus has Down syndrome or another genetic abnormality, ensure that the couple has complete information about the condition, its range of possible manifestations, and its developmental implications.

Evaluation

Expected outcomes of nursing care include the following:

- The woman and her partner are knowledgeable about the pregnancy and express confidence in their ability to make appropriate healthcare choices.
- The expectant parents (and their children) are able to cope with the pregnancy and its implications for the future.
- The woman receives effective health care throughout her pregnancy and during birth and the postpartum period.
- The woman and her partner develop skills in child care and parenting.

Critical Concept Review

LEARNING OUTCOME 11.1: Describe the most appropriate nursing care to help maintain the well-being of the expectant father and siblings during a family's pregnancy.

1. Father:
   - Provide information about expected changes (physical and emotional) during pregnancy.
   - Encourage the father to express feelings about pregnancy and other related topics such as feeding, ability to parent, and sexual activity.
   - Refer the couple to parenting classes for information about labor and birth. Also provide for support from other couples in the same situation.
   - Assess father's intended level of participation during labor and birth.

2. Siblings:
   - Discuss the possible negative feelings of siblings that may take place at the birth of a new child.
   - Teach parents to use open communication during the transition time.

LEARNING OUTCOME 11.2: Explain the causes of the common discomforts of pregnancy in each of the three trimesters.

1. In the first trimester:
   - Nausea and vomiting are caused by increased levels of hCG as well as changes in carbohydrate metabolism.
   - Urinary frequency is caused by pressure of the uterus on the bladder.
   - Fatigue may be caused by urinary frequency at night.
   - Breast tenderness is caused by increased estrogen and progesterone.
   - Increased vaginal discharge is caused by cervical hyperplasia and increased production of mucus by the endocervical gland.
   - Nasal stuffiness and epistaxis are caused by increased estrogen levels.

2. In the second and third trimesters:
   - Heartburn is caused by increased levels of progesterone as well as decreased gastric motility, increased relaxation of cardiac sphincter, and increased size of uterus, which displaces the stomach.
   - Ankle edema is caused by prolonged sitting or standing, slow venous return, increased capillary permeability, and increased level of sodium.
   - Varicose veins are caused by venous congestion and weight gain.
   - Hemorrhoids are caused by constipation and slow venous return of blood.
   - Constipation is caused by slow peristalsis due to increased level of progesterone. Constipation is also caused by decreased fluids, decreased exercise, increased level of iron, and pressure of the uterus on the intestines.
   - Backache is caused by increased lumbosacral vertebrae curve due to enlarging uterus.
   - Leg cramps are caused by an imbalance of calcium and phosphorus, fatigue, and poor lower extremity circulation.
   - Faintness is caused by a sudden change of position, which precipitates postural hypotension.
   - Dyspnea is caused by decreased vital capacity due to increasing size of uterus.
   - Flatulence is caused by decreased gastric motility and air swallowing.
   - Carpal tunnel syndrome is caused by compression of median nerve precipitated by edema.

LEARNING OUTCOME 11.3: Summarize appropriate relief measures and interventions to alleviate the common discomforts of pregnancy.

1. In the first trimester:
   - For nausea and vomiting: avoid odors and eat dry crackers before arising in a.m. Drink fluids between meals and avoid greasy foods.
   - For urinary frequency: increase fluid intake during day and decrease in the evening.
   - For fatigue: plan rest periods and ask for help from family or support persons.
   - For breast tenderness: wear a well-supporting bra.
   - For increased vaginal discharge: bathe daily and wear cotton underwear.
   - For nasal stuffiness and epistaxis: use cool mist vaporizer.
2. In the second and third trimester:
   - For heartburn: eat small, frequent meals, avoid overeating and lying down after eating.
   - For ankle edema: elevate legs while sitting or standing and dorsiflex feet frequently.
   - For varicose veins: elevate legs as much as possible and wear support hose.
   - For hemorrhoids: avoid constipation. Use ice packs or sitz baths as necessary.
   - For constipation: increase fluid and fiber in diet. Develop regular bowel habits.
   - For backache: use good body mechanics and practice pelvic tilt exercises.
   - For leg cramps: apply heat to affected muscles and dorsiflex feet.
   - For faintness: change positions slowly, avoid standing for long periods of time.
   - For dyspnea: use good posture to sit and stand, and sleep in a semi-Fowler's position.
   - For flatulence: chew food completely and avoid gas-forming foods.
   - For carpal tunnel syndrome: avoid repetitive hand movement and elevate arm as needed.

LEARNING OUTCOME 11.4: Describe self-care measures that a pregnant woman can take to maintain and promote her well-being during pregnancy.

1. Breast care:
   - Wear a bra with good support and fit.
   - If breastfeeding, avoid soap on the nipples.
2. Clothing:
   - Should be loose and nonconstricting.
   - Wear low-heeled, comfortable, well-fitting shoes.
3. Bathing (be aware of cultural norms):
   - Be careful to avoid falls or feelings of faintness.
   - Shower may be easiest way to bathe in third trimester.
4. Employment:
   - Women with low-risk pregnancy can work until labor begins.
   - Workplace should be assessed for fetotoxic hazards.
5. Travel:
   - Avoid travel if woman has history of complications or has a multiple pregnancy.
   - With car travel, stop every 2 hours and walk. Position the seat belt under the abdomen.
6. Activity and rest:
   - Maintain regular exercise in uncomplicated pregnancy.
   - Avoid supine position.
   - Drink fluids and make sure to eat adequate amount of calories.
   - Avoid exercise during hot and humid weather.
   - Stop exercising with any suspicions of complications.
   - Plan for more sleep and regular rest periods.
   - Instruct in exercises to prepare for childbirth, including the pelvic tilt, partial sit-up, Kegel exercises, and the cross-legged sitting ("tailor sit") position.
7. Dental care:
   - Maintain regular dental checkups.
   - Dental work should be done in the second trimester.
   - Dental x-rays may be done if indicated as long as the woman is covered with a lead apron with a thyroid cuff.
8. Immunizations:
   - Avoid live virus vaccines.
9. Complementary and alternative therapies:
   - The nurse should develop understanding of most common ones.
   - The nurse should provide printed information about risks and benefits of homeopathic remedies and herbs.
10. Medications:
    - Avoid all OTC medications.
    - Take only medications approved by healthcare provider.
11. Substances to avoid during pregnancy:
    - All of the following should be avoided completely or decrease the amount of substance used: tobacco, alcohol, marijuana, and cocaine.
    - Caffeine has not been proven to impact pregnancy so women should be advised concerning common sources of caffeine and advised to moderate its use.

LEARNING OUTCOME 11.5: Examine the concerns that an expectant couple might have about sexual activity.

1. Traditional positions for intercourse may be uncomfortable; consider alternative positions.
2. Sexual desire may change during pregnancy.
3. Partners need to communicate feelings and needs.
4. Intercourse is contraindicated in:
   - Multiple pregnancy.
   - Threatened abortion.
   - Incompetent cervix.
   - Sexually transmitted infection.
   - Miscarriage following orgasm.
   - Rupture of membranes.
   - Preterm labor.

LEARNING OUTCOME 11.6: Discuss the medical risks and special concerns of expectant women older than age 35.

1. Medical risks:
   - Fetal death risk is increased for all women older than age 35.
   - Mother is more likely to have chronic medical conditions such as diabetes and hypertension that could pose a risk to the fetus.
   - Increased risk for cesarean birth.
   - Increased risk for autism when the mother and father are older, especially for first-born children.
   - Increased risk for Down syndrome and all autosomal dominant inherited disorders.

2. Special concerns:
   - Parents' ability to meet needs of child.
   - Not doing same things as peers, which could lead to social isolation.
   - Concern that "biological clock" continues to tick.
   - Fear of own mortality.

Clinical Reasoning in Action

Thirty-seven-year-old Cathy Sommers, G1, P0000, presents to you, with her husband, at the OB physician's office at 32 weeks' gestation. Cathy tells you that she and her husband are practicing lawyers with their own firm. The couple delayed starting a family because it has been important to them to advance their careers and establish their firm. Cathy had an amniocentesis at 18 weeks' gestation because of her advanced maternal age, and the results ruled out chromosomal abnormalities. The couple knows that the baby is a boy, and are anticipating a vaginal birth. Cathy tells you that she is experiencing more fatigue, leg cramps, and shortness of breath when climbing stairs. The physical exam including a negative Homans' sign is within normal limits with the exception of slight ankle edema. Her weight is 150 lb, temperature 98.6°F, pulse 88, respirations 16, BP 126/70. You discuss pregnancy discomforts in the third trimester with Cathy and her husband.

1. What measures can you suggest to cope with fatigue?
2. Discuss measures to decrease leg cramps.
3. Discuss the physiologic changes underlying dyspnea.
4. Review Braxton Hicks contractions.
5. Develop a concept map that could be used to assess whether leg pain in a pregnant woman is related to cramps or to thromboembolism.

See www.nursing.pearsonhighered.com for possible responses and an interactive template for a concept map.

References

American College of Obstetricians and Gynecologists (ACOG). (2009a). *Air travel during pregnancy* (Committee Opinion No. 443). Washington, DC: Author.

American College of Obstetricians and Gynecologists (ACOG). (2009b). *Exercise during pregnancy and the postpartum period* (Reaffirmation of Technical Bulletin No. 267). Washington, DC: Author.

American College of Obstetricians and Gynecologists (ACOG). (2010a). *Moderate caffeine consumption during pregnancy* (Committee Opinion No. 462). Washington, DC: Author.

American College of Obstetricians and Gynecologists (ACOG). (2010b). *Smoking cessation during pregnancy* (Committee Opinion No. 471). Washington, DC: Author.

Bayrampour, H., & Heaman, M. (2010). Advanced maternal age and the risk of cesarean birth: A systematic review. *Birth, 37*(3), 219–226.

Ben Itzchak, E., Lahat, E., & Zachor, D. A. (2011). Advanced parental ages and low birth weight in autism spectrum disorders—Rates and effect on functioning. *Research in Developmental Disabilities, 32*(5), 1776–1781.

Cunningham, F. G., Leveno, K. J., Bloom, S. L., Hauth, J. C., Rouse, D. J., & Spong, C. Y. (2010). *Williams obstetrics* (23rd ed.). New York, NY: McGraw-Hill.

Dechanet, C., Belaisch-Allart, J., & Hédon, B. (2010). Prognosis criteria for the management of the infertile couple. *Journal of Gynecology, Obstetrics, and Biology of Reproduction (Paris), 39*(8 Suppl 2), S9–S26.

Fontaine, K. L. (2011). *Complementary and alternative therapies for nursing practice* (3rd ed.). Upper Saddle River, NJ: Prentice Hall Health.

Franz, M. B., & Hussein, P. W. (2010). Obstetrical management of the older gravida. *Women's Health, 6*(3), 463–468.

Frederikson, M. C. (2011). The new FDA pregnancy labeling requirements for drugs. *Journal of Midwifery & Women's Health, 56*(3), 303–307.

Gouin, K., Murphy, K., & Shah, P. S. (2011). Effects of cocaine use during pregnancy on low birthweight and preterm birth: Systematic review and metaanalysis. *American Journal of Obstetrics and Gynecology, 204*(4), pp. 340. e1–12.

Gregory, K. D., Niebyl, J. R., & Johnson, T. R. B. (2012). Preconception and prenatal care: Part of the continuum. In S. G. Gabbe, J. R. Niebyl, J. L. Simpson, M. B. Landon, H. L. Galan, E. R. M. Jauniaux, & D. A. Driscoll (Eds.), *Obstetrics: Normal and problem pregnancies* (6th ed.). Philadelphia, PA: Elsevier Saunders.

Gyllstrom, M. E., Hellerstedt, W. L., & Hennrikus, D. (2012). The association of maternal mental health with prenatal smoking cessation and postpartum relapse in a population-based sample. *Maternal & Child Health Journal, 16*(3), 685–693. doi:10.1007/ s10995-011-0764-2

Homish, G., Eiden, R., Leonard, K., & Kozlowski, L. (2012). Social-environmental factors related to prenatal smoking. *Addictive Behaviors, 37*(1), 73–77.

Keegan, J., Parva, M., Finnegan, M., Gerson, A., & Belden, M. (2010). Addiction in pregnancy. *Journal of Addictive Diseases, 29*(2), 175–191.

Kimberly, D. G., Niebyl, J. R., & Johnson, T. R. B. (2012). Preconception and prenatal care: Part of the continuum. In S. G. Gabbe, J. R. Niebyl, J. L. Simpson, M. B. Landon, H. L. Galan, E. R. M. Jauniaux, & D. A. Driscoll (Eds.), *Obstetrics: Normal and problem pregnancies* (6th ed.). Philadelphia, PA: Elsevier Saunders.

Manant, A., & Dodgson, J. E. (2011). CenteringPregnancy: An integrative literature review. *Journal of Midwifery & Women's Health, 56*(2), 94–102.

March of Dimes (MOD). (2009). *Pregnancy after 35.* Retrieved from http://www.marchofdimes.com/ printableArticles/14332_1155.asp

Martin, J. A., Hamilton, B. E., Ventura, S. J., Osterman, M. J. K., Wilson, E. C., & Mathews, T. J. (2012).

Births: Final data for 2010. *National Vital Statistics Reports, 61*(1), 1–72.

Martin, L. T., McNamara, M., Milot, A., Bloch, M., Hair, E. C., & Halle, T. (2008). Correlates of smoking before, during, and after pregnancy. *American Journal of Health Behavior, 32*(3), 272–282.

Maxon, P., Edwards, S., Ingram, A., & Mirando, M. (2012). Psychosocial differences between smokers and non-smokers during pregnancy. *Addictive Behaviors, 37*(2), 153–159.

Melzer, K., Schutz, Y., Boulvain, Y., & Kayser, B. (2010). Physical activity and pregnancy: cardiovascular adaptations, recommendations and pregnancy outcome. *Sports Medicine, 40*(6), 493–507.

National Center for Complementary and Alternative Medicine (NCCAM). (2012). *Herbs at a glance: Ginger.* Retrieved from http://nccam.nih.gov/health/ginger

Niebyl, J. R., & Simpson, J. L. (2012). Drugs and environmental agents in pregnancy and lactation: Embryology, teratology, epidemiology. In S. G. Gabbe, J. R. Niebyl, J. L. Simpson, M. B. Landon, H. L. Galan, E. R. M. Jauniaux, & D. A. Driscoll (Eds.), *Obstetrics: Normal and problem pregnancies* (6th ed.). Philadelphia, PA: Elsevier Saunders.

Page, R., Padilla, Y., & Hamilton, E. (2012). Psychosocial factors associated with patterns of smoking surrounding pregnancy in fragile families. *Maternal & Child Health Journal, 16*(1), 249–257.

Purnell, L. D. (2009). *Guide to culturally competent health care.* Philadelphia, PA: F. A. Davis.

Spector, R. E. (2009). *Cultural diversity in health and illness* (7th ed.). Upper Saddle River, NJ: Prentice Hall Health.

Wisner, K. L., Sit, D. K. Y., Altemus, M., Bogen, D. L., Famy, C. S., Pearlstein, T. B., . . . Perel, J. M. (2012). Mental health and behavioral disorders in pregnancy. In S. G. Gabbe, J. R. Niebyl, J. L. Simpson, M. B. Landon, H. L. Galan, E. R. M. Jauniaux, & D. A. Driscoll (Eds.), *Obstetrics: Normal and problem pregnancies* (6th ed.). Philadelphia, PA: Elsevier Saunders.

Yankowitz, J. (2008). Drugs in pregnancy. In R. Gibbs, B. Karlan, A. Haney, & Y. I. Nygaard (Eds.), *Danforth's obstetrics and gynecology* (10th ed., pp. 122–136). Philadelphia, PA: Lippincott Williams & Wilkins.

Zavorsky, G. S., & Longo, L. D. (2011). Adding strength training, exercise intensity, and caloric expenditure to exercise guidelines in pregnancy. *Obstetrics & Gynecology, 117*(6), 1399–1402.

Maternal Nutrition

When I was young I thought nutrition was boring. Now that I am pregnant I find it endlessly fascinating. I realize how important good nutrition is for me, for my husband, and for the well-being of our child. My mother just laughs and reminds me about the times I resisted her efforts to help me develop better eating habits. Oh well, it is just another example of how smart our parents get as we get older! —Maria, 26

Monart Designs/Fotolia

LEARNING OUTCOMES

12.1 Describe the recommended levels of weight gain during pregnancy when providing nursing care for pregnant women.

12.2 Explain the significance of specific nutrients in the diet of the pregnant woman.

12.3 Compare nutritional needs during pregnancy, the postpartum period, and lactation with nonpregnant requirements.

12.4 Plan adequate prenatal vegetarian diets based on the nutritional requirements of pregnancy.

12.5 Explain the ways in which various physical, psychosocial, and cultural factors can affect nutritional intake and status in the nursing management of pregnant women.

12.6 Compare recommendations for weight gain and nutrient intakes in the pregnant adolescent with those for the mature pregnant adult.

12.7 Describe basic factors a nurse should consider when offering nutritional counseling to a pregnant adolescent.

12.8 Compare nutritional counseling issues for breastfeeding and formula-feeding mothers.

A woman's nutritional status before and during pregnancy can significantly influence her health and the health of her fetus. In most prenatal clinics and offices, nurses offer nutritional counseling directly or work closely with the nutritionist in providing nutritional assessment and teaching. This chapter focuses on the nutritional needs of the pregnant woman. Special sections consider the nutritional needs of the pregnant adolescent and the woman after giving birth.

Fetal growth occurs in three overlapping stages: (1) growth by increase in cell number, (2) growth by increase in cell number and cell size, and (3) growth by increase in cell size alone. Nutritional problems that interfere with cell division may have permanent consequences. If the nutritional deficit occurs when cells are mainly enlarging, the changes are usually reversible when normal nutrition resumes.

Growing fetal and maternal tissues require increased quantities of essential dietary components. These are listed in the **Dietary Reference Intakes (DRIs)**, a broad array of dietary reference values developed jointly by the United States and Canada, as either the *Recommended Dietary Allowance (RDA)* or *Adequate Intake (AI)*. An RDA is the daily dietary intake that is considered sufficient to meet the nutritional requirements of nearly all individuals in a specific life stage and gender group. An AI is a value cited for a nutrient when there is insufficient data to calculate an estimated average requirement. Women can get most of the recommended nutrients by eating a well-balanced diet each day. The basic food groups and recommended amounts during pregnancy and lactation are presented in Table 12–1.

MATERNAL WEIGHT GAIN

Maternal weight gain is an important factor in fetal growth and infant birth weight. Optimal weight gain depends on the woman's body mass index (BMI) (a measure of body fat based on height and weight) and her prepregnant nutritional state. An adequate weight gain indicates an adequate caloric intake. However, it does not ensure that the woman has a good diet nutritionally. The pregnant woman must maintain the nutritional quality of her diet as her weight gain progresses.

The Institute of Medicine (IOM) (2009) has established optimum ranges of weight gain based on a woman's BMI, and the American College of Obstetricians and Gynecologists (ACOG) (2013a) supports these recommendations. The IOM's optimum ranges of weight gain are as follows:

- *Underweight woman:* BMI less than 18.5: 28 to 40 lb (12.5 to 18 kg)
- *Normal-weight woman:* BMI between 18.5 and 24.9: 25 to 35 lb (11.5 to 16 kg)
- *Overweight woman:* BMI between 25 and 29.9: 15 to 25 lb (7 to 11.5 kg)
- *Obese woman:* BMI equal to or greater than 30: 11 to 20 lb (5 to 9.1 kg)

The average maternal weight gain is distributed as follows:

11 lb (5 kg)	Fetus, placenta, amniotic fluid
2 lb (0.9 kg)	Uterus
4 lb (1.8 kg)	Increased blood volume
3 lb (1.4 kg)	Breast tissue
5 to 10 lb (2.3 to 4.5 kg)	Maternal stores

The pattern of weight gain is important. For women of normal weight, the IOM recommendations are based on a first-trimester weight gain of 1.1 to 4.4 lb (0.5 to 2 kg) followed by a gain of about 1 lb (0.45 kg) per week during the second and third trimesters. The rate of weight gain in the second and third trimesters needs to be slightly higher for underweight women and slightly lower for women who are overweight (0.6 lb) or obese (0.5 lb) (IOM, 2009).

Table 12–1 Daily Food Plan for Pregnancy and Lactation

Food Group	Nutrients Provided	Food Source	Recommended Daily Amount During Pregnancy	Recommended Daily Amount During Lactation
Dairy products	Protein; riboflavin; vitamins A, D, and others; calcium; phosphorus; zinc; magnesium	Milk—whole, 2%, skim, dry, buttermilk Cheeses—hard, semisoft, cottage Yogurt—plain, low-fat Soybean milk—canned, dry	Four 8-oz cups (five for teenagers) used plain or with flavoring, in shakes, soups, puddings, custards, cocoa Calcium in 1 cup milk equivalent to 1½ cups cottage cheese, 1½ oz hard or semisoft cheese, 1 cup yogurt, 1½ cups ice cream (high in fat and sugar)	Four 8-oz cups (five for teenagers); equivalent amount of cheese, yogurt, etc.
Meat and meat alternatives	Protein; iron; thiamine, niacin, and other vitamins; and minerals	Beef, pork, veal, lamb, poultry, animal organ meats, fish, eggs; legumes; nuts, seeds, peanut butter, grains in proper vegetarian combination (vitamin B$_{12}$ supplement needed)	Three servings (one serving = 2 oz), combination in amounts necessary for same nutrient equivalent (varies greatly)	Two servings
Grain products, whole grain or enriched	B vitamins; iron; whole grain also has zinc, magnesium, and other trace elements; provides fiber	Breads and bread products such as cornbread, muffins, waffles, hotcakes, biscuits, dumplings, cereals, pastas, rice	Six to 11 servings daily: one serving = one slice bread, ¾ cup or 1 oz dry cereal, ½ cup rice or pasta	Same as for pregnancy
Fruits and fruit juices	Vitamins A and C; minerals; raw fruits for roughage	Citrus fruits and juices, melons, berries, all other fruits and juices	Two to four servings (one serving for vitamin C): one serving = one medium fruit, ½–1 cup fruit, 4 oz orange or grapefruit juice	Same as for pregnancy
Vegetables and vegetable juices	Vitamins A and C; minerals; provides roughage	Leafy green vegetables; deep yellow or orange vegetables such as carrots, sweet potatoes, squash, tomatoes; green vegetables such as peas, green beans, broccoli; other vegetables such as beets, cabbage, potatoes, corn, lima beans	Three to five servings (one serving of dark green or deep yellow vegetable for vitamin A): one serving = ½–1 cup vegetable, two tomatoes, one medium potato	Same as for pregnancy
Fats	Vitamins A and D; linoleic acid	Butter, cream cheese, fortified table spreads; cream, whipped cream, whipped toppings; avocado, mayonnaise, oil, nuts	As desired in moderation (high in calories): one serving = 1 tbsp butter or enriched margarine	Same as for pregnancy
Sugar and sweets		Sugar, brown sugar, honey, molasses	Occasionally, if desired	Same as for pregnancy
Desserts		Nutritious desserts such as puddings, custards, fruit whips, and crisps; other rich, sweet desserts and pastries	Occasionally, if desired	Same as for pregnancy
Beverages	Fluid	Coffee, decaffeinated beverages, tea, bouillon, carbonated drinks	As desired, in moderation	Same as for pregnancy
Miscellaneous		Iodized salt, herbs, spices, condiments	As desired	Same as for pregnancy

Note: The pregnant woman should eat regularly: three meals a day, with nutritious snacks of fruit, cheese, milk, or other foods between meals if desired. (More frequent but smaller meals are also recommended.) Four to six 8-oz glasses of water and a total of eight to ten 8-oz cups total fluid intake should be consumed daily. Water is an essential nutrient.

Evidence-Based Practice Optimal Weight Gain During Pregnancy

Clinical Question
What prenatal nursing interventions will help mothers reach an optimal weight gain goal?

The Evidence
Three studies focused on the characteristics of women and their prenatal care that resulted in optimal weight gain during pregnancy. The studies were of different designs, including a cross-sectional descriptive study, a randomized controlled trial, and a secondary data analysis. In all, the studies involved 756 women. The large sample, replication of findings, and variety of methodologies make this the strongest evidence for practice.

One of the studies focused on lifestyle modification programs, such as individual nutrition counseling, in-home reference materials, telephone-based feedback, and support for exercise. These interventions were found to result in a decreased percentage of women who exceeded normal weight gain, and also were related to a postpartum return to normal weight (Phelan, Phipps, Abrams, et al., 2011). One study focused on goal setting, with the nurse and mother setting realistic goals for pregnancy weight gain early in the prenatal period. In both of these studies, women who set realistic and explicit goals for weight gain during pregnancy gained an appropriate amount of weight more often than women who did not (Tuvar, Guthrie, Platek, et al., 2011). Women who were nonwhite, of advanced gestational age, and previous smokers were more likely to get the prenatal counseling they needed to achieve optimal prenatal weight gain (Stotland, Tsoh, & Gerbert, 2012).

Best Practice
Helping women set realistic goals for a healthy weight gain during pregnancy can help mothers achieve them. The nurse should focus on lifestyle modifications, for example, health counseling, exercise, and nutrition information, to support achievement of weight gain goals.

Clinical Reasoning
What are the components of an effective lifestyle modification plan for the prenatal period? How can the nurse help motivate the mother to set realistic goals and adhere to lifestyle modifications?

The IOM (2009) recommends that women be within a normal BMI when they become pregnant but that has become a true challenge because of the increasing prevalence of obesity in the United States and in many developed countries. In the United States, for example, more than half of pregnant women are classified as overweight or obese (ACOG, 2013b). Pregnant women who are obese are at risk for many pregnancy complications including gestational diabetes mellitus, preeclampsia, and cesarean birth. Their fetuses are at increased risk for congenital anomalies, stillbirth, prematurity, macrosomia, and childhood obesity. Thus it is recommended that these women receive counseling on strategies to move toward and to remain at a healthful weight prior to conceiving (ACOG, 2013b). If a woman's weight gain during pregnancy is inadequate or excessive, the healthcare provider should work closely with the woman to identify the reasons and develop an appropriate management plan (Siega-Riz, Deierlein, & Stuebe, 2010).

● **Figure 12–1** It is important to monitor a pregnant woman's weight over time.

Clinical Tip
Weight varies with time of day, amount of clothing, inaccurate scale adjustment, or weighing error. Do not overemphasize a single weight, but pay attention to the overall pattern of weight gain.

Because of the association between maternal weight gain and pregnancy outcome, most caregivers pay close attention to weight gain during pregnancy (Figure 12–1 ●). Weight gain charts can be useful in monitoring the rate and pattern of weight gain over time.

Counseling the pregnant woman to eat a variety of nutrients from each of the food groups places less emphasis on the amount of her weight gain and more on the quality of her intake. It may also be helpful to encourage her to begin a simple exercise program such as walking.

MyPlate, which replaced MyPyramid in 2011, is part of a federal initiative to encourage people to eat healthfully. It illustrates the five food groups and encourages people to make half their plates fruits and vegetables (U.S. Department of Agriculture [USDA], 2011b). See Figure 12–2 ●.

● **Figure 12–2** MyPlate is part of an initiative to encourage healthy eating. It illustrates the five food groups and encourages people to fill half their plates with fruits and vegetables.
Source: U.S. Department of Agriculture and U.S. Department of Health and Human Services.

NUTRITIONAL REQUIREMENTS

The RDA for almost all nutrients increases during pregnancy, although the amount of increase varies with each nutrient. These increases reflect the additional requirements of both the mother and the developing fetus.

Calories

The term **calorie (cal)** designates the amount of heat required to raise the temperature of 1 g of water 1°C. The **kilocalorie (kcal)** is equivalent to 1000 cal and is the unit used to express the energy value of food.

The RDA for energy requirements during pregnancy is as follows: no increase during the first trimester but an increase of 300 kcal/day during the second and third trimesters. Prepregnant weight, height, maternal age, health status, and activity level all influence caloric needs, and weight should be monitored regularly during the pregnancy. See *Teaching Highlights: Adding 300 kcal During Pregnancy.*

Carbohydrates

Carbohydrates provide the body's main source of energy as well as the fiber necessary for proper bowel functioning. If the total caloric intake is not adequate, the body uses protein for energy. Protein then becomes unavailable for growth needs. In addition, protein breakdown leads to ketosis.

The carbohydrate and caloric needs of the pregnant woman increase, especially during the last two trimesters. Carbohydrate intake promotes weight gain and growth of the fetus, placenta, and other maternal tissues. Dairy products, fruits, vegetables, and whole-grain cereals and breads all contain carbohydrates and other important nutrients.

Teaching Highlights Adding 300 kcal During Pregnancy

- The notion of "eating for two" may result in overeating.
- The additional 300 kcal/day recommended during pregnancy can be achieved by adding two milk servings and one serving of meat or alternative.
- MyPlate is designed to represent the food groups needed to make a balanced diet. Following MyPlate recommendations, women should aim to have half their plate consist of fruits and vegetables, make at least half their grains whole grains, and switch to fat-free or low-fat (1%) milk. Women are encouraged to drink water rather than sugary drinks and compare the sodium content of foods and choose foods that are lower in sodium (USDA, 2011b). A balanced diet includes the following:
  - *Grains:* Six to eleven servings (one serving = 1 slice bread, ½ hamburger roll, 1 oz dry cereal, 1 tortilla, ½ cup pasta, rice, grits)
  - *Fruits:* Two to four servings; one should be a good source of vitamin C (one serving = 1 medium-sized piece of fruit, ½ cup juice)
  - *Vegetables:* Three to five servings (one serving = 1 cup raw vegetable, 1 cup green leafy vegetable, ½ cup cooked vegetable)
  - *Dairy:* Two to three servings (one serving = 1 cup milk or yogurt, 1.5 oz hard cheese, 2 cups cottage cheese, 1 cup pudding made with milk)
  - *Meats and alternatives:* Two to three servings (one serving = 2 oz cooked lean meat, poultry, or fish; 2 eggs; ½ cup cottage cheese; 1 cup cooked legumes [kidney, lima, garbanzo, or soybeans, split peas]; 6 oz tofu; 2 oz nuts or seeds; 4 tbsp peanut butter)
- Not all foods that are nutritionally equivalent have the same number of calories; it is important to consider that when making food choices.
- Consider using low-fat milk, lean cuts of meat, or fish broiled or baked instead of fried.
- Foods can be combined. For example, 1 cup spaghetti with a 2-oz meatball would count as 1 serving meat, ¾ cup spaghetti = 1 grain, and ¼ cup tomato sauce = ½ serving vegetable.
- Use a calorie-counting guide to compare the calories in a variety of foods that are equivalent, such as 2 oz beef and 2 oz fish or 1 cup low-fat milk and 1 cup whole milk.

Protein

Protein supplies the amino acids required for the growth and development of maternal tissues, such as the uterus and breasts, and to meet fetal needs. This is especially important during the last half of pregnancy, when fetal growth is greatest.

The protein requirement for a pregnant woman is 60 g/day, an increase of 14 g over nonpregnant levels. Animal products such as meat, fish, poultry, and eggs provide high-quality protein. Dairy products are also important protein sources. A quart of milk supplies 32 g of protein, more than half the average daily protein requirement. A woman can incorporate milk into her diet in a variety of dishes, including soups, puddings, custards, sauces, and yogurt. Beverages such as hot chocolate and milk-and-fruit drinks can also be included, but they are high in calories. Various kinds of hard and soft cheeses and cottage cheese are excellent protein sources, although cream cheese is considered a fat source only. Women who have allergies to milk, are lactose intolerant, or practice vegetarianism may find soy milk acceptable. It can be used in cooked dishes or as a beverage. Tofu, or soybean curd, can replace cottage cheese.

Fat

Fats are valuable sources of energy for the body and aid in the absorption of fat-soluble vitamins. Fats are more completely absorbed during pregnancy, resulting in a marked increase in serum lipids, lipoproteins, and cholesterol, and decreased elimination of fat through the bowel. Fat deposits in the fetus increase from about 2% at midpregnancy to almost 12% at term. However, fat requirements are unchanged during pregnancy and should account for about 30% of daily caloric intake, of which 10% or less should be saturated fat.

Essential fatty acids are important for the development of the central nervous system of the fetus. Of particular interest are the omega-3 fatty acids and their derivative, docosahexaenoic acid (DHA). Maternal dietary intake of DHA during pregnancy may reduce the risk of preterm birth, preeclampsia, and low birth weight, and may enhance fetal and infant brain development (Jordan, 2010). Oily fish provide the best source of DHA (however, see the *Mercury in Fish* section later in this chapter); other sources include fortified dairy products, and even some fortified soymilk. Plant sources of omega-3 fatty acids include soybean oil, canola oil, flaxseeds and their oil, and walnuts.

Minerals

Calcium and Phosphorus

Calcium and phosphorus are involved in the mineralization of fetal bones and teeth and acid–base buffering. The body absorbs and uses calcium more efficiently during pregnancy. Some calcium and phosphorus are required early in pregnancy, but most fetal bone calcification occurs during the last 2 to 3 months. Teeth begin to form at about 8 weeks' gestation and are formed by birth. The 6-year molars begin to calcify just before birth.

The identified AI for calcium for the pregnant or lactating woman, ages 19 or older, is 1000 mg/day. It is 1300 mg/day for pregnant women younger than age 19. If calcium intake is low, fetal needs will be met at the mother's expense by demineralization of bone.

A diet that includes 4 cups of milk or an equivalent dairy alternative will provide sufficient calcium. Smaller amounts of calcium are supplied by legumes, nuts, dried fruits, and dark green leafy vegetables (such as kale, cabbage, collards, and turnip greens).

The RDA for phosphorus is 700 mg/day for the pregnant or lactating woman ages 19 and older. It is 1250 mg/day for pregnant women younger than 19 years. Because phosphorus is so widely available in foods, the daily requirement is readily supplied through calcium- and protein-rich foods.

Iodine

Iodine is an essential part of the thyroid hormone thyroxine. The thyroid gland may become enlarged if iodine is not replaced by adequate dietary intake or an additional supplement. Moreover, cretinism may occur in the infant if the mother has a severe iodine deficiency. Pregnant women can meet the iodine allowance of 220 mcg/day by using iodized salt. When salt is restricted, the physician may prescribe an iodine supplement.

Sodium

Sodium is essential for proper metabolism and the regulation of fluid balance. Sodium intake in the form of salt is never entirely restricted during pregnancy, even when hypertension is present. The pregnant woman may season food to taste during cooking but should avoid using extra salt at the table. She can avoid excessive intake by eliminating salty foods such as potato chips, ham, sausages, and sodium-based seasonings.

Zinc

Zinc is needed for protein metabolism and the synthesis of DNA and RNA. It is essential for normal fetal growth and development as well as milk production during lactation. The RDA during pregnancy is 11 mg/day for women ages 19 and older. This increases to 12 mg during lactation. Sources include meats, shellfish, poultry, whole grains, and legumes.

Magnesium

Magnesium is essential for cellular metabolism and structural growth. The RDA for pregnancy is 320 mg/day for women ages 19 to 30. Good sources include milk, whole grains, dark green vegetables, nuts, and legumes.

Iron

Iron requirements increase during pregnancy because of the growth of the fetus and placenta and the increased maternal blood volume. Anemia in pregnancy is mainly caused by low iron stores, although it may also be caused by inadequate intake of other nutrients, such as vitamins B_6 and B_{12}, folic acid, ascorbic acid, copper, and zinc. Iron-deficiency anemia is generally defined as a decrease in the oxygen-carrying capacity of the blood. Anemia leads to a significant reduction in hemoglobin in the volume of packed red cells per deciliter of blood (hematocrit) or in the number of erythrocytes. Iron-deficiency anemia in pregnancy is associated with an increased incidence of preterm birth, low-birth-weight infants, and maternal and infant mortality (Hark & Catalano, 2012).

Fetal demands for iron further contribute to symptoms of anemia in the pregnant woman. The fetal liver stores iron, especially during the third trimester. The infant needs this stored iron during the first 4 months of life to compensate for the normally inadequate levels of iron in breast milk and non–iron-fortified formulas.

To prevent anemia, the woman must balance iron requirements and intake. Adequate iron intake is a problem for nonpregnant women and a greater one for pregnant women. By carefully choosing foods high in iron, the woman can increase her daily iron intake considerably. Lean meats, dark green leafy vegetables, eggs, and whole-grain and enriched breads and cereals are the usual food sources of iron. Other iron sources include dried fruits, legumes, shellfish, and molasses.

Iron absorption is usually higher for animal products than for vegetable products. However, the woman can increase absorption of iron from nonmeat sources by combining them with meat or a food rich in vitamin C. The RDA for iron during pregnancy is 27 mg/day, but this intake is almost impossible to achieve through diet alone. Thus, in the second and third trimesters the pregnant woman should take a daily supplement of 30 mg elemental iron (Hark & Catalano, 2012). Unfortunately, iron supplements often cause gastrointestinal discomfort, especially if taken on an empty stomach. Taking the iron supplement after a meal may help reduce this discomfort. Iron supplements may also cause constipation, so an adequate fluid intake is important in pregnancy.

Vitamins

Vitamins are organic substances needed for life and growth. They are found in small amounts in specific foods and generally cannot be synthesized by the body in adequate amounts.

Vitamins are grouped according to solubility. Vitamins A, D, E, and K dissolve in fat; vitamin C and the B-complex vitamins dissolve in water. An adequate intake of all vitamins is essential during pregnancy; however, several are required in larger amounts to fulfill specific needs.

Fat-Soluble Vitamins

The fat-soluble vitamins, A, D, E, and K, are stored in the liver and thus are available if the dietary intake becomes inadequate. The major complication related to these vitamins is not deficiency but toxicity due to overdose. Unlike water-soluble vitamins, excess amounts of vitamins A, D, E, and K are not excreted in the urine. Symptoms of vitamin toxicity include nausea, gastrointestinal upset, dryness and cracking of the skin, and loss of hair.

Vitamin A is involved in the growth of epithelial cells, which line the entire gastrointestinal tract and make up the skin. It also plays a role in the metabolism of carbohydrates and fats. Without vitamin A the body cannot synthesize glycogen, and the body's ability to handle cholesterol is also affected. In addition, the protective layer of tissue surrounding nerve fibers does not form properly if vitamin A is lacking.

Probably the best known function of vitamin A is its effect on vision in dim light. A person's ability to see in the dark depends on the eye's supply of retinol, a form of vitamin A. Adequate vitamin A prevents night blindness. Vitamin A is associated with the formation and development of healthy eyes in the fetus. The RDA for vitamin A is 770 mcg/day for pregnant women ages 19 and older.

Although routine supplementation with vitamin A is not recommended, supplementation with 5000 International Units is indicated for women whose dietary intake may be inadequate, such as strict vegetarians and recent emigrants from countries where deficiency of vitamin A is endemic. Rich sources of vitamin A include deep green, deep orange, and yellow vegetables; animal sources include egg yolk, cream, butter, and fortified margarine and milk.

Vitamin D is best known for its role in the absorption and use of calcium and phosphorus in skeletal development. To supply the needs of the developing fetus, the pregnant woman should have a vitamin D intake of 5 mcg/day. Main food sources of vitamin D include fortified milk, margarine, butter, and egg yolks. Drinking a quart of milk daily provides the vitamin D needed during pregnancy. Vitamin D is also obtained through the synthesis of sunlight on the skin. During the winter months, however, women who live in northern latitudes are at risk for limited sun exposure as are women who routinely wear sun protection including high SPF products and protective clothing.

Vitamin D deficiency is more common than previously recognized, affecting 40% to 80% of pregnant women (Kaludjerovic & Vieth, 2010). While universal screening for vitamin D deficiency is not currently recommended, women at risk (vegetarians, women with limited sun exposure, ethnic and racial groups with dark skin) may be screened. If a deficiency is identified, a daily dose of 1000 to 2000 International Units is safe (ACOG, 2011).

Excessive intake of vitamin D usually comes from high-potency vitamin preparations, not from the diet. Overdoses during pregnancy can cause hypercalcemia, or high blood calcium levels, due to withdrawal of calcium from the skeletal tissue. Symptoms of toxicity include excessive thirst, loss of appetite, vomiting, weight loss, irritability, and high blood calcium levels.

The major function of vitamin E, or tocopherol, is antioxidation. Antioxidants such as vitamin E protect the body's cells from the destructive effects of free radicals. Vitamin E takes on oxygen, thus preventing another substance from combining with the oxygen in a process called oxidation. For example, vitamin E helps spare vitamin A by preventing its oxidation in the intestinal tract and in the tissues. It decreases the oxidation of polyunsaturated fats, thus helping to retain the flexibility and health of the cell membrane. For this reason, vitamin E affects the health of all cells in the body.

Vitamin E is also involved in certain enzymatic and metabolic reactions. It is essential for the synthesis of nucleic acids required in the formation of red blood cells in the bone marrow. Vitamin E is useful in treating certain types of muscular pain and intermittent claudication, in surface healing of wounds and burns, and in protecting lung tissue from the damaging effects of smog. These functions may help explain the abundant claims and cures attributed to vitamin E, many of which have not been scientifically proved.

The recommended intake of vitamin E for pregnant women is unchanged at 15 mg/day. Vitamin E is widely distributed in foodstuffs, especially vegetable fats and oils, whole grains, greens, and eggs. Excessive intake of vitamin E has been associated with abnormal coagulation in the newborn.

Vitamin K, or menadione (as used synthetically in medicine), is essential for the synthesis of prothrombin, so its function is related to normal blood clotting. It is synthesized in the intestinal tract by the *Escherichia coli* bacteria normally found in the large intestine. However, the body's need for vitamin K is not totally met by synthesis. Green leafy vegetables are excellent sources. The RDA for vitamin K does not increase during pregnancy.

Intake of vitamin K is usually adequate in a well-balanced prenatal diet. Problems may arise if an illness is present that results in malabsorption of fats or if antibiotics are used for an extended period, which would inhibit vitamin K synthesis by destroying intestinal *E. coli*.

Water-Soluble Vitamins

Water-soluble vitamins are excreted in the urine. Since only small amounts are stored, adequate amounts must be consumed daily. During pregnancy the concentration of water-soluble vitamins in the maternal serum falls, whereas high concentrations are found in the fetus.

The RDA for vitamin C (ascorbic acid) increases in pregnancy from 75 to 85 mg. Vitamin C's major function is to aid in the formation and development of connective tissue and the vascular system. Ascorbic acid is essential to the formation of collagen, which binds cells together. If the collagen begins to disintegrate because of a lack of ascorbic acid, cell functioning is disturbed and cell structure breaks down, resulting in muscular weakness, capillary hemorrhage, and eventual death. These are symptoms of scurvy, the disease caused by vitamin C deficiency. Surprisingly, newborns of women who have taken megadoses of vitamin C may have a rebound form of scurvy.

Maternal plasma levels of vitamin C progressively decrease during pregnancy, with values at term being about half those found at midpregnancy. It appears that ascorbic acid concentrates in the placenta; levels in the fetus are 50% or more above maternal levels.

A nutritious diet should meet the pregnant woman's needs for vitamin C without additional supplementation. Common food sources of vitamin C include citrus fruit, tomatoes, cantaloupe, strawberries, potatoes, broccoli, and other leafy greens. Ascorbic acid is readily destroyed by water and oxidation. Therefore, foods containing vitamin C must be stored and cooked properly.

The B vitamins include thiamine (B_1), riboflavin (B_2), niacin, folic acid, pantothenic acid, vitamin B_6, and vitamin B_{12}. These vitamins serve as vital coenzyme factors in many reactions such as cell respiration, glucose oxidation, and energy metabolism. The quantities needed increase as caloric intake increases to meet the metabolic and growth needs of the pregnant woman.

- *Thiamine.* Required amount increases from the prepregnant level of 1.1 mg/day to 1.4 mg/day. *Sources:* pork, liver, milk, potatoes, and enriched breads and cereals.

- *Riboflavin.* Deficiency is manifested by *cheilosis* (fissures and cracks of the lips and corners of the mouth) and other skin lesions. During pregnancy women may excrete less riboflavin and still require more because of increased energy and protein needs. An additional 0.3 to 1.4 mg/day is recommended for pregnant women ages 19 and older. *Sources:* milk, liver, eggs, enriched breads, and cereals.

- *Niacin.* Intake should increase 4 mg/day during pregnancy to 18 mg. *Sources:* meat, fish, poultry, liver, whole grains, enriched breads, cereals, and peanuts.

- *Folic acid (folate).* Required for normal growth, reproduction, and lactation, **folic acid** prevents the macrocytic, megaloblastic anemia of pregnancy, which is rarely found in the United States, but does occur. Inadequate intake of folic acid has been associated with neural tube defects (NTDs) (spina bifida, meningomyelocele) in the fetus or newborn. Although these defects are considered multifactorial (see Chapter 7), research indicates that 50% to

70% of spina bifida and anencephaly could be prevented by adequate intake of folic acid (Centers for Disease Control and Prevention [CDC], 2010). Consequently experts recommend that all women of childbearing age (15 to 45 years) consume 400 mcg of folic acid daily because half of all U.S. pregnancies are unplanned and NTDs occur very early in pregnancy (3 to 4 weeks after conception), before most women realize they are pregnant (CDC, 2012). Folic acid can be made inactive by oxidation, ultraviolet light, and heating. To prevent unnecessary loss, foods should be stored covered to protect them from light, cooked with only a small amount of water, and not overcooked. *Sources:* fresh green leafy vegetables, liver, peanuts, and whole-grain breads and cereals.

- *Pantothenic acid.* No allowance has been set during pregnancy, but 5 mg/day is considered a safe, adequate intake. *Sources:* meats, egg yolk, legumes, and whole-grain cereals and breads.

- *Vitamin B_6 (pyridoxine).* Associated with amino acid metabolism, thus a higher-than-average protein intake requires increased pyridoxine intake. The RDA during pregnancy is 1.9 mg/day, an increase of 0.6 mg over the allowance for nonpregnant women. Generally, the slightly increased need can be supplied by diet. *Sources:* wheat germ, yeast, fish, liver, pork, potatoes, and lentils.

- *Vitamin B_{12} (cobalamin).* Plays a role in the synthesis of DNA and red blood cells, and is important in maintaining the myelin sheath of nerve cells. Vitamin B_{12} is the cobalt-containing vitamin found only in animal sources. Women of reproductive age rarely have a B_{12} deficiency. Vegetarians/vegans (see later discussion on vegetarianism) can develop a deficiency, however, so it is essential that their dietary intake be supplemented with this vitamin. Occasionally vitamin B_{12} levels decrease during pregnancy but increase again after childbirth. The RDA during pregnancy is 2.6 mcg/day, an increase of 0.2 mcg. A deficiency may be because of a congenital inability to absorb vitamin B_{12}, resulting in pernicious anemia. Infertility is a complication of this type of anemia. *Sources:* foods that come from animals.

Clinical Tip

More women are consuming over-the-counter (OTC) vitamin, mineral, and food supplements today than in the past. Ask about the use of any OTC supplements to help avoid potentially harmful excess intakes.

Fluid

Water is essential for life, and it is found in all body tissues. It is necessary for many biochemical reactions. It also serves as a lubricant, as a medium of transport for carrying substances in and out of the body, and as an aid in temperature control. A pregnant woman should consume at least eight to ten 8-oz glasses of fluid each day, of which four to six glasses should be water. Because of their sodium content, diet sodas should be consumed in

Jaya Singh, a 28-year-old, G1P0, is 14 weeks pregnant. The rate and total amount of her weight gain during the first trimester have been consistent with recommendations. She has gained an average of 0.5 kg (1 lb) per week during both of the past 2 weeks. Her appetite is good, and she consumes three meals per day and snacks between meals on occasion.

Jaya has altered her diet because she is concerned about excessive weight gain. She told you that she has decreased her intake from the bread and dairy groups in order to limit her calorie intake. Because she has omitted most dairy products, she has increased her consumption of salads and broccoli to provide calcium sources.

A diet history revealed the following:

Grain	3–4 servings, mainly cereal and rice
Fruit	2–4 servings, fresh fruit
Vegetables	3–5 servings, salads, peas, corn, broccoli
Meat	4–5 servings, beef, pork, chicken
Dairy	occasionally cheese, ice cream, pudding
Fats, oils, sweets	occasionally salad dressings, margarine, desserts
Beverages	8–10 servings, soda, juices, water

After assessing her diet history, what is your evaluation of Jaya's diet? How would you counsel her?

See www.nursing.pearsonhighered.com for possible responses.

dairy products and eggs. An adequate, pure vegan diet contains protein from unrefined grains (brown rice, whole wheat), legumes (beans, split peas, lentils), nuts in large quantities, and a variety of cooked and fresh vegetables and fruits. Complete proteins can be obtained by eating different types of plant-based proteins such as beans and rice, peanut butter on whole-grain bread, and whole-grain cereal with soy milk, either in the same meal or over the day. Seeds may provide adequate protein in the vegetarian diet if the quantity is large enough. Obtaining sufficient calories to ensure adequate weight gain may be difficult because vegan diets tend to be high in fiber and therefore filling.

Because vegans use no animal products, a daily supplement of 4 mg of vitamin B_{12} is necessary. If soy milk is used, only partial supplementation may be needed. If no soy milk is taken, daily supplements of 1200 mg of calcium and 10 mg of vitamin D are needed.

Because the best sources of iron and zinc are animal products, vegan diets may also be low in these minerals. In addition, a high fiber intake may reduce mineral (calcium, iron, and zinc) bioavailability. Nurses need to emphasize the use of foods containing these nutrients. A vegetarian food group guide appears in Table 12–2.

FACTORS INFLUENCING NUTRITION

It is important to consider the many factors that affect a patient's nutrition. What are the age, lifestyle, and culture of the pregnant woman? What food beliefs and habits does she have? What a person eats is determined by availability, economics, and symbolism. These factors and others influence the expectant mother's acceptance of dietary recommendations.

Common Discomforts of Pregnancy

Gastrointestinal functioning can be altered at times during pregnancy, resulting in discomforts such as nausea, vomiting, heartburn, and constipation. Although these changes can be uncomfortable for the woman, they are seldom a major problem. These discomforts and dietary modifications that may provide relief are discussed in Chapter 11 🔗.

Use of Artificial Sweeteners

Foods and beverages that contain artificial sweeteners are increasingly available. Sweeteners classified as Generally Recognized as Safe (GRAS) by the Food and Drug Administration

moderation. Caffeinated beverages have a diuretic effect, which is counterproductive to increasing fluid intake.

VEGETARIANISM

Vegetarianism is the dietary choice of many people for religious, health, or ethical reasons. There are several types of vegetarians. **Lacto-ovovegetarians** include milk, dairy products, and eggs in their diet. **Lactovegetarians** include dairy products but no eggs in their diets. **Vegans** are "pure" vegetarians who will not eat any food from animal sources.

The expectant mother who is vegetarian must eat the proper combination of foods to obtain adequate nutrients. If her diet allows, a woman can obtain ample and complete proteins from

Table 12–2	Vegetarian Food Groups			
Food Group	Mixed Diet	Lacto-ovovegetarian	Lactovegetarian	Vegan
Grain	Bread, cereal, rice, pasta	Bread, cereal, rice, pasta	Bread, cereal, rice, pasta	Bread, cereal, rice, pasta
Fruit	Fruit, fruit juices	Fruit, fruit juices	Fruit, fruit juices	Fruit, fruit juices
Vegetable	Vegetables, vegetable juices	Vegetables, vegetable juices	Vegetables, vegetable juices	Vegetables, vegetable juices
Dairy and dairy alternatives	Milk, yogurt, cheese	Milk, yogurt, cheese	Milk, yogurt, cheese	Fortified soy milk, rice milk
Meat and meat alternatives	Meat, fish, poultry, eggs, legumes, tofu, nuts, nut butters	Eggs, legumes, tofu, nuts, nut butters	Legumes, tofu, nuts, nut butters	Legumes, tofu, nuts, nut butters

are acceptable for use during pregnancy and include acesulfame potassium (Sweet One®), aspartame (NutraSweet™, Equal™), saccharin (Sweet'N Low®, Sugar Twin®), and sucralose (Splenda®). As with other foods, moderation should be exercised in using artificial sweeteners.

Stevia sweeteners (Truvia®, PureVia™, Sun Crystals®) are the newest low-calorie sweeteners to become available. Derived from leaves of the *Stevia rebaudiana* Bertoni plant, rebaudioside-A is FDA approved for safe consumption as a sweetener. While Stevia sweeteners are marketed as natural, at this time the sweeteners offer no additional clinical advantages over any other non-nutritive sweetener (International Food Information Council, 2009).

Energy Drinks

Energy drinks, such as Monster Energy®, Red Bull, and 5-Hour Energy®, used to boost performance and delay fatigue have become increasingly popular in recent years. These beverages are soft drinks with ingredients such as caffeine, ginseng, guarana, taurine, and sugar added to provide stimulation and increase energy. Because they are classified as dietary supplements and not food, they are not subject to the same regulations and monitoring as food (Guilbeau, 2012). The caffeine content of energy drinks can be as high as 300 mg (equivalent to about three average cups of brewed coffee). Excessive intake of energy drinks can cause a variety of symptoms including anxiety, headache, agitation, tremors, seizures, psychosis, and altered mental state (Rath, 2012).

Energy drinks have come under scrutiny for the general public because of concerns about workplace safety when drinks are used to counter the effects of inadequate sleep and reports of deaths following excessive use (Meier, 2012). Research on the effects of caffeine on pregnancy are mixed, therefore pregnant women are advised to use energy drinks cautiously and include the drink's caffeine content in calculating daily caffeine intake in order to stay within recommended levels.

Foodborne Illnesses

Because of the risk of *Salmonella* contamination in raw eggs, pregnant women are advised to avoid eating or tasting foods that may contain raw or lightly cooked eggs. Examples include cake batter, homemade eggnog, sauces made with raw eggs such as Caesar salad dressing, and homemade ice cream.

Listeria monocytogenes is another bacterium that poses a threat to an expectant mother and her fetus. *Listeria* is especially challenging because the organism can be found in refrigerated, ready-to-eat foods such as unpasteurized milk and dairy products, meat, poultry, and seafood. To prevent listeria infection (listeriosis) pregnant women should be advised to do the following (U.S. Food and Drug Administration [FDA], 2011):

- Maintain refrigerator temperature at 40°F (4°C) or below and the freezer at 0°F (−18°C).
- Refrigerate or freeze prepared foods, leftovers, and perishables within 2 hours after eating or preparation.
- Do not eat hot dogs and luncheon meats unless they are reheated until they are steaming hot.

- Avoid soft cheeses such as feta, brie, Camembert, blue-veined cheeses, queso fresco, or queso blanco (a soft cheese often used by Hispanic women in their cooking) unless the label clearly states that they are made with pasteurized milk.
- Do not eat refrigerated patés or meat spreads, foods that contain raw (unpasteurized) milk, or drink unpasteurized milk.
- Avoid eating refrigerated smoked seafood such as salmon, trout, cod, tuna, or mackerel unless it is in a cooked dish such as a casserole. Canned or shelf-stable patés, meat spreads, and smoked seafood are considered safe to eat.

Mercury in Fish

Fish and shellfish are important parts of a healthy diet, but nearly all contain traces of mercury. Although this is not a concern for most people, some fish and shellfish contain higher levels of mercury than others, and mercury can pose a serious threat to the developing nervous system of an unborn baby or a young child.

SAFETY ALERT!

Women who are pregnant or who may become pregnant, breastfeeding mothers, and young children should not eat swordfish, shark, tilefish, or king mackerel because these fish contain high levels of methyl mercury.

Many pregnant women are aware of the mercury warning, but are far less aware of the important nutritional value of fish, especially fish high in DHA. Consequently, fish consumption has declined but a strong body of evidence supports the nutritional value of fish during pregnancy (Jordan, 2010; Newman, 2011). Thus, pregnant women need to be encouraged to eat at least 8 oz and up to 12 oz/week (two average meals) of shellfish and fish that are lower in mercury (USDA, 2011a). Commonly eaten fish that are lower in mercury include canned light tuna, shrimp, salmon, catfish, and pollack. Albacore (white) tuna has more mercury than canned light tuna; therefore only 6 oz/week of albacore tuna is recommended (USDA & U.S. Department of Health and Human Services, 2010).

Lactase Deficiency (Lactose Intolerance)

Some individuals have difficulty digesting milk and milk products. This condition, known as **lactase deficiency (lactose intolerance)**, results from an inadequate amount of the enzyme lactase, which breaks down the milk sugar lactose into smaller digestible substances.

Lactase deficiency is found in most adults of African, Mexican, Native American, Ashkenazi Jewish, and Asian descent and, indeed, in many other adults worldwide. People of northern European heritage are usually not affected. Symptoms include abdominal distention, discomfort, nausea, vomiting, loose stools, and cramps.

In counseling pregnant women who might be intolerant of milk and milk products, be aware that even one glass of milk can produce symptoms. Milk in cooked form, such as custards, is sometimes tolerated, as are cultured or fermented dairy products such as buttermilk, some cheeses, kefir, and yogurt.

Lactase deficiency need not be a problem for pregnant women because the enzyme is available over the counter in tablets or drops. Lactase-treated milk is also available commercially in some grocery stores.

Cultural, Ethnic, and Religious Influences

Cultural, ethnic, and religious backgrounds determine people's experiences with food and influence food preferences and habits (Figure 12–3 ●). People of different nationalities are accustomed to eating different foods because of the kinds of foodstuffs available in their countries of origin. The way food is prepared varies, depending on the customs and traditions of the ethnic and cultural group. In addition, the laws of certain religions forbid the use of some foods and direct the preparation and serving of meals. (See *Developing Cultural Competence: The Kosher Diet* as an example.)

In each culture certain foods have symbolic meaning. Generally these symbolic foods are related to major life experiences such as birth, death, or developmental milestones. Although generalizations have been made about the food practices of ethnic and religious groups, there are many variations. The extent to which people continue to eat traditional ethnic foods and follow food-related ethnic customs is affected by their exposure to other cultures and the availability, quality, and cost of traditional foods.

When working with pregnant women from any ethnic background, it is important to understand the impact of the woman's cultural beliefs on her eating habits and to identify any beliefs she may have about food and pregnancy. Talking with the patient can help determine the level of influence that traditional food

● **Figure 12–3** Cultural factors affect food preferences and habits.
Source: © Arto/Fotolia.

Developing Cultural Competence
The Kosher Diet

The kosher diet followed by many Jewish people forbids the eating of pork products and shellfish. Certain cuts of meat from sheep and cattle are allowed as are fish with fins and scales. In addition, meat and dairy products should not be mixed and eaten at the same meal, according to kosher dietary rules.

customs exert. It is then possible to give dietary advice in a way that is meaningful to the woman and her family.

Psychosocial Factors

Various psychosocial factors may influence a woman's food choices. The sharing of food has long been a symbol of friendliness, warmth, and social acceptance in many cultures. Some foods and food practices are associated with status. Some foods are prepared "just for company"; others are served only on special occasions or holidays.

Socioeconomic level may be a determinant of nutritional status. Poverty-level families cannot afford the same foods that higher income families can. Thus, pregnant women with low incomes are frequently at risk for poor nutrition.

Knowledge about the basic components of a balanced diet is essential. Often educational level is related to economic status, but even people on very limited incomes can prepare well-balanced meals if they know enough about nutrition.

The expectant mother's attitudes and feelings about her pregnancy influence her nutritional status. For example, foods may be used as a substitute for the expression of emotions, such as anger or frustration, or as a way of expressing feelings of joy. The woman who is depressed or does not wish to be pregnant may manifest these feelings in loss of appetite or overindulgence in certain foods.

Eating Disorders

Two serious eating disorders, anorexia nervosa and bulimia nervosa, affect millions of men and women, although they develop most commonly in adolescent girls and young women. Both conditions are psychologic disorders that can have a major impact on physiologic well-being.

Anorexia nervosa is an eating disorder characterized by an extreme fear of weight gain and fat. People with this problem have distorted body images and perceive themselves as fat even when they are extremely underweight. Their dietary intake is very restrictive in both variety and quantity. They may also engage in excessive exercise to prevent weight gain.

Bulimia is characterized by binge eating (secretly consuming large amounts of food in a short time) and purging. Self-induced vomiting is the most common method of purging; laxatives or diuretics may also be used. Individuals with bulimia nervosa often maintain normal or near-normal weight for their height, so it is difficult to know whether bingeing and purging occur.

Women with anorexia nervosa do not often become pregnant because of the physiologic changes that affect their reproductive systems. Women with bulimia can become pregnant. Their self-induced vomiting may produce many of the same complications as hyperemesis gravidarum (see Chapter 16 🔴). In both anorexia nervosa and bulimia, a multidisciplinary approach to treatment, involving medical, nursing, psychiatric, and dietetic practitioners, is indicated. Pregnant women with eating disorders need to be closely monitored and supported throughout their pregnancies.

Pica

Pica is the persistent eating of substances, such as soil or clay (geophagia), powdered laundry starch or corn starch (amylophagia), soap, baking powder, ice (pagophagia), freezer frost, burned matches, or ashes that are not ordinarily considered edible or nutritionally valuable. Most women who eat such substances do so only during pregnancy.

Women who practice pica may have nutrient deficiencies because they often consume a less varied diet than they might otherwise eat. Iron-deficiency anemia is the most common concern in pica. Eating laundry starch or certain types of clay may contribute to iron deficiency because they interfere with iron absorption. The ingestion of large quantities of clay could fill the intestine and cause fecal impaction; eating starch may be associated with excessive weight gain.

Assessment for pica is an important part of a nutritional history. However, a woman may be embarrassed about her cravings or reluctant to discuss them for fear of criticism. Using a nonjudgmental approach, give the woman information that can help her decrease or eliminate this practice. Some women are able to switch to eating nonfat powdered milk instead of powdered laundry starch and frozen fruit juice instead of ice. Others find that sucking on hard lemon or mint candies helps decrease the craving.

NUTRITIONAL CARE OF THE PREGNANT ADOLESCENT

Nutritional care of the pregnant adolescent is of particular concern to healthcare professionals. Many adolescents are nutritionally at risk because of a variety of complex emotional, social, and economic factors. Important nutrition-related factors to assess in pregnant adolescents include low prepregnant weight, low weight gain during pregnancy, young age at menarche, smoking, excessive prepregnant weight, anemia, unhealthy lifestyle (drugs or alcohol use), chronic disease, and history of an eating disorder.

The nutritional needs of adolescents are generally estimated by using the Dietary Reference Intakes (DRIs) for nonpregnant teenagers (ages 11 to 14 or 15 to 18) and adding nutrient amounts recommended for all women. If she is mature (more than 4 years since menarche), the pregnant adolescent's nutritional needs approach those reported for pregnant adults. However, adolescents who become pregnant less than 4 years after menarche are at risk due to their physiologic and anatomic immaturity. They are more likely than older adolescents to still be growing, which can affect the fetus's development. Thus, young adolescents (ages 14 and younger) need to gain more

weight than older adolescents (18 years and older) to produce babies of equal size.

In determining the optimal weight gain for the pregnant adolescent, add the recommended weight gain for an adult pregnancy to that expected during the postmenarchal year in which the pregnancy occurs. If the teenager is underweight, additional weight gain is recommended to bring her to a normal weight for her height.

Specific Nutrient Concerns

Caloric needs of pregnant adolescents vary widely. Major factors in determining caloric needs include whether growth has been completed and the physical activity level of the individual. Figures as high as 50 kcal/kg have been suggested for young, growing teens who are very active physically. A satisfactory weight gain usually confirms an adequate caloric intake.

An inadequate iron intake is a major concern with the adolescent diet. Iron needs are high for the pregnant teen due to the requirement for iron by the enlarging maternal muscle mass and blood volume. Iron supplements are definitely indicated.

Calcium is another important nutrient for pregnant adolescents. Inadequate intake of calcium is often a problem in this age group. Adequate calcium intake is necessary to support normal growth and development of the fetus as well as growth and maintenance of calcium stores in the adolescent. An extra serving of dairy products is usually suggested for teenagers. Calcium supplementation is indicated for teens who dislike milk, unless they consume enough other dairy products or significant calcium sources.

Because folic acid plays a role in cell reproduction, it is also an important nutrient for pregnant teens. As previously indicated, a supplement is usually recommended for pregnant females of all ages.

Other nutrients and vitamins must be considered when evaluating the overall nutritional quality of the teenager's diet. Nutrients that have frequently been found to be deficient in this age group include zinc and vitamins A, D, and B_6. Eating a variety of foods—especially fresh and lightly processed foods—helps the teen get adequate amounts of trace minerals, fiber, and other vitamins.

Dietary Patterns

Healthy adolescents often have irregular eating patterns. Many skip breakfast, and most tend to be frequent snackers. Teens rarely follow the traditional three-meals-a-day pattern. Their day-to-day intake often varies drastically, and they eat food combinations that may seem bizarre to adults. Despite these practices, adolescents usually achieve a better nutritional balance than most adults would expect.

In assessing the diet of the pregnant adolescent, it is important to consider the eating pattern over time, not simply a single day's intake. Once the pattern is identified, counseling can be directed toward correcting deficiencies.

Counseling Issues

Counseling about nutrition and healthy eating practices is an important element of care for pregnant teenagers. Nurses can effectively provide this counseling in a community setting. It may be individualized, involve other teens, or provide a combination of both approaches. If an adolescent's family member does most of the meal preparation, it may be useful to include that person in the discussion if the adolescent agrees. Involving the expectant father in counseling may also be helpful. Clinics and schools often offer classes and focused activities designed to address this topic.

The pregnant teenager's understanding of nutrition will influence not only her well-being but also that of her child. However, teens tend to live in the present, and counseling that stresses long-term changes may be less effective than more concrete approaches. In many cases, group classes are effective, especially those with other teens.

NURSING MANAGEMENT *For the Pregnant Woman Desiring Optimum Nutrition*

Nursing Assessment and Diagnosis

To plan an optimal diet with each woman, it is essential to assess nutritional status. The woman's chart and a patient interview provide information about the following:

- Woman's height and weight, as well as her weight gain during pregnancy
- Pertinent laboratory values, especially hemoglobin and hematocrit
- Clinical signs that have possible nutritional implications, such as constipation, anorexia, or heartburn
- Dietary history to evaluate the woman's views on nutrition as well as her specific nutrient intake

While gathering data, seek information about psychologic, cultural, and socioeconomic factors that may influence food intake. Also use the opportunity to discuss important aspects of nutrition within the context of the family's needs and lifestyle. A nutritional questionnaire is often useful in gathering and recording important facts. This information can be used to develop an intervention plan to fit the woman's individual needs. The sample questionnaire shown in Figure 12–4 ● has been filled in to demonstrate this process.

Once information is obtained, begin to analyze the information, formulate appropriate nursing diagnoses, and, with the woman, develop goals and desired outcomes. Nursing diagnoses might include the following (NANDA-I © 2012). For a woman during the first trimester, the diagnosis may be **Nutrition, Imbalanced: Less than Body Requirements** *related to nausea and vomiting.* If a woman has excessive weight gain, the diagnosis might be **Nutrition, Imbalanced: More than Body Requirements** *related to excessive caloric intake.* Be specific in addressing issues such as inadequate intake of nutrients, including iron, calcium, or folic acid; problems with nutrition because of a limited food budget; problems related to physiologic alterations, including anorexia, heartburn, or nausea; and behavioral problems related to excessive dieting, binge eating, and so on. At other times the diagnosis **Knowledge, Readiness for Enhanced,** *related to nutrition* may seem most appropriate, especially if the woman asks for information about nutrition.

Planning and Implementation

After determining the nursing diagnosis, plan an approach to address any nutritional deficiencies or improve the overall quality of the diet. To be truly effective, this plan must be made in cooperation with the woman. The following example demonstrates ways to plan with the woman based on the nursing diagnosis (NANDA-I © 2012):

- *Nutrition, Imbalanced: Less than Body Requirements* related to low intake of calcium
- *Goal:* The woman will increase her daily intake of calcium to the minimum DRI level.
- *Implementation:*
  1. Plan with the woman how to add more milk or dairy products to the diet (specify amounts).
  2. Encourage the use of other calcium sources such as leafy greens and legumes.
  3. Plan for the addition of powdered milk in cooking and baking.
  4. If none of the preceding options are realistic or acceptable, consider the use of calcium supplements.

Most families can benefit from guidance about food purchasing and preparation. Advise women to plan food purchases thoughtfully by preparing general menus and a list before shopping. It is also helpful to monitor sales, compare brands, and be cautious when purchasing convenience foods, which tend to be expensive. Other techniques for keeping food costs down without jeopardizing quality include buying food in season, using bulk foods when appropriate, using whole-grain or enriched products, buying lower grade eggs (grading has no relation to the egg's nutritional value but indicates color of the shell, delicacy of flavor, and so forth), and avoiding foods from specialty shops and foods in elaborate packaging.

Health Promotion: Optimizing Maternal–Fetal Health summarizes key actions pregnant women can take to optimize maternal health and reduce the risk of birth defects.

Evaluation

Once a plan has been developed and implemented, the nurse and patient may wish to identify ways of evaluating its effectiveness. Evaluation may involve keeping a food journal, writing out weekly menus, returning for weekly weigh-ins, and the like. If anemia is a special problem, periodic hematocrit assessments are indicated.

Health Promotion Optimizing Maternal–Fetal Health

- Achieve appropriate weight gain.
- Participate in regular physical activity (at least 30 minutes of moderate, safe activity on most, if not all, days).
- Consume a variety of healthy foods using MyPlate as a guideline.
- Take appropriate vitamin and mineral supplements.
- Avoid alcohol, tobacco, and other harmful substances.
- Follow safe food handling practices.

Source: Adapted from the American Dietetic Association (2008) position statement.

NUTRITIONAL QUESTIONNAIRE

Name Susan Longmont   Date 2-18-13

Age 20

Ethnic group Caucasian

Religion Protestant

Gravida 1   Para 0   EDB 9-12-13

Age of youngest child? NA

Birth weights of previous children? NA

Usual nonpregnant weight 119   Present weight 125

Weight gain during last pregnancy? NA

Vitamin or herbal supplements? none

Current medications? aspirin for headache

Do you smoke? yes   How much per day? 1-1½ packs

Have you ever had anorexia or bulimia? Please describe the circumstances.

Eating patterns:

1. How many meals per day? 2   when 12:30 pm 6:30 pm
2. How many snacks per day? 3   when 10:30 am 4:00 pm 10:00 pm
3. What other foods are important to your usual diet? chocolate and candy bars
4. Amount per day 4 bars/week
5. Do you have any different food preferences now? no
6. Do you eat nonfoods such as: Amount

   laundry starch   no   NA
   ice   yes   10 cubes/day
   other (name)   no   NA

7. What foods do you dislike or do not eat? spinach and dried beans
8. For added information complete a typical daily intake (24-hour recall is suggested).

Do you have special problems in food preparation such as:

1. Physical disability   yes ____ no ✔ Explain _____
2. Cooking appliances   yes ____ no ✔ Explain _____
3. Refrigeration of food   yes ____ no ✔ Explain _____

Who does the meal planning? I do.   shopping? We both do.

cooking? I do most of the time but my husband likes to help.

Are there transportation problems? We have only one car but we go in the evening.

Financial situation: My husband is working and going to school.

I am not working.   Food Stamps yes   WIC no

Do you have any previous nutritional problems? No. I have never paid much attention

to food before, but now I have lots of questions.

Are there any problems with this pregnancy? Nausea Yes, in the morning.

Constipation No   Other NA

Assessment by the nurse following the completion of the questionnaire.

Basic estimated nutrient and caloric value of typical daily intake.

Please circle one of the following:

Protein intake was   low   (adequate)   high
Caloric intake was   low   adequate   (high)
Calcium intake was   (low)   adequate   high
Iron intake was   (low)   adequate   high
Vitamin C intake was   low   (adequate)   high

● **Figure 12–4** The form shown here is a sample nutritional questionnaire used in the nursing management of a pregnant woman.

POSTPARTUM NUTRITION

Nutritional needs change following childbirth. Nutrient requirements vary depending on whether the mother decides to breastfeed. An assessment of postpartum nutritional status is necessary before nutritional guidance is given.

Postpartum Nutritional Status

Postpartum nutritional status is determined by assessing the new mother's weight, hemoglobin and hematocrit levels, clinical signs, and dietary history. As mentioned previously, an ideal weight gain during pregnancy is 25 to 35 lb (11.5 to 16 kg). After birth there is a weight loss of approximately 10 to 12 lb (4.5 kg to 5.4 kg). Additional weight loss is most rapid during the next few weeks as the body adjusts to the end of pregnancy. The mother's weight then begins to stabilize. This weight stabilization may take 6 months or longer.

The mother's weight should be considered in terms of ideal weight, prepregnancy weight, and weight gain during pregnancy. Refer women who want information about weight reduction to a dietitian or community-based nutritional program.

Hemoglobin and erythrocyte levels should return to normal within 2 to 6 weeks after childbirth. Iron supplements are generally continued for 2 to 3 months following childbirth to build stores depleted by pregnancy.

Constipation is a common problem following birth. To prevent it the woman should maintain a high fluid intake, which helps keep the stool soft. Dietary sources of fiber, such as whole grains, fruits, and vegetables, also help prevent constipation.

It is important to get specific information on dietary intake and eating habits directly from the woman. Visiting the mother during mealtimes provides an opportunity for unobtrusive nutritional assessment. Which foods has the woman selected? Is her diet nutritionally sound? A comment focusing on a positive aspect of her meal selection may initiate a discussion of nutrition.

Notify the dietitian about any woman whose cultural or religious beliefs require specific foods so that appropriate meals can be prepared for her. Also consider referring women with unusual eating habits or numerous questions about good nutrition to the dietitian. In addition, providing literature on nutrition ensures that the woman has a source of information at home.

During the childbearing years the risk for obesity becomes especially problematic for women. Consequently it is critical to use the postpartum period to change behaviors and help promote effective weight management in women.

Nutritional Care of Formula-Feeding Mothers

After birth the formula-feeding mother's dietary requirements return to prepregnancy levels. If the mother has a good understanding of nutritional principles, it is sufficient to advise her to reduce her daily caloric intake by about 300 kcal and to return to prepregnancy levels for other nutrients. If the mother has a limited understanding of nutrition, now is the time to teach her the basic principles and the importance of a well-balanced diet. Her eating habits and dietary practices will eventually be reflected in the diet of her child.

If the mother has gained excessive weight during pregnancy (or perhaps was overweight before pregnancy) and wishes to lose weight, a referral to the dietitian is appropriate. The dietitian can design weight reduction diets to meet nutritional needs and food preferences. Weight loss goals of 1 to 2 lb (0.45 to 0.9 kg)/week are usually suggested.

In addition to meeting her own nutritional needs, the new mother is usually interested in learning how to provide for her infant's nutritional needs. A discussion of infant feeding that includes topics such as selecting infant formulas, formula preparation, and vitamin and mineral supplementation are appropriate and generally well received.

Nutritional Care of Breastfeeding Mothers

A breastfeeding woman needs increased nutrients. Table 12–1 provides a sample daily food guide for lactating women. It is especially important for the breastfeeding mother to consume sufficient calories, because inadequate caloric intake can reduce milk volume. However, milk quality generally remains unaffected. The breastfeeding mother should increase her calories by about 200 kcal over her pregnancy requirement, or 500 kcal over her prepregnancy requirement. This results in a total of about 2500 to 2700 kcal/day for most women.

Because protein is an important ingredient in breast milk, an adequate intake while breastfeeding is essential. An intake of 65 g/day during the first 6 months of breastfeeding and 62 g/day during the second 6 months is recommended. As in pregnancy, it is important to consume adequate nonprotein calories to prevent the use of protein as an energy source.

Calcium is an important ingredient in milk production. Requirements during lactation remain the same as during pregnancy—an increase of 1000 mg/day. If the intake of calcium from food sources is not adequate, calcium supplements are recommended.

Iron is not a principal mineral component of milk; thus, the needs of lactating women are not substantially different from those of nonpregnant women. However, supplementation for 2 to 3 months after childbirth is advisable to replenish maternal stores depleted by pregnancy.

 Clinical Tip

Explain to breastfeeding mothers that liquids are especially important during lactation, because inadequate fluid intake may decrease milk volume. Encourage them to drink at least eight to ten 8-oz glasses of fluid daily, including water, juice, milk, and soups.

In addition to counseling breastfeeding mothers on how to meet their increased nutrient needs, the nurse should discuss a few issues related to infant feeding. For example, many mothers are concerned about how specific foods they eat will affect their babies during breastfeeding. Generally the breastfeeding mother need not avoid any foods except those to which she might be allergic. Occasionally, however, some breastfeeding mothers find that their babies are affected by certain foods. Onions, turnips, cabbage, chocolate, spices, and seasonings are commonly listed as offenders. The best advice to give the breastfeeding mother is to avoid those foods she suspects cause distress in her infant. For the most part, however, she should be able to eat any nourishing food she wants without fear that her baby will be affected. For further discussion of successful infant feeding, see Chapter 26 🔗.

COMMUNITY RESOURCES

Food is a significant portion of a family's budget, and meeting nutritional needs may be a challenge for families on limited incomes. Community-based services offered through clinics, local agencies, schools, and volunteer organizations address these needs. Increasingly nurses play an important role in managing such community-based services, especially services focusing on patient education.

Most communities offer special assistance to qualifying families to meet their nutritional needs. The Food Stamp Program provides stamps or coupons for participating households whose net monthly income is below a specified level. These stamps can be used to purchase food for the household each month.

The Special Supplemental Nutrition Program for Women, Infants, and Children (WIC) is designed to assist pregnant or breastfeeding women with low incomes and their children younger than 5 years of age. The program provides food assistance, nutrition education, and referrals to healthcare providers. The food distributed, including dried beans and peas, peanut butter, eggs, cheese, milk, fortified adult and infant cereals, juice, and iron-fortified formula, is designed to provide good sources of iron, protein, and certain vitamins and minerals for people with an inadequate diet.

Critical Concept Review

LEARNING OUTCOME 12.1: Describe the recommended levels of weight gain during pregnancy when providing nursing care for pregnant women.

1. Weight gain recommendations depend on the woman's prepregnancy weight:
   - Underweight: 28–40 lb (12.5–18 kg).
   - Normal weight: 25–35 lb (11.5–16 kg).
   - Overweight: 15–25 lb (7–11.5 kg).
   - Obese: less than or equal to 15 lb (less than or equal to 7 kg).

LEARNING OUTCOME 12.2: Explain the significance of specific nutrients in the diet of the pregnant woman.

1. Carbohydrates: The body's primary source of energy. Promotes weight gain and growth of the fetus and placenta.
2. Protein: Supplies needed amino acids for growth of tissue.
3. Fat: Source of maternal energy; also promotes fetal fat deposits.
4. Calcium and phosphorus: Promotes mineralization of fetal bones and teeth.
5. Iodine: Promotes fetal thyroid gland function.
6. Sodium: Regulates fluid balance and metabolism in the mother.
7. Zinc: Promotes growth of fetus and sufficient lactation.
8. Magnesium: Promotes cellular metabolism and bone mineralization.
9. Iron: Prevents maternal anemia and contributes to fetal and infant stores of iron.
10. Vitamins: Maintain good maternal health. Folic acid, taken prior to conception, may prevent neural tube defects in the fetus.

LEARNING OUTCOME 12.3: Compare nutritional needs during pregnancy, the postpartum period, and lactation with nonpregnant requirements.

1. During pregnancy and lactation, nutritional requirements increase significantly from nonpregnant requirements:
   - Calories in second and third trimester increase by 300 kcal/day, and during lactation, by another 200 kcal/day.
   - Protein increases by 14 mg to 60 g/day.
   - Calcium requirements for the pregnant or lactating woman increase to 1000–1300 mg/day depending on the age of the woman.
   - Magnesium increases to 350 mg/day.
   - Iron increases to 27 mg/day. (It is very difficult to eat enough iron-rich foods in the regular diet, so iron supplements are commonly prescribed.)
   - Iodine increases to 220 mcg/day.
   - Zinc increases to 11 mg/day during pregnancy and 12 mg/day during lactation.
   - Vitamin A increases to 770 mcg/day.
   - Vitamin D increases to 5 mcg/day.
   - Vitamin C increases from 75 to 85 mg/day.
   - Thiamine increases from 1.1 to 1.4 mg/day.
   - Riboflavin increases from 1.1 to 1.4 mg/day.
   - Niacin increases from 14 to 18 mg/day.
   - Pantothenic acid increases to 5 mg/day.
   - Vitamin B_{12} increases from 2.4 to 2.6 mcg/day.
   - Fluid needs increase to 8–10 glasses of noncaffeinated beverages/day.
2. For nonbreastfeeding mothers, during the postpartum period, nutritional requirements return to prepregnancy levels.

LEARNING OUTCOME 12.4: Plan adequate prenatal vegetarian diets based on the nutritional requirements of pregnancy.

1. There are different types of vegetarian diets, which differ in the types of animal-based products that are eaten.
2. Vegans do not eat any animal-based products, but can obtain protein from beans, rice, peanut butter, soy products, and seeds. Most vegans need additional supplementation of vitamins B12 and D and calcium.
3. Vegetarians' daily food requirements are:
   - 6–11 servings of whole grains, cereal, pasta, and rice.
   - 2–4 servings of fruit.
   - 3–5 servings of vegetables.
   - 2–3 servings of legumes, nuts, seeds, and meat alternatives.
   - 2–3 servings of milk products (unless vegan).

LEARNING OUTCOME 12.5: Explain the ways in which various physical, psychosocial, and cultural factors can affect nutritional intake and status in the nursing management of pregnant women.

1. Nausea, vomiting, constipation, and heartburn can limit a woman's intake of nutritional foods especially during the first trimester.
2. Lactose intolerance may cause diarrhea or bloating after intake of dairy products.
3. Cultural, ethnic, and religious influences may prohibit use of certain foods that are needed for adequate nutrition.
4. Socioeconomic level may limit amounts of nutritional foods available to the woman.

5. Lack of knowledge about proper nutrition may limit the woman's ability to prepare nutritional foods.
6. Patients with eating disorders may have nutritional and electrolyte imbalances due to starvation or vomiting.
7. Pica may result in iron-deficiency anemia.

LEARNING OUTCOME 12.6: Compare recommendations for weight gain and nutrient intakes in the pregnant adolescent with those for the mature pregnant adult.

1. Weight gain: Add recommended weight gain of the adult pregnancy to the expected gain of the adolescent.

2. Nutrient needs: Adolescent needs more iron, calcium, and folic acid than the adult pregnant woman.

LEARNING OUTCOME 12.7: Describe basic factors a nurse should consider when offering nutritional counseling to a pregnant adolescent.

1. Basic factors to consider:
   - Number of years since adolescent reached menarche.
   - Whether growth has been completed.
   - Most adolescents have irregular eating patterns.
   - Adolescent may not be the one who regularly prepares meals, so the individual who prepares meals should be included in nutritional counseling.
   - Teens are present, not future, oriented, which impacts nutritional counseling.

LEARNING OUTCOME 12.8: Compare nutritional counseling issues for breastfeeding and formula-feeding mothers.

1. Formula-feeding mothers:
   - Eat a well-balanced diet.
   - Dietary requirements are the same as before pregnancy.
   - Weight loss of 1–2 lb/week is acceptable.
2. Breastfeeding mothers:
   - Calorie requirements increase by 200 kcal/day over needs during pregnancy.
   - Need 2500–2700 kcal/day.
   - Need 65 g/day of protein.
   - Need 1000 mg/day of calcium.
   - Should avoid foods that irritate the infant.

Clinical Reasoning in Action

Sandra Hill is a 17-year-old at 19 weeks' gestation with her first pregnancy. She presents to you accompanied by her mother. Her mother tells you that Sandra is an active teenager who plays sports and has been taking dance lessons for 5 years. She maintains a B+ average in school. Sandra voices concern about potential weight gain during pregnancy. She tells you that this was not a planned pregnancy and she has ambivalent feelings about it. You become concerned as she tells you that she has reduced her caloric intake over the past few months to try to keep her weight down and camouflage her pregnancy. You do a nutritional assessment and find that she is deficient in calcium, iron, and protein. Sandra seems to have irregular eating patterns and she admits to skipping breakfast often. She asks why she has to gain so much weight when you explain the nutritional needs of her baby during the pregnancy.

1. Discuss weight distribution in pregnancy.
2. Discuss foods that will increase calcium, protein, and iron in her diet.
3. Explain why folate supplementation is important.
4. What criteria will measure adequate caloric intake during pregnancy?

See www.nursing.pearsonhighered.com for possible responses.

References

American College of Obstetricians and Gynecologists (ACOG). (2011). *Vitamin D: Screening and supplementation during pregnancy* (Committee Opinion No. 495). Washington, DC: Author.

American College of Obstetricians and Gynecologists (ACOG). (2013a). *Obesity in pregnancy* (Committee Opinion No. 549). Washington, DC: Author.

American College of Obstetricians and Gynecologists (ACOG). (2013b). *Weight gain during pregnancy* (Committee Opinion No. 548). Washington, DC: Author.

American Dietetic Association. (2008). Position of the American Dietetic Association: Nutrition and lifestyle for a healthy pregnancy outcome. *Journal of the American Dietetic Association, 108*(3), 553–561.

Centers for Disease Control and Prevention (CDC). (2010). *Folic acid: Data and statistics.* Retrieved from http://www.cdc.gov/ncbddd/folicacid/data.html

Centers for Disease Control and Prevention (CDC). (2012). *Folic acid: Recommendations.* Retrieved from http://www.cdc.gov/ncbddd/folicacid/recommendations.html

Guilbeau, J. R. (2012). Health risks of energy drinks. *Nursing for Women's Health, 16*(5), 423–428.

Hark, L., & Catalano, P. M. (2012). Nutritional management during pregnancy. In S. G. Gabbe, J. R. Niebyl, J. L. Simpson, M. B. Landon, H. L. Galan, E. R. M. Jauniaux, & D. A. Driscoll (Eds.), *Obstetrics: Normal and problem pregnancies* (6th ed.). Philadelphia, PA: Elsevier Saunders.

Institute of Medicine (IOM). (2009). *Weight gain during pregnancy: Reexamining the guidelines.* Washington, DC: National Academies Press.

International Food Information Council. (2009). Stevia sweeteners: Another low-calorie option. *Food Insight*. Retrieved from http://www.foodinsight.org/Newsletter/Detail.aspx?topic=Stevia_Sweeteners_Another_Low_Calorie_Option

Jordan, R. G. (2010). Prenatal omega-3 fatty acids: Review and recommendations. *Journal of Midwifery and Women's Health, 55*(6), 520–528.

Kaludjerovic, J., & Vieth, R. (2010). Relationship between vitamin D during perinatal development and health. *Journal of Midwifery & Women's Health, 55*(6), 550–560.

Meier, B. (2012). F.D.A. may tap experts on energy drinks. *New York Times*. Retrieved from http://www.nytimes.com/2012/11/28/business/fda-may-tap-experts-on-energy-drinks.html?_r=0

Newman, R. (2011). How much fish should I eat during pregnancy? *Contemporary OB/GYN, 56*(5), 56–60.

Phelan, S., Phipps, M., Abrams, B., Darroch, F., Schaffner, A., & Wing, R. (2011). Randomized trial of a behavioral intervention to prevent excessive gestational weight gain: The Fit for Delivery study. *American Journal of Clinical Nutrition, 93*(4), 772–779.

Rath, M. (2012). Energy drinks: What is all the hype? The dangers of energy drink consumption. *Journal of the American Academy of Nurse Practitioners, 24*(2), 70–76.

Siega-Riz, A. M., Deierlein, A., & Stuebe, A. (2010). Implementation of the new Institute of Medicine gestational weight gain guidelines. *Journal of Midwifery & Women's Health, 55*(6), 512–519.

Stotland, N., Tsoh, J., & Gerbert, B. (2012). Prenatal weight gain: Who gets counseled? *Journal of Women's Health, 21*(6), 695–701.

Tuvar, A., Guthrie, L., Platek, D., Stuebe, A., Herring, S., & Oken, E. (2011). Modifiable predictors associated with having a gestational weight gain goal. *Maternal & Child Health Journal, 15*(7), 1119–1126.

U.S. Department of Agriculture (USDA). (2011a). *Eating fish while you are pregnant or breastfeeding*. Retrieved from http://www.choosemyplate.gov/pregnancy-breastfeeding/eating-fish.html

U.S. Department of Agriculture (USDA). (2011b). *MyPlate home page*. Retrieved from http://www.cnpp.usda.gov/MyPlate.htm

U.S. Department of Agriculture (USDA) & U.S. Department of Health and Human Services. (2010). *Dietary guidelines for Americans, 2010* (7th ed.). Washington, DC: U.S. Government Printing Office.

U.S. Food and Drug Administration (FDA). (2011). *Food safety for moms-to-be*. Retrieved from http://www.fda.gov/Food/ResourcesForYou/HealthEducators/ucm081785.htm

Pearson Nursing Student Resources Find additional review materials at: **nursing.pearsonhighered.com**

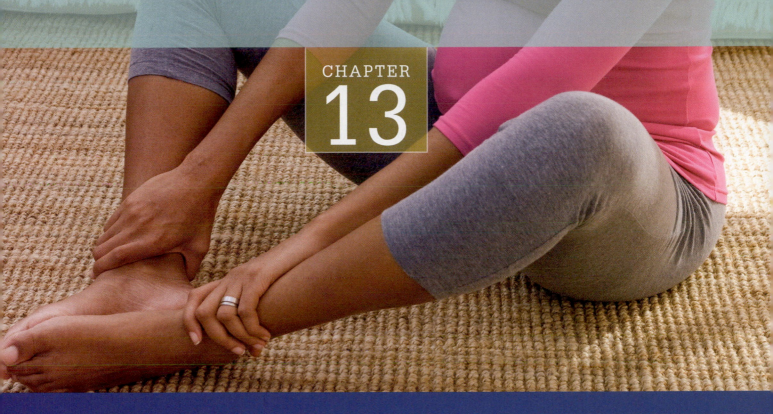

CHAPTER

13

Adolescent Pregnancy

I was a child when I had my daughter—just 16—and so afraid. I was one of the lucky ones though. My parents were wonderfully supportive and I went to a special teen clinic for my pregnancy. The nurses really taught me a lot about my body and about taking care of my baby. With help and encouragement from mom and dad, I got by. Last spring, at age 28 I graduated with a degree in nursing. I wanted a job with real security and opportunity, but more important, I want to give something back, to give others a little of the support I received. —Joanna, 29

Kevin Peterson/Getty Images

LEARNING OUTCOMES

13.1 Describe the scope of the problem and the impact of adolescent pregnancy.

13.2 Describe the major factors that contribute to adolescent pregnancy.

13.3 Identify the physical, psychologic, and sociologic risks a pregnant adolescent faces.

13.4 Delineate the characteristics of the fathers of children of adolescent mothers.

13.5 Discuss the possible reactions of the adolescent's family and social network to her pregnancy.

13.6 Formulate a plan of care to meet the needs of a pregnant adolescent.

13.7 Describe successful community approaches to prevention of adolescent pregnancy.

Pregnancy can be challenging, especially for the adolescent expectant mother. In the United States each year about 750,000 teenage girls (ages 15 to 19) become pregnant. Of these pregnancies, about one fourth (26%) are terminated by therapeutic abortion (Alan Guttmacher Institute [AGI], 2012a). A portion of pregnancies end in miscarriage but more than half of teens who become pregnant give birth and keep their babies.

In 2010, the birth rate (number of births per 1000 women) for adolescents ages 15 to 19 fell to 34.3, a historic low level, specifically the lowest rate reported in the past seven decades. See Figure 13–1 ●. Equally significant, these declines occurred for all race and Hispanic origin groups, although rates for Hispanic teens (55.7) and non-Hispanic black teens (51.5) remain considerably higher than the rates for non-Hispanic white teens (23.5) (Hamilton & Ventura, 2012). The United States continues to have the highest adolescent birth rates among industrialized nations (National Campaign to Prevent Teen and Unplanned Pregnancy [NCPTUP], 2012a). The incidence of sexual activity among teens in many other countries is as high as it is in the United States. However, these countries may have lower adolescent pregnancy rates because of family influences, a greater openness about sexuality, better access to contraceptives, and a more comprehensive approach to sex education.

This chapter explores the issue of adolescent pregnancy and the role of the nurse in meeting the special needs and concerns of pregnant adolescents and their families. It concludes with a discussion of efforts to prevent adolescent pregnancy.

OVERVIEW OF THE ADOLESCENT PERIOD

Physical Changes

Puberty—that period during which an individual becomes capable of reproduction—is a maturational process that can last from 1.5 to 6 years. The major physical changes of puberty include a growth spurt, weight change, and the appearance of secondary sexual characteristics. Menarche, or the time of the first menstrual period, usually occurs in the last half of this maturational process, with the average age between 12 and 13. The initial menstrual cycles are usually irregular and often anovulatory, although not always. Thus, contraception is important for all sexually active adolescents.

Psychosocial Development

Many writers have described the developmental tasks of adolescence, based on a variety of classic theories. The following are major developmental tasks of this period (Steinberg, 2010):

- Developing a sense of identity
- Gaining autonomy and independence
- Developing intimacy in a relationship
- Developing comfort with one's own sexuality
- Developing a sense of achievement

Resolution of these tasks is a developmental process that occurs over time. Although average ages for the completion of tasks have been identified, these ages are somewhat arbitrary and are affected by many factors, including culture, religion, and socioeconomic status.

In **early adolescence** (ages 14 and under) the teen still sees authority in his/her parents. However, he or she begins the process of gaining independence from the family by spending more time with friends. Conformity to peer group standards is important. The adolescent in this phase is very egocentric and is a concrete thinker, with only minimal ability to see him- or herself in the future or to foresee the consequences of his or her behavior. Teens perceive their locus of control as external;

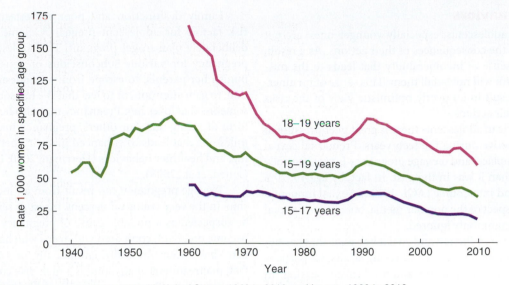

● **Figure 13–1** Birth rates for women ages 15 to 19: United States, 1940 to 2010, and by age, 1960 to 2010.

Source: Centers for Disease Control and Prevention (2012). Retrieved from http://www.cdc.gov/nchs/data/databriefs/db89.htm#citation.

that is, their destinies are controlled by others such as parents and school authorities.

Middle adolescence (ages 15 to 17 years) is the time for challenging; experimenting with drugs, alcohol, and sex are common avenues for rebellion. Middle adolescents seek independence and turn increasingly to their peer groups. They begin to move from concrete thinking to formal operational thought but are not yet able to anticipate the long-term implications of all their actions. These years are often a time of great turmoil for the family as the adolescent struggles for independence and challenges the family's values and expectations.

In **late adolescence** (ages 18 to 19 years) teens are more at ease with their individuality and decision-making ability. They can think abstractly and anticipate consequences. Late adolescents are capable of formal operational thought. They learn to solve problems, to conceptualize, and to make decisions. These abilities help them see themselves as having control, which leads to the ability to understand and accept the consequences of their behavior.

FACTORS CONTRIBUTING TO ADOLESCENT PREGNANCY

Socioeconomic and Cultural Factors

Poverty is a major risk factor for adolescent pregnancy. Adolescents who do not have access to middle-class opportunities tend to maintain their pregnancies, because they see pregnancy as their only option for adult status. Kearney and Levine (2012) suggest that teens who are on a low economic trajectory are more likely to become pregnant because of the lack of economic opportunity and the social marginalization that comes with poverty. Specifically, these girls are more likely to "drop out" of the economic mainstream and opt for early parenthood instead of investing in their own economic progress because they feel that they have little chance of advancing.

In the United States, the adolescent birth rate is higher among African American teens and Hispanic teens than among white teens. To some degree, the higher teenage pregnancy rate in these groups reflects the impact of poverty, because a disproportionately high number of African American and Hispanic youths live in poverty.

Higher levels of competence cognitively, behaviorally, and socially tend to have a protective effect on adolescent sexuality and reproductive health (House, Bates, Markham, et al., 2010). Intelligence and academic ability are positively associated with delayed sexual activity, greater use of contraception, and lower rates of pregnancy (Katz, 2011). Teens with future goals (i.e., college or job) tend to use birth control more consistently compared with other teens; if they become pregnant, they are also more likely to have abortions.

The younger the teen when she first gets pregnant, the more likely she is to have another pregnancy in her teens. Moreover, the likelihood of repeat pregnancies increases when the teen is living with her sexual partner and has dropped out of school. Then, too, girls whose sister had a baby in her early teens and girls whose mother and sister both gave birth as teens are significantly more likely to have a teenage pregnancy themselves (East, Reyes, & Horn, 2007).

Internationally, adolescent women are more likely to welcome a pregnancy in a country in which Islam is the predominant religion, where large families are desired, where social change is slow in coming, and where most childbearing occurs within marriage. Early pregnancy is less desired in countries in which the reverse is true.

Developing Cultural Competence
Impact of Education on Marriage and Childbearing

Throughout the world, the higher a woman's educational level, the more likely she is to delay marriage and childbirth.

High-Risk Behaviors

Developmentally, adolescents, especially younger ones, are not yet able to foresee the consequences of their actions. As a result, they may have a sense of invulnerability that leads to the mistaken idea that harm will not befall them. This sense of invulnerability may also result in an overly optimistic view of the risks associated with their actions.

Among American adolescents there is great peer pressure to become sexually active during the teen years. Premarital sexual activity is commonplace, and teenage pregnancy is more socially acceptable today than it was in the past. In fact, by age 19, 70% of all teens have had intercourse (AGI, 2012a). Sexual innuendo permeates every aspect of the popular media, but issues of sexual responsibility are commonly ignored.

Texting is a form of flirting and social behavior that has become commonplace among teens and young adults. Of particular note is the current blend of "sex and text" called "sexting" in which teens and young adults share semi-nude or nude pictures of themselves or others using cell phones, websites, and social media networks. When surveyed, an overwhelming majority of teens (71%) believe that sexting does lead to more sex in real life (Albert, 2010).

High-risk sexual behaviors including multiple partners and lack of contraceptive use are of concern. Research indicates that young people 15 to 24 years of age comprise 25% of the sexually experienced population in the United States. However, they account for nearly half of the new cases of sexually transmitted infections (STIs) (Centers for Disease Control and Prevention, 2011). This is particularly worrisome because many STIs, including human immunodeficiency virus (HIV), are asymptomatic. Thus, apparently healthy young people who are infected may not have a reason to seek health care.

Statistics have demonstrated an increased use of condoms among the adolescent population, probably because of the tremendous educational efforts related to HIV. Adolescents, however, remain inconsistent contraceptive users. Many teens lack accurate and adequate knowledge about contraceptive options. This is a common topic of sex education programs; nevertheless, debate continues about the appropriateness of such programs in schools. Proponents advocate early sex education to provide teens with the knowledge they need to avoid unwanted pregnancy and the risk of STIs. Opponents feel that sex education is the responsibility of parents and worry that sex education in the schools will promote sexual activity. However, a review of research on sex education reveals that it does not increase initiation of sexual activity at an earlier age. Other factors affecting the use of contraception include access or availability, cost of supplies, and concern about confidentiality.

Psychosocial Factors

Pregnancy desire tends to be higher among teens who are older, who were younger when they became sexually active, who are in a short-term relationship (which may be romanticized and intense), and who have greater perceived stress in their lives (Sipsma, Ickovics, Lewis, et al., 2011).

Family dysfunction and poor self-esteem are also major risk factors for adolescent pregnancy. Some young teenagers deliberately plan to get pregnant. The adolescent girl may use pregnancy for various subconscious or conscious reasons: to punish her parents, to escape from an undesirable home situation, to gain attention, or to feel that she has someone to love and someone that loves her. Pregnancy may also be a young woman's form of acting out. For others, pregnancy marks an important milestone that leads to enhanced maturity, better decision making, and healthier behaviors (Herrman, 2010; Pinkleton, Austin, Cohen, et al., 2008).

Teenage pregnancy can result from an incestuous relationship. In the very young adolescent, incest or sexual abuse should be suspected as a possible cause of pregnancy. More teens who become pregnant, compared with teens who have not been pregnant, have been physically, emotionally, or sexually abused. In fact, maltreatment of any kind is a high-risk contributor to early teen pregnancy. Teenage pregnancy could also be caused by other nonvoluntary sexual experiences such as acquaintance rape.

RISKS TO THE ADOLESCENT MOTHER

Physiologic Risks

Adolescents older than 15 years who receive early, thorough prenatal care are at no greater risk during pregnancy than women older than age 20. Unfortunately, adolescents often begin prenatal care later in pregnancy than other age groups. Thus, risks for pregnant adolescents include preterm births, low-birth-weight infants, cephalopelvic disproportion, iron-deficiency anemia, and preeclampsia and its sequelae. In the adolescent age group, prenatal care is the critical factor that most influences pregnancy outcome.

Teenagers ages 15 to 19 have a high incidence of STIs, including herpes virus, syphilis, and gonorrhea. The incidence of chlamydial infection is also increased in this age group. The presence of such infections during a pregnancy greatly increases the risk to the fetus. Other problems seen in adolescents are cigarette smoking and drug use. By the time pregnancy is confirmed, the fetus may already have been harmed by these substances.

Psychologic Risks

The major psychologic risk to the pregnant adolescent is the interruption of her developmental tasks. Adding the tasks of pregnancy to her own developmental tasks creates a huge amount of psychologic work, the completion of which will affect the adolescent's and her newborn's futures. Table 13–1 suggests typical behaviors of the adolescent when she becomes aware of her pregnancy. In reviewing these behaviors, the nurse should realize that other factors may influence individual response.

Sociologic Risks

Being forced into adult roles before completing adolescent developmental tasks causes a series of events that may result in prolonged dependence on parents, lack of stable relationships with the opposite sex, and lack of economic and social stability. Many teenage mothers drop out of school during their pregnancy and

Table 13–1	Initial Reaction to Awareness of Pregnancy	
Age	**Adolescent Behavior**	**Nursing Implications**
Early adolescent (14 years and younger)	Fears rejection by family and peers. Enters healthcare system with an adult, most likely mother (parents still seen as locus of control). Value system closely reflects that of parents, so teen turns to parents for decisions or approval of decisions. Pregnancy probably not a result of intimate relationship. Is self-conscious about normal adolescent changes in body. Self-consciousness and low self-esteem likely to increase with rapid breast enlargement and abdominal enlargement of pregnancy.	Be nonjudgmental in approach to care. Focus on needs and concerns of adolescent, but if parent accompanies daughter, include parent in plan of care. Encourage both to express concerns and feelings regarding pregnancy and options: abortion, maintaining pregnancy, adoption. Be realistic and concrete in discussing implications of each option. During physical exam of adolescent, respect increased sense of modesty. Explain in simple and concrete terms physical changes that are produced by pregnancy versus puberty. Explain each step of physical exam in simple and concrete terms.
Middle adolescent (15–17 years)	Fears rejection by peers and parents. Unsure of whom to confide in. May seek confirmation of pregnancy on own with increased awareness of options and services, such as over-the-counter pregnancy kits and Planned Parenthood. If in an ongoing, caring relationship with partner (peer), may choose him as confidant. Economic dependence on parents may determine if and when parents are told. Future educational plans and perception of parental support or lack of support are significant factors in decision regarding termination or maintenance of the pregnancy. Possible conflict between parental and own developing value system.	Be nonjudgmental in approach to care. Reassure the adolescent that confidentiality will be maintained. Help adolescent identify significant individuals in whom she can confide to help make a decision about the pregnancy. Be aware of state laws regarding requirement of parental notification if abortion intended. Also be aware of state laws regarding requirements for marriage: usually, minimum age for both parties is 18; 16- and 17-year-olds are, in most states, allowed to marry only with consent of parents. Encourage adolescent to be realistic about parental response to pregnancy.
Late adolescent (18–19 years)	Most likely to confirm pregnancy on own and at an earlier date due to increased acceptance and awareness of consequences of behavior. Likely to use pregnancy kit for confirmation. Relationship with father of baby, future educational plans, and personal value system are among significant determinants of decision about pregnancy.	Be nonjudgmental in approach to care. Reassure the adolescent that confidentiality will be maintained. Encourage adolescent to identify significant individuals in whom she can confide. Refer to counseling as appropriate. Encourage adolescent to be realistic about parental response to pregnancy.

then are less likely to complete their schooling. Similarly, they are less likely to go to college. In fact, fewer than 2% of teenagers who give birth before age 18 attain a college degree by age 30 (AGI, 2012a). In addition, teenage mothers are more likely to have big families and more likely to be single. Lack of education in turn reduces the quality of jobs available and leads to more tenuous employment and increased poverty (Hermann, 2010; Kirby, 2007).

Some pregnant adolescents choose to marry the father of the baby, who may also be a teenager. Unfortunately, most adolescent marriages end in divorce. This fact should not be surprising because pregnancy and marriage interrupt the adolescents' childhood and basic education. Lack of maturity in dealing with an intimate relationship also contributes to marital breakdown.

Dating violence is often an issue for teens. When surveyed, almost 10% of adolescents report some level of dating violence. The violence increases to 21% in pregnant teens. However, research suggests that this number is significantly lower than reality because teens are far less likely to report domestic violence than are adults (Herrman, 2009).

The increased incidence of maternal complications, preterm birth, and low-birth-weight babies among teen mothers also affects society because many of these mothers are on welfare. The need for increased financial support for good prenatal care and nutritional programs remains critical.

Table 13–2 identifies the early adolescent's response to the developmental tasks of pregnancy. Middle and older adolescents respond differently, reflecting their progression through developmental tasks. In addition to her maturational level, the amount of nurturing the pregnant adolescent receives is a critical factor in the way she handles pregnancy and motherhood.

Risks for the Child

Children of adolescent parents are at a disadvantage in many ways because teens are not developmentally or economically prepared to be parents. In general, children of teenage mothers are found to be at a developmental disadvantage compared with children whose mothers were older at the time of their birth. Many factors contribute to these differences, especially the adverse social and economic conditions many teenage mothers face. These factors

Table 13–2	The Early Adolescent's Response to the Developmental Tasks of Pregnancy		
Stage	**Developmental Tasks of Pregnancy**	**Early Adolescent's Response to Pregnancy**	**Nursing Implications**
First trimester	Pregnancy confirmation. Seeks early prenatal care as a confirmation tool. Begins to evaluate her diet and general health habits. Initial ambivalence common. Usually supportive partner.	May delay confirmation of pregnancy until late first trimester or later. Reasons for delay may include lack of awareness that she is pregnant, fear of confiding in anyone, and/or denial. Rapid enlargement and sensitivity of breasts are embarrassing and frightening to early adolescents—may be perceived as changes of puberty. If confiding in mother, may be experiencing family turmoil in response to pregnancy.	Explain physiologic changes of pregnancy versus those associated with puberty. Explain that ambivalence is normal with any pregnancy, but recognize it as a much greater concern with adolescent pregnancy. Emphasize need for good nutrition as important for her well-being as much as infant's (prevention of preeclampsia and anemia). Use simple explanations and lots of audiovisual aids. Have adolescent listen to fetal heart rate with Doppler.
Second trimester	Changes in physical appearance begin, and fetal movement is experienced, causing pregnancy to be experienced as a reality. Begins wearing maternity clothes to accommodate the physical changes. As a result of quickening, she perceives her fetus as a real baby and begins preparing for the maternal role and new relationships with her partner and members of her family.	Some teenagers may delay validation of pregnancy until now, with family turmoil occurring at this time. Abdominal enlargement and quickening may be perceived as loss of control over body image. May try to maintain prepregnant weight and wear restrictive clothing to control and conceal changing body. Becomes dependent on her own mother for support. Egocentric; unable to develop a maternal role at this time.	Continue to discuss importance of good nutrition and adequate weight gain as noted above. Discuss ways of wearing common teenage clothing (large sweatshirts, blouses) to promote comfort but preserve adolescent image to some degree. Discuss plans being made for baby, continued educational plans, and role of teen's parents. Explain physiologic changes of pregnancy versus those associated with puberty. Explain that ambivalence is normal with any pregnancy, but recognize it as a much greater concern with adolescent pregnancy.
Third trimester	At end of second trimester, begins to view fetus as separate from self. Buys baby clothes and supplies. Prepares a place for the baby. Realistic about what baby is like. Prepares to give birth to infant. Anxiety increases as labor and birth approach and has concerns about well-being of fetus.	May focus on "wanting it to be over." May have trouble individuating fetus. May have fantasies, dreams, or nightmares about childbirth. Natural fears of labor and birth greater than with older primigravida. Probably has not been in a hospital, and may associate this with negative experiences.	Assess whether adolescent is preparing for baby by buying supplies and preparing a place in the home. Childbirth education is important. Provide hospital tour. Assess for discomforts of pregnancy, such as heartburn and constipation. Adolescent may be uncomfortable mentioning these and other problems.

result in high rates of family instability, disadvantaged neighborhoods, and high rates of behavior problems. In addition, these children do not do as well in school and are less likely to complete high school. Children born to adolescent mothers also have higher rates of abuse and neglect.

PARTNERS OF ADOLESCENT MOTHERS

Approximately half of the fathers of infants born to adolescent mothers are not teens but 20 years of age or older (Herrman, 2010). Teens in poor, recently immigrated populations are especially likely to have older partners. Adolescent males tend to become sexually active at an earlier age than females, and they have more sexual partners in their teenage years. When the father is an adolescent, he too has uncompleted developmental tasks for his age group and is no better prepared psychologically than his female counterpart to deal with the consequences of pregnancy. Teenage fatherhood may lead to a decrease in the years of schooling the male receives, and increases the rate of cohabitation and early marriage. It also is associated with full-time and military employment status (Fletcher & Wolfe, 2012).

In general, adolescent males tend to view an unintended pregnancy as negative because of the impact on their aspirations, life goals, and current freedoms. Attitudes toward teen pregnancy tend to be more favorable among adolescent men of lower socioeconomic status and/or lower educational level (Lohan, Cruise, O'Halloran, et al., 2010).

The adolescent who attempts to assume his responsibility as a father faces many of the same psychologic and sociologic risks as the adolescent mother. The mother and father are generally from similar socioeconomic backgrounds and have similar educational levels.

Although they may not be married, many adolescent couples have meaningful relationships. The male partners may be very involved in the pregnancy and may be present for the birth. In situations in which the adolescent father wants to assume some responsibility, healthcare providers should support him in his decision. It is also important to ensure that the pregnant adolescent has the opportunity to decide for herself whether she wants the father to participate in her health care.

Fathers are included on birth certificates far more frequently today than in the past. This inclusion helps ensure the fathers' rights and encourages them to meet their responsibilities to their children. In addition, legal paternity gives children access to military and Social Security benefits and to medical information about their fathers.

In some situations the pregnant adolescent may not want to identify or contact the father of the baby, and the male may not readily acknowledge paternity. Those situations include rape, exploitative sexual relations, incest, and casual sexual relations. If healthcare providers suspect any of the first three causes, further investigation into the situation is important for the well-being of the pregnant adolescent, and referral to other resources should be made as appropriate.

Even if the adolescent father has been included in the health care of the young woman throughout the pregnancy, it is not unusual for her to want her mother as her primary support person during labor and birth. Younger adolescents are especially likely to choose their mothers for this role. It is important to support the pregnant adolescent's wishes and to acknowledge and support the adolescent father's wishes as appropriate.

As a part of counseling, the nurse should assess the young man's stressors, his support systems, his plans for involvement in the pregnancy and childbearing, and his future plans. He should be referred to social services for counseling about his educational and vocational future. When the father is involved in the pregnancy, the young mother feels less deserted, more confident in her decision making, and better able to discuss her future.

Relationships among fathers, teenage mothers, and their infants appear prone to deterioration over time. Many young fathers genuinely want to be involved with their children and would have more contact and input if they could. Issues such as conflicts with the teen mother or maternal grandparents and a lack of financial resources may act as barriers for the young father.

REACTIONS OF FAMILY AND SOCIAL NETWORK TO ADOLESCENT PREGNANCY

The reactions of families and support groups to adolescent pregnancy vary widely. In families that foster children's educational and career goals, adolescent pregnancy is often a shock. Anger, shame, and sorrow are common reactions. The majority of pregnant adolescents from these families are likely to choose abortion, with the exception of teens whose cultural and religious beliefs prevent them from seeking abortions.

In populations in which adolescent pregnancy is more prevalent and more socially acceptable, family and friends may be more supportive of the adolescent parents. In many cases the teen's friends and mother are present at the birth. The expectant parents may also have friends who are already teen parents. Some male partners of these adolescent mothers see pregnancy and the birth of a baby as signs of adult status and increased sexual prowess—a source of pride.

The mother of the pregnant adolescent is usually among the first to be told about the pregnancy. She typically becomes involved with decision making, especially with the young

adolescent, about issues such as maintaining the pregnancy, abortion, and dealing with the father-to-be and his family.

Once the pregnant adolescent decides how to proceed, it is often her mother who helps her access health care and accompanies her to her first prenatal visit. If the pregnancy is maintained, the mother may participate in prenatal care and classes and can be an excellent source of support for her daughter. She should be encouraged to participate if the mother–daughter relationship is positive. If the baby's father is involved in the pregnancy, he and the pregnant adolescent's mother may be able to work together to support the teenage mother. The nurse can update the pregnant adolescent's mother on current childbearing practices to clarify any misconceptions she might have. During labor and birth, the mother may be a key figure for her daughter, offering reassurance and instilling confidence in the teen.

The younger the adolescent when she gives birth, the more she needs her mother's support. Children of adolescent parents experience more negative outcomes, including more aggressive behavior at a younger age, when the adolescent is in constant conflict with her mother and becomes less involved in parenting.

NURSING MANAGEMENT *For the Adolescent Mother-to-Be*

Nursing Assessment and Diagnosis

Establish a knowledge base to plan interventions for the adolescent mother-to-be and family. Areas of assessment include history of family and personal physical health, developmental level and impact of pregnancy, and emotional and financial support. Also assess the family and social support network and the father's degree of involvement in the pregnancy.

As with all pregnant women, it is important to have information on the teen's general physical health. This may be the first time the adolescent has ever provided a health history. Consequently it may be helpful to ask specific questions and give examples if the young woman appears confused about a question. The teen's mother may be best able to answer questions about family history because the adolescent is often unaware of this information.

The following areas should be assessed:

- Family and personal health history
- Medical history
- Menstrual history
- Obstetric and gynecologic history
- Substance abuse history

It is important to assess the maturational level of each person. The adolescent's development level and the impact of pregnancy are reflected in the degree of recognition of the realities and responsibilities involved in teenage pregnancy and parenting. Also assess the mother's self-concept (including body image), her relationship with the significant adults in her life, her attitude toward her pregnancy, and her coping methods in the situation, as well as the teen's knowledge of, attitude toward, and anticipated ability to care for the coming baby. Ask specifically about dating violence. Teens are not likely to reveal dating violence unless they are asked about it.

The socioeconomic status of the pregnant adolescent often places the baby at risk throughout life, beginning with conception. It is essential to assess family and social support systems, as well as the extent of financial support available.

The nursing diagnoses applicable to pregnant women in general apply to the pregnant adolescent. Other nursing diagnoses are influenced by the adolescent's age, support systems, socioeconomic situation, health, and maturity. Examples of nursing diagnoses specific to the pregnant adolescent may include the following (NANDA-I © 2012):

- *Nutrition, Imbalanced: Less than Body Requirements,* related to poor eating habits
- *Self-Esteem, Situational Low, Risk for,* related to unanticipated pregnancy

Planning and Implementation

Community-Based Nursing Care

If pregnancy occurs, early, thorough prenatal care is the strongest and most critical determinant for reducing risk for the adolescent mother and her newborn. The nurse needs to understand the special needs of the adolescent mother to meet this challenge successfully.

Many new and innovative community-based programs have evolved to provide care for high-risk patients and their partners throughout the childbearing experience and beyond. Nurses in community-based agencies can help adolescents access the healthcare system as well as social services and other support services (e.g., food banks and the Special Supplemental Nutrition Program for Women, Infants, and Children [WIC]). These nurses are also involved extensively in counseling and patient teaching.

Teaching adolescents in groups according to their ages is often more effective for learning. In addition, many teens prefer teaching aids that are visual and that they can handle, such as realistic fetal models. Pregnant teens with low reading levels tend to prefer handouts and posters that have visual interest, short sentences, bulleted items, and white space (Broussard & Broussard, 2010).

Issue of Confidentiality

Most states have passed legislation that confirms the right of some minors to assume the rights of adults; they are then called **emancipated minors**. An adolescent may be considered emancipated if he or she is self-supporting and living away from home, married, pregnant, a parent, or in the military service. Even if a minor has not become formally "emancipated," all 50 states permit confidential testing and treatment for sexually transmitted infections (STIs) but only 21 states and the District of Columbia explicitly permit all minors to consent to contraception without a parent's knowledge or consent; 25 states permit minors to consent in certain circumstances (AGI, 2012e). Currently 36 states and the District of Columbia explicitly allow some minors to consent to prenatal care; of that group 28 allow all minors to give consent, while 13 states have no relevant law or policy (AGI, 2012c). All states either explicitly allow minors to give consent for their children's medical care or have no policy about it (AGI, 2012d).

Development of a Trusting Relationship with the Pregnant Adolescent

The first visit to the clinic or caregiver's office may make the young woman feel anxious and vulnerable. Making this first experience as positive as possible for the young woman will encourage the adolescent to return for follow-up care and to cooperate with her caregivers and will help her recognize the importance of health care for her and her baby. Developing a trusting relationship with the pregnant adolescent is essential. Honesty, respect, and a caring attitude promote self-esteem.

Clinical Tip

During the initial pelvic examination, with the consent of the examiner, offer the teen a handheld mirror. A mirror is helpful in enabling the young woman to see her cervix, thus educating her about her anatomy. It also gives her an active role in the exam if she so desires.

Depending on the adolescent's age, this may be her first pelvic examination, an anxiety-provoking experience for any woman. Provide explanations during the procedure. A gentle and thoughtful examination technique will help the young woman to relax.

Promotion of Self-Esteem and Problem-Solving Skills

Assist the adolescent in her decision-making and problem-solving skills so that she can proceed with her developmental tasks and begin to assume responsibility for her life and that of her newborn. Many adolescents are not aware of the legally available options for handling an unplanned pregnancy. In an open, nonjudgmental way, without imposing personal values, educate the teen about her alternatives: terminating the pregnancy, maintaining the pregnancy and parenting the infant, or relinquishing the infant for adoption. The nurse can also provide information about community resources available to help with each alternative. Once the teen has decided on a course of action, healthcare providers should respect her decision and support her efforts to achieve her goals.

If the adolescent chooses to continue her pregnancy, describe what she can expect over the prenatal period and provide an explanation and rationale for each procedure as it occurs. This overview fosters the adolescent's understanding and gives her some control.

Early adolescents tend to be egocentric and oriented to the present. They may not think it is important that their health and habits affect the fetus. Thus, it is often helpful to emphasize how these practices affect the teens themselves. Early adolescents also need help in problem solving and in visualizing the future so they can plan effectively.

Middle adolescents are developing the ability to think abstractly and can recognize that actions may have long-term consequences. They may not yet have acquired assertive communication skills, however, and may be reluctant to ask questions. Therefore, ask teens directly if they have questions. Middle adolescents can absorb more detailed health teaching and apply it.

Late adolescents can usually think abstractly, plan for the future, and function in a manner comparable to older pregnant women. They can also handle complex information and apply it.

Promotion of Physical Well-Being

Baseline weight and blood pressure measurements are valuable in assessing weight gain and predisposition to preeclampsia (Figure 13–2 ●). Encourage the adolescent to take part in her care by measuring and recording her own weight. Use this time as an opportunity for assisting the young woman in problem solving. Encourage her to ask herself the following questions: "Have I gained too much or too little weight?" "What influence does my diet have on my weight?" "How can I change my eating habits?"

Also introduce the subject of nutrition during measurement of baseline and subsequent hemoglobin and hematocrit values. Because the adolescent is at risk for anemia, she needs education about the importance of iron in her diet. Indeed, basic education about nutrition is a critical component of care for pregnant teens.

Preeclampsia is the most prevalent medical complication of pregnant adolescents. Blood pressure readings of 140/90 mm Hg are not acceptable as the determinant of preeclampsia in adolescents. Women ages 14 to 20 years without evidence of high blood pressure usually have diastolic readings between 50 and 66 mm Hg. Gradual increases from the prepregnant diastolic readings, along with excessive weight gain, must be evaluated as precursors to preeclampsia. Establishment of baseline readings is one reason early prenatal care is vital to management of the pregnant adolescent.

Adolescents have an increased incidence of STIs. The initial prenatal examination should include gonococcal and chlamydial cultures; wet-mount prep for *Candida, Trichomonas,* and *Gardnerella;* and tests for syphilis. Although today's teens are knowledgeable about HIV/AIDS, they know much less about other STIs, especially with regard to symptoms and risk reduction, so education is important. If the adolescent's history indicates that she is at increased risk for HIV, she should be given information about it and offered HIV screening.

Discuss substance abuse with the adolescent. It is important to review the risks associated with the use of tobacco, caffeine,

● **Figure 13–2** The nurse carefully assesses this pregnant teen.
Source: © Auremar/Fotolia.

drugs, and alcohol. The young woman should be aware of how these substances affect both her and her fetus's development.

Ongoing care should include the same assessments that an older pregnant woman receives. Pay special attention to evaluating fetal growth by determining when quickening occurs and by measuring fundal height, fetal heart rate, and fetal movement. If there is a question of size–date discrepancy by 2 cm either way when assessing fundal height, an ultrasound is warranted to establish fetal age so that instances of intrauterine growth restriction can be detected early.

Promotion of Family Adaptation

Assess the family situation during the first prenatal visit and find out the level of involvement the adolescent wants from each of her family members and the father of the child, as well as her perception of their present support. If the mother and daughter agree, the mother should be included in the patient's care. Pregnancy may change a teen's relationship with her mother from one of antagonism to one of understanding and empathy. The opportunity to renew or establish a positive relationship with their mothers is welcomed by most teens. Help the teen's mother assess and meet her daughter's needs. Some adolescents become more dependent during pregnancy, and some become more independent. The mother can ease and encourage her daughter's self-growth by understanding how best to respond to and support the adolescent.

The adolescent's relationship with her father is also affected by her pregnancy. Provide information to the adolescent's father and encourage his involvement to whatever degree is acceptable to both daughter and father.

The father of the adolescent's infant should not be forgotten in promoting the family's adaptation to the pregnancy. He should be included in prenatal visits, classes, health teaching, and the birth itself to the extent that he wishes and that is acceptable to the teenage mother. He should also have the opportunity to express his feelings and concerns and to have his questions answered.

Health Promotion Education

School systems attempt to meet prenatal education needs in many ways. The most effective method appears to be mainstreaming the pregnant adolescent in academic classes with her peers and adding classes appropriate to her needs during pregnancy and postpartum. Classes about growth and development beginning with the newborn and early infancy periods can help teenage parents to develop realistic expectations of their infants and may help decrease child abuse. Mainstreaming is an ideal way to help teens complete their education while learning the skills they need to cope. Vocational guidance in this setting is also beneficial as they plan for their futures.

Most childbirth educators believe that prenatal classes with other teens are best, even though they can be challenging to teach (Figure 13–3 ●). The pregnant teen may be accompanied by her mother, her boyfriend, or her girlfriends. Those who bring girlfriends may bring a different one each time, and giggling and side conversations may occur. Such activity reflects the short attention span of the teen and is fairly typical.

Goals for prenatal classes may include some or all of the following:

- Providing anticipatory guidance about pregnancy
- Preparing participants for labor and birth
- Helping participants identify the problems and conflicts of teenage pregnancy and parenting
- Promoting increased self-esteem
- Providing information about available community resources
- Helping participants develop adaptive coping skills

Although parenting topics are sometimes included in prenatal classes for adolescents, teens may not retain the information because they tend to be present oriented. Parenting skills are crucial, but adolescents generally are not ready to learn about these skills until birth makes the newborn—and thus parenting—a reality.

Hospital-Based Nursing Care

As mentioned earlier, the adolescent's mother is often present during the teen's labor and birth. The father of the baby may

---

| Health Promotion | Adolescent Childbirth Classes |

To keep the attention of adolescent participants in childbirth preparation classes, it is important to use a variety of teaching strategies including audiovisual aids, demonstrations, and games.

● **Figure 13–3** Prenatal classes for adolescents. Young adolescents may benefit from prenatal classes designed for them.

---

also be involved. Close girlfriends may arrive soon after the teen is admitted. At admission, ask the teen who will be her primary support person in labor and who she wants involved in the labor and birth. This information may also be included on her prenatal record.

The adolescent in labor has the same care needs as any pregnant woman. However, she may require more sustained care. Be readily available and answer questions simply and honestly, using lay terminology. Also help the adolescent's support people understand their roles in assisting the teen. If the father of the baby is involved, encourage him, at his own level of comfort, to play an active role in all phases of the birth process, perhaps by supporting the teen's relaxation techniques, feeding her ice chips, timing her contractions, and coaching her with her breathing. Recommend hand-holding, back rubs, and supportive touching.

During the postpartum period, most teens do not foresee that they will become sexually active in the near future and are often adamant that they will not become pregnant again for a long time. However, the statistics demonstrate a different reality. Consequently, predischarge teaching should include information about the resumption of ovulation and the importance of contraception.

Several safe and effective contraceptive options are available for adolescents. Condoms are by far the most common method of contraception among teens and, when used consistently and correctly, they offer the added advantage of protection against STIs. Increasingly, experts are recommending a dual approach to prevent pregnancy and STIs—a condom combined with a second method of contraception, typically a hormonal method such as a combined oral contraceptive, the contraceptive patch, or the vaginal ring (Hatcher, Trussell, Nelson, et al., 2011). The intrauterine device (IUD) is now considered a safe, first-line contraceptive choice for adolescents. Research indicates that the IUD does not increase the adolescent's risk of pelvic inflammatory disease (PID) or affect her fertility (American College of Obstetricians and Gynecologists, 2007; Hatcher et al., 2011), and the levonorgestrel-releasing intrauterine system (LNG-IUS) can be beneficial in teens by reducing heavy menstrual bleeding and alleviating symptoms of dysmenorrhea (Forcier & Harel, 2011).

SAFETY ALERT!
Nurses need to be certain that adolescents who are prescribed combined oral contraceptives clearly understand the correct use, possible complications, warning signs, and implications of missed pills.

As part of discharge planning, ensure that the teen is aware of community resources available to assist her and her family. Postpartum classes, especially with peers, can be particularly beneficial. Such classes address a variety of topics, including postpartum adaptation, infant and child development, and parenting skills.

Evaluation

Expected outcomes of nursing care include the following:

- A trusting relationship is established with the pregnant adolescent.
- The adolescent is able to use her problem-solving abilities to make appropriate choices.

- The adolescent follows the recommendations of the healthcare team and receives effective health care throughout her pregnancy, the birth, and the postpartum period.

- The adolescent, her partner (if he is involved), and their families are able to cope successfully with the effects of the pregnancy.

- The adolescent is able to discuss pregnancy, prenatal care, and childbirth.

- The adolescent develops skill in child care and parenting.

PREVENTION OF ADOLESCENT PREGNANCY

At the individual level, balanced and realistic sexual education, which includes information on both abstinence and contraception, can delay teens' onset of sexual activity, increase the use of contraception by sexually active teens, and reduce the number of their sexual partners. In 2007, the American Academy of Pediatrics (AAP) issued a policy statement on contraception and adolescents that addresses the role of healthcare providers in working with adolescents. The statement stresses the importance of encouraging abstinence while also providing counseling on risk-reduction approaches, including the use of latex condoms for every act of sexual intercourse. It also emphasizes the need to ensure ready access to contraceptive services and appropriate follow-up. In 2012, AAP issued a policy statement on emergency contraception. It recommends prescribing levonorgestrel 1.5 mg (Plan B or Next Choice) for teens needing emergency contraception. The policy also recommends that caregivers provide prescriptions/supplies for teens to have available in case of future need, and states that both male and female teens should be counseled about emergency contraception as part of routine anticipatory guidance about safer sex and family planning.

At the national level, the National Campaign to Prevent Teen and Unplanned Pregnancy (NCPTUP), a private, nonprofit organization made up of a broad spectrum of religious, political, social, human services, health, and academic organizations, is working to reduce teenage pregnancy by one third between 2006 and 2015 (NCPTUP, 2012c). The Association of Women's Health, Obstetric and Neonatal Nurses (AWHONN) is one of the many professional organizations that joined this group and made a commitment to focus on adolescent pregnancy prevention. Not surprisingly, the National Campaign has found that adolescent pregnancy is a multifaceted problem with no easy answers. The best approaches are local ones based on strong, community-wide involvement with a variety of programs directed at the multiple causes of the problem.

A problem in local communities continues to be conflict among different groups about how to approach adolescent pregnancy prevention. Most teens and adults believe that teens should be strongly encouraged to avoid having sex until they have completed high school, but both groups also favor providing young people with information about both abstinence and contraception (Albert, 2010). Nevertheless, some parents favor an abstinence-only approach. No evidence to date supports the effectiveness of this approach and it may have the unintended consequence of deterring teens from using contraceptives, thereby increasing the risk of sexually transmitted infections (STIs) or unintended pregnancy

 Evidence-Based Practice   Preventing Pregnancy in High-Risk Adolescents

Clinical Question

What interventions can prevent pregnancy among young women who are at risk?

The Evidence

Two studies evaluated the effectiveness of a clinic-based intervention aimed at reducing the incidence of pregnancy in high-risk adolescents. The intervention is based on the developmental stages of adolescence, and the primary elements are focused on building protective functions—such as stress management—and addressing risk of pregnancy through the use of contraception. The intervention was tested in two randomized controlled trials with more than 250 subjects. This type of study design, when replicated, forms the strongest evidence for practice. Adolescent girls who participated in more than a year of the program reported more consistent use of contraception than a group of controls (Seiving, McMorris, Beckman, et al., 2011). In addition, the adolescents exhibited better stress management skills and better use of social supports than their counterparts (Sieving, Resnick, Garwick, et al., 2011). A third study used a matched comparison group to study the effectiveness of a healthy relationship program that is customized to specific cultures. In this study of a Native American population, adolescent pregnancies were lower and contraception use higher than a comparison group (Hagen, Skenadore, Scow, et al., 2012).

Best Practice

Prevention of adolescent pregnancy relies on a combination of building protective factors in adolescent girls while emphasizing the appropriate use of contraception when sexually active. Individualized case management and peer leadership can be effective in preventing pregnancy among high-risk adolescents. Applying interventions that are culturally appropriate will be more effective for specific subgroups.

Clinical Reasoning

What are some of the considerations in designing individualized case management services for adolescents? How can the nurse provide support for adolescents in appropriately using contraception?

(AGI, 2012b). Most Americans support providing education in junior and senior high schools with information about protection against unplanned pregnancy and STIs. Evidence suggests that comprehensive programs that support both abstinence and the use of contraceptives and condoms have a positive effect in delaying or reducing sexual activity or in increasing the use of condoms or other contraceptives (AGI, 2012b). Youth development programs that meet the needs of adolescents by building on young people's abilities, assisting them to cultivate their talents and increase their feelings of self-worth, and ease their transition into adulthood can reduce sexual risk behaviors and unintended teen pregnancy (Advocates for Youth, 2008).

The National Campaign's task forces have identified characteristics shared by all successful programs, regardless of the type of offering or community. Effective adolescent pregnancy prevention programs are long term and intensive. They also involve adolescents in program planning, include good role models from the same cultural and racial backgrounds, and focus on the adolescent male.

The National Campaign has identified a list of recommendations for parents that are designed to help teens avoid pregnancy (see Table 13–3). Nurses can use this information when working with parents (NCPTUP, 2012b).

Table 13–3	Recommendations for Parents to Help Their Teens Avoid Pregnancy

- Parents should be clear about their own sexual attitudes and values in order to communicate clearly with children.
- Parents need to talk with their children about sex early and often and be specific in the discussions.
- Parents should supervise and monitor their children and teens with well-established rules, expectations, curfews, and standards of behavior.
- Parents should know their children's friends and their families.
- Parents need to clearly discourage early dating as well as frequent and steady dating.
- Parents should take a strong stand against allowing a daughter to date a much older boy; similarly, they should not allow a son to develop an intense relationship with a much younger girl.
- Parents need to help children set goals for their future and have options that are more attractive than early pregnancy and childrearing.
- Parents should show their children that they value education and take school performance seriously.
- Parents need to monitor what their children are reading, listening to, and watching.
- It is especially important for parents to build a strong, loving relationship with their children from an early age by showing affection clearly and regularly, spending time with them doing age-appropriate activities, building children's self-esteem, and have meals together as a family often.

Critical Concept Review

LEARNING OUTCOME 13.1: Describe the scope of the problem and the impact of adolescent pregnancy.

1. The adolescent birth rate for 2010 is 34.3, a historic low. Significantly these declines occurred for all race and ethnic origin groups.

2. Despite the decline, the United States continues to have one of the highest levels of adolescent childbearing among industrialized nations.

LEARNING OUTCOME 13.2: Describe the major factors that contribute to adolescent pregnancy.

1. Many factors contribute to the high teenage pregnancy rate:
   - Earlier age at first experience with sexual intercourse.
   - Lack of knowledge about conception.
   - Lack of easy access to contraception.
   - Lessened stigma associated with adolescent pregnancy in some populations.
   - Poverty.
   - Early school failure.
   - Early childhood sexual abuse.

LEARNING OUTCOME 13.3: Identify the physical, psychologic, and sociologic risks a pregnant adolescent faces.

1. Physical risks:
   - Preterm birth.
   - Low birth weight of infant.
   - Cephalopelvic disproportion of mother.
   - Iron-deficiency anemia.
   - Preeclampsia.
2. Psychologic risks:
   - Interruption of the developmental tasks of adolescence.
3. Sociologic risks:
   - More likely to drop out of school.
   - Need for public assistance.
   - Low-paying employment.
   - Single parenthood.
   - Increased domestic violence.

LEARNING OUTCOME 13.4: Delineate the characteristics of the fathers of children of adolescent mothers.

1. Fathers of children of adolescent mothers:
   - 50% are greater than 20 years of age.
   - Generally from same socioeconomic and educational level as adolescent mother.
   - Often have experienced early school failure.

LEARNING OUTCOME 13.5: Discuss the possible reactions of the adolescent's family and social network to her pregnancy.

1. Families with high educational and career goals for their children experience:
   - Anger.
   - Shock.
   - Shame.
   - Sorrow.
2. Teen often chooses abortion unless cultural or religious beliefs prohibit this.

3. Teen receives more support from family and friends where adolescent pregnancy is more common and more socially acceptable.
4. Some adolescent fathers may view pregnancy as:
   - Sign of adult status.
   - Sign of increased sexual prowess.
5. The mother of the adolescent usually provides the most support.

LEARNING OUTCOME 13.6: Formulate a plan of care to meet the needs of a pregnant adolescent.

1. Nursing care of the pregnant adolescent includes:
   - Obtaining consent for care.
   - Developing a trusting relationship with the adolescent.
   - Promoting self-esteem and problem-solving skills in the adolescent.
   - Promoting the physical health of the adolescent, especially with information concerning:
     - Regular prenatal visits.
     - Signs of complications.
     - Sexually transmitted infections.
     - Substance abuse.
     - Promoting family adaptation.
     - Facilitating prenatal education.

LEARNING OUTCOME 13.7: Describe successful community approaches to prevention of adolescent pregnancy.

1. Effective adolescent pregnancy prevention programs:
   - Are long term and intensive.
   - Involve adolescents in program planning.
   - Include good role models from the same cultural and racial backgrounds.
   - Include a focus on the adolescent male.

Clinical Reasoning in Action

Sixteen-year-old Linda Perez and her mother present to you at the OB clinic for Linda's first prenatal visit. You determine that Linda is 20 weeks pregnant. Her weight is 135 lb, height 5′4′′, T 98°F, P 80, R 14, BP 100/64. You assess that Linda's mother has type 2 diabetes, and that her siblings are healthy. Linda admits to having one sexual partner and says she has never been hospitalized. Her immunizations are up to date and she's never used tobacco or recreational drugs. To date, the father of the baby is not involved. Mrs. Perez is clearly upset that Linda's pregnancy is so far advanced without her knowledge. Linda is quiet and speaks only when questioned directly. You do your best to try to establish a trusting relationship with Linda and her mother by providing an atmosphere where issues can be discussed.

1. What psychologic factors contribute to teenage pregnancy?
2. Explore reasons why teenagers delay prenatal care.
3. Linda's mother asks you what factors facilitate adolescent pregnancies.
4. You assess that Linda has some anxiety concerning the birth process. She states she is not interested in prenatal classes because she is single and does not want to have natural childbirth. What would be your best response?
5. Develop a concept map to help Linda decide whether to try to involve the baby's father in the birth.

See www.nursing.pearsonhighered.com for possible responses and an interactive template for a concept map.

References

Advocates for Youth. (2008). *Teenage pregnancy, the case for prevention: An updated analysis of recent trends and federal expenditures associated with teenage pregnancy* (2nd ed.). Retrieved from http://www.advocatesforyouth.org/index.php?option=com_content&task=view&id=387&I

Alan Guttmacher Institute (AGI). (2012a). *Facts on American teens' sexual and reproductive health.* Retrieved from http://www.guttmacher.org/pubs/FB-ATSRH.pdf

Alan Guttmacher Institute (AGI). (2012b). *Facts on American teens' sources of information about sex.* Retrieved from http://www.guttmacher.org/pubs/FB-Teen-Sex-Ed.pdf

Alan Guttmacher Institute (AGI). (2012c). *Minors' access to prenatal care.* Retrieved from http://www.guttmacher.org/statecenter/spibs/spib_MAPC.pdf

Alan Guttmacher Institute (AGI). (2012d). *Minors' rights as parents.* Retrieved from http://www.guttmacher.org/statecenter/spibs/spib_MRP.pdf

Alan Guttmacher Institute (AGI). (2012e). *State policies in brief: Minors' access to contraceptive services.* Retrieved from http://www.guttmacher.org/statecenter/spibs/spib_MACS.pdf

Albert, B. (2010). *With one voice: America's adults and teens sound off about teen pregnancy.* Retrieved from http://www.thenationalcampaign.org/resources/pdf/pubs/wov_2010.pdf

American Academy of Pediatrics (AAP). (2007). Policy statement: Contraception and adolescents. *Pediatrics, 120*(5), 1135–1148.

American Academy of Pediatrics (AAP). (2012). Policy statement: Emergency contraception. *Pediatrics, 130*(6), 1174–1180.

American College of Obstetricians and Gynecologists. (2007). *Intrauterine device and adolescents* (Committee Opinion No. 392). Washington, DC: Author.

Broussard, A. B., & Broussard, B. S. (2010). Teaching pregnant teens: Lessons learned. *Nursing for Women's Health, 14*(2), 104–111.

Centers for Disease Control and Prevention. (2011). *Sexually transmitted disease surveillance 2010.* Atlanta, GA: U.S. Department of Health and Human Services.

East, P. L., Reyes, B. T., & Horn, E. J. (2007). Association between adolescent pregnancy and a family history of teenage births. *Perspectives on Sexual and Reproductive Health, 39*(2), 108–115.

Fletcher, J. M., & Wolfe, B. L. (2012). The effects of teenage fatherhood on young adult outcomes. *Economic Inquiry, 50*(1), 182–201.

Forcier, M., & Harel, Z. (2011). Adolescents and the IUD: An underutilized contraception for a high-risk population. *The Female Patient, 36*(6), 22–25.

Hagen, J., Skenadore, A., Scow, B., Schanen, J., & Clary, F. (2012). Adolescent pregnancy prevention in a rural Native American community. *Journal of Family Social Work, 15*(1),19–33.

Hamilton, B. E., & Ventura, S. J. (2012). *Birth rates for U.S. teenagers reach historic lows for all age and ethnic groups* (NCHS Data Brief No. 89). Retrieved from http://www.cdc.gov/nchs/data/databriefs/db89 .htm#citation

Hatcher, R. A., Trussell, J., Nelson, A. L., Cates, Jr., W., Kowal, D., & Policar, M. S. (2011). *Contraceptive technology* (20th ed.). Boston, MA: Ardent Media.

Herrman, J. W. (2009). There's a fine line . . . adolescent dating violence and prevention. *Pediatric Nursing, 35*(3), 164–170.

Herrman, J. W. (2010). Assessing the teen parent family. *Nursing for Women's Health, 14*(3), 214–224.

House, L., Bates, J., Markham, C., & Lesesne, C. (2010). Competence as a predictor of reproductive health outcomes for youth: A systematic review. *Journal of Adolescent Health, 46*(3, Suppl. 1), S7–S22.

Katz, A. (2011). Adolescent pregnancy: The good, the bad and the promise. *Nursing for Women's Health, 14*(2), 149–152.

Kearney, M. S., & Levine, P. B. (2012). Why is the teen birth rate in the United States so high and why does it matter? *Journal of Economic Perspectives, 26*(2), 141–166.

Kirby, D. (2007). *Emerging answers: Research findings on programs to reduce teen pregnancy and sexually transmitted diseases*. The National Campaign to Prevent Teen and Unplanned Pregnancy. Retrieved from http://www.thenationalcampaign.org/EA2007/ EA2007_sum.pdf

Lohan, M., Cruise, S., O'Halloran, P., Alderdice, F., & Hyde, A. (2010). Adolescent men's attitudes in relation to pregnancy and pregnancy outcomes: A systematic review of the literature from 1980–2009. *Journal of Adolescent Health, 47*, 327–345.

National Campaign to Prevent Teen and Unplanned Pregnancy (NCPTUP). (2012a). *Fast facts: Teen birth rates: How does the United States compare?* Retrieved from http://www.thenationalcampaign.org/ resources/pdf/FastFacts_InternationalComparisons.pdf

National Campaign to Prevent Teen and Unplanned Pregnancy (NCPTUP). (2012b). *Ten tips for parents*. Retrieved from http://www.thenationalcampaign.org/ parents/ten_tips.aspx

National Campaign to Prevent Teen and Unplanned Pregnancy (NCPTUP). (2012c). *Our mission: Goal*. Retrieved from http://www.thenationalcampaign.org/ about-us/our-mission.aspx

Pinkleton, B., Austin, E., Cohen, M., Chen, Y.-C., & Fitzgerald, E. (2008). Effects of a peer-led media literacy curriculum on adolescents' knowledge and attitudes toward sexual behavior and media portrayals of sex. *Health Communication, 23*, 462–472.

Sieving, R., McMorris, B., Beckman, K., Pettingell, S., Secor-Turner, M., & Kugler, K. (2011). Prime time: 12 month sexual health outcomes of a clinic-based intervention to prevent pregnancy risk behaviors. *Journal of Adolescent Health, 49*(2), 172–179.

Sieving, R., Resnick, M., Garwick, A., Bearinger, L., Beckman, K., & Oliphant, J. (2011). A clinic-based youth development approach to teen pregnancy prevention. *American Journal of Health Behavior, 35*(3), 346–358.

Sipsma, H. L., Ickovics, J. R., Lewis, J. B., Ethier, K. A., & Kershaw, T. S. (2011). Adolescent pregnancy desire and pregnancy incidence. *Women's Health Issues, 21*(2), 110–116.

Steinberg, L. (2010). *Adolescence* (9th ed.). New York, NY: McGraw-Hill.

Assessment of Fetal Well-Being

My first pregnancy was so tenuous that I didn't know from one moment to the next how it would end. I hoped for our baby's safety, but in the end the baby died. When I became pregnant the next time, I was very nervous. Being able to see the baby on ultrasound helped me so much. I knew then that our baby was alive and growing. —Sharon, 29

Peter Bowter/Science Source

LEARNING OUTCOMES

14.1 Identify pertinent information to be discussed with the woman regarding her own assessment of fetal activity and methods of recording fetal activity.

14.2 Describe the methods, clinical applications, and results of ultrasound in the nursing management of the pregnant woman.

14.3 Describe the use, procedure, information obtained, and nursing considerations for the following: first trimester combined screening, MaterniT21, Doppler velocimetry, nonstress test, fetal acoustic and vibroacoustic stimulation tests, biophysical profile, and contraction stress test.

14.4 Explain the use of amniocentesis as a diagnostic tool.

14.5 Describe the tests that can be performed using amniotic fluid.

14.6 Compare the advantages and disadvantages of chorionic villus sampling (CVS).

The past few decades have produced a notable increase in the number of techniques used to assess fetal well-being. From the relatively simple maternal assessment of fetal movement to more complex diagnostic tests guided by ultrasound, each technique is used to obtain accurate and helpful data about the developing fetus. For example, specialized diagnostic tests can provide information about the normal growth of the fetus, the presence of congenital anomalies, the location of the placenta, and fetal lung maturity (Table 14–1). At times just one test is done, and in other circumstances a combination of testing is needed.

Some of these assessment techniques pose risks to the fetus and possibly to the pregnant woman; the risk to both should be considered before deciding to perform the test. The healthcare provider must be certain that the advantages outweigh the potential risks and added expense. In addition, the diagnostic accuracy and applicability of these tests may vary.

Although some tests are for screening purposes, meaning that they indicate the fetus *may* be at risk for a certain disorder or abnormality, others are diagnostic, meaning that they can diagnose the abnormality. Certainly not all high-risk pregnancies require the same tests. Factors that indicate a pregnancy at risk include the following:

- Maternal age less than 16 or more than 35 years
- Chronic maternal hypertension, preeclampsia, diabetes mellitus, or heart disease
- Presence of Rh alloimmunization
- A maternal history of unexplained stillbirth
- Suspected intrauterine growth restriction (IUGR)
- Pregnancy prolonged past 42 weeks' gestation
- Multiple gestation
- Maternal history of preterm labor
- Previous cervical incompetence

See Chapter 9 🔗 for further discussion of prenatal at-risk factors and Chapters 15 🔗 and 16 🔗 for descriptions of various conditions that may threaten the successful completion of pregnancy.

Nursing care for the woman who is undergoing diagnostic testing focuses on outcomes to ensure that she understands the reasons for the test and its results and receives adequate support during the test (see Table 14–2). In addition, other objectives include completing the tests without complications and ensuring that the safety of the mother and her unborn child has been maintained.

MATERNAL ASSESSMENT OF FETAL ACTIVITY

Clinicians now generally agree that vigorous fetal activity provides reassurance of fetal well-being and that marked decrease in activity or cessation of movement may indicate possible fetal compromise (or even death) requiring immediate follow-up (Blackburn, 2013). Fetal activity is typically used to monitor fetal well-being beginning at approximately 28 gestational weeks. Fetal activity monitoring has been used for some time as a low-technology, inexpensive means to evaluate fetal well-being. One study of mothers with perceived decreased fetal movement identified 80% of those fetuses with intrauterine growth restriction (Saastad, Winje, Stray, et al., 2011). A reduction of fetal movement has been associated with fetal hypoxia, fetal growth restriction, and fetal death (Saastad et al., 2011). Although more research is needed to determine if fetal activity assessment improves neonatal outcomes, the literature does suggest that maternal monitoring does result in a decrease in perinatal mortality and decreases maternal anxiety (Saastad et al., 2011; Saastad, Winje, Israel, et al., 2012).

Table 14-1	Summary of Screening and Diagnostic Tests	
Goal	**Test**	**Timing**
To validate the pregnancy	Ultrasound: gestational sac volume	5 and 6 weeks after last menstrual period (LMP) by transvaginal ultrasound
To determine how advanced the pregnancy is	Ultrasound: crown–rump length Ultrasound: biparietal diameter, femur length, abdomen circumference	6 to 10 weeks' gestation 13 to 40 weeks' gestation
To identify normal growth of the fetus	Ultrasound: biparietal diameter Ultrasound: head/abdomen ratio Ultrasound: estimated fetal weight	Most useful from 20 to 30 weeks' gestation 13 to 40 weeks' gestation About 24 to 40 weeks' gestation
To detect congenital anomalies and problems	Nuchal translucency testing Ultrasound Chorionic villus sampling Amniocentesis Fetoscopy First-trimester combination screening test Quadruple test Materni21Plus	11 to 13 weeks' gestation 18 to 40 weeks' gestation 10 to 12 weeks' gestation 15 to 20 weeks' gestation 18 weeks' gestation 11 to 13 weeks' gestation Generally 15 to 20 weeks' gestation After 10 weeks' gestation
To localize the placenta	Ultrasound	Usually in third trimester or before amniocentesis
To assess fetal status	Biophysical profile Maternal assessment of fetal activity Nonstress test Contraction stress test	Approximately 28 weeks to birth Approximately 28 weeks to birth Approximately 28 weeks to birth After 28 weeks
To diagnose cardiac problems	Fetal echocardiography	Second and third trimesters
To assess fetal lung maturity	Amniocentesis L/S ratio Phosphatidylglycerol Phosphatidylcholine Lamellar body counts	33 to 40 weeks 33 weeks to birth 33 weeks to birth 33 weeks to birth 33 weeks to birth
To obtain more information about breech presentation	Ultrasound	Just before labor is anticipated or during labor

Table 14-2	Suggested Nursing Approaches to Pretest Teaching

Assess if the woman knows the reason the screening or diagnostic test is being recommended.
Examples:
  "What has your doctor or nurse-midwife told you about why this test is necessary?"
  "Sometimes tests are done for many different reasons. Can you tell me why you are having this test?"
  "What is your understanding about what the test will show?"

Provide an opportunity for questions.
Examples:
  "What questions do you have about the test?"
  "Is there anything that is not clear to you?"

Explain the test procedure, paying particular attention to any preparation the woman needs before the test.
Example:
  "The test that has been ordered for you is designed to _____ _____." (Add specific information about the particular test.
    Give the explanation using simple language.)

Validate the woman's understanding of the preparation.
Example:
  "Tell me what you will have to do to get ready for this test."

Give permission for the woman to continue to ask questions if needed.
Example:
  "I'll be with you during the test. If you have any questions at any time, please don't hesitate to ask."

A variety of methods for obtaining a **fetal movement count (FMC)** have been developed. They focus on having the woman keep a **fetal movement record (FMR)** using a technique such as the Cardiff Count-to-Ten method (see Figure 14–1 ●).

An FMR is noninvasive and lets the pregnant woman monitor and record movements easily and without expense. See *Teaching Highlights: What to Tell the Pregnant Woman About Assessing Fetal Activity.*

Sample Cardiff Count–to–Ten scoring card
Month: _____ **Week of gestation at beginning of month:** _____

● **Figure 14–1** An adaptation of the Cardiff Count-to-Ten scoring card for fetal movement assessment.

Teaching Highlights What to Tell the Pregnant Woman About Assessing Fetal Activity

- Explain that fetal movements are first felt around 18 weeks' gestation. From that time, the fetal movements get stronger and easier to detect. A slowing or stopping of fetal movement may be an indication that the fetus needs some attention and evaluation.
- Explain the procedure for the Cardiff Count-to-Ten method or for the daily fetal movement record. For both methods, advise the woman to:

  - Keep a daily record of fetal movement, beginning at about 27 weeks' gestation.
  - Try to begin counting at about the same time each day, about 1 hour after a meal if possible.
  - Lie quietly in a side-lying position.

- Using the Cardiff card, have the woman place an X for each fetal movement until she has recorded 10. Movement varies considerably, but most women feel fetal movement at least 10 times in 3 hours.
- Using the daily fetal movement record, have the woman count three times a day for 20 to 30 minutes each session. If there are fewer than 3 movements in a session, have the woman count for 1 hour or more.
- Explain when to contact the care provider:

  - If there are fewer than 10 movements in 3 hours
  - If overall the fetus's movements are slowing, and it takes much longer each day to note 10 movements
  - If there are no movements in the morning
  - If there are fewer than 3 movements in 8 hours

- Describe procedures and demonstrate how to assess fetal movement. Sit beside the woman and show her how to place her hand on the fundus to feel fetal movement.
- Provide a written teaching sheet for the woman's use at home.
- Demonstrate how to record fetal movements on the Cardiff Count-to-Ten scoring card or on the daily fetal movement record.

  - Watch the woman fill out the record as examples are provided. Encourage her to complete the record each day and bring it with her to each prenatal visit. Assure her that the record will be discussed at each prenatal visit, and questions may be addressed at that time if desired.
  - Provide the woman with a name and phone number in case she has further questions.
  - Evaluate learning by having the woman explain the method and by asking the woman to fill the card in using a fictitious situation. At each prenatal visit, the expectant mother's record is reviewed. This provides another opportunity for evaluation of learning and for questions and clarification.

 Clinical Tip

Families undergoing fetal testing experience a wide range of emotions based on personal expectations, past experiences, fears, and cultural norms. Encouraging the family to verbalize concerns, ask questions, and express any apprehensions or fears can help put the family at ease.

Fetuses spend approximately 10% of their time making gross body movements. Fetal movements are directly related to the infant's sleep–wake cycles and vary from the maternal sleep–wake cycle (Blackburn, 2013). After 38 weeks, the fetus spends 75% of its time in a quiet sleep or active sleep state. In women with a multiple gestation, daily fetal movements are significantly higher. The expectant mother's perception of fetal movements and her commitment to completing a fetal movement record may vary. When a woman understands the purpose of the assessment, how to complete the form, whom to call with questions, and what to report—and has the opportunity for follow-up during each visit—she generally views completing the fetal movement record as an important activity. The nurse is available to answer questions and clarify areas of concern.

ULTRASOUND

Valuable information about the fetus may be obtained from **ultrasound** testing. Intermittent ultrasonic waves (high-frequency sound waves) are transmitted by an alternating current to a transducer, which is applied to the woman's abdomen. The ultrasonic waves deflect off tissues within the woman's abdomen, showing structures of varying densities (Figures 14–2 ● and 14–3 ●).

● **Figure 14–2** Ultrasound scanning permits visualization of the fetus in utero.
Source: © Amy Etra/Photoedit.

● **Figure 14–3** Ultrasound of fetal face.

Diagnostic ultrasound has several advantages. It is noninvasive, is painless for both the woman and the fetus, and has no known harmful effects to either. Serial studies (several ultrasound tests done over a span of time) may be done for assessment and comparison. Soft-tissue masses (such as tumors) can be differentiated, the fetus can be visualized, fetal growth can be followed (especially in the presence of multiple gestation), cervical length and impending cervical insufficiency can be detected, and a number of other potential problems can be averted (Solt, Acuna, Ogunyemi, et al., 2011). In addition, the ultrasonographer or physician immediately obtains results.

Future research in fetal well-being will be generated and enhanced by the use of *four-dimensional ultrasound*. Four-dimensional ultrasound combines the components of three-dimensional ultrasound with a fourth dimension, time, because it monitors live action. The technology produces images of photolike quality, allowing healthcare providers to better visualize fetal structures, and providing better guidance during invasive intrauterine procedures such as amniocentesis and chorionic villus sampling (CVS) (discussed later in this chapter). Although ultrasound serves as a useful tool in monitoring the fetus throughout pregnancy, ultrasound has limitations and it cannot guarantee that a fetus does not have certain disorders or defects. Ultrasound is limited by fetal positioning and by technician or physician skill. Even though fetal problems can be diagnosed via the technology, abnormalities may, at times, go unrecognized. A "normal" ultrasound is reassuring for the parents and healthcare team, but it is important that parents realize the ultrasound or sonogram is not 100% reliable.

Procedures

The two most common methods of ultrasound scanning are transabdominal and transvaginal.

Transabdominal Ultrasound

In the transabdominal approach, a transducer is moved across the woman's abdomen. The woman is often scanned with a full bladder. When the bladder is full, the examiner can assess other structures, especially the vagina and cervix, in relation to the bladder. The ability to see the lower portion of the uterus and cervix is particularly important when vaginal bleeding is noted and placenta previa is the suspected cause. The woman is advised to drink 1 to 1.5 quarts of water approximately 2 hours before the examination, and she is asked to refrain from emptying her bladder. If the bladder is not sufficiently filled, she is asked to drink three to four 8-oz glasses of water and is rescanned 30 to 45 minutes later.

Transmission gel is generously spread over the woman's abdomen, and the sonographer slowly moves a transducer over the abdomen to obtain a picture of the uterine contents. Ultrasound testing takes 20 to 30 minutes. The woman may feel discomfort caused by pressure applied over a full bladder. In addition, if the woman lies on her back during the test, shortness of breath can develop. This may be relieved by elevating her upper body during the test.

Transvaginal Ultrasound

The transvaginal approach uses a probe inserted into the vagina. Once inserted, the transvaginal probe is close to the structures being imaged and so produces a clearer, more defined image than is possible with the transabdominal approach. The improved images obtained by transvaginal ultrasound have enabled sonographers to identify structures and fetal characteristics earlier in pregnancy. Internal visualization can also be used as a predictor for preterm birth in high-risk cases. Use of the ultrasound to detect shortened cervical length or funneling (a cone-shaped indentation in the cervical os) is helpful in predicting preterm labor, especially in women who have a history of preterm birth (American College of Obstetricians & Gynecologists [ACOG], 2009).

After the procedure is fully explained to the woman, she is prepared in the same manner as for a pelvic examination: in the lithotomy position, with appropriate drapes to provide privacy and a female attendant in the room. It is important for her buttocks to be at the end of the table so that, once inserted, the probe can be moved in various directions. A small, lightweight vaginal transducer is covered with a specially fitted sterile sheath, a condom, or one finger of a glove. Ultrasound coupling gel is then applied to both the inside and outside of the covering, making insertion into the vagina easier and providing a medium for enhancing the ultrasound image. The transvaginal procedure can be accomplished with an empty bladder, and most women do not feel discomfort during the exam. The probe is smaller than a speculum, so insertion is usually completed with ease. The woman may feel the movement of the probe during the exam as various structures are imaged. Some women may want to insert the probe themselves to enhance their comfort, whereas others would feel embarrassed even to be asked. The certified nurse-midwife, physician, or ultrasonographer offers the choice based on personal rapport with the woman.

Clinical Applications

Ultrasound testing can be of benefit in the following ways:

- *Early identification of pregnancy.* Pregnancy may be detected as early as the fifth or sixth week after the last menstrual period (LMP) by assessing the gestational sac and the presence of a fetal heart rate (FHR) after 6 gestational weeks.

- *Observation of fetal heartbeat and fetal breathing movements (FBMs).* FBMs have been observed as early as week 11 of gestation.
- *Identification of more than one embryo or fetus.*
- *Measurement of the biparietal diameter of the fetal head or the fetal femur length to assess growth patterns.* These measurements help determine the gestational age of the fetus and identify intrauterine growth restriction (IUGR).
- *Clinical estimations of birth weight. This assessment helps to* identify macrosomia (infants greater than 4000 g at birth) and low-birth-weight infants (infants less than 2500 g at birth). Macrosomia has been identified as a predictor of birth-related trauma and is a risk factor for both maternal and fetal morbidity (ACOG, 2009).
- *Detection of fetal anomalies such as facial anomalies, anencephaly, and hydrocephalus (ACOG, 2009).*
- *Examination of nuchal translucency in the first trimester to assess for trisomy 21 (Down syndrome) and other fetal structural anomalies (ACOG, 2009).* Nuchal translucency describes an area in the back of the fetal neck that is measured via ultrasound during the first trimester of pregnancy. Fetuses with a nuchal translucency measurement of greater than 3 mm are at risk for certain birth defects, including trisomies 13, 18, and 21.
- *Examination of fetal cardiac structures (echocardiography).* The presence of fetal cardiac defects during the first-trimester nuchal translucency screening test increases the risk that the fetus has a chromosomal disorder (Miguelez, De Lourdes Brizot, Liao, et al., 2012).
- *Length of fetal nasal bone.* The length of the fetal nasal bone during the nuchal translucency test is used to indicate a risk factor for Down syndrome. Fetuses with a nonvisualized or shortened nasal bone are more likely to have trisomy 21 than those with a normal length nasal bone (Sonek, Molina, Hiett, et al., 2012).
- *Identification of amniotic fluid volume (AFV) and amniotic fluid index (AFI).* Amniotic fluid volume parameters measure the single largest pocket of amniotic fluid on ultrasonography, free of cord and fetal parts, and then measure either the greatest vertical dimension or the greatest vertical and horizontal dimensions. The vertical diameter of the largest amniotic fluid pocket in each of four quadrants is measured for AFI. The measurements are totaled to obtain the AFI in centimeters. Women with an AFI of more than 24 cm and amniotic fluid volume of equal to or greater than 8 cm are considered to have hydramnios, and women with less than 5 cm at term and the deepest vertical pocket of AFV of less than 2 cm are considered to have oligohydramnios (ACOG, 2009). After 39 weeks, the amniotic fluid volume begins to decline (Cunningham, Leveno, Bloom, et al., 2010). Both hydramnios and oligohydramnios are associated with increased risk to the fetus, including nonreassuring fetal status, intrauterine growth restriction, meconium-stained amniotic fluid, and an increase in admissions to the neonatal intensive care unit.
- *Location of the placenta.* The placenta is located before amniocentesis to avoid puncturing the placenta.

Ultrasound also is valuable in identifying and evaluating placenta previa in the following ways:

- *Placental grading.* As the fetus matures, the placenta calcifies. These changes can be detected by ultrasound and graded according to the degree of calcification. Placenta grading can be used to identify internal placenta vasculature, which can be associated with preeclampsia and chronic hypertension. It can also identify disorders such as fetal growth abnormalities, triploidy, non-immune hydrops, and infections.
- *Detection of fetal death.* Inability to visualize the fetal heart beating and the separation of the bones in the fetal head are signs of fetal death.
- *Determination of fetal position and presentation.*
- *Accompanying procedures.* Ultrasound is used to assist with conducting amniocentesis, chorionic villus sampling, intrauterine procedures, and other procedures that will be discussed shortly.

Risks of Ultrasound

Ultrasound has been used clinically for over 40 years; to date no clinical studies verify harmful effects to the mother, the fetus, or the newborn. Many pregnant patients themselves received diagnostic ultrasound in utero with no adverse effects.

Nursing Management

It is important for the nurse to ascertain whether the woman understands why the ultrasound is being suggested and that the ultrasound is an extremely valuable tool although it is not 100% reliable. The nurse provides an opportunity for the woman to ask questions and acts as an advocate if there are questions or concerns that need to be addressed before the ultrasound examination. The nurse discusses the options available to the woman and her partner for fetal evaluation. The option of fetal evaluation should be offered to all women, regardless of age. This includes both invasive testing, such as amniocentesis and chorionic villus sampling (CVS), and ultrasound screening. The nurse explains the preparation needed and ensures that adequate preparation is done. After the test is completed, the nurse can assist with clarifying or interpreting test results for the woman and her partner.

FIRST-TRIMESTER COMBINED SCREENING

First-trimester combined screening is comprehensive screening testing that includes **nuchal translucency testing (NTT)** and serum screening for pregnancy-associated plasma protein-A (PAPP-A) and free beta human chorionic gonadotropin (β-hCG) to determine if a fetus is at risk for trisomies 13, 18, and 21. The combined test is more accurate than an NTT alone because it provides additional data. Using both the NTT and serum testing, the accuracy rates for diagnosis improve to 91% for assessing the risk of trisomy 21 and 98% for assessing trisomy 18 (Conner, Westgren, Marsk, et al., 2012).

Nuchal translucency testing (NTT), also known as nuchal testing (NT) or the nuchal fold test, is performed at 11 1/7 to

13 6/7 gestational weeks to screen for trisomies 13, 18, and 21 and is a component of the first-trimester combined screening (Mogra, Alabbad, & Hyett, 2012). Although women over the age of 35 have a higher risk of chromosomal disorders, universal screening is recommended for all women in the United States in their first and second trimesters. The test uses ultrasound to scan the translucent or clear area on the back of the fetal neck, measuring the diameter of the area. Fetuses with certain genetic disorders often have an excess accumulation of fluid that can be seen at the end of the first trimester. The results are computed using the nuchal measurement, exact gestational age, and maternal age. Fetuses that have a nuchal translucency measurement of greater than 3 mm are at risk for trisomies 13, 18, and 21 and their mothers should be offered an amniocentesis (to be discussed later). The NTT is a *screening test,* meaning it indicates that a fetus is at risk. Diagnostic testing, such as an amniocentesis, is a *diagnostic test,* which indicates that the fetus has or does not have the specific diagnosis.

The NTT test has several advantages over other testing options. It can be performed in the first trimester, early in a pregnancy, to determine if a fetus is *at risk* for chromosomal disorders. Unlike chorionic villus sampling (CVS) or amniocentesis, it has no risk of spontaneous abortion because it is a noninvasive test. The NTT accurately detects 90% of fetuses with Down syndrome (DS) (Conner et al., 2012). When combined with serum testing, the accuracy level increases. Many women feel anxious during pregnancy. A normal result can provide reassurance to the woman that her baby most likely does not have a chromosome disorder.

The disadvantage is that it can provide false positives and is not diagnostic. The combined test has a 5% false-positive rate, meaning the test will indicate that the fetus is at risk for Down syndrome when in fact the fetus has normal chromosomes. Women who receive an abnormal test are then counseled to determine if they would like to have an amniocentesis for diagnostic purposes. The choice to proceed with testing is a very personal one. Some women will wish to obtain the test so they will be more prepared for the diagnosis; other women will want to discontinue the pregnancy. Some women may decide not to have additional testing.

Fetuses that have a nuchal translucency measurement above the 99th percentile are also at risk for congenital heart disease (Mogra et al., 2012). A fetal echocardiogram is ordered in these cases to determine if a cardiac anomaly is also present. These fetuses have been found to have various cardiac diseases including "tricuspid regurgitation and abnormal flow in the 'a' wave of the ductus venosus" (Mogra et al., 2012, p. 264). The presence of tricuspid regurgitation provides a 55% detection rate for trisomy 21, whereas the presence of ductus venous flow provides a detection rate of 65% (Dias, 2011).

Fetuses that lack a nasal bone have a Down syndrome detection rate of 65%, and those with an abnormal facial angle as measured on ultrasound have a 45% detection rate. Clearly, combining all of these ultrasound findings and serum testing parameters dramatically increases the rate of detection. More literature is needed to move toward standardization of these testing techniques because currently the biochemical markers and nuchal translucency imaging remain the gold standard of screening testing.

Clinical Tip

When advising patients that a screening test, such as the NTT, is abnormal, be sure to explain that this does not mean their baby definitely has the disorder, but rather indicates that the baby may be at risk. It is imperative for parents to understand that an abnormal NTT, or any type of screening test, is only an indication that more testing is needed to make the actual diagnosis. Advise parents that some women with abnormal test results have normal fetuses and that because the test only screens and does not actually diagnose the fetus, a fetus that screens within the normal criteria could have an unrecognized anomaly.

MATERNIT21

In late 2011, *MaterniT21* was introduced as a maternal screening blood test that can be obtained to test for trisomies 13, 18, and 21. The test detects circulating fetal DNA within the maternal serum, which is as high as 6% to 10%. The test is noninvasive and detects 98.6% of fetuses affected with Down syndrome (trisomy 21) (ACOG, 2012). At this time, the test is not yet FDA approved but is available in the United States and is being marketed by a single distributor. In laboratory testing, false positives did occur in 0.5% of testing samples and an additional 0.6% of samples could not be definitively tested (Palomaki et al., 2012).

DOPPLER BLOOD FLOW STUDIES (UMBILICAL VELOCIMETRY)

Umbilical velocimetry, a noninvasive ultrasound test, measures blood flow changes that occur in maternal and fetal circulation in order to assess placental function. An ultrasound beam, like that provided by the pocket Doppler (a handheld ultrasound device), is directed at the umbilical artery (in some cases a maternal vessel such as the arcuate can also be used). The signal is reflected off the red blood cells moving within the vessels and creates a "picture" (waveform) that looks like a series of waves. The highest velocity peak of the waves is the systolic measurement, and the lowest point is the diastolic velocity. To interpret the waveforms, the systolic (S) peak is divided by the end-diastolic (D) component. This calculation is called the S/D ratio. The normal S/D ratio is below 2.6 by 26 weeks' gestation and below 3 at term. A decrease in uteroplacental perfusion (because of narrowing of the vessels) causes an increase in placental bed resistance and a decrease in diastolic flow, resulting in an elevated S/D ratio (Blackburn, 2013). Elevations of 3 and above are considered

Health Promotion   Infants with Down Syndrome

Healthy People 2020 strives to reduce the mortality of infants with Down syndrome at 1 year of age. Early detection and intensive treatment of identified comorbidities can help reduce infant mortality for this group.

abnormal. Doppler blood flow studies are helpful in assessing and managing pregnancies with suspected uteroplacental insufficiency before asphyxia occurs (Blackburn, 2013). Abnormal Doppler flow studies accompanied by a decrease in amniotic fluid have been associated with small-for-gestational-age fetuses, cesarean section for nonreassuring fetal status, 5-minute Apgar score of less than 7 (7 to 10 is the normal range), respiratory distress syndrome, NICU admission, and perinatal death (Blackburn, 2013).

Doppler blood flow studies are relatively easy to obtain. The woman lies supine with a wedge under the right hip (to promote uteroplacental perfusion). Warmed transducer gel is applied to the abdomen, and a pulsed-wave Doppler device is used to ascertain the blood flow. The Doppler flow study takes about 15 to 20 minutes. Doppler flow studies can be initiated at 16 to 18 weeks' gestation and are then scheduled at regular intervals for women at risk.

NONSTRESS TEST

The **nonstress test (NST)**, a widely used method of evaluating fetal status, may be used alone or as part of a more comprehensive diagnostic assessment called a biophysical profile (BPP) (discussed later in this chapter). The nonstress test is based on the knowledge that when the fetus has adequate oxygenation and an intact central nervous system, there are accelerations of the fetal heart rate (FHR) with fetal movement (FM). An NST requires an electronic fetal monitor to observe and record these fetal heart rate accelerations. (See discussion of accelerations in Chapter 18 .) A nonreactive NST is fairly consistent in identifying at-risk fetuses (Cunningham et al., 2010). The advantages of the NST are as follows:

- It is quick to perform, permits easy interpretation, and is inexpensive.
- It can be done in an office or clinic setting.
- There are no known side effects.

The disadvantages of the NST include the following:

- It is sometimes difficult to obtain a suitable tracing.
- The woman has to remain relatively still for at least 20 minutes.

Procedure

The NST can be done with the woman in a reclining chair or in bed in a left-tilted semi-Fowler's or side-lying position. Research has shown that certain maternal positions can help produce more favorable results. Women in left-tilted semi-Fowler's, reclining, and left lateral positions have more fetal movement and are more likely to have a reactive tracing. Women should not be placed in a supine position because it is associated with less fetal movement, maternal back pain, and maternal shortness of breath. The nurse places the electronic fetal monitor under the woman's clothing. Privacy should be provided. The examiner places two elastic belts on the woman's abdomen. Some facilities utilize disposable mesh sashes to hold the devices in place. One belt (tocodynamometer) holds a device that detects uterine or fetal movement; the other belt holds the ultrasound transducer that detects the FHR. As the NST is done, each fetal movement is documented, so that associated or simultaneous FHR changes can be evaluated. See Skill 2–6 in the *Clinical Skills Manual* SKILLS .

Interpretation of NST Results

Women with a high-risk factor will probably begin having NSTs at 30 to 32 weeks' gestation and at frequent intervals for the remainder of the pregnancy. The results of the NST are interpreted as follows:

- *Reactive test.* A reactive NST shows at least two accelerations of FHR with fetal movements of 15 beats per minute (beats/min), lasting 15 seconds or more, over 20 minutes (Figure 14–4 ●). This is the desired result. (See Table 14–3.) Some practitioners may begin NSTs at 28 weeks and utilize

● **Figure 14–4** Example of a reactive nonstress test (NST). The test shows accelerations of 15 beats/min lasting 15 seconds with each fetal movement (FM). Top of strip shows fetal heart rate (FHR); bottom of strip shows uterine activity tracing. Note that FHR increases (above the baseline) at least 15 beats and remains at that rate for at least 15 seconds before returning to the former baseline.

Table 14–3	Nonstress Test

Diagnostic value: Demonstrates fetus's ability to respond to its environment by acceleration of FHR with movement.

Results:
- *Reactive test:* Accelerations (at least 2) of 15 beats/min above the baseline, lasting 15 seconds or more in a 20-minute window, are present, indicating fetal well-being.
- *Nonreactive test:* Accelerations are not present or do not meet the above criteria, indicating that the fetus is at risk or asleep.

a 10-beat increase criteria at this gestational age (Glantz & Bertoia, 2011). Central nervous system maturity is required to execute a nonstress test, which is why earlier testing is not performed.

- *Nonreactive test.* In a nonreactive test, the reactive criteria are not met. For example, the accelerations do not meet the requirements of 15 beats/min or do not last 15 seconds (Figure 14–5 ●).

- *Unsatisfactory test.* An NST is unsatisfactory if the data cannot be interpreted or there was inadequate fetal activity.

It is important that anyone who performs the NST understand the significance of any decelerations of the FHR during testing. If decelerations are noted, the certified nurse-midwife (CNM) or physician should be notified for further evaluation of fetal status. (See Chapter 18 🔗 for further discussion of FHR decelerations.)

Clinical Management

The clinical management of potential nonreassuring fetal status may vary depending on the clinical judgment of the care provider. One commonly used protocol is as follows: If the NST is reactive in less than 30 minutes, the test is concluded and rescheduled as indicated by the high-risk condition that is present.

If it is nonreactive, the test time is extended for 30 minutes until the results are reactive, and then the test is rescheduled as indicated. It is estimated that 80% to 90% of nonreactive NSTs happen because of fetal sleep states (Cunningham et al., 2010). If the FHR remains nonreactive for longer than 30 minutes, the test is typically repeated after the woman eats or the fetus is stimulated via vibroacoustic stimulation or palpation. Such measures often wake a fetus, so a reactive NST can be obtained. If a reactive test is not obtained within 30 minutes, additional testing (such as diagnostic ultrasound and biophysical profile [BPP]) or immediate birth is considered; if the NST is nonreactive and spontaneous decelerations of the FHR are present, diagnostic ultrasound and BPP are performed and birth is recommended. Many testing guidelines vary in frequency, recommending a retest either once or twice a week, depending on the at-risk condition that exists.

Nursing Management

The nurse evaluates the woman's understanding of the NST and the possible results. The patient should be reassured that more frequent evaluation is used to ensure the well-being of the fetus and that reassuring fetal status means that uteroplacental circulation is providing adequate oxygenation to the fetus. The reasons for the NST and the procedure are reviewed before beginning the test. The nurse administers the NST, interprets the results, and reports the findings to the CNM or physician and the expectant woman.

FETAL ACOUSTIC AND VIBROACOUSTIC STIMULATION TESTS

Acoustic (sound) and vibroacoustic (vibration and sound) stimulation of the fetus can be used as an adjunct to the nonstress test (NST). A handheld, battery-operated device is applied to the woman's abdomen over the area of the fetal head. This device generates a low-frequency vibration and a buzzing sound. These are intended to induce movement and associated accelerations of the fetal heart rate (FHR) in fetuses with a nonreactive NST

● **Figure 14–5** Example of a nonreactive NST. There are no accelerations of fetal heart rate (FHR) with fetal movement (FM). Baseline FHR is 130 beats/min. The tracing of uterine activity is on the bottom of the strip.

and in fetuses with decreased variability of FHR during labor. (See discussion of variability in Chapter 18 🔗.) The sound stimulus persists for 2 to 5 seconds; if no accelerations occur, it is then repeated at 1-minute intervals up to three times. Whether the fetus responds more to the vibration or to the sound is not known. Two FHR accelerations of 15 beats/min, lasting 15 seconds, in a 20-minute period indicate a reactive test (Cunningham et al., 2010). Although no evidence-based clinical trials have examined the safety and efficiency of this technique, it continues to be used, although somewhat infrequently, in clinical practice (East, Smyth, Reader, et al., 2009).

Advantages of the fetal acoustic stimulation test (FAST) and the vibroacoustic stimulation test (VST) are as follows:

- Both are noninvasive techniques and are easy to perform.
- Results are rapidly available.
- Time for the NST is shortened.

BIOPHYSICAL PROFILE

The **biophysical profile (BPP)** is a comprehensive assessment of five biophysical variables and can be performed after 28 weeks (Buonocore, Bracci, & Weindling, 2012):

1. Fetal breathing movement
2. Fetal movements of body or limbs
3. Fetal tone (extension and flexion of extremities)
4. Amniotic fluid volume (visualized as pockets of fluid around the fetus)
5. Reactive fetal heart rate (FHR) with activity (reactive nonstress test [NST])

The first four variables are assessed by ultrasound scanning; FHR reactivity is assessed with the NST. By combining these five assessments, the BPP helps to either identify the compromised fetus or confirm the healthy fetus and provides an assessment of placental functioning. Specific criteria for normal and abnormal assessments are presented in Table 14–4. A score of 2 is assigned to each normal finding, and a score of 0 to each abnormal one, for a maximum score of 10. The absence of a specific activity

is difficult to interpret, because it may indicate central nervous system (CNS) depression or simply the resting state of a healthy fetus. Scores of 8/10 (with normal amniotic fluid) and 10/10 are considered normal. Such scores have the least chance of being associated with a compromised fetus unless a decrease in the amount of amniotic fluid is noted, in which case the infant's birth may be indicated. The use of maximum vertical pocket depth, and not the four-quadrant AFI (amniotic fluid index), in traditional BPS is validated by current research (Jelsema, 2012). See Skill 2–8 in the *Clinical Skills Manual* SKILLS.

The BPP is indicated when there is risk of placental insufficiency or fetal compromise because of the following:

- Intrauterine growth restriction (IUGR)
- Maternal diabetes mellitus
- Maternal heart disease
- Maternal chronic hypertension
- Maternal preeclampsia or eclampsia
- Maternal sickle cell disease
- Suspected fetal postmaturity (more than 42 weeks' gestation)
- History of previous stillbirths
- Rh sensitization
- Abnormal estriol excretion
- Hyperthyroidism
- Renal disease
- Nonreactive NST

CONTRACTION STRESS TEST

The **contraction stress test (CST)** is a means of evaluating the respiratory function (oxygen and carbon dioxide exchange) of the placenta. It enables the healthcare team to identify the fetus at risk for intrauterine asphyxia by observing the response of the FHR to the stress of uterine contractions (spontaneous or induced). During contractions, intrauterine pressure increases. Blood flow to the intervillous space of the placenta is reduced

Table 14–4	Criteria for Biophysical Profile Scoring	
Component	**Normal (score = 2)**	**Abnormal (score = 0)**
Fetal breathing movements	≥1 episode of rhythmic breathing lasting ≥30 sec within 30 min	≤30 sec of breathing in 30 min
Gross body movements	≥3 discrete body or limb movements in 30 min (episodes of active continuous movement considered as single movement)	≤2 movements in 30 min
Fetal tone	≥1 episode of extension of a fetal extremity with return to flexion, or opening or closing of hand	No movements or extension/flexion
Amniotic fluid volume	Single vertical pocket > 2 cm amniotic fluid index (AFI) > 5 cm	Largest single vertical pocket ≤2 cm AFI < 5 cm
Nonstress test	≥2 accelerations of ≥15 beats/min for ≥15 sec in 20 min	0 or 1 acceleration in 20 min

momentarily, thereby decreasing oxygen transport to the fetus. A healthy fetus usually tolerates this reduction well and maintains a steady heart rate. If the placental reserve is insufficient, fetal hypoxia, depression of the myocardium, and a decrease in fetal heart rate (FHR) occur.

In many areas, the CST has given way to the biophysical profile. CST is still used in areas where the availability of other technology is reduced (such as during night shifts) or limited (such as at small community hospitals or birthing centers). It may also be used as an adjunct to other forms of fetal assessment. Often, a nurse will document CST results as part of her assessment if the criteria for a CST are met; however, they are rarely ordered in standard practice due to the wide availability of ultrasound technology.

SAFETY ALERT!

Because CST is contraindicated in cases of third-trimester bleeding from placenta previa, marginal abruptio placentae or unexplained vaginal bleeding, previous cesarean with classical incision (vertical incision in the fundus of the uterus), premature rupture of the membranes, incompetent cervix, cerclage in place, anomalies of the maternal reproductive organs, history of preterm labor (if being done before term), or multiple gestation, the need to obtain a complete and comprehensive patient history prior to starting the test is imperative.

Procedure

The critical component of the CST is the presence of uterine contractions. They may occur spontaneously (which is unusual before the onset of labor), or they may be induced (stimulated) with oxytocin (Pitocin) administered intravenously (also known as an oxytocin challenge test [OCT]). A natural method of obtaining oxytocin is through the use of breast stimulation (either via nipple self-stimulation or application of an electric breast pump); the posterior pituitary produces oxytocin in response to stimulation of the breasts or nipples (Angelini & Lafontaine, 2013).

An electronic fetal monitor is used to provide continuous data about the fetal heart rate and uterine contractions. After a 15-minute baseline recording of uterine activity and FHR, the tracing is evaluated for evidence of spontaneous contractions. If three spontaneous contractions of good quality and lasting 40 to 60 seconds occur in a 10-minute window, the results are evaluated, and the test is concluded. If no contractions occur or they are insufficient for interpretation, oxytocin is administered intravenously or breast self-stimulation or application of an electric breast pump is done to produce contractions of good quality. (See Chapter 23 🔗 for more information on nursing care management of oxytocin induction.) The CST should be conducted only in a setting where tocolytic medications are available if a hyperstimulation pattern occurs or if labor is stimulated from the test. See Skill 2–7 in the *Clinical Skills Manual* SKILLS .

Interpretation of CST Results

The CST is classified as follows:

- *Negative.* A negative CST shows three contractions of good quality lasting 40 or more seconds in 10 minutes without evidence of late decelerations. This is the desired result. It implies that the fetus can handle the hypoxic stress of uterine contractions.

- *Positive.* A positive CST shows repetitive persistent late decelerations with more than 50% of the contractions (Figure 14–6 ●). This is not a desired result. The hypoxic stress of the uterine contraction causes a slowing of the FHR. The pattern will not improve and will most likely get worse with additional contractions.

- *Equivocal or suspicious.* An equivocal or suspicious test has nonpersistent late decelerations or decelerations associated with hyperstimulation (contraction frequency of every 2 minutes or duration lasting longer than 90 seconds). When this test result occurs, more information is needed.

● **Figure 14–6** Example of a positive contraction stress test (CST). Repetitive late decelerations occur with each contraction. Note that there are no accelerations of fetal heart rate (FHR) with three fetal movements (FM). The baseline FHR is 120 beats/min. Uterine contractions (bottom half of strip) occurred four times in 12 minutes.

Clinical Application

A negative CST implies that the placenta is functioning normally, fetal oxygenation is adequate, and the fetus will probably be able to withstand the stress of labor. If labor does not occur in the ensuing week, further testing is done.

A positive CST with a nonreactive NST presents evidence that the fetus will not likely withstand the stress of labor. A positive CST may be able to identify compromised fetuses earlier than a nonreactive NST because of the stimulated interruption of intervillous blood flow (Blackburn, 2013). Although a negative CST is reliable in predicting fetal status, a positive result needs to be verified, such as with a biophysical profile (see Table 14–5).

Nursing Management

The nurse ascertains the woman's understanding of the CST, the reasons for the test, and the possible results before the test begins. Written consent is required in some settings. In this case, the certified nurse-midwife (CNM) or physician is responsible for fully informing the woman about the test. The nurse administers the CST and reports the findings to the physician/CNM and the expectant woman. In some settings, the presence of the physician/CNM is required because there is a risk of initiating labor or hypertonic uterine contractions. Throughout the procedure, the nurse performs critical assessments and provides continual reassurance to the woman and her support person.

AMNIOTIC FLUID ANALYSIS

Amniocentesis is a procedure used to obtain amniotic fluid for genetic testing (early in pregnancy or between 15 and 16 weeks of pregnancy) for fetal abnormalities or to determine fetal lung maturity in the third trimester of pregnancy. During an amniocentesis, the physician scans the uterus using ultrasound to identify the fetal and placental positions and to identify adequate pockets of amniotic fluid. The skin is then cleaned with a Betadine solution. The use of a local anesthetic at the needle insertion site is optional. A 22-gauge needle is then inserted into the uterine cavity to withdraw amniotic fluid (Figure 14–7 ●). After 15 to 20 mL of fluid has been removed, the needle is withdrawn and the site is assessed for streaming (movement of fluid), which is an indication of bleeding. The fetal heart rate and maternal vital signs are then assessed. Rh immune globulin is given to all Rh-negative women. The analysis of amniotic fluid provides valuable information about fetal status. Amniocentesis is a fairly simple procedure, although complications do occur on rare occasions (fewer than 0.5% of cases). For nursing interventions during amniocentesis, see Clinical Skill 2–5 in the *Clinical Skills Manual* SKILLS .

Diagnostic Uses of Amniocentesis

A number of studies can be performed on amniotic fluid. These tests can provide information about fetal health, fetal lung maturity, and genetic disorders.

Table 14–5	Contraction Stress Test

Diagnostic value: Demonstrates reaction of FHR to stress of uterine contraction.

Results:
- *Negative test:* Stress of uterine contraction shows three contractions of good quality lasting 40 or more seconds in 10 minutes without evidence of late decelerations.
- *Positive test:* Stress of uterine contraction shows repetitive persistent late deceleration with more than 50% of the uterine contractions.
- *Equivocal or suspicious:* Nonpersistent late decelerations or decelerations associated with hyperstimulation.

● **Figure 14–7** Amniocentesis. The woman is usually scanned by ultrasound to determine the placenta site and to locate a pocket of amniotic fluid. As the needle is inserted, three levels of resistance are felt when the needle penetrates the skin, fascia, and uterine wall. When the needle is placed within the amniotic cavity, amniotic fluid is withdrawn.

Evaluation of Fetal Health

Concentrations of certain substances in amniotic fluid provide information about the health status of the fetus. The **quadruple screen** is another test that can be used to screen for Down syndrome (trisomy 21), trisomy 18, and neural tube defects (NTDs). The serum test assesses for appropriate levels of alpha-fetoprotein (AFP), human chorionic gonadotropin (hCG), and unconjugated estriol (UE3) and dimeric inhibin-A. The quadruple screen offers the advantage of being noninvasive but is only a screening test. The quadruple screen is less accurate and has higher false positive rates than a first-trimester combined screening test and should be offered to women for whom the first-trimester combined screening is unavailable (Kwon, Park, Kwon, et al., 2012). It is less invasive than an amniocentesis and may be used as a screening tool prior to the administration of an amniocentesis (Kwon et al., 2012). An amniocentesis is 99% accurate in diagnosing genetic abnormalities.

NTD's
&
spina
bifida
&
mylomenin
gocele

Evaluation of Fetal Lung Maturity

Because gestational age, birth weight, and the rate of development of organ systems do not necessarily correspond, amniotic fluid may also be analyzed to determine the maturity of the fetal lungs.

Health Promotion   Reducing the Rate of Preterm Births

Healthy People 2020 goals include reducing the rate of preterm births. Fetal lung maturity testing can reduce the number of infants born prematurely related to incorrect dating in earlier stages of pregnancy and reduce the rates of late preterm infants.

Fetal lung maturity determination in conjunction with gestational age is important when making clinical decisions regarding the timing of birth for women who may have complications, such as preeclampsia or diabetes. Women with pregnancies that are affected by diabetes have slower fetal lung maturation than other pregnancies not complicated by diabetes.

Lecithin/Sphingomyelin (L/S) Ratio.   The alveoli of the lungs are lined with a substance called **surfactant**, which is composed of phospholipids. Surfactant lowers the surface tension of the alveoli when the newborn exhales. When a newborn with mature pulmonary function takes its first breath, a tremendously high pressure is needed to open the lungs. By lowering the alveolar surface tension, surfactant stabilizes the alveoli, and a certain amount of air always remains in the alveoli during expiration. Thus when the infant exhales, the lungs do not collapse. An infant born before synthesis of surfactant is complete is unable to maintain lung stability. Each breath requires the same effort as the first. This results in underinflation of the lungs and the development of respiratory distress syndrome (RDS).

Fetal lung maturity can be ascertained by determining the **lecithin/sphingomyelin (L/S) ratio**; lecithin and sphingomyelin are two components of surfactant. Early in pregnancy, the sphingomyelin concentration in amniotic fluid is greater than the concentration of lecithin, and so the L/S ratio is low (lecithin levels are low and sphingomyelin levels are high). At about 32 weeks' gestation, sphingomyelin levels begin to fall and the amount of lecithin begins to increase. By 35 weeks' gestation, an L/S ratio of 2:1 (also reported as 2.0) is usually achieved in the normal fetus. A 2:1 L/S ratio indicates that the risk of RDS is very low. Under certain conditions of stress (a physiologic problem in the mother, placenta, and/or fetus, such as hypertension or placental insufficiency), the fetal lungs mature more rapidly (Angelini & Lafontaine, 2012).

Evidence-Based Practice   Pharmacologic and Nonpharmacologic Interventions During Amniocentesis

Clinical Question

Do pharmacologic and nonpharmacologic interventions have an effect on perceived pain during amniocentesis?

The Evidence

In addition to the known risks for mother and fetus associated with amniocentesis, women are often concerned that the procedure will be painful. A Cochrane systematic review of the Pregnancy and Childbirth Group's Trials Register was conducted to determine if either pharmacologic or nonpharmacologic pain reduction techniques affected the perception of pain during amniocentesis. Five randomized trials involving 805 women were reviewed for this recommendation. These types of systematic reviews, particularly those published according to the rigorous standards of the Cochrane Library, form the strongest level of evidence. Three primary pain reduction techniques were evaluated in this review: (1) local anesthesia at the needle insertion site, including infiltrative lidocaine or superficial lidocaine-prilocaine cream; (2) massage during the procedure; and (3) use of a subfreezing-temperature needle for the procedure. Pain was measured in all five studies using a Visual Analog Scale. None of the procedures provided

pain relief greater than placebo (Mujezinovic & Alfirevic, 2011). Actual pain was reported as minor regardless of treatment. A repeated measure study demonstrated that women who received pre-procedure counseling about what to expect during the amniocentesis reported lowered pain and anxiety levels during the procedure (Balci, Acar, Mahmoud, et al., 2011).

Best Practice

Women should be reassured that the pain associated with an amniocentesis is minor, and any pain reduction techniques should be optional. Pre-procedure counseling about what to expect during the procedure can help prevent both pain and anxiety. When women request pain reduction, noninvasive procedures such as massage should be offered to minimize the potential side effects of pharmacologic agents.

Clinical Reasoning

Should women be asked about their concerns regarding pain during amniocentesis when the procedure results in only minor pain? If a woman requests pain reduction techniques, what counsel can the nurse provide?

Table 14–6	Fetal Lung Maturity Values

Diagnostic value: Provides information to help determine fetal lung maturity.

Results:
- An L/S ratio of 2:1 and presence of PG correlate with 35 weeks' gestation.
- An L/S ratio lower than 2:1 and/or an absence of PG may indicate underinflation of lungs and an increased risk for development of RDS.
- An LBC of over 50,000 counts/mcL is predictive of fetal lung maturity.

Fetuses whose mothers are administered corticosteroids have an acceleration in fetal lung maturity.

Phosphatidylglycerol. **Phosphatidylglycerol (PG)** is another phospholipid in surfactant. Phosphatidylglycerol is not present in the fetal lung fluid early in gestation. It appears when fetal lung maturity has been attained, at about 35 weeks' gestation. Because the presence of PG is associated with fetal lung maturity, when it is present the risk of RDS is low. Phosphatidylglycerol determination is also useful in blood-contaminated specimens. Because PG is not present in blood or vaginal fluids, its presence is reliable in predicting fetal lung maturity. (See Table 14–6.)

Lamellar Body Count. **Lamellar body counts (LBCs)** are present in amniotic fluid when phosphatidylglycerol (PG) is present (Ridsdale, Lewis, Weaver, et al., 2012). When the LBC is 30,000 to 40,000 counts/mcL probable lung maturity is assumed. The laboratory analysis for LBC is considerably less costly than the previously discussed tests and can usually be performed at the acute care facility rather than a reference laboratory (Ridsdale et al., 2012).

Future Advances in Fetal Lung Maturity Testing. Some researchers are now examining the use of Doppler ultrasound as a means of identifying fetuses whose lungs have matured by using the measurement of the fetal pulmonary artery Doppler wave acceleration time/ejection time ratio (PATET) (Schenone, Samson, Suhag, et al., 2012). Although further research is needed, research in noninvasive screening tools continues to evolve and could potentially reduce risk factors for mothers and fetuses.

SAFETY ALERT!
When an amniocentesis is being done for fetal lung maturity, continuous fetal monitoring should be performed to assess for nonreassuring fetal status.

CHORIONIC VILLUS SAMPLING

Chorionic villus sampling (CVS) involves obtaining a small sample of chorionic villi from the developing placenta. Chorionic villus sampling is performed in some medical centers for first-trimester diagnosis of genetic, metabolic, and deoxyribonucleic acid (DNA) studies. Chorionic villus sampling can be performed either transabdominally or transcervically. The fetal loss rate is the same regardless of the approach used, although vaginal spotting is more common with the transcervical approach (Cunningham et al., 2010).

The advantages of this procedure are early diagnosis and short waiting time for results. Whereas amniocentesis is not done until at least 16 weeks' gestation, CVS is typically performed between 10 and 12 weeks. Previous studies that evaluated the use of CVS at 9 weeks found a possible association between limb reduction birth defects and early CVS. Based on these findings, most practitioners do not recommend early CVS before 10 gestational weeks (Cunningham et al., 2010). Risks of CVS include failure to obtain tissue, rupture of membranes, leakage of amniotic fluid, bleeding, intrauterine infection, maternal tissue contamination of the specimen, and Rh alloimmunization. Because CVS testing is performed so early in the pregnancy, it cannot detect neural tube defects. Women who desire testing for neural tube defects would need a quadruple screening at 15 to 20 weeks' gestation.

Nursing Management

The nurse assists the physician during the amniocentesis or CVS and supports the woman undergoing the procedure. Although the physician has explained the procedure in advance so that the woman can give informed consent, the woman is likely to be apprehensive both about the procedure itself and about the information it may reveal. She may become anxious during the procedure and need additional emotional support. The nurse can provide support by further clarifying the physician's instructions or explanations, by relieving the woman's physical discomfort when possible, and by responding verbally and physically to the woman's need for reassurance.

Following the procedure, the nurse reiterates explanations given by the physician and provides opportunities for questions. The nurse reviews the experience with the woman and presents self-care measures. Typically, the woman is monitored for a short time following the procedure. The nurse observes for contraction or uterine activity, amniotic fluid leakage, bleeding, or pain. The woman is advised of the warning signs of complications following the procedure.

Following an amniocentesis, approximately 1% of women develop complications such as amniotic fluid leakage from the puncture site or vaginal spotting. Approximately 1 in 1000 women develop infection. Needle puncture of the fetus rarely occurs during amniocentesis because of the use of ultrasound technology, which allows for continuous visualization of the fetus (Cunningham et al., 2010). Women should be reassured that although the complication rates are low, notification of her healthcare provider is necessary if any of these symptoms develop.

 Clinical Tip

When explaining genetic testing options to expectant parents, inform the mother that even if a CVS shows no chromosomal abnormality, it cannot screen for neural tube defects. Women who have a normal CVS and an abnormal quadruple screen test would be offered amniocentesis. Women with risk factors for neural tube defects may want to consider amniocentesis instead of CVS because it screens for both types of disorders.

Because fetal loss occurs more commonly before 15 weeks, many practitioners theorize that the loss rates associated with CVS are higher than those associated with amniocentesis. Early amniocentesis before 15 weeks is associated with an increased risk of fetal loss when compared with performing the procedure after 15 weeks. Approximately 1 in 200 fetal losses occurs with CVS.

When an amniocentesis is performed between 15 and 20 weeks, the risk of fetal loss is 1% (Corrado, Cannata, La Galia, et al., 2012). When any invasive procedure, such as an amniocentesis or a CVS, is performed, the nurse administers RhoGAM to the woman if she is Rh negative to prevent alloimmunization. Documentation should be charted and provided to the woman for future reference.

Critical Concept Review

LEARNING OUTCOME 14.1: Identify pertinent information to be discussed with the woman regarding her own assessment of fetal activity and methods of recording fetal activity.

1. Pertinent information to be discussed with the woman:
   - The purpose of the assessment.
   - How to complete the fetal activity form.
   - Whom to call with questions.
   - What to report.
2. Provide the opportunity for follow-up during each visit.

LEARNING OUTCOME 14.2: Describe the methods, clinical applications, and results of ultrasound in the nursing management of the pregnant woman.

1. Ultrasound offers a valuable means of assessing intrauterine fetal growth because the growth can be followed over a period of time.
2. It is noninvasive and painless.
3. It allows the certified nurse-midwife or physician to study the gestation serially.
4. It is nonradiating to both the woman and her fetus. It has no known harmful effects.

LEARNING OUTCOME 14.3: Describe the use, procedure, information obtained, and nursing considerations for the following: first trimester combined screening, MaterniT21, Doppler velocimetry, nonstress test, fetal acoustic and vibroacoustic stimulation tests, biophysical profile, and contraction stress test.

1. First trimester combined screening includes nuchal translucency testing and serum screening for pregnancy-associated plasma protein-A (PAPP-A) and free beta human chorionic gonadotropin (β-hCG) to determine if a fetus is at risk for trisomies 13, 18, and 21.
2. MaterniT21 is a noninvasive maternal screening blood test that identifies trisomies 13, 18, and 21 by detecting circulating fetal DNA within the maternal serum. It detects 98.6% of fetuses affected with Down syndrome (trisomy 21).
3. Doppler blood flow studies are used to assess placental function and sufficiency.
   - It is noninvasive. The woman lies supine and the Doppler is placed on the abdomen.
4. A nonstress test is based on the knowledge that the FHR normally increases in response to fetal activity and to sound stimulation.
   - The woman is attached to an electronic fetal monitor for approximately 20 minutes. She is required to lie still during the test.
   - Desired result is a reactive test.
5. Fetal acoustic and vibroacoustic stimulation of the fetus can be used as an adjunct to the nonstress test.
   - A battery-operated device is applied to the woman's abdomen over the area of the fetal head and generates a low-frequency vibration and a buzzing sound.
   - The intention is to induce movement and associated accelerations of the fetal heart rate in fetuses with a nonreactive NST and in fetuses with decreased variability of FHR during labor.
6. A biophysical profile is a combination of an ultrasound and a nonstress test to assess a fetus at risk for intrauterine compromise. It includes five variables:
   - Fetal breathing movement.
   - Fetal body movement.
   - Fetal tone.
   - Amniotic fluid volume.
   - Fetal heart rate reactivity.
7. A contraction stress test evaluates respiratory function of the placenta.
   - The woman is attached to an electronic fetal monitor and contractions are stimulated. This evaluates the ability of the fetus to handle contractions. The procedure may precipitate labor prematurely.
   - Desired result is a negative test.

LEARNING OUTCOME 14.4: Explain the use of amniocentesis as a diagnostic tool.

1. Amniocentesis assesses amniotic fluid for the presence of genetic disorders, fetal health status, and evaluation of fetal maturity.

LEARNING OUTCOME 14.5: Describe the tests that can be performed using amniotic fluid.

1. The quadruple screen measures substances contained in the amniotic fluid that provide information regarding the presence of fetal anomalies such as neural tube defects and Down syndrome.
2. The lecithin/sphingomyelin ratio, presence of phosphatidylglycerol, and level of lamellar body counts can be assessed to determine fetal lung maturity.

LEARNING OUTCOME 14.6: Compare the advantages and disadvantages of chorionic villus sampling (CVS).

1. Advantages:
   - Early detection of fetal disorders.
   - Decreased waiting time for results.
2. Disadvantages:
   - Increased risk of injury to fetus.
   - Inability to detect neural tube defects.
   - Potential for repeated invasive procedures.

Clinical Reasoning in Action

Patricia Adams is a 20-year-old, married, G2, P0010 at 36 weeks' gestation with gestational diabetes. She presents to you during her prenatal visit with a complaint of decreased fetal movement for the "last day or so." Her OB history includes a 13-lb weight gain, hematocrit of 29%, diastolic BP ranging 80–96 mm Hg, and 1+ proteinuria. A 19-week ultrasound demonstrated no fetal anatomic defects. A hemoglobin A$_{1c}$ at 23 weeks was 5.8%. Patricia has had weekly NSTs since 28 weeks' gestation. You place Patricia on the fetal monitor for an NST. You obtain vital signs of T 97°F, P 88, R 14, BP 130/88. After 30 minutes you observe that the fetal heart rate baseline is 160–165, variability is decreased, and repetitive variable decelerations are occurring. No contractions are noted. The fetus is very active.

You notify the physician of the fetal heart rate baseline and unsatisfactory NST. The physician orders a biophysical profile (BPP) for fetal well-being. You describe and explain the biophysical profile test to Patricia.

1. How would you describe and explain the biophysical profile test?
2. To heighten Patricia's awareness of fetal movement, how would you instruct her to do a daily fetal movement record (FMR)?
3. Explain when Patricia should contact her care provider.
4. Discuss the significance of fetal movement.
5. Explore factors that decrease fetal movements.
6. Create a concept map for Patricia's care based on her diagnosis of gestational diabetes. Patricia will be undergoing multiple tests including an NST and a BPP, which should be incorporated into her concept map.

See www.nursing.pearsonhighered.com for possible responses and an interactive template for a concept map.

References

American College of Obstetricians & Gynecologists (ACOG). (2009). Ultrasonography in pregnancy (ACOG Practice Bulletin No. 101). *Obstetrics & Gynecology, 113*(2) Part 1, 451–461.

American College of Obstetricians & Gynecologists (ACOG). (2012). Ultrasonography in pregnancy. Noninvasive prenatal testing for fetal aneuploidy (ACOG Committee Opinion No. 545). Washington, DC: Author.

Angelini, D. J., & Lafontaine, D. (2013). *Obstetric triage and emergency care protocols*. New York, NY: Springer.

Balci, O., Acar, A., Mahmoud, A., & Colakoglu, M. (2011). Effect of pre-amniocentesis counseling on maternal pain and anxiety. *Journal of Obstetrics and Gynaecology Research, 37*(12), 1828–1832.

Blackburn, S. T. (2013). *Maternal, fetal, & neonatal physiology: A clinical perspective* (4th ed.). St. Louis, MO: Saunders.

Buonocore, G., Bracci, R., & Weindling, M. (2012). *Neonatology: A practical review of neonatal management*. New York, NY: Springer.

Conner, P., Westgren, M., Marsk, A., Gustafsson, S., & Kublickas, M. (2012). Combined ultrasound and biochemistry for risk evaluation in the first trimester. *Acta Obstetricia et Gynecologica Scandinavica, 91*, 34–38. doi:10.1111/j.1600-0412.2011.01268.x

Corrado, F., Cannata, M. L., La Galia, T., Magliarditi, M., Imbruglia, L., D'anna, R., & Carlo Stella, R. (2012). Pregnancy outcome following mid-trimester amniocentesis. *Journal of Obstetrics & Gynecology, 32*(2), 117–119. doi: abs/10.3109/01443615.2011.633717

Cunningham, F. G., Leveno, K. J., Bloom, S. L., Hauth, J. C., Rouse, D. J., & Spong, C. Y. (2010). *William's obstetrics* (23rd ed.). New York, NY: McGraw-Hill.

Dias, T. (2011). Screening for chromosomal defects. *Sri Lanka Journal of Obstetrics and Gynaecology, 33*, 124–128.

East, C., Smyth, R., Reader, L., Henshell, N., Coditz, C., & Tan, K. (2009). Vibroacoustic stimulation for fetal assessment in labour in the presence of a nonreassuring fetal heart rate trace. *Cochrane Review*. doi:10.1002/14651858.CD004664.pub2

Glantz, J. C., & Bertoia, N. (2011). Preterm nonstress testing: 10-beat compared with 15-beat criteria. *Obstetrics & Gynecology, 118*(1), 87–93. doi:10.1097/AOG.0b013e31821d85e5

Jelsema, R. (2012). In the measurement of amniotic vertical pockets, are all pockets of similar depth the same? *Journal of Ultrasound in Medicine, 31*, 666.

Kwon, J., Park, I., Kwon, S., & Shin. J. (2012). The quadruple test for Down syndrome screening in pregnant women of advanced maternal age. *Archives of Gynecology and Obstetrics, 285*(3), 629–633. doi:10.1007/s00404-011-2052-1

Miguelez, J., De Lourdes Brizot, M., Liao, A. W., De Carvalho, M. H. B., & Zugaib, M. (2012). Second-trimester soft markers: Relation to first-trimester nuchal translucency in unaffected pregnancies. *Ultrasound Obstetrics & Gynecology, 39*, 274–278. doi:10.1002/uog.9024

Mogra, R., Alabbad, N., & Hyett, J. (2012). Increased nuchal translucency and congenital heart disease. *Early Human Development, 88*(5), 261–267. doi:10.1016/j.earlhumdev.2012.02.009

Mujezinovic, F., & Alfirevic, Z. (2011). Analgesia for amniocentesis or chorionic villus sampling. *Cochrane Database of Systematic Reviews*. Issue 11. Art. No.: CD008580.

Palomaki, G. E., Deciu, C., Kloza, E. M., Lambert-Messerlian, G. M., Haddow, J. E., Neveux, L. M., Ehrich, M., van den Boom, D., Bombard, A. T., Grody, W. W., Nelson, S. F., & Canick, J. A. (2012). DNA sequencing of maternal plasma reliably identifies trisomy 18 and trisomy 13, as well as Down syndrome: An international collaborative study. *Genetics Medicine, 14*(3), 296–305.

Ridsdale, R., Lewis, D. F., Weaver, T. E., & Akinbi, H. T. (2012). Proteomic analysis of lamellar bodies isolated from amniotic fluid: Implications for function. *American Journal of Perinatology, 29*(4), 19–28.

Saastad, E., Winje, B. A., Israel, P. and Frøen, J. F. (2012). Fetal movement counting: Maternal concern and experiences: A multicenter, randomized, controlled trial. *Birth, 39*, 10–20. doi:10.1111/j.1523-536X.2011.00508.x

Saastad, E., Winje, B. A., Stray, P. B., & Frøen, J. F. (2011) Fetal movement counting improved identification of fetal growth restriction and perinatal outcomes: A multi-centre, randomized, controlled trial. *PLoS ONE 6*(12), e28482. doi:10.1371/journal.pone.0028482

Schenone, M., Samson, J., Suhag, A., Jenkins, L., &, Mari, G. (2012). *A non-invasive method to predict fetal lung maturity using fetal pulmonary artery Doppler wave acceleration time/ejection time ratio*. Retrieved from http://www.eventkaddy.com/smfm2012/pdfs/363.pdf

Solt, I., Acuna, J. G., Ogunyemi, D., Rotmensch, S., & Kim, M. J. (2011). Teaching 3-dimensional fetal ultrasound: A randomized study. *Journal of Maternal–Fetal and Neonatal Medicine, 24*(6), 837–841. doi: http://dx.doi.org/10.3109/14767058.2010.531322

Sonek, J., Molina, F., Hiett, A. K., & Glover, M. (2012). Prefrontal space ratio: Comparison between trisomy 21 and euploid fetuses in the second trimester. *Ultrasound in Obstetrics & Gynecology, 40*(3), 293–296. doi:10.1002/uog.11120

Pregnancy at Risk: Pregestational Problems

When I learned I had gestational diabetes I felt panicky. My grandmother died of diabetes and it has always scared me. However, by taking each day as it came, cooperating with my doctors and nurses, and watching my diet, I did fine and gave birth to a beautiful 7 pound 10 ounce daughter. One good thing has come of the experience—I'm no longer so terrified of developing diabetes. I have become far more careful about taking care of myself, and I now think of diabetes as a chronic disease to be controlled. —Ayisha, 34

Bruce Ayres/Getty Images

LEARNING OUTCOMES

15.1 Discuss the pathology, treatment, and nursing care of pregnant women with diabetes mellitus.

15.2 Distinguish among the major types of anemia associated with pregnancy with regard to signs, treatment, and implications for pregnancy.

15.3 Summarize the effects of alcohol and illicit drugs on the childbearing woman and her fetus/newborn.

15.4 Explain the possible implications of maternal psychologic factors and disorders in caring for the childbearing family.

15.5 Describe acquired immunodeficiency syndrome (AIDS), including care of the pregnant woman with HIV/AIDS, fetal/neonatal implications, and ramifications for the childbearing family.

15.6 Describe the effects of various heart disorders on pregnancy, including their implications for nursing care.

15.7 Compare the effects of selected pregestational medical conditions on pregnancy.

Even though it is a normal process, for women with preexisting (pregestational) conditions, pregnancy may become a life-threatening event because of factors such as age, parity, blood type, socioeconomic status, psychologic health, or preexisting chronic illnesses. This chapter focuses on women with pregestational medical disorders and their possible effects on the pregnancy.

CARE OF THE WOMAN WITH DIABETES MELLITUS

Diabetes mellitus (DM), an endocrine disorder of carbohydrate metabolism, results from inadequate production or use of insulin. Insulin, produced by the β-cells of the islets of Langerhans in the pancreas, lowers blood glucose levels by enabling glucose to move from the blood into muscle and adipose tissue cells.

Carbohydrate Metabolism in Normal Pregnancy

In early pregnancy the rise in serum levels of estrogen, progesterone, and other hormones stimulates increased insulin production by the maternal pancreas and increased tissue response to insulin. Thus, an anabolic (building-up) state exists during the first half of pregnancy, with storage of glycogen in the liver and other tissues.

In the second half of pregnancy, placental secretion of human placental lactogen (hPL) and prolactin (from the decidua), as well as elevated cortisol and glycogen levels, causes increased resistance to insulin and decreased glucose tolerance. This decreased effectiveness of insulin results in a catabolic (destructive) state during fasting periods, such as during the night or after meal absorption. Because increasing amounts of circulating maternal glucose and amino acids are diverted to the fetus, maternal fat is metabolized much more readily during fasting periods than in a nonpregnant woman. As a result of this lipolysis (maternal metabolism of fat), ketones may be present in the urine.

The delicate system of checks and balances between glucose production and glucose use is stressed by the growing fetus, who derives energy from glucose taken solely from maternal stores. This stress is known as the *diabetogenic effect of pregnancy*. Thus, any preexisting disruption in carbohydrate metabolism is augmented by pregnancy, and any diabetic potential may precipitate gestational diabetes mellitus.

Pathophysiology of Diabetes Mellitus

In DM the pancreas fails to produce insulin or does not produce enough insulin to allow necessary carbohydrate metabolism. Without adequate insulin, glucose does not enter the cells and they become energy depleted. Blood glucose levels remain high (hyperglycemia), and the cells break down their stores of fats and protein for energy. Protein breakdown results in a negative nitrogen balance; fat metabolism causes ketosis.

These pathologic developments cause the four cardinal signs and symptoms of DM: polyuria, polydipsia, polyphagia, and weight loss. Polyuria (frequent urination) results because water is not reabsorbed by the renal tubules due to the osmotic activity of glucose. Polydipsia (excessive thirst) is caused by dehydration from polyuria. Polyphagia (excessive hunger) is caused by tissue loss and a state of starvation, which results from the inability of the cells to use the blood glucose. Weight loss (seen with marked hyperglycemia) is due to the use of fat and muscle tissue for energy.

Classification

The primary classification of diabetes is based on cause and includes four main categories (American Diabetes Association [ADA], 2012):

■ *Type 1 diabetes:* This type develops because of β-cell destruction and generally results in an absolute insulin deficiency.

- *Type 2 diabetes:* This is the most common form of diabetes and results from a combination of an insulin secretory defect and insulin resistance.

- *Other specific types:* There are eight subcategories including genetic defects, drug-induced diabetes, and endocrine disorders. (*Note:* The complete list can be found in medical-surgical textbooks and through ADA original sources.)

- *Gestational diabetes mellitus.*

Gestational diabetes mellitus (GDM) is defined as any degree of glucose intolerance that has its onset or is first diagnosed during pregnancy. It occurs in about 7% of all pregnancies in the United States (American College of Obstetricians and Gynecologists [ACOG], 2011b). Women who are markedly obese, have a prior history of GDM, have glycosuria, or have a strong family history of diabetes are at high risk (ADA, 2012). Diagnosis of GDM is very important because even mild diabetes causes increased risk for perinatal morbidity and mortality. Furthermore, many women with GDM progress over time to overt type 2 diabetes mellitus.

Influence of Pregnancy on Diabetes

Pregnancy can affect diabetes significantly because the physiologic changes of pregnancy can drastically alter insulin requirements. Pregnancy may also alter the progress of vascular disease secondary to DM. Pregnancy can affect diabetes in the following ways:

- DM may be difficult to control because insulin requirements are changeable.

- During the first trimester, the need for insulin frequently decreases. Levels of hPL, an insulin antagonist, are low; fetal needs are minimal; and the woman may consume less food because of nausea and vomiting.

- Nausea and vomiting may cause dietary fluctuations and increase the risk of hypoglycemia, formerly called insulin shock.

- Insulin requirements begin to rise in the second trimester as glucose use and glucose storage by the woman and fetus increase. Insulin requirements may double or quadruple by the end of pregnancy as a result of placental maturation and hPL production.

- Increased energy needs during labor may require increased insulin to balance IV glucose.

- Usually an abrupt decrease in insulin requirement occurs after passage of the placenta and the resulting loss of hPL in maternal circulation.

- A decreased renal threshold for glucose leads to a higher incidence of glycosuria.

- The risk of ketoacidosis, which may occur at lower serum glucose levels in the pregnant woman with DM than in the nonpregnant woman with diabetes, increases.

- The vascular disease that accompanies DM may progress during pregnancy.

- Hypertension may occur, contributing to vascular changes.

- Nephropathy may result from renal impairment, and retinopathy may develop.

Influence of Diabetes on Pregnancy Outcome

The pregnancy of a woman who has diabetes carries a higher risk of complications, especially perinatal mortality and congenital anomalies. Tight metabolic control (fasting blood glucose level of 95 mg/dL or less, pre-meal values of 100 mg/dL or less, and a 2-hour postprandial glucose level of 120 mg/dL or less) reduces this risk (ACOG, 2012b). New techniques for monitoring blood glucose level, delivering insulin, and monitoring the fetus have also helped reduce perinatal mortality.

Maternal Risks

The prognosis for the pregnant woman with gestational, type 1, or type 2 diabetes without significant vascular damage is positive.

Case Study · *Patient with Gestational Diabetes*

 Evidence-Based Practice Modifiable Risk Factors for Gestational Diabetes

Clinical Question

What are the modifiable risk factors for gestational diabetes?

The Evidence

Understanding the risk factors for gestational diabetes is key to its prevention. If the nurse can identify those women most at risk for gestational onset of diabetes, interventions can be designed to minimize those risks. Risk factors associated with gestational diabetes were determined via a systematic epidemiologic review, a longitudinal study, and a prospective comparative study. Thirty-nine studies were included in the review and nearly 17,000 women were included in the prospective analyses. These kinds of reviews and replicated comparative studies form the strongest level of evidence. Risk factors were grouped into modifiable and nonmodifiable, with a focus on risk that could be mediated with behavior change. A concurrent systematic review determined the effectiveness of lifestyle modification interventions in preventing the onset of gestational

diabetes (Ferrara, Hedderson, Albright, et al., 2011). Nonmodifiable risk factors were advanced maternal age, previous episodes of gestational diabetes, and longer than average menstrual cycles (Dishi, Enquobahrie, Abetew, et al., 2011). Modifiable risk factors were body mass index greater than 29, high dietary fat intake, and low levels of physical activity (Baker & Haeri, 2012; Bower, Tobias, Yeung, et al., 2012).

Best Practice

Evaluation of modifiable risk factors should be a part of each prenatal visit. Healthy lifestyle interventions should be offered to women with risk factors before signs of gestational diabetes appear.

Clinical Reasoning

What should be included in the prenatal history to determine modifiable risk factors for gestational diabetes? What should be included in the lifestyle modification intervention plan?

However, diabetic pregnancy still carries a higher risk of complications than normal pregnancy.

Hydramnios, or an increase in the volume of amniotic fluid, occurs in 10% to 20% of pregnant women with diabetes. It is thought to be a result of excessive fetal urination because of fetal hyperglycemia. Premature rupture of membranes and onset of labor may occasionally be a problem with hydramnios.

Preeclampsia/eclampsia occurs more often in diabetic pregnancies than in normal pregnancies, especially when vascular changes already exist.

Hyperglycemia, due to insufficient amounts of insulin, can lead to *ketoacidosis* as a result of the increase in ketone bodies (which are acidic) released in the blood from the metabolism of fatty acids. Decreased gastric motility and the anti-insulin effects of hPL also predispose the woman to ketoacidosis. Ketoacidosis usually develops slowly but, if untreated, can lead to coma and death for mother and fetus.

Pregnancy can also worsen *retinopathy* in women with diabetes. However, good control of blood glucose levels lessens the impact. Hence, women with preexisting diabetes should be referred to an ophthalmologist for evaluation during pregnancy.

The pregnant woman with diabetes is also at increased risk for monilial vaginitis and urinary tract infections because of increased glycosuria, which contributes to a favorable environment for bacterial growth.

Fetal/Neonatal Risks

Many of the problems of the newborn result directly from high maternal plasma glucose levels. In the presence of untreated maternal ketoacidosis, the risk of fetal death increases dramatically.

The incidence of *congenital anomalies* in diabetic pregnancies is 6% to 12% and is the major cause of death of infants born to women with diabetes. Research suggests that this increased incidence is related to multiple factors including high glucose levels in early pregnancy (ACOG, 2012b). Most anomalies involve the heart, central nervous system, and skeletal system. One anomaly, *sacral agenesis,* appears almost exclusively in infants of mothers with diabetes. In sacral agenesis, the sacrum and lumbar spine fail to develop and the lower extremities develop incompletely. Preconception counseling and strict diabetes control before conception help reduce the incidence of congenital anomalies.

Characteristically, infants of mothers with diabetes on insulin therapy are *large for gestational age (LGA)* as a result of the high maternal levels of blood glucose, from which the fetus derives its glucose. These elevated levels continually stimulate the fetal islets of Langerhans to produce insulin. This hyperinsulin state causes the fetus to use the available glucose, which leads to excessive growth (known as **macrosomia**) and fat deposits. If born vaginally, the macrosomic infant is at increased risk for shoulder dystocia and traumatic birth injuries; thus, cesarean birth may be considered if birth weight is expected to exceed 4500 g.

Once the umbilical cord is cut after birth, the generous maternal blood glucose supply stops. However, continued islet cell hyperactivity leads to high insulin levels and depleted blood glucose (hypoglycemia) in 2 to 4 hours. Macrosomia can be significantly reduced by strict maternal blood glucose control.

Infants of mothers with advanced diabetes (vascular involvement) may demonstrate *intrauterine growth restriction (IUGR),* which occurs because vascular changes in the mother decrease the efficiency of placental perfusion and the fetus is not as well sustained.

Respiratory distress syndrome (RDS) appears to result from high levels of fetal insulin, which inhibit some fetal enzymes necessary for surfactant production. *Polycythemia* (excessive number of red blood cells) in the newborn is mainly due to the diminished ability of glycosylated hemoglobin in the mother's blood to release oxygen. *Hyperbilirubinemia* is a direct result of the inability of immature liver enzymes to metabolize the increased bilirubin resulting from the polycythemia.

Clinical Therapy

All pregnant women, regardless of risk factors, should have their risk for undiagnosed type 2 diabetes assessed at the first prenatal visit. Women at high risk (non-Caucasian, prior history of GDM or birth of an LGA infant, marked obesity, diagnosis of polycystic ovarian syndrome, hypertension, presence of glycosuria, or a strong family history of type 2 DM) should be screened for diabetes as soon as possible. Various screening approaches may be used. An HbA_{1c} level equal to or greater than 6.5% would be considered diagnostic, as would a fasting plasma glucose level equal to or greater than 126 mg/dL or a 2-hour plasma glucose level equal to or greater than 200 mg/dL during an oral glucose tolerance test (OGTT) (see following discussion). Women determined to have diabetes at this visit should be diagnosed as having overt diabetes and not GDM (ADA, 2012).

The ADA (2012) recommends that pregnant women at average risk be screened at 24 to 28 weeks' gestation using a 75-g 2-hour OGTT. To do the test, the woman ingests a 75-g oral glucose solution in the morning after an overnight fast. Plasma glucose levels are determined fasting and at 1 and 2 hours. Gestational diabetes is diagnosed if any of the following values are equaled or exceeded:

Fasting	92 mg/dL
1 hour	180 mg/dL
2 hour	153 mg/dL

ACOG (2011b) does not currently support the one-step, 75-g approach. It recommends a two-step approach in which all pregnant women are screened for diabetes. Women at average risk are given a 50-g, 1-hour OGTT at 24 to 28 weeks' gestation. The oral glucose load can be given at any time of the day with no requirement for fasting. One hour later plasma glucose is measured. If plasma glucose levels are elevated (greater than 130 to 140 mg/dL, depending on the laboratory used), a 100-g, 3-hour glucose test is done.

Laboratory Assessment of Long-Term Glucose Control

Measurement of glycosylated hemoglobin levels provides information about the long-term (previous 4 to 8 weeks) control of hyperglycemia. The test measures the percentage of glycohemoglobin in the blood. Glycohemoglobin, or HbA_{1c}, is the hemoglobin to which a glucose molecule is attached. Because glycosylation is a rather slow and essentially irreversible process, the test is not reliable for screening for gestational diabetes or for close daily control. However, in women with known pregestational DM, abnormal HbA_{1c} values correlate directly with the frequency of spontaneous abortion and fetal congenital anomalies. Consequently, women with preexisting diabetes who plan to become pregnant should work to achieve HbA_{1c} levels at target levels (less than 6%) without significant hypoglycemia (ADA, 2012).

Antepartum Management of Diabetes Mellitus

To ensure an optimally healthy mother and newborn, good prenatal care using a team approach must be a top priority. The woman with gestational diabetes may find the diagnosis shocking and upsetting. She needs clear explanations and teaching to gain her cooperation in ensuring a good outcome. The nurse-educator plays a major role in this counseling.

The woman with pregestational diabetes needs to understand what changes she can expect during pregnancy; she should receive such teaching during preconception counseling. In addition, preconception care focuses on stringent blood glucose control prior to conception and during the first trimester. A pregnant woman with preexisting diabetes may also require referral to specialists such as an ophthalmologist or nephrologist.

Dietary Regulation

The pregnant woman with diabetes needs to increase her caloric intake by about 300 kcal/day. During the first trimester, the normal-weight woman generally requires about 30 kcal/kg of ideal body weight. During the second and third trimesters, she needs about 35 kcal/kg of ideal body weight. Approximately 40% to 50% of the calories should come from complex carbohydrates, 15% to 20% from protein, and 20% to 30% from fats. The food is divided among three meals and three snacks. The bedtime snack is the most important and should include both protein and complex carbohydrates to prevent nighttime hypoglycemia. A nutritionist should work out meal plans with the woman based on the woman's lifestyle, culture, and food preferences. The woman needs to be familiar with the use of food exchanges so she can plan her own meals.

Glucose Monitoring

Glucose monitoring is essential to determine the need for insulin and to assess glucose control. Many physicians have the woman come in for weekly assessment of her fasting glucose levels and one or two postprandial levels. In addition, frequent self-monitoring of glucose levels is paramount in maintaining good glucose control. Self-monitoring is discussed later in the chapter.

Insulin Administration

Many women with gestational diabetes need insulin to maintain normal glucose levels. Those with pregestational diabetes typically have type 1 diabetes and are already on insulin. In either case, human insulin should be used because it is the least likely to cause an allergic reaction. Insulin is given either in multiple injections or by continuous subcutaneous infusion. Multiple injections are more common and generally produce excellent results. Many women receive a combination of intermediate and regular insulin.

Recently, clinicians have moved away from the use of regular human insulin, replacing it with an insulin analog (either lispro or aspart), which is associated with better glucose control and a decreased risk of delayed postprandial hypoglycemia (Reece, 2011). Often a four-dose approach is used, with regular insulin or an analog taken before each meal and NPH or Lente insulin added at bedtime. Other clinicians vary the NPH and regular insulin patterns slightly but still prefer a four-dose approach.

Until recently oral hypoglycemics were not generally used during pregnancy because they cross the placenta and had not been well studied. Recent research suggests that glyburide, a second-generation sulfonylurea, and metformin, a biguanide, may be safe to use in women with gestational diabetes (Moore, 2012; Reece, 2011).

Evaluation of Fetal Status

Information about the well-being, size, and maturation of the fetus is important for planning the course of pregnancy and the timing of birth. In pregnancies complicated by diabetes, the fetus is at increased risk of neural tube defects such as spina bifida, so maternal serum alpha-fetoprotein (MSAFP) screening is offered at 16 to 20 weeks' gestation.

Ultrasound done at 18 weeks confirms gestational age and detects anomalies. It is repeated at 28 weeks to monitor fetal growth for IUGR or macrosomia. Some physicians do *fetal biophysical profiles* (ultrasound evaluations of fetal well-being that assess fetal breathing movements, fetal activity, reactivity, muscle tone, and amniotic fluid volume) as part of an ongoing evaluation of fetal status.

Daily maternal evaluation of *fetal activity* is begun at about 28 weeks. Nonstress testing (NST) is usually begun weekly at 28 weeks and increased to twice weekly at 32 weeks' gestation. If the NST is nonreactive, a fetal biophysical profile or *contraction stress test* is performed. (For an explanation of these tests, see Chapter 14 🔗.) If the woman requires hospitalization for complications or to control blood glucose levels, NSTs may be done weekly.

Intrapartum Management of Diabetes Mellitus

During the intrapartum period, medical therapy focuses on the following:

- *Timing of birth.* Most pregnant women with diabetes, regardless of the type, are allowed to go to term, with spontaneous labor. Some clinicians, however, opt to induce labor in a woman at term to avoid problems related to decreased perfusion as the placenta ages. Cesarean birth may be indicated if signs of fetal distress exist. Birth before term may be indicated for women with diabetes who are experiencing vascular changes and worsening hypertension or if evidence of IUGR exists. To determine fetal lung maturity, amniotic fluid (obtained by amniocentesis) is evaluated using the lecithin/sphingomyelin (L/S) ratio, fluorescent polarization, and/or the presence of phosphatidylglycerol (see Chapter 14 ●). Preterm birth, often by cesarean, is considered if prenatal testing indicates that the fetus is deteriorating.

■ *Labor management.* Frequently, maternal insulin requirements decrease dramatically during labor. Consequently maternal glucose levels are measured hourly to determine insulin need (Figure 15–1 ●). The primary goal in controlling maternal glucose levels intrapartally is to prevent neonatal hypoglycemia (American Academy of Pediatrics [AAP] & ACOG, 2012). (Often two IV lines are used, one with a 5% dextrose solution and one with a saline solution. The saline solution is then available for piggybacking insulin or if a bolus is needed.) Because insulin clings to plastic IV bags and tubing, the tubing should be flushed with insulin before the prescribed amount is added. During the second stage of labor and the immediate postpartum period, the woman may not need additional insulin. The IV insulin is discontinued at the end of the third stage of labor.

Postpartum Management of Diabetes Mellitus

Generally maternal insulin requirements fall significantly during the postpartum period because hormone levels fall after placental separation and their anti-insulin effect ceases, resulting in decreased blood glucose levels. For the first 24 hours postpartum,

● **Figure 15–1** Maternal glucose levels. During labor the nurse closely monitors the blood glucose levels of the woman with diabetes mellitus.

women with preexisting diabetes typically require very little insulin and are usually managed with a sliding scale. Afterward a more regular insulin dosage pattern can be reestablished based on blood glucose testing.

Women with GDM seldom need insulin during the postpartum period. Clinicians routinely decrease the dose significantly for women with preexisting DM to avoid hypoglycemia and then monitor blood glucose levels. Breastfeeding can be encouraged, but the nurse needs to remember that insulin requirements do decrease with breastfeeding, so a prenursing snack may be indicated (Hood, 2012). If elevated glucose levels develop, oral antihyperglycemic agents may be tried if the woman is not breastfeeding. The woman should be reassessed 6 weeks postpartum to determine whether her glucose levels are normal. If the levels are normal, she should be reassessed at a minimum of 3-year intervals (ADA, 2012).

If the newborn requires a special care nursery, the nurse should provide the parents with ongoing information, support, and encouragement to visit and be involved in the newborn's care, since establishing parent–child relationships is a high priority during the postpartum period.

The nurse should encourage breastfeeding as beneficial to both mother and baby. Maternal calorie needs increase during lactation to 500 to 800 kcal above prepregnant requirements, and insulin must be adjusted accordingly. Home blood glucose monitoring should continue for the woman with type 1 diabetes.

The woman and her partner, if he is involved, should also receive information on family planning. Barrier methods of contraception (diaphragm, cervical cap, condom) used with a spermicide are safe, effective, economical, and the method of choice for women with insulin-dependent diabetes. The use of combined oral contraceptives (COCs) by women with diabetes is somewhat controversial. Many physicians who prescribe low-dose COCs to women with diabetes restrict them to women who have no vascular disease and do not smoke. The progesterone-only pill may also be used as may Depo-Provera. Many couples who have completed their families choose elective sterilization.

NURSING MANAGEMENT *For the Woman with Diabetes Mellitus or GDM*

The *Nursing Care Plan: The Woman with Diabetes Mellitus* on pages 299–301 summarizes nursing management.

Nursing Assessment and Diagnosis

Whether diabetes has been diagnosed before pregnancy occurs or the diagnosis is made during pregnancy (GDM), careful assessment of the disease process and the woman's understanding of diabetes is important. Thorough physical examination—including assessment for vascular complications of the disease, any signs of infectious conditions, and urine and blood testing for glucose—is essential on the first prenatal visit. Follow-up visits are usually scheduled twice a month during the first two trimesters and once a week during the last trimester.

Assessment provides information about the woman's ability to cope with the combined stress of pregnancy and diabetes and to follow a recommended regimen of care. Determine the

Nursing Care Plan The Woman with Diabetes Mellitus

Intervention	Rationale	Expected Outcome

1. Nursing Diagnosis: *Nutrition, Imbalanced: Less than Body Requirements*, related to poor carbohydrate metabolism (NANDA-I © 2012)

Intervention	Rationale	Expected Outcome
NIC Priority Intervention: *Nutrition management:* Assistance with or provision of a balanced dietary intake of foods and fluids		**NOC Suggested Outcome:** *Nutritional status:* Extent to which nutrients are available to meet metabolic needs
Goal: The patient will maintain adequate nutrition throughout pregnancy.		
■ Emphasize importance of regular prenatal visits for assessment of weight gain, blood sugar levels, fetal heart tones, urine ketones, and fundal height measurement.	■ Regular follow-up and assessment of weight, blood sugar levels, fetal heart tones, urine ketones, and fundal height will promote a healthy pregnancy and outcome and also allow for modifications in the treatment regimen if necessary.	■ Patient will maintain adequate nutrition as evidenced by adequate weight gain, controlled blood sugar levels, verbalization of understanding of personal treatment regimen, and appropriate fetal growth and development during pregnancy.
■ Coordinate care with a dietitian to assist patient in meal planning and educate patient on the daily caloric needs of pregnancy.	■ A daily intake of high-quality foods promotes fetal growth and controls maternal glucose levels.	
■ Instruct patient on signs and symptoms of hyperglycemia: polyphagia, nausea, hot flushes, polydipsia, polyuria, fruity breath, abdominal cramps, rapid deep breathing, headache, weakness, drowsiness, and general malaise. Instruct patient on signs and symptoms of hypoglycemia: hunger, clammy skin, irritability, slurred speech, seizures, tachycardia, headache, pallor, sweating, disorientation, shakiness, blurred vision, and, if untreated, coma or convulsions.	■ Maintaining a euglycemic state throughout pregnancy aids in preventing diabetic complications and promotes a positive pregnancy outcome.	
■ Instruct patient on management of hyperglycemia and hypoglycemia.		
■ Include family members in meal planning.	■ Gives the family member a sense of involvement and an understanding of the importance of adequate nutrition in pregnancy.	■ Patient will recognize signs and intervene appropriately.

2. Nursing Diagnosis: *Injury, Risk for,* to the fetus related to possible complications associated with altered tissue perfusion secondary to maternal diagnosis of diabetes mellitus (NANDA-I © 2012)

Intervention	Rationale	Expected Outcome
NIC Priority Intervention: *High-risk pregnancy care:* Identification and management of a high-risk pregnancy to promote healthy outcomes for mother and baby		**NOC Suggested Outcome:** *Risk control:* Actions to eliminate or reduce actual, personal, and modifiable health threats
Goal: Uncomplicated birth of a healthy newborn.		
■ Assess fetal heart tones for reassuring variability and accelerations.	■ Reassuring fetal heart rate variability and accelerations are interpreted as adequate placental oxygenation.	■ Fetus will not exhibit signs and symptoms of altered tissue perfusion as evidenced by positive fetal activity, reassuring fetal heart rate patterns, a biophysical profile score between 8 and 10, negative CST, L/S ratio indicating fetal lung maturity, and a reactive nonstress test.
■ Instruct mother on how to lie in a left recumbent position after eating and record how many fetal movements she feels in an hour.	■ More than five fetal kicks in an hour are indicative of fetal well-being.	
■ **Collaborative:** Perform oxytocin challenge test (OCT)/contraction stress test (CST) and nonstress tests as determined by physician.	■ Fetal surveillance testing assesses fetal well-being and adequate placental perfusion.	

(continued)

Nursing Care Plan   The Woman with Diabetes Mellitus—continued

Intervention	Rationale	Expected Outcome
■ Prepare patient for frequent ultrasound assessments.	■ Ultrasonography is indicated at 18 and 28 weeks per physician order to confirm gestational age and fetal well-being. More frequent ultrasounds may be ordered depending on the woman's status.	
■ Prepare patient for amniocentesis procedure.	■ A sample of amniotic fluid contains two phospholipids (lecithin/sphingomyelin) that can be used to detect fetal lung maturity and enables medical personnel to prepare for a potential preterm birth.	
■ Assist physician with biophysical profile assessment.	■ Helps ensure fetal well-being and a positive fetal outcome.	

3. Nursing Diagnosis: *Knowledge, Readiness for Enhanced,* related to information about the effects of blood sugar on pregnancy related to an expressed desire to maintain stable blood glucose levels (NANDA-I © 2012)

NIC Priority Intervention:
Health education: Developing and providing instruction and learning experiences to facilitate voluntary adaptation of behavior conducive to health in individuals, families, groups, or communities

NOC Suggested Outcome:
Health-seeking behavior: Actions to promote optimal wellness, recovery, and rehabilitation

Goal: The patient and her family will verbalize the importance of maintaining blood sugar within prescribed ranges during pregnancy.

■ Assess the patient and family's cognitive level and develop a teaching strategy that will facilitate learning at that level.	■ Behavior changes occur when teaching strategies are appropriate for the patient and family's cognitive level.	■ Patient and family members will verbalize understanding of the effects of blood sugar fluctuations on pregnancy as evidenced by asking questions and seeking health information when necessary. The patient adheres to personal treatment regimen throughout pregnancy.
■ Teach blood glucose monitoring, insulin administration, and predicted insulin needs throughout pregnancy, and then have patient and family members repeat the discussion.	■ Basic understanding of the relationship between blood sugar levels and how insulin needs change throughout pregnancy will foster compliance with prescribed regimen.	
■ Emphasize the importance of maintaining a healthy diet and exercise program during pregnancy. Encourage patient and family to develop a sample diabetic diet and exercise regimen that is appropriate for pregnancy while present in the clinic or hospital and evaluate for appropriateness.	■ Involves the patient and her family members in her care, and the evaluation method promotes positive reinforcement and a time for modifications of regimen if necessary.	
■ Emphasize the importance of prenatal care for the purpose of maternal and fetal surveillance.	■ Frequent prenatal visits allow for modifications in regimen and promote a healthy pregnancy outcome.	

4. Nursing Diagnosis: *Infection, Risk for,* related to increased levels of glucose in urine (NANDA-I © 2012)

NIC Priority Intervention:
Infection control: Minimizing the acquisition and transmission of infectious agents

NOC Suggested Outcome:
Knowledge: infection control: Extent of understanding conveyed about prevention and control of infection

Goal: The patient will have no urinary tract infections (UTIs) during pregnancy.

■ Encourage patient to use preventive measures to prevent UTIs: increasing intake of water and cranberry juice, wearing cotton underwear, wiping perineum from front to back, voiding frequently, and voiding before and immediately after sexual intercourse.	■ Using preventive measures decreases the likelihood of patient acquiring a UTI.	■ Patient will remain free of UTIs during pregnancy as evidenced by verbalizing and complying with appropriate preventive measures, increasing fluid intake, and negative urine samples during prenatal visits.

Nursing Care Plan The Woman with Diabetes Mellitus—continued

Intervention	Rationale	Expected Outcome
■ Instruct patient on the signs and symptoms of UTIs: urinary frequency, dysuria, cloudy urine, hematuria, lower back pain, and foul-smelling urine.	■ Patient will be aware of signs and symptoms of UTIs and report to physician for immediate intervention.	
■ **Collaborative:** Instruct patient on how to obtain a clean-catch urine sample and send to lab for culture and sensitivity per physician's orders.	■ A clean-catch urine sample will contain bacteria if a UTI is present.	
■ Administer prescribed antibiotic therapy and teach patient about medication, adverse effects, and appropriate dosage.	■ Antibiotic therapy is the appropriate treatment for a UTI. Compliance increases when a patient fully understands medication regimen.	
■ Encourage patient to drink 8–10 glasses of water each day.	■ Increased fluid intake assists in flushing bacteria out of the urinary tract system.	

5. Nursing Diagnosis: *Anxiety*, related to unfamiliarity with diagnosis (NANDA-I © 2012)

NIC Priority Intervention:
Anxiety reduction: Minimizing apprehension, dread, foreboding, or uneasiness related to an unidentified source of anticipated danger

Goal: The patient will express less anxiety.

NOC Suggested Outcome:
Anxiety control: Ability to eliminate or reduce feelings of apprehension and tension from an unidentifiable source

Intervention	Rationale	Expected Outcome
■ Assess patient's level of anxiety (mild–1, moderate–2, or severe–3) and have patient verbalize causes of anxiety.	■ Verbalization of anxiety provokers encourages expression of feelings and questions.	■ Patient will demonstrate appropriate coping strategies as evidenced by utilizing resources efficiently and verbalizing feelings of anxiety and the ways to deal with them.
■ Share information on diabetes care such as nutrition, exercise, and glucose control in a clear and concise manner.	■ Accurate information gives the patient a sense of control and comfort.	
■ Instruct patient on anxiety-reducing techniques used in pregnancy such as imagery, breathing exercises, and massage.	■ Gives patient the tools necessary for decreasing anxiety.	
■ Refer patient to a diabetes support group.	■ A support group allows patients with similar problems to express concerns and share information with each other.	

woman's knowledge about diabetes and self-care before developing a teaching plan.

Nursing diagnoses that may apply to the pregnant woman with diabetes include the following (NANDA-I © 2012):

■ *Nutrition, Imbalanced: More than Body Requirements, Risk for,* related to imbalance between intake and available insulin

■ *Injury, Risk for,* related to possible complications secondary to hypoglycemia or hyperglycemia

■ *Family Processes, Interrupted,* related to the need for hospitalization secondary to DM

Planning and Implementation

For the woman with preexisting diabetes, a nurse and a physician may provide prepregnancy counseling using a team approach. Ideally they see the couple before pregnancy so that the DM can be evaluated. The outlook for pregnancy is good if the diabetes is of recent onset without vascular complications, provided that glucose levels can be controlled.

For women with GDM, nursing care focuses heavily on patient education about the condition, its implications, and its management.

Community-Based Nursing Care

In many cases, women with GDM are stabilized in the hospital and necessary teaching for self-care is begun. Women with preexisting diabetes may also require hospitalization for stabilization of their diabetes. In either case the majority of ongoing teaching and supervision of pregnant women with diabetes is then carried out by nurses in clinics, community agencies, and the women's homes.

Effective Insulin Use

Ensure that the woman and her partner understand the purpose of insulin, the types of insulin to be used, and the correct procedure for administering it. Instruct the woman's partner

Clinical Reasoning Glucose Intolerance

Patti Chang, a 35-year-old G3P2, is a well-educated, active Chinese American woman with no history of glucose intolerance. Her two children were born healthy at 36 weeks' gestation. She receives the usual 50-g glucose tolerance test at 26 weeks' gestation, and her plasma level is 160 mg/dL. She seems irritated and frustrated when her obstetrician tells her that it would be best to perform a 3-hour fasting glucose tolerance test. After the physician leaves the room, Patti asks you the following questions: "Will the glucose hurt my baby? What will the treatment be?" How will you answer the questions? Why does Patti seem so upset?

See www.nursing.pearsonhighered.com for possible responses.

Clinical Tip

Have a woman with GDM who is learning to test her blood glucose do a fingerstick while you watch. For many women, actually sticking their finger can be a challenge to overcome. This also enables you to verify that correct technique is used.

possibility of exercise-induced hypoglycemia), to monitor her blood glucose levels regularly, and to avoid injecting insulin into an extremity that will soon be used during exercise.

If the woman has not been following a regular exercise plan, encourage her to begin gradually. Due to alterations in metabolism with exercise, the woman's blood glucose should be well controlled before she begins an exercise program. *See Health Promotion: The Pregnant Woman with Diabetes.*

Hospital-Based Nursing Care

Hospitalization may become necessary during the pregnancy to evaluate blood glucose levels and adjust insulin dosages. In such cases, monitor the woman's status and provide teaching so that she is knowledgeable about her condition and its management.

SAFETY ALERT!

Insulin is a high-risk medication that carries significant potential risks. Like all medications, nurses should use two patient identifiers, administer it at the correct time, and monitor the patient afterward. Nurses should have documented knowledge about insulin administration and demonstrate competency in administering, storing, and handling it and in the key assessments and findings indicated for maternity patients receiving insulin (Hurst, 2011).

During the intrapartum period, continue to monitor the woman's status, maintain her IV fluids, remain alert for signs of hypoglycemia, and provide the care indicated for any woman in labor. If a cesarean birth becomes necessary, provide appropriate care, as described in Chapter 22 ✪.

Evaluation

Expected outcomes of nursing care include the following:

- The woman is able to discuss her condition and its possible impact on her pregnancy, labor and birth, and postpartum period.

- The woman participates in developing a healthcare regimen to meet her needs and follows it throughout her pregnancy.

- The woman avoids developing hypoglycemia or hyperglycemia.

- The woman gives birth to a healthy newborn.

- The woman is able to care for her newborn.

CARE OF THE WOMAN WITH ANEMIA

Anemia indicates inadequate levels of hemoglobin (Hb) in the blood. During pregnancy, *anemia* is defined as hemoglobin less than 11 g/dL (Samuels, 2012). The common anemias of pregnancy are due either to insufficient hemoglobin production

about insulin administration in case it becomes necessary for the partner to give it. For some highly motivated women whose glucose levels are not well controlled with multiple injections, a continuous infusion pump may improve glucose control.

Teach the woman how and when to monitor her blood glucose level, the desired range of blood glucose levels, and the importance of good control (Figure 15–2 ●). Most women use a glucose meter to monitor blood sugar level because the meter is more accurate. Teach the woman to follow the manufacturer's directions exactly; to wash her hands thoroughly before puncturing her finger; to touch the blood droplet, not her finger, to the test pad on the strip; and to store the test strips as directed and discard them after the expiration date. Patients with diabetes need to keep a record of each blood sugar reading. Specific record sheets are available for this purpose.

Planned Exercise Program

Regardless of the type of diabetes, unless otherwise medically contraindicated, exercise is important for the woman's overall well-being. If she is used to a regular exercise program, encourage her to continue. Advise the woman to exercise after meals when blood sugar levels are high, to wear diabetic identification, to carry a simple sugar such as hard candy (because of the

● **Figure 15–2** Home glucose monitoring. The nurse teaches the pregnant woman with gestational diabetes mellitus how to do home glucose monitoring.

Health Promotion The Pregnant Woman with Diabetes

Glucose Monitoring

Home monitoring of blood glucose levels is the most accurate and convenient method to determine insulin dose and assess control.

- Teach the woman self-monitoring techniques that are done according to a specified schedule. Women with GDM typically measure their blood glucose 4 times a day (fasting and 1 to 2 hours after meals). Women with preexisting DM should monitor their blood in the fasting state, before each meal, 1 to 2 hours after each meal, and at bedtime (ACOG, 2012b).
- Instruct the woman to regulate her insulin dosage based on blood glucose values and anticipated activity level.
- Encourage her to maintain blood glucose levels in normal ranges as follows: fasting (before eating or taking insulin), equal to or less than 95 mg/dL; and either 1 hour after a meal, less than or equal to 140 mg/dL; or 2 hours after each meal, less than or equal to 120 mg/dL (ADA, 2012).

Review Symptoms of Hypoglycemia or Hyperglycemia

- Teach the pregnant woman with diabetes to recognize symptoms of changing glucose levels and to take appropriate action by immediately checking her capillary blood glucose level.
- If blood glucose is less than 60 mg/dL, advise her to drink one 8-oz cup of milk or ½ cup of orange juice, apple juice, or regular soft drink, or eat four to six pieces of hard candy, or consume 1 tablespoon of honey, brown sugar, or corn syrup. Wait 15 minutes and recheck blood glucose (Cleveland Clinic, 2012). (*Note:* Many people overtreat their symptoms by continuing to eat, but doing so can cause rebound hyperglycemia.)
- Have the woman carry a snack at all times and have other fast sources of glucose (simple carbohydrates) at hand to treat an insulin reaction when milk or juice is not available.

- Ensure that family members learn how to inject glucagon in case food does not work or is not feasible (e.g., in the presence of severe morning sickness).

Smoking

- Ensure that the woman knows that smoking has harmful effects on both the maternal vascular system and the developing fetus and thus is contraindicated for both pregnancy and diabetes.

Travel

- Insulin can be kept at room temperature while traveling. Instruct woman to keep insulin supplies with her; they should not be packed in the baggage.
- Special meals can be arranged by notifying most airlines a few days before departure.
- Have her wear a diabetic identification bracelet or necklace and check with her physician for any instructions or advice before traveling.

Support Groups

- Many communities have diabetes support groups or education classes that are helpful to women with newly diagnosed diabetes. Refer her to them.

Cesarean Birth

- Chances for a cesarean birth increase if the pregnant woman is diabetic. Anticipate the possibility and suggest enrollment in cesarean birth preparation classes. The couple may prefer simply to discuss cesarean birth with the nurse and their obstetrician and read some books on the topic.

related to nutritional deficiency in iron or folic acid during pregnancy or to hemoglobin destruction in an inherited disorder such as sickle cell disease (Figure 15–3 ●). Table 15–1 describes these common anemias.

● **Figure 15–3** Health teaching is an important part of nursing care for the pregnant woman with sickle cell disease.
Source: © Mark Richards/PhotoEdit, Inc.

CARE OF THE WOMAN WITH SUBSTANCE ABUSE PROBLEMS

Substance abuse occurs when a person experiences difficulties with work, family, social relations, and health as a result of alcohol or drug use. In general, the rate of illicit drug use among pregnant women is significantly less than half the rate among nonpregnant women. Approximately 4.4% of pregnant women ages 15 to 44 report having used an illicit drug in the past month as compared to 10.9% of nonpregnant women. However, illicit drug use varies significantly by age with the highest rate among the youngest pregnant women, specifically 16.2% among females ages 15 to 17; the rate was 7.4% among those ages 18 to 25, and 1.9% among prepregnant women ages 26 to 44 (Substance Abuse and Mental Health Services Administration [SAMHSA], 2011).

Drugs that are commonly misused include tobacco, alcohol, cocaine, marijuana, amphetamines, barbiturates, hallucinogens, club drugs, heroin, and other narcotics. (Tobacco is discussed in Chapter 11 ✇ as a teratogenic substance.) Polydrug use involving multiple substances such as alcohol, tobacco, and illicit drugs is fairly common and contributes to the risks a pregnant

Table 15–1	Anemia and Pregnancy		
Condition	**Brief Description**	**Maternal Implications**	**Fetal/Neonatal Implications**
Iron deficiency anemia	Most common medical complication of pregnancy. Condition caused by inadequate iron intake resulting in hemoglobin levels below 11 g/dL. To prevent this, most women are advised to take supplemental iron during pregnancy and to eat an iron-rich diet.	A pregnant woman with this anemia tires easily, is more susceptible to infection, has increased chance of preeclampsia/eclampsia and postpartum hemorrhage, and cannot tolerate even minimal blood loss during birth. Healing of episiotomy or incision may be delayed.	Risk of low birth weight, preterm birth, nonreassuring fetal status, and perinatal mortality increases in women with severe iron deficiency anemia (maternal Hb less than 6 g/dL). Fetus may be hypoxic during labor due to impaired uteroplacental oxygenation.
Sickle cell disease (also referred to as sickle cell anemia)	Recessive autosomal disease in which normal adult hemoglobin, hemoglobin A, is abnormally formed. It occurs primarily in people of African descent and occasionally in people of Southeast Asian or Mediterranean descent. The disease is characterized by sickling of the red blood cells (RBCs) in the presence of decreased oxygenation. Because the woman maintains her Hb levels by intense erythropoiesis, additional folic acid supplements (1 mg/day) are necessary. Condition may be marked by crisis with profound anemia, jaundice, high temperature, infarction, and acute pain. Crisis is treated by rehydration with intravenous fluids, administration of oxygen, antibiotics, and analgesics. The fetus is monitored throughout.	Pregnancy may aggravate sickle cell disease and bring on a vaso-occlusive crisis. Maternal mortality is rare but there is a significant risk of pyelonephritis, acute chest syndrome, and gestational hypertension (Cunningham, Leveno, Bloom, et al., 2010). Congestive heart failure or acute renal failure may also occur. Maternal infections are treated aggressively because dehydration and fever can trigger sickling and crisis. Oxygen supplementation is used throughout labor, and IV fluids are given to maintain hydration. Fetal heart rate (FHR) is monitored closely. Antiembolism stockings may be used postpartum.	Fetal death due to maternal complications, preterm labor, prematurity, intrauterine growth restriction (IUGR), and low birth weight (MacMullen & Dulski, 2011).
Folic acid deficiency anemia	Folic acid deficiency is the most common cause of megaloblastic anemia. In the absence of folic acid, immature RBCs fail to divide, become enlarged (megaloblastic), and are fewer in number. Increased folic acid metabolism during pregnancy and lactation can result in deficiency. All women who could become pregnant should take a multivitamin containing 400 mcg daily (generally found in prenatal vitamins) before conception and through at least the first trimester of pregnancy. The condition is treated with 1 mg folate daily (see Chapter 12).	Folate deficiency is the second most common cause of anemia in pregnancy. Severe deficiency increases the risk that the mother may need a blood transfusion following birth due to anemia. She also has an increased risk of hemorrhage due to thrombocytopenia and is more susceptible to infection. Folic acid is readily available in foods such as fresh leafy green vegetables, red meat, fish, poultry, and legumes, but it is easily destroyed by overcooking or cooking with large quantities of water.	Maternal folic acid deficiency has been associated with an increased risk of neural tube defects (NTDs) such as spina bifida, meningomyelocele, and anencephaly in the newborn. Women who have already had one baby with a NTD are generally advised to take a larger dose of folic acid daily.

woman faces. Table 15–2 identifies common addictive drugs and their effects on the fetus or newborn.

Drug use during pregnancy, particularly in the first trimester, may have a negative effect on the health of the woman and the growth and development of the fetus. Unfortunately, prenatal drug use may be the most frequently missed diagnosis in all of maternity care. Physicians and nurses may fail to ask women about drug and alcohol use because of their own lack of knowledge, discomfort, or biases. Often substance-abusing women wait until late in pregnancy to seek health care. Moreover, the substance-abusing woman who seeks early prenatal care may not voluntarily reveal her addiction, so healthcare providers should be alert for a history or physical signs that might indicate substance abuse.

Providing effective prenatal care to chemically dependent women is often challenging for clinicians. However, pregnancy is a time when most women are receptive to caring interventions.

Clinical Tip

Keep in mind that at least 1 of 10 women in the United States, regardless of socioeconomic status or ethnic background, is currently abusing a substance. If you consider that possibility with every woman, you will ask the important questions about drug use and be alert for signs of substance abuse.

Table 15–2   Possible Effects of Selected Drugs of Abuse/Addiction on Fetus and Newborn

Maternal Drug	Effect on Fetus/Newborn
DEPRESSANTS	
Alcohol	Mental retardation, microcephaly, midfacial hypoplasia, cardiac anomalies, intrauterine growth restriction (IUGR), potential teratogenic effects, fetal alcohol syndrome (FAS), fetal alcohol effects (FAE).
NARCOTICS	
Heroin	Withdrawal symptoms, known as *neonatal abstinence syndrome (NAS)*, include tremors, irritability, sneezing, vomiting, fever, diarrhea, abnormal respiratory function, and possible seizures.
Methadone	Neonates may present with NAS and be small for gestational age (SGA).
BARBITURATES	
Phenobarbital	Withdrawal symptoms. Fetal growth restriction.
TRANQUILIZERS	
Diazepam (Valium)	Withdrawal symptoms.
ANTIANXIETY DRUGS	
Lithium	Congenital anomalies.
STIMULANTS	
Amphetamines Amphetamine sulfate (Benzedrine)	Low birth weight; withdrawal symptoms (B. L. Thompson, Levitt, & Stanwood, 2009).
Cocaine	Cerebral infarctions, microcephaly, learning disabilities, poor state organization, decreased interactive behavior, CNS anomalies, cardiac anomalies, genitourinary anomalies, sudden infant death syndrome (SIDS).
Methamphetamine	SGA, low birth weight, decreased arousal, lower scores on tests of attention, verbal memory, and visual motor integration (ACOG, 2011a).
Nicotine (half to one pack cigarettes/day)	Increased rate of spontaneous abortion, increased incidence of placental abruption, SGA, small head circumference, decreased length, SIDS, attention deficit hyperactivity disorder (ADHD) in school-age children.
PSYCHOTROPICS	
PCP ("angel dust")	Withdrawal symptoms. Newborn behavioral and developmental abnormalities.
Marijuana	Possible association with structural and neurobehavioral defects (Hurt et al., 2009).

Substances Commonly Abused During Pregnancy

Alcohol

Alcohol is a central nervous system (CNS) depressant and a potent teratogen. Among pregnant women ages 15 to 44, estimates suggest that 10.8% use alcohol in a given month. This rate is significantly lower than the rate for nonpregnant women of that age (54.7%) (SAMHSA, 2011). This figure is of concern, however, because birth defects that are related to fetal alcohol exposure can occur in the first 3 to 8 weeks' gestation, often before the woman even knows she is pregnant. Alcohol use among pregnant women tends to decrease by trimester.

The effects of alcohol on the fetus may result in a group of signs known as *fetal alcohol spectrum disorders* (FASD). FASD has characteristic physical and mental abnormalities that vary in severity (see discussion in Chapter 27 ⊘). There is no final answer to how much alcohol a woman can safely drink during pregnancy. Consequently the expectant woman should avoid alcohol completely. Even low levels of alcohol cannot be recommended (O'Leary et al., 2009).

Chronic abuse of alcohol can undermine maternal health by causing malnutrition (especially folic acid and thiamine deficiencies), bone marrow suppression, increased incidence of infections, and liver disease. As a result of alcohol dependence, a woman may have withdrawal seizures in the intrapartum period as early as 12 to 48 hours after she stops drinking. Delirium tremens may occur in the postpartum period, and the newborn may suffer a withdrawal syndrome. Nurses in the maternal–newborn unit must be aware of the manifestations of alcohol abuse so they can prepare for the woman's special needs. Care includes sedation to decrease irritability and tremors, seizure precautions, intravenous (IV) fluid therapy for hydration, and preparation for an addicted newborn. Although high doses of sedatives and analgesics may be necessary for the woman, caution is advised because these medications can cause fetal depression.

Breastfeeding generally is not contraindicated, although alcohol is excreted in breast milk. Excessive alcohol consumption may intoxicate the infant and inhibit the maternal letdown reflex. Discharge planning for the alcohol-addicted mother and newborn needs to be correlated with the social service department of the hospital.

Cocaine and Crack

Cocaine acts at the nerve terminals to prevent the reuptake of dopamine and norepinephrine, which in turn results in vasoconstriction, tachycardia, and hypertension. Placental vasoconstriction decreases blood flow to the fetus. The onset of cocaine effects occurs rapidly, but the euphoria lasts only about 30 minutes. Euphoria and excitement are usually followed by irritability, depression, pessimism, fatigue, and a strong desire for more cocaine. This pattern often leads the user to take repeated doses to sustain the effect. Cocaine metabolites may be present in the urine of a pregnant woman for as long as 4 to 7 days after use.

Cocaine can be taken by IV injection or by snorting the powdered form. *Crack*, a form of freebase cocaine that is made up of baking soda, water, and cocaine mixed into a paste and microwaved to form a rock, can be smoked. Smoking crack leads to a quicker, more intense high because the drug is absorbed through the large surface area of the lungs.

The cocaine user is difficult to identify prenatally. Because cocaine is illegal, many women are reluctant to admit that they use it. The nurse may recognize subtle signs of cocaine use, including mood swings and appetite changes, and withdrawal symptoms such as depression, irritability, nausea, lack of motivation, and psychomotor changes.

Major adverse maternal effects of cocaine use include seizures and hallucinations, pulmonary edema, cerebral hemorrhage, respiratory failure, and heart problems. Women who use cocaine have an increased incidence of spontaneous abortion, abruptio placentae, preterm birth, and stillbirth (Niebyl & Simpson, 2012).

Fetal exposure to cocaine increases the risk of intrauterine growth restriction (IUGR), microcephaly, altered brain development, shorter body length, congenital anomalies, and neurobehavioral abnormalities (Niebyl & Simpson, 2012). Newborns exposed to cocaine in utero may have neurobehavioral disturbances, marked irritability, an exaggerated startle reflex, labile emotions, and an increased risk of sudden infant death syndrome (SIDS). (See Chapter 27 🔗 for further discussion.) Most children who were exposed to cocaine in utero have normal intelligence. In some cases, cocaine-exposed children have subtle behavioral and learning problems; however, a good home environment seems to help reduce these effects (March of Dimes, 2008).

Cocaine crosses into breast milk and may cause symptoms in the breastfeeding infant, including extreme irritability, vomiting, diarrhea, dilated pupils, and apnea. Thus, women who continue to use cocaine after childbirth should avoid breastfeeding.

Methamphetamine

Methamphetamine use has increased in the United States and is the only illicit drug that can be made easily from ingredients that are legally obtained. It is a powerful stimulant that can be ingested, injected, smoked, snorted, or taken anally (Della Grotta et al., 2010). Infants of women who use methamphetamine are at increased risk of being small for gestational age (SGA). Other risks include low birth weight, decreased arousal, and lower scores on tests of attention, verbal memory, and visual motor integration (ACOG, 2011a).

Marijuana

Marijuana is the most widely used illicit drug among women, both pregnant and nonpregnant. To date, there is no strong evidence that marijuana has teratogenic effects on the fetus (Niebyl & Simpson, 2012). In reality, the impact of heavy marijuana use on pregnancy is difficult to evaluate because of the variety of social factors that may influence the impact of marijuana itself.

MDMA (Ecstasy)

Methylenedioxymethamphetamine (MDMA), better known as Ecstasy, is the most commonly used of a group of drugs referred to as *club drugs,* so called because they have become popular among adolescents and young adults who frequent dance clubs and "raves." Other club drugs include flunitrazepam (Rohypnol), gamma hydroxybutyrate (GHB), and ketamine hydrochloride. Phencyclidine (PCP) and LSD are sometimes classified as club drugs as well.

A stimulant, MDMA is taken by mouth, usually as a tablet. It produces euphoria and feelings of empathy for others. It has been widely perceived as a "safe" drug because of a relatively low incidence of adverse reactions. However, adverse responses are very unpredictable and the incidence is growing. MDMA can cause sleep problems, confusion, depression, drug cravings, memory deficits, and severe anxiety. In high doses it can lead to severe hyperthermia by interfering with the body's temperature regulation. This can lead to organ failure and even death (National Institute on Drug Abuse, 2010).

Little is yet known about the effects of MDMA on pregnancy. Preliminary research using rats suggests that prenatal use of MDMA may be associated with long-term impaired memory and learning in the child. However, the impact of the timing of Ecstasy use by the pregnant woman during fetal brain development may be a critical issue (V. B. Thompson et al., 2009).

Heroin

Heroin is an illicit CNS depressant narcotic that alters perception and produces euphoria. It is an addictive drug that is generally administered IV (Figure 15–4 ●). Pregnancy in women who use heroin is considered high risk because of the increased incidence in these women of poor nutrition, iron deficiency anemia, and preeclampsia. Women addicted to heroin also have a higher incidence of sexually transmitted infections because many rely on prostitution to support their drug habit.

● **Figure 15–4** The use of illicit drugs puts the pregnant woman and her unborn child at increased risk for a variety of complications.

Source: © Diego Cervo/Fotolia.

The fetus of a woman who is addicted to heroin is at increased risk for preterm birth, IUGR, meconium aspiration, and withdrawal symptoms (neonatal abstinence syndrome) after birth such as restlessness; shrill, high-pitched cry; irritability; fist sucking; vomiting; and seizures. Signs of withdrawal usually appear within 72 hours and may last for several days. These behaviors may interfere with successful maternal attachment and increase the risk for parenting problems or abuse in an already high-risk mother (Vucinovic et al., 2009).

Methadone is the most commonly used therapy for women dependent on opioids such as heroin. Methadone blocks withdrawal symptoms and reduces or eliminates the craving for narcotics. Dosage should be individualized at the lowest possible therapeutic level. Methadone does cross the placenta, and, consequently, newborns are at risk for neonatal abstinence syndrome (NAS). However, various studies have demonstrated inconsistent long-term effects on the newborn (ACOG, 2012a). Buprenorphine, a partial opioid agonist, is an acceptable alternative because it may decrease the severity of NAS in the infant (Niebyl & Simpson, 2012).

Clinical Therapy

A team approach to the care of the pregnant woman with substance abuse problems ensures the management necessary to provide safe labor and birth for the woman and her child.

The management of drug addiction may include hospitalization if necessary to start detoxification. "Cold turkey" withdrawal is not advisable during pregnancy because of the possible risk to the fetus. Maintenance and support therapy are best individualized to the woman's history and condition. Urine screening is also done regularly throughout pregnancy if the woman has a known or suspected substance abuse problem and should include maternal informed consent. This testing helps to identify the type and amount of drug being abused.

NURSING MANAGEMENT *For the Pregnant Woman with a Substance Abuse Problem*

Nursing Assessment and Diagnosis

Because of the prevalence of substance abuse, it is important to screen all pregnant women for substance abuse during the health history. Several simple screening tools are available. In addition, be alert for clues in the history or appearance of the woman that suggest substance abuse. If abuse is suspected, ask direct questions, beginning with less threatening questions about use of tobacco, caffeine, and over-the-counter medications. Then progress to questions about alcohol intake and finally to questions focusing on past and current use of illegal drugs. A matter-of-fact, nonjudgmental approach is more likely to elicit honest responses.

When assessing a woman with a known substance abuse problem, focus on the woman's general health status, with specific attention to nutritional status, susceptibility to infections, and evaluation of all body systems. Also assess the woman's understanding of the impact of substance abuse on herself and on her pregnancy.

Nursing diagnoses that may apply to a woman at risk because of substance abuse include the following (NANDA-I © 2012):

- *Nutrition, Imbalanced: Less than Body Requirements*, related to inadequate food intake secondary to substance abuse
- *Infection, Risk for,* related to use of inadequately cleaned syringes and needles secondary to IV drug use
- *Health Maintenance*, *Ineffective,* related to a lack of information about the impact of substance abuse on the fetus

Planning and Implementation

Prevention of substance abuse during pregnancy is the ideal nursing goal and is best accomplished through education. Unfortunately, many women who abuse substances do not receive regular health care and may not seek care until they are far along in pregnancy.

Thus it is important to focus on ongoing assessment and patient teaching. Consider providing information about the relationship between substance abuse and existing health problems and the implications for the woman's unborn child. Establishing a relationship of trust and support helps ensure the woman's cooperation. If possible, discuss strategies to help the woman quit (addiction treatment programs, 12-step programs, individual counseling) and suggest a referral for more in-depth assessment by a specialist.

Preparation for labor and birth should be part of prenatal planning. Nonnarcotic psychologic support and careful explanation of the labor process may help relieve the woman's fear, tension, and discomfort. If pain medication is necessary, it should not be withheld; the notion that it will contribute to further addiction is mistaken. Preferred methods of pain relief include the use of psychoprophylaxis and regional blocks, such as epidurals, or local anesthetics, such as pudendal block and local infiltration. Immediate intensive care should be available for the newborn, who is often depressed, small for gestational age (SGA), and premature. (For care of the addicted newborn, see Chapter 27 🔗.)

Evaluation

Expected outcomes of nursing care include the following:

- The woman is able to describe the impact of her substance abuse on herself and her unborn child.
- The woman gives birth to a healthy infant.
- The woman accepts a referral to social services (or another appropriate community agency) for follow-up care after discharge.

CARE OF THE WOMAN WITH A PSYCHOLOGIC DISORDER

The prevalence of psychologic disorders among adults in the United States is 26.2% or roughly one in four adults (National Institute of Mental Health, 2010). **Psychologic disorders** are characterized by alterations in thinking, mood, or behavior. Although many such disorders can affect labor and birth, only the most common are discussed here. Because an in-depth discussion of psychologic disorders is beyond the scope of this text, students are encouraged to consult a mental health nursing textbook for further reference. Postpartum psychologic disorders are discussed in Chapter 31 🔗.

Maternal Implications

Depression, a common disorder that affects many pregnant women, often goes undiagnosed or untreated. Estimates suggest that 9.4% to 12.7% of pregnant women will have a major depression (Shade et al., 2011). Research findings are mixed, but women with depression may be more likely to have a preterm birth, a small-for-gestational age (SGA) newborn, or a low-birth-weight (LBW) infant (Smith, Shao, Howell, et al., 2011).

Depression can reduce the woman's ability to concentrate or process information being provided by healthcare team members. Untreated depression can lead to poor self-care, inadequate nutrition, self-medication, poor maternal–infant bonding, and maternal suicide (Khan & Lusskin, 2010). The labor process may feel overwhelming to a woman with depression and she may feel hopelessness about the outcome of her labor. However, she may not be able to articulate these feelings and may appear irritable or withdrawn.

Women with *bipolar disorder* experience the symptoms of depression during the depressive phase. A pregnant woman experiencing a manic episode may engage in behaviors that are dangerous to herself or her fetus including alcohol or drug use, reckless driving, driving without a seat belt, and unprotected sexual intercourse. If labor occurs during a manic phase, the woman may be hyperexcitable and exhibit poor judgment.

Anxiety disorders include a cluster of diagnoses such as panic disorder, obsessive-compulsive disorder (OCD), post-traumatic stress disorder (PTSD), general anxiety disorder, and other specific phobias. These disorders can cause a wide range of symptoms in pregnant women and laboring women. For example, women with OCD may need to repeat specific rituals as a means of coping, while women with PTSD may experience flashbacks and avoidance behaviors. Anxiety may cause the laboring woman to experience physical symptoms such as chest pain, shortness of breath, faintness, fear, or even terror. In general, laboring women with psychologic disorders tend to exhibit the behaviors characteristic of their disorders, but these behaviors may be somewhat exaggerated because of the intense emotions that are evoked in the women's memories. Women with a past history of abuse, including physical and sexual abuse, are often fearful of losing control.

Clinical Therapy

The goal of clinical therapy is to provide strategies that will help decrease the woman's anxiety (as well as that of her partner), keep her oriented to reality, and promote optimal functioning during pregnancy and while in labor. Pharmacologic measures such as sedatives, analgesics, or antianxiety medications are determined on an individual basis following careful assessment.

NURSING MANAGEMENT *For the Pregnant Woman with a Psychologic Disorder*

Use therapeutic communication and sharing of information to allay anxiety for both the woman and her support person during each prenatal visit and during labor and childbirth. Consistency in her care enables the woman to adjust to new experiences and begin to establish a relationship with her caregivers.

Nursing Assessment and Diagnosis

Research suggests that perinatal mood and anxiety disorders are often underdetected in clinical practice unless a formal screening program is in place (Shade et al., 2011). At the first prenatal visit, begin the assessment by reviewing the woman's background. Factors such as age, marital and socioeconomic status, culture, methods of coping, support system, and understanding of the labor process contribute to the woman's psychologic response to pregnancy and birth. It is important to ask all women if they have ever been diagnosed with a psychologic disorder. If the woman has, ask her if she is currently receiving any treatment, including medications or psychotherapy. Also ask if she has ever had a psychiatric hospitalization or if she has ever had thoughts of hurting herself or others.

This same attention to detail is important when the woman goes into labor. The prenatal record should be reviewed for additional information regarding any psychiatric illnesses. During labor, assess the woman for objective cues indicating a psychologic disorder. Monotone replies and/or a flat affect may indicate depression. Women with schizophrenia may lack orientation to person, time, and place. Objective cues indicating acute anxiety or signs of a panic attack include tachycardia and hyperventilation.

As labor progresses, remain alert to the woman's verbal and nonverbal behavioral responses to the pain and anxiety. The woman who is too quiet and compliant, is disoriented, is agitated and seems uncooperative, or is experiencing acute anxiety symptoms may require further appraisal for psychologic disorders. These rare circumstances require one-on-one nursing care. A consult with a psychiatrist is often warranted.

Nursing diagnoses that may apply to the woman with a psychologic disorder include the following (NANDA-I © 2012):

- *Anxiety,* related to stress of the labor process, unfamiliar environment, and unknown caregivers
- *Fear,* related to unknown outcome of labor and invasive medical procedures
- *Coping, Ineffective,* related to increased anxiety and stress

Planning and Implementation

The primary nursing interventions center on providing support to the pregnant woman and her partner or family. During labor, families that have had the opportunity to attend prenatal classes may benefit from encouragement as they employ some of the coping techniques they have learned. If the woman begins to lose her ability to cope or her orientation to reality, assist her in regaining control and orientation by explaining where she is, why she is there, and what is currently happening; providing reassurance; decreasing stimuli; and acknowledging her fears, concerns, and symptoms.

Your ability to help the woman and her partner cope with the stress of labor is directly related to the rapport you have established with them. By employing a calm, caring, confident, nonjudgmental approach, you may be able not only to acknowledge the anxiety or other emotions the woman is feeling but also to identify the source of the distress. Once the causative factors are known, implement appropriate interventions such as offering information, comfort measures, touch, or therapeutic communication. Some women with severe psychologic disorders may have excessive symptoms during their labor and birth. Although providing emotional support is imperative, care of these women should focus on maintaining a safe environment and ensuring maternal and fetal well-being. Pharmacologic interventions may be necessary for excessive symptoms. See Chapter 31 🔗 for a discussion of medications commonly used.

Evaluation

Anticipated outcomes of nursing care include the following:

- The woman experiences a decrease in physiologic and psychologic stress and an increase in physical and psychologic comfort.
- The woman remains oriented to person, time, and place.
- The woman uses effective coping mechanisms to manage her stress and anxiety in labor.
- The woman is able to verbalize feelings about her labor.
- The woman's and her family's fear is decreased.

CARE OF THE WOMAN WITH HIV INFECTION

AIDS (acquired immunodeficiency syndrome), caused by the virus known as **HIV** (human immunodeficiency virus), is one of today's major health concerns. As of the end of 2009, an estimated 784,701 persons ages 13 or older in the United States were living with HIV/AIDS (Centers for Disease Control and Prevention [CDC], 2012). Male adults and adolescents are the largest groups of infected individuals. Of these groups, infection occurred as follows: male-to-male sexual contact (68%), IV drug use (13%), high-risk heterosexual contact (11%), and 8% through both male-to-male sexual contact and IV drug use. Among females with HIV/AIDS, 74% were infected through high-risk heterosexual contact and 26% were infected because of IV drug use (CDC, 2012).

Of the estimated 10,805 children living with HIV/AIDS in the United States, 88% were exposed perinatally (CDC, 2012). Fortunately, the incidence of new pediatric AIDS cases is declining rapidly.

Pathophysiology of HIV and AIDS

HIV-1, which causes most cases of AIDS worldwide, typically enters the body through blood, blood products, or other body fluids such as semen, vaginal fluid, and breast milk. HIV affects specific T cells, thereby decreasing the body's immune responses. This makes the affected person susceptible to opportunistic infections such as *Pneumocystis carinii,* which causes a severe pneumonia, candidiasis, cytomegalovirus, tuberculosis, and toxoplasmosis.

Once infected with the virus, the individual develops antibodies that can be detected with the enzyme-linked immunoabsorbent assay (ELISA) and confirmed with the Western blot test. A confirmed case is then categorized into one of four HIV infection stages for adults and adolescents over age 13. These stages are used for public health surveillance and not as a guide for diagnosis and therapy.

The diagnosis of AIDS is made when a person is HIV positive and has one of several specific opportunistic infections.

Maternal Risks

Recent advances and the availability of antiretroviral therapy (ART) have led women who are HIV positive and who adhere to their ART to consider pregnancy because of their increased life expectancy. If pregnancy is considered, priorities should focus on maintaining the health of the mother before, during, and after the pregnancy; preventing transmission to a potentially

---

Developing Cultural Competence Variations in the Prevalence Rates of New HIV Infections

The prevalence rates per 100,000 of HIV/AIDS–infected individuals vary significantly among races and ethnic groups: 62 per 100,000 in the black/African American population, 20.4 in the Hispanic/Latino population, 19.3 in the Native Hawaiian/Pacific Islander population, 9.7 in the American Indian/Alaska Native population, 7.3 in the white population, and 6.5 in the Asian population (CDC, 2012).

seronegative father; and preventing mother-to-child transmission. Reproductive assisted technology is one possibility along with further interventions including cesarean birth to reduce the risk of transmission to the fetus (Matthews & Mukherjee, 2009).

For women who have not had access to ART or who are noncompliant, AIDS-defining symptoms that are more common in women than men include wasting syndrome, esophageal candidiasis, and herpes simplex virus disease. Kaposi's sarcoma is rare in women. Non–AIDS-defining gynecologic conditions, such as vaginal *Candida* infections and cervical pathology, are prevalent among women at all stages of HIV infection.

Fetal/Neonatal Risks

HIV transmission can occur during pregnancy and through breast milk; however, it is believed that the majority of all infections occur during labor and birth. In the United States, the rate of transmission has dropped dramatically and is now less than 2% for pregnant women infected with HIV who receive prophylactic antiretroviral therapy, give birth by elective cesarean at 38 weeks before rupture of membranes, and avoid breastfeeding (Panel on Treatment of HIV-Infected Pregnant Women and Prevention of Perinatal Transmission [Panel on Treatment], 2011). These decreases in transmission are dramatic and impressive.

Following birth, HIV infection in infants should be diagnosed using HIV virologic assays as soon as possible, with initiation of infant antiretroviral prophylaxis immediately if the test is positive. For further discussion of the infant who is HIV positive, see Chapter 27 🔗.

Clinical Therapy

The revised CDC HIV testing guidelines indicate that HIV screening should be emphasized as a routine part of prenatal care while continuing to ensure that the testing of pregnant women is voluntary and informed (Panel on Treatment, 2011). Initial testing is done using enzyme-linked immunoabsorbent assay (ELISA). If the results are positive, the Western blot test is used to confirm the diagnosis. Women who test positive should be counseled about the implications of the diagnosis for themselves and their fetus to ensure an informed reproductive choice.

Antiretroviral therapy should be recommended to all infected pregnant women regardless of CD4 count to reduce the rate of perinatal transmission. As more antiretroviral medications have been developed, a wide array of options exists. Highly active antiretroviral therapy (HAART) is recommended during pregnancy and should include ZDV (Retrovir or zidovudine). Longer duration therapy is preferable to shorter duration approaches. Thus it is best to start prophylaxis after the first trimester and no later than 28 weeks' gestation in women who do not require immediate therapy for their own health (Panel on Treatment, 2011).

Treatment recommendations have also been developed for the mother and infant for the intrapartum and postpartum periods. The decision about which regimen is most appropriate should be determined following discussion with the woman about the risks and benefits based on her individual HIV status.

Women with HIV infection should be evaluated and treated for other sexually transmitted infections and for conditions occurring more commonly in women with HIV, such as tuberculosis, cytomegalovirus, toxoplasmosis, and cervical dysplasia. Women with HIV infection with no history of hepatitis B should receive the hepatitis vaccine, which is not contraindicated prenatally, as well as the pneumococcal vaccine and an annual flu shot. In addition to routine prenatal laboratory tests, a platelet count and a complete blood count with differential should be obtained at the first prenatal visit and repeated each trimester to identify anemia, thrombocytopenia, and leukopenia, which are associated both with HIV infection and with antiviral therapy.

The woman with HIV also should be assessed regularly for serologic changes that indicate the disease is progressing. This is determined by the absolute CD4+ T-lymphocyte count, which provides the number of helper T4 cells. When the CD4+ counts fall to 200/mm^3 or lower, opportunistic infections such as *Pneumocystis carinii* pneumonia are more likely to develop, and prophylaxis may need to be instituted (Panel on Treatment, 2011).

At each prenatal visit, women with asymptomatic HIV infection are monitored for early signs of complications, such as weight loss in the second or third trimesters or fever. The clinician inspects the mouth for signs of infections such as thrush (candidiasis) or hairy leukoplakia; the lungs are auscultated for signs of pneumonia; and the lymph nodes, the liver, and the spleen are palpated for signs of enlargement. Each trimester the woman should have a visual examination and examination of the retina to detect such complications as toxoplasmosis retinitis.

A pregnancy complicated by HIV infection, even if asymptomatic, is considered high risk, and the fetus is monitored closely. Weekly nonstress testing is begun at 32 weeks' gestation, and serial ultrasounds are done to detect IUGR. Biophysical profiles are also indicated (see Chapter 14 🔗). Invasive procedures such as amniocentesis are avoided when possible to prevent the contamination of a noninfected fetus.

Scheduled cesarean birth is indicated for women with HIV RNA levels greater than 1000 copies/mL and for women with unknown HIV RNA levels near the time of birth, whether they are on antiretroviral therapy or not (Panel on Treatment, 2011). The cesarean may be done as early as 38 weeks' gestation to decrease the risk of rupture of the membranes or onset of labor.

Women who are HIV positive are at increased risk for complications such as intrapartum or postpartum hemorrhage, postpartum infection, poor wound healing, and infections of the genitourinary tract. Thus they need careful monitoring and appropriate therapy as indicated. Following childbirth, the woman who is HIV positive should be referred to a physician knowledgeable about treating individuals with HIV infection.

NURSING MANAGEMENT *For the Pregnant Woman Who Is HIV Positive*

The *Nursing Care Plan: The Woman with HIV Infection* on pages 311–312 addresses nursing management.

Nursing Assessment and Diagnosis

A woman who tests positive for HIV may be asymptomatic or may present with any of the following signs or symptoms: fatigue,

Nursing Care Plan The Woman with HIV Infection

Intervention	Rationale	Expected Outcome

1. Nursing Diagnosis: *Infection, Risk for,* related to inadequate defenses (leukopenia, suppressed inflammatory response) secondary to HIV-positive status (NANDA-I © 2012)

NIC Priority Intervention:
Infection control: Minimizing the acquisition of infection

Goal: The patient will remain free of opportunistic infection during the course of pregnancy.

NOC Suggested Outcome:
Risk control: Actions taken to eliminate or reduce risk of exposure to infection

Intervention	Rationale	Expected Outcome
■ Obtain a complete health history and physical examination during first prenatal visit.	■ A complete health history will help determine risk factors for the development of opportunistic infections, and a physical examination will assist in identifying any underlying problem symptoms or illnesses that may compromise the pregnancy or complicate the treatment of HIV.	■ Patient will remain free of opportunistic infection as evidenced by CD4+ T-lymphocyte count within normal limits; no complaints of chills, fever, or sore throat; normal weight gain throughout pregnancy.
■ Educate the woman as to the signs and symptoms of infection.	■ Early recognition of signs and symptoms of infection will allow for immediate treatment, which may decrease the severity of the infection. Signs and symptoms of infections include fever, weight loss, fatigue, persistent candidiasis, diarrhea, cough, and skin lesions (Kaposi's sarcoma and hairy leukoplakia in the mouth).	
■ Obtain nutritional history and monitor weight gain at each prenatal visit.	■ The woman with HIV infection needs to maintain optimal nutritional intake. A compromised nutritional status may affect maternal and fetal well-being. Depleted reserves of protein and iron may decrease the patient's ability to fight infection, thereby making her more susceptible to opportunistic infections.	
■ **Collaborative:** Monitor the absolute CD4+ T-lymphocyte count, erythrocyte sedimentation rate (ESR), complete blood count (CBC) with differential, and hemoglobin and hematocrit (H&H) at each prenatal visit.	■ Lab results provide information about the woman's immune system and the potential for disease progression. Opportunistic infections are more likely to occur when the CD4+ T-lymphocyte count drops below a level of 200/mm^3. ESR can rise above 20 mm/hr with anemia and with acute and chronic inflammation. CBC with differential and platelet count helps identify anemia, thrombocytopenia, and leukopenia. H&H can also identify anemia.	

2. Nursing Diagnosis: *Health Maintenance, Ineffective,* related to lack of information about HIV/AIDS and its long-term implications for the woman, her unborn child, and her family (NANDA-I © 2012)

NIC Priority Intervention:
Health information: Providing instruction and learning experiences to facilitate the woman's understanding of her condition and to enhance her self-care activities

Goal: The patient and her family will verbalize the importance of following her medication regimen and of obtaining regular prenatal care.

NOC Suggested Intervention:
Health-promoting behavior: Actions to promote optimal wellness and a healthy pregnancy and birth

Intervention	Rationale	Expected Outcome
■ Assess the patient's and family's level of understanding of HIV infection, its methods of spread, and the long-term implications.	■ Knowledge of the woman's (and her family's) level of understanding about her HIV infection forms a starting point for further health teaching.	■ Woman will actively seek information about her condition, her treatment regimen, and her pregnancy and will cooperate with her caregivers.

(continued)

Nursing Care Plan The Woman with HIV Infection—continued

Intervention	Rationale	Expected Outcome
■ Explain the risks of mother-to-child transmission of HIV infection.	■ In untreated women the risk of transmission is 21%. That risk has been reduced dramatically because of the availability of antiretroviral therapy, the use of cesarean birth when indicated, and formula-feeding rather than breastfeeding.	
■ Describe antiretroviral therapy. Include the regimen prescribed, its purposes, and the procedures for taking it.	■ Highly active antiretroviral therapy (HAART) is indicated for all pregnant women to reduce the risk of perinatal transmission. Generally it includes oral ZDV daily, IV ZDV during labor and until birth, and ZDV therapy for the infant for 6 weeks following birth.	
■ Discuss signs the woman should be alert for, including fever, fatigue, weight loss, persistent candidiasis, diarrhea, cough, skin lesions, and behavior changes.	■ These symptoms may indicate that the woman is developing symptomatic HIV infection.	

3. Nursing Diagnosis: *Family Processes, Dysfunctional,* related to the implications of positive maternal HIV status on fetal/neonatal well-being and long-term family functioning (NANDA-I © 2012)

NIC Priority Intervention: *Emotional support:* Provision of reassurance, acceptance, and encouragement during times of stress		NOC Suggested Outcome: *Family coping:* Family actions to manage stressors that tax family resources
Goal: The family is able to manage stressors related to the maternal diagnosis.		
■ Assess ability and readiness of family to learn about HIV and its long-term implications.	■ Readiness is a key element in the teaching–learning process.	■ Family members will actively participate in the treatment plan, be involved in planning for labor and birth in light of a positive HIV status, and be able to express unresolved feelings about the diagnosis.
■ Provide woman and her family with accurate, reliable information about her diagnosis, its prognosis for her and for her baby, and the immediate and long-term implications for her care.	■ Fear and anxiety will lessen when the woman and her family understand her health status and the implications of the HIV diagnosis and can then plan for the future.	
■ Assess interactions between the woman and her family. Be alert for potentially destructive behaviors.	■ If the HIV diagnosis was not expected, the couple may have to deal with issues of blame, concerns about mortality, and worries about the status of the baby. If the HIV diagnosis was known, concerns may focus on fetal/neonatal well-being. In either case, negative responses can lead to destructive behaviors.	
■ Assist family in realistically identifying the needs of the woman and family unit.	■ Once needs are identified realistically, it is possible to plan interventions to meet the needs.	
■ **Collaborative:** Explore available community resources and family support systems.	■ Because HIV is a long-term condition, the family may require ongoing assistance.	

anemia, malaise, progressive weight loss, lymphadenopathy, diarrhea, fever, neurologic dysfunction, cell-mediated immunodeficiency, or evidence of Kaposi's sarcoma (purplish, reddish brown lesions either externally or internally). If a woman tests positive for HIV or is involved in a relationship that places her at high risk, assess the woman's knowledge level about the disease, its implications for her and her fetus, and self-care measures the woman can take.

Examples of nursing diagnoses that might apply to a pregnant woman who tests positive for HIV include the following (NANDA-I © 2012):

- *Health Maintenance, Ineffective,* related to lack of information about HIV/AIDS and its long-term implications for the woman and her unborn child
- *Infection, Risk for,* related to altered immunity secondary to HIV infection
- *Family Processes, Interrupted,* related to the implications of a positive HIV test in one of the family members

Planning and Implementation
Community-Based Nursing Care

Women need to understand that HIV/AIDS is often a fatal disease. HIV infection can be avoided if women practice safe sex, including insisting that their partners wear a latex condom for each act of intercourse and avoiding sharing IV drug needles. Women at high risk for HIV/AIDS should be offered premarital and prepregnancy screening for HIV antibodies.

In monitoring the asymptomatic pregnant woman who is HIV positive, be alert for nonspecific symptoms such as fever, weight loss, fatigue, persistent candidiasis, diarrhea, cough, skin lesions, and behavior changes. These may be signs of developing symptomatic HIV infection. Laboratory findings such as increased viral load; decreased hemoglobin, hematocrit, and CD4+ T lymphocytes; elevated erythrocyte sedimentation rate (ESR); and abnormal complete blood count, differential, and platelets may indicate complications such as infection or progression of the disease.

Education about optimal nutrition and maintenance of wellness is important; review the information frequently with the woman. Give her information about her HAART regimen during pregnancy and for her newborn after birth.

Hospital-Based Nursing Care

Protocols have been established for postexposure treatment of a healthcare worker who experiences a needlestick or exposure to the body fluids of a person with positive or unknown HIV status. The effectiveness of the therapy, usually a combined drug approach, depends on starting rapidly. Thus, such exposure should be reported immediately.

SAFETY ALERT!

In 1987, the CDC stated that the increasing prevalence of HIV/AIDS and the risk of exposure faced by healthcare workers is significant enough that *precautions should be taken with all patients* (not only those with known HIV infection), especially when dealing with blood and body fluids. These precautions are called *standard precautions.*

Health Promotion   The Pregnant Woman with HIV Infection

The psychologic implications of HIV/AIDS for the childbearing family are staggering.

- The woman is faced with the knowledge that she and her newborn, if infected, have a decreased life expectancy. If her infant is not infected, she must face the possibility that others will raise her child. She must also face the reality that she can only hope to lengthen her life by carefully following an expensive, exacting medical regimen.
- The couple must deal with the impact of the illness on the partner, who may or may not be infected, and on other children. The woman and her family may feel fearful, helpless, angry, and isolated.
- It is essential to provide complete, accurate information about the condition, transmission prevention, and ways of coping using language that is well understood by the woman and her partner.
- Ensure that the woman is referred to a comprehensive program that includes social services, psychologic support, and appropriate health care.

Evaluation

Expected outcomes of nursing care include the following:

- The woman discusses the implications of her HIV infection (or diagnosis of AIDS), its implications for her unborn child and for herself, the method of transmission, and the treatment options.
- The woman uses information about social services (or other agency referral) for follow-up assistance and counseling.
- The woman begins to verbalize her feelings about her condition and its implications for her and her family.

CARE OF THE WOMAN WITH HEART DISEASE

Pregnancy results in increased cardiac output, heart rate, and blood volume. The normal heart is able to adapt to these changes without difficulty. The woman with heart disease, however, has decreased cardiac reserve, making it more difficult for her heart to handle the higher workload of pregnancy.

Cardiac disease complicates about 1% of pregnancies (Cunningham et al., 2010). The pathology found in a pregnant woman with heart disease varies with the type of disorder. The more common conditions are discussed briefly here.

Congenital heart defects have become more common in pregnant women as improved surgical techniques enable females born with heart defects to live to childbearing age. Congenital heart defects most commonly seen in pregnant women include atrial septal defect, ventricular septal defect, patent ductus arteriosus, coarctation of the aorta, and tetralogy of Fallot.

For women with congenital heart disease, the impact of pregnancy depends on the specific defect. If the heart defect has been surgically repaired and no evidence of heart disease remains, the woman may undertake pregnancy with confidence. Women with chronic cyanosis are at increased risk for complications and so are their fetuses. A few conditions such as Eisenmenger syndrome, pulmonary hypertension, uncorrected coarctation of the aorta, severe symptomatic aortic stenosis, and Marfan syndrome in certain instances carry such great risk of complications and death that they can be considered absolute contraindications (Harris, 2011).

Rheumatic fever, which may develop in untreated Group A β-hemolytic streptococcal infections, is an inflammatory connective tissue disease that can involve the heart, joints, central nervous system, skin, and subcutaneous tissue. Once it occurs, rheumatic fever can recur; it is serious primarily because of the permanent damage it can do to the heart—rheumatic heart disease. Fortunately, rheumatic heart disease has declined rapidly in the past half century, primarily because of the availability of antibiotics for treatment.

Rheumatic heart disease results when recurrent inflammation from bouts of rheumatic fever causes scar tissue to form on the valves. The scarring results in stenosis (failure of the valve to open completely), regurgitation due to failure of the valve to close completely, or a combination of both, thereby increasing the workload of the heart. Although mitral valve stenosis is most common, the aortic and tricuspid valves may also be affected.

The increased blood volume of pregnancy, coupled with the pregnant woman's need for increased cardiac output, stresses the heart of a woman with mitral stenosis and increases her risk of developing congestive heart failure. Even the woman who has no symptoms at the onset of her pregnancy is at risk.

Mitral valve prolapse (MVP) is usually asymptomatic and commonly found in women of childbearing age. The condition is more common in women than in men and seems to run in families. In MVP the mitral valve leaflets tend to prolapse into the left atrium during ventricular systole because the chordae tendineae that support them are long, stretched, and thin. This produces a characteristic systolic click on auscultation. In more pronounced cases of MVP, mitral valve regurgitation occurs, producing a systolic murmur.

Women with MVP usually tolerate pregnancy well. Most women require assurance that they can continue with normal activities. A few women experience symptoms—primarily palpitations, chest pain, and dyspnea—which are often due to arrhythmias. They are usually treated with propranolol hydrochloride (Inderal). Limiting caffeine intake also helps decrease palpitations. *Peripartum cardiomyopathy* is a relatively rare but serious dysfunction of the left ventricle that occurs in the last month of pregnancy or the first 5 months postpartum in a woman with no previous history of heart disease. The cause is unknown, but mortality is increased with maternal age, in women who have had four or more live births, and in women of African descent (Elkayam, 2011). The symptoms are similar to those of congestive heart failure: dyspnea, orthopnea, fatigue, cough, chest pain, palpitations, and edema. The condition usually presents with anemia and infection; consequently, treatment focuses on underlying abnormalities. Digitalis, diuretics,

vasodilators, anticoagulants, sodium restriction, and strict bed rest are often part of the treatment. In over half of women, heart function returns to normal within 2 to 6 months with bed rest and careful monitoring (Elkayam, 2011). Subsequent pregnancy is strongly discouraged because the disease tends to recur during pregnancy.

Clinical Therapy

The primary goal of clinical therapy is early diagnosis and ongoing management of the woman with cardiac disease. Echocardiogram, chest x-ray, auscultation of heart sounds, and sometimes cardiac catheterization are essential for establishing the type and severity of the heart disease. The severity of the disease can also be determined by the individual's ability to perform ordinary physical activity. Table 15–3 outlines the classification of functional capacity that has been standardized by the Criteria Committee of the New York Heart Association (1994).

Women in classes I and II usually experience a normal pregnancy and have few complications, whereas those in classes III and IV are at risk for more severe complications. Because anemia increases the work of the heart, it should be diagnosed early and treated if present. Infections, even if minor, also increase cardiac workload and should be treated. As pregnancy progresses, the woman's activity should be limited to minimize cardiac workload. Similarly, weight gain and sodium intake may also be restricted.

Drug Therapy

Besides the iron and vitamin supplements prescribed during pregnancy, the pregnant woman with heart disease may need additional drug therapy to maintain health. Antibiotic prophylaxis is not indicated for uncomplicated vaginal or cesarean birth unless infection is suspected. If the woman develops coagulation problems, the anticoagulant heparin may be used. Heparin is safest for the fetus because it does not cross the placenta. The thiazide diuretics and furosemide (Lasix) may be used to treat congestive heart failure if it develops. Digitalis glycosides and common antiarrhythmic drugs may be used to treat cardiac failure and arrhythmias. These agents cross the placenta but have no reported teratogenic effect.

Table 15–3	Severity of Heart Disease by Functional Capacity
Class	Functional Capacity
I	Asymptomatic. No limitation of physical activity.
II	Slight limitation of physical activity. Asymptomatic at rest; symptoms occur with ordinary physical activity.
III	Marked limitation of physical activity. Comfortable at rest but symptomatic during less-than-ordinary physical activity.
IV	Inability to carry on any physical activity without discomfort. Even at rest the person experiences symptoms of cardiac insufficiency or anginal pain; discomfort increases with any physical activity.

Labor and Birth

Spontaneous natural labor with adequate pain relief is usually recommended for women in classes I and II. Special attention should be given to the prompt recognition and treatment of any signs of heart failure (Figure 15–5 ●). Those in classes III and IV may have labor induced and may need to be hospitalized before the onset of labor for cardiac stabilization. They also require invasive cardiac monitoring during labor.

Vaginal birth with low-dose regional analgesia (epidural) is recommended with the use of forceps or vacuum assistance if necessary to limit maternal pushing. The regional analgesia helps decrease maternal cardiac output and oxygen demand by reducing pain and related maternal anxiety. Cesarean birth is used only if fetal or maternal indications exist, not on the basis of heart disease alone.

NURSING MANAGEMENT *For the Pregnant Woman with Heart Disease*

Nursing Assessment and Diagnosis

Assess the stress of pregnancy on the heart's functioning during every antepartum visit. Note the category of functional capacity assigned to the woman; take the woman's pulse, respirations, and blood pressure; and compare the findings with the normal values expected during pregnancy. Then determine the woman's activity level, including rest, and any changes in the pulse and respirations since previous visits. Identify and evaluate other factors that would increase strain on the heart. These factors might include anemia, infection, anxiety, lack of a support system, and household and career demands.

The following signs and symptoms, if they are progressive, indicate congestive heart failure:

- Cough (frequent, with or without blood-stained sputum [hemoptysis])
- Dyspnea (progressive, on exertion)
- Edema (progressive, generalized, including extremities, face, eyelids)
- Heart murmurs (heard on auscultation)
- Palpitations
- Rales (auscultated in lung bases)
- Weight gain (related to fluid retention)

Progressiveness of the cycle is the critical factor because some of these same signs and symptoms are seen to a minor degree in a pregnancy without cardiac problems.

Nursing diagnoses that might apply to the pregnant woman with heart disease include the following (NANDA-I © 2012):

- *Cardiac Output, Decreased,* resulting in easy fatigability
- *Gas Exchange, Impaired,* related to pulmonary edema secondary to cardiac decompensation
- *Fear,* related to the effects of the maternal cardiac condition on fetal well-being

Planning and Implementation

Nursing care is directed toward maintaining a balance between cardiac reserve and cardiac workload.

Antepartum Nursing Care

The priority of nursing action varies based on the severity of the disease process and the individual needs of the woman determined by the nursing assessment. Ensure that the woman and her family thoroughly understand her condition and its management and that they recognize signs of potential complications; this level of understanding will decrease their anxiety. Providing thorough explanations, using printed material, and giving frequent opportunities to ask questions and discuss concerns lets the woman better meet her own healthcare needs and seek assistance appropriately.

As part of health teaching, explain the purposes of the required dietary and activity changes. A diet high in iron, protein, and essential nutrients but low in sodium, with adequate calories to ensure normal weight gain, best meets the nutrition needs of the woman with cardiac disease. To help preserve her cardiac reserves, the woman may need to restrict her activities. In addition, 8 to 10 hours of sleep, with frequent daily rest periods, are essential. Because upper respiratory infections may tax the heart and lead to decompensation, the woman must avoid contact with sources of infection.

During the first half of pregnancy, the woman is seen approximately every 2 weeks to assess cardiac status. During the second half of pregnancy, the woman is seen weekly. These

● **Figure 15–5** Monitoring for signs of heart failure. When a woman with heart disease begins labor, the nursing students and instructor monitor her closely for signs of congestive heart failure.

Activity | Care Plan: Antepartum Patient at Risk

assessments are especially important between weeks 28 and 30, when the blood volume reaches its maximum. If symptoms of cardiac decompensation occur, prompt medical intervention is indicated to correct the cardiac problem.

Intrapartum Period

Labor and birth exert tremendous stress on the woman and her fetus. This stress could be fatal to the fetus of a woman with cardiac disease, because the fetus may be receiving a decreased oxygen and blood supply. Thus, the intrapartum care of a woman with cardiac disease is aimed at reducing physical exertion and the accompanying fatigue.

Evaluate maternal vital signs frequently to determine the woman's response to labor. A pulse rate greater than 100 beats per minute (beats/min) or respirations greater than 25 per minute may indicate the onset of cardiac decompensation and require further evaluation. Auscultate the woman's lungs frequently for evidence of rales and carefully observe for other signs that she is developing decompensation.

To ensure cardiac emptying and adequate oxygenation, encourage the laboring woman to assume either a semi-Fowler's or side-lying position, with her head and shoulders elevated. Oxygen by mask, diuretics to reduce fluid retention, sedatives and analgesics, prophylactic antibiotics, and digitalis may also be used as indicated by the woman's status. Remain with the woman to support her. It is essential to keep the woman and her family informed of labor progress and management plans, collaborating with them to fulfill their wishes for the birth experience as much as possible. Maintain an atmosphere of calm to lessen the anxiety of the woman and her family.

Continuous electronic fetal monitoring provides ongoing assessment of the fetal response to labor. To prevent overexertion and the accompanying fatigue, encourage the woman to sleep and relax between contractions and give her emotional support and encouragement. Epidural anesthesia is often used to decrease exertion. During pushing, encourage the woman to use shorter, more moderate open-glottis pushing, with complete relaxation between pushes. Forceps or vacuum extraction may be used if pushing is too difficult. Monitor vital signs closely during the second stage.

Postpartum Period

The postpartum period is a significant time for the woman with cardiac disease. As extravascular fluid returns to the bloodstream for excretion, cardiac output and blood volume increase. This physiologic adaptation places great strain on the heart and may lead to decompensation, especially in the first 48 hours after birth.

To detect any possible problems, the woman may remain in the hospital postpartum longer than the low-risk woman.

Monitor her vital signs frequently, and assess for signs of decompensation. She stays in the semi-Fowler's or side-lying position, with her head and shoulders elevated, and begins a gradual, progressive activity program. Appropriate diet and stool softeners facilitate bowel movement without undue strain.

Give the woman opportunities to discuss her birth experience and help her deal with any feelings or concerns that distress her. Encourage maternal–infant attachment by providing frequent opportunities for the mother to interact with her child.

No evidence exists that breastfeeding stresses the heart. Thus, the only concern about breastfeeding for women with cardiovascular disease is related to medications the mother may be taking. These should be evaluated for the likelihood of passing into the milk or affecting lactation. Assist the breastfeeding mother to a comfortable side-lying position, with her head moderately elevated, or to a semi-Fowler's position. To conserve the mother's energy, position the newborn at the breast and be available to burp the baby and reposition him or her at the other breast.

In addition to providing the normal postpartum discharge teaching, ensure that the woman and her family understand the signs of possible problems from her heart disease or other postpartum complications. Work with the woman and her family to plan an activity schedule. Visiting nurse referrals may be necessary, depending on the woman's health status.

Evaluation

Expected outcomes of nursing care include the following:

- The woman participates in developing an appropriate healthcare regimen and follows it throughout her pregnancy.
- The woman gives birth to a healthy infant.
- The woman avoids congestive heart failure, thromboembolism, and infection.
- The woman is able to identify signs and symptoms of possible postpartum complications.
- The woman is able to care effectively for her newborn infant.

OTHER MEDICAL CONDITIONS AND PREGNANCY

A woman with a preexisting medical condition needs to be aware of the possible impact of pregnancy on her condition, as well as the impact of her condition on the successful outcome of her pregnancy. Table 15–4 discusses some less common medical conditions in relation to pregnancy.

Table 15–4   Less Common Medical Conditions and Pregnancy

Brief Description	Maternal Implications	Fetal/Neonatal Implications
ASTHMA		
Asthma, an obstructive lung condition, is the most common respiratory disease found in pregnancy, complicating approximately 8% of all pregnancies (Whitty & Dombrowski, 2012). Typical symptoms include wheezing, dyspnea, and episodic coughing. A severe asthmatic attack may require hospitalization. It is managed by long-term comprehensive drug therapy to prevent airway inflammation, combined with drug treatment to manage attacks or exacerbations. Patient education focuses on triggers (such as cold air, dust, smoke, exercise, food additives), methods of prevention, and treatment options.	The severity of asthma may improve, worsen, or remain unchanged during pregnancy. The mechanisms associated with these variations remain undefined; however, poor asthma control is associated with increased maternal and neonatal complications, most likely from poor adherence to the treatment regime. Maternal complications include preeclampsia, growth restriction, and preterm birth. Asthma management during labor and birth focuses on maintenance of adequate hydration and analgesia as well as continuing asthma medications (Whitty & Dombrowski, 2012).	Preeclampsia, preterm birth, low birth weight, and perinatal mortality are more common among the infants of women who have asthma (Whitty & Dombrowski, 2012). The goal of therapy is to prevent maternal exacerbations because even a mild exacerbation can cause severe hypoxia-related complications in the fetus. If an exacerbation occurs, it should be managed in the same way as for a nonpregnant woman because the asthma drugs used are less of a threat to the fetus than a serious asthma attack.
EPILEPSY		
Chronic disorder characterized by seizures; may be idiopathic or secondary to other conditions, such as head injury, metabolic and nutritional disorders such as phenylketonuria (PKU) or vitamin B_6 deficiency, encephalitis, neoplasms, or circulatory interferences. Treated with anticonvulsants.	Vast majority of pregnancies in women with seizure disorders are uneventful and have an excellent outcome. Women with more frequent seizures before pregnancy may have exacerbations during pregnancy, but this may be related to lack of cooperation with drug regimen or sleep deprivation. During pregnancy the woman should continue to be treated with the medication that best controls her seizures. Folic acid therapy should be started prior to conception if possible. Folic acid and vitamin D are indicated throughout pregnancy (Tomson & Battino, 2009).	Certain anticonvulsant medications are associated with increased incidence of congenital anomalies, especially cleft lip and heart defects, although the incidence has decreased in recent years. The lowest dose of a single effective medication is the goal of treatment to decrease the potential for fetal anomalies (Samuels & Niebyl, 2012). Multiple medications and valproic acid should also be avoided for women planning pregnancy when possible (Tomson & Battino, 2009).
HEPATITIS B		
Hepatitis B, caused by the hepatitis B virus (HBV), is a major, growing health problem. Groups at risk include those from areas with a high incidence (primarily developing countries), injection drug users, prostitutes, homosexuals, those with multiple sex partners, individuals who are HIV positive, and those with occupational exposure to blood. HBV transmission is bloodborne, primarily sexually and perinatally transmitted. Because of the dramatic increase and the difficulty of vaccinating high-risk individuals before they become infected, the CDC now recommends (1) testing all pregnant women for the presence of hepatitis B surface antigen (HBsAg) and prophylactic treatment for all infants born to women who are HBsAg positive or whose status is unknown; (2) routine infant vaccination; (3) vaccination of children and adolescents through age 18 years who have not been vaccinated; and (4) vaccination of unvaccinated adults who are at risk for hepatitis B (CDC, 2010).	In the United States estimates suggest 1% to 2% of the population has chronic hepatitis B (Apuzzio et al., 2012a). Hepatitis B does not usually affect the course of pregnancy. However, chronic HBV carriers have a great potential for infecting others when exposure to blood and body fluids occurs. In addition, chronic carriers may develop long-term sequelae, such as chronic liver disease and liver cancer. It is now recommended that all pregnant women be tested for the presence of HBsAg. A woman who is negative may be given the hepatitis vaccine.	Perinatal transmission most often occurs at or near the time of childbirth. In fact, women who are positive for HBsAG have almost a 100% chance of transmitting HBV to their newborn at birth (Apuzzio et al., 2012a). More important, the risk of becoming a chronic carrier of the HBV is inversely related to the age of the individual at the time of initial infection. Therefore, infants infected perinatally have the highest risk of becoming chronically infected if not treated. Routine vaccination of all neonates born to HBsAg-negative women is indicated. Infants born to HBsAg-positive mothers should receive hepatitis B immune globulin at birth or at least within the first 12 hours and should also receive the hepatitis B vaccine (Apuzzio et al., 2012b).

(continued)

Table 15–4	Less Common Medical Conditions and Pregnancy—continued	
Brief Description	**Maternal Implications**	**Fetal/Neonatal Implications**
HYPERTHYROIDISM (THYROTOXICOSIS)		
Enlarged, overactive thyroid gland; increased T_4:TBG ratio and increased basal metabolic rate (BMR). Symptoms include muscle wasting, tachycardia, excessive sweating, and exophthalmos. Treatment by antithyroid drug propylthiouracil (PTU) while monitoring free T_4 levels. Surgery used only if drug intolerance exists.	Mild hyperthyroidism is not dangerous. Increased incidence of preeclampsia and postpartum hemorrhage if not well controlled. Serious risk related to thyroid storm characterized by high fever, tachycardia, sweating, and congestive heart failure. Now occurs rarely. When diagnosed during pregnancy, may be transient or permanent.	Neonatal thyrotoxicosis is rare. Even low doses of antithyroid drug in mother may produce a mild fetal/neonatal hypothyroidism; higher dose may produce a goiter or mental deficiencies. Fetal loss not increased in euthyroid women. If untreated, rates of abortion, intrauterine death, and stillbirth increase. Breastfeeding contraindicated for women on antithyroid medication because it is excreted in the milk (may be tried by woman on low dose if neonatal T_4 levels are monitored).
HYPOTHYROIDISM		
Characterized by inadequate thyroid secretions (decreased T_4:TBG ratio), elevated TSH, lowered BMR, and enlarged thyroid gland (goiter). Iodine deficiency is the most common cause worldwide (Abel, 2011). Symptoms include lack of energy, excessive weight gain, cold intolerance, dry skin, and constipation. Treated by thyroxine replacement therapy.	Long-term replacement therapy continues; at least half of pregnant women need an increase in their thyroxine dose (Abel, 2011). Serial ultrasounds are done to monitor fetal growth; nonstress tests are not necessary in well-controlled disease but are considered beginning at 32 to 34 weeks' gestation in cases of poorly controlled disease (Abel, 2011).	If mother untreated, fetal loss is high; newborn is at risk for severe neurologic problems and congenital goiter (Sullivan, 2011). Therefore newborns are screened for T_4 level. Mild TSH elevations present little risk because TSH does not cross the placenta.
MATERNAL PHENYLKETONURIA (PKU) (HYPERPHENYLALANINEMIA)		
Inherited recessive single gene anomaly causing a deficiency of the liver enzyme needed to convert the amino acid phenylalanine to tyrosine, resulting in high serum levels of phenylalanine. Brain damage and mental retardation occur if not treated early.	Low phenylalanine diet is mandatory before conception and during pregnancy. The woman should be counseled that her children will either inherit the disease or be carriers, depending on the zygosity of the father for the disease. Treatment at a PKU center is recommended.	Risk to fetus if maternal treatment not begun preconception. In untreated women increased incidence of fetal mental retardation, microcephaly, congenital heart defects, and growth retardation. Fetal phenylalanine levels are approximately 50% higher than maternal levels.
MULTIPLE SCLEROSIS		
Neurologic disorder characterized by destruction of the myelin sheath of nerve fibers. The condition occurs primarily in young adults, more commonly in females, and is marked by periods of remission; progresses to marked physical disability in 10 to 20 years.	Exacerbation rate is reduced during the second and third trimester but increased during the 3 months following birth. Exclusive breastfeeding has recently been reported to reduce postpartum exacerbation (Franklin & Tremlett, 2009). Rest is important; help with child care should be planned. Uterine contraction strength is not diminished, but because sensation is frequently lessened, labor may be almost painless.	Some evidence for slightly lower birth weight infants (3%–4%). Increased evidence of a genetic predisposition. Therefore reproductive counseling is recommended.
RHEUMATOID ARTHRITIS		
Chronic inflammatory disease believed to be caused by a genetically influenced antigen–antibody reaction. Symptoms include fatigue, low-grade fever, pain and swelling of joints, morning stiffness, pain on movement. Treated with salicylates, physical therapy, and rest. Corticosteroids used cautiously if not responsive to above.	Usually there is remission of rheumatoid arthritis symptoms during pregnancy, often with a relapse postpartum. Anemia may be present due to blood loss from salicylate therapy. Mother needs extra rest, particularly to relieve weight-bearing joints, but needs to continue range-of-motion exercises. If in remission, may stop medication during pregnancy.	Women taking prednisone during pregnancy give birth slightly earlier (38 wks vs. 39 wks) and have corresponding lower birth weights (de Man et al., 2009).

Table 15–4	Less Common Medical Conditions and Pregnancy—continued	
Brief Description	**Maternal Implications**	**Fetal/Neonatal Implications**

SYSTEMIC LUPUS ERYTHEMATOSUS (SLE)

Chronic autoimmune collagen disease, characterized by exacerbations and remissions; symptoms range from characteristic rash to inflammation and pain in joints, fever, nephritis, depression, cranial nerve disorders, and peripheral neuropathies.	SLE during pregnancy needs to be actively managed with careful surveillance of blood pressure, proteinuria, and placental blood flow. SLE medications may be necessary to control exacerbations and lupus flare. Preeclampsia, prematurity, and fetal growth restriction are common complications. Women with severe disease may be counseled to avoid pregnancy (Ruiz-Irastorza & Khamashta, 2009).	Increased incidence of spontaneous abortion, stillbirth, prematurity, intrauterine growth restriction (IUGR), and neonatal lupus. Neonatal lupus is characterized by a photosensitive skin rash, thrombocytopenia, neutropenia, or anemia, all of which resolve by about 6 months of age. Complete congenital heart block is the most serious complication of SLE, typically diagnosed in utero. When diagnosed, the mother is given corticosteroids that cross the placenta and decrease fetal heart inflammation. The prognosis for these infants varies based on the extent of the cardiac damage. Live-born infants may require a pacemaker (Akin, Baykan, Sezer, et al., 2011).

TUBERCULOSIS (TB)

Tuberculosis (TB) is a major health problem. Two billion people (approximately one third of the population of the world) carry the TB bacteria. Worldwide more women die from TB than from any other infection (Nhan-Chang & Jones, 2010). Infection is caused by *Mycobacterium tuberculosis;* an inflammatory process causes destruction of lung tissue, increased sputum, and coughing. Associated primarily with poverty and malnutrition, 80% of new cases are found in developing countries primarily in Asia and Africa. In the United States the majority of cases occur in foreign-born people (Nhan-Chang & Jones, 2010). Treated with isoniazid and either ethambutol or rifampin, or both.	The incidence of pregnancy complications may be higher in women with TB. TB skin test screening is recommended for women in high-risk groups: healthcare workers; foreign-born women from countries with a high TB risk; women who have had known contact with an infectious person, those who are HIV infected, alcoholics, or illicit drug users; women living or working in homeless shelters; or prisoners and detainees (Cunningham et al., 2010). If TB is inactive due to prior treatment, isoniazid therapy is delayed until the postpartum period unless the woman is HIV positive, has close contact with a person with active TB, or has had a skin test convert to positive within the last 2 years. For those women, isoniazid is started during pregnancy (Nhan-Chang & Jones, 2010). Women with active TB are treated with isoniazid, rifampin, and ethambutol during pregnancy (Cunningham et al., 2010). Extra rest and limited contact with others is required until disease becomes inactive.	If maternal TB is inactive, mother may breastfeed and care for her infant. If TB is active, newborn should not have direct contact with mother until she is noninfectious. Isoniazid crosses the placenta, but most studies show no teratogenic effects. Rifampin crosses the placenta. Possibility of harmful effects is still being studied.

Critical Concept Review

LEARNING OUTCOME 15.1: Discuss the pathology, treatment, and nursing care of pregnant women with diabetes mellitus.

1. The key point in the care of the pregnant woman with diabetes is scrupulous maternal plasma glucose control. This is best achieved by home blood glucose monitoring, multiple daily insulin injections, and a careful diet.

LEARNING OUTCOME 15.2: Distinguish among the major types of anemia associated with pregnancy with regard to signs, treatment, and implications for pregnancy.

1. Anemia indicates inadequate levels of hemoglobin in the blood.
2. Signs include fatigue, paleness, and lack of energy.
3. Iron deficiency anemia is the most common form of anemia. Treatment is done through iron replacement by diet, iron supplement, or both.
4. Other common forms of anemia include folic acid deficiency and sickle cell disease.
5. Implications for the infant include low birth weight, prematurity, and stillbirth.

LEARNING OUTCOME 15.3: Summarize the effects of alcohol and illicit drugs on the childbearing woman and her fetus/newborn.

1. Substance abuse (either drugs or alcohol) not only is detrimental to the mother's health but also may have profound, lasting effects on the fetus.

LEARNING OUTCOME 15.4: Explain the possible implications of maternal psychologic factors and disorders in caring for the childbearing family.

1. Psychologic disorders are characterized by alterations in thinking, mood, or behavior.
2. Depression is a common disorder that can reduce the woman's ability to concentrate or process information and, if untreated, can lead to poor self-care, inadequate nutrition, self-medication, poor maternal–infant bonding, and maternal suicide.
3. Women with bipolar disorder may experience symptoms of depression during the depressive state; during the manic stage the woman may engage in behaviors that pose a risk to herself or her fetus.
4. *Anxiety disorders* include a cluster of diagnoses such as panic disorder, obsessive-compulsive disorder (OCD), posttraumatic stress disorder (PTSD), general anxiety disorder, and other specific phobias.
5. Therapy is aimed at keeping the woman oriented to reality and promoting optimal functioning during pregnancy, labor, and birth.
6. The need for pharmacologic measures such as sedatives, analgesics, or antianxiety medications is determined on an individual basis following careful assessment.

LEARNING OUTCOME 15.5: Describe acquired immunodeficiency syndrome (AIDS), including care of the pregnant woman with HIV/AIDS, fetal/neonatal implications, and ramifications for the childbearing family.

1. HIV infection, which is transmitted via blood and body fluids, may also be transmitted vertically from the mother to the fetus.
2. Vertical transmission of HIV infection has been reduced dramatically with the administration of ZDV to the mother prenatally and during labor, and to the newborn.
3. Nurses should employ blood and body fluid precautions in caring for all women to avoid potential spread of infection.

LEARNING OUTCOME 15.6: Describe the effects of various heart disorders on pregnancy, including their implications for nursing care.

1. Cardiac disease during pregnancy requires careful assessment, limitation of activity, and reporting signs of impending cardiac decompensation by both patient and nurse.

LEARNING OUTCOME 15.7: Compare the effects of selected pregestational medical conditions on pregnancy.

1. All women with chronic medical conditions require increased vigilance of their condition during pregnancy.
2. Most chronic medical conditions will have some effect on the mother because pregnancy increases the stress on the mother's body.
3. Many chronic medical conditions in the mother increase risks to the newborn, such as premature birth, low birth weight, and growth retardation.

Clinical Reasoning in Action

Jane Adams, a 23-year-old G3P2, at 37 weeks' gestation, presents to you in the birthing unit complaining of "vaginal pressure" but no contractions. You assess her and find that her history includes being HIV positive for 2 years, second-trimester cocaine and marijuana use, missed appointments, anemia (HCT 28%), and a positive syphilis serology. Jane tells you that she has other children and that they are being cared for by her mother, who has legal custody of them. You admit Jane and place her on the fetal monitor for evaluation of fetal well-being and contraction patterns. The monitor shows you that the fetal heart rate baseline is 120 to 130 with no decelerations; contractions are mild and irregular, lasting 20 to 30 seconds. You obtain vital signs of BP 130/88, temperature 97.0°F, P 88, R 14. A vaginal exam determines that Jane is 7 cm dilated at +1 station with intact membranes. She asks you if being HIV positive will affect her labor.

1. Discuss the prophylactic regimen for the prevention of HIV transmission to the fetus during labor.
2. Discuss the transmission of HIV to the fetus during pregnancy and birth.
3. Identify the emotional impact of HIV infection or other STIs on the woman.
4. On postpartum day 2 you inform Jane that her infant is HIV antibody positive. How would you clarify the results?
5. Develop a concept map that correlates Jane's stage of labor with her care and her existing HIV.

See www.nursing.pearsonhighered.com for possible responses and an interactive template for a concept map.

References

Abel, D. E. (2011). Thyroid disease during pregnancy: Part 1. Thyroid function testing and hypothyroidism. *The Female Patient, 36*(1), 16–22.

Akin, M. A., Baykan, A., Sezer, S., & Gunes, T. (2011). Review of literature for the striking clinic picture seen in two infants of mothers with systemic lupus erythematosus. *Journal of Maternal–Fetal and Neonatal Medicine, 24*(8), 1022–1026.

American Academy of Pediatrics (AAP) and American College of Obstetricians and Gynecologists (ACOG). (2012). *Guidelines for perinatal care* (7th ed.). Elk Grove Village, IL: American Academy of Pediatrics.

American College of Obstetricians and Gynecologists (ACOG). (2011a). *Methamphetamine abuse in women of reproductive age* (ACOG Committee Opinion No 479). Washington, DC: Author.

American College of Obstetricians and Gynecologists (ACOG). (2011b). *Screening and diagnosis of gestational diabetes mellitus* (Committee Opinion No. 504). Washington, DC: Author.

American College of Obstetricians and Gynecologists (ACOG). (2012a). *Opioid abuse, dependence, and addiction in pregnancy* (ACOG Committee Opinion No. 524). Washington, DC: Author.

American College of Obstetricians and Gynecologists (ACOG). (2012b). *Pregestational diabetes mellitus* (ACOG Practice Bulletin No. 60, issued 2005, reaffirmed 2012). Washington, DC: Author.

American Diabetes Association (ADA). (2012). Position statement: Standards of Medical Care in Diabetes—2012. *Diabetes Care, 35*(Suppl. 1), S11–S63.

Apuzzio, J., Block, J. M., Cullison, S., Cohen, C., Leong, S. L., London, W. T., . . . McMahon, B. J. (2012a). Chronic hepatitis B in pregnancy: A workshop consensus statement on screening, evaluation, and management, Part 1. *The Female Patient, 37*(4), 22–27.

Apuzzio, J., Block, J. M., Cullison, S., Cohen, C., Leong, S. L., London, W. T., . . . McMahon, B. J. (2012b). Chronic hepatitis B in pregnancy: A workshop consensus statement on screening, evaluation, and management, Part 2. *The Female Patient, 37*(5), 30–34.

Baker, A. M., & Haeri, S. (2012). Estimating risk factors and perinatal outcomes for gestational diabetes and impaired glucose tolerance in teen mothers. *Diabetes/Metabolism Research and Reviews, 28*(8), 688–691. doi:10.1002/dmrr.2338

Bower, K., Tobias, D., Yeung, E., Hu, F., & Zhang, C. (2012). A prospective study of prepregnancy dietary fat intake and risk of gestational diabetes. *American Journal of Clinical Nutrition, 95*(2), 446–453.

Centers for Disease Control and Prevention (CDC). (2010). Sexually transmitted diseases treatment guidelines, 2010. *Mortality and Morbidity Weekly Report, 59*(RR-12), 1–114.

Centers for Disease Control and Prevention (CDC). (2012). *HIV Surveillance Report, 2010,* Vol. 221. Retrieved from http://www.cdc.gov/hiv/surveillance/resources/reports/2010report/pdf/2010_HIV_Surveillance_Report_vol_22.pdf

Cleveland Clinic. (2012). *Gestational diabetes.* Retrieved from http://my.clevelandclinic.org/disorders/Diabetes_Gestational/hic_Gestational_Diabetes.aspx

Criteria Committee of the New York Heart Association. (1994). *Nomenclature and criteria for diagnosis of diseases of the heart and great vessels* (9th ed.). Dallas, TX: American Heart Association.

Cunningham, F. G., Leveno, K. J., Bloom, S. L., Hauth, J. C., Rouse, D. J., & Spong, C. Y. (2010). *Williams obstetrics* (23rd ed.). New York, NY: McGraw-Hill.

de Man, Y. A., Hazes, J. M., van der Heide, H., Willemsen, S. P., de Groot, C. J., Steegers, E. A., & Dolhain, R. J. (2009). Association of higher rheumatoid arthritis disease activity during pregnancy with lower birth weight: Results of a national prospective study. *Arthritis Rheumatology, 60*(11), 3196–3206.

Della Grotta, S., LaGasse, L. L., Arria, A. M., Derauf, C., Grant, P., Smith, L. M., . . . Lester, B. M. (2010). Patterns of methamphetamine use during pregnancy: Results from the Infant Development, Environment, and Lifestyle (IDEAL) Study. *Maternal Child Health Journal, 14,* 519–527.

Dishi, M., Enquobahrie, D. A., Abetwe, D. F., Qiu, C., Rudra, C. B., & Williams, M. A. (2011). Age at menarche, menstrual cycle characteristics, and risk of gestational diabetes. *Diabetes Research and Clinical Practice, 93*(3), 437–442.

Elkayam, U. (2011). Clinical characteristics of peripartum cardiomyopathy in the United States. *Journal of the American College of Cardiology, 58*(7), 659–670.

Ferrara, A., Hedderson, M., Albright, C., Ehrlich, S., Quesenberry, C., & Peng, T. (2011). A pregnancy and postpartum lifestyle intervention in women with gestational diabetes mellitus reduces diabetes risk factors: A feasibility randomized control trial. *Diabetes Care, 34*(7), 1519–1525.

Franklin, G. M., & Tremlett, H. (2009). Multiple sclerosis and pregnancy: What should we be telling our patients? *Neurology, 73* (22), 1820–1822.

Harris, I. S. (2011). Management of pregnancy in patients with congenital heart disease. *Progress in Cardiovascular Diseases, 53,* 305–311.

Hood, D. G. (2012). Continuous subcutaneous insulin infusion for managing diabetes. *Nursing for Women's Health, 16*(4), 310–317.

Hurst, H. (2011). Insulin revisited: Safety in the maternity setting. *Nursing for Women's Health, 15*(3), 244–248.

Hurt, H., Betancourt, L. M., Malmud, E. K., Shera, D. M., Giannetta, J. M., Brodsky, N. L., & Farah, M. J. (2009). Children with and without gestational cocaine exposure: A neurocognitive systems analysis. *Neurotoxicology Teratology, 31*(6), 334–341.

Khan, S. J., & Lusskin, S. I. (2010). Update on depression in pregnancy. *The Female Patient, 35*(6), 27–31.

MacMullen, N. J., & Dulski, L. A. (2011). Perinatal implications of sickle cell disease. *MCN, 36*(4), 232–238.

March of Dimes. (2008). *Illicit drug use in pregnancy.* Retrieved from http://www.marchofdimes.com/pregnancy/alcohol_illicitdrug.html

Matthews, L. T., & Mukherjee, J. S. (2009). Strategies for harm reduction among HIV-infected couples who want to conceive. *AIDS and Behavior, 13*(Suppl. 1), 5–11.

Moore, L. E. (2012). Gestational diabetes: Should you use oral agents? *Contemporary OB/GYN, 57*(2), 28–32.

National Institute on Drug Abuse. (2010). *DrugFacts: MDMA (Ecstasy).* Retrieved from http://www.drugabuse.gov/publications/drugfacts/mdma-ecstasy

National Institute of Mental Health. (2010). *Any disorder among adults.* Retrieved from http://www.nimh.nih.gov/statistics/1ANYDIS_ADULT.shtml

Nhan-Chang, C., & Jones, T. B. (2010). Tuberculosis in pregnancy. *Clinical Obstetrics and Gynecology, 53*(2), 311–321.

Niebyl, J. R., & Simpson, J. L. (2012). Drugs and environmental agents in pregnancy and lactation: Embryology, teratology, epidemiology. In S. G. Gabbe, J. R. Niebyl, J. L. Simpson, M. B. Landon, H. L. Galan, E. R. M. Jauniaux, & D. A. Driscoll (Eds.), *Obstetrics: Normal and problem pregnancies* (6th ed.). Philadelphia, PA: Elsevier Saunders.

O'Leary, C. M., Nassar, N., Zubrick, S. R., Kurinczuk, J. J., Stanley, F., & Bower, C. (2009). Evidence of a complex association between dose, pattern and timing of prenatal alcohol exposure and child behaviour problems. *Addiction, 105*(1), 74–86. doi:10.1111/j.1360-0443.2009.02756.x

Panel on Treatment of HIV-Infected Pregnant Women and Prevention of Perinatal Transmission. (2011, September 14). *Recommendations for use of antiretroviral drugs in pregnant HIV-1-infected women for maternal health and interventions to reduce perinatal HIV transmission in the United States* (pp. 1–207). Retrieved from http://aidsinfo.nih.gov/contentfiles/PerinatalGL.pdf

Reece, E. A. (2011). How to improve outcomes in gestational diabetes—For mother and baby. *OBG Management, 23*(3), 37–45.

Ruiz-Irastorza, G., & Khamashta, M. A. (2009). Managing lupus patients during pregnancy. *Best Practice and Research. Clinical Rheumatology, 23*(4), 575–582.

Samuels, P. (2012). Hematologic complications of pregnancy. In S. G. Gabbe, J. R. Niebyl, J. L. Simpson, M. B. Landon, H. L. Galan, E. R. M. Jauniaux, & D. A. Driscoll (Eds.), *Obstetrics: Normal and problem pregnancies* (6th ed.). Philadelphia, PA: Elsevier Saunders.

Samuels, P., & Niebyl, J. R. (2012). Neurologic disorders. In S. G. Gabbe, J. R. Niebyl, J. L. Simpson, M. B. Landon, H. L. Galan, E. R. M. Jauniaux, & D. A. Driscoll (Eds.), *Obstetrics: Normal and problem pregnancies* (6th ed.). Philadelphia, PA: Elsevier Saunders.

Shade, M., Miller, L., Borst, J., English, B., Valliere, J., Downs, K., . . . Hare, I. (2011). Statewide innovations to improve services for women with perinatal depression. *Nursing for Women's Health, 15*(2), 127–136.

Smith, M. V., Shao, L., Howell, H., Lin, H., & Yonkers, K. A. (2011). Perinatal depression and birth outcomes in a Healthy Start project. *Maternal–Child Nursing Journal, 15*(3), 401–409.

Substance Abuse and Mental Health Services Administration (SAMHSA). (2011). *Results from the 2010 National Survey on Drug Use and Health: Summary of National Findings* (NSDUH Series H-41, DHHS Publication No. SMA 11–4658). Rockville, MD: Office of Applied Studies.

Sullivan, S. A. (2011). Subclinical hypothyroidism: Identification and treatment in pregnancy. *Contemporary OB/GYN, 56*(6), 46–53.

Thompson, B. L., Levitt, P., & Stanwood, G. D. (2009). Prenatal exposure to drugs: Effects on brain development and implications for policy and education. *Nature Reviews Neuroscience, 10*(4), 303–312.

Thompson, V. B., Heiman, J., Chambers, J. B., Benoit, S. C., Buesing, W. R., Norman, M. K., . . . Lipton, J. W. (2009). Long-term behavioral consequences of prenatal MDMA exposure. *Physiology & Behavior, 96*(4–5), 593–601.

Tomson, T., & Battino, D. (2009). Teratogenic effects of antiepileptic medications. *Neurology Clinics, 27*(4), 993–1002.

Vucinovic, M., Roje, D., Vucinovic, Z., Capkun, V., Bucat, M., & Banovic, I. (2009). Maternal and neonatal effects of substance abuse during pregnancy: Our ten-year experience. *Yonsei Medical Journal, 49*(5), 705–713.

Whitty, J. E., & Dombrowski, M. P. (2012). Respiratory diseases in pregnancy. In S. G. Gabbe, J. R. Niebyl, J. L. Simpson, M. B. Landon, H. L. Galan, E. R. M. Jauniaux, & D. A. Driscoll (Eds.), *Obstetrics: Normal and problem pregnancies* (6th ed.). Philadelphia, PA: Elsevier Saunders.

Pearson Nursing Student Resources Find additional review materials at: **nursing.pearsonhighered.com**

Pregnancy at Risk: Gestational Onset

When we decided to have children we were so excited, so ready. I never expected that I would have two miscarriages. I can't tell you how hard that was to handle. Even today, with two healthy children, I remember the pain, the loss, the sense of failure, and I grieve for the children we will never know. —Jasmine, 36

Chris Baker/Getty Images

LEARNING OUTCOMES

16.1 Contrast the etiology, medical therapy, and nursing interventions for the various bleeding problems associated with pregnancy.

16.2 Discuss the medical therapy and nursing care of a woman with hyperemesis gravidarum.

16.3 Describe the maternal and fetal/neonatal risks, clinical manifestations, and nursing care of a pregnant woman with a hypertensive disorder.

16.4 Summarize the risks and implications of surgical procedures performed during pregnancy.

16.5 Relate the impact of trauma caused by an accident to the nursing care of the pregnant woman or her fetus.

16.6 Discuss the needs and care of the pregnant woman who experiences abuse.

16.7 Contrast the effects of various infections on the pregnant woman and her unborn child.

16.8 Relate the cause, fetal/neonatal risks, prevention, and clinical therapy to the nursing care of the woman at risk for Rh alloimmunization.

16.9 Compare Rh incompatibility to ABO incompatibility with regard to occurrence, clinical treatment, and implications for the fetus or newborn.

In some pregnancies, problems arise that place the woman and her unborn child at risk. Regular prenatal care helps detect these complications quickly so that effective care can be provided. This chapter focuses on problems that develop during pregnancy, those with a *gestational onset*. (*Note:* Conditions such as diabetes mellitus and anemia, which may occur prior to pregnancy or develop during pregnancy, are discussed in Chapter 15 🔗.)

CARE OF THE WOMAN WITH A BLEEDING DISORDER

During the first and second trimesters, the major cause of bleeding is abortion. **Abortion** is the expulsion of the fetus prior to viability, which is considered to be 20 weeks' gestation or weight of less than 500 g. Definitions of viability vary somewhat according to state reporting laws (Cunningham et al., 2010). Abortions are either *spontaneous* (occurring naturally) or *induced* (occurring as a result of medical or surgical means). **Miscarriage** is a lay term used for spontaneous abortion.

Other complications that can cause bleeding in the first half of pregnancy are ectopic pregnancy and gestational trophoblastic disease. In the second half of pregnancy, particularly in the third trimester, the two major causes of bleeding are placenta previa and abruptio placentae (see Chapter 21 🔗 for more information). Regardless of the cause of bleeding, however, the nurse has certain general responsibilities in providing nursing care.

General Principles of Nursing Intervention

Spotting is relatively common during pregnancy and usually occurs following sexual intercourse or exercise because of trauma to the highly vascular cervix. However, the woman is advised to report any spotting or bleeding that occurs during pregnancy so that it can be evaluated.

It is often the nurse's responsibility to make the initial assessment of bleeding. In general, the following nursing measures are indicated:

- Monitor blood pressure and pulse frequently. The frequency is determined by the extent of the bleeding and the stability of the woman's condition.
- Observe the woman for behaviors indicative of shock, such as pallor, clammy skin, perspiration, dyspnea, or restlessness.
- Count and weigh pads to assess amount of bleeding over a given time period; save any tissue or clots expelled.
- If pregnancy is of 12 weeks' gestation or beyond, assess fetal heart tones with a Doppler.
- Prepare for intravenous (IV) therapy. There may be standing orders to begin IV therapy on patients who are bleeding.
- Prepare equipment for examination and have oxygen available.
- Collect and organize all data, including antepartum history, onset of bleeding episode, and laboratory studies (hemoglobin, hematocrit, Rh status, hormonal assays) for analysis.
- Obtain an order to type and cross-match for blood if evidence of significant blood loss exists.
- Assess coping mechanisms of the woman in crisis. Give emotional support to enhance her coping abilities by continuous, sustained presence; by clear explanation of procedures; and by communicating her status to her family. Prepare the woman for possible fetal loss. Assess her expressions of anger, denial, silence, guilt, depression, or self-blame.
- Assess the family's response to the situation.

Spontaneous Abortion (Miscarriage)

The incidence of spontaneous abortion is about 15% in clinically recognized pregnancies (Richards, 2012). However, advanced maternal age increases the risk significantly.

A majority of early miscarriages are related to chromosomal abnormalities. Other causes include teratogenic drugs, faulty implantation caused by abnormalities of the female reproductive tract, a weakened cervix, placental abnormalities, chronic maternal diseases, endocrine imbalances, and maternal infections. Women who use hot tubs or jacuzzis may be at increased risk for miscarriage because of the hyperthermia resulting from increased core body temperature (Harms, 2010).

Classification

Spontaneous abortions are subdivided into the following categories:

- *Threatened abortion* (Figure 16–1A ●). The embryo or fetus is jeopardized by unexplained bleeding, cramping, and backache. The cervix is closed. Bleeding may persist for days. It may be followed by partial or complete expulsion of the embryo or fetus, placenta, and membranes (sometimes called the "products of conception").

- *Imminent abortion* (Figure 16–1B ●). Bleeding and cramping increase. The internal cervical os dilates. Membranes may rupture. The term *inevitable abortion* also applies.

- *Complete abortion.* All the products of conception are expelled.

- *Incomplete abortion* (Figure 16–1C ●). Some of the products of conception are retained, most often the placenta. The internal cervical os is dilated slightly.

- *Missed abortion.* The fetus dies in utero but is not expelled. Uterine growth ceases, breast changes regress, and the woman may report a brownish vaginal discharge. The cervix is closed. If the fetus is retained beyond 6 weeks, the breakdown of fetal tissues results in the release of thromboplastin, and disseminated intravascular coagulation (DIC) may develop.

- *Recurrent pregnancy loss (formerly called habitual abortion).* Abortion occurs consecutively in three or more pregnancies.

- *Septic abortion.* Infection is present. It may occur with prolonged, unrecognized rupture of the membranes, pregnancy with an intrauterine device (IUD) in place, or attempts by unqualified individuals to end a pregnancy.

Clinical Therapy

Pelvic cramping and backache are reliable indicators of potential spontaneous abortion. These symptoms are usually absent in bleeding caused by polyps, ruptured cervical blood vessels, or cervical erosion.

● **Figure 16–1** Types of spontaneous abortion. *A,* Threatened. The cervix is not dilated, and the placenta is still attached to the uterine wall, but some bleeding occurs. *B,* Imminent. The placenta has separated from the uterine wall, the cervix has dilated, and the amount of bleeding has increased. *C,* Incomplete. The embryo or fetus has passed out of the uterus, but the placenta remains.

Speculum examination is done to determine the presence of cervical polyps or cervical erosion. Ultrasound scanning may detect the presence of cardiac activity and a gestational sac, or may reveal a crown-to-rump length that is small for gestational age. Laboratory determination of the human chorionic gonadotropin (hCG) level can confirm a pregnancy, but because the hCG level falls slowly after fetal death, it cannot confirm a live embryo/fetus. Serial hCG levels may be indicated to confirm a diagnosis. Hemoglobin and hematocrit levels are obtained to assess blood loss. Blood is typed and cross-matched for possible replacement needs.

The therapy prescribed for the pregnant woman with bleeding is bed rest, abstinence from coitus, and emotional support. If bleeding persists and abortion is imminent or incomplete, the woman may be hospitalized, IV therapy or blood transfusions may be started to replace fluid, and dilation and curettage (D&C) or suction evacuation is performed to remove the remainder of the products of conception. If the woman is Rh negative and not sensitized, Rh immune globulin (RhoGAM) is given within 72 hours (see discussion on Rh alloimmunization later in this chapter).

In missed abortions, the products of conception usually are expelled spontaneously. Diagnosis is based on history, pelvic examination, and a negative pregnancy test and may be confirmed by ultrasound if necessary. If this does not occur within 4 to 6 weeks after embryo or fetal death, hospitalization is necessary. If in the first trimester, D&C or suction evacuation is done. In the second trimester, labor is induced or dilation and evacuation (D&E) may be used.

NURSING MANAGEMENT *For the Woman Experiencing Spontaneous Abortion*

Nursing Assessment and Diagnosis

Assess the woman's vital signs, amount and appearance of any bleeding, level of comfort, and general physical health. The woman's blood type and antibody status should be identified to determine the need for Rh immune globulin. If the pregnancy is 10 to 12 weeks or more, determine fetal heart rates with a Doppler. It is also important to assess the responses of the woman and her family to this crisis, their coping mechanisms, and their ability to comfort each other.

Examples of nursing diagnoses that may apply include the following (NANDA-I © 2012):

- *Pain, Acute,* related to abdominal cramping secondary to threatened abortion
- *Fluid Volume, Deficient,* related to excessive bleeding secondary to spontaneous abortion

Planning and Implementation

Community-Based Nursing Care

If a woman in her first trimester of pregnancy begins cramping or spotting, she is often evaluated on an outpatient basis. Provide analgesics for pain relief if the woman's cramps are severe, and explain what is occurring throughout the process.

Feelings of shock or disbelief are normal. Couples who approached the pregnancy with joy and excitement now feel grief, sadness, and possibly anger. Because many women, even with

---

Developing Cultural Competence
Individual Responses to Fetal Loss

Remember that individual responses to fetal loss following miscarriage may vary greatly and may be influenced by ethnic or cultural norms.

- Miscarriage may be viewed in many ways. For example, it may be seen as a punishment from God, as the result of the evil eye or of a hex or curse by an enemy, or as a natural part of life.
- When grieving over a pregnancy loss, women from some cultures and ethnic groups may show their emotions freely, crying and wailing, whereas other women may hide their feelings behind a mask of stoicism.
- In some cultures the woman's partner is her primary source of support and comfort. In others, the woman turns to her mother or close female relatives for comfort.
- Avoid falling into the trap of stereotyping women according to culture. Individual responses are influenced by many factors, including the degree of assimilation into the dominant culture.

---

planned pregnancies, feel some ambivalence initially, guilt is also a common emotion. These feelings may be even stronger for women who were negative about their pregnancies. The women may even believe that the miscarriage is a punishment for some wrongdoing.

Offer psychologic support to the woman and her family by encouraging them to talk about their feelings, allowing them the privacy to grieve, and listening sympathetically to their concerns about this pregnancy and future ones. To help decrease feelings of guilt or blame, inform the woman and her family about the causes of miscarriage. If the woman has older children, she may need guidance in how to help them understand and cope with what has occurred. Refer them to other healthcare professionals for additional help as necessary.

The grieving period following a miscarriage usually lasts 6 to 24 months. Many couples can be helped during this period by an organization or support group established for parents who have lost a fetus or newborn.

Hospital-Based Nursing Care

A woman with an incomplete or missed abortion may need a D&C or other procedure, which is typically done on an outpatient basis. Barring any complications, the woman can return home a few hours after the procedure. Monitor the woman's condition closely and provide instruction for self-care. Administer Rh immune globulin if it is indicated.

Health Promotion   After a Miscarriage

Provide information about community resources to help the woman and her loved ones cope with the loss and advise her to:

- Report heavy or bright red vaginal bleeding, fever, chills, foul-smelling vaginal discharge, or abdominal tenderness.
- Take the full course of antibiotics if any are prescribed.
- Delay pregnancy for at least 2 months to allow sufficient time for healing.

Evaluation

Expected outcomes of nursing care include the following:

- The woman is able to explain spontaneous abortion, the treatment measures employed in her care, and long-term implications for future pregnancies.
- The woman suffers no complications.
- The woman and her partner begin verbalizing their grief and acknowledge that the grieving process lasts several months.

Ectopic Pregnancy

Ectopic pregnancy (EP) is the implantation of the fertilized ovum in a site other than the endometrial lining of the uterus. It has many causes, including tubal damage from pelvic inflammatory disease (PID), previous tubal surgery, congenital anomalies of the tube, endometriosis, previous EP, presence of an IUD, and in utero exposure to diethylstilbestrol (DES).

Ectopic pregnancy occurs in about 2% of diagnosed pregnancies. Although the incidence of EP has increased, the mortality rate in the United States has decreased to 0.5 deaths per 100,000. This decline can be credited to improved recognition of early signs and symptoms and better diagnostic methods, which allow detection before tubal rupture. Nevertheless, EP accounts for approximately 9% of maternal deaths today (Marion & Meeks, 2012).

EP occurs when the fertilized ovum is prevented or slowed in its passage through the tube and thus implants before it reaches the uterus, usually in the ampulla of the fallopian tube. *Pathophysiology Illustrated: Ectopic Pregnancy* identifies other implantation sites.

Initially symptoms of pregnancy may be present, including amenorrhea, breast tenderness, and nausea. The hormone hCG is present in the blood and urine. As the pregnancy progresses, the chorionic villi grow into the tube wall or implantation site and establish a blood supply. When the embryo outgrows this space, the tube ruptures and there is bleeding into the abdominal cavity. This bleeding irritates the peritoneum, causing the characteristic symptoms of sharp, one-sided pain, syncope, and referred right shoulder pain. The woman may also have lower abdominal pain. Vaginal bleeding occurs because of fluctuations in hormone levels.

Physical examination usually reveals adnexal (area over each ovary and fallopian tube) tenderness. An adnexal mass is palpable about half the time. Bleeding is slow and chronic, and the abdomen gradually becomes rigid and very tender. With bleeding into the abdominal cavity, pelvic examination is very painful, and a mass of blood may be palpated in the lower abdomen. Laboratory tests may reveal low hemoglobin and hematocrit levels and rising leukocyte levels.

Clinical Therapy

The following measures are used to establish the diagnosis of ectopic pregnancy and assess the woman's status:

- A careful assessment of menstrual history, particularly the last menstrual period (LMP), is completed.
- A pelvic exam is conducted to identify any abnormal pelvic masses and tenderness.
- Transvaginal ultrasound is the initial test of choice to detect an intrauterine pregnancy or an adnexal mass (Jurkovic & Wilkinson, 2011). Confirming an intrauterine pregnancy nearly eliminates the diagnosis of ectopic pregnancy.
- Serial measurements of serum hCG values are taken, which should increase significantly every 2 days. Women with an ectopic pregnancy often have serial serum hCG values that

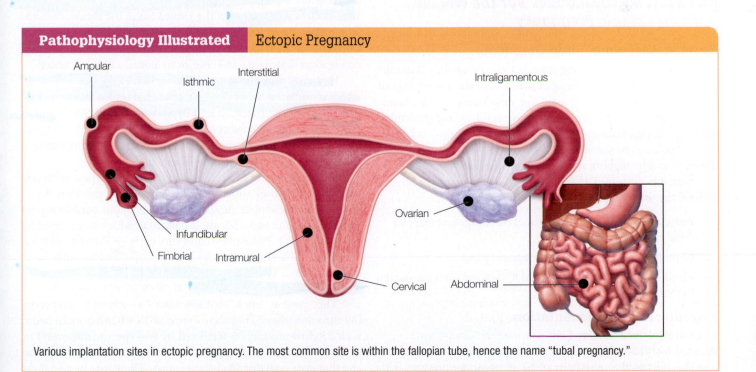

Pathophysiology Illustrated | Ectopic Pregnancy

Various implantation sites in ectopic pregnancy. The most common site is within the fallopian tube, hence the name "tubal pregnancy."

increase more slowly than expected with a viable intrauterine pregnancy (Visconti & Zite, 2012).

■ Laparoscopic intervention may be necessary for both diagnosis and treatment if the presence or absence of an ectopic pregnancy cannot be confirmed by other measures.

Treatment may be medical or surgical. Methotrexate is used for the woman who desires future pregnancy, if her ectopic pregnancy is unruptured and of 4 cm size or less, and if her condition is stable. In addition, there must be no fetal heart motion and the woman must have no evidence of a blood disorder or kidney or liver disease.

Methotrexate is a folic acid antagonist that interferes with the proliferation of trophoblastic cells. It is administered intramuscularly (IM) using either a single-dose or multiple-dose regimen. As an outpatient, the woman is monitored for increasing abdominal pain and β-hCG titers are determined. β-hCG titers are assessed on day 4 and day 7. If hCG levels do not decrease at least 15% from day 4 to day 7 after the initial injection, an additional dose of methotrexate is given on day 7 (Lipscomb, 2012). The multidose regimen includes methotrexate given IM and leucovorin administered orally on alternate days for up to 8 days (Visconti & Zite, 2012). This regimen is far more care intensive and is reserved for patients who present with high hCG levels.

If surgery is indicated and the woman desires future pregnancies, a laparoscopic linear salpingostomy will be performed to gently evacuate the ectopic pregnancy and preserve the tube. If the tube is ruptured or if future childbearing is not an issue, laparoscopic salpingectomy (removal of the tube) is performed, leaving the ovary in place unless it is damaged. If the woman is in shock and unstable, an abdominal incision will be made. With both medical and surgical therapies for EP, the Rh-negative nonsensitized woman is given Rh immune globulin to prevent sensitization.

NURSING MANAGEMENT *For the Woman with an Ectopic Pregnancy*

Nursing Assessment and Diagnosis

When the woman with a suspected ectopic pregnancy is admitted to the hospital, assess the appearance and amount of vaginal bleeding and monitor vital signs for developing shock. Assess the woman's emotional state and coping abilities, and determine the couple's informational needs. Determine the woman's level of pain, which can be significant. If surgery is necessary, complete the appropriate ongoing assessments postoperatively.

Nursing diagnoses that may apply for a woman with EP include the following (NANDA-I © 2012):

■ *Pain, Acute,* related to abdominal bleeding secondary to tubal rupture

■ *Grieving* related to expected pregnancy loss

■ *Fluid Volume, Deficient,* related to hypovolemia secondary to maternal blood loss

Planning and Implementation
Community-Based Nursing Care
Women with EP are often seen initially in a clinic or office setting. Be alert to the possibility of EP if a woman presents with complaints of abdominal pain and lack of menses for 1 to 2 months. A woman receiving medical treatment using methotrexate is followed as an outpatient. Advise the woman that some abdominal pain is common following the injection, but generally it is mild and lasts only 24 to 48 hours. More severe pain might indicate treatment failure and should be evaluated. The woman should also report heavy vaginal bleeding, dizziness, or tachycardia. Stress the need to return for follow-up β-hCG testing.

Hospital-Based Nursing Care
Once a diagnosis of EP is made and surgery is scheduled, start an IV as ordered and begin preoperative teaching. Immediately report signs of developing shock. If the woman experiences severe abdominal pain, administer analgesics and evaluate their effectiveness.

Regardless of the treatment used, the woman and her family will need emotional support during this difficult time. Their feelings and responses to this crisis are generally similar to those that occur in cases of spontaneous abortion; similar nursing actions are required.

Evaluation
Expected outcomes of nursing care include the following:

■ The woman is able to explain ectopic pregnancy, treatment alternatives, and implications for future childbearing.

■ The woman and her caregivers detect possible complications early and manage them successfully.

■ The woman and her partner are able to begin verbalizing their loss.

Gestational Trophoblastic Disease

Gestational trophoblastic disease (GTD) is the pathologic proliferation of trophoblastic cells (the trophoblast is the outermost layer of embryonic cells). In the United States the incidence is approximately 1 per 1000 to 1500 live births (Salani, Eisenhauer, & Copeland, 2012). It includes hydatidiform mole, invasive mole (chorioadenoma destruens), and choriocarcinoma, a form of cancer.

Hydatidiform mole (molar pregnancy) is a condition in which a proliferation of trophoblastic cells results in the formation of a placenta characterized by *hydropic* (fluid-filled) grapelike clusters. The disease results in the loss of the pregnancy and the possibility, though remote, of developing choriocarcinoma, a form of cancer, from the trophoblastic tissue.

Molar pregnancies are classified into two types, complete and partial, both of which meet the previously mentioned criteria. A *complete mole* develops from an ovum containing no maternal genetic material, an "empty egg," which is fertilized by a normal sperm. The embryo dies very early, no circulation is established, the hydropic vesicles are avascular, and no embryonic tissue is found. Choriocarcinoma seems to be associated exclusively with the complete mole.

The *partial mole* usually has a triploid karyotype (69 chromosomes). This occurs most often when a normal ovum with 23 chromosomes is fertilized by two sperm (dispermy) or by a sperm that has failed to undergo the first meiotic division and therefore contains 46 chromosomes. There may be a fetal sac or even a fetus with a heartbeat. The fetus has multiple anomalies and little chance for survival. Often partial moles are recognized only after miscarriage, and they may go unnoticed even then.

Invasive mole (chorioadenoma destruens) is similar to a complete mole, but it involves the uterine myometrium. Treatment is the same as for complete mole.

Clinical Therapy

With hydatidiform mole, the following signs may be present:

- Vaginal bleeding occurs almost universally. It is often brownish (like prune juice) because of liquefaction of the uterine clot, but it may be bright red.

- Uterine enlargement greater than expected for gestational age is a classic sign of a complete mole, which is present in about half of cases.

- Hydropic vesicles (grapelike clusters) may be passed; if so, they are diagnostic (Figure 16–2 ●). With a partial mole the vesicles are often smaller and may not be noticed.

- Serum human chorionic gonadotropin (hCG) levels are markedly elevated because of continued secretion by the proliferating trophoblastic tissue.

- Hyperemesis gravidarum is present because of the elevated hCG level.

- Anemia occurs frequently because of blood loss.

- Symptoms of preeclampsia are observed before 24 weeks' gestation.

- Fetal heart tones are absent despite other signs of pregnancy.

Transvaginal ultrasound is used for diagnosis. Therapy begins with suction evacuation of the mole and curettage of the uterus to remove all fragments of the placenta. Early evacuation decreases the possibility of other complications. Rh immune globulin is administered to women with an Rh-negative blood type. If the woman is older and has completed her childbearing, or if there is excessive bleeding, hysterectomy may be the treatment of choice to reduce the risk of choriocarcinoma.

Because of the risk of choriocarcinoma, the woman treated for hydatidiform mole should receive extensive follow-up therapy. Follow-up care includes a baseline chest x-ray to detect lung metastasis and a physical examination including a pelvic examination. Approaches to ongoing monitoring vary somewhat. Typically serum β-hCG levels are monitored weekly until negative results are obtained three consecutive times, then monthly for 6 to 12 months (Salani et al., 2012). The woman should avoid pregnancy during that time because the elevated hCG levels associated with pregnancy would cause confusion as to whether cancer had developed. If, after a year of monitoring, the hCG serum titers are within normal limits, a couple may be assured that a normal pregnancy can be anticipated, with a low risk of recurring hydatidiform mole.

If hCG levels plateau for 3 consecutive weeks or rise, pregnancy must be ruled out and then the woman should be evaluated for metastatic disease and treated appropriately (Salani et al., 2012). Treatment at a center specializing in GTD is advised.

NURSING MANAGEMENT *For the Woman with Gestational Trophoblastic Disease*

Nursing Assessment and Diagnosis

Observe for symptoms of hydatidiform mole at each antepartum visit. The classic symptoms are found more frequently with the complete mole. Before evacuation the partial mole may be difficult to distinguish from a missed abortion. If a molar pregnancy is diagnosed, assess the woman's (or the couple's) understanding of the condition and its implications.

Nursing diagnoses that may apply include the following (NANDA-I © 2012):

- *Fear* related to the possible development of choriocarcinoma

- *Grieving* related to the loss of the pregnancy secondary to GTD

Planning and Implementation

Community-Based Nursing Care

When a molar pregnancy is suspected, the woman needs emotional support. Answer questions about the condition and explain what ultrasound and other diagnostic procedures will entail. If a molar pregnancy is diagnosed, support the parents as they deal with their grief about the lost pregnancy and their fear about the possibility of having a serious illness (DiGiulio, Wiedaseck, & Monchek, 2012). Healthcare counselors, a member of the clergy, or a professional counselor may also be of help.

Hospital-Based Nursing Care

When the woman is hospitalized for removal of the mole, monitor vital signs and vaginal bleeding for signs of hemorrhage. Determine the presence of abdominal pain and evaluate the woman's emotional state and coping ability. Have typed and cross-matched blood available for surgery. Administer oxytocin as ordered to keep the uterus contracted and to prevent hemorrhage. If the woman is Rh negative and not sensitized, give Rh immune globulin to prevent antibody formation.

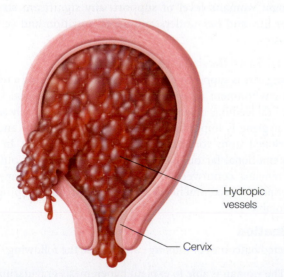

Hydropic vesicles

Cervix

● **Figure 16–2** Hydatidiform mole. A common sign is vaginal bleeding, often brownish (the characteristic "prune juice" appearance) but sometimes bright red. In this figure, some of the hydropic vessels are being passed. This occurrence is diagnostic for hydatidiform mole.

> **Health Promotion** Hydatidiform Mole
>
> - Stress the importance of follow-up visits.
> - Advise the woman to delay another pregnancy until the follow-up program has been completed.

Evaluation

Expected outcomes of nursing care include the following:

- The woman has a smooth recovery following successful evacuation of the mole.
- The woman is able to explain GTD and its treatment, follow-up, and long-term implications for pregnancy.
- The woman and her partner are able to begin talking about their grief at the loss of their anticipated child.
- The woman can discuss the importance of follow-up care and indicates her willingness to cooperate with the regimen.

CARE OF THE WOMAN WITH HYPEREMESIS GRAVIDARUM

Hyperemesis gravidarum, which is excessive vomiting during pregnancy, occurs in 0.3% to 2% of pregnancies (Nayeri, 2012). It may be mild at first, but true hyperemesis may progress to a point at which the woman not only vomits everything she swallows but also retches between meals.

Although the exact cause of hyperemesis is unclear, increased levels of human chorionic gonadotropin (hCG) may play a role. Other mechanisms that may relate to hyperemesis are displacement of the gastrointestinal tract, hypofunction of the anterior pituitary gland and adrenal cortex, abnormalities of the corpus luteum, and psychologic factors. Research suggests that genetics may also play a role in its development (Zhang, Cantor, MacGibbon, et al., 2011).

In severe cases, hyperemesis causes dehydration, which leads to fluid–electrolyte imbalance and alkalosis from loss of hydrochloric acid. Hypovolemia, hypotension, tachycardia, increased hematocrit and blood urea nitrogen (BUN), and decreased urine output can also occur. If untreated, metabolic acidosis may develop. Severe potassium loss interferes with the ability of the kidneys to concentrate urine and may disrupt cardiac functioning. Starvation causes muscle wasting and severe protein and vitamin deficiencies. Fetal or embryonic death may result, and the woman may suffer irreversible metabolic changes or death. The diagnostic criteria for hyperemesis include a history of intractable vomiting in the first half of pregnancy, dehydration, ketonuria, and a weight loss of 5% of prepregnancy weight.

Clinical Therapy

The goals of treatment include control of vomiting and dehydration, restoration of electrolyte balance, and maintenance of adequate nutrition. If the woman does not respond to standard approaches to the control of nausea and vomiting in pregnancy (see Chapter 11 🔗), she may require IV fluids on an outpatient basis. If her symptoms do not improve, hospitalization may be indicated. Initially the woman is given nothing by mouth (NPO), and IV fluids are administered. Potassium chloride is often added to the IV to prevent hypokalemia. Phenothiazines such as prochlorperazine and chlorpromazine, antihistamines, and metoclopramide (an antiemetic) are considered safe for the treatment of hyperemesis, as is pyridoxine (vitamin B_6) (Sonkusare, 2011). Typically the woman remains NPO for 48 hours. If her condition does not improve, total parenteral nutrition may be needed. She then begins controlled oral feedings.

NURSING MANAGEMENT *For the Woman with Hyperemesis Gravidarum*

Nursing Assessment and Diagnosis

When a woman is hospitalized for control of vomiting, assess the amount and character of any emesis, intake and output, fetal heart rate, signs of jaundice or bleeding, and her emotional state.

Nursing diagnoses that may apply include the following (NANDA-I © 2012):

- *Nutrition, Imbalanced: Less than Body Requirements* related to persistent vomiting secondary to hyperemesis
- *Fluid Volume, Deficient,* related to severe dehydration secondary to persistent vomiting

Planning and Implementation
Community-Based Nursing Care

Parenteral therapy provided at home in collaboration with a physician and a registered dietitian is sometimes used to enable the woman to remain in her home. This therapy also gives an opportunity to observe family interactions and evaluate the home environment. This assessment helps determine the pregnant woman's level of support, any significant stressors in her life, and her understanding of nutrition and self-care measures.

Hospital-Based Nursing Care

Nursing care is supportive and directed at maintaining a relaxed, quiet environment away from food odors or offensive smells. Once oral feedings resume, food needs to be attractively served. Oral hygiene is important because the mouth is dry and may be irritated from vomitus. Monitor weight regularly. In some cases emotional factors have appeared to play a role, although that remains controversial. Nevertheless, psychotherapy may sometimes be recommended. With proper treatment, prognosis is favorable.

Evaluation

Expected outcomes of nursing care include the following:

- The woman is able to explain hyperemesis gravidarum, its therapy, and its possible effects on her pregnancy.
- The woman's condition is corrected and complications are avoided.

CARE OF THE WOMAN WITH A HYPERTENSIVE DISORDER

Hypertensive disorders, which affect 5% to 10% of pregnant women, are the most common medical complications in pregnancies (Sibai, 2012). For clinical purposes, the following classification of hypertensive disorders is used (Cunningham et al., 2010):

- Preeclampsia/eclampsia
- Chronic hypertension
- Chronic hypertension with superimposed preeclampsia or eclampsia
- Gestational hypertension

Preeclampsia and Eclampsia

Preeclampsia, the most common hypertensive disorder in pregnancy, is defined as an increase in blood pressure after 20 weeks' gestation accompanied by proteinuria in a previously normotensive woman. Previously, edema was included in the definition but was removed because it is such a common finding in pregnancy. However, sudden onset of severe edema warrants close evaluation to rule out preeclampsia or other pathologic processes such as renal disease.

Preeclampsia, typically categorized as mild or severe, is a progressive disorder. In its most severe form, **eclampsia** (generalized seizures or coma) develops. Most often preeclampsia occurs in the last 10 weeks of gestation, during labor, or in the first 48 hours after childbirth. Although birth of the fetus and removal of the placenta are the only known cure for preeclampsia, it can be controlled with early diagnosis and careful management. Preeclampsia is seen more often in teenagers and in women over age 35, especially if they are primigravidas. Women with a history of preeclampsia are at increased risk, as are women with gestational trophoblastic disease (GTD), Rh incompatibility, diabetes, and a large placental mass associated with multiple gestation.

Pathophysiology of Preeclampsia/Eclampsia

The cause of preeclampsia/eclampsia remains unknown, despite decades of research. Preeclampsia affects all the major systems of the body. The following pathophysiologic changes are associated with the disease:

- In normal pregnancy the lowered peripheral vascular resistance and the increased maternal resistance to the pressor effects of angiotensin II result in lowered blood pressure. In preeclampsia, blood pressure begins to rise after 20 weeks' gestation, probably in response to a gradual loss of resistance to angiotensin II. This response has been linked to the ratio between the prostaglandins prostacyclin and thromboxane. Prostacyclin is a potent vasodilator that decreases blood pressure, prevents platelet aggregation, and promotes uterine blood flow. Thromboxane, produced by platelets, causes vessels to constrict and platelets to clump together. Prostacyclin is decreased in preeclampsia, allowing the potent vasoconstrictor and platelet-aggregating effects of thromboxane to dominate. These hormones are produced partially by the placenta, which helps explain the reversal of the condition when the placenta is removed and why the incidence is increased when there is a larger than normal placental mass.

- The loss of normal vasodilation of uterine arterioles and the concurrent maternal vasospasm result in decreased placental perfusion (see *Pathophysiology Illustrated: Preeclampsia*). The effect on the fetus may be growth restriction, decrease in fetal movement, and chronic hypoxia or fetal distress.

Activity | Case Study: Patient with Preeclampsia

Pathophysiology Illustrated | Preeclampsia

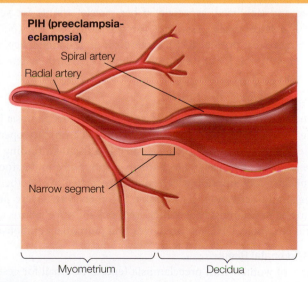

A, In a normal pregnancy, the passive quality of the spiral arteries permits increased blood flow to the placenta.
B, In preeclampsia, vasoconstriction of the myometrial segment of the spiral arteries occurs.

■ In preeclampsia, normal renal perfusion is decreased. With a reduction of the glomerular filtration rate, serum levels of creatinine, BUN, and uric acid begin to rise from normal pregnant levels, while urine output decreases. Sodium is retained in increased amounts, which results in increased extracellular volume, increased sensitivity to angiotensin II, and edema. Stretching of the capillary walls of the glomerular endothelial cells allows the large protein molecules, primarily albumin, to escape in the urine, decreasing serum albumin levels. The decreased serum albumin concentration causes decreased plasma colloid osmotic pressure. This lowered pressure results in a further movement of fluid to the extracellular spaces, which also contributes to the development of edema.

■ The decreased intravascular volume causes increased viscosity of the blood and a corresponding rise in hematocrit.

HELLP syndrome (**h**emolysis, **e**levated **l**iver enzymes, and **l**ow **p**latelet count) is sometimes associated with severe preeclampsia. Women who experience this multiple-organ-failure syndrome have high morbidity and mortality rates, as do their offspring.

The hemolysis that occurs is termed *microangiopathic hemolytic anemia*. It is thought that red blood cells are fragmented during passage through small, damaged blood vessels. Elevated liver enzymes occur from blood flow that is obstructed by fibrin deposits. Hyperbilirubinemia and jaundice may also be seen. Liver distention causes epigastric pain. Thrombocytopenia (platelet count less than 100,000/mm^3) is a frequent finding in preeclampsia. It occurs when platelets aggregate at the sites of vascular damage associated with vasospasm. Symptoms may include nausea, vomiting, flulike symptoms, or epigastric pain. HELLP syndrome is sometimes complicated by disseminated intravascular coagulation (DIC).

Women with HELLP syndrome are best cared for in a tertiary care center. Initially the mother's condition should be assessed and stabilized, especially if her platelet counts are very low. The fetus is also assessed, using a nonstress test (NST) and biophysical profile (BPP). Regardless of gestational age, all women with true HELLP syndrome should give birth as expeditiously as possible.

Maternal Risks

Central nervous system changes associated with preeclampsia include hyperreflexia, headache, and seizures. Thrombocytopenia (platelet count less than 100,000/mm^3) is a frequent finding in preeclampsia. The exact mechanism is not fully understood, but platelet consumption is believed to be related to endothelial damage and activation of thrombin. Women with severe preeclampsia or eclampsia are at increased risk for renal failure, abruptio placentae, DIC, ruptured liver, and pulmonary embolism.

Fetal/Neonatal Risks

Infants of women with preeclampsia tend to be small for gestational age (SGA). The cause is related specifically to maternal vasospasm and hypovolemia, which result in fetal hypoxia and malnutrition. In addition, the newborn may be premature because of the necessity for early birth. At birth, the newborn may be oversedated because of medications given to the mother. The newborn may also have hypermagnesemia resulting from treatment of the woman with large doses of magnesium sulfate.

Clinical Manifestations and Diagnosis

Mild Preeclampsia. Women with mild preeclampsia may exhibit few, if any, symptoms. The blood pressure is elevated to 140/90 mm Hg or higher, 1+ proteinuria may occur, and liver enzymes may be elevated minimally. Although no longer considered a diagnostic sign of preeclampsia, edema may be present.

Severe Preeclampsia. Severe preeclampsia may develop suddenly. Blood pressure is 160/110 mm Hg or higher on two occasions at least 6 hours apart while the woman is on bed rest. Proteinuria of 5 g or higher is found in a 24-hour urine collection, while a dipstick urine protein measurement is 3+ to 4+ on two random samples obtained at least 4 hours apart. Oliguria is present with urine output equal to or less than 500 mL in 24 hours. Additional characteristic symptoms include visual or cerebral disturbances (frontal headaches, blurred vision, scotomata [spots before the eyes]), cyanosis or pulmonary edema, epigastric or right upper quadrant pain, impaired liver function, thrombocytopenia or evidence of hemolysis or both, and intrauterine fetal growth restriction. Other signs or symptoms may include nausea, vomiting, irritability, hyperreflexia, and retinal edema (retinas appear wet and glistening), with narrowed segments on the retinal arterioles when examined with an ophthalmoscope. Epigastric pain is often the sign of impending convulsion and is thought to be caused by increased vascular engorgement of the liver.

Eclampsia. Eclampsia, characterized by a grand mal convulsion, may occur before labor, during labor, or early in the postpartum period. Some women experience only one seizure; others have several.

Clinical Therapy

The goals of medical management are prevention of cerebral hemorrhage, convulsion, hematologic complications, and renal and hepatic diseases, and birth of an uncompromised newborn as close to term as possible.

Antepartum Management. The clinical therapy for preeclampsia/eclampsia depends on the severity of the disease.

Home care of mild preeclampsia. For some women with mild preeclampsia, home care is an option. The woman monitors her blood pressure, weight, and urine protein daily. Weight gains of 1.4 kg (3 lb) in 24 hours or 1.8 kg (4 lb) in a 3-day period are generally a cause for concern. Remote nonstress tests (NSTs) are performed twice per week or biophysical profiles (BPPs) are done weekly. Nursing contact varies from daily to weekly, depending on physician request. It is extremely important to advise the woman to report to the doctor if she develops signs of worsening preeclampsia.

Hospital care of mild preeclampsia. The woman is placed on bed rest, primarily on her left side, to decrease pressure on the vena cava, thereby increasing venous return, circulatory volume, and placental and renal perfusion. She is weighed daily and evaluated for worsening edema, persistent headache, visual changes, or epigastric pain. Urine dipstick is done daily to assess for protein; blood pressure is checked at least 4 times per day. The woman's diet should be well balanced and moderate to high in protein (80 to 100 g/day, or 1.5 g/kg/day) to replace protein lost in the urine. Sodium intake should be moderate, not to exceed 6 g/day. Excessively salty foods should be avoided, but sodium restriction and diuretics are no longer used in treating preeclampsia.

To achieve a safe outcome for the fetus, tests to evaluate fetal status are done more frequently as preeclampsia progresses. The following tests are used:

- Fetal movement record
- Nonstress test
- Ultrasonography every 3 or 4 weeks for serial determination of growth
- Biophysical profile
- Amniocentesis to determine fetal lung maturity
- Doppler velocimetry beginning at 30 to 32 weeks to screen for fetal compromise

Hospital care of severe preeclampsia. In severe cases, birth may be the treatment of choice for both mother and fetus, even if the fetus is immature. Other medical therapies for severe preeclampsia include the following:

- *Bed rest.* Bed rest must be complete. Stimuli that may bring on a seizure should be reduced.
- *Diet.* A high-protein, moderate-sodium diet is given as long as the woman is alert and has no nausea or indication of impending seizure.
- *Anticonvulsants.* Magnesium sulfate is the treatment of choice for eclamptic seizure prevention and treatment because of its depressant action on the central nervous system. (See *Drug Guide: Magnesium Sulfate* on page 448 in Chapter 21 .)
- *Fluid and electrolyte replacement.* The goal of fluid intake is to achieve a balance between correcting hypovolemia and preventing circulatory overload. Fluid intake may be oral or supplemented with IV therapy. IV fluids may be started "to keep lines open" in case they are needed for drug therapy even when oral intake is adequate. Electrolytes are replaced as indicated by daily serum electrolyte levels.
- *Corticosteroids.* Betamethasone or dexamethasone is often administered to the woman whose fetus has an immature lung profile. Corticosteroids may also have a beneficial effect in women with HELLP syndrome.
- *Antihypertensives.* Antihypertensive medications are the most commonly used methods of treatment. Antihypertensive therapy is generally given for sustained systolic blood pressure of at least 160 mm Hg or diastolic blood pressures of 110 mm Hg or higher (Magee, Abalos, von Dadelszen, et al., 2011). Labetalol and hydralazine are first-line medications for the treatment of acute-onset, severe hypertension in pregnancy and are generally administered

by IV boluses. Labetalol should be avoided in women with asthma or heart failure (American College of Obstetricians and Gynecologists [ACOG], 2011a). Oral nifedipine acts rapidly and has favorable hemodynamic effects and fewer side effects than IV hydralazine. Methyldopa is often used for long-term control of mild to moderate hypertension in pregnancy because it is safe and effective.

Hospital care of eclampsia. An eclamptic seizure requires immediate, effective treatment. A bolus of 4 to 6 g magnesium sulfate is given intravenously in 100 mL IV fluid over 15 to 20 minutes followed by 2 g/hr IV infusion (Cunningham et al., 2010). Antihypertensive agents are used to keep the diastolic blood pressure between 90 and 100 mm Hg, thus avoiding a potential reduction in uteroplacental blood flow or cerebral perfusion. A sedative such as diazepam or amobarbital is used only if the seizures are not controlled by magnesium sulfate. The lungs are auscultated for pulmonary edema. The woman is observed for circulatory and renal failure and signs of cerebral hemorrhage. Furosemide (Lasix) may be given for pulmonary edema; digitalis may be given for circulatory failure. An indwelling Foley catheter is often inserted and intake and output are monitored hourly.

The woman is assessed for signs of labor. She is also checked every 15 minutes for evidence of vaginal bleeding and abdominal rigidity, which might indicate abruptio placentae. While she is comatose, she is positioned on her side with the side rails up.

Because of the severity of her condition, the woman is often cared for in an intensive care unit. Invasive hemodynamic monitoring of either central venous pressure or pulmonary artery wedge pressure may be started using a Swan-Ganz catheter. Both of these procedures carry risk to the woman, and the decision to use them should be made judiciously. When the condition of the woman and the fetus have been stabilized, induction of labor is considered, because birth is the only known cure for preeclampsia/eclampsia. The woman and her partner should be given a careful explanation about her status and that of her unborn child and the treatment they are receiving. Plans for further treatment and for birth must be discussed with them.

Intrapartum Management. Labor may be induced by IV oxytocin when there is evidence of fetal maturity and cervical readiness. In very severe cases, cesarean birth may be necessary even if the fetus is immature.

Assessment for signs of worsening preeclampsia continues. The woman may receive IV oxytocin and magnesium sulfate simultaneously. Infusion pumps should be used, and bags and tubing must be carefully labeled.

Narcotics may be given IV for pain relief in labor. An epidural, spinal, or combined spinal-epidural can be safely administered to the woman with preeclampsia in the absence of thrombocytopenia.

Electronic fetal monitoring is used to assess fetal status continuously. Birth in the Sims' or semisitting position should be considered. If the lithotomy position is used, a wedge should be placed under the right buttock to displace the uterus. The wedge should also be used if birth is by cesarean. Oxygen is administered to the woman during labor if the need is indicated by fetal response to the contractions.

A pediatrician or neonatal nurse practitioner must be available to care for the newborn at birth. This caregiver must be informed of all amounts and times of medication the woman has received during labor.

Postpartum Management. The woman with preeclampsia usually improves rapidly after giving birth, although seizures can still occur during the first 48 hours postpartum. When the hypertension is severe, the woman may continue to receive antihypertensives or magnesium sulfate postpartum.

NURSING MANAGEMENT *For the Woman with Preeclampsia/Eclampsia*

See *Nursing Care Plan: The Woman with Preeclampsia* on pages 336–338 for information on nursing care.

Nursing Assessment and Diagnosis

Take and record the blood pressure during each antepartum visit. If the blood pressure rises, or if the normal slight decrease in blood pressure expected between 8 and 28 weeks of pregnancy does not occur, the woman should be followed closely. Also check the woman's urine for proteinuria at each visit.

If hospitalization becomes necessary, assess the following:

- *Blood pressure.* Assess every 1 to 4 hours, or more frequently if indicated by medication or other changes in the woman's status.

- *Temperature.* Take every 4 hours, or every 2 hours if elevated or if premature rupture of the membranes (PROM) has occurred.

- *Pulse and respirations.* Determine pulse rate and respirations along with blood pressure.

- *Fetal heart rate (FHR).* Check the fetal heart rate with the blood pressure, or monitor continuously with the electronic fetal monitor if the situation indicates.

- *Urinary output.* Measure every voiding. The woman frequently has an indwelling catheter. In this case, urine output can be assessed hourly. Output should be 700 mL or greater in 24 hours, or at least 30 mL/hr.

- *Urinary protein.* Evaluate urinary protein hourly if an indwelling catheter is in place or with each voiding. Readings of 3+ or 4+ indicate loss of 5 g or more of protein in 24 hours.

- *Urine specific gravity.* Check specific gravity of the urine hourly or with each voiding. Readings over 1.040 correlate with oliguria and proteinuria.

- *Weight.* Weigh the woman daily at the same time. She should be wearing the same robe or gown and slippers. Weighing may be omitted if the woman is to maintain strict bed rest.

- *Pulmonary edema.* Observe the woman for coughing, shortness of breath, or difficulty breathing. Auscultate the lungs for moist respirations.

- *Deep tendon reflexes.* Assess the woman for evidence of hyperreflexia in the brachial, wrist, patellar, or Achilles' tendons (Table 16–1). The patellar reflex is the easiest

Table 16–1	Deep Tendon Reflex Rating Scale
Rating	**Assessment**
4+	Hyperactive; very brisk, jerky, or clonic response; abnormal
3+	Brisker than average; may not be abnormal
2+	Average response; normal
1+	Diminished response; low normal
0	No response; abnormal

to assess (Figure 16–3 ●). Clonus, an abnormal finding, is assessed by vigorously dorsiflexing the foot while the knee is held in a fixed position. Normally, no clonus is present. Clonus is present if the foot "jerks" or taps the examiner's hand, at which time the examiner counts the number of taps or beats and records it as such. See Skill 2–3 in the *Clinical Skills Manual* SKILLS .

- *Placental separation.* Assess hourly for vaginal bleeding and uterine rigidity.

- *Headache.* Ask about the existence and location of any headache.

- *Visual disturbance.* Ask about any visual blurring or changes or scotomata. The results of the daily funduscopic examination should be recorded on the chart.

- *Epigastric pain.* Ask about any epigastric pain. It is important to differentiate it from simple heartburn, which tends to be familiar and less intense.

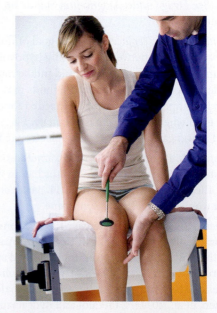

● **Figure 16–3** Correct position for eliciting patellar reflex: sitting.
Source: © BSIP SA/Alamy.

- *Laboratory blood tests.* Daily tests of hematocrit to measure hemoconcentration; blood urea nitrogen (BUN), creatinine, and uric acid levels to assess kidney function; clotting studies for signs of thrombocytopenia or DIC; liver enzymes; and electrolyte levels are all indicated. Magnesium levels are monitored regularly in women receiving magnesium sulfate.
- *Level of consciousness.* Observe the woman for alertness, mood changes, and any signs of impending convulsion.
- *Emotional response and level of understanding.* Carefully assess the woman's emotional response so that support and teaching can be planned accordingly.

In addition, assess the effects of any medications administered. Become familiar with the more commonly used medications and their purpose, implications, and associated untoward or toxic effects.

Examples of nursing diagnoses that might apply include the following (NANDA-I © 2012):

- *Fluid Volume, Deficient,* related to fluid shift from intravascular to extravascular space secondary to vasospasm
- *Injury, Risk of,* related to the possibility of seizure secondary to cerebral vasospasm or edema

Planning and Implementation
Community-Based Nursing Care

A woman with preeclampsia may fear losing her fetus, worry about her personal relationship with her other children and her personal and sexual relationship with her partner because of the limitations placed on her activities, be concerned about finances, and feel bored and a little resentful if she faces prolonged bed rest. If she has small children, she may have trouble providing for their care. Help couples identify and discuss these concerns. Offer information and explanations if certain aspects of therapy cause difficulty. Refer the woman and her family to community resources such as support groups or homemaker services as appropriate.

Health Promotion Preeclampsia

- The woman needs to know which symptoms are significant and should be reported at once.
- She is usually seen once or twice weekly. Explain that she may need to come in earlier than her next appointment if symptoms indicate that her condition is progressing.

Hospital-Based Nursing Care

The development of severe preeclampsia/eclampsia is a cause for increased concern about the prognosis for the woman and her fetus. Explain medical therapy and its purpose and offer honest, hopeful information. Keep the couple informed of fetal status and discuss other concerns the couple may express. Provide as much information as possible and seek other sources of information or aid for the family as needed. Offer to contact a member of the clergy or hospital chaplain for additional support if the couple so chooses.

Maintain a quiet, low-stimulus environment for the woman. She should be in a private room in a quiet location where she can be watched closely. Limit visitors to close family members or main support persons. The woman should maintain the left lateral recumbent position most of the time, with side rails up for her protection.

Eliminate phone calls except for those that are planned because the phone ringing unexpectedly may be too jarring. To avoid a sense of isolation, however, some women find it preferable to take calls, but limit them to a certain time of day. Bright lights and sudden loud noises may precipitate seizures in the woman with severe preeclampsia.

Monitor the effectiveness of medications administered. Be alert for signs of untoward effects or developing toxic levels.

The occurrence of a convulsion is frightening to any family members who may be present, although the woman will not be able to recall it when she becomes conscious. Therefore, it is essential to offer explanations to the family members and the woman herself later.

SAFETY ALERT!

When caring for a woman with preeclampsia who is receiving IV magnesium sulfate, it is imperative to follow protocols for monitoring blood levels of magnesium. You are probably already aware of the common signs of increasing magnesium levels, such as diminished reflexes and decreased respiratory rate. However, you can also watch for some subtle clues that may suggest either the therapeutic or toxic range. When a woman's magnesium level is in the therapeutic range, she usually has some slurring of speech, awkwardness of movement, and decreased appetite. If the woman begins to have difficulty swallowing and begins to drool, she may be approaching the toxic range.

A grand mal seizure has both a tonic phase, marked by pronounced muscular contraction and rigidity, and a clonic phase, marked by alternate contraction and relaxation of the muscles, which causes the woman to thrash about wildly. When the tonic phase of the contraction begins, turn the woman to her side (if she is not already in that position) to aid circulation to the placenta. Turn her head face down to allow saliva to drain from her mouth. Attempting to insert a padded tongue blade is no longer advocated in many facilities; in others, it is used if it can be inserted without force because it may prevent injury to the woman's mouth. The side rails should be padded or a pillow put between the woman and each side rail.

After 15 to 20 seconds, the clonic phase starts. When the thrashing subsides, intensive monitoring and therapy begin. An oral airway is inserted, the woman's nasopharynx is suctioned, and oxygen is administered by nasal catheter. Fetal heart tones are monitored continuously. Monitor maternal vital signs every 5 minutes until they are stable, then every 15 minutes.

Nursing Management During Labor and Birth

Keep the woman positioned on her left side as much as possible. Carefully monitor both the woman and the fetus throughout labor. Note the progress of labor and remain alert for signs of worsening preeclampsia or its complications.

Nursing Care Plan   The Woman with Preeclampsia

Intervention	Rationale	Expected Outcome

1. Nursing Diagnosis: *Fluid Volume, Deficient,* related to fluid shift from intravascular to extravascular space secondary to vasospasm (NANDA-I © 2012)

NIC Priority Intervention:
Fluid management: Promotion of fluid balance and prevention of complications related to fluid shifts

NOC Suggested Outcome:
Fluid balance: Balance of fluid in the intracellular and extracellular compartments of the body

Goal: The patient will be restored to normal fluid volume levels.

Intervention	Rationale	Expected Outcome
■ Encourage woman to lie in the left lateral recumbent position.	■ The left lateral recumbent position decreases pressure on the vena cava, thereby increasing venous return, circulatory volume, and placental and renal perfusion. Angiotensin II levels are decreased when there is improved renal blood flow, which helps to promote diuresis and lower blood pressure.	■ The signs and symptoms of preeclampsia will diminish as evidenced by decreased blood pressure, urine protein levels of zero, and a return of the deep tendon reflexes to normal.
■ Assess blood pressure every 1 to 4 hours as necessary.	■ Frequent monitoring will assess for progression of the disorder and allow for early intervention to ensure maternal and fetal health and well-being.	
■ Monitor urine for volume and proteinuria every shift or every hour per agency protocol.	■ Monitoring provides information to assess renal perfusion. Proteinuria is the last cardinal sign of preeclampsia to appear. As the disorder worsens, the capillary walls of the glomerular endothelial cells stretch, allowing protein molecules to pass into the urine. Normal urine does not contain protein. Readings of 3+ and 4+ indicate loss of 5 g or more protein in 24 hours. Urinary output decreases when there is a reduction of the glomerular filtration rate. Urinary output that falls below 30 mL/hr or less than 700 mL in a 24-hour period should be reported.	
■ Assess deep tendon reflexes and clonus.	■ Hyperreflexia may occur as preeclampsia worsens. Eliciting deep tendon reflexes provides information about CNS status and is also used to assess for magnesium sulfate toxicity. Reflexes are graded on a scale of 0 to 4+ using the deep tendon reflex rating scale. A rating of 4+ is abnormal and indicates hyperreflexia. A rating of 0 or no response is also abnormal and is seen with high maternal serum magnesium levels. The presence of clonus is an abnormal finding that indicates a more pronounced hyperreflexia and is indicative of CNS irritability.	
■ Assess for edema.	■ Edema develops as fluid shifts from the intravascular to the extravascular spaces. Edema is assessed either by weight gain (more than 3.3 lb/month in the second trimester or more than 1.1 lb/week in the third trimester) or by assessing for pitting edema (assessed by using finger pressure to a swollen area, usually the lower extremities, and grading on a scale of 1+ to 4+).	

Nursing Care Plan   The Woman with Preeclampsia—continued

Intervention	Rationale	Expected Outcome
■ Administer magnesium sulfate per infusion pump as ordered.	■ As preeclampsia worsens, the risk of an eclamptic seizure increases. Magnesium sulfate is the treatment of choice for seizures because of its CNS depressant action. As a secondary effect, magnesium sulfate relaxes smooth muscles and may therefore decrease the blood pressure.	
■ Assess for magnesium sulfate toxicity.	■ Side effects of magnesium sulfate are dose related. Therapeutic levels are in the range of 4.8–9.6 mg/dL. As maternal serum magnesium levels increase, toxicity may occur. Signs of toxicity include decreased or absent deep tendon reflexes (DTRs), urine output below 30 mL/hr, respirations below 12, and confusion.	
■ Provide a balanced diet that includes 80–100 g/day or 1.5 g/kg/day of protein.	■ A diet rich in protein is necessary to replace protein that is excreted in the urine.	

2. Nursing Diagnosis: *Injury, Risk for* (fetal), related to uteroplacental insufficiency secondary to vasospasm (NANDA-I © 2012)

NIC Priority Intervention:
High-risk pregnancy care: Identification and management of preeclampsia to promote healthy outcomes for mother and baby

NOC Suggested Outcome:
Risk control: Actions to manage signs and symptoms of preeclampsia and thereby reduce fetal risk

Goal: The fetus will avoid complications related to uteroplacental insufficiency.

Intervention	Rationale	Expected Outcome
■ Instruct woman to count fetal movements 3 times a day for 20 to 30 minutes.	■ Fetal activity provides reassurance of fetal well-being. Decrease in fetal movement or cessation of movement may indicate fetal compromise.	■ Fetus will have an adequate supply of oxygen and nutrients as evidenced by absence of signs of fetal distress and fetal diagnostic test results within normal limits.
■ Encourage woman to rest in the left lateral recumbent position.	■ Lying in the left lateral recumbent position decreases pressure on the vena cava, which increases venous return, circulatory volume, and placental and renal perfusion. Blood flow to the fetus is increased, thereby reducing the risk of fetal hypoxia and malnutrition.	
■ **Collaborative:** Assist with serial ultrasounds.	■ Maternal vasospasm and hypovolemia result from preeclampsia, which may lead to SGA newborns. Ultrasound provides assessment of fetal growth by measuring the biparietal diameter of the fetal head or the fetal femur length.	
■ Perform nonstress test as ordered.	■ A nonstress test (NST) is performed to assess the fetal heart rate in response to fetal movement. Accelerations of fetal heart rate with fetal movement may indicate the fetus has adequate oxygenation and an intact central nervous system. (Refer to Chapter 14 🔴 for interpretation of NST results.)	

(continued)

Nursing Care Plan The Woman with Preeclampsia—continued

Intervention	Rationale	Expected Outcome
■ Describe for the woman the purposes of a biophysical profile (BPP).	■ Preeclampsia or eclampsia places the woman at risk for uteroplacental insufficiency resulting from the loss of normal vasodilation of uterine arterioles and maternal vasospasm. This results in decreased uteroplacental perfusion, which may lead to fetal hypoxia. A BPP is one assessment tool used to evaluate fetal well-being. Providing explanation of the diagnostic test helps relieve anxiety and ensures the woman understands what the test evaluates and what the results mean. (See discussion of BPP in Chapter 14 🔗.)	
■ Assist with amniocentesis to obtain lecithin/ sphingomyelin (L/S) ratio.	■ Women with preeclampsia may give birth before term. Amniotic fluid may be analyzed to determine the maturity of the fetal lungs. An L/S ratio of 2:1 or greater indicates fetal lung maturity and is usually achieved by 35 weeks' gestation.	
■ Explain the purpose of Doppler flow studies.	■ Doppler flow studies (umbilical velocimetry) help to assess placental function and sufficiency. Uteroplacental insufficiency is a risk for a woman with preeclampsia. (See Chapter 14 🔗.)	

3. Nursing Diagnosis: *Health Maintenance, Ineffective,* related to deficient knowledge about new diagnosis (preeclampsia) (NANDA-I © 2012)

NIC Priority Intervention:		NOC Suggested Outcome:
Disease process teaching: Assisting the woman to understand information related to the diagnosis of preeclampsia		*Knowledge: Treatment regimen:* Extent of understanding conveyed about treatment regimen for preeclampsia

Goal: The woman will describe the condition and treatment regimen.

■ Assess the woman and family's understanding of preeclampsia and its implications for pregnancy.	■ This assessment provides information about the woman's cognitive level and her understanding of her diagnosis. Behavior changes occur when teaching strategies are appropriate for the woman and family's cognitive level.	■ Woman will demonstrate understanding of preeclampsia and its implications as evidenced by verbalization of basic condition, signs and symptoms of progression, importance of sufficient rest in side-lying position, and need to follow prescribed diet.
■ Provide information about the disease process, impact on maternal well-being, risks of progression, implications for the fetus, and dangers of eclampsia.	■ Basic understanding of the condition and its implications is necessary for the woman to understand the treatment plan. A woman who shows signs of early preeclampsia often feels well and may have difficulty accepting the need to rest.	
■ Emphasize the importance of self-monitoring for signs that her condition is worsening and the importance of regular prenatal care for the purpose of maternal and fetal surveillance.	■ The woman should be able to identify signs of disease progression, including evidence of increasing edema, decreased urine output, signs of cerebral disturbance (frontal headache, blurred vision, scotomata), epigastric or right upper quadrant pain, nausea or vomiting, and increased irritability.	

During the second stage of labor, encourage the woman to push in the side-lying position if possible. If she is unable to do so comfortably or effectively, she can be helped to a semisitting position for pushing and can then resume the lateral position between contractions. Birth is in the side-lying position or in the lithotomy position with a wedge placed under the woman's right hip. Encourage a family member or other support person to stay with the woman as much as possible. Keep the woman and her support person informed of the progress and plan of care. Whenever possible, respect their wishes concerning the birth experience.

Nursing Management During the Postpartum Period

Because the woman with preeclampsia is hypovolemic, even normal blood loss can be serious. Assess the amount of vaginal bleeding and observe the woman for signs of shock. Monitor blood pressure and pulse every 4 hours for 48 hours. Check hematocrit daily. Assess the woman for any further signs of preeclampsia. Measure intake and output. Normal postpartum diuresis helps eliminate edema and is a favorable sign.

Postpartum depression can develop after such a difficult pregnancy. To help prevent it, provide opportunities for frequent maternal–infant contact and encourage family members to visit. The couple may have many questions, so be available for discussion. Give the couple family-planning information. Combined oral contraceptives may be used if the woman's blood pressure has returned to normal by the time they are prescribed (usually 4 to 6 weeks after birth).

Evaluation

Expected outcomes of nursing care include the following:

- The woman is able to explain preeclampsia/eclampsia, its implications for her pregnancy, the treatment regimen, and possible complications.

- The woman suffers no eclamptic seizures.

- The woman and her caregivers detect early evidence of increasing severity of the preeclampsia or possible complications so that treatment measures can be instituted.

- The woman gives birth to a healthy newborn.

Chronic Hypertension

Chronic hypertension exists when the blood pressure is 140/90 mm Hg or higher before pregnancy or before the 20th week of gestation, or when hypertension persists longer than 12 weeks following childbirth, which is also considered diagnostic (ACOG, 2012a). The cause of chronic hypertension has not been determined. In most women the disease is mild.

The woman is seen regularly for prenatal care (every 2 to 3 weeks during the first two trimesters and then weekly until birth). She is taught the importance of daily rest periods in the left lateral recumbent position and also learns to monitor her blood pressure at home. Sodium is limited to about 2.4 g/day.

Antihypertensive medication is generally used only for women with blood pressure over 150–160/100–110. Labetalol, nifedipine, and methyldopa are the antihypertensives most commonly used in pregnancy when medication is required (ACOG, 2012a).

SAFETY ALERT!

Before administering labetalol, be certain to check the patient's health history. Labetalol is contraindicated for people with bronchial asthma.

Twenty-four-hour urines, serum creatinine, uric acid, hematocrit, and ultrasound examinations are repeated at least once in the second and third trimesters.

Nursing care is directed at providing information so that the woman can meet her healthcare needs. Provide information about her diet, the need for regular rest, her medications, the need for blood pressure control, and any procedures used to monitor the well-being of her fetus.

Chronic Hypertension with Superimposed Preeclampsia

Preeclampsia may develop in women with chronic hypertension. After 20 weeks' gestation the onset of proteinuria and worsening hypertension are suggestive of superimposed preeclampsia. A rise in the serum uric acid level is helpful in identifying preeclampsia, which frequently occurs late in the second trimester or early in the third.

Gestational Hypertension

Gestational hypertension is characterized by hypertension occurring for the first time after midpregnancy without proteinuria. If preeclampsia does not develop and if the blood pressure returns to normal within 12 weeks following childbirth, the diagnosis of gestational hypertension may be assigned. If the blood pressure elevation persists after 12 weeks' postpartum, the woman is diagnosed with chronic hypertension.

Disseminated Intravascular Coagulation

Disseminated intravascular coagulation (DIC) occurs more often in pregnancies complicated by preeclampsia, abruptio placentae, intrauterine fetal demise, amniotic fluid embolism, maternal liver disease, and septic abortion. Although DIC is not considered a component of severe preeclampsia, eclampsia, or HELLP syndrome, it can occur as a complication when any of these conditions exist.

Clinical Reasoning Pregnancy Complication

Jillian Rundus is a 31-year-old G1P0 who is 35 weeks pregnant. She presents for a routine office visit with complaints of nausea and abdominal pain rating 7/10. She has had a headache and general malaise for 2 days. She denies visual changes. Upon examination, you find her to be alert and oriented and her physical exam is unremarkable with the exception of abdominal tenderness and a blood pressure of 170/110. She has had no previous history of hypertension. Fetal heart rate ranges from 140 to 150 beats per minute.

What should the nurse do at this time?

See www.nursing.pearsonhighered.com for possible responses.

DIC occurs when the normal clotting process is overactivated. In most instances, tissue factor entering the circulation is the primary trigger for DIC. When this occurs, there is an imbalance between the coagulation and the fibrinolytic systems. This mechanism leads to hemorrhage and shock. During these events, clots are being formed and fibrin is being deposited into the microcirculation, resulting in cell or tissue damage. This triggers further coagulation, which eventually depletes the plasma clotting factors. These fibrin clots can lead to intravascular obstruction and infarctions. In addition the fibrinolytic system is activated, which results in the formation of fibrin-fibrinogen degradation products or fibrin split products. The release of these products decreases platelet functioning and further inhibits coagulation (Blackburn, 2013).

DIC is diagnosed when thrombocytopenia, low fibrinogen levels, and elevated fibrin split products are found in the laboratory findings. Serial platelet and serum fibrin degradation product counts are performed to monitor the mother's hematologic status. Supportive measures and reversing the causative factors are the primary interventions used to manage DIC.

CARE OF THE WOMAN REQUIRING SURGERY DURING PREGNANCY

Although elective surgery should be delayed until the postpartum, essential surgery can generally be done during pregnancy. Surgery poses some risks, however. The early second trimester is the best time to operate because there is less risk of spontaneous abortion or early labor, and the uterus is not so large as to impinge on the abdominal field.

General preoperative and postoperative care is similar for pregnant and nonpregnant women; however, special considerations must be kept in mind whenever the surgical patient is pregnant. If a chest x-ray is done, the fetus should be shielded from radiation.

To prevent uterine compression of major blood vessels while the woman is supine, the caregiver must place a wedge under the woman's right hip to tilt the uterus during both surgery and recovery. The decreased intestinal motility and delayed gastric emptying that occur in pregnancy increase the risk of vomiting when anesthetics are given and during the postoperative period. Thus, a nasogastric tube may be recommended before major surgery. An indwelling urinary catheter prevents bladder distention, decreases risk of injury to the bladder, and permits monitoring of output. Fetal heart rate (FHR) must be monitored electronically before, during, and after surgery.

Pregnancy causes increased secretions of the respiratory tract and engorgement of the nasal mucous membrane, often making breathing through the nose difficult. Consequently, pregnant women often need an endotracheal tube to maintain an airway during surgery. Caregivers must guard against maternal hypoxia during surgery because uterine circulation will be decreased and fetal oxygenation can decline quickly. Blood loss is also monitored throughout the procedure and following it.

Postoperatively, encourage the woman to turn, breathe deeply, and cough regularly and to use any ventilation therapy, such as incentive spirometry, to avoid developing pneumonia. Sequential compression devices (SCDs) or support stockings during and after surgery help prevent venous stasis and the development of thrombophlebitis. Encourage leg exercises while the woman is confined to bed, and introduce ambulation as soon as possible.

Discharge teaching is very important. The woman and her family should understand what to expect regarding activity level, discomfort, diet, medications, and any special considerations. In addition, they should know the warning signs they need to report to the physician immediately.

CARE OF THE WOMAN SUFFERING MAJOR TRAUMA

Trauma complicates from 6% to 8% of pregnancies; trauma from motor vehicle accidents is the leading cause of fetal and maternal death (Mozurkewich & Pearlman, 2012). Falls and violence—including domestic violence—are the next most common causes of injury.

Late in pregnancy, when balance and coordination are affected, the woman may fall. Her protruding abdomen is vulnerable to a variety of minor injuries. The fetus is usually well protected by the amniotic fluid, which distributes the force of a blow equally in all directions, and by the muscle layers of the uterus and abdominal wall. In early pregnancy, while the uterus is still in the pelvis, it is shielded from blows by the surrounding pelvic organs, muscles, and bones.

Trauma that causes concern includes blunt trauma, penetrating abdominal injuries, and the complications of maternal shock, premature labor, and spontaneous abortion. Maternal mortality most often occurs from head trauma or hemorrhage. Uterine rupture is a rare but life-threatening complication of trauma. It may result from strong deceleration forces in an automobile accident, with or without seat belts. Traumatic separation of the placenta can occur, which causes a high rate of fetal mortality. Premature labor, often following rupture of membranes during an accident, is another serious hazard to the fetus. Premature labor can begin even if the woman is not injured. To help prevent trauma from automobile accidents, all pregnant women should wear both lap seat belts and shoulder harnesses.

Penetrating trauma most often results from gunshot wounds and stab wounds. The mother generally fares better than the fetus if the penetrating trauma involves the abdomen, as the enlarged uterus is likely to protect the mother's bowel from injury. Unfortunately, the fetal injury rate is high.

Treatment of major injuries during pregnancy focuses initially on lifesaving measures for the woman. Such measures include establishing an airway, controlling external bleeding, and administering IV fluid to alleviate shock. The woman must be kept on her left side to prevent further hypotension. Oxygen is administered. Fetal heart rate (FHR) and fetal movement are monitored. Exploratory surgery may be necessary following abdominal trauma to determine the extent of injuries. If the fetus is near term and the uterus has been damaged, cesarean birth is indicated. If the fetus is still immature, the uterus can often be repaired, and the pregnancy can continue until term.

In cases of trauma in which the mother's life is not directly threatened, fetal monitoring for a minimum of 4 hours is

Evidence-Based Practice   Safe Radiologic Procedures for the Evaluation of Trauma During Pregnancy

Clinical Question

What radiologic procedures are safe to use for the evaluation of trauma during pregnancy?

The Evidence

Accurately diagnosing the extent and effects of trauma often requires radiologic examination. Exposure to radiologic materials during pregnancy requires a careful balancing of risks and benefits, and may cause significant concern for the mother. A systematic review of the evidence regarding radiologic examination during pregnancy was conducted, and 17 studies and practice guidelines were evaluated, including the recommendations from the American College of Obstetricians and Gynecologists. A review that includes both studies and guidelines forms the strongest level of evidence for practice. The review concluded that most contemporary diagnostic imaging procedures are associated with little significant fetal risk. Radiation exposure of less than 5 rads has not been shown to exert any fetal effects (Puri et al., 2011). Radiography of the chest, head, neck, teeth, or extremity exposes the developing embryo to insignificant amounts of radiation except when radionuclides are used. However, the use of contrast materials should

be avoided during pregnancy (Brent, 2011). Ultrasound and magnetic resonance imaging (MRI) should be considered first, because they have not been shown to exert any ill effects. If multiple radiologic studies are anticipated, a dosimetrist (an expert in calculating radiologic exposure) should be consulted. Placing a radiation badge on the patient to monitor total sequential radiation and using lead apron shielding whenever possible should be a part of routine care. The radiation badge can also reassure the mother that her exposure to harmful radiation remains acceptably low.

Best Practice

The mother can be reassured that radiologic examination during pregnancy, particularly ultrasound and MRI, carries low levels of risk for the fetus. Applying a radiation badge can both monitor exposure and reassure the mother that risks to the fetus are minimized.

Clinical Reasoning

What are traumatic conditions for which radiologic examination may be indicated? How can the nurse reassure the mother that risks and benefits have been balanced?

---

suggested if there are no contractions, vaginal bleeding, uterine tenderness, or leaking amniotic fluid. Abruptio placentae may occur following a blow to the abdomen. Increased uterine irritability in the first few hours after trauma helps identify women who may be at risk for this potentially catastrophic complication.

When cardiopulmonary resuscitation (CPR) is performed on the pregnant woman late in gestation, perimortem cesarean birth is advocated if CPR is unsuccessful in the first 5 minutes. Chest compressions are less effective in the third trimester because of compression of the inferior vena cava by the gravid uterus. Cesarean birth alleviates this compression and improves resuscitation efforts in both the fetus and the mother.

CARE OF THE PREGNANT WOMAN WHO HAS EXPERIENCED DOMESTIC VIOLENCE

Domestic violence, also called *intimate partner violence,* most often the intentional injury of a woman by her partner, frequently begins or increases during pregnancy. Estimates suggest that approximately 25% of women in the United States have experienced physical and/or sexual violence by a current or former intimate partner (Devi, 2012). Physical abuse may result in loss of pregnancy, preterm labor, low-birth-weight infants, and fetal death. Abused women have significantly higher rates of complications such as anemia, infection, low weight gain, pelvic fracture, and placental abruption. Violence may escalate during pregnancy, and homicide by an intimate partner is a significant cause of maternal mortality (ACOG, 2012b).

The first step toward helping the battered woman is to identify her. Asking every woman about abuse at various times

during pregnancy is crucial because a woman may not disclose abuse until she knows her caregivers better. Screening for abuse should be done at the first prenatal visit, at least once each trimester, and then again during the postpartum period (ACOG, 2012b).

Chronic psychosomatic symptoms can be an indicator of abuse. The woman may have nonspecific or vague complaints. It is important to assess old scars around the head, chest, arms, abdomen, and genitalia. Any bruising or evidence of pain is also evaluated. Be especially alert for signs of bruising or injury to the woman's breasts, abdomen, or genitalia because these areas are common targets of violence during pregnancy. Other indicators include a decrease in eye contact; silence when the partner is in the room; and a history of nervousness, insomnia, drug overdose, or alcohol problems. Frequent visits to the emergency department and a history of accidents without understandable causes are possible indicators of abuse.

The goals of treatment are to identify the woman at risk, to increase her decision-making abilities to decrease the risk for further abuse, and to provide a safe environment for the woman and her unborn child. She needs to be aware of community resources available to her, such as emergency shelters; police, legal, and social services; and counseling. Ultimately it is the woman's decision to either seek assistance or return to old patterns.

Because abuse often begins during pregnancy, it may be a new, unexpected experience for the woman, one she believes is an isolated incident. She needs to know that battering may continue after childbirth and may extend to the child as well. This is an important time to provide information and establish a trusted link for the woman with a healthcare professional. (For further discussion see Chapter 5 .)

CARE OF THE WOMAN WITH A PERINATAL INFECTION AFFECTING THE FETUS

Fetal infection may develop at any time during pregnancy. In general, perinatal infections are most likely to cause harm when the embryo is exposed during the first trimester when organ development is occurring. Infections that occur later in pregnancy create other concerns such as growth restriction, preterm birth, and neurologic changes. (The acronym TORCH—to identify **to**xoplasmosis, **r**ubella, **c**ytomegalovirus, and **h**erpes—is occasionally used to identify the most common of these infections.) This section addresses several of the most commonly occurring viral and parasitic infections that may have an impact on the fetus if acquired during pregnancy.

Toxoplasmosis

Toxoplasmosis is caused by the protozoan *Toxoplasma gondii*. It is barely noticeable in adults, but, when contracted in pregnancy, it can profoundly affect the fetus. The pregnant woman may contract the organism by eating raw or undercooked meat, by drinking unpasteurized goat's milk, or by contact with the feces of infected cats, either through the cat litter box or by gardening in areas frequented by cats.

Fetal/Neonatal Risks

The likelihood of fetal infection increases with each trimester of pregnancy, but the risk of serious impact on the fetus decreases. Thus, maternal infection contracted during the first trimester is associated with the lowest incidence of fetal infection but the highest risk of severe fetal disease or death. The highest rate of fetal infection (72%) occurs when the mother contracts the infection in the third trimester, but most of these infants are born without clinical signs of infection (Duff, 2012). However, up to half of these infants will develop signs and symptoms if left untreated (Johnson, 2009). In mild cases, retinochoroiditis (inflammation of the retina and choroid of the eye) may be the only recognizable damage, and it and other manifestations may not appear until adolescence or young adulthood. Severe neonatal disorders associated with congenital infection include convulsions, coma, microcephaly, and hydrocephalus. The infant with a severe infection may die soon after birth. Survivors are often blind, deaf, and have severe intellectual disabilities. Treatment of the mother who develops acute toxoplasmosis during pregnancy can reduce the incidence of fetal infection and decrease the late sequelae of the infection (Duff, 2012).

Clinical Therapy

Diagnosis can be made by serologic testing of antibody titers, specifically the IgG and IgM fluorescent antibody (IFA) tests. A positive IgG and negative IgM in the third trimester or any positive IgM result should be followed by confirmatory testing. The toxoplasmosis polymerase chain reaction (PCR) test of amniotic fluid is useful in diagnosing congenital toxoplasmosis. Ultrasound may be useful in detecting signs of fetal infection such as ascites, microcephaly, intracranial calcifications, and fetal growth restriction.

Pregnant women in whom maternal infection is established should receive spiramycin in the first and early second trimester and pyrimethamine/sulfadiazine and folinic acid (leucovorin) in the late second and third trimesters (Centers for Disease Control and Prevention [CDC], 2010a). Spiramycin is not commercially available in the United States, but it can be obtained for treatment through the CDC. Newborns with congenital infection are treated with pyrimethamine, sulfadiazine, and leucovorin (Duff, 2012).

NURSING MANAGEMENT *For the Pregnant Woman with Toxoplasmosis*

Nursing Assessment and Diagnosis

The incubation period for the disease is 10 days. The woman with acute toxoplasmosis may be asymptomatic, or she may develop myalgia, malaise, rash, splenomegaly, and enlarged posterior cervical lymph nodes. Symptoms usually disappear in a few days or weeks.

Nursing diagnoses that might apply include the following (NANDA-I © 2012):

- *Knowledge, Readiness for Enhanced,* related to a desire to understand the ways in which a pregnant woman can contract toxoplasmosis
- *Grieving* related to potential effects on infant of maternal toxoplasmosis

Planning and Implementation

During the antepartum period, discuss methods of preventing toxoplasmosis. The woman must understand the importance of avoiding poorly cooked or raw meat, especially pork, beef, lamb, and, in the Arctic region, caribou. Fruits and vegetables should be washed. She should avoid contact with the cat litter box and have someone else clean it frequently, since it takes approximately 48 hours for a cat's feces to become infectious. Stress the importance of wearing gloves when gardening and of avoiding garden areas frequented by cats.

Evaluation

Expected outcomes of nursing care include the following:

- The woman is able to discuss toxoplasmosis, its methods of transmission, the implications for her fetus, and measures she can take to avoid contracting it.
- The woman implements health measures to avoid contracting toxoplasmosis.
- The woman gives birth to a healthy newborn.

Rubella

The effects of rubella (German measles) on the fetus and newborn are great, because rubella causes a chronic infection that begins in the first trimester of pregnancy and that may persist for months after birth. Fortunately, the success of the rubella vaccination program in the United States has led to a dramatic decrease in the incidence of rubella.

Fetal/Neonatal Risks

The period of greatest risk for the effects of rubella on the fetus is the first trimester. The most common clinical signs of congenital infection include congenital cataracts, sensorineural deafness, and congenital heart defects, particularly patent ductus arteriosus. Other abnormalities, such as mental retardation or cerebral palsy, may become evident in infancy. Diagnosis in the newborn can be made in the presence of these conditions and with an elevated rubella IgM antibody titer at birth. Infants born with congenital rubella syndrome are infectious and should be isolated.

Clinical Therapy

The best therapy for rubella is prevention. Live attenuated vaccine is available and should be given to all children. Women of childbearing age should be tested for immunity and vaccinated if susceptible once it is established that they are not pregnant.

As part of the prenatal laboratory screen, the woman is evaluated for rubella using hemagglutination inhibition (HAI), a serology test. The presence of a 1:8 titer or greater is evidence of immunity. A titer less than 1:8 indicates susceptibility to rubella. Because the vaccine is made with attenuated virus, pregnant women are not vaccinated. However, it is considered safe for newly vaccinated children to have contact with pregnant women. Women whose titers indicate that they are susceptible to rubella should be given the rubella vaccine postpartally.

If a woman becomes infected during the first trimester, therapeutic abortion is a legally available alternative.

NURSING MANAGEMENT *For the Woman Who Develops Rubella During Pregnancy*

Nursing Assessment and Diagnosis

The woman may be asymptomatic or may show signs of a mild infection including a maculopapular rash, lymphadenopathy, muscular achiness, and joint pain. The presence of IgM antirubella antibody is diagnostic of a recent infection. These titers remain elevated for approximately 1 month after infection.

Nursing diagnoses that may apply to the woman who develops rubella early in her pregnancy include the following (NANDA-I © 2012):

- *Coping, Ineffective,* resulting from an inability to accept the possibility of fetal anomalies secondary to maternal rubella exposure
- *Health Maintenance, Ineffective,* related to lack of knowledge about the importance of rubella immunization before becoming pregnant

Planning and Implementation

Support is vital for the couple considering abortion because of a diagnosis of rubella. Such a decision may trigger a crisis for the couple. The parents need objective data to understand the possible effects on their unborn fetus and the long-term prognosis.

Evaluation

Expected outcomes of nursing care include the following:

- The woman is able to describe the implications of rubella exposure during the first trimester of pregnancy.
- If exposure occurs in a woman who is not immune, she is able to identify her options and make a decision about continuing her pregnancy that is acceptable to her and her partner.

- The nonimmune woman receives the rubella vaccine during the early postpartum period.
- The woman gives birth to a healthy infant.

Cytomegalovirus

Cytomegalovirus (CMV) belongs to the herpes virus group and causes both congenital and acquired infections that are referred to as cytomegalic inclusion disease (CID). This virus can be transmitted by asymptomatic women across the placenta to the fetus or by the cervical route during birth.

The virus can be found in virtually all body fluids. It can be passed between humans by any close contact, such as kissing, breastfeeding, and sexual intercourse Asymptomatic CMV infection is particularly common in children and pregnant women. It is a chronic, persistent infection in that the individual may shed the virus continually over many years. The cervix can harbor the virus, and an ascending infection can develop after birth. Although the virus is usually innocuous in adults and children, it may be fatal to the fetus.

Accurate diagnosis in the pregnant woman is best documented by seroconversion. Identification of the virus in amniotic fluid by PCR or culture is the most specific way of diagnosing congenital infection (Bernstein, 2012). Ultrasound findings may include fetal hydrops, growth restriction, hydramnios, cardiomegaly, and fetal ascites.

CMV is the most frequent cause of viral infection in the human fetus. Subclinical infections in the newborn can produce intellectual disability and hearing loss, sometimes not recognized for several months, or learning disabilities not seen until childhood. In children, congenital CMV is the leading cause of hearing loss (Bernstein, 2012).

For the fetus/newborn, serious long-term complications most often follow a primary maternal infection in the first half of pregnancy (Bernstein, 2012). For the fetus, this infection can result in extensive intrauterine tissue damage that leads to fetal death; to survival with microcephaly, hydrocephaly, cerebral palsy, or mental retardation; or to survival with no damage at all. The infected newborn is often small for gestational age (SGA).

At present, no treatment exists for maternal CMV or for the congenital disease in the newborn although a vaccine against CMV is under development and has shown promise (Bernstein, 2012). Thus, prevention is important. The pregnant woman should be advised to avoid areas with high concentrations of young children such as daycare centers, if possible, and to practice good handwashing techniques.

Herpes Simplex Virus

Herpes simplex virus (HSV-1 or HSV-2) infection can cause painful lesions in the genital area. Lesions may also develop on the cervix. (This condition and its implications for nonpregnant women are discussed in Chapter 6 🔗.)

Fetal/Neonatal Risks

Primary infection poses the greatest risk to both the mother and her infant. Primary infection has been associated with spontaneous abortion, low birth weight, and preterm birth. Transmission to the fetus almost always occurs after the membranes rupture and the virus ascends or during birth through an infected birth canal. Transplacental infection is rare. The risk of transmission to the newborn is 30% to 50% if a woman develops a primary infection near birth; the risk is less than 1% for women who acquire HSV early in pregnancy or who have a recurrent lesion near the time of childbirth (CDC, 2010c).

The infected infant is often asymptomatic at birth but develops symptoms of fever (or hypothermia), jaundice, seizures, and poor feeding any time after birth and up to 4 weeks of age. Approximately half of infected infants develop the characteristic vesicular skin lesions. All infants who have neonatal herpes should be evaluated promptly and treated with acyclovir (CDC, 2010c).

Clinical Therapy

The vesicular lesions of herpes have a characteristic appearance, and they rupture easily. Definitive diagnosis is made by culturing active lesions.

Women with a primary HSV infection during pregnancy can be treated with oral acyclovir, valacyclovir, or famciclovir. Currently, there is no evidence that there are any adverse fetal effects related to exposure to any of these drugs during any trimester but their safety has not been established definitively (CDC, 2010c). For a woman with either a primary or a secondary outbreak of genital herpes during labor, or symptoms that may indicate an impending outbreak, the preferred method of childbirth is cesarean birth (CDC, 2010c). Although fetal transmission with recurrent outbreaks is low, a cesarean birth is warranted because of the serious nature of the disease in the newborn. Women who do not have any signs or symptoms of herpes or its prodromal symptoms at the onset of labor can give birth vaginally (CDC, 2010c).

NURSING MANAGEMENT *For the Pregnant Woman with Herpes Simplex Virus Infection*

Nursing Assessment and Diagnosis

During the initial prenatal visit, it is important to learn whether the woman or her partner has had previous herpes infections. If so, ongoing assessment is indicated as pregnancy progresses.

Nursing diagnoses that may apply include the following (NANDA-I © 2012):

- *Pain, Acute,* related to the presence of lesions secondary to herpes infection
- *Coping, Ineffective,* related to depression secondary to the risk to the fetus if herpes lesions are present at birth

Planning and Implementation

Patient education about this fast-spreading disease is crucial. Inform women of the association of HSV infection with spontaneous abortion, newborn mortality and morbidity, and the possibility of cesarean birth. A woman needs to inform all healthcare providers of her infection. She should also know of the possible association of genital herpes with cervical cancer and the importance of a yearly Pap smear.

The woman who acquired HSV infection as an adolescent may be devastated as a mature adult who wants to have a family. Counseling that allows her to express the negative feelings she may have about the infection may help. Literature may also help and is available from many public health agencies.

Evaluation

Expected outcomes of nursing care include the following:

- The woman is able to describe her infection with regard to its method of spread, therapy and comfort measures, implications for her pregnancy, and long-term implications.
- The woman gives birth to a healthy infant.

Group B Streptococcal Infection

Group B streptococcus (GBS) is a bacterial infection found in the vagina or rectum of 10% to 30% of pregnant women (ACOG, 2011b). Women may transmit GBS to their fetus in utero or during childbirth. GBS is one of the major causes of early-onset neonatal infection. Newborns become infected in one of two ways: by vertical transmission from the mother during birth or from horizontal transmission from colonized nursing personnel or colonized infants. GBS causes severe, invasive disease in infants. In newborns the majority of cases occur within the first week of life and are thus designated as early-onset disease. Late-onset disease occurs 1 week or more after birth.

Early-onset GBS is often characterized by signs of serious illness, including pneumonia, apnea, and shock. Late-onset GBS often manifests as meningitis or pneumonia. Long-term neurologic complications are common in both types of GBS.

Risk factors for GBS neonatal sepsis include young maternal age, African American or Hispanic race, preterm labor, maternal intrapartum fever, prolonged rupture of the membranes, previous birth of an infected infant, and GBS bacteriuria in the current pregnancy. Guidelines for the detection and preventive treatment of newborns at risk include the following (CDC, 2010b):

- All pregnant women should be screened for both vaginal and rectal GBS colonization at 35 to 37 weeks' gestation. Treatment should be based on these results, even if cultures were done earlier in pregnancy.
- Women identified as GBS carriers should receive antibiotic prophylaxis at the onset of labor or the rupture of membranes.
- Women with GBS in their urine should be treated according to guidelines for treating urinary tract infections (UTIs) during pregnancy and should receive antibiotic prophylaxis intrapartally. These women do not need vaginal and rectal cultures at 35 to 37 weeks because therapy is already indicated.
- Women who have already given birth to a newborn with invasive GBS disease should receive intrapartum antibiotic prophylaxis. Culture-based screening is not necessary for them.
- If the results of GBS screening are not known when labor begins, prophylaxis is indicated for women with any of the following risk factors: gestation less than 37 weeks, membranes ruptured 18 hours or longer, temperature equal to or greater than 38.0°C (100.4°F).

Intrapartum antibiotic therapy is recommended as follows: initial dose of penicillin G, 5 million units IV followed by 2.5 to 3 million units IV every 4 hours until childbirth. Alternatively, ampicillin 2 g initial dose IV followed by 1 g IV every 4 hours until childbirth may be used. In women at high risk for an anaphylactic reaction to penicillin because of marked allergy, testing is done to see if the organism is susceptible to clindamycin and erythromycin. If the organism is susceptible, clindamycin 900 mg IV every 4 hours until birth may be used. If the organism is resistant or if susceptibility testing is not done, vancomycin is administered 1 g IV every 12 hours until birth (ACOG, 2011b; CDC, 2010b).

Other Infections in Pregnancy

Table 16–2 summarizes other urinary tract, vaginal, and sexually transmitted infections that contribute to risk during pregnancy. (These are described in more detail in Chapter 6 🔗.) Spontaneous abortion is frequently the result of a severe maternal infection. Some evidence links infection and prematurity. If the pregnancy is carried to term in the presence of infection, the risk of maternal and fetal morbidity and mortality increases. Thus, it is essential to maternal and fetal health that infection be diagnosed and treated promptly.

Table 16–2   Infections That Put Pregnancy at Risk

Condition and Causative Organism	Signs and Symptoms	Treatment	Implications for Pregnancy
URINARY TRACT INFECTIONS (UTIs)			
Asymptomatic bacteriuria (ASB): *Escherichia, Klebsiella, Proteus* most common	Bacteria present in urine on culture with no accompanying symptoms.	Oral sulfonamides early in pregnancy, ampicillin and nitrofurantoin (Furadantin) in late pregnancy. Antibody sensitivity results will guide the selection of an appropriate antibiotic.	Women with ASB in early pregnancy may go on to develop cystitis or acute pyelonephritis by third trimester if not treated. Oral sulfonamides taken in the last few weeks of pregnancy may lead to neonatal hyperbilirubinemia and kernicterus.
Cystitis (lower UTI): causative organisms same as for ASB	Dysuria, urgency, frequency; low-grade fever and hematuria may occur. Urine culture (clean catch) shows ↑ leukocytes. Presence of 10^5 (100,000) or more colonies bacteria/mL urine.	Same as for ASB.	If not treated, infection may ascend and lead to acute pyelonephritis.
Acute pyelonephritis: causative organisms same as for ASB	Sudden onset. Chills, high fever, flank pain. Nausea, vomiting, malaise. May have decreased urine output, severe colicky pain, dehydration. Increased diastolic BP, positive fluorescent antibody (FA) test, low creatinine clearance. Marked bacteremia in urine culture, pyuria, white blood cell (WBC) casts.	Hospitalization; IV antibiotic therapy. Other antibiotics safe during pregnancy include carbenicillin, methenamine, cephalosporins. Catheterization if output is ↓. Supportive therapy for comfort. Follow-up urine cultures are necessary.	Increased risk of premature birth and intrauterine growth restriction (IUGR). Antibiotics used for treatment interfere with urinary estriol levels and can cause false interpretations of estriol levels during pregnancy.
VAGINAL INFECTIONS			
Vulvovaginal candidiasis (yeast infection): *Candida albicans*	Often thick, white, curdy discharge, severe itching, dysuria, dyspareunia. Diagnosis based on presence of hyphae and spores in a wet-mount preparation of vaginal secretions.	Intravaginal insertion of miconazole, butoconazole, or other topical azole preparation, clotrimazole vaginal tablets at bedtime for 1 week (CDC, 2010c).	If the infection is present at birth and the fetus is born vaginally, the fetus may contract thrush.
Bacterial vaginosis: *Gardnerella vaginalis*	Thin, watery, yellow-gray discharge with foul odor often described as "fishy." Wet-mount preparation reveals "clue cells." Application of potassium hydroxide (KOH) to a specimen of vaginal secretions produces a pronounced fishy odor.	Metronidazole 500 mg PO BID × 7 days or metronidazole 250 mg PO TID × 7 days or clindamycin 300 mg PO BID × 7 days (CDC, 2010c).	CDC (2010c) reports that multiple studies have failed to demonstrate a teratogenic effect from metronidazole.

(continued)

Table 16–2   Infections That Put Pregnancy at Risk—continued

Condition and Causative Organism	Signs and Symptoms	Treatment	Implications for Pregnancy
Trichomoniasis: *Trichomonas vaginalis*	Occasionally asymptomatic. May have frothy greenish gray vaginal discharge, pruritus, urinary symptoms. Strawberry patches may be visible on vaginal walls or cervix. Wet-mount preparation of vaginal secretions shows motile flagellated trichomonads.	Single 2-g dose of metronidazole orally (CDC, 2010c).	Increased risk for premature rupture of the membranes (PROM), preterm birth, and low birth weight.

SEXUALLY TRANSMITTED INFECTIONS

Chlamydial infection: *Chlamydia trachomatis*	Women are often asymptomatic. Symptoms may include thin or purulent discharge, urinary burning and frequency, or lower abdominal pain. Lab test available to detect monoclonal antibodies specific for *Chlamydia*.	Doxycycline, ofloxacin, and levofloxacin are contraindicated during pregnancy. Thus, pregnant women are treated with azithromycin or amoxicillin followed by repeat culture in 3 weeks (CDC, 2010c).	Infant of woman with untreated chlamydial infection may develop newborn conjunctivitis, which can be treated with erythromycin eye ointment (but not silver nitrate). Infant may also develop chlamydial pneumonia. May be responsible for premature labor and fetal death.
Syphilis: *Treponema pallidum*, a spirochete	Primary stage: chancre, slight fever, malaise. Chancre lasts about 4 weeks, then disappears. Secondary stage: occurs 6 weeks to 6 months after infection. Skin eruptions (condyloma lata); also symptoms of acute arthritis, liver enlargement, iritis, chronic sore throat with hoarseness. Diagnosed by blood tests such as VDRL, RPR, FTA, ABS. Dark-field examination for spirochetes may also be done.	For syphilis less than 1 year in duration: single dose of 2.4 million units benzathine penicillin G IM. For syphilis of more than 1 year's duration or latent syphilis of unknown duration: 2.4 million units benzathine penicillin G once a week for 3 weeks. Sexual partners should also be screened and treated (CDC, 2010c)	Syphilis can be passed transplacentally to the fetus. If untreated, one of the following can occur: second-trimester abortion, stillborn infant at term, congenitally infected infant, uninfected live infant.
Gonorrhea: *Neisseria gonorrhoeae*	Majority of women asymptomatic; disease often diagnosed during routine prenatal cervical culture. If symptoms are present they may include purulent vaginal discharge, dysuria, urinary frequency, inflammation, and swelling of the vulva. Cervix may appear eroded.	Pregnant women are treated with a cephalosporin (ceftriaxone, cefixime); Spectinomycin is not available in the United States; thus, azithromycin 2 g PO may be used if the woman cannot tolerate a cephalosporin. Also treated for chlamydia using azithromycin or amoxicillin (CDC, 2010c). All sexual partners are also treated.	Infection at time of birth may cause ophthalmia neonatorum in the newborn.
Condyloma acuminata (genital warts): caused by the human papilloma virus (HPV)	Soft, grayish pink lesions on the vulva, vagina, cervix, or anus.	Podophyllin, podofilox, sinecatechins, and imiquimod are contraindicated during pregnancy. Some caregivers recommend removing warts by surgical methods or laser because the warts can proliferate and become friable (bleed easily) during pregnancy but the results may be poor or incomplete (CDC, 2010c).	Possible teratogenic effect of podophyllin. Large doses have been associated with fetal death. Cesarean birth is only indicated for women with warts that obstruct the pelvic outlet or if vaginal birth would result in significant bleeding (CDC, 2010c).

Clinical Reasoning Preventing Cystitis

Your friend Jena Yoo, G1P0, is 6 months pregnant and mentions to you that she is developing symptoms of a bladder infection. She has had several bladder infections over the past few years and feels she has warded off others by increasing her fluid intake and drinking acidic juices. Jena tells you that she plans to use the same approach this time because she just had her prenatal appointment last week. She assures you that if symptoms persist, she will discuss it with her care provider at her next prenatal visit. What advice would you give her? *See www.nursing.pearsonhighered.com for possible responses.*

CARE OF THE WOMAN AT RISK FOR Rh ALLOIMMUNIZATION

The Rh blood group is present on the surface of erythrocytes of most of the population. When it is present, a person is said to be Rh positive. Those without the factor are Rh negative. If an Rh-negative individual is exposed to Rh-positive blood (antigen Rh[D]), an antigen–antibody response occurs, and the person forms anti-Rh agglutinin and is said to be sensitized. Subsequent exposure to Rh-positive blood can then cause a serious reaction that results in agglutination and hemolysis of red blood cells (RBCs). In the United States about 15% to 18% of white Americans, 3% to 7% of African Americans, and 1% of Asian and Native Americans are Rh negative (Taylor, Uhlmann, Meyer, et al., 2011).

Rh alloimmunization (sensitization), also called *isoimmunization,* most often occurs when an Rh-negative woman carries an Rh-positive fetus, either to term or to termination by miscarriage or induced abortion. It can also occur if an Rh-negative nonpregnant woman receives an Rh-positive blood transfusion.

The red blood cells (RBCs) from the fetus invade the maternal circulation, thereby stimulating the production of Rh antibodies. Because this transfer of RBCs usually occurs at birth, the first child is not affected. In a subsequent pregnancy, however, Rh antibodies cross the placenta and enter the fetal circulation, causing severe hemolysis. The destruction of fetal RBCs causes anemia in the fetus (Figure 16–4 ●).

Fetal-Neonatal Risks

Although maternal sensitization can now be prevented by administration of **Rh immune globulin (RhoGAM**, WinRho-SDF), the incidence of alloimmunization has increased in recent years because of the migration of Rh-negative sensitized women from countries with lower healthcare standards or limited resources

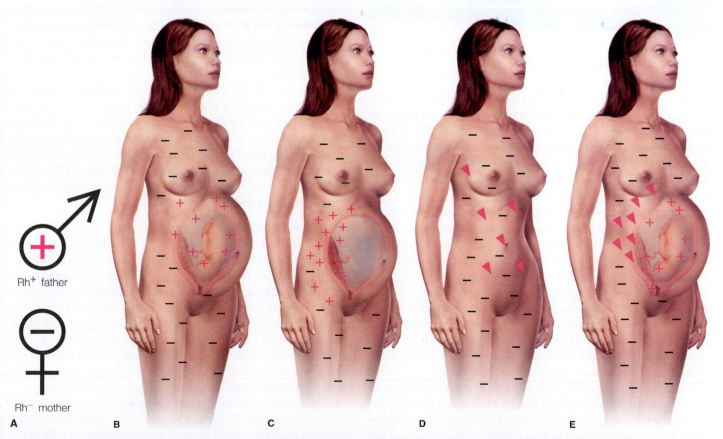

Rh⁺ father

Rh⁻ mother

A   B   C   D   E

● **Figure 16–4** Rh alloimmunization sequence. *A,* Rh-positive father and Rh-negative mother. *B,* Pregnancy with Rh-positive fetus. Some Rh-positive blood enters the mother's bloodstream. *C,* As the placenta separates, the mother is further exposed to the Rh-positive blood. *D,* Anti-Rh-positive antibodies (triangles) are formed. *E,* In subsequent pregnancies with an Rh-positive fetus, Rh-positive red blood cells are attacked by the anti-Rh-positive maternal antibodies, causing hemolysis of the red blood cells in the fetus.

to developed countries (Bettelheim et al., 2010). If treatment with Rh immune globulin is not initiated, the anemia resulting from this disorder can cause marked fetal edema, called **hydrops fetalis**. Congestive heart failure may result; marked jaundice (called *icterus gravis*), which can lead to neurologic damage (*kernicterus*), is also possible. This severe hemolytic syndrome is known as **erythroblastosis fetalis**.

Screening for Rh Incompatibility and Sensitization

At the first prenatal visit, healthcare providers should do the following:

1. Take a history of past pregnancies, previous sensitization, abortions, blood transfusions, or children who developed jaundice or anemia during the newborn period.

2. Determine maternal blood type (ABO) and Rh factor and do a routine Rh antibody screen.

3. Identify other medical complications such as diabetes, infections, or hypertension.

An antibody screen (*indirect Coombs' test*) is done to determine whether an Rh-negative woman is sensitized (has developed isoimmunity) to the Rh antigen. The test measures the number of antibodies in the maternal blood. If the pregnant woman is not sensitized, a second antibody screening test is done at 28 weeks' gestation. If the maternal antibody screen is positive, a maternal antibody titer is obtained. A woman with an elevated antibody titer should be considered sensitized and her pregnancy should be managed closely.

Clinical Therapy

Antepartum Management

If the antibody screen obtained at 28 weeks' gestation is negative, the woman is given an IM injection of 300 mcg Rh immune globulin as a prophylactic (preventive) measure. The Rh immune globulin provides passive antibody protection against Rh antigens. This "tricks" the body, which does not then produce antibodies of its own (active immunity). As discussed later, Rh immune globulin is also given postpartum.

When the woman is Rh negative and not sensitized and the father is Rh positive or unknown, Rh immune globulin is also given after each abortion (whether spontaneous or induced), ectopic pregnancy, hydatidiform mole, chorionic villus sampling (CVS), amniocentesis, placenta previa with bleeding, percutaneous umbilical blood sampling (PUBS), blunt trauma to the abdomen, external cephalic version, suspected abruption, or stillbirth.

Two primary interventions can help the fetus whose blood cells are being destroyed by maternal antibodies: early birth and intrauterine transfusion. Both carry risks. Ideally, birth should be delayed until fetal maturity is confirmed at about 36 to 37 weeks.

Ultrasound should be done at 14 to 16 weeks to determine gestational age. Ultrasound can also be used to detect ascites and subcutaneous edema, which are signs of severe fetal involvement. Other indicators of the fetal condition include an increase in fetal heart size and hydramnios.

Doppler ultrasound to measure peak systolic velocity in the middle cerebral artery (MCA-PSV) of the fetus is now the

standard of care to detect fetal anemia (Taylor et al., 2011). The decreasing fetal red cell mass and concurrent decrease in blood viscosity result in an increase in fetal cardiac output and an increase in the velocity of blood flow through the middle cerebral artery, which is demonstrated by an increase in the peak systolic velocities. MCA-PSV trends over time correlate well with increasing levels of bilirubin in the amniotic fluid and should be monitored regularly starting at 15 to 18 weeks. After 35 weeks' gestation, the false-positive rate for the prediction of anemia increases (Taylor et al., 2011).

Historically, management of Rh disease was done with ΔOD (delta optical density) analysis, a test that determines the amount of bilirubin pigment found in the amniotic fluid. Normally the concentration of bilirubin pigments in the amniotic fluid declines during pregnancy. Elevated bilirubin levels are significant. Because the amount of bilirubin found in the amniotic fluid correlates roughly with the extent of the hemolysis, the ΔOD analysis serves as an indirect predictor of the severity of the fetal anemia. It should only be used if MCA screening is not available.

Negative antibody titers can consistently identify the fetus not at risk. However, the titers cannot reliably point out the fetus in danger, because titer level does not always correlate with the severity of the disease. Thus, if the maternal antibody titer is 1:16 or greater, further testing is indicated.

If MCA-PSV indicates severe fetal anemia or if fetal hydrops is present, percutaneous umbilical blood sampling (PUBS) may be performed to determine fetal hematocrit. If the hematocrit is low (generally less than 30%), the fetus is given an intrauterine blood transfusion either intravascularly through PUBS or intraperitoneally. Severely sensitized fetuses may require birth at 32 to 34 weeks.

Previously, PUBS was the only direct method of assessing the Rh status of a fetus in planning the care of a woman who is Rh negative and sensitized. Fetal genotyping from maternal blood is now available and has been shown to be highly accurate in determining whether the fetus of an Rh-negative mother is Rh positive (Amaral, Credidio, Pellegrino, et al., 2011). As the methodology improves, DNA typing of the fetus may replace amniocentesis for this purpose.

Postpartum Management

The Rh-negative mother who has no antibody titer (indirect Coombs' test negative, nonsensitized) and has given birth to an Rh-positive fetus (direct Coombs' test negative) is given an injection of Rh immune globulin within 72 hours of childbirth so that she does not have time to produce antibodies to fetal cells that entered her bloodstream when the placenta separated. A standard dose of Rh immune globulin can prevent sensitization after exposure of up to 30 mL of Rh(D) positive blood. Rh immune globulin provides her with temporary passive immunity, which prevents the development of permanent active immunity (antibody formation).

Rh immune globulin is not given to the newborn or the father. It should not be given to a previously sensitized woman. However, sometimes after birth or an abortion, the results of the blood test do not clearly show whether the mother is already sensitized to the Rh antigen. In such cases the Rh immune globulin is given; it will cause no harm (Table 16–3).

Table 16–3	Rh Alloimmunization

When trying to work through Rh problems, remember the following:

- A potential problem exists when an Rh-negative mother and an Rh-positive father conceive a child who is Rh positive.
- In this situation, the mother may become sensitized or produce antibodies to her fetus's Rh-positive blood.

The following tests are used to detect sensitization:

- Indirect Coombs' test—done on the mother's blood to measure the number of Rh-positive antibodies.
- Direct Coombs' test—done on the infant's blood to detect antibody-coated Rh-positive red blood cells.

Based on the results of these tests, the following may be done:

- If the mother's indirect Coombs' test is negative and the infant's direct Coombs' test is negative (confirming that sensitization has not occurred), the mother is given Rh immune globulin within 72 hours of birth.
- If the mother's indirect Coombs' test is positive and her Rh-positive infant has a positive direct Coombs' test, Rh immune globulin is not given; in this case the infant is carefully monitored for hemolytic disease.
- It is recommended that Rh immune globulin be given at 28 weeks antenatally to decrease possible transplacental bleeding concerns.

Rh immune globulin is also administered after each abortion (spontaneous or therapeutic), antepartum hemorrhage, mismatched blood transfusion, ectopic pregnancy, amniocentesis, chorionic villi sampling (CVS), percutaneous umbilical blood sampling (PUBS), fetal cephalic version, or maternal trauma.

NURSING MANAGEMENT *For the Pregnant Woman at Risk for Rh Sensitization*

Nursing Assessment and Diagnosis

As part of the initial prenatal history, ask the mother if she knows her blood type and Rh factor. Many women are aware that they are Rh negative and that this status has implications for pregnancy. Ask the woman if she has ever received Rh immune globulin, if she has had any previous pregnancies and their outcomes, and if she knows her partner's Rh factor. If the partner is Rh negative, there is no risk to the fetus, who will also be Rh negative. If the woman does not know what Rh type she is, intervention begins after the initial laboratory data are obtained. Plan care based on the findings.

If the woman becomes sensitized during her pregnancy, nursing assessment focuses on the knowledge and coping skills of the woman and her family. After birth, review data about the Rh type of the fetus. If the newborn is Rh positive, the mother is Rh negative, and no sensitization has occurred, it is necessary to administer Rh immune globulin.

Nursing diagnoses that might apply include the following (NANDA-I © 2012):

- *Knowledge, Readiness for Enhanced,* information about the purpose of Rh immune globulin related to an expressed desire to understand the treatment of Rh incompatibility.
- *Coping, Ineffective,* related to depression secondary to the development of indications of the need for fetal exchange transfusion

Planning and Implementation

During the antepartum period, explain the mechanisms involved in alloimmunization (isoimmunization) and answer any questions the woman and her partner have. It is imperative that the woman understand the importance of receiving Rh immune globulin after every miscarriage, abortion, or ectopic pregnancy. In addition, explain the purpose of the Rh immune globulin administered at 28 weeks' gestation if the woman is not sensitized.

If the woman is sensitized to the Rh factor, it poses a threat to any Rh-positive fetus she carries. Provide emotional support to the family to help the members deal with their concern and any feelings of guilt about the infant's condition. If an intrauterine transfusion becomes necessary, provide support while also assuming responsibility as part of the healthcare team. During labor, when caring for an Rh-negative woman who has not been sensitized, ensure that the woman's blood is assessed for any antibodies and that it has also been cross-matched for Rh immune globulin. The postpartum nurse is usually responsible for administering the Rh immune globulin IM if the newborn is Rh positive. See Skill 2–4 in the *Clinical Skills Manual* SKILLS.

Evaluation

Expected outcomes of nursing care include the following:

- The woman is able to explain the process of Rh sensitization and its implications for her unborn child and for subsequent pregnancies.
- If the woman has not been sensitized, she is able to discuss the importance of receiving Rh immune globulin when necessary and cooperates with the recommended dosage schedule.
- The woman gives birth to a healthy newborn.
- If complications develop for the fetus or newborn, they are detected quickly and therapy is instituted.

CARE OF THE WOMAN AT RISK FROM ABO INCOMPATIBILITY

ABO incompatibility is somewhat common (occurring in 15% to 25% of pregnancies) but rarely causes significant hemolysis (Black & Maheshwari, 2009). In most cases, ABO incompatibility is limited to type O mothers with a type A or B fetus. The group B fetus of a group A mother and the group A fetus of a group B mother are only occasionally affected. Group O infants, because they have no antigenic sites on the red blood cells (RBCs), are never affected regardless of the mother's blood type. The incompatibility occurs as a result of the maternal antibodies present in her serum and interaction between the antigen sites on the fetal RBCs.

Anti-A and anti-B antibodies are naturally occurring; that is, women are naturally exposed to the A and B antigens through the foods they eat and through exposure to infection by gram-negative bacteria. As a result, some women have high serum anti-A and anti-B titers before they become pregnant. Once they become pregnant, the maternal serum anti-A and anti-B antibodies cross the placenta and produce hemolysis of the fetal red blood cells.

With ABO incompatibility, the first infant is often involved, and no relationship exists between the appearance of the disease and repeated sensitization from one pregnancy to the next.

Unlike Rh incompatibility, antepartum treatment is not warranted. As part of the initial assessment, however, note whether the potential for an ABO incompatibility exists (type O mother and type A or B father). This alerts caregivers so that, following birth, the newborn can be assessed carefully for the development of hyperbilirubinemia. (For a discussion of hyperbilirubinemia, see Chapter 28 🔗.)

Critical Concept Review

LEARNING OUTCOME 16.1: Contrast the etiology, medical therapy, and nursing interventions for the various bleeding problems associated with pregnancy.

1. Several health problems associated with bleeding arise from the pregnancy itself:
   - Spontaneous abortion (SAB).
   - Ectopic pregnancy.
   - Gestational trophoblastic disease (GTD).
2. Medical treatment determined by etiology:
   - SAB: D&C if needed; Rh immune globulin if indicated.
   - Ectopic: medical or surgical intervention.
   - GTD: suction evacuation of mole; yearlong monitoring for signs of choriocarcinoma.

3. The nurse needs to be alert to early signs of these situations:
   - Guard the woman against heavy bleeding and shock.
   - Facilitate the medical treatment.
   - Provide educational and emotional support.

LEARNING OUTCOME 16.2: Discuss the medical therapy and nursing care of a woman with hyperemesis gravidarum.

1. Treatment of hyperemesis gravidarum is aimed at:
   - Controlling the vomiting.
   - Correcting fluid and electrolyte imbalance.
   - Correcting dehydration.
   - Improving nutritional status.

2. Nursing care includes:
   - Maintain a relaxed, quiet environment.
   - Monitor weight.
   - Encourage vigilant oral hygiene.

LEARNING OUTCOME 16.3: Describe the maternal and fetal/neonatal risks, clinical manifestations, and nursing care of a pregnant woman with a hypertensive disorder.

1. Hypertension may exist before pregnancy or, more often, may develop during pregnancy.
2. Preeclampsia can lead to growth retardation for the fetus.
3. Untreated preeclampsia may lead to seizures and death of the mother and infant.

4. It is important to educate the mother about the disease process. This may help motivate her to maintain the required rest periods in the left lateral recumbent position.
5. Antihypertensive and anticonvulsive drugs may be used.

LEARNING OUTCOME 16.4: Summarize the risks and implications of surgical procedures performed during pregnancy.

1. During surgery, a wedge is placed under the mother's hip to prevent compressing vessels while the mother is supine.
2. Pregnancy may hinder diagnosis because of the risk x-rays pose to the developing fetus.

3. Surgery increases the risk of miscarriage, preterm labor, and growth retardation in the fetus.

LEARNING OUTCOME 16.5: Relate the impact of trauma caused by an accident to the nursing care of the pregnant woman or her fetus.

1. Trauma during pregnancy increases the risk of bleeding, a result of the increased blood volume of the mother.
2. The types of trauma that are of most concern are blunt trauma, penetrating injuries, and gunshot wounds.

3. Treatment centers on lifesaving measures to the mother.
4. Mother and fetus should be monitored after an accident even if no injury is apparent.

LEARNING OUTCOME 16.6: Discuss the needs and care of the pregnant woman who experiences abuse.

1. The nurse needs to be alert for signs of abuse, including bruising or injury to the breasts, abdomen, or genitalia.

2. The woman should be given information about female partner abuse and about community resources available to assist her.

LEARNING OUTCOME 16.7: Contrast the effects of various infections on the pregnant woman and her unborn child.

1. Toxoplasmosis, rubella, cytomegalovirus, herpes, GBS, and other perinatal infections pose a grave threat to the fetus.
2. Prevention is the best therapy.

3. There is no known treatment for rubella or CMV, but antimicrobial drugs are available for toxoplasmosis, herpes, and GBS.

LEARNING OUTCOME 16.8: Relate the cause, fetal/neonatal risks, prevention, and clinical therapy to the nursing care of the woman at risk for Rh alloimmunization.

1. Rh incompatibility can occur when an Rh-negative woman and an Rh-positive partner conceive a child who is Rh positive.

2. Use of Rh immune globulin has greatly decreased the incidence of severe complications resulting from Rh incompatibility, because the drug "tricks" the body into thinking antibodies have been produced in response to the Rh antigens.

LEARNING OUTCOME 16.9: Compare Rh incompatibility to ABO incompatibility with regard to occurrence, clinical treatment, and implications for the fetus or newborn.

1. ABO incompatibility occurs when the mother has type O blood and the infant has A, B, or AB.

2. Unlike Rh incompatibility, no treatment exists to prevent the occurrence.

3. It creates hyperbilirubinemia in the infant, which is treated with phototherapy.

Clinical Reasoning in Action

Carol Smith, a 40-year-old, single, G2P0010, presents to you at 32 weeks' gestation while you are working in the birthing unit. Her chief complaint is severe headache, nausea, and trouble seeing. She describes "blackened areas" in her visual fields bilaterally. Her prenatal record reveals long-term substance abuse, depression, and hypertension currently treated with nifedipine 60 mg by mouth once in the morning. You note that she has had two prenatal visits with this pregnancy. You determine her blood pressure to be 170/110; deep tendon reflexes are 3+, clonus negative. She has general edema and 3+ proteinuria. You place Carol on the external fetal monitor to observe for fetal well-being and any contractions. You position her on her left side with her head elevated and use pillows for comfort.

You observe that the fetal heart rate is 143–148 with decreased variability. No fetal heart rate decelerations or accelerations are noted. The uterus is soft, and no contractions are palpated or noted on the fetal monitor.

Carol asks you why she should stay on her left side.

1. How would you explain the importance of the left side-lying position when on bed rest?

2. You administer nifedipine 10 mg sublingual and a loading dose of magnesium sulfate 4 g IV piggyback to the main IV line of Ringer's lactate. What findings would indicate that Carol has therapeutic levels of magnesium?

3. What signs of magnesium toxicity should you monitor Carol for?

4. Carol asks if magnesium sulfate will affect her infant. How would you answer her?

5. Which signs of premature labor would you ask Carol to notify you of if she experiences them?

6. Develop a concept map that relates nursing care for a woman receiving magnesium sulfate to her physical findings on assessment.

See www.nursing.pearsonhighered.com for possible responses and an interactive template for a concept map.

References

Amaral, D. R., Credidio, D. C., Pellegrino, J., Jr., & Castilho, L. (2011). Fetal RHD genotyping by analysis of maternal plasma in a mixed population. *Journal of Clinical Laboratory Analysis, 25*(2), 100–104.

American College of Obstetricians and Gynecologists (ACOG). (2011a). *Emergent therapy for acute-onset, severe hypertension with preeclampsia or eclampsia* (Committee Opinion No. 514). Washington, DC: Author.

American College of Obstetricians and Gynecologists (ACOG). (2011b). *Prevention of early-onset group B streptococcal disease in newborns* (Committee Opinion No. 485). Washington, DC: Author.

American College of Obstetricians and Gynecologists (ACOG). (2012a). *Chronic hypertension in pregnancy* (Practice Bulletin No. 125). Washington, DC: Author.

American College of Obstetricians and Gynecologists (ACOG). (2012b). *Intimate partner violence* (Committee Opinion No. 518). Washington, DC: Author.

Bernstein, H. B. (2012). Maternal and perinatal infection—Viral. In S. G. Gabbe, J. R. Niebyl, J. L. Simpson, M. B. Landon, H. L. Galan, E. R. M. Jauniaux, & D. A. Driscoll (Eds.), *Obstetrics: Normal and problem pregnancies* (6th ed.). Philadelphia, PA: Elsevier Saunders.

Bettelheim, D., Panzer, S., Reesink, H. W., Csapo, B., Pessoa, C., Guerra, F., Wendel, S., . . . Holzgreve, W. (2010). Monitoring and treatment of anti-D in pregnancy. *Vox Sanguinis: The International Journal of Transfusion Medicine, 99*, 177–192.

Black, V. L., & Maheshwari, A. (2009). Disorders of the feto-maternal unit: Hematologic manifestations in the fetus and neonate. *Seminars in Perinatology, 33,* 12–19.

Blackburn, S. T. (2013). *Maternal, fetal, and neonatal physiology: A clinical perspective* (4th ed.). St. Louis, MO: Saunders.

Brent, R. (2011). The pulmonologist's role in caring for pregnant women with regard to the reproductive risks of diagnostic radiological studies or radiation therapy. *Clinics in Chest Medicine, 32*(1), 33–42.

Centers for Disease Control and Prevention (CDC). (2010a). *Diagnostic findings: Toxoplasmosis.* Retrieved from http://www.cdc.gov/parasites/toxoplasmosis/health_professionals/index.html

Centers for Disease Control and Prevention (CDC). (2010b). Prevention of perinatal group B streptococcal disease: Revised guidelines from CDC, 2010. *Morbidity and Mortality Weekly Report, 59* (RR10), 1–32.

Centers for Disease Control and Prevention (CDC). (2010c). Sexually transmitted diseases treatment guidelines, 2010. *Morbidity and Mortality Weekly Report, 59*(RR-12), 1–109.

Cunningham, F. G., Leveno, K. J., Bloom, S. L., Hauth, J. C., Rouse, D. J., & Spong, C. Y. (2010.) *Williams obstetrics* (23rd ed.). New York, NY: McGraw-Hill Medical.

Devl, S. (2012). US guidelines for domestic violence screening spark debate. *The Lancet, 379*, 506.

DiGiulio, M., Wiedaseck, S., & Monchek, R. (2012). Understanding hydatidiform mole. *American Journal of Maternal–Child Nursing, 37*(1), 30–34.

Duff, P. (2012). Maternal and perinatal infection—Bacterial. In S. G. Gabbe, J. R. Niebyl, J. L. Simpson, M. B. Landon, H. L. Galan, E. R. M. Jauniaux, & D. A. Driscoll (Eds.), *Obstetrics: Normal and problem pregnancies* (6th ed.). Philadelphia, PA: Elsevier Saunders.

Harms, R. W. (2010). *Is it safe to use a hot tub during pregnancy?* Retrieved from http://www.mayoclinic.com/health/pregnancy-and-hot-tubs/an02109

Johnson, K. E. (2009*). Overview of TORCH infections.* Retrieved from http://www.uptodate.com

Jurkovic, D., & Wilkinson, H. (2011). Diagnosis and management of ectopic pregnancy. *British Medical Journal, 342*, d3397. doi:10.1136/bmj.d3397

Lipscomb, G. H. (2012). Medical management of ectopic pregnancy. *Clinical Obstetrics and Gynecology, 55*(2), 424–432.

Magee, L. A., Abalos, E., von Dadelszen, P., Sibai, B., Easterling, T., & Walkinshaw, S. (2011). How to manage hypertension in pregnancy effectively. *British Journal of Clinical Pharmacology, 72*(3), 394–401.

Marion, L. B., & Meeks, G. R. (2012). Ectopic pregnancy: History, incidence, epidemiology, and risk factors. *Clinical Obstetrics and Gynecology, 55*(2), 376–386.

Mozurkewich, E. L., & Pearlman, M.D. (2012). Trauma and related surgery in pregnancy. In S. G. Gabbe, J. R. Niebyl, J. L. Simpson, M. B. Landon, H. L. Galan, E. R. M. Jauniaux, & D. A. Driscoll (Eds.), *Obstetrics: Normal and problem pregnancies* (6th ed.). Philadelphia, PA: Elsevier Saunders.

Nayeri, U. A. (2012). Hyperemesis in pregnancy: Taking a tiered approach. *Contemporary OB/GYN, 57*(7), 22–31.

Puri, A., Khadem, P., Ahmed, S., Yadav, P., & Al-Dulaimy, K. (2011). Imaging of trauma in a pregnant patient. *Seminars in Ultrasound, CT, and MRI, 33*(1), 37–45.

Richards, D. S. (2012). Obstetrical ultrasound: Imaging, dating, and growth. In S. G. Gabbe, J. R. Niebyl, J. L. Simpson, M. B. Landon, H. L. Galan, E. R. M. Jauniaux, & D. A. Driscoll (Eds.), *Obstetrics: Normal and problem pregnancies* (6th ed.). Philadelphia, PA: Elsevier Saunders.

Salani, R., Eisenhauer, E. L., & Copeland, L. J. (2012). Malignant diseases and pregnancy. In S. G. Gabbe, J. R. Niebyl, J. L. Simpson, M. B. Landon, H. L. Galan, E. R. M. Jauniaux, & D. A. Driscoll (Eds.), *Obstetrics: Normal and problem pregnancies* (6th ed.). Philadelphia, PA: Elsevier Saunders.

Sibai, B. M. (2012). Hypertension. In S. G. Gabbe, J. R. Niebyl, J. L. Simpson, M. B. Landon, H. L. Galan, E. R. M. Jauniaux, & D. A. Driscoll (Eds.), *Obstetrics: Normal and problem pregnancies* (6th ed.). Philadelphia, PA: Elsevier Saunders.

Sonkusare, S. (2011). The clinical management of hyperemesis gravidarum. *Archives of Gynecology and Obstetrics.* doi:10.1007/s00404-011-1877-y

Taylor, M., Uhlmann, R. A., Meyer, N. L., & Mari, G. (2011). Hemolytic disease: Diagnosis, counseling, and management. *Contemporary OB/GYN, 56*(6), 34–45.

Visconti, K., & Zite, N. (2012). hCG in ectopic pregnancy. *Clinical Obstetrics and Gynecology, 55*(2),410–417.

Zhang, Y., Cantor, R. M., MacGibbon, K., Romero, R., Goodwin, T. M., Mullin, P. M., & Fejzo, M. S. (2011). Familial aggregation of hyperemesis gravidarum. *American Journal of Obstetrics and Gynecology, 204*(3), 230–233.

Pearson Nursing Student Resources Find additional review materials at: **nursing.pearsonhighered.com**

Processes and Stages of Labor and Birth

Leanne Temme/Getty Images

I think experts refer to us as a blended family. I have two sons, ages 12 and 9, from a previous marriage. They live part-time with us and part-time with their father. My husband has a 15-year-old daughter who lives with her mother. Here I am, 6 months pregnant with our first child together. It has been quite the time, getting used to the idea of a baby and trying to include our children in the pregnancy. They have all heard the heartbeat and felt the baby move. My sons are pretty blasé about it. I didn't know how Jack's daughter would respond but she has been great. Maybe this new baby will help us all grow closer together. I sure hope so. —Letetia, 34

LEARNING OUTCOMES

17.1 Describe the five critical factors that influence labor in the assessment of an expectant woman's and fetus's progress in labor and birth.

17.2 Examine an expectant woman's and fetus's response to labor based on the physiologic processes that occur during labor.

17.3 Assess for the premonitory signs of labor when caring for the expectant woman.

17.4 Differentiate between false and true labor.

17.5 Describe the physiologic and psychologic changes that occur in an expectant woman during each stage of labor in the nursing care management of the expectant woman.

17.6 Explain the maternal systemic responses to labor in the nursing care of the expectant woman.

17.7 Examine fetal responses to labor.

I n the final weeks of pregnancy, both mother and baby begin to prepare for birth. The onset of labor begins a remarkable change in the relationship between the woman and her baby. In those hours and moments, the birth process may seem to carry all the power in the universe. The mother-to-be and her partner may feel stretched beyond their normal limits of concentration, purpose, endurance, and pain as they work to bring forth a precious new life.

This chapter focuses on the processes and stages of labor. Subsequent chapters describe intrapartum assessment and nursing care.

CRITICAL FACTORS IN LABOR

Five factors are of critical importance in the process of labor and birth: the passage, the fetus, the relationship between the passage and the fetus, the physiologic forces of labor, and the psychosocial considerations. Abnormalities that affect any component of these critical forces can alter the outcome of labor and jeopardize both the expectant woman and her baby. The five factors are summarized in Table 17–1 and the first four are described in this section. Psychosocial factors are discussed in detail in Chapter 18 🔗. Labor-related complications are discussed in Chapter 22 🔗.

The Birth Passage

The true pelvis, which forms the bony canal through which the fetus must pass, is divided into three sections: the inlet, the pelvic cavity (midpelvis), and the outlet. (See Chapter 3 🔗 for discussion of the pelvis and Chapter 10 🔗 for assessment techniques.)

The Caldwell-Moloy classification of pelvises is widely used to differentiate bony pelvis types. The four classic types of pelvis are *gynecoid, android, anthropoid,* and *platypelloid* (Caldwell & Moloy, 1933) (Figure 17–1 ●). The gynecoid, or female, pelvis is most common. All diameters of the gynecoid are adequate for childbirth. Implications of each type of pelvis for childbirth are summarized in Table 17–2.

Table 17–1	Critical Factors in Labor
Critical Factors	**Components**
THE BIRTH PASSAGE	■ Size of the pelvis (diameters of the pelvic inlet, midpelvis or pelvic cavity, and outlet) ■ Type of pelvis (gynecoid, android, anthropoid, platypelloid, or a combination) ■ Ability of the cervix to dilate and efface and ability of the vaginal canal and the external opening of the vagina (the introitus) to distend
THE FETUS	■ Fetal head (size and presence of molding) ■ Fetal attitude (flexion or extension of the fetal body and extremities) ■ Fetal lie ■ Fetal presentation (the part of the fetal body entering the pelvis first in a single- or multiple-gestation pregnancy)
RELATIONSHIP BETWEEN THE PASSAGE AND THE FETUS	■ Engagement of fetal presenting part ■ Station (location of fetal presenting part within the maternal pelvis) ■ Fetal position (relationship of the presenting part to one of the four quadrants of the maternal pelvis)
PHYSIOLOGIC FORCES OF LABOR	■ Frequency, duration, and intensity of uterine contractions as the fetus moves through the birth passage ■ Effectiveness of the maternal pushing effort ■ Duration of labor
PSYCHOSOCIAL CONSIDERATIONS (see Chapter 18 🔗 for an in-depth discussion)	■ Physical preparation for childbirth ■ Sociocultural values and beliefs ■ Previous childbirth experience(s) ■ Support from significant others ■ Emotional status

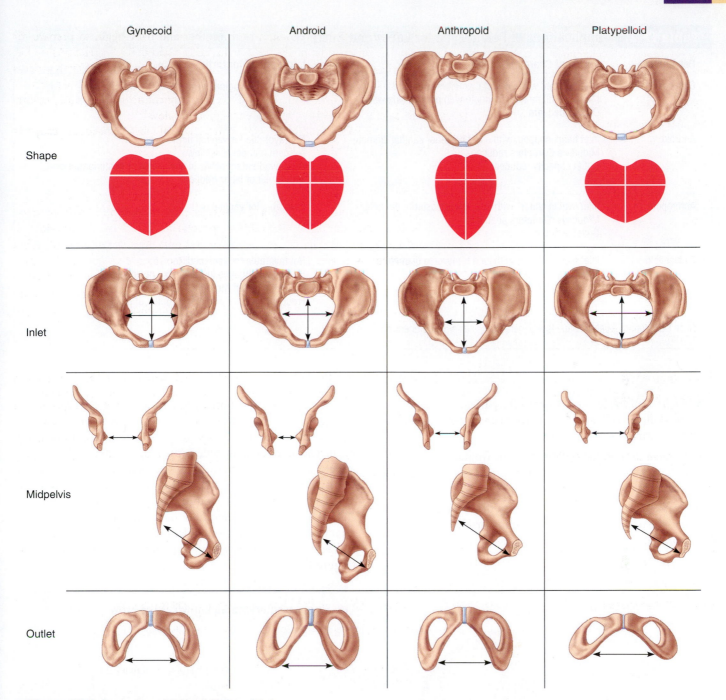

| Gynecoid | Android | Anthropoid | Platypelloid |

Shape

Inlet

Midpelvis

Outlet

● **Figure 17–1** Comparison of Caldwell-Moloy pelvic types.

The Fetus

Fetal Head

The fetal skull (cranium) has three major parts: the face, the base of the skull, and the vault of the cranium (roof). The bones of the face and cranial base are well fused and essentially fixed. The base of the cranium is composed of the two temporal bones, each with a sphenoid and ethmoid bone. The bones composing the vault are the two frontal bones, the two parietal bones, and the occipital bone (Figure 17–2 ●). These bones are not fused, so this portion of the head can adjust in shape as the presenting part passes through the narrow portions of the pelvis. The cranial bones overlap under pressure of the powers of labor and the demands of the unyielding pelvis. This overlapping is called **molding**. Once the head (the least compressible and largest part of the fetus) has been born, the birth of the rest of the body is rarely delayed.

The **sutures** of the fetal skull are membranous spaces between the cranial bones. The intersections of the cranial sutures are called **fontanelles**. These sutures allow for molding of the fetal head and help the clinician to identify the position of the fetal head during vaginal examination. The important sutures of the cranium are as follows (see Figure 17–2):

■ *Frontal (mitotic) suture:* located between the two frontal bones; becomes the anterior continuation of the sagittal suture

Table 17–2	Implications of Pelvic Type for Labor and Birth	
Pelvic Type	**Pertinent Characteristics**	**Implications for Birth**
Gynecoid	Inlet rounded with all inlet diameters adequate Midpelvis diameters adequate with parallel side walls Outlet adequate	Favorable for vaginal birth
Android	Inlet heart-shaped, with short posterior sagittal diameter Midpelvis diameters reduced Outlet capacity reduced	Not favorable for vaginal birth Descent into pelvis is slow Fetal head enters pelvis in transverse or posterior position, with arrest of labor frequent
Anthropoid	Inlet oval in shape, with long anteroposterior diameter Midpelvis diameters adequate Outlet adequate	Favorable for vaginal birth
Platypelloid	Inlet oval in shape, with long transverse diameters Midpelvis diameters reduced Outlet capacity inadequate	Not favorable for vaginal birth Fetal head engages in transverse position Difficult descent through midpelvis Frequent delay of progress at outlet of pelvis

Note: Description of pelvic shape is exaggerated for easier comprehension.

- *Sagittal suture:* located between the parietal bones; divides the skull into left and right halves; runs anteroposteriorly, connecting the two fontanelles
- *Coronal sutures:* located between the frontal and parietal bones; extend transversely left and right from the anterior fontanelle
- *Lambdoidal suture:* located between the two parietal bones and the occipital bone; extends transversely left and right from the posterior fontanelle

The anterior and posterior fontanelles are clinically useful (along with the sutures) in identifying the position of the fetal head in the pelvis and in assessing the status of the newborn after birth. The anterior fontanelle is diamond shaped and measures about 2 cm by 3 cm. It permits growth of the brain by remaining unossified for as long as 18 months. The posterior fontanelle is much smaller and closes within 8 to 12 weeks after birth. It is shaped like a small triangle and marks the meeting point of the sagittal suture and the lambdoidal suture.

Following are several important landmarks of the fetal skull (Figure 17–3 ●):

- *Mentum:* fetal chin
- *Sinciput:* anterior area known as the brow

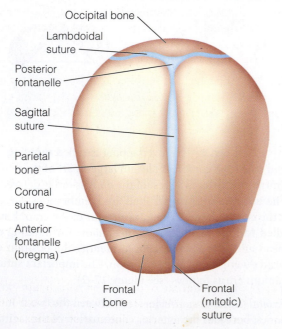

● **Figure 17–2** Superior view of the fetal skull.

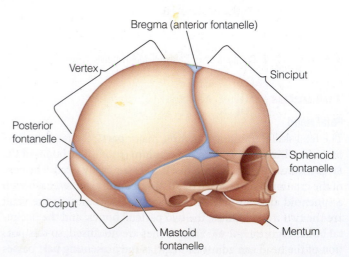

● **Figure 17–3** Lateral view of the fetal skull. This figure identifies the landmarks that have significance during birth.

● **Figure 17–4** Fetal skull measurements. *A,* Typical anteroposterior diameters of the fetal skull. When the vertex of the fetus presents and the fetal head is flexed with the chin on the chest, the smallest anteroposterior diameter (suboccipitobregmatic) enters the birth canal. *B,* Transverse diameters of the fetal skull.

● **Figure 17–5** Fetal attitude. The attitude (or relationship of body parts) of this fetus is normal. The head is flexed forward, with the chin almost resting on the chest. The arms and legs are flexed.

- *Bregma:* large diamond-shaped anterior fontanelle
- *Vertex:* area between the anterior and posterior fontanelles
- *Posterior fontanelle:* intersection between posterior cranial sutures
- *Occiput:* area of the fetal skull occupied by the occipital bone, beneath the posterior fontanelle

The diameters of the fetal skull vary considerably within normal limits. Some diameters shorten and others lengthen as the head is molded during labor. Fetal head diameters are measured between the various landmarks on the skull (Figure 17–4 ●). For example, the suboccipitobregmatic diameter is the distance from the undersurface of the occiput to the center of the bregma, or anterior fontanelle.

Fetal Attitude and Fetal Lie
Fetal attitude refers to the relation of the fetal parts to one another. The normal attitude of the fetus is one of moderate flexion of the head, flexion of the arms onto the chest, and flexion of the legs onto the abdomen (Figure 17–5 ●).

Fetal lie refers to the relationship of the cephalocaudal axis (spinal column) of the fetus to the cephalocaudal axis of the woman. The fetus may assume either a longitudinal or a transverse lie. A *longitudinal lie* occurs when the cephalocaudal axis

of the fetus is parallel to the woman's spine. A *transverse lie* occurs when the cephalocaudal axis of the fetus is at a right angle to the woman's spine.

Fetal Presentation
Fetal presentation is determined by fetal lie and by the body part of the fetus that enters the pelvic passage first. This portion of the fetus is referred to as the **presenting part**. Fetal presentation may be cephalic, breech, or shoulder. Cephalic presentation, in which the fetal head presents itself to the passage, occurs in approximately 97% of term births. When this presentation occurs, labor and birth are likely to proceed normally. Breech and shoulder presentations are associated with difficulties during labor, and labor does not proceed as expected; therefore, they are called **malpresentations** (see Chapter 22 ✪ for discussion of malpresentations).

The cephalic presentation can be further classified according to the degree of flexion or extension of the fetal head (attitude):

- *Vertex presentation.* The most common type of presentation; the fetal head is completely flexed onto the chest, and the smallest diameter of the fetal head (suboccipitobregmatic) presents to the maternal pelvis (Figure 17–6*A* ●); the occiput is the presenting part.
- *Sinciput presentation* (also called *military presentation*). The fetal head is neither flexed nor extended; the occipitofrontal diameter presents to the maternal pelvis (Figure 17–6*B* ●); the top of the head is the presenting part.
- *Brow presentation.* The fetal head is partially extended; the occipitomental diameter, the largest anteroposterior diameter, is presented to the maternal pelvis (Figure 17–6*C* ●); the sinciput is the presenting part (see Figure 17–3).
- *Face presentation.* The fetal head is hyperextended (completely extended); the submentobregmatic diameter presents to the maternal pelvis (Figure 17–6*D* ●); the face is the presenting part.

Breech presentation is a birth in which the buttocks and/or feet are the presenting part rather than the head. It occurs in 3% to 4% of term pregnancies. These presentations are classified according to the attitude of the fetus's hips and knees. In all

| **A** Suboccipitobregmatic diameter | **B** Occipitofrontal diameter | **C** Occipitomental diameter | **D** Submentobregmatic diameter |

● **Figure 17–6** Cephalic presentation. *A*, Vertex presentation. Complete flexion of the head allows the suboccipitobregmatic diameter to present to the pelvis. *B*, Sinciput (median vertex) presentation (also called *military presentation*) with no flexion or extension. The occipitofrontal diameter presents to the pelvis. *C*, Brow presentation. The fetal head is in complete extension, and the submentobregmatic diameter presents to the pelvis. *D*, Face presentation. The fetal head is in partial (halfway) extension. The occipitomental diameter, which is the largest diameter of the fetal head, presents to the pelvis.

Activity | Care Plan: Patient in Uncomplicated Labor | Animation | Vaginal Birth

the following variations of the breech presentation, the sacrum is the landmark to be noted:

- *Complete breech.* The fetal knees and hips are both flexed; the thighs are on the abdomen, and the calves are on the posterior aspect of the thighs; the buttocks and feet of the fetus present to the maternal pelvis. (See Figure 22–7 🗗 on page 475.)

- *Frank breech.* The fetal hips are flexed, and the knees are extended; the buttocks of the fetus present to the maternal pelvis.

- *Footling breech.* The fetal hips and legs are extended, and the feet of the fetus present to the maternal pelvis. In a single footling, one foot presents; in a double footling, both feet present.

A shoulder presentation is also called a *transverse lie*. Most frequently the shoulder is the presenting part and the acromion process of the scapula is the landmark to be noted. However, the fetal arm, back, abdomen, or side may present in a transverse lie (see Chapter 22 🗗).

Relationship Between the Maternal Pelvis and Presenting Part

Engagement

Engagement of the presenting part occurs when the largest diameter of the presenting part reaches or passes through the pelvic inlet and is at the level of the ischial spines (Figure 17–7 ●). Engagement can be determined by vaginal examination. In primigravidas, engagement occurs approximately 2 weeks before term. Multiparas, however, may experience engagement several weeks before the onset of labor or during the process of labor. Engagement confirms the adequacy of the pelvic inlet. Engagement does not, however, indicate whether the midpelvis and outlet are also adequate.

Station

Station refers to the relationship of the presenting part to an imaginary line drawn between the ischial spines of the maternal pelvis. In a normal pelvis, the ischial spines mark the narrowest diameter through which the fetus must pass. These spines are not sharp protrusions that harm the fetus but blunted prominences at the midpelvis. The ischial spines as a landmark have been designated as zero station (Figure 17–8 ●). If the presenting part is higher than the ischial spines, a negative number is assigned, noting centimeters above zero station. Positive numbers indicate that the presenting part has passed the ischial spines. Station –5 is at the pelvic inlet, and station +4 is at the outlet. If the presenting part can be seen at the woman's perineum, birth is imminent. During labor the presenting part should move progressively from the negative stations to the midpelvis at zero station and into the positive stations. If the presenting part fails to descend in the presence of strong contractions, there may be disproportion between the maternal pelvis and fetal presenting part.

Fetal Position

Fetal position refers to the relationship of a designated landmark on the presenting fetal part to the front, sides, or back of the maternal pelvis. The landmark chosen for vertex presentations is the occiput, and the landmark for face presentations is the mentum. In breech presentations the sacrum is the designated landmark, and the acromion process on the scapula is the landmark in shoulder presentations. If the landmark is directed toward the side of the pelvis, fetal position is designated as *transverse*, rather than anterior or posterior. Three notations are used to describe fetal position:

1. Right (R) or left (L) side of the maternal pelvis
2. The landmark of the fetal presenting part: occiput (O), mentum (M), sacrum (S), or acromion process (A)
3. Anterior (A), posterior (P), or transverse (T), depending on whether the landmark is in the front, back, or side of the pelvis

Figure 17–7 Process of engagement in cephalic presentation. *A*, Floating. The fetal head is directed down toward the pelvis but can still easily move away from the inlet. *B*, Dipping. The fetal head dips into the inlet but can be moved away by exerting pressure on the fetus. *C*, Engaged. The biparietal diameter (BPD) of the fetal head is in the inlet of the pelvis. In most instances the presenting part (occiput) is at the level of the ischial spines (zero station).

Figure 17–8 Measuring the station of the fetal head while it is descending. In this view the station is −2/−3.

These abbreviations help the healthcare team communicate the fetal position. Thus when the fetal occiput is directed toward the back and left of the birth passage, the abbreviation used is LOP (left occiput posterior). The term *dorsal* (D) is used when denoting the fetal position in a transverse lie; it refers to the fetal back. For example, RADA indicates that the acromion process of the scapula is directed toward the woman's right, and the fetus's back is anterior.

The most frequently occurring positions are illustrated in Figure 17–9 ●. The most common fetal position is occiput anterior. When this position occurs, labor and birth are likely to proceed normally. Positions other than occiput anterior are more frequently associated with problems during labor; therefore, they are called *malpositions*. (See Chapter 22 ● for more information about malpositions.)

Assessment techniques to determine fetal position include inspection and palpation of the maternal abdomen and vaginal examination. They are discussed in Chapter 18 ●.

Physiologic Forces of Labor

Primary and secondary forces work together to achieve birth of the fetus, the fetal membranes, and the placenta. The *primary force* is uterine muscular contractions, which cause the complete effacement and dilatation of the cervix. The *secondary force* is the use of abdominal muscles to push during the second stage of labor. The pushing adds to the primary force after full dilatation.

● **Figure 17–9** Categories of presentation.

Dilatation is the process of the cervix opening during the labor process. The cervix *dilates* or opens from 0 to 10 centimeters during the first stage of labor in response to uterine contractions.

In labor, uterine contractions are rhythmic but intermittent. Between contractions a period of relaxation occurs. This allows uterine muscles to rest and provides relief for the laboring woman. It also restores uteroplacental circulation, which is important to fetal oxygenation and adequate circulation in the uterine blood vessels.

Each contraction has three phases: (1) *increment*, the building up of the contraction (the longest phase); (2) *acme*, or the peak of the contraction; and (3) *decrement*, or the letting up of the contraction. The terms *frequency, duration,* and *intensity* are used to describe uterine contractions during labor. **Frequency** refers to the time between the beginning of one contraction and the beginning of the next contraction. **Duration** is measured from the beginning of a contraction to the completion of that same contraction (Figure 17–10 ●). **Intensity** refers to the strength of the contraction during acme. In most instances, intensity is estimated by palpating the uterine fundus during a contraction, but it may be measured directly with an intrauterine catheter. When estimating intensity by palpation, the nurse determines whether it is mild, moderate, or strong by judging the amount of indentability of the uterine wall during the acme of a contraction. If the uterine wall can be indented easily, the contraction is considered mild. Strong intensity exists when the uterine wall cannot be indented. Moderate intensity falls somewhere between. When intensity is measured with an intrauterine catheter, the normal resting pressure in the uterus (between contractions) averages 10 to 12 mm Hg. During acme the intensity ranges from 25 to 40 mm Hg in early labor, 50 to 70 mm Hg in active labor, 70 to 90 mm Hg during transition, and 70 to 100 mm Hg while the woman is pushing in the second stage (Blackburn, 2013). (See Chapter 18 ⊘ for further discussion of assessment techniques.)

At the beginning of labor, contractions are usually mild. As labor progresses, the duration, intensity, and frequency of contractions increase. Contractions are involuntary; the laboring woman cannot control their duration, frequency, or intensity.

After the cervix is completely dilated, the maternal abdominal muscles contract as the woman pushes. This pushing action (called *bearing down*) aids in the expulsion of the fetus and placenta. If the cervix is not completely dilated, however, bearing down can cause cervical edema (which retards dilatation), possible tearing and bruising of the cervix, and maternal exhaustion.

The duration of labor varies considerably and is related to multiple factors including fetal factors such as presentation, position, fetal weight, number of fetuses, and the station of the presenting part; maternal factors such as age, parity, maternal body weight, pain threshold, and maternal positioning during labor; uterine factors such as the intensity, frequency, and duration of contractions; and obstetric interventions such as the use of epidural anesthesia or other medications, whether the labor was induced or augmented with Pitocin infusions, and whether instrument interventions such as forceps or vacuum delivery were performed (Ijaiya et al., 2010).

THE PHYSIOLOGY OF LABOR

Possible Causes of Labor Onset

The process of labor usually begins between the 38th and 42nd week of gestation, when the fetus is mature and ready for birth. The exact cause of labor onset is not clearly understood. However, some important aspects have been identified:

- Progesterone relaxes smooth muscle tissue.
- Estrogen stimulates uterine muscle contractions.
- Connective tissue loosens to permit the softening, thinning, and eventual opening of the cervix (Blackburn, 2013).

Currently, researchers are focusing on the role of fetal membranes (chorion and amnion), the decidua, and the effect of progesterone withdrawal, of prostaglandin, and of corticotropin-releasing hormone in relation to labor onset (Blackburn, 2013).

Progesterone Withdrawal Hypothesis

Progesterone, produced by the placenta, relaxes uterine smooth muscle by interfering with the conduction of impulses from one cell to the next. During pregnancy, progesterone exerts a quieting effect and the uterus generally does not have coordinated contractions. Toward the end of gestation, biochemical changes decrease the availability of progesterone to myometrial cells and may be associated with an antiprogestin that inhibits the relaxant effect but allows other progesterone actions such as lactogenesis. With the decreased availability of progesterone, estrogen is better able to stimulate contractions (Blackburn, 2013). Interestingly, progesterone administration is now used as a mechanism to prevent preterm labor and birth (Blackburn, 2013).

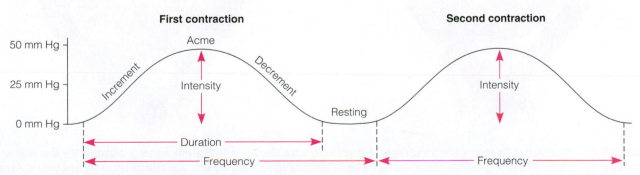

● **Figure 17–10** Characteristics of uterine contractions.

Prostaglandin Hypothesis

Although the exact relationship between prostaglandin and the onset of labor is not yet known, the effect is clinically demonstrated by the successful induction of labor after vaginal application of prostaglandin E. Preterm labor may be stopped by using an inhibitor of prostaglandin synthesis. Oxytocin may also play a role in the process in two ways: first by direct stimulation of uterine contractions and second, indirectly, by stimulating prostaglandin production by the amnion and decidua (Blackburn, 2013).

Corticotropin-Releasing Hormone

Corticotropin-releasing hormone (CRH) has a possible role in labor onset. It increases throughout pregnancy, with a sharp increase at term. Plasma CRH is also increased before preterm labor, and CRH levels are elevated in multiple gestation. CRH is known to stimulate the synthesis of prostaglandin F and prostaglandin E by amnion cells (Kalantaridos et al., 2011).

Myometrial Activity

In true labor the muscles of the upper uterine segment shorten and exert a longitudinal pull on the cervix with each contraction, causing effacement. **Effacement** is the drawing up of the internal os and the cervical canal into the side walls of the uterus. The cervix changes progressively from a long, thick structure to one that is tissue-paper thin (Figure 17–11 ●). In primigravidas, effacement usually occurs before dilatation.

● **Figure 17–11** Effacement of the cervix in the primigravida. *A*, Beginning of labor. There is no cervical effacement or dilatation. The fetal head is cushioned by amniotic fluid. *B*, Beginning cervical effacement. As the cervix begins to efface, more amniotic fluid collects below the fetal head. *C*, Cervix about one-half effaced and slightly dilated. The increasing amount of amniotic fluid exerts hydrostatic pressure. *D*, Complete effacement and dilatation.

The uterus elongates with each contraction, decreasing the horizontal diameter. This elongation causes a straightening of the fetal body, pressing the upper portion against the fundus and thrusting the presenting part down toward the lower uterine segment and the cervix. The pressure exerted by the fetus is called the *fetal axis pressure*. As the uterus elongates, the longitudinal muscle fibers are pulled upward over the presenting part. This action and the hydrostatic pressure of the fetal membranes cause cervical dilatation. The cervical os and cervical canal widen from less than 1 cm to approximately 10 cm, allowing birth of the fetus. When the cervix is completely dilated and retracted up into the lower uterine segment, it can no longer be palpated. At the same time, the round ligament pulls the fundus forward, aligning the fetus with the bony pelvis.

Musculature Changes in the Pelvic Floor

The levator ani muscle and fascia of the pelvic floor draw the rectum and vagina upward and forward with each contraction, along the curve of the pelvic floor. As the fetal head descends to the pelvic floor, the pressure of the presenting part causes the perineal structure, which was once 5 cm in thickness, to thin to less than 1 cm. The anus everts, exposing the interior rectal wall as the fetal head descends forward (Blackburn, 2013).

Premonitory Signs of Labor

Most primigravidas and many multiparas experience the following signs and symptoms of impending labor.

Lightening

Lightening describes the effects that occur when the fetus begins to settle into the pelvic inlet (engagement). With fetal descent the uterus moves downward, and the fundus no longer presses on the diaphragm, which allows breathing to become easier. However, with increased downward pressure of the presenting part, the woman may notice the following:

- Leg cramps or pains due to pressure on the nerves that pass through the obturator foramen in the pelvis
- Increased pelvic pressure
- Increased venous stasis, leading to edema in the lower extremities
- Increased vaginal secretions resulting from congestion of the vaginal mucous membranes

Braxton Hicks Contractions

Before the onset of labor, *Braxton Hicks contractions* (the irregular, intermittent contractions that have been occurring throughout the pregnancy) may become uncomfortable. The pain seems to be focused in the abdomen and groin but may feel like the "drawing" sensations experienced by some women with dysmenorrhea. When these contractions are strong enough for the woman to believe she is in labor, she is said to be in *false labor*. False labor is uncomfortable and may be exhausting. Since the contractions can be fairly regular, the woman has no way of knowing if they are true labor.

Cervical Changes

Considerable change occurs in the cervix during the prenatal and intrapartum period. At the beginning of pregnancy, the cervix is rigid and firm, and it must soften so it can stretch and dilate to allow the fetus passage. This softening of the cervix is called *ripening*.

As term approaches, collagen fibers in the cervix are broken down by certain enzymes. As the fibers change, their ability to bind together decreases, while the water content of the cervix increases. These changes result in a weakening and softening of the cervix.

Bloody Show

During pregnancy, cervical secretions accumulate in the cervical canal to form a barrier called a *mucous plug*. With softening and effacement of the cervix, the mucous plug is often expelled, resulting in a small amount of blood loss from the exposed cervical capillaries. The resulting pink-tinged secretions are called **bloody show**. Bloody show is considered a sign that labor will begin within 24 to 48 hours. Recent intercourse or vaginal examination that includes manipulation of the cervix may also result in a blood-tinged discharge, which may be confused with bloody show.

Rupture of Membranes

Approximately 10% of women at term (38 through 41 weeks' gestation) experience rupture of the amniotic membranes (ROM) before the onset of labor. Rupture of membranes occurs when the amniotic sac surrounding the fetus, amniotic fluid, and placenta ruptures or is perforated and results in the expulsion of amniotic fluid from the vagina (Cunningham et al., 2010). After the membranes rupture, 90% of women give birth within 24 hours (Jazayeri, 2011). Women who are 34 weeks' gestation or more and who present with ruptured membranes without contractions are often started on an oxytocin infusion to decrease the incidence of chorioamnionitis. Women with preterm gestations of less than 34 weeks are managed conservatively provided both the mother and the fetus are stable (Jazayeri, 2011).

When the membranes rupture, the amniotic fluid may be expelled in large amounts. If engagement has not occurred, there is danger of the umbilical cord washing out with the fluid (prolapsed cord). In addition, the open pathway into the uterus increases the risk of infection. Because of these risks, when the membranes rupture, the woman is advised to call her certified nurse-midwife or physician and proceed to the hospital or birthing center. In some instances the fluid is expelled in small amounts and may be confused with episodes of urinary incontinence associated with urinary urgency, coughing, or sneezing. The discharge should be checked to determine its source and the appropriate action. (See Chapter 18 🔴 for assessment techniques.)

Sudden Burst of Energy

Some women report a sudden burst of energy approximately 24 to 48 hours before labor. The cause of the energy spurt is unknown. In prenatal teaching it is important to warn prospective mothers not to overexert themselves during this energy burst to avoid being overtired when labor begins.

Animation
Rupturing Membranes

Case Study: Patient in First Stage of Labor

Activity

First Stage of Labor and Transition

Video

Clinical Tip

Encourage expectant mothers who experience a sudden burst of energy to eat small, frequent, nutritious meals during this period, and to rest. Encourage the pregnant woman to have her spouse or partner or a friend do chores and activities that she feels are essential to complete before the baby arrives.

Other Signs

Additional premonitory signs include the following:

- Weight loss of 1 to 3 lb resulting from fluid loss and electrolyte shifts produced by changes in estrogen and progesterone levels

- Diarrhea, indigestion, or nausea and vomiting just before onset of labor

The causes of these signs are unknown.

Differences Between True and False Labor

The contractions of true labor produce progressive dilatation and effacement of the cervix. They occur regularly and increase in frequency, duration, and intensity. The discomfort of true labor contractions usually starts in the back and radiates around to the abdomen. The pain is not relieved by ambulation (in fact, walking may intensify the pain).

The contractions of false labor do not produce progressive cervical effacement and dilatation. Classically, they are irregular and do not increase in frequency, duration, and intensity. The contractions may be perceived as a hardening or "balling up" without discomfort, or discomfort may occur mainly in the lower abdomen and groin. The discomfort may be relieved by ambulation, changes of position, drinking a large amount of water, or a warm shower or tub bath. Many times the only way to differentiate accurately between true and false labor is to assess effacement and dilatation. The woman must feel free to come in for accurate assessment of labor and should be counseled not to feel foolish if the labor is false. She can be reassured that false labor is common and that it often cannot be distinguished from true labor except by vaginal examination (Table 17–3).

STAGES OF LABOR AND BIRTH

The labor process is divided into phases and stages of labor. These represent theoretic separations in the process. A laboring woman does not usually experience distinct differences from one stage to the next.

The *first stage* begins with the onset of true labor and ends when the cervix is completely dilated to 10 cm. The *second stage* begins with complete dilatation and ends with the birth of the baby. The *third stage* begins with the birth of the baby and ends with the expulsion of the placenta. Some clinicians identify a *fourth stage*. During this stage, which lasts 1 to 4 hours after expulsion of the placenta, the uterus contracts to control bleeding at the placental site (Simkin & Ancheta, 2011).

First Stage

The first stage of labor is divided into the *latent, active,* and *transition* phases. Each phase of labor is characterized by physical and psychologic changes.

Latent Phase

The *latent phase* starts with the beginning of regular contractions, which are usually mild. The woman feels able to cope with the discomfort. She may be relieved that labor has finally started. Although she may be anxious, she is able to recognize and express those feelings of anxiety. The woman is often talkative and smiling and is eager to talk about herself and answer questions. Excitement is high, and her partner or other support person is often as elated as she is.

Uterine contractions become established during the latent phase and increase in frequency, duration, and intensity. They may start as mild contractions lasting 30 seconds with a frequency of 10 to 30 minutes and progress to moderate ones lasting 30 to 40 seconds with a frequency of 5 to 7 minutes. As the cervix begins to dilate, it also effaces, although little or no fetal descent is evident. For a woman in her first labor (nullipara), the latent (or early) phase of the first stage of labor averages 8.6 hours but should not exceed 20 hours. The latent phase in multiparas averages 5.3 hours but should not exceed 14 hours.

Table 17–3	Comparison of True and False Labor	
True Labor	**False Labor**
Contractions occur at regular intervals.	Contractions are irregular.
Interval between contractions gradually shortens.	Usually no change.
Contractions increase in duration and intensity.	Usually no change.
Discomfort begins in back and radiates around to abdomen.	Discomfort is usually in abdomen.
Intensity usually increases with walking.	Walking has no effect on or lessens contractions.
Cervical dilatation and effacement are progressive.	No change.

At the beginning of labor, the amniotic membranes bulge through the cervix in the shape of a cone. **Spontaneous rupture of membranes (SROM)** generally occurs at the height of an intense contraction with a gush of fluid out of the vagina. In many instances the membranes are ruptured by the certified nurse-midwife (CNM) or physician, using an instrument called an *amniohook*. This procedure is called an *amniotomy*, or **artificial rupture of membranes (AROM)**.

Active Phase

When a woman enters the early *active phase*, her anxiety tends to increase as she senses the intensification of contractions and pain. She begins to fear a loss of control and may use a variety of coping mechanisms. Some women show decreased ability to cope and a sense of helplessness. Women who have support people and family available may feel greater satisfaction and less anxiety than those without support. During this phase the cervix dilates from about 4 to 7 cm. Fetal descent is progressive. Cervical dilatation averages 1.2 cm/hr in nulliparas and 1.5 cm/hr in multiparas.

Transition Phase

The *transition phase* is the last part of the first stage of labor. When the woman enters transition, she may show significant anxiety. She becomes acutely aware of the increasing force and intensity of the contractions. She may become restless, frequently changing position. By the time the woman enters the transition phase, she is inner directed and often tired. She may fear being left alone at the same time the support person may be feeling the need for a break. The nurse should reassure the woman that she will not be left alone. It is important to be available as relief support at this time and to keep the woman informed about where her labor support people are, if they leave the room.

During the active and transition phases, contractions become more frequent and longer in duration, and they increase in intensity. During transition, contractions have a frequency of about every 1½ to 2 minutes, a duration of 60 to 90 seconds, and strong intensity. Cervical dilatation slows as it progresses from 8 to 10 cm, and the rate of fetal descent dramatically increases. The average rate of descent is 1.6 cm/hr and at least 1 cm/hr in nulliparas; the average rate is 5.4 cm/hr and at least 2.1 cm/hr in multiparas. The transition phase does not usually last longer than 3 hours for nulliparas or longer than 1 hour for multiparas (Simkin & Ancheta, 2011).

As dilatation approaches 10 cm, the woman may feel increased rectal pressure and an uncontrollable desire to bear down, the amount of bloody show may increase, and the membranes may rupture (if it has not already occurred). The woman may also fear that she will be "torn open" or "split apart" by the force of the contractions. With the peak of a contraction, she may experience a sensation of pressure so great that it seems to her that her abdomen will burst open with the force. The nurse should inform the woman that what she is feeling is normal. The woman may doubt her ability to cope with labor and may become apprehensive, irritable, and withdrawn. She may be terrified of being left alone, though she does not want anyone to talk to or touch her. However, with the next contraction she may ask for verbal and physical support. Other characteristics of this phase may include the following:

- Increasing bloody show
- Hyperventilation, as the woman increases her breathing rate
- Generalized discomfort, including low backache, shaking and cramping in legs, and increased sensitivity to touch
- Increased need for partner's or nurse's presence and support
- Restlessness
- Increased apprehension and irritability
- Difficulty understanding directions
- A sense of bewilderment, frustration, and anger at the contractions
- Requests for medication
- Hiccuping, belching, nausea, or vomiting
- Beads of perspiration on the upper lip or brow
- Increasing rectal pressure and an urge to bear down

The woman in this phase is anxious to "get it over with." She may be amnesic and sleep between her frequent contractions. Her support persons may start to feel helpless and may turn to the nurse for increased help as their efforts to alleviate her discomfort seem less effective.

Second Stage

The second stage of labor begins with complete cervical dilatation and ends with birth of the infant. The second stage is usually completed within 3 hours after the cervix becomes fully dilated for primigravidas; the stage averages 15 minutes for multiparas. Contractions continue with a frequency of about every 1½ to 2 minutes, duration of 60 to 90 seconds, and strong intensity. Descent of the fetal presenting part continues until it reaches the perineal floor.

Some authors have further subdivided the second stage into two phases including the latent/passive fetal descent stage in which the woman may initially experience the urge to push. During this time, passive fetal descent occurs in response to the uterine contractions. Nursing tasks during this phase include (Association of Women's Health, Obstetric and Neonatal Nurses [AWHONN], 2007):

- Assessing the woman's perception of the need or urge to push
- Evaluating the maternal–fetal oxygenation status to ensure adequate uteroplacental perfusion is occurring
- Assessing fetal status through recommended monitoring protocols

Developing Cultural Competence
Presence of the Father

The presence of the father during labor and at birth, although common in countries such as the United States, Canada, and Australia, is not a universal norm. Rather it is strongly influenced by cultural practices. The father is not present at the birth in many countries, including Algeria, Brazil, China, Ethiopia, and Korea. Similarly, Orthodox Jews do not allow men to attend the labor and birth (Spector, 2012).

Video | Second Stage of Labor

The second phase (within the second stage of labor) is known as the active pushing phase and occurs once the urge to push has been established and the woman begins to actively push with her contractions. Nursing tasks during this phase include (AWHONN, 2007):

- Assessing the effectiveness of the maternal pushing efforts
- Providing encouragement and direction to obtain a more adequate pushing effort
- Assessing fetal response that occurs as maternal pushing is performed including continued fetal assessment measures

While some women may be encouraged to begin pushing immediately after the identification of complete dilatation, others may be encouraged to delay pushing and allow for passive fetal descent, an act known as "laboring down." A recent systematic review comparing both methods of pushing did not identify any differences in maternal or fetal outcomes; however, women in the passive descent or laboring down group experienced a longer second stage of labor that resulted in a reduction of active pushing efforts (Tuuli, Frey, Odibo, et al., 2012). Laboring down does aid the woman who is extremely fatigued and does prevent extensive pushing efforts that may occur before the urge to push is experienced by the woman.

As the fetal head descends, the woman usually has the urge to push because of pressure of the fetal head on the sacral and obturator nerves. As she pushes, contraction of the maternal abdominal muscles exerts intra-abdominal pressure. As the fetal head continues its descent, the perineum begins to bulge, flatten, and move anteriorly. The amount of bloody show may increase. The labia begin to part with each contraction. Between contractions the fetal head appears to recede. With succeeding contractions and maternal pushing effort, the fetal head descends farther. **Crowning** occurs when the fetal head is encircled by the external opening of the vagina (introitus), and it means birth is imminent.

The woman may feel some relief that the acute pain she felt during the transition phase is over (Table 17–4). She may also be relieved that the birth is near and she can push. Some women feel a sense of purpose that they can be actively involved. Others, particularly those without childbirth preparation, may become frightened and fight each contraction. Such behavior may be disconcerting to the woman's support persons. The woman may feel she has lost her ability to cope and become embarrassed, or she may demonstrate extreme irritability toward the staff or her supporters as she attempts to regain control over forces against which she feels helpless. Most women feel acute, increasingly severe pain and a burning sensation as the perineum distends.

Spontaneous Birth (Vertex Presentation)

As the fetal head distends the vulva with each contraction, the perineum becomes extremely thin and the anus stretches and protrudes. With time the head extends under the symphysis pubis and is born. When the anterior shoulder meets the underside of the symphysis pubis, a gentle push by the mother aids in the birth of the shoulders. The body then follows (see a birthing sequence in Figure 17–12 ●). (Birth of a fetus in other than a vertex presentation is discussed in Chapter 22 ⊘.)

Cardinal Movements of Labor

For the fetus to pass through the birth canal, the fetal head and body must adjust to the passage by certain positional changes. These changes, called **cardinal movements** or mechanisms of labor, are described in the order in which they occur (Figure 17–13 ●).

Descent.   Descent occurs because of four forces: (1) pressure of the amniotic fluid, (2) direct pressure of the uterine fundus on the breech, (3) contraction of the abdominal muscles, and (4) extension and straightening of the fetal body. The head enters the inlet

(left margin) Care Plan: Labor Progress | Activity

Table 17–4	Characteristics of Labor			
	First Stage			**Second Stage**
	Latent Phase	Active Phase	Transition Phase	
Nullipara	8.6 hr	4.6 hr	3.6 hr	Up to 3 hr
Multipara	5.3 hr	2.4 hr	Variable	Less than 1 hr; averages 15 min
Cervical dilatation	0–3 cm	4–7 cm	8–10 cm	
CONTRACTIONS				
Frequency	Every 10–30 min, progressing to every 5–7 min	Every 2–3 min	Every 1½–2 min	Every 1½–2 min
Duration	30–40 sec	40–60 sec	60–90 sec	60–90 sec
Intensity	Begin as mild and progress to moderate; 25–40 mm Hg by intrauterine pressure catheter (IUPC)	Begin as moderate and progress to strong; 50–70 mm Hg by IUPC	Strong by palpation; 70–90 mm Hg by IUPC	Strong by palpation; 70–100 mm Hg by IUPC

● **Figure 17–12** A birthing sequence.

● **Figure 17–13** Mechanisms of labor. *A* and *B*, Descent. *C*, Internal rotation. *D*, Extension. *E*, External rotation.

in the occiput transverse or oblique position because the pelvic inlet is widest from side to side. The sagittal suture is an equal distance from the maternal symphysis pubis and sacral promontory.

Flexion. Flexion occurs as the fetal head descends and meets resistance from the soft tissues of the pelvis, the muscles of the pelvic floor, and the cervix. As a result of the resistance, the fetal chin flexes downward onto the chest.

Internal Rotation. The fetal head must rotate to fit the diameter of the pelvic cavity, which is widest in the anteroposterior diameter. As the occiput of the fetal head meets resistance from the levator ani muscles and their fascia, the occiput rotates—usually from left to right—and the sagittal suture aligns in the anteroposterior pelvic diameter.

Extension. The resistance of the pelvic floor, and the mechanical movement of the vulva opening anteriorly and forward, assist with extension of the fetal head as it passes under the symphysis pubis. With this positional change, the occiput, then brow and face, emerge from the vagina.

Restitution. The shoulders of the fetus enter the pelvic inlet obliquely and remain oblique when the head rotates to the anteroposterior diameter through internal rotation. Because of this rotation, the neck becomes twisted. Once the head is born and is free of pelvic resistance, the neck untwists, turning the head to one side (restitution), and aligns with the position of the back in the birth canal.

External Rotation. As the shoulders rotate to the anteroposterior position in the pelvis, the head turns farther to one side (external rotation).

Expulsion. After the external rotation, and through the pushing efforts of the laboring woman, the anterior shoulder meets the undersurface of the symphysis pubis and slips under it. As lateral flexion of the shoulder and head occurs, the anterior shoulder is born before the posterior shoulder. The body follows quickly.

Third Stage

Placental Separation

After the infant is born, the uterus contracts firmly, decreasing its capacity and the surface area of placental attachment. The placenta begins to separate because of this decreased surface area. As separation occurs, bleeding results in the formation of a hematoma between the placental tissue and the remaining decidua. This hematoma speeds the separation process. The membranes are the last to separate. They are peeled off the uterine wall as the placenta descends into the vagina. Signs of placental separation usually appear about 5 minutes after the birth of the newborn. These signs are (1) a globular-shaped uterus, (2) a rise of the fundus in the abdomen, (3) a sudden gush or trickle of blood, and (4) further protrusion of the umbilical cord out of the vagina.

Placental Delivery

When the signs of placental separation appear, the woman may bear down to aid in placental expulsion. If this fails and the certified nurse-midwife or physician has ascertained that the fundus is firm, gentle traction may be applied to the cord while pressure is exerted on the fundus. The weight of the placenta as it is guided into the placental collection pan aids in the removal of the membranes from the uterine wall. A placenta is considered to be retained if 30 minutes have elapsed from completion of the second stage of labor.

A

Bleeding

B

Bleeding

● **Figure 17–14** Placental separation and expulsion. *A*, Schultze mechanism. *B*, Duncan mechanism.

If the placenta separates from the inside to the outer margins, it is expelled with the fetal (shiny) side presenting (Figure 17–14 ●). This is known as the Schultze mechanism of placental delivery or, more commonly, "shiny Schultze" (also see Figure 4–9 🔗 on page 71). If the placenta separates from the outer margins inward, it rolls up and presents sideways with the maternal surface expelled first. This is known as the Duncan mechanism and is commonly called "dirty Duncan" because the placental surface is rough (also see Figure 4–8 🔗 on page 71). (Interventions for the third stage are discussed in Chapter 19 🔗.)

Fourth Stage

The fourth stage of labor is the time, from 1 to 4 hours after birth, during which physiologic readjustment of the mother's body begins. With the birth, hemodynamic changes occur. Blood loss ranges from 250 to 500 mL. With this blood loss and removal of the weight of the pregnant uterus from the surrounding vessels, blood is redistributed into venous beds. This results in a moderate drop in both systolic and diastolic blood pressure, increased pulse pressure, and moderate tachycardia (Cunningham et al., 2010).

The uterus remains contracted in the midline of the abdomen. The fundus is usually midway between the symphysis pubis and umbilicus. Its contracted state constricts the vessels at the site of placental implantation. Immediately after expulsion of the placenta, the cervix is widely spread and thick.

Nausea and vomiting usually cease. The woman may be thirsty and hungry. She may experience a shaking chill, which is thought to be associated with the ending of the physical exertion of labor. The bladder is often hypotonic due to trauma during the second stage or the administration of anesthetics that decrease sensations. Hypotonic bladder can lead to urinary retention.

SAFETY ALERT!

During the fourth stage of labor, women should be assisted during their initial attempt to ambulate since dizziness and syncope can lead to falls. The woman should be advised not to hold the baby with ambulation when first attempting ambulation after the birth.

MATERNAL SYSTEMIC RESPONSE TO LABOR

The process of labor and birth affects almost all maternal physiologic systems.

Cardiovascular System

Uterine contractions and the pain, anxiety, and apprehension a laboring woman experiences stress her cardiovascular system. With each contraction, 300 to 500 mL of blood volume is forced back into the maternal circulation, which results in an increase in cardiac output of as much as 10% to 15% over the typical third-trimester levels (Blackburn, 2013). Cardiac output increases more as the laboring woman experiences pain with uterine contractions and her anxiety and apprehension increase.

Maternal position also affects cardiac output. In the supine position, cardiac output decreases, heart rate increases, and stroke volume decreases. When the woman turns to a lateral (side-lying) position, cardiac output increases (Blackburn, 2013).

Blood Pressure

As a result of increased cardiac output, blood pressure rises during uterine contractions. In the first stage, systolic pressure increases by 35 mm Hg and diastolic pressure increases by about

25 mm Hg. There may be further increases in the second stage during pushing (Blackburn, 2013).

Respiratory System

Oxygen demand and consumption increase when labor begins because of the presence of uterine contractions. As anxiety and pain from contractions increase, hyperventilation frequently occurs. With hyperventilation there is a fall in $PaCO_2$, and respiratory alkalosis results (Powrie, Greene, & Camann, 2012).

By the end of the first stage, most women have developed a mild metabolic acidosis compensated by respiratory alkalosis. As they push in the second stage of labor, their $PaCO_2$ levels may rise along with blood lactate levels (due to muscular activity), and mild respiratory acidosis occurs. By the time the baby is born (end of second stage), the woman has metabolic acidosis uncompensated for by respiratory alkalosis. The changes in acid–base status that occur in labor are quickly reversed in the fourth stage because of changes in women's respiratory rates. Acid–base levels return to pregnancy levels by 24 hours after birth, and to nonpregnant values a few weeks after birth (Powrie et al., 2012).

Renal System

During labor there is an increase in maternal renin, plasma renin activity, and angiotensinogen. This elevation is thought to be important in the control of uteroplacental blood flow during birth and the early postpartum period. Structurally the base of the bladder is pushed forward and upward when engagement occurs. The pressure from the presenting part may impair blood and lymph drainage from the base of the bladder, leading to edema (Cunningham et al., 2010).

Gastrointestinal System

During labor, gastric motility and absorption of solid food are reduced. Gastric emptying time is prolonged, and gastric volume (amount of contents that remain in the stomach) remains increased, regardless of the time the last meal was taken. Some narcotics also delay gastric emptying time and add to the risk of aspiration if general anesthesia is used.

Immune System and Other Blood Values

The white blood cell (WBC) count increases to 25,000 to 30,000/mm³ during labor and the early postpartum period. The change in WBC count is mostly due to increased neutrophils resulting from a physiologic response to stress. The increased WBC count makes it difficult to identify an infection. Maternal blood glucose levels decrease because the body uses glucose as an energy source during contractions. Decreased blood glucose levels lead to a decrease in insulin requirements.

Pain

Pain during labor comes from a complexity of physical causes. Each woman will experience and cope with pain differently. Multiple factors affect a woman's reaction to labor pain.

Causes of Pain During Labor

The pain associated with the first stage of labor is unique in that it accompanies a normal physiologic process. Even though perception of the pain of childbirth varies among women, there is a physiologic basis for discomfort during labor. Pain during the first stage of labor arises from (1) dilatation of the cervix, which is the primary source of pain; (2) stretching of the lower uterine segment; (3) pressure on adjacent structures; and (4) hypoxia of the uterine muscle cells during contraction (Blackburn, 2013). The areas of pain include the lower abdominal wall and the areas over the lower lumbar region and the upper sacrum (Figure 17–15 ●).

During the second stage of labor, discomfort is due to (1) hypoxia of the contracting uterine muscle cells, (2) distention of the

● **Figure 17–15** Area of reference of labor pain during the first stage. Pain is most intense in the darkened areas.

vagina and perineum, and (3) pressure on adjacent structures. The area of pain increases as shown in Figures 17–16 ● and 17–17 ●.

Pain during the third stage results from uterine contractions and cervical dilatation as the placenta is expelled. This stage of labor is short, and after it anesthesia is needed primarily for episiotomy repair.

Factors Affecting Response to Pain

Many factors affect the individual's perception of and response to pain. For example, research shows that childbirth preparation classes often reduce the need for analgesia during labor. People tend to respond to painful stimuli in the way that is acceptable in their culture. In some cultures it is natural to communicate pain,

● **Figure 17–16** Distribution of labor pain during the later phase of the first stage and early phase of the second stage. The darkest colored areas indicate the location of the most intense pain, moderate color indicates moderate pain, and lighter color indicates mild pain. The uterine contractions, which at this stage are very strong, produce intense pain.

● **Figure 17–17** Distribution of labor pain during the later phase of the second stage and actual birth. The perineal component is the primary cause of discomfort. Uterine contractions contribute much less to the level of pain.

Complementary Care Music During Childbirth

The therapeutic use of music to help with pain management is becoming increasingly popular. Research suggests that soft music can help decrease both the sensation of labor pain and a woman's response to it. With this in mind, the woman should choose her music selections in advance so that she is prepared when labor begins. She can also be advised to bring her own MP3, MP4, or CD player, so she does not have to rely on the availability of equipment in the birthing area.

no matter how mild, whereas members of other cultures stoically accept pain. Fatigue and sleep deprivation may also influence response to pain. The tired woman has less energy and ability to use such strategies as distraction or imagination to deal with pain. As a result she may lose her ability to cope with labor and choose analgesics or other medications to relieve the discomfort.

The woman's previous experience with pain and her anxiety level also affect her ability to manage current and future pain. Those who have had experience with pain seem more sensitive to painful stimuli than those who have not. Unfamiliar surroundings and events can increase anxiety, as does separation from family and loved ones. Anticipation of discomfort and questions about whether she can cope with the contractions may also increase anxiety.

Both attention and distraction influence the perception of pain. When pain sensation is the focus of attention, the perceived intensity is greater. A sensory stimulus such as a back rub can be a distraction that focuses the woman's attention on the stimulus rather than on the pain.

FETAL RESPONSE TO LABOR

When the fetus is healthy, the mechanical and hemodynamic changes of normal labor have no adverse effects. Certain physiologic responses do occur, however:

- *Heart rate changes.* Early fetal heart rate decelerations can occur with intracranial pressures of 40 to 55 mm Hg, as the head pushes against the cervix. This early deceleration is believed to be due to hypoxic depression of the central nervous system, which is under vagal control. The absence of head compression decelerations in some fetuses during labor is explained by a threshold reached more gradually in the presence of intact membranes and lack of maternal resistance. These early decelerations are harmless in a normal fetus.

- *Acid–base status in labor.* Blood flow is decreased to the fetus at the peak of each contraction, which leads to a slow decrease in pH. During the second stage of labor, as uterine contractions become longer and stronger and the woman holds her breath to push, the fetal pH decreases more rapidly. The base deficit increases, and fetal oxygen saturation drops about 10% (Blackburn, 2013).

- *Hemodynamic changes.* The adequate exchange of nutrients and gases in the fetal capillaries and intervillous spaces depends in part on the fetal blood pressure. Fetal blood pressure protects the normal fetus during the anoxic periods caused by the contracting uterus during labor. The fetal and placental reserve is usually enough to see the fetus through these anoxic periods unharmed (Blackburn, 2013).

- *Fetal sensation.* Beginning at about 37 or 38 weeks' gestation, the fetus is able to experience sensations of light, sound, and touch. The full-term fetus is able to hear music and the maternal voice. Even in utero the fetus is sensitive to light and will move away from a bright light source. The term baby is aware of pressure sensations during labor such as the touch of the care provider during a vaginal examination or pressure on the head as a contraction occurs. Although the fetus may not be able to process this input, the fetus is experiencing labor as the woman labors.

Critical Concept Review

LEARNING OUTCOME 17.1: Describe the five critical factors that influence labor in the assessment of an expectant woman's and fetus's progress in labor and birth.

1. Birth passage:
   - The ability of the pelvis and cervix to accommodate the passage of the fetus.
2. Fetus:
   - The ability of the fetus to complete the birth process.
3. Relationship between the passage and the fetus:
   - The position of the fetus in relation to the pelvis.
4. Physiologic forces of labor:
   - Characteristics of contractions and the effectiveness of expulsion methods.
5. Psychosocial considerations:
   - Understanding and preparing for the childbirth experience.
   - Amount of support from others.
   - Present emotional status.
   - Beliefs and values.

LEARNING OUTCOME 17.2: Examine an expectant woman's and fetus's responses to labor based on the physiologic processes that occur during labor.

1. Progesterone causes relaxation of smooth muscle tissue.
2. Estrogen causes stimulation of uterine muscle contractions.
3. Connective tissue loosens and permits the softening, thinning, and opening of the cervix.
4. Muscles of the upper uterine segment shorten and cause the cervix to thin and flatten.
5. Fetal body is straightened as the uterus elongates with each contraction.
6. Pressure of the fetal head causes cervical dilatation.
7. Rectum and vagina are drawn upward and forward with each contraction.
8. During the second stage, the anus everts.

LEARNING OUTCOME 17.3: Assess for the premonitory signs of labor when caring for the expectant woman.

1. Lightening:
   - Fetus descends into the pelvic inlet.
2. Braxton Hicks contractions:
   - Irregular, intermittent contractions that occur during pregnancy.
   - Cause more discomfort closer to onset of labor.
3. Cervical changes:
   - Cervix begins to soften and weaken (ripening).
4. Bloody show:
   - Loss of the cervical mucous plug.
   - Causes blood-tinged discharge.
5. Rupture of membranes:
   - If membranes rupture prior to the onset of labor, there is a good chance labor will begin within 24 hours.
6. Sudden burst of energy:
   - Known as nesting.
   - Usually occurs 24–48 hours before the start of labor.
7. Other signs:
   - Loss of 1–3 pounds.
   - Diarrhea, indigestion, nausea, and vomiting may occur prior to the onset of labor.

LEARNING OUTCOME 17.4: Differentiate between false and true labor.

1. True labor is characterized by:
   - Contractions that occur at regular intervals and increase in duration and intensity.
   - Discomfort that begins in the back and radiates to the front of the abdomen.
   - Walking intensifies contractions.
   - Resting or relaxing in warm water does not decrease the intensity of contractions.
   - Contractions that produce cervical dilatation.
2. False labor is characterized by:
   - Irregular contractions that do not increase in duration or intensity.
   - Contractions that may be lessened by walking, rest, or warm water.
   - Discomfort that is felt primarily in the abdomen.
   - Contractions that produce no effect on cervix.

LEARNING OUTCOME 17.5: Describe the physiologic and psychologic changes that occur in an expectant woman during each stage of labor in the nursing care management of the expectant woman.

1. Latent phase physiologic changes:
   - Regular, mild contractions begin and increase in intensity and frequency.
   - Cervical effacement and dilatation begin.
2. Active phase physiologic changes:
   - Contractions increase in intensity, frequency, and duration.
   - Cervical dilatation increases from 4 to 7 cm.
   - Fetus begins to descend into the pelvis.
3. Transition phase physiologic changes:
   - Contractions continue to increase in intensity, duration, and frequency.
   - Cervix dilates from 8 to 10 cm.
   - Fetus descends rapidly into the birth passage.
   - Woman may experience rectal pressure.
   - Woman may experience nausea, vomiting, or both.
4. Second stage physiologic changes:
   - Stage begins with complete cervical dilatation and ends with the birth of the infant.
   - Woman pushes due to pressure of fetal head on sacral and obturator nerves.
   - Woman uses intra-abdominal pressure.
   - Perineum begins to bulge, flatten, and move anteriorly as fetus descends.
5. Third stage physiologic changes:
   - Placental separation: Uterus contracts and the placenta begins to separate.
   - Placental expulsion: Woman bears down and expels the placenta. Physician may put slight traction on the cord to assist the expulsion of the placenta.
6. Fourth stage physiologic changes:
   - Woman experiences increased pulse and decreased blood pressure due to redistribution of blood from uterus and blood loss.
   - Uterus remains contracted and is located between umbilicus and symphysis pubis.
   - Woman may experience a shaking chill.
   - Urine may be retained due to decreased bladder tone and possible trauma to the bladder.

LEARNING OUTCOME 17.6: Explain the maternal systemic responses to labor in the nursing care of the expectant woman.

1. Cardiovascular changes:
   - Increase in cardiac output.
2. Blood pressure:
   - Rises with each contraction.
   - May rise further with pushing.
3. Respiratory system:
   - Increase in oxygen demand and consumption.
   - Mild respiratory acidosis usually occurs by time of birth.
4. Renal system:
   - Increase in renin, plasma renin activity, and angiotensinogen.
   - Edema may occur at base of bladder due to pressure of fetal head.
5. Gastrointestinal system:
   - Gastric motility decreased.
   - Gastric emptying is prolonged.
   - Gastric volume remains increased.
6. Immune system and other blood values:
   - WBC count increases.
   - Blood glucose decreases.
7. Pain:
   - In the first stage: Arises from dilatation of cervix, stretching of lower uterine segment, pressure, and hypoxia of uterine muscle cells during contractions.
   - In the second stage: Arises from hypoxia of contracting uterine muscle cells, distention of the vagina and perineum, and pressure.
   - In the third stage: Arises from contractions and dilatation of cervix as placenta is expelled.

LEARNING OUTCOME 17.7: Examine fetal responses to labor.

1. Labor may cause no adverse effects in the healthy fetus.
2. FHR may decrease as the head pushes against the cervix.
3. Blood flow decreases to the fetus at the peak of each contraction, leading to a decrease in pH.
4. Further decrease of pH occurs during pushing due to the woman holding her breath.

Clinical Reasoning in Action

Ann Nelson, a 28-year-old, G2P0010 at 41 weeks' gestation, is admitted to the birthing unit where you are working. She is here for cervical ripening and induction of labor due to postdate pregnancy and decreased amniotic fluid volume. A review of her prenatal chart reveals a pertinent history of infertility (Clomid-induced pregnancy) and asthma (treated with inhalers on a PRN basis). The Doppler picks up a fetal heart rate of 120 beats/min. You place Ann on the electronic fetal monitor and obtain the following data: BP 126/76, T 98°F, P 82, R 16; vaginal exam reveals a 20% effaced cervix, 1 cm dilatation in the posterior position, and vertex at −2 station. The fetal monitor shows a fetal heart rate baseline of 120 to 128 with occasional variable decelerations, accelerations to 140 with fetal activity. No contractions are noted on the monitor or palpated. Ann asks you what to expect with "cervical ripening" using prostaglandin gel.

1. Discuss the action of prostaglandin gel.
2. Ann asks you why cervical ripening and induction of labor are recommended for her and her baby. How would you best respond to her?
3. Ann asks how she will know if she is getting contractions. How would you answer her?
4. Discuss the difference between mild, moderate, and strong contractions.
5. Describe the latent phase of labor.
6. Create a concept map for Ann's care based on the need for cervical ripening and induction of labor due to postdate pregnancy and decreased amniotic fluid volume. Ann also has a history of asthma that warrants consideration in her plan of care.

See www.nursing.pearsonhighered.com for possible responses and an interactive template for a concept map.

References

Association of Women's Health, Obstetric and Neonatal Nurses (AWHONN). (2007). *Evidence-based clinical practice guideline: Nursing care and management of the second stage of labor* (2nd ed.). Washington, DC: Author.

Blackburn, S. T. (2013). *Maternal, fetal, and neonatal physiology: A clinical perspective* (4th ed.). Philadelphia, PA: Saunders.

Caldwell, W. E., & Moloy, H. C. (1933). Anatomical variation in the female pelvis and their effect on labor with a suggested classification. *American Journal of Obstetrics and Gynecology, 26*, 479–487.

Cunningham, F. G., Leveno, K. J., Bloom, S. L., Hauth, J. C., Rouse, D. J., & Spong, C. Y. (2010). *Williams obstetrics* (23rd ed.). New York, NY: McGraw-Hill.

Ijaiya, M. A., Adesina, K. T., Raji, H. O., Aboyeji, A. P., Olatinwo, A. O., Adeniran, A. S., . . . Isiaka-Lawal, S. (2010). Duration of labour with spontaneous onset at the University of Ilorin Teaching Hospital, Ilorin, Nigeria. *Research Journal of Medical Sciences, 4*(3), 195–198. doi:10.3923/rjmsci.2010.195.198

Jazayeri, A. (2011). Premature rupture of membranes. *eMedicine.* Retrieved from http://emedicine.medscape.com/article/261137-overview#aw2aab6b3

Kalantaridos, S., Zoumakis, E., Makrigiannakis, A., Lavasidis, L., Vrekoussis, G. P., & Chrousos, K. (2011). Corticotropin-releasing hormone, stress and human reproduction: An update. *Journal of Reproductive Immunology, 85*(1), 33–39. doi:10.1016/j.jri.2010.02.005

Powrie, R., Greene, M., & Camann, V. (2012). *De Swiet's medical disorders in obstetric practice* (5th ed.). New York, NY: John Wiley & Sons.

Simkin, P., & Ancheta, L. (2011). *The labor progress handbook: Early interventions to prevent and treat dystocia.* New York, NY: John Wiley & Sons.

Spector, R. E. (2012). *Cultural diversity in health and illness* (8th ed.). Upper Saddle River, NJ: Pearson.

Tuuli, M. G., Frey, H. A., Odibo, A. O., Macones, G. A., & Cahill, A. G. (2012). Immediate compared with delayed pushing in the second stage of labor: A systematic review and meta-analysis. *Obstetrics & Gynecology, 120*(3), 660–668. doi:10.1097/AOG.0b013e3182639fae

Intrapartum Nursing Assessment

It was strange. After months of waiting for my baby's birth, labor took me by surprise. I wasn't quite ready to move from being pregnant to being a mother. Not that I had any choice! —Malika, 23

LEARNING OUTCOMES

18.1 Describe a maternal assessment of the laboring woman that includes the patient history, high-risk screening, and physical and psychosociocultural factors.

18.2 Evaluate the progress of labor by assessing the laboring woman's contractions, cervical dilatation, and effacement.

18.3 Delineate the procedure for performing Leopold's maneuvers and the information that can be obtained, including the importance of identifying accurate fetal position prior to performing a fetal heart rate assessment.

18.4 Describe the steps and frequency for performing auscultation of fetal heart rate.

18.5 Distinguish between baseline and periodic changes in fetal heart rate monitoring, and the appearance and significance of each.

18.6 Evaluate fetal heart rate tracings using a systematic approach.

18.7 Compare nonreassuring fetal heart rate patterns to appropriate nursing responses.

18.8 Explain the family's responses to electronic fetal monitoring in nursing management.

The physiologic events during labor call for many adaptations by the mother and the fetus. Thus, frequent and accurate assessments are crucial. The woman's partner or chosen support person is also an integral part of the childbirth experience. Moreover, the traditional assessment techniques of observation, palpation, and auscultation are augmented by the judicious use of technology such as ultrasound and electronic monitoring. However, the technology only provides data; it is the nurse who monitors the mother and her baby.

MATERNAL ASSESSMENT

History

Obtain a brief oral history when the woman is admitted to the birthing area. Each agency has its own admission forms, but they usually include the following information:

- Woman's name and age
- Last menstrual period (LMP) and estimated date of birth (EDB)
- Attending physician or certified nurse-midwife (CNM)
- Personal data: blood type; Rh factor; results of serology testing; prepregnant and present weight; allergies to medications, foods, or other substances; prescribed and over-the-counter medications taken during pregnancy; and history of drug and alcohol use and smoking during the pregnancy
- History of previous illness, such as tuberculosis, heart disease, diabetes, and other serious conditions that could influence the pregnancy
- Problems in the prenatal period, such as elevated blood pressure, bleeding problems, recurrent urinary tract infections, other infections
- Pregnancy data: gravida, para, abortions, and perinatal deaths
- The method chosen for infant feeding
- Type of prenatal education classes (childbirth education classes)
- Woman's preferences about labor and birth, such as no episiotomy, no analgesics or anesthetics, or the presence of the father or others at the birth
- Pediatrician or family practice physician
- Additional data: history of special tests such as nonstress test (NST), biophysical profile (BPP), or ultrasound; history of any preterm labor; onset of labor; amniotic fluid membrane status; and brief description of previous labor and birth
- Onset of labor
- Status of amniotic membranes (Are they intact or ruptured? If ruptured, time of rupture, color of fluid, and odor.)

Psychosocial Considerations

Assessment of psychosocial history is a critical component of intrapartum nursing assessment. The parents' psychosocial readiness, including their fears, anxieties, birth fantasies, excitement level, feelings of joy and anticipation, and level of social support, can be a critical factor in a successful birth experience. Some mothers may fear having a bowel movement during the second stage of labor and experiencing embarrassment related to this normal physiologic process. Other mothers may feel a sense of failure if they desire an unmedicated birth and then use pain medication at the actual time of labor or birth. Both the mother and father are making a transition into a new role, and both have expectations of themselves during the labor and birth experience, and as caregivers for their child and their new family. Psychosocial factors affecting labor and birth include the couple's accomplishment of the tasks of pregnancy, usual coping mechanisms in response to stressful life events, support system, preparation for childbirth, and cultural influences. Even mothers and fathers who attend childbirth preparation classes and have a solid support system can be concerned about what labor will be like, whether they will be able to perform the way they expect, whether the pain will be more than the mother expects or can cope with, and whether the father can provide helpful support. The physical and emotional stress of birth can impact a couple's responses to the labor itself.

Some women may fear the pain of contractions, whereas others welcome the opportunity to feel the birth process. Some women view the pain as threatening and associate it with a loss of control over their bodies and emotions. Other women see pain as a rite of passage into motherhood and a necessary means to an end. It is helpful for women to realize that the pain of labor is natural. Assurances that labor is progressing normally can go a long way toward reducing anxiety and thereby reducing pain, and providing positive reinforcement that the mother is doing "a good job." In one study, empowerment and having control over one's body played key roles in determining whether a woman viewed her labor and birth positively (Lee-Rife, 2010). Women who viewed their births as a positive experience were also more likely to have a sense of well-being about themselves after the experience (Lee-Rife, 2010). A wide variety of coping techniques to assist both the laboring woman and her partner are discussed in Chapter 19 🔗 and Chapter 20 🔗.

How the woman views the birth experience in hindsight may affect her mothering behaviors. It appears that any activities by the expectant woman or by healthcare providers that enhance the birth experience will be beneficial to the mother–baby connection and improve bonding. Some studies have shown that when some women are disappointed with their birth experience or have negative feelings during the third trimester, they may have some initial difficulties and be more prone to postpartum mood disorders (Weisman et al., 2010). Psychosocial factors associated with a positive birth experience are summarized in Table 18–1.

The laboring woman's support system also influences the course of labor and birth. Some women prefer not to have a support person or family member with them. They may feel that the birth process is a private moment that they wish to reserve for themselves. However, most women choose to have significant persons (father or partner, family members, friends) with them during labor and birth. Social support tends to have a positive effect. For some families, the birth event is a celebration, and they want to create a joyful, festive atmosphere with many loved ones present. Some facilities may limit the number of family members present during labor and birth, so the nurse needs to be familiar with specific facility policies. Generally, the presence of the laboring woman's partner at the bedside provides a means to enhance communication and to demonstrate feelings of love.

Psychosocial Risk Factors. The psychosocial history is a critical component of assessment. An estimated one-third of all pregnant women are exposed to some type of psychotropic medication during their pregnancies. There are growing concerns that some psychotropic medications may cause fetal and neonatal side effects, such as a shortened gestational period, short-term neonatal irritability, neurobehavioral changes, and, rarely, persistent pulmonary hypertension of the newborn. There have been reports of congenital anomalies although no specific patterns have been noted with the exception of the use of Paxil, which is known to cause cardiac anomalies. In 2012, the American Psychological Association and the American College of Obstetricians and Gynecologists issued a joint statement indicating that these side effects cannot be attributed solely to medication administration and can also be related to the impact of depression and psychiatric illness on the pregnancies of affected mothers (Yonkers et al., 2012).

It is estimated that 10% of pregnant women meet the criteria for major depressive disorder during pregnancy and another 18% have depressive symptoms during the gestational period (Marcus, 2009). It is also not uncommon for women to be diagnosed with other mental illnesses that may impact the labor and birth process. These may include (Davidson, 2012):

- Eating disorders
- Autism
- Learning disabilities
- Attention deficit or attention deficit hyperactivity disorder
- Anxiety
- Mood disorders

Any of these diagnoses can play a role in how the woman copes with labor and birth and should be assessed by the admitting nurse. Women with identified disorders will need ongoing assessment during the labor and birth. In addition, they are at greater risk for postpartum mood disorders and posttraumatic stress disorders (PTSDs) and warrant additional evaluation in the immediate, intermediate, and extended postpartum periods.

Because of the prevalence of intimate partner and domestic violence in our society (see Chapter 5 🔗), the nurse needs to consider the possibility that the woman may have experienced abuse at some point in her life. Many victims of domestic violence, sexual assault, or childhood abuse may have anxiety about the labor process before it begins, or the anxiety may arise during labor. Therefore, it is essential to be alert for information that may indicate abuse or a history of victimization of violence.

Table 18–1	Factors Associated with a Positive Birth Experience

- Motivation for the pregnancy
- Attendance at childbirth education classes
- A sense of competence or mastery
- Self-confidence and self-esteem
- Positive relationship with mate
- Perception of maintaining control during labor
- Support from mate or other person during labor
- Not being left alone in labor
- Trust in the medical and nursing staff
- Having personal control of breathing patterns, comfort measures
- Choosing a physician or certified nurse-midwife who has a similar philosophy of care
- Receiving clear information regarding procedures

SAFETY ALERT!

If a woman feels unsafe in the clinical environment and fears for her safety due to past intimate partner violence, alert security and the charge nurse ahead of time to deny access to the birthing area for that partner. Antepartum assessment for domestic violence is discussed in Chapter 10 🔗.

Clinical Tip

Many nurses have difficulty asking questions about domestic violence, sexual abuse, sexual intercourse/sexual practices, and drug or alcohol use during pregnancy. However, this information is necessary to provide effective care. To create a relationship of trust with the woman, the following tips may be helpful:

- Explore your own beliefs and values.
- Use open-ended questions.
- Be receptive to the answers.
- Be accepting of others' life experiences.

Intrapartum High-Risk Screening

Screening for intrapartum high-risk factors is an integral part of assessment. As the history is obtained, note the presence of any factors that may be associated with a high-risk condition. For example, the woman who reports a physical symptom such as intermittent bleeding needs further assessment to rule out abruptio placentae or placenta previa before the admission process continues. In such a case, the woman should be asked the amount of bleeding that occurred, the onset, duration, and if she needed to wear a sanitary pad. If a pad was placed, the time between pad saturation should be assessed. In cases of unknown vaginal bleeding, patient teaching includes advising the woman that she should never have a vaginal examination performed if bleeding is present. It is also important to recognize the implications of a high-risk condition for the laboring woman and her fetus. For example, if there is an abnormal fetal presentation, labor may be prolonged, prolapse of the umbilical cord is more likely, and the possibility of a cesarean birth is increased.

Although physical conditions are major factors that increase risk in the intrapartum period, sociocultural variables may also increase risk; these include:

- Poverty
- Nutrition
- Degree of prenatal care received
- Cultural beliefs about pregnancy
- Communication patterns
- Social support
- Alcohol, tobacco, and drug use
- Presence of PTSD (Davidson, 2012)

Begin gathering data about sociocultural factors as the woman enters the birthing area. Observe the communication pattern between the woman and her support person or people and their responses to admission questions and initial teaching. If the woman and those supporting her do not speak English and translators are not available among the birthing unit staff, the course of labor and the ability of caregivers to interact and provide support and education are affected. The couple must receive information in their primary language to make informed decisions. Communication may also be affected by cultural practices such as beliefs about when to speak, who should ask questions, or whether it is acceptable to let others know about discomfort. In some countries such as Algeria, Brazil, China, and Korea, and among orthodox Jews, the father is not expected to be in the birthing area. Culturally sensitive nurses realize that this should not be interpreted as a lack of interest in the mother, the infant, or the birth itself (Spector, 2012).

Table 18–2 provides a partial list of intrapartum risk factors to keep in mind during the intrapartum assessment.

Table 18–2	Intrapartum High-Risk Factors	
Factor	**Maternal Implications**	**Fetal/Neonatal Implications**
Abnormal presentation	↑ Incidence of cesarean section (C/S) birth ↑ Incidence of prolonged labor	↑ Incidence of placenta previa Prematurity ↑ Risk of congenital abnormality Neonatal physical trauma ↑ Risk of intrauterine growth restriction (IUGR)
Multiple gestation	↑ Uterine distention → ↑ risk of postpartum hemorrhage ↑ Risk of C/S ↑ Risk of preterm labor	Low birth weight Prematurity ↑ Risk of congenital anomalies Twin-to-twin transfusion
Hydramnios/polyhydramnios	↑ Discomfort ↑ Dyspnea ↑ Risk of preterm labor Edema of lower extremities Increases risk of cord prolapse with AROM/SROM	↑ Risk of esophageal or other high-alimentary-tract atresias ↑ Risk of CNS anomalies (myelocele)
Oligohydramnios	Maternal fear	↑ Incidence of congenital anomalies ↑ Incidence of renal lesions ↑ Risk of IUGR ↑ Risk of fetal acidosis ↑ Risk of cord compression Postmaturity
Meconium staining of amniotic fluid	Psychologic stress due to fear for baby	↑ Risk of fetal asphyxia ↑ Risk of meconium aspiration ↑ Risk of pneumonia due to aspiration of meconium

Table 18–2	Intrapartum High-Risk Factors—continued	
Factor	Maternal Implications	Fetal/Neonatal Implications
Premature rupture of membranes	↑ Risk of infection (chorioamnionitis) ↑ Risk of preterm labor ↑ Anxiety Fear for the baby Prolonged hospitalization ↑ Incidence of tocolytic therapy	↑ Perinatal morbidity Prematurity ↑ Birth weight ↑ Risk of respiratory distress syndrome Prolonged hospitalization
Induction of labor	↑ Risk of hypercontractility of uterus ↑ Risk of uterine rupture Length of labor if cervix not ready ↑ Anxiety	Prematurity if gestational age not assessed correctly Hpoxia if hyperstimulation occurs Nonreassuring fetal status can occur
Abruptio placentae	Hemorrhage Uterine atony ↑ Incidence of C/S Severe maternal abdominal pain	Fetal hypoxia/acidosis Fetal exsanguination ↑ Perinatal mortality
Placenta previa	Hemorrhage Uterine atony Increased incidence of C/S Painless vaginal bleeding	Fetal hypoxia/acidosis Fetal exsanguination Increased perinatal mortality
Failure to progress in labor	Maternal exhaustion ↑ Incidence of augmentation of labor ↑ Incidence of C/S	Fetal hypoxia/acidosis Intracranial birth injury
Precipitous labor (less than 3 hr)	Perineal, vaginal, cervical lacerations ↑ Risk of postpartum hemorrhage Maternal hematomas	Tentorial tears
Prolapse of umbilical cord	↑ Fear for baby C/S birth	Acute fetal hypoxia/acidosis
Fetal heart aberrations	↑ Fear for baby ↑ Risk of C/S, forceps, vacuum Continuous electronic monitoring and intervention in labor	Tachycardia, chronic asphyxic insult, bradycardia, acute asphyxic insult Chronic hypoxia Congenital heart block
Uterine rupture	Maternal hemorrhage Cesarean birth for hysterectomy ↑ Risk of death	Fetal anoxia Fetal hemorrhage Neonatal morbidity and mortality Fetal neurologic sequelae
Postdates (greater than 42 weeks)	↑ Anxiety ↑ Incidence of induction of labor ↑ Incidence of C/S ↑ Use of technology to monitor fetus ↑ Risk of shoulder dystocia Placenta calcifications/advanced placental grading	Postmaturity syndrome ↑ Risk of fetal/neonatal mortality and morbidity ↑ Risk of antepartum fetal death ↑ Incidence or risk of large baby ↑ Risk of intrauterine growth restriction Fetal hypoxia Increased nonreassuring fetal status
Diabetes	↑ Risk of hydramnios ↑ Risk of hypoglycemia or hyperglycemia ↑ Risk of preeclampsia/eclampsia	↑ Risk of malpresentation ↑ Risk of macrosomia ↑ Risk of IUGR ↑ Risk of respiratory distress syndrome ↑ Risk of congenital anomalies ↑ Risk of fetal death Neonatal hypoglycemia
Preeclampsia/eclampsia	↑ Risk of seizures ↑ Risk of stroke ↑ Risk of HELLP Syndrome (**h**emolysis, **e**levated **l**iver enzymes, and **l**ow **p**latelet count) and DIC (disseminated intravascular coagulation)	↑ Risk of small-for-gestational-age baby ↑ Risk of preterm birth ↑ Risk of mortality
AIDS/sexually transmitted infection (STI)	↑ Risk of additional infections	↑ Risk of transplacental transmission ↑ Risk of infection during birth process or with invasive medical procedures

---

Clinical Reasoning Identifying Domestic Violence

You are the birthing center nurse and you have reason to suspect that Lynn Ling, who has just been admitted in labor, may be in an abusive relationship. How could you set up an interview so that the partner would leave the room (and take any accompanying children) without feeling that you are possibly increasing the risk to the woman? What communication techniques would you use to encourage Lynn to reveal if her partner is abusive?

See www.nursing.pearsonhighered.com for possible responses.

Complementary Care Aromatherapy in Childbirth

Aromatherapy is the use of aromas for physical, mental, and emotional healing. The primary sources of healing aromas are essential oils distilled from herbs and flowers. During labor, essential oils such as jasmine or lavender may be used as an environmental fragrance or added to a hydrotherapy bath. They may also be diluted with a carrier oil or lotion for massage. Therapeutic grade oils may help promote relaxation, improve a woman's ability to cope, and decrease the perception of pain (Datta, Kodeli, & Sega, 2010).

Intrapartum Physical and Psychosociocultural Assessment

A physical examination is part of the admission procedure and part of the ongoing care of the woman. Although the intrapartum physical assessment is not as complete and thorough as the initial prenatal physical examination (see Chapter 10 🔴), it does involve assessment of some body systems and of the actual labor process. See *Assessment Guide: Intrapartum—First Stage of Labor* on pages 393–398 for a framework to use when examining the laboring woman.

The physical assessment portion includes assessments performed immediately on admission as well as ongoing assessments. When labor is progressing very quickly, there may not be time for a complete nursing assessment. In that case the critical physical assessments include significant pregnancy history, high-risk factors/problems that occurred during pregnancy, maternal vital signs, labor status, fetal status, and laboratory findings.

The cultural assessment portion provides a starting point for this increasingly important aspect of assessment. Individualized nursing care can best be planned and implemented when the values and beliefs of the laboring woman are known and honored. It is sometimes challenging to achieve a balance between cultural awareness and the risk of stereotyping because cultural responses are influenced by so many factors. Nurses are most effective when they combine an awareness of the major cultural values and beliefs of a specific group with the recognition that individual differences have an impact.

The final section of the assessment guide addresses psychosocial factors. The laboring woman's psychosocial status is an important part of the total assessment. The woman has previous ideas, knowledge, and fears about childbearing. By assessing her psychosocial status, the nurse can meet the woman's needs for information and support.

While performing the intrapartum assessment, it is crucial to follow the Centers for Disease Control and Prevention (CDC) guidelines to prevent exposure to body substances. Provide information about the precautions in a factual manner.

Developing Cultural Competence
Use of Protective Amulets

Placing a protective amulet on the baby or in the crib is common practice among people from many countries, including Greece, Iran, Iraq, Israel, Italy, Malaysia, and Russia (Spector, 2012).

Methods of Evaluating Labor Progress

The nurse assesses the woman's contractions and cervical dilatation and effacement to evaluate labor progress.

Contraction Assessment

Uterine contractions may be assessed by palpation or continuous electronic monitoring.

Clinical Tip

Uterine contractions are documented in frequency by the number of minutes, whereas duration is expressed in seconds.

Palpation.   Assess contractions for frequency, duration, and intensity by placing one hand on the uterine fundus. Keep the hand relatively still because excessive movement may stimulate contractions or cause discomfort. Determine the frequency of the contractions by noting the time from the beginning of one contraction to the beginning of the next. If contractions begin at 7:00, 7:04, and 7:08, for example, their frequency is every 4 minutes. To determine contraction duration, note the time when tensing of the fundus is first felt (beginning of contraction) and again as relaxation occurs (end of contraction). During the acme of the contraction, intensity can be evaluated by estimating the indentability of the fundus. Assess at least three successive contractions to gain enough data to determine the contraction pattern. See Table 18–3 for a review of contraction characteristics in different phases of labor.

This is also a good time to assess the laboring woman's perception of pain. How does she describe the pain? What is her affect? Is this contraction more uncomfortable than the last one? Note and chart the woman's affect and response to the contractions.

Electronic Monitoring of Contractions.   Electronic monitoring of uterine contractions provides continuous data. In many birth settings, electronic monitoring is routine for high-risk patients and women having oxytocin-induced labor. Other facilities monitor all laboring women.

Electronic monitoring may be done externally with a device placed against the maternal abdomen, or internally with an **intrauterine pressure catheter**. When monitoring by external means, the portion of the monitoring equipment called a tocodynamometer, or "toco," is positioned against the fundus of

Table 18–3	Contraction and Labor Progress Characteristics

CONTRACTION CHARACTERISTICS

Latent phase:	Every 10–30 min × 30 sec; mild, progressing to Every 5–7 min × 30–40 sec; moderate
Active phase:	Every 2–5 min × 40–60 sec; moderate to strong
Transition phase:	Every 1 1/2–2 min × 60–90 sec; strong

LABOR PROGRESS CHARACTERISTICS

Primipara:	At least 1.2 cm/hr dilatation At least 1 cm/hr descent Less than 2 hr in second stage
Multipara:	At least 1.5 cm/hr dilatation At least 2.1 cm/hr descent Less than 1 hr in second stage

● **Figure 18–1** Woman in labor with external monitor applied. The tocodynamometer placed on the uterine fundus is recording uterine contractions. The lower belt holds the ultrasonic device that monitors the fetal heart rate. The belts can be adjusted for comfort.

Source: Courtesy of Wilson Garcia.

the uterus and held in place with an elastic belt (Figure 18–1 ●). The toco contains a flexible disk that responds to pressure. When the uterus contracts, the fundus tightens and the change in pressure against the toco is amplified and transmitted to the electronic fetal monitor. The monitor displays the uterine contraction as a pattern on graph paper.

External monitoring provides a continuous recording of the frequency and duration of uterine contractions and is noninvasive. However, it does not accurately record the intensity of the uterine contraction, and it is difficult to obtain an accurate fetal heart rate (FHR) in some women, such as those who are very obese, those who have polyhydramnios/hydramnios (an abnormally large amount of amniotic fluid), those whose fetus is very active, and in the case of premature fetuses. In addition, the belt may bother the woman if it requires frequent readjustment when she changes position.

Internal intrauterine monitoring provides the same data and also provides accurate measurement of uterine contraction intensity (the strength of the contraction and the actual pressure within the uterus). After membranes have ruptured, the physician/CNM inserts the intrauterine pressure catheter (IUPC) into the uterine cavity and connects it by a cable to the electronic fetal monitor. In some facilities, labor and delivery nurses may obtain specialized training to perform IUPC insertions. A small micropressure device located in the tip of the catheter measures the pressure within the uterus in the resting state and during each contraction. Internal electronic monitoring is used when it is imperative to have accurate intrauterine pressure readings to evaluate the stress on the uterus.

In addition, it is important to evaluate the woman's labor status by palpating the intensity and resting tone of the uterine fundus during contractions.

Cervical Assessment

Cervical dilatation and effacement are evaluated directly by vaginal examination (see Skill 3–1 in the *Clinical Skills Manual* SKILLS). The vaginal examination can also provide information about membrane status, characteristics of amniotic fluid, fetal position, and station. Refer to *Assessment Guide: Intrapartum—First Stage of Labor* on pages 393–398.

See Figures 18–2 ●, 18–3 ●, and 18–4 ●.

● **Figure 18–2** Gauging cervical dilatation. To gauge cervical dilatation, the nurse places the index and middle fingers against the cervix and determines the size of the opening. Before labor begins, the cervix is long (approximately 2.5 cm), the sides feel thick, and the cervical canal is closed, so an examining finger cannot be inserted. During labor the cervix begins to dilate, and the size of the opening progresses from 1 to 10 cm in diameter.

 Clinical Tip

Many experienced nurses note that when palpating a woman's uterus, mild contractions feel similar in consistency to the tip of the nose, moderate contractions feel more like the chin, and with strong contractions, there is little indentability, much like the forehead. When palpating during a contraction, compare the consistency to your nose, chin, and forehead to determine the intensity.

● **Figure 18–3** Palpating the presenting part (portion of the fetus that enters the pelvis first). *A,* Left occiput anterior (LOA). The occiput (area over the occipital bone on the posterior part of the fetal head) is in the left anterior quadrant of the woman's pelvis. When the fetus is LOA, the posterior fontanelle (located just above the occipital bone and triangular in shape) is in the upper left quadrant of the maternal pelvis. *B,* Left occiput posterior (LOP). The posterior fontanelle is in the lower left quadrant of the maternal pelvis. *C,* Right occiput anterior (ROA). The posterior fontanelle is in the upper right quadrant of the maternal pelvis. *D,* Right occiput posterior (ROP). The posterior fontanelle is in the lower right quadrant of the maternal pelvis.

Note: The anterior fontanelle is diamond shaped. Because of the roundness of the fetal head, only a portion of the anterior fontanelle can be seen in each of the views, so it appears to be triangular in shape.

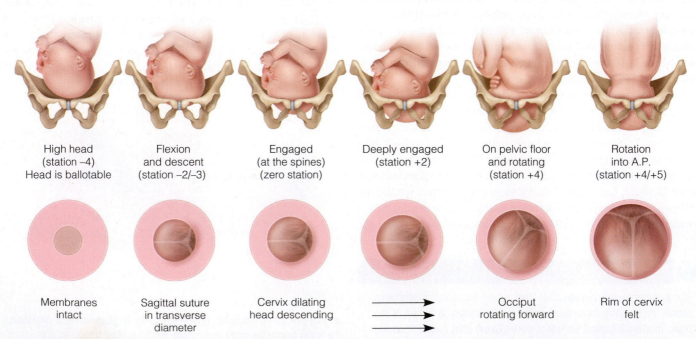

● **Figure 18–4** Assessing fetal position and station. *Top:* The fetal head progressing through the pelvis. *Bottom:* The changes the nurse will detect on palpation of the occiput through the cervix while doing a vaginal examination.

Alisa is fascinated with baby Lydia's tiny fingers and toes. I love being with parents as they explore their baby. Each new baby is such a wonder . . . such a miracle.

Now my attention turns to Alisa. As part of my assessment, I check the position and tone of her fundus. All is well. I head home after a busy, but rewarding, day.

Photographer: Jenny Thomas

CONCEPTION

0

4 WEEKS

1

FETAL DEVELOPMENT

The sperm fertilizes the ovum, which then divides and burrows into the uterus.

From the embryonic disk (ectoderm, entoderm, mesoderm), the first body segments appear that will eventually become the spine, brain, and spinal cord. Heart, blood circulation, and digestive tract take shape. Embryo is less than a quarter-inch long.

MATERNAL CHANGES

Mother misses first period; breasts become tender, may enlarge. Chronic fatigue and urinary frequency begin, may persist for three or more months. hCG in urine and serum 9 days after conception.

CLIENT TEACHING/ ANTICIPATORY GUIDANCE

Supportive bra may ease discomfort. Increased rest and relaxation necessary now and throughout pregnancy. Increase fluids during the day; decrease fluid intake only at night to help prevent nocturia; sleep on side to decrease pressure on bladder. Avoid using any medications unless prescribed. Avoid use of social drugs; check with caregiver before using any OTC preparations.

Darnell and Ayisha are expecting their first baby. Ayisha calls to tell me her labor has begun, and I meet with them at the birth center. After the electronic fetal monitor is applied, we talk about the fetal heart tracing. I want to be sure they understand the monitor and have the opportunity to ask questions.

I do an exam to see how labor is progressi my findings with them.

During the active phase of Ayisha's labor, Darnell lovingly provides comfort and support.

It's time to push. Ayisha wants to stand comfortable on the bed. Darnell stands b provides support. I continue to talk with vide encouragement. After an hour of Kinshasha is born.

e infor-
els and

to
as
the
and
and

ects the body; fine hair (lanugo)
ody and keeps the oil on the
ows, eyelashes, and head hair
tus develops a regular schedule
, sucking, and kicking.

Skeleton develops rapidly as bone-forming cells increase activity. Respiratory movements begin. Fetus weighs about 1 lb, 10 oz.

Fetus can breathe, swallow, regulate temperature. Surfactant forms in lungs. Eyes begin to open and close. Baby is ⅔ the size it will be at birth.

ches level of
Breasts begin
olostrum.
ac holds about
d. Faintness and
ay occur, espe-
sudden po-
ges. Varicose
egin to
oman
fetal
and
may sud-
more
la darken.
ness may de-
cramps may
cur. Constipa-
evelop.

Fundus above umbilicus. Backache and leg cramps may begin. Skin changes can include striae gravidarum, chloasma, linea nigra, acne, redness on palms of hands and soles of feet. Nosebleeds can occur. May experience abdominal itching as uterus enlarges; will continue until end of pregnancy.

Fundus halfway between umbilicus and xiphoid process. May develop hemorrhoids. Thoracic breathing replaces abdominal breathing. Fetal outline palpable. May be tired of pregnancy and eager for the mothering role. Heartburn may begin to occur. May begin taking childbirth preparation classes with partner or support person.

t elevated when possible;
and carefully. Avoid
lower thighs. Support
ay be helpful. Cool-air
nay help. Eat foods con-
r, such as raw fruits,
cereals with bran; drink
exercise frequently.
ast care. Discuss dorsiflex-
to relieve cramps; heat to
uscle.

Assure woman that skin changes generally subside soon after birth. Discuss specific exercises such as pelvic tilt to help strengthen back and abdominal muscles, and stress importance of good body mechanics. Reiterate importance of avoiding medications, caffeine, alcohol, and smoking. Woman may choose to apply petroleum jelly in nostrils to relieve nosebleeds. Cool vaporizer may also help. Lanolin-based cream can relieve itching. Mild soap can remove excess oil associated with acne.

Avoid constipation; use sitz baths, gentle reinsertion of hemorrhoids with a fingertip as necessary. Topical anesthetic agents may offer relief of hemorrhoids. Stool softeners may be prescribed by caregiver. Elevate legs and assume sidelying position when resting. Eat small, more frequent meals; avoid fatty foods, lying down after eating. Maalox or Mylanta may be helpful; Avoid sodium bicarbonate. Discuss expectations about labor and delivery, caring for an infant.

Brown fat deposits are developing beneath the skin to insulate the baby following birth. Baby has grown to about 15–17 in. Begins storing iron, calcium, and phosphorus.

The entire uterus is occupied by the baby, thus restricting its activity. Maternal antibodies are transferred to the baby. This provides immunity for about 6 months until the infant's own immune system can take over.

Prentice Hall Health
Upper Saddle River, New Jersey 07458
Illustrations by Imagineering Media Services, Inc.

Fundus reaches xiphoid process; breasts full and tender. Urinary frequency may return. Swollen ankles and sleeping problems may develop. Dyspnea may develop.

The fetus descends deeper into the mother's pelvis (lightening). The placenta is nearly 4 times as thick as it was 20 weeks ago, weighing nearly 20 oz. Mother is eager for birth, may have final burst of energy. Backaches, urinary frequency increase. Braxton Hicks contractions intensify as cervix and lower uterine segment prepare for labor. Couple may tour labor and delivery area.

Wear well-fitting supportive bra. Elevate legs once or twice daily for an hour or so. Sleep on left side if possible. Use naturally occurring diuretics such as 2 tbsp lemon juice in 1 cup water or a generous serving of watermelon if available. Avoid most diuretics unless specifically prescribed. Maintain proper posture; use extra pillows at night for severe dyspnea. Following culture and personal preference, may begin preparing nursery now.
Review signs of labor. Discuss plans for other children (if any), transportation to agency.

Continue pelvic tilt exercises. Wear low-heeled shoes or flats. Avoid heavy lifting. Sleep on side to relieve bladder pressure. Urinate frequently. Avoid all analgesics except acetaminophen. Pack suitcase for delivery.

Discuss postpartum period including decisions such as circumcision, rooming-in. Discuss common postpartum discomforts; mention postpartum blues. Discuss family planning methods, infant care. Stress need for adequate rest post-partally. Provide support, especially if baby is overdue.

A Day in the Life of a Nurse-Midwife

TO ME, PREGNANCY IS A WONDERFUL, normal experience—part of the cycle of life. That's why I love the fact that I can participate in all aspects of it, from pregnancy through birth and into the postpartal period. My practice enables me to ensure that a family's childbirth experience incorporates their personal beliefs and meets their expectations as much as possible. Come along with me for a day.

Cherrene has come for contraceptiv mation. I find it helpful to use mod examples during the discussion.

Dianne and her family come together for every appointment. We all enjoy listening to the fetal heartbeat.

Gretchen's pregnancy is progressing well. She asks what her baby looks like now. I like to use a visual device as I talk with her about her baby's development.

I measure the height of the fundu determine if the baby is growin expected. Gretchen and I talk abou impact of her nutrition, exercise, healthy lifestyle habits on her baby the outcome of her pregnancy.

Development is rapid; heart begins to pump blood; limb buds are well developed. Facial features and major divisions of the brain are discernible. Ears develop from skin folds; tiny bones and muscles are formed beneath the thin skin.

Embryo becomes a fetus, its beating heart discernible by ultrasound. Assumes a more human shape as lower body develops. At week 12, first movements begin. Sex is determinable. Kidneys produce urine.

Musculoskeletal system has matured; nervous system begins to exert control. Blood vessels rapidly develop. Fetal hands can grasp; legs kick actively. All organs begin to mature and grow. Fetus weighs about 7 oz (½ lb). FHT discernible with Doppler. Pancreas produces insulin.

Ve co ski de of

Morning sickness, may persist to 12 weeks. Uterus changes from pear to globular shape. Hegar's, Goodell's and Piskacek's signs appear. Cervix flexes; leukorrhea increases. Surprise and ambivalence about pregnancy may occur. No noticeable weight gain.

Chadwick's sign appears. Uterus rises above pelvic brim by 12 weeks. Braxton Hicks contractions may begin and continue throughout pregnancy. Potential for urinary tract infection (UTI) increases and exists throughout pregnancy. Weight gain of about 2 ½ to 4 lb during first trimester.

Placenta now fully functioning and producing hormones.

Fundus halfway between symphysis and umbilicus. Woman gains slightly less than 1 lb per wk for remainder of pregnancy. May feel more energetic. BPD measurement on ultrasound. Vaginal secretions increase. Itching, irritation, malodor suggest infection. Woman may begin wearing maternity clothes. Pressure on bladder lessens and urinary frequency decreases.

Fu un sec An 40 dia cia sit vei de exp me pre de "re Na vel be tio

Eat dry crackers before arising; try frequent small, dry, low-fat meals with fluids taken between meals. Avoid use of hot tubs, saunas, and steam rooms throughout pregnancy.

Discuss attitudes toward pregnancy. Discuss value of early pregnancy classes that focus on what to expect during pregnancy. Provide information about childbirth preparation classes.

Adequate fluid intake and frequent voiding (every 2 hr while awake) help prevent UTI. Also helpful to void following intercourse. Wipe from front to rear.

Discuss nutrition and appropriate weight gain. Stress value of regular physical exercise, especially non-weightbearing activities or walking. Discuss possible effects of pregnancy on sexual relationship.

Daily shower or bath and thorough drying of vulva helpful; avoid douching during pregnancy. Consult caregiver if infection suspected; use only prescribed medications.

Review danger signs of pregnancy. Discuss infant feeding options; provide information on the value of breastfeeding. Provide information about clothing, shoes.

Sit ris pre sto va tai ve liq Di ior aff

share

While I'm at the birth center, I check in on Alisa and Richard. Their baby, Lydia Rose, was born 6 hours ago. Alisa has asked for help with breastfeeding. Baby Lydia is a sleepy little one and needs encouragement to latch on and begin feeding.

After baby Lydia has finished nursing, I do a physical assessment. I prefer to do an assessment in the room with the parents. It is such a wonderful opportunity for them to learn about their baby.

is most
her and
nd pro-
g, baby

FETAL ASSESSMENT

Fetal Position and Presentation

Fetal position and presentation are determined by inspecting the woman's abdomen, palpating it, performing a vaginal examination, and auscultating fetal heart rate (FHR). Ultrasound may also be used.

Inspection

Observe the size and shape of the woman's abdomen. Assess the lie of the fetus by noting whether the uterus projects up and down (longitudinal lie) or left to right (transverse lie).

Palpation: Leopold's Maneuvers

Leopold's maneuvers are a systematic way to evaluate the maternal abdomen. Frequent practice increases the examiner's skill in determining fetal position by palpation. Leopold's maneuvers may be difficult to perform on an obese woman or on a woman who has excessive amniotic fluid (hydramnios). Before performing Leopold's maneuvers, have the woman empty her bladder and lie on her back with her feet on the bed and her knees bent. (See Figure 18–5 ● for technique. Also see Skill 3–3 in the *Clinical Skills Manual* SKILLS.)

First maneuver

A

Second maneuver

B

Third maneuver

C

Fourth maneuver

D

● **Figure 18–5** Leopold's maneuvers for determining fetal position and presentation. *A,* First maneuver: Facing the woman, palpate the upper abdomen with both hands. Note the shape, consistency, and mobility of the palpated part. The fetal head is firm and round and moves independently of the trunk. The buttock feels softer, and it moves with the trunk. *B,* Second maneuver: Moving the hands on the pelvis, palpate the abdomen with gentle but deep pressure. The fetal back, on one side of the abdomen, feels smooth, and the fetal extremities on the other side feel knobby. *C,* Third maneuver: Place one hand just above the symphysis. Note whether the part palpated feels like the fetal head or the breech and whether it is engaged. *D,* Fourth maneuver: Facing the woman's feet, place both hands on the lower abdomen and move hands gently down the sides of the uterus toward the pubis. Note the cephalic prominence or brow.

Vaginal Examination and Ultrasound

During a vaginal examination, the examiner can palpate the presenting part if the cervix is dilated. The examination also provides information about the position of the fetus and the degree of flexion of its head (in cephalic presentations). Visualization by ultrasound is used when the fetal position cannot be determined by abdominal palpation.

Auscultation of Fetal Heart Rate

The handheld Doppler ultrasound (a device that operates using ultrasound waves that transmit the sounds made by the fetal heart rate) is used to auscultate the FHR between, during, and immediately after uterine contractions. Fetoscopes, which are modern combinations of both the stethoscope and the Pinard horn, can also be used to auscultate the FHR after 20 weeks. Fetoscopes are being used with decreasing frequency in modern obstetric practice, although some practitioners or patients may prefer this assessment method. Instead of listening haphazardly over the woman's abdomen for the FHR, it is useful to perform Leopold's maneuvers first. Leopold's maneuvers not only indicate the probable location of the FHR but also help determine the presence of multiple fetuses, fetal lie, and fetal presentation. The FHR is heard most clearly at the fetal back (Figure 18–6 ●). Thus, in a cephalic presentation, the FHR is best heard in the lower quadrant of the maternal abdomen. In a breech presentation, it is heard at or above the level of the maternal umbilicus. In a transverse lie, the FHR may be heard best just above or just below the umbilicus. As the presenting part descends and rotates through the pelvic structure during labor, the location of the FHR tends to descend and move toward the midline.

After the FHR is located, it is usually counted for 30 seconds and multiplied by 2 to obtain the number of beats per minute (beats/min). Check the woman's pulse against the fetal sounds. If the rates are the same, readjust the Doppler or fetoscope. Occasionally listen for a full minute, through and just after a contraction, to detect any abnormal heart rate, especially if the FHR is over 160 beats/min (tachycardia), under 110 beats/min (bradycardia), or irregular. If the FHR is irregular or has changed markedly from the last assessment, listen for a full minute through and immediately after a contraction. In these situations, continuous electronic fetal monitoring is warranted (American College of Obstetricians and Gynecologists [ACOG], 2009). (See Skill 3–4 in the *Clinical Skills Manual* SKILLS and Table 18–4 for guidelines on how often to auscultate the FHR.) Refer to *Assessment Guide: Intrapartum—First Stage of Labor* on pages 393–398.

Intermittent auscultation has been found to be as effective as the electronic method for fetal surveillance. A growing number of healthcare professionals, physicians and nurses alike, are beginning to question the widespread use of a technology that has not proven its overall worth. Figure 18–7 ● shows the use of a Doppler to auscultate the FHR.

Electronic Monitoring of Fetal Heart Rate

Electronic fetal monitoring (EFM) produces a continuous tracing of the FHR, which allows visual assessment of many characteristics of the FHR (see Skill 3–5 in the *Clinical Skills Manual* SKILLS).

Indications for Electronic Monitoring

If one or more of the following factors are present, the FHR and contractions are monitored by electronic fetal monitoring:

- Previous history of a stillborn (fetus dies in the uterus) at 38 or more weeks' gestation
- Presence of a complication of pregnancy (e.g., preeclampsia/eclampsia, placenta previa, abruptio placentae, multiple gestation, prolonged or premature rupture of membranes)

LSA
LOP
RSA
LOA
ROP
ROA

Location of FHR in LOA position

● **Figure 18–6** Location of FHR in relation to the more commonly seen fetal positions.

Table 18–4	Frequency of Auscultation: Assessment and Documentation

Low-Risk Women	High-Risk Women
First stage of labor: q30 min	First stage of labor: q15 min
Second stage of labor: q15 min	Second stage of labor: q5 min

Labor Events

Assess FHR before:
- Initiation of labor-enhancing procedures (e.g., artificial rupture of membranes)
- Periods of ambulation
- Administration of medications
- Administration or initiation of analgesia or anesthesia

Assess FHR following:
- Rupture of membranes
- Recognition of abnormal uterine activity patterns, such as increased basal tone or tachysystole
- Evaluation of oxytocin (maintenance, increase, or decrease of dosage)
- Administration of medications (at time of peak action)
- Expulsion of enema
- Urinary catheterization
- Vaginal examination
- Periods of ambulation
- Evaluation of analgesia and/or anesthesia (maintenance, increase, or decrease of dosage)

Source: Adapted from American College of Obstetricians & Gynecologists. (2009). *Intrapartum fetal heart rate monitoring: Nomenclature, interpretation, and general management principles* (ACOG Practice Bulletin, No. 106). Washington, DC: Author.

● **Figure 18–7** The nurse uses a Doppler to assess the fetal heart rate. Doppler monitors can be used for intermittent labor monitoring or in the outpatient or community setting.

Source: © Artur Steinhagen/Fotolia.

- Induction of labor (labor that is begun as a result of some type of intervention such as an intravenous infusion of oxytocin [Pitocin])

- Preterm labor (gestation less than 37 completed weeks)

- Decreased fetal movement

- Nonreassuring fetal status

- Meconium staining of amniotic fluid (meconium has been released into the amniotic fluid by the fetus, which may indicate a problem)

- Trial of labor after cesarean birth (TOLAC) (ACOG, 2010a). For a complete discussion of TOLAC, see Chapter 23 ●.

Methods of Electronic Monitoring of FHR

External monitoring of the fetus is usually accomplished by ultrasound. A transducer, which emits continuous sound waves, is placed on the maternal abdomen. When the transducer is placed correctly, the sound waves bounce off the fetal heart and are picked up by the electronic monitor. The actual moment-by-moment FHR is displayed graphically on a screen (Figure 18–8 ●). In some instances the monitor may track the maternal heart rate instead of the fetal heart rate. Avoid this error by palpating the maternal pulse or using a pulse oximeter to compare to the rate of the FHR.

Recent advances in technology have led to the development of new ambulatory methods of external monitoring. Using a telemetry system, a small, battery-operated transducer transmits signals to a receiver connected to the monitor. This system, held in place with a shoulder strap, allows the woman to ambulate, helping her to feel more comfortable and less confined during labor. In contrast, the system depicted in Figure 18–8 requires the woman to remain close to the electrical power source for the monitor.

Internal monitoring requires an internal spiral electrode. To place the spiral electrode on the fetal occiput, the amniotic membranes must be ruptured, the cervix must be dilated at least 2 cm, the presenting part must be down against the cervix, and the presenting part must be known (that is, the examiner must be able to detect the actual part of the fetus that is down against the cervix). If all these factors are present, the labor and birth nurse, the physician, or the certified nurse-midwife inserts a sterile internal spiral electrode into the vagina and places it against the fetal presenting part. The spiral electrode is rotated clockwise until it is attached to the presenting part. Wires that extend from the spiral electrode are attached to a leg plate (which is placed on the woman's thigh) and then attached to the electronic fetal monitor (see Skill 3–6 in the *Clinical Skills Manual* SKILLS). This method of monitoring the FHR provides more accurate continuous data than external monitoring, because the signal is clearer and movement of the fetus or the woman does not interrupt it (Figure 18–9 ●). The FHR tracing at the top of Figure 18–10 ● was obtained by internal monitoring with a spiral electrode; the uterine contraction tracing at the bottom of the figure was obtained by external monitoring with a toco.

Baseline Fetal Heart Rate

The **baseline rate** refers to the average FHR rounded to increments of 5 beats/min observed during a 10-minute period of monitoring. Normal FHR (baseline rate) ranges from 110 to 160 beats/min. This excludes periodic or episodic changes,

● **Figure 18–8** Electronic fetal monitoring by external technique. The tocodynamometer ("toco") is placed over the uterine fundus. The toco provides information that can be used to monitor uterine contractions. The ultrasound device is placed over the area of the fetal back. This device transmits information about the FHR. Information from both the toco and the ultrasound device is transmitted to the electronic fetal monitor. The FHR is displayed in a digital display (as a blinking light), on the special monitor paper, and audibly (by adjusting a button on the monitor). The uterine contractions are displayed on the special monitor paper as well.

periods of marked variability, greater than 25 beats/min. Episodic patterns are those not associated with uterine contractions, whereas periodic patterns are those associated with uterine contractions, including early, late, and variable decelerations. The duration should be at least 2 minutes (Goodwin, Montoro, Muderspach, et al., 2010). There are two abnormal variations of the baseline rate: those above 160 beats/min (tachycardia) and those below 110 beats/min (bradycardia). Another change affecting the baseline is called *variability,* a change in FHR over a few seconds to a few minutes.

Fetal tachycardia is a sustained rate of 161 beats/min or above. *Marked tachycardia* is 180 beats/min or above. Causes of tachycardia include the following (Cunningham et al., 2010):

■ Early fetal hypoxia, which leads to stimulation of the sympathetic system as the fetus compensates for reduced blood flow

■ Maternal fever, which accelerates the metabolism of the fetus

■ Maternal dehydration

■ Beta-sympathomimetic drugs such as ritodrine, terbutaline, atropine, and isoxsuprine, which have a cardiac stimulant effect (ACOG, 2012).

■ Amnionitis (fetal tachycardia may be the first sign of developing intrauterine infection)

■ Maternal hyperthyroidism (thyroid-stimulating hormones may cross the placenta and stimulate FHR)

■ Fetal anemia (the heart rate is increased to improve tissue perfusion)

Tachycardia is considered an ominous sign if it is accompanied by decreases in the FHR characterized as late decelerations, severe variable decelerations, or decreased variability (to be discussed shortly.) If tachycardia is associated with maternal fever, treatment may include antipyretics and/or antibiotics.

Fetal bradycardia is a rate less than 110 beats/min during a 10-minute period or longer. Causes of fetal bradycardia include the following (Cunningham et al., 2010):

■ Late (profound) fetal hypoxia (depression of myocardial activity)

■ Maternal hypotension, which results in decreased blood flow to the fetus

■ Prolonged umbilical cord compression; fetal baroreceptors are activated by cord compression and this produces vagal stimulation, which results in decreased FHR

■ Fetal arrhythmia, which is associated with complete heart block in the fetus

■ Uterine hyperstimulation

■ Abruptio placentae

■ Uterine rupture

■ Vagal stimulation in the second stage (since this does not involve hypoxia, the fetus can recover)

■ Congenital heart block

■ Maternal hypothermia

Bradycardia may be a benign or an ominous sign. If average long-term variability exists, the bradycardia is considered benign. When bradycardia is accompanied by decreased long-term

Electrode wires

Grip

Guide tube

Electrode tip

Electrode

A

B

C

● **Figure 18–9** Technique for internal, direct fetal monitoring. *A,* Spiral electrode. *B,* Attaching the spiral electrode to the scalp. *C,* Attached spiral electrode with the guide tube removed.

variability and late decelerations, it is considered a sign of non-reassuring fetal status (Cunningham et al., 2010).

Baseline Variability

Baseline variability is a measure of the interplay (the push–pull effect) between the sympathetic and parasympathetic nervous systems over a 10-minute period. It reflects baseline fluctuations that are irregular in frequency and amplitude.

Fetal heart rate variability is defined as follows (Goodwin et al., 2010) (see Figure 18–11 ●):

- *Absent:* amplitude undetectable
- *Minimal:* amplitude detectable but 5 beats/min or less
- *Moderate:* amplitude 6 to 25 beats/min
- *Marked:* amplitude greater than 25 beats/min

Reduced variability is the best single predictor for determining fetal compromise (Cunningham et al., 2010). Fetal acidosis and subsequent hypoxia are highest in fetuses that have absent or minimal variability (Goodwin et al., 2010).

Causes of decreased variability include the following (Cunningham et al., 2010):

- Hypoxia and acidosis (decreased blood flow to the fetus)
- Administration of drugs such as meperidine hydrochloride (Demerol), diazepam (Valium), or hydroxyzine (Vistaril), which depress the fetal central nervous system
- Fetal sleep cycle (during fetal sleep, variability is decreased; fetal sleep cycles usually last for 20 to 40 minutes each hour)
- Fetus of less than 32 weeks' gestation (fetal neurologic control of heart rate is immature)

No FHR slowing with contractions

Beginning of contraction — End of contraction

←1 minute→

● **Figure 18–10** Normal FHR pattern obtained by internal monitoring. Note normal FHR, 140 to 158 beats/min, presence of long- and short-term variability, and absence of deceleration with adequate contractions. The bottom portion depicts uterine contractions obtained by external monitoring. Each dark vertical line marks 1 minute, and each small rectangle represents 10 seconds. The contraction frequency is about every 2½ minutes, and the duration of the contractions is 50 to 60 seconds. Arrows on the bottom of the tracing indicate beginnings of uterine contractions.

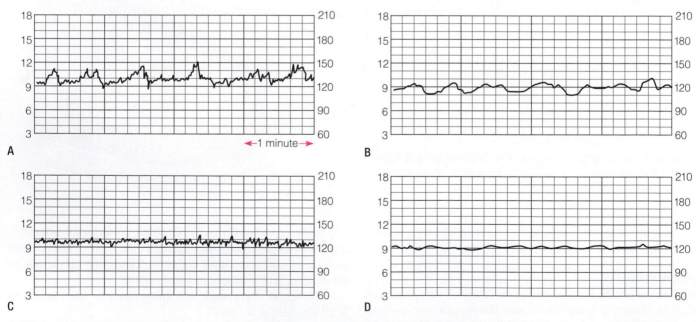

A

←1 minute→

B

C

D

● **Figure 18–11** Variability. *A,* Marked variability. *B,* Moderate variability. *C,* Minimal variability. *D,* Absent variability.

- Fetal anomalies affecting the heart, central nervous system, or autonomic nervous system
- Fetal dysrhythmias or fetal anomalies affecting the heart, central nervous system, or autonomic nervous system
- Previous neurologic insult
- Tachycardia

Causes of marked variability include the following (Goodwin et al., 2010):

- Early mild hypoxia (variability increases as a result of compensatory mechanism)
- Fetal stimulation or activity (stimulation of autonomic nervous system because of abdominal palpation, maternal

vaginal examination, application of spiral electrode on fetal head, or acoustic stimulation)

■ Fetal breathing movements

■ Advancing gestational age (greater than 30 weeks' gestation)

■ Stimulant medications

Absent variability that does not appear to be associated with a fetal sleep cycle or the administration of drugs is a warning sign of nonreassuring fetal status. It is especially ominous if absent or minimal variability is accompanied by late decelerations, explained shortly.

External electronic fetal monitoring is not an adequate method to assess variability. If decreased variability is noted on monitoring, application of a spiral electrode should be considered to obtain more accurate information.

Accelerations

Accelerations are transient increases in the FHR normally caused by fetal movement. When the fetus moves, the heart rate increases, just as the heart rates of adults increase during exercise. Often, accelerations accompany uterine contractions, usually due to fetal movement in response to the pressure of the contractions. Accelerations of this type are thought to be a sign of fetal well-being and adequate oxygen reserve. The accelerations with fetal movement form the basis for nonstress tests (discussed further in Chapter 16 ●).

Decelerations

Decelerations are periodic decreases in FHR from the normal baseline. They are categorized as early, late, and variable according to the time of their occurrence in the contraction cycle and their waveform (Figure 18–12 ●). When the fetal head is compressed, cerebral blood flow is decreased, which leads to central

	Early deceleration	**Late deceleration**	**Variable deceleration**
	Head compression (HC)	Uteroplacental insufficiency (UPI)	Umbilical cord compression (CC)
FHR pattern	Uniform shape	Uniform shape	Variable shape
Shape	Waveform consistently uniform; inversely mirrors contraction	Waveform uniform; shape reflects contraction	Waveform variable; generally sharp drops and returns
Onset	Just prior to or early in contraction	Late in contraction	Abrupt with fetal insult; not related to contraction
Lowest level	Consistently at or before midpoint of contraction	Consistently after the midpoint of the contraction	Variable around midpoint
Range	Usually within normal range of 120–160 beats/min	Usually within normal range of 120–130 beats/min	Not usually within normal range
Ensemble	Can be single or repetitive	Occasional, consistent, gradual increase—repetitive	Variable—single or repetitive

● **Figure 18–12** Types and characteristics of early, late, and variable decelerations.

vagal stimulation and results in early deceleration. The onset of **early deceleration** occurs before the onset of the uterine contraction. This type of deceleration is of uniform shape, is usually considered benign, and does not require intervention.

Late deceleration is caused by uteroplacental insufficiency resulting from decreased blood flow and oxygen transfer to the fetus through the intervillous spaces during uterine contractions. The most common causes of late decelerations are maternal hypotension resulting from the administration of epidural anesthesia and uterine hyperstimulation associated with oxytocin infusion (Reich, 2011). The onset of the deceleration occurs after the onset of a uterine contraction and is of a uniform shape that tends to reflect associated uterine contractions. The late deceleration pattern is considered a nonreassuring sign but does not necessarily require immediate childbirth. However, if they continue and birth is not imminent, a cesarean birth may be indicated.

Variable decelerations occur if the umbilical cord becomes compressed, thus reducing blood flow between the placenta and fetus. The resulting increase in peripheral resistance in the fetal circulation causes fetal hypertension. The fetal hypertension stimulates the baroreceptors in the aortic arch and carotid sinuses, which slow the FHR. The onset of variable decelerations varies in timing with the onset of the contraction, and the decelerations are variable in shape. This pattern requires further assessment. Nursing interventions for late and variable decelerations in FHR are presented in Table 18–5.

A *sinusoidal pattern* appears similar to a waveform. The characteristics of this pattern include absence of variability and the presence of a smooth, wavelike undulating shape. This pattern is associated with Rh alloimmunization, fetal anemia, severe fetal hypoxia, or a chronic fetal bleed. It may also occur with the administration of medications such as meperidine (Demerol) or butorphanol tartrate (Stadol). When it appears in association with medication, the pattern is usually temporary and is commonly referred to as *pseudosinusoidal* (Reich, 2011).

Decelerations are also classified based on the rate in which the FHR leaves the baseline FHR. *Episodic decelerations* occur independently of the uterine contractions and are frequently the result of external stimulations, such as vaginal exams. *Intermittent decelerations* refer to decelerations that occur with less than 50% of contractions and are considered recurrent if they occur with 50% or more of the contractions (Reich, 2011). Decelerations that leave the baseline for more than 2 minutes but less than 10 minutes are known as *prolonged decelerations*.

Psychologic Reactions to Electronic Monitoring

Responses to electronic fetal monitoring can be varied and complex. Many women have little knowledge of monitoring unless they have attended a prenatal class that dealt with this subject. Some women react to electronic monitoring positively, viewing it as a reassurance that "the baby is OK." They may also feel that the monitor helps identify problems that develop in labor. Other women may have ambivalent or even negative feelings about the monitor and may feel powerless to move and react in a way that feels natural to them. They may think that the monitor is interfering with a natural process, and they do not want the intrusion.

Clinical Tip

The presence of repetitive early decelerations may be a sign of advanced dilatation or the beginning of the second stage of labor. If the monitoring strip shows recurring early decelerations, ask the laboring woman if she is experiencing any pressure. Pressure that occurs only with the contractions typically indicates advanced dilatation. Intense pressure that does not change or ease up when the contractions cease may indicate the beginning of the second stage. A vaginal examination may be performed to establish the dilatation.

Some women may find that the equipment, wires, and sounds increase their anxiety. The discomfort of lying in one position and fear of injury to the baby are other objections.

Nursing Management

A key strength of technology is its ability to explain and possibly predict health patterns or problems. However, this advantage has the potential to dehumanize the nurse–patient relationship. It is crucial that nurses balance technology with holistic nursing practice. Therefore, it is important to recognize that every encounter with the childbearing family offers an opportunity to provide education and empowerment to the laboring woman and her partner. Helping to provide information when needed, answering questions, and encouraging the woman to make decisions establishes a trusting nurse–patient relationship.

Before using the electronic fetal monitor, explain the reason for its use and the information that it can provide. After applying the monitor, record basic information on the monitor strip. These data should include the date, patient's name, physician or certified nurse-midwife's name, hospital identification number, age, gravida, para, estimated date of birth, membrane status, and maternal vital signs. As the monitor strip runs and care is provided, occurrences during labor should be recorded not only in the medical record but also on the monitor strip. This information helps the healthcare team assess current status and evaluate the tracing.

Note the following information on the tracing (Murray, Huelsmann, & Koperski, 2011):

- Vaginal examination (dilatation, effacement, station, position)
- Amniotomy or spontaneous rupture of membranes, color and amount of amniotic fluid, presence of any odor
- Maternal vital signs
- Maternal position in bed and changes of position
- Application of spiral electrode or intrauterine pressure catheter
- Medications given
- Oxygen administration
- Maternal behaviors (emesis, coughing, hiccups)
- Fetal scalp stimulation or fetal scalp blood sampling
- Vomiting
- Pushing
- Administration of anesthesia blocks

Table 18–5   Guidelines for Management of Variable, Late, and Prolonged Deceleration Patterns

Pattern	Nursing Interventions
Variable decelerations Isolated or occasional Moderate	Report findings to physician or CNM and document in chart. Provide explanation to woman and partner. Change maternal position to one in which FHR pattern is most improved. Discontinue oxytocin if it is being administered and other interventions are unsuccessful. Perform vaginal examination to assess for prolapsed cord or change in labor progress. Monitor FHR continuously to assess current status and for further changes in FHR pattern.
Variable decelerations Severe and uncorrectable	Administer oxygen at 7 to 10 L/min. Report findings to physician or CNM and document in chart. Provide explanation to woman and partner. Prepare for probable cesarean birth. Follow interventions listed above. Prepare for vaginal birth unless baseline variability is decreasing or FHR is progressively rising—then cesarean, forceps, or vacuum birth is indicated. Assist physician with fetal scalp sampling if ordered. Prepare for cesarean birth if scalp pH shows acidosis or downward trend.
Late decelerations	Administer oxygen by face mask at 7 to 10 L/min. Report findings to physician or CNM and document in chart. Provide explanation to woman and partner. Monitor for further FHR changes. Maintain maternal position on left side. Maintain good hydration with IV fluids (normal saline or lactated Ringer's). Discontinue oxytocin if it is being administered and late decelerations persist despite other interventions. Monitor maternal blood pressure and pulse for signs of hypotension; possibly increase flow rate of IV fluids to treat hypotension. Follow physician's orders for treatment for hypotension if present. Assess labor progress (dilatation and station). Assist physician with fetal blood sampling: If pH stays above 7.25, physician will continue monitoring and resample; if pH shows downward trend (between 7.25 and 7.2) or is below 7.2, prepare for birth by most expeditious means.
Late decelerations with tachycardia or decreasing variability	Report findings to physician or CNM and document in chart. Maintain maternal position on left side. Administer oxygen by face mask at 7 to 10 L/min. Discontinue oxytocin if it is being administered. Assess maternal blood pressure and pulse. Increase IV fluids (normal saline or lactated Ringer's). Assess labor progress (dilatation and station). Prepare for immediate cesarean birth. Explain plan of treatment to woman and partner. Assist physician with fetal blood sampling (if ordered).
Prolonged decelerations	Perform vaginal examination to rule out prolapsed cord or to determine progress in labor status. Change maternal position as needed to try to alleviate decelerations. Discontinue oxytocin if it is being administered. Notify physician or CNM of findings and initial interventions and document in chart. Provide explanation to woman and partner. Increase IV fluids (normal saline or lactated Ringer's). Administer tocolytic if hypertonus noted and ordered by physician or CNM. Anticipate normal FHR recovery following deceleration if FHR previously normal. Anticipate intervention if FHR previously abnormal or deceleration lasts more than 3 minutes.

If the monitor does not automatically add the time on the strip at specific intervals, include the time when recording any information on the strip. If more than one nurse is adding information to the monitor strip, it is essential to initial each note. The tracing is considered a legal part of the woman's medical record and is submissible as evidence in court.

The fetal monitoring strip should be reviewed regularly—at least every 30 minutes in the first stage and every 15 minutes during the second stage (Murray et al., 2011).

The laboring woman needs to feel that what is happening to her is the central focus. Acknowledge this need by always speaking to and looking at the woman when entering the room, before looking at the monitor.

Evaluation of FHR Tracings

With a systematic approach to evaluating FHR tracings, the nurse can make a more accurate and rapid assessment, avoid interpreting findings on the basis of inadequate or erroneous data, and easily communicate data to the woman, physician or CNM, and staff. A universal language for documentation should be used consistently within the facility to avoid errors.

Evaluation of the electronic monitor tracing begins by looking at the uterine contraction pattern. To evaluate the contraction pattern, the nurse should do the following:

1. Determine the uterine resting tone.

2. Assess the contractions: What is the frequency? What is the duration? What is the intensity?

After evaluating the FHR tracing for the contraction pattern, the nurse may categorize the tracing according to the Three-Tier FHR Interpretation System (Table 18–6). The three-tier system for the categorization of FHR patterns is recommended by ACOG, AWHONN, and the National Institute of Child Health and Human Development (ACOG, 2010b; Macones, Hankins, Spong, et al., 2008). Categorization of the FHR tracing evaluates the fetus at that point in time; tracing patterns can and will change. A FHR tracing may move back and forth between categories depending on the clinical situation and management strategies employed.

Category I FHR tracings are normal. They are strongly predictive of normal fetal acid–base status at the time of observation. The FHR tracings may be followed in a routine manner, and no specific action is required.

Category II FHR tracings are indeterminate. They are not predictive of abnormal fetal acid–base status, yet there is not enough adequate evidence at present to classify these as Category I or Category III. Category II tracings require evaluation and continued surveillance and reevaluation, taking into account the entire associated clinical circumstances.

Category III FHR tracings are abnormal. They are predictive of abnormal fetal acid–base status at the time of observation if they continue. They require prompt evaluation. Depending on the clinical situation, efforts to expeditiously resolve the abnormal FHR pattern may include, but are not limited to, provision of maternal oxygen, change in maternal position, discontinuation of labor stimulation, and treatment of maternal hypotension. If they are not immediately corrected, acidemia will occur; therefore, birth is required via the fastest route possible.

Provision of Emotional Support

It is vital to provide information to the laboring woman about the FHR pattern and the interventions, if necessary, that will help her fetus. Most women are aware that something is happening. Sharing information with them provides reassurance that a potential or actual problem is identified and that they are active participants in the interventions. Occasionally a problem arises that requires immediate intervention. In that case it may be helpful to say something like, "It is important for you to turn on your left side right now because the baby is having a little difficulty. I'll explain what is happening in just a few moments." This type of response lets the woman know that although an action needs to be accomplished rapidly, information will soon be provided. In the haste to act quickly, nurses and other caregivers must not forget that it is the woman's body and her baby.

Table 18–6	Three-Tier Fetal Heart Rate Interpretation System	
Category 1	**Category 2**	**Category 3**
Reassuring Fetal Heart Rate Tracings	**Patterns Warranting Continual Assessment**	**Patterns of Nonreassuring Fetal Status That Warrant Immediate Intervention**
■ Normal range FHR 110–160 beats/min ■ Normal FHR variability in the moderate range ■ Absence of variable or late decelerations ■ Accelerations may be present or may be absent ■ Early decelerations may be present or may be absent; they do not represent a nonreassuring status	■ Baselines that include bradycardia with continued variability, or tachycardia ■ Baseline changes in variability that include minimal variability, absent variability without decelerations, or marked baseline variability ■ Lack of accelerations with scalp stimulation ■ Episodic decelerations that include recurrent variable decelerations with minimal or moderate variability, prolonged decelerations lasting >2 minutes but <10 minutes in duration, or recurrent late decelerations that maintain moderate variability ■ Variable deceleration patterns that include overshoots, shoulders, or slow return to baseline status	■ Absent variability in baseline FHR with recurrent late decelerations, recurrent variable decelerations, and/or bradycardia ■ Sinusoidal FHR patterns

Source: Data from Macones, G. A., Hankins, G. D. V., Spong, C. Y., Hauth, J., & Moore, T. (2008). The 2008 National Institute of Child Health and Human Development workshop report on electronic monitoring: Update on definitions, interpretation, and research guidelines. *Journal of Obstetrics, Gynecology and Neonatal Nursing, 37*(5), 510–515.

Scalp Stimulation Test

When there is a question about fetal status, a scalp stimulation test can be used before the more invasive **fetal blood sampling**. In this test the examiner applies pressure to the fetal scalp while doing a vaginal examination. The fetus who is not in any stress or distress responds with an acceleration of the FHR. Fetuses that fail to respond have an increased incidence of acidosis, hypoxia, and lower Apgar scores (Rathore et al., 2011).

Fetal vibroacoustic stimulation using a handheld artificial larynx applied to the maternal abdomen may also be used to assess fetal status. As with scalp stimulation, fetal heart rate accelerations in response are a sign of fetal well-being (Murray et al., 2011).

SAFETY ALERT!

If there is no fetal reaction to the scalp stimulation test and a Category II or Category III fetal heart rate tracing persists, the nurse should contact the physician/CNM to come to the woman's bedside and perform further evaluation.

Cord Blood Analysis at Birth

In some cases, when the practitioner wishes to determine if acidosis was present, a cord blood analysis will be obtained. Indications for cord blood analysis include:

- Meconium-stained amniotic fluid
- Significantly abnormal FHR patterns
- Infant is depressed at birth
- Apgar scores are less than 7 at 5 minutes of age

The cord is clamped before the infant takes the first breath. A small amount of blood is aspirated with a syringe from one of the umbilical arteries. If the cord blood will not be analyzed immediately, a heparinized syringe should be used. Normal fetal blood pH should be above 7.25 (Blackburn, 2013). Lower levels indicate acidosis and hypoxia. Many practitioners obtain cord blood analysis to minimize medicolegal exposure.

Assessment Guide Intrapartum—First Stage of Labor

Physical Assessment/Normal Findings	Alterations and Possible Causes*	Nursing Responses to Data†
Vital Signs		
Blood pressure (BP): less than or equal to 120 systolic and 80 diastolic in adult 18 years of age or older or no more than 15–20 mm Hg rise in systolic pressure over baseline BP during early pregnancy	High BP (essential hypertension, preeclampsia, renal disease, apprehension or anxiety) Low BP (supine hypotension)	Evaluate history of preexisting disorders and check for presence of other signs of preeclampsia or other hypertensive disorders. Assess for previous history of BP issues. Ensure blood pressure is being obtained with a proper cuff size because using a cuff that is too small will result in falsely abnormal elevated blood pressure readings. Do not assess during contractions; implement measures to decrease anxiety and reassess. Turn woman on her side and recheck BP. Provide quiet environment. Have O_2 available.
Pulse: 60–100 beats per minute (beats/min)	Increased pulse rate (excitement or anxiety, cardiac disorders, early shock)	Evaluate cause, reassess to see if rate continues; report to physician.
Respirations: 12–20/minute (or pulse rate divided by 4) (may be higher during labor)	Marked tachypnea (respiratory disease), hyperventilation in transition phase Hyperventilation (anxiety)	Assess between contractions; if marked tachypnea continues, assess for signs of respiratory disease.
Pulse oximeter (if used) 95% or greater	Less than 90% (hypoxia, hypotension, hemorrhage)	Encourage slow breaths if woman is hyperventilating. Apply O_2; notify physician.
Temperature: 36.2–37.6°C (98–99.6°F)	Elevated temperature (infection, dehydration, prolonged rupture of membranes, epidural regional block)	Assess for other signs of infection or dehydration.
Weight		
25–35 lb greater than prepregnant weight	Weight gain greater than 35 lb (fluid retention, obesity, large infant, diabetes mellitus, preeclampsia), weight gain less than 15 lb (small for gestational age [SGA], substance abuse, psychosocial problems)	Assess for signs of edema. Evaluate pattern from prenatal record.
Lungs		
Normal breath sounds, clear and equal	Rales, rhonchi, friction rub (infection), pulmonary edema, asthma	Reassess; refer to physician.

(continued)

Assessment Guide Intrapartum—First Stage of Labor—continued

Physical Assessment/Normal Findings	Alterations and Possible Causes*	Nursing Responses to Data†
Fundus At 40 weeks' gestation fundus is located just below xiphoid process	Uterine size not compatible with estimated date of birth (SGA, large for gestational age [LGA], hydramnios, multiple pregnancy, placental/fetal anomalies, malpresentation)	Reevaluate history regarding pregnancy dating. Refer to physician for additional assessment.
Edema Nondependent/nonpitting edema	Pitting edema of face, hands, legs, abdomen, sacral area (preeclampsia)	Check deep tendon reflexes for hyperactivity; check for clonus; refer to physician.
Hydration Normal skin turgor, elastic	Poor skin turgor (dehydration)	Assess skin turgor; refer to physician for deviations.
Perineum Tissues smooth, pink color (see *Assessment Guide: Initial Prenatal Assessment* in Chapter 10 🔗)	Varicose veins of vulva, herpes lesions, genital warts	Exercise care while doing a perineal prep; note on patient record need for follow-up in postpartum period; reassess after birth; refer to physician/CNM. If herpes lesions are present, do not assess the cervix if prophylaxis therapy has not been started as this increases transmission of infection.
Clear mucus; may be blood tinged with earthy or human odor	Profuse, purulent, foul-smelling drainage	Suspected gonorrhea or chorioamnionitis; report to physician/CNM; initiate care to newborn's eyes; notify neonatal nursing staff and pediatrician.
Presence of small amount of bloody show that gradually increases with further cervical dilatation	Hemorrhage	Assess BP and pulse, pallor, diaphoresis; report any marked changes. (*Note:* Gaping of vagina or anus and bulging of perineum are signs that suggest the onset of the second stage of labor.) Follow universal precautions.
Labor Status *Uterine contractions:* regular pattern	Failure to establish a regular pattern, prolonged latent phase; hypertonicity; hypotonicity; dehydration	Evaluate whether woman is in true labor; ambulate if in early labor. Evaluate patient status and contractile pattern. Obtain a 20-minute electronic fetal monitor (EFM) strip. Notify physician/CNM. Provide hydration.
Cervical dilatation: progressive cervical dilatation from size of fingertip to 10 cm (see Skill 3–1 in the *Clinical Skills Manual* SKILLS)	Rigidity of cervix (frequent cervical infections, scar tissue, failure of presenting part to descend)	Evaluate contractions, fetal engagement, position, and cervical dilatation. Inform woman of progress.
Cervical effacement: progressive thinning of cervix (see Skill 3–1 SKILLS)	Failure to efface (rigidity of cervix, failure of presenting part to engage); cervical edema (pushing effort by woman before cervix is fully dilated and effaced	Evaluate contractions, fetal engagement, and position. Notify physician/CNM if cervix is becoming edematous; work with woman to prevent pushing until cervix is completely dilated. Keep vaginal exams to a minimum.
Fetal descent: progressive descent of fetal presenting part from station −5 to +4 (see Skill 3–1 SKILLS)	Failure of descent (abnormal fetal position or presentation, macrosomic fetus, inadequate pelvic measurement)	Evaluate fetal position, presentation, and size. Evaluate maternal pelvic measurements. If descent is slow, offer birthing ball or assist with squatting position.
Membranes: may rupture before or during labor	Rupture of membranes more than 12–24 hours before onset of labor	Assess for ruptured membranes using Nitrazine test tape before doing vaginal exam. Follow universal precautions. Instruct woman with ruptured membranes to remain on bed rest if presenting part is not engaged and firmly down against the cervix. Keep vaginal exams to a minimum to prevent infection. When membranes rupture in the birth setting, *immediately assess fetal heart rate* to detect changes associated with prolapse of umbilical cord (FHR slows).

Assessment Guide Intrapartum—First Stage of Labor—continued

Physical Assessment/Normal Findings	Alterations and Possible Causes*	Nursing Responses to Data†
Findings on Nitrazine test tape: Membranes probably intact Yellow pH 5.0 Olive pH 5.5 Olive green pH 6.0 Membranes probably ruptured Blue-green pH 6.5 Blue-gray pH 7.0 Deep blue pH 7.5	False-positive results may be obtained if large amount of bloody show is present, previous vaginal examination has been done using lubricant, sweat or sperm is present, or tape is touched by nurse's fingers.	Assess fluid for consistency, amount, odor; assess FHR frequently. Assess fluid at regular intervals for presence of meconium staining. Follow universal precautions while assessing amniotic fluid. Reassure woman that amniotic fluid is continually produced. Teach woman that she may feel amniotic fluid trickle or gush with contractions. Change chux pads often.
Amniotic fluid clear, with earthy or human odor, no foul-smelling odor	Greenish amniotic fluid (fetal stress) Bloody fluid (abruptio placentae)	Assess FHR; do vaginal exam to evaluate for prolapsed cord; apply fetal monitor for continuous data; report to physician/CNM.
	Strong or foul odor (amnionitis)	Take woman's temperature and report to physician/CNM.

Fetal Status

Fetal heart rate (FHR): 110–160 beats/min	Less than 110 or greater than 160 beats/min (nonreassuring fetal status); abnormal patterns on fetal monitor: decreased variability, late decelerations, variable decelerations, absence of accelerations with fetal movement	Initiate interventions based on particular FHR pattern.
Presentation: Cephalic, 97% Breech, 3%	Face, brow, breech, or shoulder presentation	Report to physician/CNM; after presentation is confirmed as face, brow, breech, or shoulder, woman may be prepared for cesarean birth.
Position: left occiput anterior (LOA) most common	Persistent occipital posterior (OP) position; transverse arrest	Carefully monitor maternal and fetal status. Reposition mother to side-lying or hands and knees to promote rotation of fetal head.
Activity: fetal movement	Hyperactivity (may precede fetal hypoxia) Complete lack of movement (fetal distress or fetal demise)	Carefully evaluate FHR; apply fetal monitor. Carefully evaluate FHR; apply fetal monitor. Report to physician/CNM.

Laboratory Evaluation

Hematologic tests: Hemoglobin: 12–16 g/dL	Less than 11 g/dL (anemia, hemorrhage)	Evaluate woman for problems due to decreased oxygen-carrying capacity caused by lowered hemoglobin.

Complete blood count (CBC):
Hematocrit: 38%–47%
Red blood cell count
    (RBC): 4.2–5.4 million/mm³
White blood cell count
    (WBC): 4500–11,000/mm³, although leukocytosis to 20,000/mm³ is not unusual
Platelets: 150,000–400,000/mm³
	Presence of infection or blood dyscrasias, loss of blood (hemorrhage, disseminated intravascular coagulation [DIC])	Evaluate for other signs of infection or for petechiae, bruising, or unusual bleeding.

Serologic testing: Serologic test for syphilis (STS) or Venereal Disease Research Laboratory (VDRL) test: nonreactive	Positive reaction (see *Assessment Guide: Initial Prenatal Assessment* in Chapter 10)	For reactive test, notify newborn nursery and pediatrician.
Rh factor	Rh-positive fetus in Rh-negative woman	Assess prenatal record for titer levels during pregnancy. Obtain cord blood for direct Coombs' at birth.
Urinalysis Glucose: negative	Glycosuria (low renal threshold for glucose, diabetes mellitus)	Assess blood glucose level; test urine for ketones; ketonuria and glycosuria require further assessment of blood sugar levels.‡

(continued)

Assessment Guide Intrapartum—First Stage of Labor—continued

Physical Assessment/Normal Findings	Alterations and Possible Causes*	Nursing Responses to Data†
Ketones: negative	Ketonuria (starvation ketosis), vomiting, hyperemesis gravidarum	
Proteins: negative	Proteinuria (urine specimen contaminated with vaginal secretions, fever, kidney disease); proteinuria of 2+ or greater found in uncontaminated urine may be a sign of ensuing preeclampsia	Instruct woman in collection technique; incidence of contamination from vaginal discharge is common. Report any increase in proteinuria to physician/CNM.
Red blood cells: negative	Blood in urine (calculi, cystitis, glomerulonephritis, neoplasm)	Assess collection technique (may be bloody show).
White blood cells: negative	Presence of white blood cells (infection in genitourinary tract)	Assess for signs of urinary tract infection.
Casts: none	Presence of casts (nephrotic syndrome)	

Cultural Assessment§	Variations to Consider	Nursing Responses to Data†
Cultural influences determine customs and practices regarding intrapartum care.	Individual preferences may vary.	
Ask the following questions: Who would you like to remain with you during your labor and birth?	She may prefer only her partner/significant other to remain or may also want family and/or friends.	Provide support for her wishes by encouraging desired people to stay. Provide information to others (with the woman's permission) who are not in the room.
What would you like to wear during labor?	She may be more comfortable in her own clothes if permitted by facility policy.	Offer supportive materials such as chux pad if needed to protect her own clothing. Avoid subtle signals to the woman that she should not have chosen to remain in her own clothes. Have other clothing available if the woman desires. If her clothing becomes contaminated, it will be simple to place it in a plastic bag. The nurse can soak soiled clothing in cool water. The nurse needs to remember to wear disposable gloves and a plastic apron if splashing is anticipated.
What activity would you like during labor?	She may want to ambulate most of the time, stand in the shower, sit in the Jacuzzi, sit in a chair or on a stool, remain on the bed, and so forth. These activities may be impacted by facility policy.	Support the woman's wishes; provide encouragement and complete assessments in a manner so her activity and positional wishes are disturbed as little as possible.
What position would you like for the birth?	She may feel more comfortable in lithotomy with stirrups and her upper body elevated, or side-lying or sitting in birthing bed, or standing, or squatting, or on hands and knees.	Collect any supplies and equipment needed to support her in her chosen birthing position. Provide information to the coach regarding any changes that may be needed based on the chosen position.
Is there anything special you would like?	She may want the room darkened or to have curtains and windows open, music playing, a Leboyer birth (waterbirth), certain scents, her coach to cut the umbilical cord, to save a portion of the umbilical cord, to save the placenta, to videotape the birth, and so forth.	Support requests and communicate requests to any other nursing or medical personnel (so requests can continue to be supported and not questioned). If another nurse or physician does not honor the request, act as advocate for the woman by continuing to support her unless her desire is truly unsafe.
Ask the woman if she would like fluids and ask what temperature she prefers.	She may prefer clear fluids other than water (tea, clear juice). She may prefer iced, room-temperature, or warmed fluids.	Provide fluids as desired.

Assessment Guide Intrapartum—First Stage of Labor—continued

Physical Assessment/Normal Findings	Alterations and Possible Causes*	Nursing Responses to Data†
Observe the woman's response when privacy is difficult to maintain and her body is exposed.	Some women do not seem to mind being exposed during an exam or procedure; others feel acute discomfort.	Maintain privacy and respect the woman's sense of privacy. If the woman is unable to provide specific information, the nurse may draw from general information regarding cultural variation: a Southeast Asian woman may not want any family member in the room during exams or procedures. Her partner may not be involved with coaching activities during labor or birth. Muslim women may need to remain covered during the labor and birth and avoid exposure of any body part. The husband may need to be in the room but remain behind a curtain or screen so he does not view his wife at this time.
If the woman is to breastfeed, encourage her to feed her baby immediately after birth while the baby is in a more alert state.	She may want to feed her baby right away or may want to wait a little while if she feels too fatigued. However, the nurse should encourage immediate feeding when possible.	
Preparation for Childbirth Woman has some information regarding process of normal labor and birth.	Some women do not have any information regarding childbirth.	Add to present information base.
Woman has breathing and/or relaxation techniques to use during labor.	Some women do not have any method of relaxation or breathing to use, and some do not desire them.	Support breathing and relaxation techniques that patient is using; provide information if needed.
Response to Labor *Latent phase* (0–3 cm): relaxed, excited, anxious for labor to be well established	May feel unable to cope with contractions because of fear, anxiety, or lack of information	Provide support and encouragement; establish trusting relationship.
Active phase (4–7 cm): becomes more intense, begins to tire *Transitional phase* (8–10 cm): feels tired, may feel unable to cope, needs frequent coaching to maintain breathing patterns	May remain quiet and without any sign of discomfort or anxiety, may insist that she is unable to continue with the birthing process	Provide support and coaching if needed.
Coping mechanisms: ability to cope with labor through utilization of support system, breathing, relaxation techniques	May feel marked anxiety and apprehension, may not have coping mechanisms that can be brought into this experience, or may be unable to use them at this time.	Support coping mechanisms if they are working for the woman; provide information and support if she exhibits anxiety or needs alternative to present coping methods.
	Survivors of sexual abuse may demonstrate fear of IVs or needles, may recoil when touched, may insist on a female caregiver, may be very sensitive to body fluids and cleanliness, and may be unable to labor lying down.	Encourage participation of coach or significant other if a supportive relationship seems apparent. Establish rapport and a trusting relationship. Provide information that is true and offer your presence.
Anxiety Some anxiety and apprehension is within normal limits	May show anxiety through rapid breathing, nervous tremors, frowning, grimacing, clenching of teeth, thrashing movements, crying, increased pulse and blood pressure.	Provide support, encouragement, and information. Teach relaxation techniques; support controlled breathing efforts. May need to provide a paper bag to breathe into if woman says her lips are tingling. Note FHR.
Sounds During Labor	Some women are very quiet; others moan or make a variety of noises.	Provide a supportive environment. Encourage woman to do what is right for her.

(continued)

Assessment Guide Intrapartum—First Stage of Labor—continued

Physical Assessment/Normal Findings	Alterations and Possible Causes*	Nursing Responses to Data†
Support System		
Physical intimacy between mother and father (or mother and support person); caretaking activities such as soothing conversation, touching	Some women would prefer no contact; others may show clinging behaviors.	Encourage caretaking activities that appear to comfort the woman; encourage support to the woman; if support is limited, the nurse may take a more active role.
Support person stays in proximity	Limited interaction may come from a desire for quiet.	Encourage support person to stay close (if this seems appropriate).
Relationship between mother and father (or support person): involved interaction	The support person may seem to be detached and maintain little support, attention, or conversation.	Support interactions; if interaction is limited, the nurse may provide more information and support. Ensure that coach or significant other has short breaks, especially prior to transition.

*Possible causes of alterations are placed in parentheses.
†This column provides guidelines for further assessment and initial nursing intervention.
‡Glycosuria should not be discounted. The presence of glycosuria necessitates follow-up.
§These are only a few suggestions. We do not mean to imply that this is a comprehensive cultural assessment; rather, it is a tool to encourage cultural sensitivity.

Critical Concept Review

LEARNING OUTCOME 18.1: Describe a maternal assessment of the laboring woman that includes the patient history, high-risk screening, and physical and psychosociocultural factors.

1. High-risk screening is completed to determine if there are any factors present that may be associated with a high-risk condition.
2. Maternal physical factors include:
   - Vital signs.
   - Labor status.
   - Fetal status.
   - Laboratory findings.
3. Cultural assessment:
   - Individual beliefs and preferences.
4. Psychosocial factors:
   - Childbearing fears.
   - Childbearing knowledge and fantasies.
   - Previous history of psychologic disorders.

LEARNING OUTCOME 18.2: Evaluate the progress of labor by assessing the laboring woman's contractions, cervical dilatation, and effacement.

Progress of labor is evaluated by:
1. Assessment of strength and frequency of contractions:
   - Hand palpation.
   - Electronic monitoring.
   - External and internal pressure catheters.
2. Cervical assessment:
   - Determination of cervical dilatation—from 1 to 10 cm
   - Determination of effacement—measured in percentage. Full effacement is 100%.

LEARNING OUTCOME 18.3: Delineate the procedure for performing Leopold's maneuvers and the information that can be obtained, including the importance of identifying accurate fetal position prior to performing a fetal heart rate assessment.

1. Leopold's maneuvers evaluate the position, presentation, and lie of the fetus by palpation of the woman's abdomen:
   - Woman empties her bladder and lies on her back with her knees flexed.
   - The practitioner palpates the abdomen gently but deeply using the palms of the hands.
   - One hand is held steady while the other explores one side of the abdomen, then the action of the hands is switched.
2. The FHR is heard most clearly at the fetal back; therefore, fetal position should be identified.
   - In a cephalic presentation, the FHR is best heard in the lower quadrant of the maternal abdomen.
   - In a breech presentation, it is heard at or above the level of the maternal umbilicus.
   - In a transverse lie, the FHR may be heard best just above or just below the umbilicus.

LEARNING OUTCOME 18.4: Describe the steps and frequency for performing auscultation of fetal heart rate.

1. Location of fetal heart rate:
   - Heard best at the fetal back.
2. Assessment may be intermittent:
   - Handheld Doppler ultrasound auscultates the FHR between, during, and after a contraction.
   - Fetoscope may be used.

3. Most assessment is continuous:
   - External.
   - Internal scalp electrode.

LEARNING OUTCOME 18.5: Distinguish between baseline and periodic changes in fetal heart rate monitoring, and the appearance and significance of each.

1. Baseline fetal heart rate:
   - Average FHR observed during a 10-minute period of monitoring.
   - Should be between 110 and 160 beats/min.
   - Baseline changes of the FHR include tachycardia, bradycardia, and variability.

Periodic changes:
1. Accelerations:
   - Usually caused by fetal movement.
   - Reassuring sign of fetal well-being when it occurs during a contraction.

2. Decelerations:
   - Early deceleration occurs before a contraction and usually requires no intervention.
   - Later deceleration occurs during and after a contraction and indicates insufficient blood flow to the fetus. It is a nonreassuring sign.
   - Variable decelerations occur due to umbilical cord compression and require further assessment.
   - Sinusoidal pattern appears when there are no periods of normal fetal heart rate. It is associated with Rh problems, fetal anemia, severe fetal hypoxia, or a chronic fetal bleed.

LEARNING OUTCOME 18.6: Evaluate fetal heart rate tracings using a systematic approach.

1. Evaluate the uterine contraction pattern.
2. Determine the baseline FHR.
3. Determine FHR variability.
4. Determine if a sinusoidal pattern is present.
5. Determine if there are periodic changes.

LEARNING OUTCOME 18.7: Compare nonreassuring fetal heart rate patterns to appropriate nursing responses.

1. Severe variable decelerations.
2. Late decelerations of any magnitude.
3. Absence of variability.
4. Prolonged deceleration.

Nursing responses include:
1. Notify the physician or CNM.
2. Administer maternal oxygen.

3. Turn mother to the left side.
4. Discontinue oxytocin if being administered.
5. Monitor FHR continuously.
6. Provide explanation to the mother and partner.

LEARNING OUTCOME 18.8: Explain the family's responses to electronic fetal monitoring in nursing care management.

1. Explain the use of EFM.
2. Look at mother prior to looking at monitor.

3. Record pertinent data on monitor strip.

Clinical Reasoning in Action

Cindy Bell, a 20-year-old gravida 2, para 1, at 40 weeks' gestation, presents to you in the birthing unit with contractions every 5 to 7 minutes. She is accompanied by her husband. Spontaneous rupture of membranes occurred 2 hours prior to admission. Cindy tells you that the fluid was colorless and clear. You orient Cindy and her family to the birthing room and perform a physical assessment, documenting the following data: vital signs are normal. A vaginal exam demonstrates the cervix is 75% effaced, 4 cm dilated with a vertex at –1 station in the LOP position. You place Cindy on an external fetal monitor. The fetal heart rate baseline is 140–147 with accelerations to 156; no decelerations are noted. Contractions are 5–6 minutes apart, moderate intensity, and lasting 40–50 seconds. Cindy states she would like to stay out of bed as long as possible because lying down seems to make the contractions more painful, especially in her back.

1. Discuss the benefits of ambulation in labor.
2. Cindy would like her daughter to be present for the baby's birth. What would you discuss with her about the impact of having a young sibling present during labor and birth?
3. What fetal heart rate assessment will best ensure fetal well-being during the period Cindy is ambulating?
4. When a nonreassuring fetal heart pattern is detected, what remedial nursing intervention is carried out?
5. What are indications for continuous fetal monitoring in labor?
6. Create a concept map for Cindy's care based on her current labor status.

See www.nursing.pearsonhighered.com for possible responses and an interactive template for a concept map.

References

American College of Obstetricians and Gynecologists (ACOG). (2009). *Intrapartum fetal heart rate monitoring: Nomenclature, interpretation, and general management principles* (ACOG Practice Bulletin, No. 106). Washington, DC: Author.

American College of Obstetricians and Gynecologists (ACOG). (2010a). *Appropriateness of trial of labor after previous cesarean delivery* (Patient Safety Checklist No. 8). Washington, DC: ACOG.

American College of Obstetricians and Gynecologists (ACOG). (2010b). *Management of fetal heart rate tracings* (Practice Bulletin No. 116). Washington, DC: Author.

American College of Obstetricians and Gynecologists (ACOG). (2012). *Prevention and prediction of preterm birth.* (Practice Bulletin No. 130). Washington, DC: Author.

Blackburn, S. T. (2013). *Maternal, fetal, and neonatal physiology: A clinical perspective* (4th ed.). Philadelphia, PA: Saunders.

Cunningham, F. G., Leveno, K. J., Bloom, S. L., Hauth, J. C., Rouse, D. J., & Spong, C. Y. (2010). *Williams obstetrics* (23rd ed.). New York, NY: McGraw-Hill.

Datta, S., Kodeli, B., & Sega, S. (2010). Non-pharmacological methods for relief of labor pain. *Obstetric Anesthesia Handbook*, 85–93. doi:10.1007/978-0-387-88602-2_7

Davidson, M. R. (2012). *A nurse's guide to women's mental health.* New York, NY: Springer.

Goodwin, T. M., Montoro, M. N., Muderspach, L., Paulson, R., & Roy, S. (2010). *Management of common problems in obstetrics and gynecology.* New York, NY: Wiley-Blackwell.

Lee-Rife, S. M. (2010). Women's empowerment and reproductive experiences over the life course. *Social Science & Medicine, 71*(3), 634–642. doi:10.1016/j.socscimed.2010.04.019

Macones, G. A., Hankins, G. D. V., Spong, C. Y., Hauth, J., & Moore, T. (2008). The 2008 National Institute of Child Health and Human Development workshop report on electronic monitoring: Update on definitions, interpretation, and research guidelines. *Journal of Obstetrics, Gynecology and Neonatal Nursing, 37*(5), 510–515.

Marcus, S. (2009). Depression during pregnancy: Rates, risks and consequences. *Canadian Journal of Clinical Pharmacology, 16*(1), e15–e22.

Murray, M., Huelsmann, G., & Koperski, N. (2011). *Essentials of fetal monitoring* (4th ed.). New York, NY: Springer.

Rathore, A. M., Ramji, S., Devi, C. B., Saini, S., Manaktala, U., & Batra, S. (2011). Fetal scalp stimulation test: An adjunct to intermittent auscultation in non-reassuring fetal status during labor. *Journal of Obstetrics and Gynaecology Research, 37*, 819–824. doi:10.1111/j.1447-0756.2010.01442.x

Reich, D. L. (2011). *Monitoring in anesthesia and perioperative care.* Cambridge, UK: Cambridge University Book Press.

Spector, R. E. (2012). *Cultural diversity in health and illness* (8th ed.). Upper Saddle River, NJ: Pearson.

Weisman, O., Granat, A., Gilboa-Schechtman, E., Singer, M., Gordon, I., Azulay, H., . . . Feldman, R. (2010). The experience of labor, maternal perception of the infant, and the mother's postpartum mood in a low-risk community cohort. *Archives of Women's Mental Health, 13*(6), 505–513. doi:10.1007/s00737-010-0169-z

Yonkers, K. A., Wisner, K. L., Stewart, D. E., Oberlander, T. F., Dell, D. L., Stotland, N., . . . Lockwood, C. (2012). The management of depression during pregnancy: A report from the American Psychiatric Association and the American College of Obstetricians and Gynecologists. *FOCUS 2012, 10*, 78–89. doi:10.1176/appi.focus.10.1.78

Pearson Nursing Student Resources Find additional review materials at: **nursing.pearsonhighered.com**

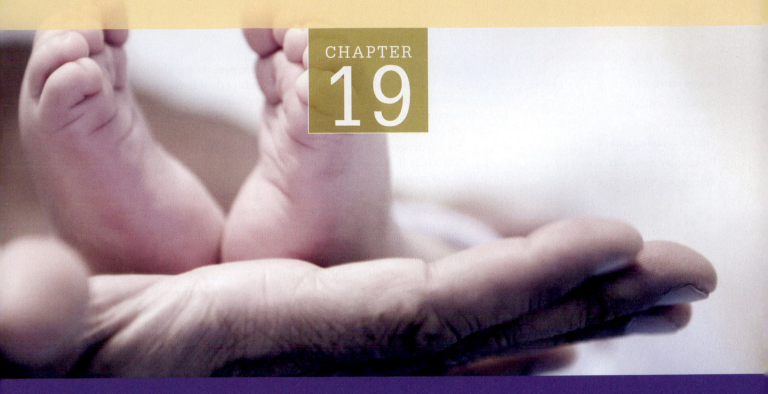

The Family in Childbirth: Needs and Care

For as long as I can remember, I have been fascinated with birth. Currently, I am a labor and delivery nurse at our town's only hospital. I'm still fascinated with birth but a little nervous, too. You see, I was just admitted in early labor with my first child. Before I got here I worried that I would be a "bad" patient or that I would lose my cool. How silly I was. All that matters is that my baby is healthy and that I am able to take care of him effectively. (Yes. We know it is a boy!) —Amanda, 31

Jonathan Nourok/PhotoEdit

LEARNING OUTCOMES

19.1   Identify admission data that should be noted when a woman is admitted to the birthing area.

19.2   Describe the nursing care of a woman and her partner/family upon admission to the birthing area.

19.3   Use assessment data to determine the nursing interventions to meet the psychologic, social, physiologic, and spiritual needs of the woman and her partner/family during each stage of labor.

19.4   Compare methods of promoting comfort during the first and second stages of labor.

19.5   Explain the immediate needs and physical assessment of the newborn following birth in the provision of nursing care.

19.6   Examine the unique needs of the adolescent during birth in the provision of nursing care.

19.7   Describe the role and responsibilities of the nurse in the management of a precipitous labor and birth.

It is time for a child to be born. The parents are about to undergo one of the most meaningful and stressful events of their lives. The adequacy of their preparation for childbirth, including the coping mechanisms, communication, and support systems that they have established, will be put to the test. Like Amanda, the childbearing woman may feel that her psychologic and physical limits are about to be challenged. These events may be even more challenging for the single woman, especially if she lacks a strong support system.

Family-centered care is a model of care based on the philosophy that the physical, sociocultural, spiritual, and economic needs of the family are combined and considered collectively when planning care for the childbearing family (Institute for Patient and Family-Centered Care, 2012). To reflect the consumer demand for family-centered care, most birthing centers now have **birthing rooms**, single rooms where the woman and her partner or other family members will stay for the labor, birth, recovery, and possibly the postpartum period. These rooms may be called *labor–delivery–recovery–postpartum (LDRP) rooms* or *single-room maternity care (SRMC)*.

The birthing room atmosphere is more relaxed than a traditional labor room, and families seem to feel more comfortable in it. Not having to be transferred from one area to another for birth helps the laboring woman create her own space to labor in and enhances the family's involvement. Birthing rooms usually have beds that can be adapted for birth by removing a small section near the foot. The room's decor is designed to produce a homelike atmosphere in which families can feel both safe and at ease.

The previous two chapters provided information about physiologic and psychologic changes during labor and birth and necessary nursing assessments. This chapter focuses on nursing care during labor and birth.

NURSING DIAGNOSIS DURING LABOR AND BIRTH

When devising a plan of care for the intrapartum period, the nurse can develop a general plan that encompasses the total process, from the beginning of labor through the fourth stage, or a more specific plan that identifies nursing diagnoses for each stage of labor and birth.

Examples of appropriate nursing diagnoses may include the following (NANDA-I © 2012):

- *Fear* related to uncertainty about the outcome of the birth process
- *Pain, Acute,* related to uterine contractions, cervical dilatation, and fetal descent
- *Knowledge, Readiness for Enhanced,* related to information about the fetal monitor and an expressed desire to understand equipment used
- *Family Processes, Readiness for Enhanced,* related to opportunity to incorporate newborn into the family

NURSING CARE DURING ADMISSION

During prenatal visits, instruct the woman to come to the birthing unit if any of the following occurs:

- Rupture of membranes (ROM)
- Regular, frequent uterine contractions (nulliparas, 5 minutes apart for 1 hour; multiparas, 6 to 8 minutes apart for 1 hour)
- Vaginal bleeding
- Decreased fetal movement

The woman in labor and her partner or support person(s) tend to be concerned about arriving at the birth center in time for the birth. Sometimes the labor is advanced and birth is imminent, but usually the woman is in early labor at admission. If time permits and the family is not familiar with what will occur during labor, provide necessary information. (See *Teaching Highlights: What to Expect During Labor.*)

Teaching Highlights   What to Expect During Labor

- Describe aspects of the admission process:
  - Abbreviated history
  - Physical assessment (maternal vital signs, fetal heart rate, contraction status, status of membranes)
  - Assessment of uterine contractions (frequency, duration, intensity)
  - Orientation to surroundings
  - Introductions to other staff
  - Determination of the woman's and support person's expectations of the nurse
- Present aspects of ongoing physical care, such as when to expect assessment of maternal vital signs, fetal heart rate, and contractions.
- If an electronic fetal monitor is used, describe how it works and the information it provides. Orient the woman to sights and sounds of the monitor.
- Explain what "normal" data look like and what characteristics are being watched for.
- Be sure to note that assessments will increase as the labor progresses, especially during the transition phase, to help keep the mother and baby safe by noting any changes from the normal course.
- Explain the vaginal examination and the information it can provide.
- Review comfort techniques that may be used in labor and ascertain what the woman thinks will promote comfort.
- Review breathing techniques the woman has learned so that you can support her technique.
- Review comfort and support measures such as positioning, back rub, effleurage, touch, distraction techniques, and ambulation.
- If the woman is in early labor, offer her a tour of the birthing area.
- Have printed materials available for reference, especially for the partner or support person.
- If time permits, a brief video describing procedures may be helpful.

The way the maternity nurse greets the woman and her partner influences the course of the woman's hospital stay. The sudden environmental change and the sometimes impersonal and technical aspects of admission can produce significant stress. If women and their families are greeted in a brusque, harried manner, they are less likely to look to the nurse for support. A calm, pleasant manner indicates to the woman that she is important. It helps to instill a sense of confidence in the staff's ability to provide quality care during this critical time.

Following the initial greeting, escort the woman to the birthing room and provide a quick yet thorough orientation to the facility, including the location of the restrooms, public phones, and nurse-call or emergency-call system. These simple steps can go a long way toward helping the woman and her partner feel more at ease. Explain the monitoring equipment or other unfamiliar technology and make every effort to make the environment less frightening for the laboring woman and her support person(s).

Some women prefer that their partner remain with them during the admission process, and others prefer to have the partner wait outside. While helping the woman undress and get into a hospital gown, begin to develop rapport and establish a nursing database. The experienced labor and birth nurse can obtain essential information about the woman and her pregnancy within a few minutes after admission, initiate any immediate interventions needed, and establish individualized priorities.

The woman may be facing a number of unfamiliar procedures that seem routine for healthcare providers. Remember that all women have the right to determine what happens to their bodies. The woman's informed consent should be obtained prior to any procedure that involves touching her.

If indicated, assist the woman into bed. A side-lying or semi-Fowler's position rather than a supine position is most comfortable and avoids supine hypotensive syndrome (vena caval syndrome). After obtaining the essential information from the woman and her records, begin the intrapartum assessment (see Chapter 18 🔗). Once the assessment is complete, it is possible to make effective nursing decisions about care, such as the following:

- Should ambulation, bed rest, or a combination of both be encouraged?
- Is more frequent or continuous electronic fetal monitoring needed?
- What does the woman want during her labor and birth?
- Is a support person available?
- What special needs do this woman and her partner have?

Auscultate the fetal heart rate (FHR). Determine the woman's blood pressure, pulse, respirations, and oral temperature and assess contraction frequency, duration, and intensity (possibly while gathering other data). Before the vaginal examination, inform the woman about the procedure and its purpose; afterward, report the findings. If signs of advanced labor exist (frequent contractions, an urge to bear down, and so on), a vaginal examination must be done immediately. If there are signs of excessive bleeding or if the woman reports episodes of painless bleeding in the last trimester, suspect placenta previa. *Do not do a vaginal examination, and notify the physician or certified nurse-midwife (CNM) immediately.*

Results of FHR assessment, uterine contraction evaluation, and the vaginal examination help determine whether the rest of the admission process can proceed at a leisurely pace or whether additional interventions are required. For example, an FHR of less than 110 beats per minute (beats/min) on auscultation indicates that a fetal monitor should be applied immediately to obtain additional data. The woman's vital signs can be assessed once the monitor is in place.

After obtaining admission data, collect a clean voided midstream urine specimen. The woman with intact membranes may collect her specimen in the bathroom. If the membranes are ruptured and the presenting part is not engaged, the woman generally remains in bed to avoid prolapse of the umbilical cord. Views vary about the wisdom of ambulation once the membranes are ruptured. The decision is generally based on history and physical findings (for example, history of precipitous labors, indications for continuous fetal monitoring, presence of meconium), clinician orders, the woman's desires, agency policy, and safety concerns.

Use a dipstick to test the woman's urine for the presence of protein, ketones, and glucose before sending the sample to the laboratory. This procedure is especially important if edema or elevated blood pressure is noted on admission. Proteinuria of 1+ or more may be a sign of impending preeclampsia. Glycosuria (sugar in the urine) is found frequently in pregnant women because of the increased glomerular filtration rate in the proximal tubules and the inability of these tubules to increase reabsorption of glucose. However, it may also be associated with gestational diabetes, so do not discount it. Ketones can be associated with inadequate calorie intake, dehydration, vomiting, skipping meals, insulin resistance, or gestational diabetes. While the woman is collecting the urine specimen, gather the equipment needed for any procedures ordered by the CNM or physician.

Laboratory tests are done during early admission. Hemoglobin and hematocrit values help determine the oxygen-carrying capacity of the circulatory system and the woman's ability to withstand blood loss at birth. Elevation of the hematocrit may reveal hemoconcentration of blood, which occurs with edema or dehydration. A low hemoglobin, in the absence of other evidence of bleeding, suggests anemia. Blood may be typed and cross-matched if the woman is in a high-risk category. Platelets are also evaluated because low platelets can lead to bleeding problems. Additional serologic testing may be performed as indicated. HIV testing should be offered to all women who have not been previously screened (Centers for Disease Control & Prevention [CDC], 2012).

Depending on how rapidly labor is progressing, notify the CNM or physician before or after completing the admission procedures. The report should include the following information: parity, cervical dilatation and effacement, station, presenting part, status of the membranes, contraction pattern, FHR, vital signs that are not in the normal range, any significant prenatal history, the woman's birth preferences, and her reaction to labor.

Enter a nursing admission note into the computer or the charting system. The admission note should include the reason for admission, the date and time of the woman's arrival and notification of the CNM or physician, the condition of the woman and her baby, and labor and membrane status.

NURSING CARE DURING THE FIRST STAGE OF LABOR

After completing the nursing assessment and diagnosis steps, create a plan of care to achieve identified nursing goals. For instance, if the woman and her support person did not have the opportunity to attend childbirth preparation classes, the nursing goal would be to provide desired information. To accomplish this goal, the nurse would assess the current level of the couple's understanding and then plan to provide brief explanations as labor progresses.

Integration of Family Expectations

Families come into the birth setting with basic expectations that they will not be harmed and that the labor and birth will be safe for the mother and baby. In addition, women look for the following from their nurses:

- Emotional support, which includes sustained presence of the nurse, praise, encouragement, reassurance, and companionship
- Comfort measures such as the use of touch, provision of ice chips and fluids, massage, assistance with care, and a bath or shower
- Information and advice, which includes offering information about procedures, interventions as they occur, and reports of labor progress
- Advocacy to help the woman and her partner achieve their goals, hopes, and dreams for their labor and birth experience
- Support of the partner, including encouragement, praise for his or her efforts, an opportunity for rest breaks, and role modeling

Integration of Cultural Beliefs

Knowledge of values, customs, and practices of different cultures is as important during labor as it is in the prenatal period. Without this knowledge a nurse is less likely to understand a family's behavior and may attempt to impose personal values and beliefs on them. As cultural sensitivity increases, so does the likelihood of providing high-quality care.

The following sections briefly present a few possible cultural responses to labor. General examples about any culture or belief system should be viewed as background information only. An individual example of a birthing practice will never be pertinent to all women in a given group. Within every culture, each person develops his or her own beliefs, values, and behaviors. Culture is also discussed in Chapter 2 🔴.

Modesty

Modesty is an important consideration for women regardless of culture. However, some women may be more uncomfortable than others with the degree of exposure needed for certain procedures during labor and the birth process. Some women may be particularly uncomfortable when men are present and feel more comfortable with women; others may be uncomfortable with exposure of personal body parts regardless of the gender of the caregivers. The nurse should be alert to the woman's responses to examinations and procedures and provide the draping and privacy the woman needs. It is more prudent to assume that embarrassment will occur with exposure and take measures to provide privacy than to assume that it will not matter to the woman if she is exposed during procedures.

Pain Expression

The manner in which a woman chooses to deal with the discomfort of labor varies widely. Some women seem to turn inward and remain very quiet during the whole process. They speak only to ask others to leave the room or cease conversation. Others may be very vocal, with behaviors such as counting out loud, moaning quietly, crying, or use of loud vocalization. They may also turn from side to side or change positions frequently.

In many Asian cultures, it is important for individuals to act in a way that will not bring shame on the family. Therefore, the Korean woman may not express pain outwardly for fear of shaming herself or her family. Silence is valued in Chinese society, so a woman of that heritage is usually quiet and stoic to avoid dishonoring herself or her family. Mexican women often chant the phrase "Aye yie yie" while in labor, which is actually a form of "folk lamaze." Repeating the phrase in succession several times necessitates taking long, slow, deep breaths. Thus, it is a cultural method for alleviating pain (Spector, 2012). European Americans demonstrate a wide variety of behaviors in response to pain, from silence to shouting. It is important to support a woman's individual expression, whatever it may be (as long as harm is not done to another), in order to enhance the birthing experience for mother, baby, and family.

Cultural Beliefs: Some Examples

It is essential to avoid stereotyping in providing care. The four examples that follow give insight into the variety of responses nurses may encounter.

Squatting during labor is common for Hmong women from Laos. They may also prefer to be active and move about. The husband is frequently present and involved in providing comfort. The woman may ask that the amniotic membranes not be ruptured until just before birth. It is thought that the escape of fluid at this time makes the birth easier. During labor the woman usually prefers only "hot" foods and warm water to drink (Spector, 2012). As soon as the baby is born, the family may request that a soft-boiled egg be given to the mother to restore her energy.

Vietnamese women usually maintain self-control and may even smile throughout labor. They may prefer to walk about and to give birth in a squatting position. In labor the woman may prefer cold beverages because pregnancy is viewed as a "hot" condition. However, during the postpartum, which is viewed as a "cold" condition, she may prefer warm liquids (Spector, 2012). The newborn is protected from praise to prevent jealousy (Spector, 2012).

Latina women have identified expectations of their partners during labor and birth such as wanting their partners to stay with them and to reassure them that everything will be all right. As they labor, the women want their partners to show their love and to speak using affectionate words.

Muslim women may have their husband, a female friend or relative, or a male relative with them during childbirth. If a specialist such as an anesthesiologist or neonatologist is needed, it is best to speak to the husband first and obtain his permission. Family support is important but does not preclude the importance of the nurse's presence. The woman may want to retain her head covering (khimar) and may prefer to wear two long-sleeved gowns to enhance modesty. It is important for a female nurse, physician, or CNM to perform examinations whenever possible. After the birth Muslim fathers may call praise to Allah (adhan) in the newborn's right ear and clean the newborn.

Maternity nurses can provide culturally sensitive care by first becoming acquainted with the beliefs and practices of the various cultures in their communities. In the birthing situation, the truly effective nurse supports the family's cultural practices as long as it is safe to do so.

Provision of Care in the First Stage of Labor
Latent Phase

As discussed in Chapter 18 🔗, it is important to assess the physical well-being of the woman and her fetus. Monitor maternal temperature every 4 hours unless the temperature is over 37.5°C (99.6°F); in such cases take it every hour. Monitor blood pressure, pulse, and respirations every hour. If the woman's blood pressure is over 120/80 mm Hg or her pulse is more than 100, notify the CNM or physician and reevaluate the blood pressure and pulse more frequently.

Palpate uterine contractions for frequency, intensity, and duration every 30 minutes. Auscultate the fetal heart rate (FHR) every 60 minutes for low-risk women and every 30 minutes for high-risk women as long as it remains between 110 and 160 beats/min and is reassuring (American College of Obstetricians and Gynecologists [ACOG], 2010). Auscultate the FHR throughout one contraction and for about 15 seconds after the contraction to ensure that there are no decelerations. If the FHR baseline is not in the 110 to 160 range or if decelerations are heard, continuous electronic monitoring is recommended. See Table 19–1 for nursing assessments during the four stages of labor.

Offer the woman fluids in the form of clear liquids or ice chips frequently, unless complications exist that may result in a cesarean birth. Some certified childbirth educators advise the woman to bring lollipops to help combat the dryness that occurs with some of the labor breathing patterns. Avoiding both liquids and solids during labor, which was once a standard of practice, is no longer deemed necessary. Evidence-based practice research and new guidelines indicate that clear fluids can be consumed throughout labor and up to 2 hours before an elective cesarean birth. Current guidelines suggest avoiding solids for 6 to 8 hours before an elective cesarean birth (ACOG, 2009b). Eating during labor has not been associated with an increase in aspiration

---

Developing Cultural Competence
Native American Women and Labor

Native American women typically view labor pain as natural, and may use meditation, self-control, or indigenous plants or herbs, such as black cohosh, throughout their labor as well as to aid them during birth (Spector, 2012).

Clinical Reasoning   Gender-Specific Care Preference

Fatima Al Ahala is a 22-year-old, G1 who presents in labor. Fatima and her husband Samir are from Pakistan. The couple has stated that they can accept care only from female providers. The couple is being attended by a female nurse-midwife, and the backup physician is also a female. When her labor intensifies, Fatima requests an epidural. The only anesthesiologist available is a male physician. What actions can you take to help this family meet their cultural preferences?
See www.nursing.pearsonhighered.com for possible responses.

Table 19–1	Nursing Assessments During the Stages of Labor	
Stage	**Maternal Assessments**	**Fetal Assessments**
FIRST STAGE *Latent phase*	Blood pressure (BP), respirations each hour if in normal range. Temperature every 4 hours unless over 37.5°C (99.6°F) or membranes ruptured, then every 2 hours. Uterine contractions every 30 minutes.	Fetal heart rate (FHR) every 30 minutes for low-risk women and every 15 minutes for high-risk women if normal characteristics present (average variability, baseline in the 110 to 160 beats/min range, without late or variable decelerations). Note fetal activity. If electronic fetal monitor is in place, assess for reactive nonstress test (NST).
Active phase	BP, pulse, respirations every hour if in normal range. Uterine contractions palpated every 15 to 30 minutes.	FHR every 30 minutes for low-risk women and every 15 minutes for high-risk women if normal characteristics are present.
Transition phase	BP, pulse, respirations every 30 minutes. Contractions palpated at least every 15 minutes.	FHR every 30 minutes for low-risk women and every 15 minutes for high-risk women if normal characteristics are present.
SECOND STAGE	BP, pulse, and respirations every 5 to 15 minutes. Temperature every 2 hours. Uterine contractions palpated continuously.	FHR every 15 minutes for low-risk women and every 5 minutes for high-risk women.
THIRD STAGE	BP, pulse, and respirations every 5 minutes. Palpate uterine contractions intermittently to assess for signs of placenta separation.	Newborn assessment at time of birth, gestational age assessment, and neurologic assessment within first hour of birth. Apgars at 1 and 5 minutes. Assess initial BP, apical pulse, respirations, and temperature. Assess for umbilical cord for the presence of three vessels.
FOURTH STAGE	Assess maternal vital signs including temperature, BP, pulse, and respirations every 15 minutes for first hour. Assess fundus, lochia, perineum, laceration/episiotomy site, bladder distention, and rectum every 15 minutes.	Perform complete exam to include vital signs, gestational age assessment, physical examination, and neurologic reflexes once between 1 and 4 hours postbirth. After initial 8 hours, assess vitals and perform assessment every 8 hours. Skin color should be assessed every 4 hours.

but some institutions continue to limit oral intake during labor (ACOG, 2009b). Previously, it was believed that drinking fluids should be avoided because it can lead to vomiting caused by the decreased gastric emptying time. Although vomiting is common during the first stage of labor, many women have more energy and tolerate labor better with oral intake and have higher satisfaction with their labor and birth experience (ACOG, 2009b).

Active Phase

During the active phase, contractions have a frequency of 2 to 5 minutes, a duration of 40 to 60 seconds, and a moderate to strong intensity. Palpate contractions every 15 to 30 minutes. As the contractions become more frequent and intense, vaginal exams assess cervical dilatation and effacement and fetal station and position. During the active phase, the cervix dilates from 4 to 7 cm, and vaginal discharge and bloody show increase. Monitor maternal blood pressure, pulse, and respirations every hour for low-risk women (unless elevated, as previously noted) and every 30 minutes for high-risk women. Auscultate the FHR every 30 minutes for low-risk women and every 15 minutes for high-risk women (ACOG, 2009a).

A woman who has been ambulatory up to this point may wish to sit in a chair or on a bed. If the woman wants to lie on the bed, encourage her to assume a side-lying position, help her into a comfortable position, and place pillows to support her body. To increase comfort, offer a back rub or effleurage or place a cool cloth on the woman's forehead or across her neck. Because vaginal discharge increases, change the chux pad frequently. Washing the perineum with warm soapy water removes secretions and increases comfort. During such procedures it is essential to wear disposable gloves to avoid exposure to vaginal discharge.

If the amniotic membranes have not ruptured previously, they may do so during this phase. When the membranes rupture, immediately note the FHR on the monitor if one is being used (if the woman is not on a monitor, auscultate FHR) and then note the color, odor, and consistency of the amniotic fluid and the time of rupture. The fluid should be clear, with no odor. The presence of any frank bright red vaginal bleeding should be noted because it is not considered a normal finding. Fetal stress leads to intestinal and anal sphincter relaxation, and meconium may be released into the amniotic fluid, which turns the fluid greenish brown. Whenever meconium-stained fluid is present, apply an electronic monitor to assess the FHR continuously. Note the time of rupture because infection increases as the duration of ruptured membranes is prolonged.

Prolapse of the umbilical cord is a possible risk when membranes rupture and the fetus is not engaged, because the amniotic fluid coming through the cervix might wash the umbilical cord out through the cervix. With each contraction the cord would then become trapped between the presenting part and the maternal pelvis. The FHR is auscultated because a drop in the rate might indicate an undetected prolapsed cord. Immediate

Table 19–2	Deviations from Normal Labor Process Requiring Immediate Intervention
Problem	**Immediate Action**
Woman admitted with vaginal bleeding or history of painless vaginal bleeding	Do not perform vaginal examination. Assess fetal heart rate (FHR). Evaluate amount of blood loss and initiate a pad count. Evaluate labor pattern. Notify physician or certified nurse-midwife (CNM) immediately.
Presence of greenish or brownish amniotic fluid	Continuously monitor FHR. Evaluate dilatation of cervix and determine if umbilical cord is prolapsed. Evaluate presentation (vertex or breech). Maintain woman on complete bed rest on left side. Notify physician or CNM immediately.
Absence of FHR and fetal movement	Notify physician or CNM. Provide truthful information and emotional support to laboring couple. Remain with the couple.
Prolapse of umbilical cord	Relieve pressure on cord manually. Continuously monitor FHR; watch for changes in FHR pattern. Notify physician or CNM. Assist woman into knee-chest position or place in Trendelenburg position. Administer oxygen. Prepare for possible emergency cesarean birth.

Woman admitted in advanced labor; birth imminent	Prepare for immediate birth.
	Obtain critical information:
	    Estimated date of birth (EDB)
	    History of bleeding problems
	    History of medical or obstetric problems
	    Past or present use or abuse of prescription, over-the-counter (OTC), or illicit drugs
	    Problems with this pregnancy
	    FHR and maternal vital signs
	    Whether membranes are ruptured and how long since rupture
	    Blood type and Rh.
	Direct another person to contact physician or CNM.
	Do not leave woman alone.
	Provide support to couple.
	Put on gloves.

intervention is necessary to remove pressure on a prolapsed umbilical cord (see Chapter 21 🔗). (See Table 19–2 for additional deviations from the normal labor process.)

Transition

During transition the contraction frequency is every 1½ to 2 minutes, duration is 60 to 90 seconds, and intensity is strong. Cervical dilatation increases from 8 to 10 cm, effacement is complete (100%), and there is usually a heavy amount of bloody show. Palpate contractions at least every 15 minutes. Sterile vaginal examinations may be done more frequently because this stage of labor usually is accompanied by rapid change. Take the maternal blood pressure, pulse, and respirations at least every 30 minutes, and auscultate FHR every 15 minutes.

Comfort measures are important in this phase of labor, but continual assessment is required to intervene appropriately. The woman may rapidly change from wanting a back rub and other hands-on care to wanting to be left completely alone. The support person and the nurse need to follow her cues and change interventions as needed. Because the woman is breathing more

rapidly, increase her comfort by offering small spoonfuls of ice chips to moisten her mouth or offer an emollient for her dry lips. Encourage the woman to rest between contractions. If analgesics have been administered, a quiet environment enhances the quality of rest between contractions. Awaken the woman just before a contraction begins so that she can begin patterned breathing.

Some women have difficulty coping during this time and need help with their breathing. Either the support person or the nurse can breathe along with the woman during each contraction to help her maintain her pattern. It is helpful to encourage the woman and to assure her that she is doing a good job. The woman will begin to feel increased rectal pressure as the fetal presenting part moves down the birth canal. To help prevent cervical edema, encourage the woman to refrain from pushing until the cervix is completely dilated.

The end of transition and the beginning of the second stage may be indicated by a change in the woman's voice or the sounds she is making. As the fetus moves down and she feels increased pressure and a bearing-down sensation, her voice tends to deepen. A moan during a contraction takes on a more guttural quality.

Promotion of Comfort in the First Stage

The first step in planning care is to talk with the woman and her partner or support person to identify their goals. Usually the woman or couple is concerned with discomfort, so it is helpful to identify factors that may contribute to it. These factors include uncomfortable positions, diaphoresis, continual leaking of amniotic fluid, a full bladder, a dry mouth, anxiety, and fear. Nursing interventions can minimize the effects of these factors. These interventions are described later in this section.

As the intensity of contractions increases with the progress of labor, the woman becomes less aware of the environment and may have difficulty hearing and understanding verbal instructions. The pattern of coping with labor contractions ranges from the use of highly structured breathing techniques to turning inward. Low moaning that begins deep in the throat, rocking or swaying, facial grimacing, and using loud vocalizations are all effective means of dealing with the power of labor and birth. Some women feel that making sounds helps them cope and do the work of labor, whereas others make loud sounds only as they lose their perception of control.

The most frequent physiologic manifestations of pain are increased pulse and respiratory rates, dilated pupils, increased blood pressure, and muscle tension. In labor these reactions are transitory because the pain is intermittent. Increased muscle tension is most significant because it may impede the progress of labor. Women in labor often tighten skeletal muscles voluntarily during a contraction and remain motionless. This method of dealing with the contractions may actually increase the level of discomfort because of muscular tension, but the women may believe it is the only acceptable way to cope with the pain.

A woman generally wants touching, massage, effleurage, and other forms of physical contact during the first part of labor, but when she moves into the transition phase, she may pull away. Women may provide verbal and nonverbal signs such as crying, moaning, and beseeching the coach or nurse to hold their hand or rub their back. Some women are uncomfortable with being touched at all, regardless of the phase of labor. It is important to confirm the woman's preferences and to meet each family on its own terms, always keeping in mind that this is their experience.

Nonpharmacologic Pain Relief

The nurse can introduce the following nonpharmacologic pain relief techniques in labor to encourage maternal comfort and facilitate coping: massage, hydrotherapy, position changes, hypnosis, aromatherapy, sitting in a rocking chair/glider/birthing ball, walking, leaning against the bed or her partner, use of a TENS unit, visualization, relaxation techniques, the use of prayer or meditation, and breathing techniques. See *Complementary Care: Acupressure During Labor.*

Many nurses readily respond to the woman's needs. As the nurse and woman or couple work together to increase comfort during contractions, a ritual of supportive measures begins to develop. The nurse watches for cues and nonverbal behaviors and asks for feedback from the woman. As labor progresses, the nurse and couple use their experience and growing rapport to change comfort measures as needed. Nursing measures used to decrease pain are discussed next.

Complementary Care Acupressure During Labor

Acupressure is an ancient Chinese medical treatment that involves using the fingers to press key pressure points on the surface of the skin. This pressure ultimately stimulates the immune system to promote healing by triggering the release of endorphins, reducing stress through muscle relaxation, and promoting circulation. The specific acupressure point used in laboring women is the San Yin-Jiao (SP-6) acupressure point. The SP-6 acupressure point is located on the medial side of the leg, in the calf region, approximately 3 cm (1.2 in.) superior to the prominence of the inner malleus. The use of acupressure in labor has been associated with shorter labors and lower subjective and objective pain scores. Women who receive acupressure typically use less pain medication than those who do not receive acupressure (Simpkin, Bolding, Keppler, et al., 2010).

General Comfort

General comfort measures are of great importance during labor. By relieving minor discomforts, the nurse helps the woman optimize her ability to cope with pain. Encourage the woman to ambulate as long as there are no contraindications, such as vaginal bleeding or rupture of membranes before the fetus is engaged in the pelvis. Ambulation can increase comfort and aid in fetal descent (Figure 19–1 ●).

Even if the woman prefers not to walk around, upright positions such as sitting in a rocker or leaning against a wall or bed can enhance comfort. If she stays in bed, encourage the woman to assume positions that she finds comfortable (Figure 19–2 ●). A side-lying position is generally the most advantageous for the laboring woman, although frequent position changes seem to achieve more efficient contractions. It is important to support all body parts, with the joints kept slightly flexed. For instance,

● **Figure 19–1** Increasing comfort and aiding in fetal descent. This woman and her partner are walking in the hospital during labor.

A   **B**   **C**

● **Figure 19–2** The laboring woman is encouraged to choose a comfortable position. *A, B,* The nurse modifies assessments and interventions as necessary. *C,* While often promoting maternal comfort during labor, the birthing ball also facilitates fetal descent and rotation and helps increase the diameter of the pelvis.

Source: A, © olly/Fotolia. *B,* © BSIP SA/Alamy.

when the woman is in a side-lying position, pillows may be placed against her chest and under the uppermost arm. Place a pillow or folded bath blanket between her knees to support the uppermost leg and relieve tension or muscle strain. A pillow placed at the woman's midback also helps provide support. If the woman is more comfortable on her back, elevate the head of the bed to relieve the pressure of the uterus on the vena cava.

Pillows may be placed under each arm and under the knees to provide further support. Because a pregnant woman is at increased risk for thrombophlebitis, excessive pressure behind the knee and calf should be avoided. Assess pressure points frequently.

Back rubs and frequent changes of position contribute to comfort and relaxation. Wearing socks or slippers may alleviate cold feet, just as adjusting the room's thermostat can offset excessive warmth. Attention to such details allows the woman to focus on the more important issues of giving birth.

Diaphoresis and the constant leaking of amniotic fluid can dampen the woman's gown and bed linen. Fresh, smooth, dry bed linen promotes comfort. To avoid having to change the bottom sheet following rupture of the membranes, replace chux pads at frequent intervals (following body substance isolation precautions). Keep the woman's perineal area as clean and dry as possible to promote comfort and to prevent infection.

A full bladder adds to the discomfort during a contraction and may prolong labor by interfering with the descent of the fetus. The bladder should be kept as empty as possible. Even if the woman is voiding, urine may be retained because of the pressure of the fetal presenting part. To detect a full bladder, palpate directly over the symphysis pubis. Some regional analgesia procedures contribute to the inability to void, and catheterization may be necessary. Encourage the woman to empty her bladder every 1 to 2 hours.

Clinical Tip

Support persons and family members need to be encouraged to maintain their own comfort. Because they are paying attention to the laboring woman, they may forget their own needs. It may be necessary to encourage them to take breaks, to eat and drink, and to rest. However, they may be reluctant to leave the woman unattended while they meet their own personal needs. Offer to stay with the woman during their absence. This provides reassurance that the woman will be well cared for in their absence.

Handling Anxiety

A woman's anxiety as she begins labor is related to a combination of factors inherent to the process. A moderate amount of anxiety about the pain enhances the woman's ability to deal with it. In contrast, an excessive degree of anxiety decreases her ability to cope. Women who have increased anxiety about safety and their ability to cope are much more likely to describe their pain as unbearable.

To decrease anxiety not related to pain, give information (which eases fear of the unknown), establish rapport with the couple (which helps them preserve their personal integrity), and express confidence in the couple's ability to work with the labor process. Remaining with the woman as much as possible conveys a caring attitude and dispels fears of abandonment. Praise for breathing, relaxation, and pushing efforts not only encourages repetition of the behavior but also decreases anxiety about the ability to cope with labor.

Patient Teaching

Providing truthful information about the nature of the discomfort that will occur during labor is important. Stressing the intermittent nature and maximum duration of the contractions can be most helpful. The woman can cope with pain better when she knows that a period of relief will follow.

Descriptions of sensations are best accompanied by information on specific comfort measures. Some women experience the urge to push during transition, when the cervix is not fully dilated and effaced. Pushing prior to complete dilatation and effacement can result in cervical edema, which in turn slows down the effacement/dilation process, or in cervical lacerations. Panting can control this sensation (it is difficult to pant and bear down at the same time). If time permits, explain the purpose of panting and have the woman practice before the technique is needed.

Thorough orientation and explanation of surroundings, procedures, and equipment being used also decrease anxiety, thereby reducing pain. Explain beeps, clicks, and other strange noises and give a simplified explanation of the monitor strip, emphasizing that the use of the fetal monitor provides a way to assess the well-being of the fetus during labor. It helps to show the woman and her partner or support person how the monitor can identify the beginnings of contractions. At the onset of each contraction, encourage the woman to begin her breathing technique to lessen her perception of pain.

Labor and childbirth may be a critical time for the woman with a history of childhood sexual abuse or rape. All women entering the healthcare arena need to be evaluated for a history of sexual abuse or rape. However, a woman may or may not be able to address this issue with the nurse, because sharing such personal information with a stranger is difficult. It is especially important to be alert for nonverbal cues, such as unexplained anxiety, unrelenting pain, or fear during vaginal examinations, and to be prepared to offer additional teaching and relaxation support to help offset the woman's anxiety.

Supportive Relaxation Techniques

Tense muscles increase resistance to the descent of the fetus and contribute to maternal fatigue. This fatigue increases pain perception and decreases the woman's ability to cope with the pain. Comfort measures, massage, water therapy using immersion in a whirlpool tub, techniques for decreasing anxiety, and patient teaching can contribute to relaxation. Adequate sleep and rest are also important. Encourage the laboring woman to use the periods between contractions for rest and relaxation. A prolonged prodromal phase of labor may have kept her awake. Moreover, a woman beginning labor is naturally excited, making it difficult for her to sleep even if her contractions are mild and infrequent.

Distraction helps increase relaxation and ability to cope with discomfort. During early labor, conversation or activities such as light reading or playing cards or other games serve as

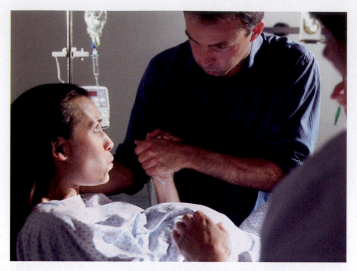

● **Figure 19–3** The woman's partner provides support and encouragement during labor.
Source: © Hans Neleman/Getty Images.

distractions. It may be helpful to have the woman concentrate on a pleasant experience she has had in the past. Other techniques include the use of a specific visual or mental focal point, breathing techniques, counting or humming, or visualization.

Touch is another type of distraction (Figure 19–3 ●). Although some women regard touching as an invasion of privacy or threat to their independence, many want to touch and be touched during a painful experience. Nurses can make themselves available to the woman who desires touch by placing a hand on the side of the bed within the woman's reach. The person who needs touch will reach out for contact. (See *Complementary Care: Intuitive Touch.*)

Mild to moderate abdominal discomfort during contractions may be relieved or lessened by effleurage. Firm pressure on the lower back or sacral area may relieve back pain associated with labor. To apply firm pressure, place a hand or a rolled, warmed towel or blanket in the small of the woman's back. In addition to the measures just described, enhance the woman's relaxation by providing encouragement and support for her controlled breathing techniques.

Complementary Care Intuitive Touch

Intuitive touch is the nurse's intentional use of physical contact with the woman with the intent of helping to slow down and regulate the breathing pattern. (*Note:* Therapeutic Touch, a complementary therapy that focuses on energy fields, is a different process. See discussion in Chapter 2 ●.) Evidence suggests that touch induces the relaxation response, which is mediated through the neuroendocrine and sympathetic nervous systems.

A variety of techniques can be used. These include hand-holding; stroking or patting of a woman's arm, face, or legs; placing one hand on her shoulder; putting an arm around her shoulders; and hugging. To implement intuitive touch, use long, slow, up-and-down strokes on the woman's limbs. You do not need special training to use this intervention; all that is needed is the intention to help regulate the breathing pattern and the willingness to use a little time to achieve this goal.

Evidence-Based Practice Pharmacologic and Nonpharmacologic Pain Management Interventions During Labor

Clinical Question
How do pharmacologic and nonpharmacologic pain management interventions compare in terms of effectiveness and satisfaction?

The Evidence
Much study has been given to pain management during labor. A range of both pharmacologic and nonpharmacologic interventions has been posed as helping mothers cope with pain during the birthing process. However, studies have seldom compared the various pain relief measures. Therefore, a Cochrane meta-review was conducted to compare various pain relief measures for laboring mothers. A meta-review is a compilation and evaluation of systematic reviews and forms the strongest level of evidence for practice. This review identified 15 Cochrane reviews and 3 non-Cochrane reviews including 310 individual studies. The results were grouped into three sets of recommendations: (1) what a preponderance of evidence shows is effective, (2) studies that suggest a pain relief measure may work for some women in certain situations, and (3) studies that reveal insufficient evidence to draw a conclusion about effectiveness. Evidence showed that epidural, combined spinal-epidural, and inhaled analgesia effectively manage pain in labor, but may cause adverse effects. Of the pain relief measures, these were the most effective. There is evidence that water immersion or warm showers (Shu-Ling, Chieh-Yu, Yu-Yin, et al., 2013), relaxation techniques (including guided imagery and breathing), acupuncture, massage, and nonopioid drugs may improve management of labor pain with few or no side effects. There is insufficient evidence to support TENS, hypnosis, biofeedback, aromatherapy, or parenteral opioids as effective in managing the pain of labor (Jones, Othman, Dowswell, et al., 2012).

Best Practice
It is important to tailor pain relief methods to each woman's wishes, needs, and circumstances, as well as the anticipated duration of labor, the infant's condition, and induction methods. Pharmacologic methods are the most effective, but carry with them adverse effects. Many nonpharmacologic methods provide pain relief with little or no side effects.

Clinical Reasoning
How can the nurse assess the mother's specific needs for pain relief? What are the elements of a pain relief teaching plan?

Breathing Techniques
Breathing techniques may help the laboring woman. Used correctly they increase the woman's pain threshold, permit relaxation, enhance the woman's ability to cope with the uterine contractions, and allow the uterus to function more efficiently.

Many women learn patterned-paced breathing during childbirth preparation classes. This type of controlled breathing often has three levels. The woman tends to begin with the first level and then proceed to the next when she feels the need. Regardless of the level of breathing used, a cleansing breath begins and ends each pattern. A cleansing breath involves only the chest. It consists of inhaling through the nose and exhaling through pursed lips.

1. The first pattern may also be called slow, deep breathing or slow-paced breathing. During the breathing movements, only the chest moves. The woman inhales slowly through her nose. She moves her chest up and out during the inhalation. She exhales through pursed lips. The breathing rate is 6 to 9 breaths a minute.

2. The second pattern is called shallow or modified-paced breathing. The woman begins with a cleansing breath and at the end of the cleansing breath pushes out a short breath. She then inhales and exhales through the mouth at a rate of about 4 breaths every 5 seconds. This pattern can be altered into a more rapid rate that does not exceed 2 to 2½ breaths every second.

3. The third pattern is called pant–blow or patterned-paced breathing. It is similar to modified-paced breathing except the breathing is punctuated every few breaths by a forceful exhalation through pursed lips. A pattern of 4 breaths may be used to begin. All breaths are kept equal and rhythmic. As the contraction becomes more intense, the woman may adjust the pattern as needed to 3:1, 2:1, and finally 1:1.

If the woman has not learned a controlled breathing technique, teaching her may be difficult when she is admitted in active labor. In this instance, teach abdominal and pant–pant–blow breathing. In abdominal breathing the woman moves the abdominal wall upward as she inhales and downward as she exhales. This method tends to lift the abdominal wall off the contracting uterus and thus may provide some pain relief. The breathing is deep and rhythmic. As transition approaches, the woman may feel the need to breathe more rapidly. To avoid breathing too rapidly, the woman can use the pant–pant–blow breathing pattern.

Hyperventilation is the result of an imbalance of oxygen and carbon dioxide (i.e., too much carbon dioxide is exhaled, and too much oxygen remains in the body). Hyperventilation may occur when a woman breathes very rapidly over a prolonged period. The signs and symptoms of hyperventilation are tingling or numbness in the tip of the nose, lips, fingers, or toes; dizziness; spots before the eyes; or spasms of the hands or feet (carpal-pedal spasms). If hyperventilation occurs, encourage the woman to slow her breathing rate and take shallow breaths. With instruction and encouragement, many women are able to change their breathing to correct the problem. It may also help to count out loud for the woman so she can pace her breathing during contractions. If the signs and symptoms continue or become more severe (i.e., they progress from numbness to spasms), the woman can breathe into a paper surgical mask or a paper bag until symptoms go away. Breathing into a mask or bag causes rebreathing of carbon dioxide. During this time, remain with the woman to reassure her.

In some instances, analgesics or regional anesthetic blocks may be used to increase comfort and relaxation during labor. (See Chapter 20 🔗 for a discussion of pharmacologic pain management.) Table 19–3 summarizes labor progress, possible responses of the laboring woman, and support measures.

Table 19–3   Normal Progress, Psychologic Characteristics, and Nursing Support During the First and Second Stages of Labor

Phase	Cervical Dilatation	Uterine Contractions	Woman's Response	Support Measures
STAGE 1 *Latent phase*	1–4 cm	Every 10–20 minutes, 15–20 seconds' duration Mild intensity *progressing to* Every 5–7 minutes, 30–40 seconds' duration Moderate intensity	Usually happy, talkative, and eager to be in labor. Exhibits need for independence by taking care of own bodily needs and seeking information.	Establish rapport on admission and continue to build during care. Assess information base and learning needs. Be available to consult regarding breathing technique if needed; teach breathing technique if needed and in early labor. Orient family to room, equipment, monitors, and procedures. Encourage woman and partner to participate in care as desired. Provide needed information. Assist woman into position of comfort; encourage frequent change of position; encourage ambulation during early labor. Offer fluids or ice chips. Keep couple informed of progress. Encourage woman to void every 1 to 2 hours. Assess need for an interest in using visualization to enhance relaxation, and teach if appropriate.
Active phase	4–7 cm	Every 2–3 minutes, 40–60 seconds' duration Moderate to strong intensity	May experience feelings of helplessness. Exhibits increased fatigue and may begin to feel restless and anxious as contractions become stronger. Expresses fear of abandonment. Becomes more dependent because she is less able to meet her needs.	Encourage woman to maintain breathing patterns. Provide quiet environment to reduce external stimuli. Provide reassurance, encouragement, support; keep couple informed of progress. Promote comfort by giving back rubs, sacral pressure, cool cloth on forehead, assistance with position changes, support with pillows, effleurage. Provide ice chips, ointment for dry mouth and lips. Encourage to void every 1 to 2 hours. Offer shower, whirlpool, or warm bath if available.
Transition phase	8–10 cm	Every 2 minutes, 60–75 seconds' duration Strong intensity	Tires and may exhibit increased restlessness and irritability. May feel she cannot keep up with labor process and is out of control. Exhibits physical discomforts. Fears being left alone. May fear tearing open or splitting apart with contractions.	Encourage woman to rest between contractions. If she sleeps between contractions, wake her at beginning of contraction so she can begin breathing pattern (increases feeling of control). Provide support, encouragement, and praise for efforts. Keep couple informed of progress; encourage continued participation of support persons. Promote comfort as listed earlier but recognize that many women do not want to be touched when in transition. Provide privacy. Provide ice chips, ointment for lips. Encourage to void every 1 to 2 hours.
STAGE 2	Complete	Every 2 minutes	May feel out of control, helpless, panicky	Assist woman in pushing efforts. Encourage woman to assume position of comfort. Provide encouragement and praise her efforts. Keep couple informed of progress. Provide ice chips. Maintain privacy as woman desires.

Role of the Doula

Throughout the first stage of labor, assess and support the interactions between the woman and her support person or partner. In the absence of a partner, or when the partner wants a less active role in the support of the laboring woman, it is becoming more common for women to employ a paid care provider, often called a **doula**, who has experience in caring for laboring women. The doula typically has received special training and may even be certified. The role of the doula is to enhance the comfort and decrease the anxiety of the laboring woman. A doula can be a valuable advocate to the laboring woman and her family, as well as an asset to the labor nurse. For example, the doula might support the woman by helping identify the beginning of each contraction and encouraging her as she breathes through it.

NURSING CARE DURING THE SECOND STAGE OF LABOR

The second stage is reached when the cervix is fully dilated (10 cm). The contractions continue as in the transition phase. Maternal pulse is assessed at the onset of the second stage. Blood pressure is assessed every 30 minutes, but may be done more frequently if fetal decelerations or bradycardia occur. The fetal heart rate (FHR) is assessed every 15 minutes in low-risk women and every 5 minutes in women with high-risk complications (ACOG, 2009a). Once the second stage is reached, the nurse remains with the woman continually and does not generally leave the room.

As the woman pushes during the second stage, she may make a variety of sounds. A low-pitched, grunting sound ("uhhh") usually indicates that the woman is working with the pushing. The nurse who feels comfortable with maternal sounds and stays sensitive to changes in the sounds may be able to detect if the woman is losing her ability to cope. For instance, if the woman feels afraid of the sensations produced by her pushing effort, her sound may change to a high-pitched cry or whimper. During the second stage, the woman may interpret rectal pressure as a need to move her bowels. The instinctive response is to resist and to tighten muscles rather than bear down (push). A sensation of splitting apart also occurs in the latter part of the second stage, and the woman may fear the urge to push. The woman who expects these sensations and understands that bearing down contributes to progress at this stage is more likely to do so effectively.

When the urge to bear down becomes uncontrollable and pushing begins, the nurse can help by encouraging the woman and by assisting with positioning (Figure 19–4 ●). Most women spontaneously push very effectively in response to messages from their body. However, in some settings sustained, forceful pushing is still advocated. In that case, when the contraction begins, the woman is told to take a cleansing breath or two, then to take a third large breath and hold it while pushing down with her abdominal muscles (called the Valsalva maneuver). A more natural approach that lets the mother wait to bear down until she feels an urge to push may shorten the pushing phase, reducing the incidence of physiologic stress in the mother and acidosis in the newborn.

A nullipara is usually prepared for birth when perineal bulging is noted. A multipara usually progresses far more quickly, so she may be prepared for the birth when the cervix is dilated 7 to 8 cm. As the birth approaches, the woman's partner or support person also prepares for the birth.

Monitor the woman's blood pressure and the FHR between contractions, and palpate the contractions at least every 5 minutes until the birth. Continue to assist the woman in her pushing efforts, keep both the woman and the coach informed of procedures and progress, and support them both throughout the birth.

Promotion of Comfort in the Second Stage

Most of the comfort measures used during the first stage remain appropriate at this time. Applying cool cloths to the face and forehead may help cool the woman involved in the intense physical exertion of pushing. The woman may feel hot and want to remove some covers. Care still needs to be taken to provide privacy even though covers are removed. Encourage the woman to rest and relax all muscles during the periods between contractions. With the support person(s), help the woman into a pushing position with each contraction. Sips of fluids or ice chips may relieve dry mouth. Continually provide encouragement and positive reinforcement.

Assisting During Birth

In addition to assisting the woman and her partner, the nurse also assists the physician/CNM in preparing for the birth. The physician/CNM dons a sterile gown and gloves and may place sterile drapes over the woman's abdomen and legs. An episiotomy may be done just before the actual birth if needed. (See the discussion of episiotomy in Chapter 23 ●.)

Shortly before the birth, the birthing room or delivery room is prepared with the equipment and materials that may be needed. Family members do not need to change into other clothing if the birth occurs in a birthing room; they don a disposable scrub suit or scrubs provided by the facility if the birth is to occur in a delivery room or surgery suite. Thorough handwashing is required of the nurses and physician/CNM. Nurses who will be in direct contact with the mother at the time of birth need to wear protective clothing such as an apron or gown with a splash apron, disposable gloves, and eye covering. The physician/CNM also needs to wear a plastic apron or a gown with a splash apron, eye covering, and sterile gloves.

If the laboring woman is to give birth in a location other than the birthing room (such as in the case of a cesarean birth), she is moved onto her bed or a stretcher shortly before birth. To ensure the woman's safety, the side rails should be raised into a locked position. It is important that the woman not be moved from one bed to another during a contraction. During a contraction the woman feels increased discomfort and may be involved in pushing efforts. Take care to preserve her privacy during the transfer. The labor bed or transfer cart must be carefully braced against the delivery table to ensure the woman's safety during the transfer.

● **Figure 19–4** The nurse provides encouragement and support during pushing efforts.

Clinical Tip

Birth is imminent if the woman shows the following changes:

- Bulging of the perineum
- Uncontrollable urge to bear down
- Increased bloody show

Even though there are differences in the delivery room setting, the family can still be together during the birth. Encourage family members to participate, because the delivery room environment may seem intimidating. The family member may hesitate to continue providing support because of fear of interfering or being in the way.

Maternal Birthing Positions

Until modern times the upright posture for birth was considered normal in most societies. Women chose to squat, kneel, stand, or sit for birth. The recumbent position (lithotomy) became more usual in the Western world because of the convenience it offers in applying technology. The lithotomy position has thus become the conventional manner in which North American women give birth in hospitals. In seeking alternative positions, consumers and professionals alike are refocusing on the comfort of the laboring woman rather than on the convenience of the physician/CNM (Figure 19–5 ● and Table 19–4).

● **Figure 19–5** Side-lying (also known as left lateral Sims') birthing position.
Source: © Angela Hampton Picture Library/Alamy.

Table 19–4	Comparison of Birthing Positions		
Position	**Advantages**	**Disadvantages**	**Nursing Actions**
Sitting on birthing stool	Gravity aids descent and expulsion of infant. Does not compromise venous return from lower extremities. Woman can view birth process.	It is difficult to provide support for the woman's back.	Encourage woman to sit in a position that increases her comfort.
Semi-Fowler's	Does not compromise venous return from lower extremities. Woman can view birth process.	If legs are positioned wide apart, relaxation of perineal tissues is decreased.	Assess that upper torso is evenly supported. Increase support of body by changing position of bed or using pillows as props.
Left lateral Sims'	Does not compromise venous return from lower extremities. Increases perineal relaxation and decreases need for episiotomy. Appears to prevent rapid descent.	It is difficult for the woman to see the birth.	Adjust position so that the upper leg lies on the bed (scissor fashion) or is supported by the partner or on pillows.
Squatting	Size of pelvic outlet is increased. Gravity aids descent and expulsion of newborn. Second stage may be shortened.	It may be difficult to maintain balance while squatting.	Help woman maintain balance. Use a birthing bar if available.
Sitting in birthing bed	Gravity aids descent and expulsion of the fetus. Does not compromise venous return from lower extremities. Woman can view the birth process. Leg position may be changed at will.		Ensure that legs and feet have adequate support.
Hands and knees	Increases perineal relaxation and decreases need for episiotomy. Increases placental and umbilical blood flow and decreases fetal distress. Improves fetal rotation. Better able to assess the perineum. Better access to fetal nose and mouth for suctioning at birth. Facilitates birth of infant with shoulder dystocia.	Woman cannot view birth. There is decreased contact with birth attendant. Caregivers cannot use instruments. There may be increased maternal fatigue.	Adjust birthing bed by dropping the foot down. Supply extra pillows for increased support.

The woman is typically positioned for birth on a bed with leg supports, in a squatting position, or perhaps on her hands and knees. If a birthing bed is used, the back is elevated 30 to 60 degrees to help the woman bear down. Stirrups, if needed and used, are padded to avoid pressure. In helping the woman place her legs in the stirrups, lift both legs simultaneously to avoid strain on abdominal, back, and perineal muscles. Adjust the stirrups to fit the woman's legs. The feet are supported in the stirrup holders. The height and angle of the stirrups are adjusted so there is no pressure on the backs of the knees or the calves, which might cause discomfort and postpartum vascular problems. When stirrups are not used for the birth, the woman's legs may be placed in stirrups after the birth to enhance visibility if a perineal repair is needed.

Cleansing the Perineum

After the woman has been positioned for the birth, her vulvar and perineal areas are cleansed to increase her comfort and to remove any bloody discharge. Depending on agency protocol or on physician or CNM orders, perineal cleansing methods range from use of soapy water to aseptic technique. Once the cleansing is completed, the woman returns to the desired birthing position.

Continued Labor Support

Both the woman's partner and the nurse who has been with the woman during the labor continue to provide support during contractions. The woman is encouraged to push with each contraction and, as the fetal head emerges, is asked to take shallow breaths or to pant to prevent pushing. While supporting the head, the physician or certified nurse-midwife assesses whether the umbilical cord is around the fetal neck and removes it if it is, then suctions the mouth and nose with a bulb syringe. The mouth is suctioned first to prevent reflex inhalation of mucus when the nostrils are touched with the bulb syringe tip. The woman is encouraged to push again as the rest of the newborn's body is born. See the birthing sequence shown in Figure 17–12 on page 367.

NURSING CARE DURING THE THIRD AND FOURTH STAGES OF LABOR

Initial Care of the Newborn

The physician/CNM places the newborn on the mother's abdomen, which promotes attachment, or in the radiant-heated unit. The newborn is maintained in a modified Trendelenburg position. In this position, gravity aids drainage of mucus from the nasopharynx and trachea. Dry the newborn immediately and help keep the infant warm by placing warmed blankets over the newborn or by placing him or her in skin-to-skin contact with the mother. If the newborn is in a radiant-heated unit, he or she is dried, placed on a dry blanket, and left uncovered. Because radiant heat warms the outer surface of objects, a newborn wrapped in blankets will receive no benefit from the unit.

Suction the newborn's nose and mouth with a bulb syringe as needed. Most immediate care of the newborn can be done while the newborn is in the parent's arms or in the radiant-heated unit.

Table 19–5	The Apgar Scoring System		
		Score	
Sign	**0**	**1**	**2**
Heart rate	Absent	Slow; less than 100 beats/min	Greater than 100 beats/min
Respiration	Absent	Slow; irregular	Good breathing with crying
Muscle tone	Flaccid	Some flexion of extremities	Active movement of extremities
Reflex response	Absent	Grimace; noticeable facial movement	Vigorous cry; coughs; sneezes; pulls away when touched
Skin color	Pale or blue	Pink body, blue extremities	Pink body and extremities

Source: Data from Apgar, V. (1966). *The newborn (Apgar) scoring system, reflections and advice.* Retrieved from http://profiles.nlm.nih.gov/ps/access/CPBBJY.pdf.

Apgar Scoring System

The Apgar scoring system (Table 19–5) evaluates the physical condition of the newborn at birth. The newborn is rated 1 minute after birth and again at 5 minutes and receives a total score (**Apgar score**) ranging from 0 to 10 based on the following assessments:

1. *Heart rate* is auscultated or palpated at the junction of the umbilical cord and skin. This is the most important assessment. A heart rate above or equal to 100 is scored as 2, a heart rate below 100 receives a 1, and a score of 0 is assigned if there is no heartbeat. A newborn heart rate of less than 100 beats per minute indicates the need for immediate resuscitation.

2. *Respiratory effort* is the second most important Apgar assessment. A vigorous cry indicates adequate respirations and is scored as 2, whereas a slow, irregular respiratory effort receives a 1. Complete absence of respirations is termed apnea (scored 0).

3. *Muscle tone* is determined by evaluating the degree of flexion and resistance to straightening of the extremities. A normal newborn's elbows and hips are flexed, with the knees positioned up toward the abdomen (scored as 2). Some flexion of the extremities is scored as 1, while a flaccid infant receives a 0.

4. *Reflex irritability* is evaluated by stroking the baby's back along the spine, by flicking the soles of the feet, or by using the bulb syringe to perform oral or nasal suctioning. A cry merits a full score of 2. A grimace is 1 point, and no response is 0.

5. *Skin color* is inspected for cyanosis and pallor. Generally, newborns have blue extremities, with a pink body, which

Video | Newborn Assessment

merits a score of 1. This condition is termed *acrocyanosis* and is present in many normal newborns at 1 minute after birth. A totally pink newborn scores a 2, and a totally cyanotic, pale infant scores 0. Newborns with darker skin are not pink in color. Their skin color is assessed for pallor and acrocyanosis.

A score of 7 to 10 indicates a newborn in good condition who requires only nasopharyngeal suctioning and perhaps some oxygen near the face (called "blow-by" oxygen). If the Apgar score is below 7, resuscitative measures may be needed. (See the discussion in Chapter 27 ⊘.) Apgar scores of less than 3 at 5 minutes postbirth may correlate with neonatal mortality (ACOG, 2009a). (See Skill 5–2 in the *Clinical Skills Manual* SKILLS .)

Care of Umbilical Cord

Delayed cord clamping is associated with positive outcomes for the infant and is now the preferred approach (ACOG, 2012). If the physician/CNM has not placed some type of cord clamp on the newborn's umbilical cord, the nurse does so. Before applying the cord clamp, examine the cut end of the cord for the presence of two arteries and one vein. The umbilical vein is the largest vessel, and the arteries are seen as smaller vessels. Record the number of vessels on the birth and newborn records. The cord is clamped approximately 1/2 to 1 inch from the abdomen to allow room between the abdomen and clamp as the cord dries. Abdominal skin must not be clamped, because this will cause necrosis of the tissue. The most common type of cord clamp is the plastic Hollister cord clamp (Figure 19–6 ●). The Hollister clamp is removed in the nursery about 24 hours after the cord has dried.

Cord Blood Collection for Banking

A growing number of parents are arranging for cord blood banking with individual cord blood registries. Cord blood banking involves collecting the newborn's umbilical cord blood immediately following expulsion of the infant. Since cord blood, like bone marrow, contains hematopoietic stem cells, it can be used to treat numerous cancers, genetic and blood disorders, cerebral palsy, and immune disorders. Cord blood has advantages over bone marrow. It is a no-risk procedure and causes no discomfort to the newborn or mother and is less likely to trigger a potentially fatal rejection response. Cord blood can also work with a less than perfect match and is more readily available than bone marrow. Although cord blood banks have been established in the United States, universal cord blood collection does not exist. While some facilities collect volunteer donations, the majority of hospitals do not. Most of the banking performed in the United States is done by for-profit agencies where the parents pay a set fee to collect the blood and have it processed followed by an annual storage fee. The main drawback of cord blood banking is the cost.

Cord blood transfusions can be utilized to treat a growing number of disorders. It is estimated that over 20,000 transfusions had been performed in the United States as of 2009 (Parent's Guide to Cord Blood Foundation, 2012). Both ACOG and the American Academy of Pediatrics have issued position statements on the importance of cord blood banking and the need to discuss the advantages and disadvantages with parents. While universal cord blood banking is not routinely recommended, parents who have an older child affected by a condition that may benefit from a cord blood transfusion should consider cord blood banking. Recent recommendations have also been made that women at risk of giving birth prematurely should consider cord blood banking since these infants are more at risk for cerebral palsy and other neurologic injuries (Parent's Guide to Cord Blood Foundation, 2012).

Once collected, the blood is tested for infectious and genetic disorders before it is frozen. Abnormal blood results are communicated to the parents. Written consent is required for both collection and storage of cord blood, preferably upon admission or prior to the onset of labor.

● **Figure 19–6** Hollister cord clamp. *A,* Clamp is positioned 0.5 to 1 inch from the abdomen and then secured. *B,* Cut cord. The one vein and two arteries can be seen. *C,* Plastic device for removing clamp after cord has dried. After the cord has dried, the nurse grasps the Hollister clamp on either side of the cut area and gently separates it.

These registries provide the parents with a special container for the cord blood, which they bring with them to the birth. The parents should have received directions from the registry about the storage and care of the container prior to the birth. Immediately after the newborn's umbilical cord is clamped and cut and the placenta is expelled, the CNM or physician withdraws blood from the remaining umbilical cord and the placenta and places it in the special container. The cord blood remains with the mother until it is picked up by the cord blood registry.

Physical Assessment of the Newborn

The nurse performs an abbreviated systematic physical assessment in the birthing area to detect any abnormalities (Table 19–6). (See Chapter 25 ❷ for an in-depth discussion of newborn assessment.) First, note the size of the newborn and the contour and size of the head in relationship to the rest of the body. The newborn's posture and movements indicate tone and neurologic functioning.

Inspect the skin for discoloration, presence of vernix caseosa and lanugo, and signs of trauma and desquamation (peeling of skin). Vernix caseosa is a white, cheesy substance found normally on newborns. It is absorbed within 24 hours after birth. Vernix is abundant on preterm infants and absent on postterm newborns. Fine hair (lanugo) is often seen on preterm newborns' shoulders, foreheads, backs, and cheeks. Desquamation is seen in postterm newborns.

Observe the nares (nostrils) for flaring and, as the newborn cries, inspect the palate for cleft palate. Look for mucus in the nose and mouth, and remove it with a bulb syringe as needed. Inspect the chest for respiratory rate and the presence of retractions. If retractions are present, assess the newborn for grunting or stridor. A normal respiratory rate is 30 to 60 per minute. Auscultate the lungs bilaterally for breath sounds. Absence of breath sounds on one side could mean pneumothorax. Crackles may be heard immediately after birth because a small amount of fluid may remain in the lungs; this fluid will be absorbed. Rhonchi indicate aspiration of oral secretions. If there is excessive mucus or respiratory distress, suction the newborn with a mucus trap. (See Figure 19–7 ● as well as Skill 5–1 in the *Clinical Skills Manual* SKILLS.) Note and record elimination of urine or meconium on the newborn record.

Newborn Identification

Place two ID bands on the newborn—one on the wrist and one on the ankle. The bands must fit snugly so they will not be lost although caution should be used to prevent constriction. To ensure correct identification, while still in the birthing or delivery room, give the mother and her partner each a band that matches that of the baby. The bands allow access to the infant care areas and must not be removed until the infant is discharged.

Some facilities use newborn alarm safety devices to prevent abduction and ensure the safety of newborns in hospital settings. Umbilical cord alarms are one type of security device that are placed at the time the cord clamp is applied. The cord clamp and alarm are left in place until the mother and baby are discharged

Table 19–6	Initial Newborn Evaluation
Assess	**Normal Findings**
Respirations	Rate 36–60, irregular No retractions, no grunting
Apical pulse	Rate 120–160 and somewhat irregular
Temperature	Skin temp above 36.5°C (97.8°F)
Skin color	Body pink with bluish extremities
Umbilical cord	Two arteries and one vein
Gestational age	Should be 38–42 weeks to remain with parents for extended time
Sole creases	Sole creases that involve the heel

In general, expect scant amount of vernix on upper back, axilla, groin; lanugo only on upper back; ears with incurving of upper 2/3 of pinnae and thin cartilage that springs back from folding; male genitals—testes palpated in upper or lower scrotum; female genitals—labia majora larger, clitoris nearly covered

In the following situations, newborns should generally be stabilized rather than remain with parents in the birth area for an extended period of time:

- Apgar less than 8 at 1 minute and less than 9 at 5 minutes or baby requires resuscitation measures (other than whiffs of oxygen)
- Respirations below 30 or above 60, with retractions and/or grunting
- Apical pulse below 120 or above 160 with marked irregularities
- Skin temperature below 36.5°C (97.8°F)
- Skin color pale blue or circumoral pallor
- Baby less than 38 weeks' or more than 42 weeks' gestation
- Baby very small or very large for gestational age
- Congenital anomalies involving open areas in the skin (meningomyelocele)

● **Figure 19–7** DeLee mucus trap being used to suction a newborn's mouth to remove excess secretions. One end of the suction tubing is connected to low suction, and the other end of the tubing is inserted 3 to 5 inches into the newborn's nose or mouth. Suction is applied as the tubing is pulled out. The process is repeated for as long as fluid is aspirated.
Source: Courtesy of Wilson Garcia.

● **Figure 19–8** A newborn infant with a security device in place on one ankle.

Source: Courtesy of Anne Garcia.

home. An alarm system that is attached to either the wrist or ankle by a band is another infant safety device that may be utilized by some facilities (Figure 19–8 ●). A newer option, a skin sensing tag alarm, is placed on the wrist or ankle and senses if the tag has been removed by monitoring changes in temperature that would occur if the tag were to be removed or become dislodged from the newborn. All three devices sound an alarm if the infant is removed from the hospital unit or if the device is cut or disengaged. The need for proper disinfection techniques for devices that are reused in clinical practice is imperative (Association of Perioperative Registered Nurses, 2013).

Additional hospital security measures are now commonplace in maternity settings. This includes mandating that all staff wear appropriate identification at all times. The nurse advises the parents to place the infant on the side of the bed away from the door, and to have the baby returned to the nursery whenever the mother naps or showers and no other family member is present.

Although hospital infant abductions are rare, they are catastrophic to the family, hospital, and community. Many abductors pose as medical personnel to gain access to the infant. Women should be advised to ask all hospital personnel for proper identification. If the mother or family feels unsure of the individual, they should immediately call on the call bell to alert the nurse and ask for other verification. If a woman is reluctant to allow a student nurse to transport her infant, the staff nurse should be asked to assist the student.

Delivery of the Placenta

After birth the CNM or physician prepares for the delivery of the placenta. The following signs suggest placental separation:

1. The uterus rises upward in the abdomen.
2. As the placenta moves downward, the umbilical cord lengthens.

3. A sudden trickle or spurt of blood appears.
4. The shape of the uterus changes from discoid to globular.

While waiting for these signs, palpate the uterus to check for ballooning caused by uterine relaxation and subsequent bleeding into the uterine cavity. After the placenta has separated, the woman may be asked to bear down to aid delivery of the placenta.

Oxytocics are frequently given at the time of the delivery of the placenta, so the uterus will contract and bleeding will be minimized. Oxytocin (Pitocin), 10 to 20 units, may be added to an intravenous (IV) infusion, or 10 units may be given intramuscularly. Some physicians order methylergonovine maleate (Methergine), 0.2 mg administered intramuscularly, or carboprost tromethamine (Hemabate), 250 mcg/mL administered intramuscularly. (See *Drug Guide: Carboprost Tromethamine (Hemabate).*) In addition to administering the ordered medications, it is essential to assess and record maternal blood pressure before and after administration of oxytocics. For further information, refer to *Drug Guide: Oxytocin (Pitocin)* (in Chapter 23 🔗 on page 501) and *Drug Guide: Methylergonovine Maleate (Methergine)* (in Chapter 30 🔗 on page 735). After expulsion of the placenta, the CNM or physician inspects the placental membranes to make sure they are intact and that all cotyledons are present. If there is a defect or a part missing from the placenta, a manual uterine examination is done. On the birth record, note the time of delivery of the placenta.

After the placenta is expelled, the physician/CNM inspects the vagina and cervix for lacerations and makes any necessary repairs. The episiotomy may be repaired if that has not been done previously (see Chapter 23 🔗).

Enhancing Attachment

The first few hours and even minutes after birth are an important period for the attachment of mother and infant. If this period of contact can occur during the first hour after birth, the newborn will be in the quiet state and able to interact with parents by looking at them. Newborns also turn their heads in response to a spoken voice. (For further discussion of newborn states, see Chapter 24 🔗.)

The first parent–newborn contact may be brief (a few minutes), to be followed by a more extended contact after uncomfortable procedures (expulsion of the placenta and suturing of the episiotomy) are completed. When the newborn is returned to the mother, help her begin breastfeeding if she so desires. The baby may seek out the mother's breast, and early contact between the two can greatly affect breastfeeding success. Even if the newborn does not actively nurse, he or she can lick, taste, and smell the mother's skin. This activity by the newborn stimulates the maternal release of prolactin, which promotes the onset of lactation.

Clinical Tip

Infant to mother skin-to-skin contact immediately following birth supports breastfeeding and bonding (Mahmood, Jamal, & Khan, 2011).

Drug Guide Carboprost Tromethamine (Hemabate)

Pregnancy Risk Category: D

Overview of Action

Carboprost tromethamine (Hemabate) is used to reduce blood loss secondary to uterine atony. It stimulates myometrial contractions to control postpartum hemorrhaging that is unresponsive to usual techniques. Carboprost tromethamine can also be used to induce labor in women desiring an elective termination of a pregnancy. The drug is also used to induce labor in cases of intrauterine fetal death and hydatidiform mole (Wilson, Shannon, & Shields, 2013).

Route, Dosage, Frequency

In cases of immediate postpartum hemorrhage the usual intramuscular dose is 250 mcg (1 mL), which can be repeated every 1.5 to 3.5 hours if uterine atony persists. The dosage can be increased to 500 mcg (2 mL) if uterine contractility is inadequate after several doses of 250 mcg. The total dosage should not exceed 12 mg. The maximum duration of use is 48 hours (Wilson et al., 2013).

Contraindications

The drug is contraindicated in women with active cardiac, pulmonary, or renal disease. It should not be administered during pregnancy or in women with acute pelvic inflammatory disease. It should be used with caution in women with asthma, adrenal disease, hypotension, hypertension, diabetes mellitus, epilepsy, fibroids, cervical stenosis, or previous uterine surgery (Wilson et al., 2013).

Side Effects

The most common side effects are nausea and diarrhea. Fever, chills, and flushing can occur. Headache, muscle, joint, abdominal, or eye pain can also occur (Wilson et al., 2013).

Nursing Considerations

- The injection should be given in a large muscle. Aspiration should be performed to avoid injection into a blood vessel, which can result in bronchospasm, tetanic contractions, and shock.
- After administration, monitor uterine status and bleeding carefully.
- Report excess bleeding to the physician/CNM.
- Check vital signs routinely, observing for an increase in temperature, elevated pulse, and decreased blood pressure.
- Breastfeeding should be delayed for 24 hours after administration (Wilson et al., 2013).

Darkening the birthing room by turning out most of the lights causes newborns to open their eyes and gaze around. This in turn enhances eye-to-eye contact with the parents. (*Note:* If the physician/CNM needs a light source, the spotlight can be left on.) Treatment of the newborn's eyes may also be delayed. Many parents who establish eye contact with the newborn are content to quietly gaze at their infant. Others may show more active involvement by touching or inspecting the newborn. Some mothers talk to their babies in a high-pitched voice, which seems to be soothing to newborns. Some couples verbally express amazement and pride when they see they have produced a beautiful, healthy baby. Their verbalization enhances feelings of accomplishment and ecstasy.

Both parents need to be encouraged to do whatever they feel most comfortable doing. Some parents prefer only limited contact with the newborn immediately after birth and instead want private time together in a quiet environment. In spite of the current zeal for providing immediate attachment opportunities, nursing personnel need to be aware of parents' wishes. The desire to delay interaction with the newborn does not necessarily imply a decreased ability of the parents to bond with their newborn. (For further discussion of parent–newborn attachment, see Chapter 26 ⊘.)

Provision of Care in the Fourth Stage

The period of 1 to 4 hours immediately following the expulsion of the placenta, during which the mother's condition stabilizes, is often referred to as the fourth stage of labor and birth. This is actually the initial recovery period.

After childbirth it is critical that the uterine fundus stay well contracted to clamp off uterine blood vessels at the placental site and thereby prevent hemorrhaging. Consequently, palpate the uterine fundus at frequent intervals for the first 4 hours to ensure that it remains firmly contracted. Normally the fundus is located in the midline and at or below the umbilicus. Palpate the fundus (Figure 19–9 ●) but do not massage it unless it is soft (boggy). When a uterus becomes boggy, pooling of blood occurs within it, causing clots. Anything left in the uterus prevents it from contracting effectively. Thus, if the uterus becomes boggy or appears to rise in the abdomen, massage the fundus until firm; then with one hand supporting the uterus at the symphysis pubis, use the other hand to exert steady pressure on the fundus to express retained clots. The uterus is very tender at this time so all palpation and massage must be done as gently as possible.

In some women the uterus becomes so relaxed that it cannot be found when palpation is attempted. In this case, place one hand in the midline of the abdomen at about the level of the umbilicus and begin to make kneading motions. This motion generally stimulates the uterus to contract, and it then feels like a firm, hard object. (See Skill 4–1 in the *Clinical Skills Manual* SKILLS .)

Wash the woman's perineum with gauze squares and warmed solution and dry the area well with a towel before placing the maternity pad. If stirrups have been used, remove both of the woman's legs from the stirrups at the same time to avoid muscle strain. Encourage the woman to move her legs gently up and down in a bicycle motion. The woman remains in the same bed or is transferred to a recovery room bed. Help her don a clean gown and offer her something to drink.

During the recovery period, it is essential to monitor maternal vital signs closely. Check the maternal blood pressure at 5- to 15-minute intervals to detect any changes. Blood pressure should return to the prelabor level as a result of an increased volume of blood returning to the maternal circulation from the uteroplacental shunt. Pulse rate should be slightly lower than it was during labor. Baroreceptors cause a vagal response, which slows

Video

Fourth Stage of Labor

● **Figure 19–9** Suggested method of palpating the fundus of the uterus during the fourth stage. The left hand is placed just above the symphysis pubis, and gentle downward pressure is exerted. The right hand is cupped around the uterine fundus.

Table 19–7	Maternal Adaptations Following Birth
Characteristic	**Normal Finding**
Blood pressure	Returns to prelabor level
Pulse	Slightly lower than in labor
Uterine fundus	In the midline at the umbilicus or one to two finger breadths below the umbilicus
Lochia	Red (rubra), small to moderate amount (from spotting on pads to ¼–½ of pad covered in 15 minutes)
	Does not exceed saturation of one pad in first hour
Bladder	Nonpalpable
Perineum	Smooth, pink, without bruising or edema
Emotional state	Wide variation, including excited, exhilarated, smiling, crying, fatigued, verbal, quiet, pensive, and sleepy

the pulse. A rise in blood pressure may be a response to oxytocic drugs or may be caused by preeclampsia. A lowered blood pressure and a rising pulse rate may reflect blood loss (Table 19–7).

Also monitor the woman's temperature. Frequently, women have tremors in the immediate postpartum period, possibly caused by a difference in internal and external body temperatures (higher temperature inside the body than outside). Another theory is that the woman is reacting to the fetal cells that have entered the maternal circulation at the placental site. A heated bath blanket placed next to the woman is helpful and can be replaced as often as the mother desires.

Inspect the bloody vaginal discharge for amount and chart it as minimal, moderate, or heavy and with or without clots. This discharge, lochia rubra, should be bright red. A soaked perineal pad contains approximately 100 mL of blood. If the perineal pad becomes soaked in a 15-minute period or if blood pools under the buttocks, continuous observation is necessary (see Skill 4–2 in the *Clinical Skills Manual* SKILLS). When the fundus is firm, a continuous trickle of blood may signal laceration of the vagina or cervix or an unligated vessel in the episiotomy.

If the fundus rises and displaces to the right, it is important to consider two factors:

1. As the uterus rises, the uterine contractions become less effective and increased bleeding may occur.

2. The most common cause of uterine displacement is bladder distention.

Palpate the bladder to determine whether it is distended. The bladder fills rapidly with the extra fluid volume returned from the uteroplacental circulation (and with any fluid received intravenously during labor and birth). The postpartum woman may not realize that her bladder is full because trauma to the bladder and urethra during childbirth and the use of regional anesthesia decrease bladder tone and the urge to void.

Use a variety of measures to help the mother to void. Place a warm towel across the lower abdomen or pour warm water over the perineum to relax the urinary sphincter and facilitate voiding. If the woman is unable to void, catheterization is necessary.

The perineum is inspected for edema and hematoma formation. An ice pack often reduces the swelling and alleviates the discomfort of an episiotomy.

The couple may be tired, hungry, and thirsty. Some agencies serve the couple a meal. The tired mother will probably drift off into a welcome sleep. The partner can also be encouraged to rest, since the supporting role is physically and mentally tiring. If the mother is not in a birthing room, she is usually transferred from the birthing unit to the postpartum or mother–baby area after 2 hours or more, depending on agency policy and whether the following criteria are met:

■ Stable vital signs

■ No bleeding

■ Undistended bladder

■ Firm fundus

■ Sensations fully recovered from any anesthetic agent received during birth

SUPPORT OF THE ADOLESCENT DURING BIRTH

As with all women, each adolescent in labor is different. Assess what each teen brings to the experience by considering the following:

- Has the young woman received prenatal care?
- What are her attitudes and feelings about the pregnancy?
- Who will attend the birth and what is the person's relationship to her?
- What preparation has she had for the experience?
- What are her expectations and fears regarding labor and birth?
- How has her culture influenced her?
- What are her usual coping mechanisms?
- Does she plan to keep the newborn?

Adolescent women are at highest risk for pregnancy and labor complications and must be assessed carefully. Fetal well-being is established by fetal monitoring. Be especially alert for any physiologic complications of labor. The young woman's prenatal record is carefully reviewed for risks, and she is screened for preeclampsia, cephalopelvic disproportion, anemia, drugs ingested during pregnancy, sexually transmitted infections, and size–date discrepancies.

The support role of the nurse depends on the young woman's support system during labor. The adolescent may not be accompanied by someone who will stay with her during childbirth, or she may have her mother, the father of the baby, or a close friend as her labor partner. Regardless of whether the teen has a support person, it is important to establish a trusting relationship with her. In this way it is possible to help the teen understand what is happening to her. The adolescent given positive reinforcement for "work well done" will leave the experience with increased self-esteem, despite the emotional problems that may accompany her situation. If a support person accompanies the adolescent, that person also needs encouragement and support. Explain changes in the young woman's behavior and describe ways the support person can be of help.

The adolescent who has taken childbirth education classes is generally better prepared for labor than the adolescent who has not. However, the younger the adolescent, the less she may be able to participate actively in the process, even if she has taken prenatal classes. See Figure 19–10 ●.

The very young adolescent (age 14 and under) has fewer coping mechanisms and less experience to draw on than her older counterparts. Because her cognitive development is incomplete, the younger adolescent may have fewer problem-solving capabilities. She may be more threatened by the experience, and she may be more vulnerable to stress and discomfort.

The very young adolescent needs someone to rely on at all times during labor. She may be more childlike and dependent than older teens. Instructions and explanations should be simple and concrete. During the transition phase, the young teenager may become withdrawn and unable to express her need to be

● **Figure 19–10** An adolescent mother receives breastfeeding assistance in the immediate postpartum period.

nurtured. Touch, soothing encouragement, and measures to provide comfort help her maintain control and meet her needs for dependence. During the second stage of labor, the young adolescent may feel as if she is losing control and may reach out to those around her. It is important to remain calm and give clear, simple directions to help the teen cope with feelings of helplessness.

The middle adolescent (ages 15 to 17 years) often attempts to remain calm and unflinching during labor. Nevertheless, a caring attitude still helps the young woman. Many older adolescents believe that they "know it all," but they may be no more prepared for childbirth than their younger counterparts. Positive reinforcement and a nonjudgmental manner will help them save face. If the adolescent has not taken childbirth preparation classes, she may require preparation and explanations. The older teenager's (ages 18 to 19) response to the stresses of labor, however, is similar to that of the adult woman.

Even if the adolescent is planning to relinquish her newborn, she should be given the option of seeing and holding the infant. She may be reluctant to do this at first, but the mother's grieving process is facilitated if she sees the infant. However, seeing or holding the newborn should be the young woman's choice. (See Chapter 30 ✐ for further discussion of the relinquishing mother and the adolescent parent.)

NURSING CARE DURING PRECIPITOUS LABOR AND BIRTH

Occasionally labor progresses so rapidly that the maternity nurse is faced with the task of managing the actual birth of the baby. The terms **precipitous labor** and **precipitous birth** are used when the labor and birth occur in 3 hours or less. The attending nurse has the primary responsibility for providing a physically and psychologically safe experience for the woman and her baby. A woman whose certified nurse-midwife (CNM) or physician is not present may feel disappointed, frightened, abandoned, angry, and cheated. She may fear what is going to happen and feel

Clinical Tip

When birth is imminent and a physician/CNM is not present, do not take the bed apart (or "break the bed") because this increases the risk that the newborn could be dropped at the time of birth. Lower the foot of the bed slightly to create space beneath the buttocks so you are able to adequately deliver the head without the risk of a newborn fall.

that everything is out of her control. In working with the woman, the nurse provides support by keeping her informed about the labor progress and assuring her that the nurse will stay with her.

If birth is imminent, the nurse must not leave the mother alone. The nurse can direct auxiliary personnel to contact the physician/CNM and retrieve the emergency birth pack ("precip pack"), which should be readily accessible to birthing rooms. A typical pack contains the following items:

- A small drape that can be placed under the woman's buttocks to provide a sterile field
- A bulb syringe to clear mucus from the newborn's mouth
- Two sterile clamps (Kelly or Rochester) to clamp the umbilical cord before applying a cord clamp
- Sterile scissors to cut the umbilical cord
- A sterile umbilical cord clamp, either Hesseltine or Hollister
- A baby blanket to wrap the newborn in after birth
- A package of sterile gloves

At all times during the birth, the nurse remains calm, provides suggestions such as when to maintain a controlled breathing pattern and when to push, supports the woman's efforts, and provides reassurance.

The nurse assists in the precipitous labor and birth as follows: The woman is encouraged to assume a comfortable position. If time permits, the nurse scrubs his or her hands with soap and water and puts on sterile gloves. Sterile drapes are placed under the woman's buttocks. The nurse may place an index finger inside the lower portion of the vagina and the thumb on the outer portion of the perineum and gently massage the area to help stretch perineal tissues and prevent perineal lacerations. This procedure is called "ironing the perineum."

When the infant's head crowns, the nurse instructs the woman to pant, which decreases her urge to push. The nurse checks whether the amniotic sac is intact. If it is, the nurse tears the sac so the newborn will not breathe in amniotic fluid with the first breath.

With one hand the nurse applies gentle pressure against the fetal head to prevent it from popping out rapidly. The nurse does not hold the head back forcibly. Rapid birth of the head may result in tears in the woman's perineal tissues. The rapid change in pressure within the fetal head may cause subdural or dural tears. The nurse supports the perineum with the other hand and allows the head to be born between contractions.

As the woman continues to pant, the nurse inserts one or two fingers along the back of the fetal head to check for the umbilical cord. If there is a nuchal cord (umbilical cord around the neck), the nurse bends his or her fingers like a fish hook, grasps the cord, and pulls it over the baby's head. It is important to check that the cord is not wrapped around the neck more than one time. If the cord is tightly looped and cannot be slipped over the baby's head, two clamps are placed on the cord, the cord is cut between the clamps, and the cord is unwound.

Immediately after birth of the head, the nurse suctions the baby's mouth, throat, and nasal passages. The nurse then places one hand on each side of the head and exerts gentle downward traction until the anterior shoulder passes under the symphysis pubis. Then gentle upward traction aids the birth of the posterior shoulder. The nurse then instructs the woman to push gently so that the rest of the body can be born quickly. The newborn must be supported as he or she emerges.

The newborn is held at the level of the uterus to facilitate blood flow through the umbilical cord. The combination of amniotic fluid and vernix makes the newborn very slippery, so the nurse must be careful to avoid dropping the baby. The nose and mouth of the newborn are suctioned again, using a bulb syringe. The nurse then dries the newborn to prevent heat loss. As soon as the nurse determines that the newborn's respirations are adequate, the infant can be placed on the mother's abdomen. The newborn's head should be slightly lower than the body to aid drainage of fluid and mucus. The weight of the newborn on the mother's abdomen stimulates uterine contractions, which aid in placental separation. The umbilical cord should not be pulled. The nurse is alert for signs of placental separation (slight gush of dark blood from the vagina, lengthening of the cord, or a change in uterine shape from discoid to globular). When these signs are present, the nurse tells the mother to push so that the placenta can be delivered. The nurse inspects the placenta to determine whether it is intact.

The nurse checks the firmness of the uterus. The fundus may be gently massaged to stimulate contractions and decrease bleeding. Putting the newborn to breast also stimulates uterine contractions through release of oxytocin from the pituitary gland.

The umbilical cord may now be cut. The nurse places two sterile Kelly clamps approximately 1 to 3 inches from the newborn's abdomen. The cord is cut between the Kelly clamps with sterile scissors. The nurse places a sterile umbilical cord clamp adjacent to the clamp on the newborn's cord, between the clamp and the newborn's abdomen. The clamp must not be placed snugly against the abdomen, because the cord will dry and shrink.

The nurse cleanses the area under the mother's buttocks and inspects her perineum for lacerations. Bleeding from lacerations may be controlled by pressing a clean perineal pad against the perineum and instructing the woman to keep her thighs together.

If the physician/CNM's arrival is delayed or if the newborn is having respiratory distress, the newborn should be transported immediately to the nursery. The newborn must be properly identified before he or she leaves the birth area. The nurse notes and places on a birth record the following information:

- Position of fetus at birth
- Presence of cord around neck or shoulder (nuchal cord)
- Time of birth
- Apgar scores at 1 and 5 minutes after birth
- Gender of newborn
- Time of expulsion of placenta
- Method of placental expulsion
- Appearance and intactness of placenta
- Mother's condition
- Any medications given to mother or newborn (per agency protocol)

EVALUATION

As a result of comprehensive nursing care during the intrapartum period, the following outcomes may be anticipated:

- The mother's physical and psychologic well-being has been maintained and supported.
- The baby's physical and psychologic well-being has been protected and supported.
- The couple have had input into the birth process and have participated as much as they desired.
- The mother and her baby have had a safe birth.

Critical Concept Review

LEARNING OUTCOME 19.1: Identify admission data that should be noted when a woman is admitted to the birthing area.

1. Information obtained during admission is used to develop a clinical care management plan for the four stages of labor:
   - Prenatal information.
   - Current assessments.
   - Expected teaching.
   - Nursing care expected for each stage.
   - Expected activity level.
   - Proposed comfort measures.
   - Elimination and nutritional needs.
   - Level of family involvement.

LEARNING OUTCOME 19.2: Describe the nursing care of a woman and her partner/family upon admission to the birthing area.

1. The nursing care at admission focuses on providing an orientation to the unit and obtaining an overall physical assessment of the mother that focuses on the well-being of the mother and fetus:
   - Assess the maternal vital signs and FHR.
   - Perform a vaginal exam to determine stage of cervical dilatation and state of membranes.
   - Determine frequency and intensity of contractions.
   - Review systems such as respiratory and neurologic.
   - Assess any recent symptoms experienced by the woman.
   - Assess the woman's understanding of the labor process and identification of the woman's support system.

LEARNING OUTCOME 19.3: Use assessment data to determine the nursing interventions to meet the psychologic, social, physiologic, and spiritual needs of the woman and her partner/family during each stage of labor.

1. First stage of labor:
   - Establish rapport with the woman and support person.
   - Discuss expectations of labor and birth.
   - Provide for privacy.
   - Discuss individual expression of pain and discomfort.
2. Second stage of labor:
   - Provide as much privacy as possible.
   - Encourage the woman and support person to decide who should be present at the birth.
   - Provide praise and encouragement of progress.
3. Third and fourth stages of labor:
   - Encourage the woman and support person to hold and look at infant as much as possible.
   - Teach the woman the care to be performed after the baby is born.
   - Provide the woman with food and fluids as allowed.

LEARNING OUTCOME 19.4: Compare methods of promoting comfort during the first and second stages of labor.

1. Comfort measures common to the first and second stages of labor include:
   - Assist the woman to reduce anxiety.
   - Teach the woman about what to expect during the labor experience.
   - Promote relaxation techniques.
   - Instruct in appropriate controlled breathing pattern.
   - Give instruction to the woman's support person.
2. Comfort measures specific to the first stage of labor:
   - Administer pharmacologic agents as ordered by the physician or certified nurse-midwife.
   - Assist with the placement of an epidural for pain control.
3. Comfort measures specific to the second stage of labor:
   - Help the woman find an effective pushing pattern.
   - Support the woman's attempt to rest between pushes.

LEARNING OUTCOME 19.5: Explain the immediate needs and physical assessment of the newborn following birth in the provision of nursing care.

1. Immediate care of the newborn includes:
   - Maintain respiration.
   - Promote warmth.
   - Prevent infection.
   - Provide accurate identification.

LEARNING OUTCOME 19.6: Examine the unique needs of the adolescent during birth in the provision of nursing care.

1. The adolescent is unique in that she has developmental needs as well as physical needs that must be addressed.

LEARNING OUTCOME 19.7: Describe the role and responsibilities of the nurse in the management of a precipitous labor and birth.

1. A precipitous labor and birth is one that occurs rapidly without a physician or certified nurse-midwife in attendance.
2. The nurse attends to the woman, guides the infant's passage through the birth canal, clamps the umbilical cord, and immediately transports the infant to the nursery for care.
3. The nurse focuses care on the woman and the expulsion of the placenta and contraction of the uterus.

Clinical Reasoning in Action

Anita Grey, a 22-year-old primigravida at 40 weeks' gestation, is admitted by you to the birthing center in labor. Anita was sent from her physician's office after being evaluated at her prenatal visit. While in the office, she was assessed to be 4 cm dilated, 100% effaced, vertex at 0 station with bulging membranes. She tells you that her husband is on his way to the birthing center and that she is anxious for him to arrive. A review of her prenatal record shows no complications affecting this pregnancy. Anita's vital signs are within normal limits. You assess the fetal heart rate and contraction pattern with the fetal monitor and observe a fetal heart rate of 140 to 150 beats/min with accelerations to 160s. Contractions are every 3 to 4 minutes × 30 seconds of moderate intensity by palpation. Anita seems to be tolerating the contractions well, but still seems anxious about her husband's arrival.

1. What steps can you take to reduce the stress and anxiety of the laboring woman and her family?
2. When you notify the physician/CNM, what pertinent information should the report contain?
3. What support measures can you give in the active phase of labor?
4. What measures can be used to decrease discomfort/pain as labor progresses?
5. What observations reflect the physiologic manifestations of pain?
6. Create a concept map for Anita's plan of care based on her current labor status. Keep in mind that Anita is a primigravida and is likely to be anxious about her upcoming admission.

See www.nursing.pearsonhighered.com for possible responses and an interactive template for a concept map.

References

American College of Obstetricians and Gynecologists. (ACOG). (2009a). *Intrapartum fetal heart rate monitoring: Nomenclature, interpretation, and general management principles* (ACOG Practice Bulletin No. 106). Washington, DC: Author.

American College of Obstetricians & Gynecologists (ACOG). (2009b). *Oral intake during labor* (ACOG Committee Opinion No. 441). Washington, DC: Author.

American College of Obstetricians & Gynecologists (ACOG). (2010). *Management of intrapartum fetal heart rate tracings monitoring* (ACOG Practice Bulletin No.116). Washington, DC: Author.

American College of Obstetricians & Gynecologists (ACOG). (2012). *Timing of umbilical cord clamping after birth* (ACOG Practice Bulletin No. 543). Washington, DC: Author.

Apgar, V. (1966). *The newborn (Apgar) scoring system, reflections and advice.* Retrieved from http://profiles.nlm.nih.gov/ps/access/CPBBJY.pdf

Association of Perioperative Registered Nurses (AORN). (2013). AORN Guidance Statement: reuse of single-use devices. *Perioperative Standards and Recommended Practices.* Denver, CO: AORN.

Centers for Disease Control and Prevention (CDC). (2012). One test, two lives: HIV screening for prenatal care. Retrieved from http://www.cdc.gov/Features/1Test2Lives

Institute for Patient and Family-Centered Care. (2012). *Family-centered care.* Retrieved from http://www.ipfcc.org/faq.html

Jones, L., Othman, M., Dowswell, T., Alfirevic, A., Gates, S., & Newburn, M. (2012). Pain management for women in labour: An overview of systematic reviews. *Cochrane Database of Systematic Reviews.* Issue 3. Art. No.: CD009234.

Mahmood, I., Jamal, M., & Khan, N. (2011). Effect of mother–infant early skin-to-skin contact on breastfeeding status:

A randomized controlled trial. *Journal of College Physicians in Surgery in Pakistan, 21*(10), 601–605.

Parent's Guide to Cord Blood Foundation. (2012). *Diseases treated.* Retrieved from http://parentsguide-cordblood.org/diseases.php

Shu-Ling, L., Chieh-Yu, L., Yu-Yin, L., & Meei-Ling, G. (2013). Efficacy of warm showers in labor pain and birth experiences during first labor stage. *Journal of Obstetric, Gynecologic & Neonatal Nursing, 42*(1),19–28.

Simpkin, P., Bolding, A., Keppler, A., & Durham, J. (2010). *Pregnancy, childbirth, and the newborn: The complete guide* (4th ed.). Hopkins, MN: Meadowbrooke.

Spector, R. E. (2012). *Cultural diversity in health and illness* (8th ed.). Upper Saddle River, NJ: Pearson.

Wilson, B. A., Shannon, M. T., & Shields, K. M. (Eds.). (2013). *Pearson's nurse's drug guide 2013.* Upper Saddle River, NJ: Prentice Hall.

Pharmacologic Pain Management

We had attended our classes and practiced through the last few weeks, but I was not ready for the amount of discomfort that I felt during my labor. I've always been able to handle pain much better, but this pain was very different. I had hoped to go through all of labor and birth without medications, but we had talked about it and I knew that if I felt I needed something, it would be all right. My nurse was also helpful and supportive of my decision. She helped me feel that I was making a good decision and that I wasn't failing somehow. —Kyung-aie, 36

Blend Images/Alamy

LEARNING OUTCOMES

20.1 Describe the use, administration, dose, onset of action, and adverse effects of systemic drugs to promote pain relief during the nursing management of the woman in labor and her fetus.

20.2 Compare the major types of regional analgesia and anesthesia, including area affected, advantages, disadvantages, techniques, and nursing management of the laboring woman and her fetus.

20.3 Explain the possible complications of regional anesthesia in nursing management of the laboring woman and her fetus.

20.4 Describe the nursing management for the laboring woman and her fetus related to general anesthesia.

20.5 Describe the major complications of general anesthesia during labor in nursing management of the woman in labor and her fetus.

Childbearing women experience varying levels of pain and other demanding sensations during labor and birth. As discussed in Chapter 19 ✆, nursing interventions directed toward pain relief begin with psychologic measures such as providing information, support, and encouragement. Measures to promote physical comfort include back rubs, showers, whirlpool baths, and the application of cool cloths. Some laboring women need no further interventions.

For other women, the progression of labor brings increasing pain that interferes with their ability to cope. These women may elect to use pharmacologic agents such as systemic medications, regional nerve blocks (epidural, spinal, or combined epidural-spinal), and local anesthetic blocks (pudendal and perineal) to decrease discomfort, increase relaxation, and reestablish their ability to participate more effectively in the labor and birth experience. The methods are not all mutually exclusive, and any of them may be used in combination with nonpharmacologic comfort measures. The use of general anesthesia has very limited use in modern obstetrics. It is occasionally used during emergency cesarean births, although this trend continues to decrease because of the associated adverse maternal and fetal effects.

Although systemic analgesics and regional anesthetic blocks may affect the fetus, so do the laboring woman's pain and stress. During labor, maternal respirations and oxygen consumption increase, and this decreases the amount of oxygen available to the fetus. In addition, the pain and stress can lead to metabolic acidosis and the release of catecholamines, which cause maternal blood vessels to constrict, lessening oxygen and nutrient supply to the fetus (Reynolds, 2010).

There is a good deal of peer pressure on expectant parents to have the "ideal" birth experience. They may plan a natural childbirth, in which case the need for analgesia may make them feel inadequate and guilty. The nurse has a special role in helping a woman and her partner accept alterations in their original plan and recognize the unique qualities of their birth experience. Reassurance that accepting analgesia for discomfort is not a failure can help maintain the woman's self-esteem. The emphasis should be on achieving a healthy, satisfying outcome for the family. Evidence has shown that women who have continuous one-to-one support during labor were more likely to have a spontaneous vaginal birth, less likely to require analgesia, and less likely to report dissatisfaction with their childbirth experience (O'Sullivan, 2009). Also, the American College of Obstetricians and Gynecologists has concluded that a woman's request is sufficient justification for pain relief during labor (Reynolds, 2010).

SYSTEMIC MEDICATIONS

Note that this discussion of obstetric analgesia and anesthesia applies only to a healthy woman and fetus. Pain relief during labor and birth for women with high-risk conditions, such as preterm labor, preeclampsia, blood disorders, or diabetes mellitus, requires skilled decision making, close observation, and awareness of all the potential threats to both the woman and her baby. The goal of pharmacologic analgesia during labor is to provide maximum pain relief at minimum risk for the mother and fetus. To reach this goal, clinicians must consider a number of factors, including the following:

- All systemic medications used for pain relief during labor cross the placental barrier by simple diffusion, but some medications cross more readily than others.

- Medication action in the body depends on the rate at which the substance is metabolized by liver enzymes and excreted by the kidneys.

- High medication doses may remain in the fetus for long periods because fetal liver enzymes and kidney excretion are inadequate for metabolizing analgesic agents.

Clinical Reasoning Anesthesia During Labor

Luisa Silva, a 33-year-old G1P0, is 32 weeks pregnant. She is trying to decide whether she should accept any analgesia during her labor. She has finished childbirth education classes and wants an unmedicated labor and birth. She says, "I want to do this on my own, but I'm afraid it may be too much. Will it be OK if I need to take something?" What will you tell her?

See www.nursing.pearsonhighered.com for possible responses.

Teaching Highlights What Women Need to Know About Pain-Relief Medications

Before receiving medications, the woman should understand the following:

- Type of medication administered
- Route of administration
- Expected effects of medication
- Implications for fetus or newborn
- Safety measures needed (e.g., remain in bed with side rails up)

Nursing Management

Analgesic medications provide pain relief for the laboring woman but also affect the fetus and the labor process. Pain medication given too early may prolong labor and depress the fetus; if given too late it is of minimal use to the woman and may lead to respiratory depression in the newborn. The nurse assesses the mother and fetus and also evaluates the contraction pattern before administering prescribed systemic medications.

Maternal assessment parameters include the following:

- The woman is willing to receive medication after being advised about the risks and benefits of the medication.
- Maternal vital signs are stable.
- Contraindications (such as specific medication allergy, respiratory compromise, or current medication dependence) are not present.

Fetal assessment parameters include:

- The fetal heart rate (FHR) baseline is between 110 and 160 beats per minute, and no late decelerations or nonreassuring FHR patterns are present.
- Variability is present.
- The fetus exhibits normal movement, and accelerations are present with fetal movement.
- The fetus is term.

Assessment of labor includes:

- Documentation of the contraction pattern
- The cervical status, including cervical position, consistency, effacement, dilatation, and station

Before administering the medication, the nurse once again ascertains whether the woman has a history of any medication reactions or allergies and provides information about the medication. (See *Teaching Highlights: What Women Need to Know About Pain-Relief Medications.*) Maternal vital signs, FHR, contraction pattern, and pain level should be assessed and documented before administering any pain medication. After giving the medication, the nurse records the medication name, dose, route, and site, as well as the woman's blood pressure (BP) and pulse, within the electronic medical record (EMR). If the woman is alone, side rails should be raised to provide safety. The nurse assesses the FHR for possible adverse effects of the medication. After the medication has been administered, the nurse should

Developing Cultural Competence
Cultural Influence on Responses to Pain

A woman's cultural background may influence her responses to pain. Following are generalizations of how some cultures perceive pain and pain responses:

- Mexican American women may moan rhythmically and massage their thighs and abdomen when in pain.
- Haitian women may prefer massage, movement, and position changes to increase comfort.
- Filipino women may lie quietly because they believe that noise and activity increase labor pain.
- Black, Puerto Rican, and Middle Eastern women are often verbally expressive of pain.
- Native American women may be viewed as stoic, using meditation, self-control, and traditional herbs.
- Thai women's silent but restless behavior can reflect high levels of pain.
- Japanese, Chinese, Vietnamese, Laotian, and other women of Asian descent may feel that crying out during labor is shameful.
- Samoan women may believe no verbal response is allowed.

document the woman's pain level, the effectiveness of the medication, and any adverse effects if they occurred.

When an analgesic medication is administered by intramuscular or subcutaneous route, it takes a few minutes for the effect to be felt. The nurse can continue with other supportive measures to enhance comfort, such as ensuring a quiet environment, providing a back rub or cool cloth, assisting with relaxation and visualization exercises, or providing Therapeutic Touch until the woman feels the effect of the medication. Often, continued reassurance and verbal praise have a calming effect. When the medication begins to take effect, the woman may sleep between contractions. This short period of rest helps her relax and can restore her energy. When the physician/CNM orders an intravenous route, the effect of the medication will be felt within a few minutes, so if any change of position is necessary or if the woman needs to void, the nurse may suggest that the woman complete these activities before receiving the medication. Some women may be so uncomfortable that they do not want anything except the medication. In this case, administering the medication first would be more helpful for the woman.

Opioid Analgesics

Opioid analgesic agents that are injected into the circulation have their primary action at sites in the brain, activating the neurons that descend to the spinal cord. The opioid analgesics used in early labor are given in either intermittent doses or, less commonly, by patient-controlled administration. It is unclear if these medications work by providing an analgesic effect or by inducing sedation; however, the medications do have a quieting effect that reduces pain for the laboring woman (Anderson, 2011). See Table 20–1 for information about analgesics used in labor.

Butorphanol Tartrate (Stadol) and Nalbuphine Hydrochloride (Nubain)

Butorphanol tartrate (Stadol) is a synthetic agonist–antagonist opioid analgesic agent. The medication has been proven effective in reducing pain intensity in laboring women. Respiratory depression of both the mother and fetus or newborn can occur if given late in the first stage of labor but can be reversed with naloxone (Narcan).

The most common side effect associated with butorphanol (Stadol) is drowsiness. Dizziness, fainting, and hypotension can also occur (Wilson, Shannon, & Shields, 2013). Urinary retention following administration of butorphanol is not common but does occur. Therefore, the nurse should be alert for bladder distention when a woman has received butorphanol for analgesia during labor, has IV fluids infusing, and receives regional anesthesia for the birth. Butorphanol needs to be protected from light and stored at room temperature (Wilson et al., 2013).

SAFETY ALERT!

Because the most common side effect of butorphanol tartrate (Stadol) is drowsiness, the mother should be advised to remain in bed with side rails up to prevent falls or injuries after administration of the medication.

Like butorphanol, nalbuphine hydrochloride (Nubain) is a synthetic agonist–antagonist opioid analgesic and may precipitate medication withdrawal if the woman is physically dependent on opioids. It also crosses the placenta to the fetus and can cause a nonreassuring fetal heart rate and neonatal respiratory depression. In the birth setting, nalbuphine may be given directly into the tubing of a running IV infusion and 10 mg should be administered over 3 to 5 minutes (Wilson et al., 2013). Both nalbuphine and butorphanol can have a ceiling effect where the pain reduction qualities do not increase, but the side effects increase. Nalbuphine is often the medication of choice because it is associated with less nausea and vomiting, and a lower incidence of respiratory depression. Nalbuphine is also associated with increased maternal sedation, which allows the mother an opportunity to rest between contractions. See *Drug Guide: Nalbuphine Hydrochloride (Nubain).*

Fentanyl (Sublimaze)

Fentanyl is a short-acting opiate that has been used during labor to relieve pain and induce sedation. Fentanyl is 50 to 100 times more potent than morphine. Fentanyl has less neonatal neurobehavioral depression than Demerol because it does not cross the placenta.

Table 20–1	Analgesics Used in Labor			
Drug/Class	Dosage, Route, Frequency	Common Side Effects	Life-Threatening Reactions	Contraindications
Stadol (butorphanol tartrate): CNS agent, analgesic, narcotic agonist/antagonist	IM 1–2 mg every 4 hours IV 0.5–2 mg every 4 hours; rapid onset; peak: 30–60 min; duration 3–4 hours Intranasal: 1 mg (1 puff) may repeat in 90 seconds (max dose every 3–4 hours)	Sedation; sweaty, clammy skin; nausea and vomiting	Respiratory depression	Narcotic dependency, breastfeeding, women with chronic hypertension or preeclampsia
Nubain (nalbuphine hydrochloride): CNS agent analgesic, narcotic agonist	10–20 mg every 3–6 hours PRN subcutaneous IM/IV	Sedation, dizziness, fainting, hypotension, hypertension	Respiratory depression	Hypersensitivity to the drug
Demerol (meperidine hydrochloride): CNS agent, analgesic, narcotic agonist	IV 2.5–15 mg every 4 hours IM/subcutaneous 5–20 mg every 4 hours	Pruritus, dizziness, sedation, nausea, constipation	Respiratory depression, convulsions, cardiovascular collapse, cardiac arrest, respiratory depression in newborn, bronchoconstriction	Hypersensitivity to the drug, convulsive disorders, breastfeeding, undiagnosed acute abdomen
Fentanyl (Sublimaze): Short-acting opiate agonist, analgesic	50–100 mcg every 2 hours IV/IM IV give over 1–2 min; immediate onset; peak 30–60 min, duration limited to 30–60 min IM onset 7–15 min	Bradycardia, hypotension, nausea, vomiting, and respiratory depression	Muscle rigidity, especially in the respiratory muscles	Women with opioid dependency

Drug Guide Nalbuphine Hydrochloride (Nubain)

Overview of Action

Nubain is a synthetic opioid analgesic with agonist and weak antagonist properties. Analgesic properties are equal to those produced by morphine. Nubain's potency is three to four times greater than that of pentazocine. The incidence of respiratory depression that occurs is equivalent to that of morphine.

Dosage, Route, Frequency

Nubain is indicated for moderate to severe pain. Adults: 10 to 20 mg every 3 to 6 hours PRN subcutaneous/IM/IV. Commonly given IV, onset in 2–3 min, peaks in 15–20 min, duration 3–6 hours. IM or subcutaneous, onset in less than 15 min, peaks 30–60 min, duration 3–6 hours (Wilson et al., 2013).

Maternal Contraindications

Hypersensitivity or allergy to nalbuphine hydrochloride, respiratory depression, acute asthma attack, bradycardia, inflammatory bowel disease, and substance abuse.

Maternal Side Effects

Sedation, clammy sweaty skin, abdominal pain with cramps, nausea and vomiting, dizziness, vertigo, fainting, nervousness, restlessness, depression; false sense of well-being, hallucinations, headache, nightmares, allergic dermatitis, allergic reactions, anorexia, blurred vision, diplopia, bradycardia, tachycardia, asthma, dyspnea, flushing, general weakness, hypertension, hypotension, impaired cognition, malaise, pruritus, urinary urgency.

Nursing Considerations

- Assess patient's allergy, sensitivity, or dependence to opioids on admission.
- Inform woman of potential side effects.
- Monitor and evaluate analgesic effect. Ask patient about comfort level and notify analgesia provider of inadequate pain relief.
- Observe for symptoms of hypersensitivity: pruritus, urticaria, and/or burning sensation.
- May produce an allergic response in patients with sulfite sensitivity.
- If allergic reaction (urticaria, edema, or respiratory difficulties) occurs, administer naloxone or diphenhydramine per physician order.
- Assess respiratory rate before administration. Notify healthcare provider if respirations are less than 12 per minute.
- Monitor urinary output and assess bladder for distention. Assist patient to void.
- Maintain bed rest or assist patient with ambulation after administration.
- Counsel patient that use with alcohol or other central nervous system depressants may increase medication effects.
- Prolonged use with abrupt discontinuation can result in symptoms consistent with opioid withdrawal in both the mother and infant.

However, neonatal depression can still occur, although at much lower rates when compared with Demerol. Fentanyl results in less sedation, nausea, vomiting, and pruritus compared with Demerol. See Table 20–1.

Analgesic Potentiators

The use of **analgesic potentiators**, also known as *ataractics*, can decrease anxiety and increase the effectiveness of analgesics when given simultaneously. These medications, which are classified as tranquilizers, have no specific properties that decrease pain; however, they do work well to potentiate the effects of opioid analgesics without increasing unwanted side effects. This enhancement enables the woman to receive a smaller dose of the opioid being administered. These medications can also be used to manage the unpleasant side effects, such as nausea or vomiting, associated with the administration of opioid analgesics.

Commonly used analgesic potentiators include promethazine (Phenergan), hydroxyzine (Vistaril), propiomazine (Largon), and promazine (Sparine). The main side effect is sedation, which may be helpful in promoting rest in women who have had a prolonged labor or who have had little sleep; however, the effect may be undesirable to other women.

Opiate Antagonist: Naloxone (Narcan)

Because naloxone is an antagonist with little or no agonistic effect, it exhibits little pharmacologic activity in the absence of opioids. Naloxone can be used to reverse the mild respiratory depression that follows administration of small doses of opiates such as fentanyl and meperidine, as well as butorphanol tartrate and nalbuphine hydrochloride. Naloxone is the medication of choice when the depressant is unknown because it will cause no further depression (Wilson et al., 2013). An initial dose of 0.4 to 2 mg may be administered intravenously to the laboring woman. If the woman is nonresponsive, the medication can be readministered every 2 to 3 minutes. The nurse should be prepared to provide basic airway management, including the chin-lift/jaw-thrust maneuver, and initiation of respirations through a bag-valve-mask device when the woman is not immediately responsive and respiratory depression is occurring. It is typically administered to mothers who have received opioids within 4 hours of the birth (Wilson et al., 2013). When naloxone is given, other resuscitative measures may be indicated, and trained personnel should be readily available. The duration of the medication's effect is shorter than that of the analgesic medication for which it is acting as an antagonist, so the nurse must be alert to the return of respiratory depression and the need for repeated doses. Naloxone should not be given in women with known or suspected opiate dependency because it may precipitate severe withdrawal (Wilson et al., 2013). Naloxone may be given to the newborn if needed after birth. The newborn dose is 0.1 mg/kg and may need to be repeated if respiratory effort remains abnormal. (See *Drug Guide: Naloxone Hydrochloride (Narcan)* on page 669 in Chapter 28 .)

Complementary Care Acupressure for Labor Pain

Acupressure can lessen pain during the first stage of labor (Cho, Lee, & Ernst, 2010). The acupressure point for labor and birth is found in the webbing between the thumb and index finger. This point should never be stimulated during pregnancy since it stimulates uterine contractions. The mother places her right thumb on the back of her left hand and her right index finger on the front of the left hand at the acupressure point. She can rub the point to stimulate labor and squeeze the point to decrease labor pain. Another acupressure point is found between the inner ankle bone and the Achilles' tendon. Squeezing for 1 minute on each ankle reduces labor pain. See www.nursing.pearsonhighered.com for more information on acupressure, including an interview with a labor and delivery nurse on her use of acupressure to relieve labor pain.

REGIONAL ANESTHESIA AND ANALGESIA

Regional anesthesia is the temporary loss of sensation produced by injecting an anesthetic agent (called a *local*) into direct contact with nervous tissue. Loss of sensation happens because the local agents stabilize the cell membrane, which prevents initiation and transmission of nerve impulses. The regional anesthetic blocks most commonly used in childbirth include the epidural, spinal, and combined epidural-spinal blocks. Epidural blocks may be used for analgesia during labor and vaginal birth and for anesthesia during cesarean birth.

An epidural relieves pain associated with the first stage of labor by blocking the sensory nerves supplying the uterus. Pain associated with the second stage of labor and with birth can be alleviated with epidural, combined epidural-spinal, and pudendal blocks (see Figure 20–1 ●).

Until recently, the same anesthetic agents used for regional epidurals were also used to produce **regional analgesia** (pain relief to a body region) during labor. This practice was problematic because the anesthetic agents used alter the transmission of impulses to the bladder, making voiding difficult. The agents also interfere with blood pressure stability and leg movement. The descent of the fetus is slowed and an increased risk of perineal lacerations occurs more commonly in women with epidural anesthesia (Gillesby et al., 2010). The process of laboring down, or delaying the maternal pushing effort until the woman feels an acute urge to push, can result in a reduction of active pushing in women who have received epidural anesthesia (Gillesby et al., 2010). To address these difficulties, regional analgesia is now obtained by injecting an opioid such as fentanyl along with only a small amount of anesthetic agent. New medication combinations relieve the woman's pain while minimizing the side effects just discussed (Anderson, 2011).

The intrathecal injection of opioids results in another type of regional analgesia. In this case, the opioid is injected into the subarachnoid space. It is important for the anesthesia provider to provide a test dose before giving the entire dose to determine that the catheter is correctly placed. Fentanyl citrate and preservative-free morphine are the most commonly used medications. This typically results in more effective pain relief over the subsequent 24 hours after birth, although the incidence of nausea may be increased in some women (Anderson, 2011).

Nursing care during administration of regional analgesia is directed toward helping the woman void before administration, assisting her with positioning during and after the procedure, monitoring and assessing vital signs and respiratory status, monitoring analgesic effect, and determining fetal well-being. Reassurance and thorough explanations help decrease anxiety and fear. Additional measures may be needed to address pruritus, nausea and vomiting, and urinary retention.

A B C

● **Figure 20–1** Schematic diagram showing pain pathways and sites of interruption. *A,* Lumbar sympathetic (spinal) block: relief of uterine pain only. *B,* Pudendal block: relief of perineal pain. *C,* Lumbar epidural block: dark area demonstrates peridural (epidural) space and nerves affected, and the gray tube represents a continuous plastic catheter.

Activity | Case Study: Relief Therapies During Birth | Video | Epidural Placement

As with other procedures, the woman needs to know how the block is given, the expected effect on her and the fetus, advantages and disadvantages, and possible complications. Many women discuss possible anesthetic blocks with their care provider at some point in the pregnancy. If they have not, it is important to give them an opportunity to ask questions and obtain information before receiving the block while in labor.

Anesthetic Agents for Regional Blocks

Local anesthetic agents block the conduction of nerve impulses from the periphery to the central nervous system by preventing the propagation of an action potential from the source of pain (Anderson, 2011). The types of nerve fibers are differentially sensitive to the various anesthetic agents. In general, the smaller the fiber, the more sensitive it is to local agents. For example, it is possible to block the small C and A delta fibers, which transmit pain and temperature, without blocking the larger A alpha, A beta, and A gamma fibers, which continue to maintain a sense of pressure, muscle tone, position sense, and motor function.

Absorption of local anesthetics depends primarily on the vascularity of the area of injection. The agents themselves contribute to increased blood flow by causing vasodilation. High concentrations of medications cause greater vasodilation. Good maternal physical condition or a high metabolic rate aids absorption. Malnutrition, dehydration, electrolyte imbalance, and cardiovascular and pulmonary problems increase the potential for toxic effects. The pH of tissues affects the rate of absorption, which has implications for fetal complications such as acidosis. The addition of vasoconstrictors such as epinephrine delays absorption and prolongs the anesthetic effect because vasoconstrictors decrease uteroplacental blood flow. The breakdown of local anesthetics in the body is accomplished by the liver and plasma esterase, and the resulting substance is eliminated by the kidneys. It is important to use the weakest concentration and the smallest amount necessary to produce the desired results.

Types of Local Anesthetic Agents

Two types of local anesthetic agents are currently available: esters and amides. The ester type includes procaine hydrochloride (Novocain), chloroprocaine hydrochloride (Nesacaine), and tetracaine hydrochloride (Pontocaine). Esters are rapidly metabolized; therefore, toxic maternal levels are not as likely to be reached, and placental transfer to the fetus is prevented. Ester-linked agents have a higher incidence of allergic reactions when compared with amides. However, they do not appear to have a higher incidence of fetal effects (Douma, Verwey, Kam-Endtz, et al., 2009).

Amide types include lidocaine hydrochloride (Xylocaine), mepivacaine hydrochloride (Carbocaine), and bupivacaine hydrochloride (Marcaine). Amide types are more powerful and longer-acting agents. They readily cross the placenta, can be measured in the fetal circulation, and affect the fetus for a prolonged period. Lidocaine (Xylocaine) has been associated with major neurologic and minor neurologic toxicity; therefore, the dose of lidocaine should not exceed 75 mg.

Ropivacaine (Naropin) is a new generation amide that is also used in labor. The pain relief effects are similar to those of other amides. However, the blockade effect is slightly lower than other amides, thus increasing the rates of vaginal births and decreasing instrument-assisted births. Levobupivacaine (Chirocaine) has less toxicity than ropivacaine and is safer in longer surgical procedures because it has decreased toxicity.

Adverse Maternal Reactions to Anesthetic Agents

Reactions to local anesthetic agents range from mild symptoms to cardiovascular collapse. Mild reactions include palpitations, tinnitus, apprehension, confusion, and a metallic taste in the mouth. Moderate reactions include more severe degrees of mild symptoms plus nausea and vomiting, hypotension, and muscle twitching, which may progress to convulsions. Severe reactions are sudden loss of consciousness, coma, severe hypotension, bradycardia, respiratory depression, and cardiac arrest. Anesthetic agents should not be used unless an intravenous line is in place.

The preferred treatment for a mild toxic reaction is administration of oxygen and IV injection of a short-acting barbiturate to diminish anxiety.

Neonatal Neurobehavioral Effects of Anesthesia and Analgesia

Many studies have focused on the neurobehavioral effects on the newborn of pharmacologic agents used during labor and birth. Although analgesic and anesthetic agents may alter the behavioral and adaptive function of the newborn, physiologic factors such as hunger, degree of hydration, and time within the sleep–wake cycle may also exert an influence (Datta, Kodali, & Sega, 2010). Note that more neurologic impairment occurs in the newborn resulting from the normal birth process than from epidural complications.

Epidural Block

A lumbar **epidural block** involves injection of an anesthetic agent into the epidural space to provide pain relief throughout labor. The epidural space, a potential space between the dura mater and the ligamentum flavum, is accessed through the lumbar area (Figure 20–2 ●). The epidural is most frequently used as a continuous block to provide analgesia and anesthesia from active labor through episiotomy repair (Figure 20–3 ●).

Epidurals have become a relatively common method of analgesia and anesthesia during labor and birth in the United States. It is estimated that 61% of all women in the United States receive an epidural during their labor. Non-Hispanic white women had the highest rates of epidural use (68.8%) followed by non-Hispanic black women (62.1%). Native American women used epidural anesthesia the least (42.1%). Epidural use decreases with maternal age (Osterman & Martin, 2011). An epidural can be given as soon as active labor is established.

Advantages

The epidural block relieves discomfort during labor and birth, and the woman is fully awake and a part of the birth process. Epidural anesthesia results in fewer adverse fetal effects when compared with intravenous analgesia or general anesthesia. It can also allow the woman to rest and regain strength before the woman needs

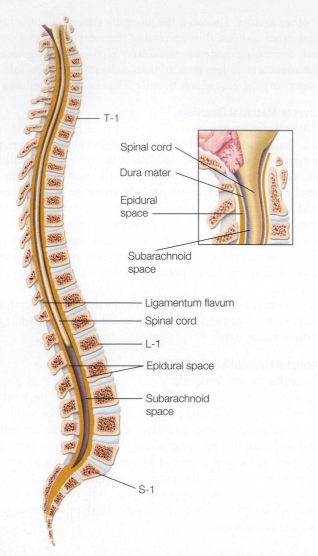

Spinal cord

Dura mater

Epidural
space

Subarachnoid
space

T-1

Ligamentum flavum
Spinal cord
L-1
Epidural space
Subarachnoid
space
S-1

● **Figure 20–2** The epidural space lies between the dura mater and the ligamentum flavum, extending from the base of the skull to the end of the sacral canal.

to push during the second stage. The continuous epidural allows different blocking for each stage of labor, so that the fetus is able to descend and rotate in the maternal pelvis; many times the woman's urge to bear down is preserved. Epidurals that combine anesthesia and an opioid agent are often effective in providing postoperative pain relief for longer periods of time.

Opioids are used with epidural blocks for labor. Some of the agents used include morphine, fentanyl, butorphanol, and meperidine (Anderson, 2011). When only opioids are used epidurally, rather than in combination with another type of agent, the amount of pain relief is not as effective, especially toward the end of labor; therefore, a combination of opioids and a low dose of local is given (Anderson, 2011).

Disadvantages

The most common complication of an epidural block is maternal hypotension, which is generally prevented by administering intravenous fluid before epidural placement, left uterine displacement, and maternal positioning on her side. In some

instances, labor progress and fetal descent may be slowed, and pushing efforts in the second stage may be less effective because of a decrease in sensation. There appears to be an increase in forceps or vacuum use or in cesarean section births related to epidural anesthesia (Cutura et al., 2011). Delay in return of bladder sensation may result in urinary retention and the need for catheterization during labor and in the fourth stage (Cutura et al., 2011). Low back pain can also occur after an epidural and is usually more common in women who underwent vaginal deliveries. Typically, epidurals do not cause chronic low back pain, although the woman can have soreness at the insertion site for a few days.

Contraindications

The absolute contraindications for epidural block are patient refusal, infection at the site of the needle puncture, maternal problems with blood coagulation (coagulopathies), raised intracranial pressure, specific medication allergy to the agent being used, and hypovolemic shock (Anderson, 2011).

Nursing Management

Assessment of the woman's knowledge level about an epidural block is essential. Before providing information, the nurse determines the woman's current knowledge and evaluates factors related to learning, such as primary language spoken, ability to hear and interpret information, and the presence of anxiety. Although the nurse is an integral person in providing information, the anesthesia provider is the essential person to provide information and to obtain written informed consent.

In preparation for the epidural, the nurse encourages the woman to empty her bladder, because the block may interfere with her ability to void. The nurse assesses the woman's pain level, maternal blood pressure, pulse, respirations, and FHR to determine that normal parameters are present and to establish a baseline. Continuous electronic fetal monitoring to assess fetal status and frequent monitoring of maternal blood pressure and pulse for hypotension are essential. An intravenous infusion is usually begun with an 18-gauge plastic indwelling catheter. A large-gauge catheter is used so that IV fluids can be administered quickly if hypotension occurs. A bolus of 500 to 1000 mL of IV fluid is given before beginning the epidural block to decrease the incidence of hypotension.

Either of two positions can be used to achieve epidural placement: side-lying or sitting. If the side-lying position is used, the nurse assists the woman to move to the edge of the bed, where the mattress is firmer and provides more support. The woman's head is supported with a small pillow so it remains in alignment with the spine. A pillow may also be placed in front of her chest to provide support for her upper arm. Her back needs to remain straight, with the shoulders square. Her legs are bent and her knees kept together so that the upper hip does not roll forward and cause the spine to twist (Figure 20–4 ●).

The block may also be given with the woman in a sitting position, with her back flexed and her feet supported on a stool (Figure 20–5 ●). The woman should be advised to push her back toward the anesthesia provider. The nurse typically stands directly in front of the woman with hands placed on the woman's shoulders. The woman is encouraged to arch her back and push

Figure 20–3 Technique for lumbar epidural block. *A*, Proper position for insertion. *B*, Needle in the ligamentum flavum. *C*, Tip of needle in epidural space. *D*, Force of injection pushing dura away from tip of needle.

Clinical Tip

Advise the woman to identify when uterine contractions are occurring. Reassure her that the anesthesiologist will administer the injection between contractions when she is comfortable. Provide encouragement and reposition the woman as needed after a contraction occurs, since it is common for the woman to slouch during intense uterine contractions.

back toward the analgesia provider. After positioning, the nurse continues to provide support and tries to ensure that the woman does not move during the procedure. After the needle and catheter are placed, the woman is assisted into a reclining position.

Maternal vital signs are assessed frequently per protocol until the block wears off. The blood pressure can be monitored

Figure 20–4 Correct maternal positioning. The back is straight and vertical, the shoulders are square, and the upper leg is prevented from rolling forward.

by a mechanical blood pressure device or directly by the nurse. The vital signs are recorded on the fetal monitor strip and/or on the patient record. The nurse encourages the woman to maintain a side-lying position to maximize uteroplacental blood flow and changes her position (from side to side) frequently to increase circulation, promote comfort, and avoid a one-sided block. The nurse assesses the woman's ability to lift her legs and her level of sensation every 30 minutes to monitor the effects of the nerve block.

The nurse assesses the woman's bladder for distention at frequent intervals because the epidural block decreases the urge to urinate. During the second stage of labor, the woman with an epidural block may need assistance with pushing. The nurse may need to tell the woman when contractions begin and give extra assistance by holding her legs during pushing efforts. The woman's legs need to be protected from pressure applied to them while sensation is diminished. If the woman has little or no control of her legs, stirrups may be needed to avoid injury.

The most common side effect of epidural regional block is hypotension. The risk can be minimized by a preload fluid bolus of crystalloid solution (Gabbe et al., 2012). If hypotension occurs, the nurse increases the IV flow rate (to increase intravascular volume and raise the blood pressure), ensures or verifies left uterine displacement (to increase circulation), and administers oxygen (to improve oxygenation). If blood pressure is not restored in 1 to 2 minutes, ephedrine 5 to 10 mg IV is administered (Gabbe et al., 2012). After ephedrine is administered, the blood pressure is continually monitored and the maternal and fetal responses are recorded.

● **Figure 20–5** Correct sitting position for woman having an epidural anesthesia block: shoulders rolled forward and back exposed for needle insertion.

The epidural may cause elevation of maternal temperature (pyrexia). Pyrexia may be confused with maternal infection and frequently results in additional testing of the newborn to rule out infection (Gabbe et al., 2012).

Headache (which may occur with spinal blocks) is not a side effect of epidural anesthesia because the dura mater of the spinal canal has not been penetrated and there is no leakage of spinal fluid. Motor control of the legs is weak but not totally absent after birth. Return of complete sensation and the ability to control the legs are essential before ambulation is attempted. Recovery may take several hours, depending on the anesthetic agent and the dose given.

To assess sensation, the nurse can touch various parts of the woman's legs and abdomen bilaterally to determine if the touch can be felt. The nurse can evaluate motor control by asking the woman to raise her knees, to lift her feet (one at a time) off the bed, or to dorsiflex her foot. Even though assessments may indicate that sensation and motor control have returned, the nurse needs to be ready to support the woman's weight as she stands and quickly return her to bed if motor control is inadequate.

In addition, blood pressure assessments help the nurse determine the safety of ambulation. The nurse assesses blood pressure while the woman is lying down, then sitting in the bed. As long as blood pressure values remain stable (no evidence of orthostatic hypotension), a standing blood pressure is assessed. To maintain safety, it is advisable to have additional assistance when the woman stands for the first time. See Skill 3–8 in the *Clinical Skills Manual* SKILLS.

Continuous Epidural Infusion

Epidural anesthesia may be given with a continuous infusion pump. Some of the benefits include good to excellent analgesia, infrequent nausea, minimal sedation, decreased anxiety, earlier mobilization, retained cough reflex, decreased risk of deep vein thrombosis, decreased myocardial oxygen demand, and ease of administration. A continuous infusion reduces the use of bolus dosages, which may provide intermittent pain control.

Ease of administration does not imply lack of need for close observation. Malfunctioning equipment with subsequent overdose is always a possibility. Fortunately, infusion pumps designed specifically for use in epidural anesthesia have safety factors incorporated. Continuous epidural infusions should be administered with the same precautions used for intermittent injections.

Some of the potential problems of epidural infusions include breakthrough pain, sedation, nausea and vomiting, pruritus, and hypotension. Breakthrough pain may occur at any time during the epidural infusion but usually occurs when the infusion rate of the agent is below the recommended therapeutic rate. It may also occur when the infusion pump rate is altered or the integrity of the epidural line is broken. When breakthrough pain occurs, the nurse checks the integrity of the epidural infusion line and notifies the analgesia provider. There may be standing orders for treatment of breakthrough pain, but it is best to inform the analgesia provider of any problems that occur. Often, breakthrough pain can be corrected with a bolus dose of medication. In rare circumstances, the epidural itself may need to be replaced.

Some women may experience *hot spots,* or areas of incomplete anesthesia coverage. Nursing interventions include position changes. If the hot spot becomes too uncomfortable, an anesthesia provider can administer additional medication. In some cases, the epidural will need to be replaced.

General sedation and resulting respiratory depression may occur from the systemic effect of the epidural agents as they are absorbed into the circulation. The respiratory rate, along with the quality of respirations, should be assessed no less frequently than every 15 to 30 minutes. The nurse should notify the anesthetist of any significant decreases in respiratory rate or respiratory pattern change. If respiratory rate decreases below 12 respirations per minute, naloxone may be given to counteract the effect of the anesthetic agent; typically respirations then return to a normal rate.

Nausea and vomiting can occur at any time during or after epidural infusion. The nurse should give an antiemetic if one is ordered and notify the analgesia provider. The nausea and

Level of anesthesia for cesarean birth

Level of anesthesia for vaginal birth

● **Figure 20–6** Levels of spinal anesthesia for vaginal and cesarean births.

vomiting can make the woman very uncomfortable, and the infusion rate of the epidural may need to be decreased or terminated to alleviate this discomfort. Nausea and vomiting can sometimes occur as a result of transition rather than as a direct side effect of the epidural infusion.

Pruritus (itching and rash) may occur at any time during the epidural infusion. It usually appears first on the face, neck, or torso and is usually the result of the agent in the epidural infusion. Treatment generally involves administration of diphenhydramine hydrochloride (Benadryl). If no standing order exists, the nurse notifies the anesthetist and identifies the problem. The epidural infusion may need to be decreased or terminated.

Hypotension may occur from hypovolemia or from the effect of the epidural. Treatment involves administering oxygen by mask, administering a bolus of crystalloid fluid, and notifying the anesthetist. Usually standing orders for treatment of hypotension are graded in terms of the degree of hypotension. The epidural infusion may have to be terminated and the woman placed in the Trendelenburg position.

Epidural Opioid Analgesia After Birth

To provide analgesia for approximately 24 hours after the birth, the analgesia provider may inject an opioid, such as morphine sulfate (Duramorph) or fentanyl (Sublimaze), into the epidural space immediately after the birth. The analgesic effect begins approximately 30 to 60 minutes after the injection. The side effects include pruritus, nausea and vomiting, and urinary retention (Wilson et al., 2013). The onset seems to occur early, and it resolves within 14 to 16 hours after the birth. (See *Drug Guide: Postpartum Epidural Morphine* on page 747 in Chapter 30 ●.)

Spinal Block

In a **spinal block**, a local anesthetic agent is injected directly into the spinal fluid in the spinal canal to provide anesthesia for cesarean birth and occasionally for vaginal birth. This technique involves passing through the epidural space and dura mater and injecting the medication directly into the cerebral spinal fluid. The technique of administration varies depending on whether the spinal block is being given for a cesarean or vaginal birth (Figure 20–6 ●).

Advantages

The advantages of spinal block are immediate onset of anesthesia, relative ease of administration, a need for smaller medication volume, and maternal compartmentalization of the medication.

Disadvantages

The primary disadvantage of spinal block is blockade of sympathetic nerve fibers, resulting in a high incidence of hypotension; maternal hypotension may lead to alterations in the fetal heart rate and fetal hypoxia. In addition, uterine tone is maintained, which makes intrauterine manipulation difficult.

Contraindications

Contraindications for spinal block include severe hypovolemia, infection over the puncture site, sepsis, coagulation problems, and patient refusal (Suresh, Segal, Preston, et al., 2013).

Nursing Management

If an intravenous infusion is not already in place, it is started with a 16- to 18-gauge plastic catheter. A bolus of 500 to 1000 mL is infused rapidly. The nurse assesses maternal vital signs, pain level, and the FHR to establish a baseline and then positions the woman in a sitting (or a side-lying) position. The woman sits on the side of the bed or operating room table and places her feet on a stool. The woman places her arms between her knees or up around the nurse's shoulders, places her head to her chest, and arches her back to widen the intervertebral spaces. The nurse supports the woman in this position and palpates the uterus to identify the beginning of uterine contractions (if labor is present). The analgesia provider injects the anesthetic agent between contractions. If the anesthetic agent is injected during a contraction, the level of anesthesia obtained is higher and may compromise respirations.

The woman remains in a sitting position for 30 seconds and then returns to a lying position, with a rolled towel or blanket under her right hip to displace the uterus from the vena cava. The nurse monitors maternal blood pressure and pulse frequently per protocol or physician's order. The blood pressure is also reassessed when the woman is moved after birth, because movement may lower blood pressure.

If the spinal block is being used during vaginal birth, the nurse monitors uterine contractions and instructs the woman to bear down during a contraction. The block may reduce the woman's ability to push, although the new combinations of medications tend to decrease this side effect. Sometimes, the birth may be assisted with forceps or vacuum extractor (see Chapter 23 🌶).

After birth, the temporary motor paralysis of the woman's legs continues. The nurse needs to exercise caution when moving the woman from the birthing bed (or operating room table) to protect her from injury. The woman remains in bed for 6 to 12 hours following the block; she may not regain sensation and control of her bladder for 8 to 12 hours and may need to be catheterized. An indwelling bladder catheter is usually inserted before surgery for women undergoing cesarean birth.

The epidural or spinal catheter is removed by either an analgesia provider or the nurse. The tape used to secure the block is removed. The catheter is then grasped between the fingers and slowly removed with gentle traction. The catheter should be inspected to ensure the tip did not break off. A bandage or gauze and tape is placed over the site. It is not unusual for a small amount of bleeding to occur initially upon removal. Continuous bleeding warrants a call to the anesthesia provider. The nurse documents removal of the catheter and any adverse effects.

Combined Spinal-Epidural Block

Spinal anesthesia may be combined with an epidural block. The combined spinal-epidural (CSE) block can be used for labor analgesia and for cesarean birth. The anesthetic and analgesic agents used differ according to the purpose of the CSE block. A CSE is accomplished by inserting an epidural needle into the epidural space. A narrow-gauge atraumatic (24- to 27-gauge pencil point) needle is inserted through the epidural needle, through the dura, and into the cerebral spinal fluid. A small amount of local anesthetic agent, opioid, or both is injected, and the atraumatic needle is withdrawn. An epidural catheter is then threaded through the epidural needle and into the epidural space. The epidural needle is removed, and the epidural catheter is secured.

An advantage of CSE block is that the spinal (intrathecal) anesthetic and/or analgesic agent has a faster onset than medications that are injected into the epidural space. Most medications are used in low dose, so spinal analgesia may be given in early labor to assist in alleviating labor pain. The epidural is activated when active labor begins. Another advantage of a CSE block is that laboring women can ambulate after the CSE is placed.

SAFETY ALERT!
Advise women with a CSE in place always to have assistance during ambulation to prevent falls.

Pudendal Block

A **pudendal block**, administered by a transvaginal method, intercepts signals to the pudendal nerve (Figure 20–7 ●). The pudendal block provides perineal anesthesia for the latter part of the first stage of labor, the second stage, birth, and episiotomy repair. The pudendal block relieves the pain of perineal distention and typically relieves pain in the lower vagina, vulva, and perineum but not the discomfort of uterine contractions (Anderson, 2011).

Advantages of the pudendal block are ease of administration and absence of maternal hypotension. It also may be used to decrease the discomfort of low forceps or vacuum-assisted birth. Because a pudendal block does not alter maternal vital signs or FHR, additional assessments are not necessary. The nurse explains the procedure and answers any questions.

The disadvantages of the pudendal block include possible broad ligament hematoma, perforation of the rectum, and trauma to the sciatic nerve. A moderate dose of anesthetic agent has minimal ill effects on the course of labor, but the urge to push may decrease.

● **Figure 20–7** Pudendal block. *A,* Pudendal block by the transvaginal approach. *B,* Area of perineum affected by pudendal block.

Local Infiltration Anesthesia

Local infiltration anesthesia is accomplished by injecting an anesthetic agent into the intracutaneous, subcutaneous, and intramuscular areas of the perineum (Figure 20–8 ●). It is generally used at the time of birth, both in preparation for an episiotomy if one is needed and for the episiotomy repair. Women who have followed some type of prepared childbirth method and want minimal analgesia and anesthesia usually do not object to local anesthesia for the episiotomy or laceration repair. The administration procedure is technically uncomplicated and is practically free from complications.

A disadvantage of local infiltration is that large amounts of local anesthetic must be used to infuse the tissues. Although any local anesthetic may be used, chloroprocaine hydrochloride (Nesacaine), lidocaine hydrochloride (Xylocaine), tetracaine hydrochloride (Pontocaine), and mepivacaine hydrochloride (Carbocaine) are the agents of choice because of their capacity for diffusion. Because local anesthetic agents have no effect on maternal vital signs or FHR, additional assessments are unnecessary.

GENERAL ANESTHESIA

Occasionally, **general anesthesia** (induced unconsciousness) may be needed for cesarean birth. The method used to achieve general anesthesia is usually a combination of intravenous injection and inhalation of anesthetic agents. Maternal complications include difficulty in maternal intubation resulting in increased incidence of vomiting and aspiration, increased blood loss because of uterine relaxation, and possible difficulty remembering events in the early postpartum period (Gabbe et al., 2012).

A common fetal complication is fetal depression. The depression in the fetus is directly proportional to the depth and duration of the anesthesia. Infants born to mothers who have received general anesthesia have lower 1-minute Apgar scores and a higher incidence of metabolic acidosis than those who are given regional anesthesia for an emergency cesarean birth (Vanita, Kajal, Babita, et al., 2011). General anesthesia is not advocated when the fetus is considered to be at high risk, particularly in preterm birth.

Nursing Management

Because pregnancy results in decreased gastric motility, and the onset of labor halts the process almost entirely, food eaten hours earlier may remain undigested in the stomach. The nurse must find out when the laboring woman last ate and record this information on the patient's chart and on her anesthesia record. Even when food and fluids have been withheld, the gastric juice produced during fasting is highly acidic and can cause chemical pneumonitis if aspirated. Prophylactic antacid therapy to reduce the acidic content of the stomach before general anesthesia is common practice. A nonparticulate antacid (such as Bicitra), H2-receptor antagonists (such as Cimetidine [Tagamet] or Famotidine), or the use of prokinetic medications (such as metoclopramide), may also help empty gastric contents.

● **Figure 20–8** Local infiltration anesthesia. *A,* Technique of local infiltration for episiotomy and repair. *B,* Technique of local infiltration showing fan pattern for the fascial planes.

Clinical Tip

Some women may wake from general anesthesia with an awareness of events that occurred during a cesarean birth. A small number of women experience unpleasant thoughts or nightmares as a result. If a woman expresses anxiety or states she has unpleasant memories of the birth, the nurse should encourage her to discuss her feelings and the experiences she remembers. The analgesia provider and physician should be notified so they can establish a therapeutic dialogue with the woman. Some women may have to be referred for counseling to prevent or treat posttraumatic stress disorder.

Before induction of anesthesia, the nurse places a wedge under the woman's right hip to displace the uterus and prevent vena caval compression in the supine position. The woman should also be preoxygenated with 3 to 5 minutes of 100% oxygen. Intravenous fluids are started so that access to the intravascular system is immediately available. During the preparation, the woman should be counseled on what to expect and should be told that the baby will have limited exposure to the anesthesia agents.

During the process of rapid induction of anesthesia, the nurse applies cricoid pressure to occlude the esophagus and prevent possible aspiration; the esophagus is occluded by applying 1 to 2 kg before the loss of consciousness and increasing that to 2 to 4 kg after the induction of anesthesia. The amount of pressure applied is critical because too much pressure can result in difficulty in performing a successful intubation. Too little pressure can result in aspiration. Cricoid pressure is maintained until the anesthesia provider has placed the endotracheal tube and indicates that the pressure can be released. Figure 20–9 ● shows the appropriate technique.

● **Figure 20–9** Cricoid pressure technique. Proper position for fingers in applying cricoid pressure until a cuffed endotracheal tube is placed by the analgesia provider or certified nurse-anesthetist. The cricoid cartilage is depressed 2 to 3 cm posteriorly so that the esophagus is occluded.

Critical Concept Review

LEARNING OUTCOME 20.1: Describe the use, administration, dose, onset of action, and adverse effects of systemic drugs to promote pain relief during the nursing management of the woman in labor and her fetus.

1. The goal is to provide maximum pain relief with minimum risk to the mother and fetus.
2. After complete assessment, an analgesia agent is generally administered when cervical change has occurred.
3. Drugs may cause fetal respiratory depression at birth if given too late in labor.
4. Maternal and fetal vital signs must be stable before systemic drugs may be administered.
5. Naloxone (Narcan) should be available at birth to treat respiratory depression in the newborn.

LEARNING OUTCOME 20.2: Compare the major types of regional analgesia and anesthesia, including area affected, advantages, disadvantages, techniques, and nursing management of the laboring woman and her fetus.

1. Epidural:
   - Injection of anesthetic agent into the epidural space.
   - Produces little or no feeling to the area from the uterus downward.
   - Pushing during second stage of labor may be impaired due to lack of sensation.
   - Hypotension is the most common side effect.
   - May preload with crystalloid solution bolus.
   - Woman may need urinary catheterization due to the loss of bladder sensation.
   - Assess sensation, motor control, and orthostatic blood pressure.
2. Continuous epidural analgesia:
   - Provides good analgesia.
   - Produces less nausea and provides a greater ability to cough.
   - May produce breakthrough pain, sedation, and respiratory depression.
   - Itching and hypotension are side effects.
3. Spinal block:
   - A local anesthetic agent is injected directly into spinal canal. The level of anesthesia is dependent on the level of administration. May be administered higher for cesarean birth or lower for vaginal birth.
   - The onset of anesthesia is immediate.
   - Side effects include maternal hypotension, which can lead to fetal hypoxia.
   - Requires frequent blood pressure monitoring with changes in position.
   - Indwelling urinary catheter is usually needed due to decreased bladder sensation and tone.
   - Woman's legs must be protected from injury for 8 to 12 hours after birth of baby due to decreased movement and sensation.
4. Pudendal block:
   - Local anesthesia is injected directly into the pudendal nerve, which produces anesthesia to the lower vagina, vulva, and perineum.
   - Produces pain relief only at the end of labor.
   - Has no effect on fetus or the progress of labor.
   - May cause hematoma, perforation of the rectum, or trauma to the sciatic nerve.
5. Local infiltration anesthesia:
   - Local anesthesia is injected into the perineum prior to an episiotomy.
   - Provides pain relief only for the episiotomy incision.
   - There is no effect on maternal or fetal vital signs.
   - Requires large amounts of local anesthetic agents.

LEARNING OUTCOME 20.3: Explain the possible complications of regional anesthesia in nursing management of the laboring woman and her fetus.

Regional anesthesia administered per spinal or epidural route has similar possible complications:

1. Maternal hypotension.
2. Bladder distention.
3. Inability to push during second stage of labor.
4. Severe headache with spinal anesthesia.
5. Elevated temperature with epidural anesthesia.
6. Possible neurologic damage.

LEARNING OUTCOME 20.4: Describe the nursing management for the laboring woman and her fetus related to general anesthesia.

The nurse should:

1. Assess when the mother ate or drank last.
2. Administer prescribed premedications such as an antacid.
3. Place a wedge under the mother's right hip to displace the uterus and prevent vena cava compression.
4. Provide oxygen prior to the start of the surgery.
5. Ensure that IV access is established.
6. Assist the anesthesiologist by applying cricoid pressure during the placement of the endotracheal tube.

LEARNING OUTCOME 20.5: Describe the major complications of general anesthesia during labor in nursing management of the woman in labor and her fetus.

Major complications of general anesthesia are:

1. Fetal depression.
2. Uterine relaxation.
3. Vomiting.
4. Aspiration.

Clinical Reasoning in Action

Sandra, a 26-year-old G1P0000, is in active labor when she presents to you at the birthing center. She has been in labor for 5 hours and is clearly tired and seems to be having difficulty coping with the pain. Her contractions are occurring every 2 to 4 minutes lasting 50 to 60 seconds, and are moderate to strong in intensity. You assess the fetal heart rate of 120 to 130 beats/min with early decelerations; moderate variability is present. Sandra's vital signs are stable and her laboratory results are within normal limits. She is requesting an epidural analgesia for pain control. A vaginal exam demonstrates the cervix is 100% effaced, 6 cm dilated with the vertex at 0 station in the left occiput transverse (LOT) position. You notify the physician of Sandra's wish for pain relief and labor progress.

You review the patient's record for written consent for regional analgesia and assist the anesthesiologist with the procedure.

1. Discuss the advantages of regional analgesia.
2. Describe the nursing responsibility during the administration of regional analgesia.
3. Discuss the side effects of regional analgesia.
4. What are the absolute contraindications for an epidural block?
5. How do you assist Sandra with the second stage of labor when she cannot feel her contractions?
6. Create a concept map for Sandra's care based on her current labor status, her coping abilities at this stage of labor, and her request for regional anesthesia.

See www.nursing.pearsonhighered.com for possible responses and an interactive template for a concept map.

References

Anderson, D. (2011). A review of systemic opioids commonly used for labor pain relief. *Journal of Midwifery & Women's Health, 56*, 222–239. doi:10.1111/j.1542-2011.2011.00061.x

Cho, S. H., Lee, H., & Ernst, E. (2010). Acupuncture for pain relief in labour: A systematic review and meta-analysis. *BJOG, 117*, 907–920. doi:10.1111/j.1471-0528.2010.02570.x

Cutura, N., Soldo, V., Milovanović, S. R., Orescanin-Dusić, Z., Curković, A., Tomović, B., & Janković-Raznatović, S. (2011). Optimal dose of an anesthetic in epidural anesthesia and its effect on labor duration and administration of vacuum extractor and forceps. *Clinical Expert in Obstetrics & Gynecology, 38*(3), 247–250.

Datta, S., Kodali, B., & Sega, S. (2010). *Obstetrical anesthesia handbook* (2nd ed.). New York, NY: Springer.

Douma, M. R., Verwey, R. A., Kam-Endtz, C. E., van der Linden, P. D., & Stienstra, R. (2009). Obstetric analgesia: A comparison of patient-controlled meperidine, remifentanil, and fentanyl in labour. *British Journal*

of Anaesthesia, 104*(2), 209–215. doi:10.1093/bja/aep359

Gabbe, S. G., Niebyl, J. R., Galan, H., Jauniaux, E. R. M., Landon, M., Simpson, J. L., & Driscoll, D. (2012). *Obstetrics: Normal & problem pregnancies* (6th ed.). Philadelphia, PA: Saunders.

Gillesby, E., Burns, S., Dempsey, A., Kirby, S., Mogensen, K., Naylor, K., . . . Whelan, B. (2010). Comparison of delayed versus immediate pushing during second stage of labor for nulliparous women with epidural anesthesia. *Journal of Obstetric, Gynecologic, & Neonatal Nursing, 39*, 635–644. doi:10.1111/j.1552-6909.2010.01195.x

Osterman, M. J. K., & Martin, J. A. (2011). Epidural and spinal anesthesia use during labor: 27-state reporting area, 2008. *National Vital Statistics Reports, 59*(5), 1–14.

O'Sullivan, G. (2009). Non-neuraxial analgesic techniques. In B. A. Bucklin, D. R. Gambling, & D. Wlody (Eds.), *A practical approach to obstetric anesthesia*

(pp. 131–142). Philadelphia, PA: Lippincott Williams & Wilkins.

Reynolds, F. (2010). The effects of maternal labour analgesia on the fetus. *Best Practice & Research Clinical Obstetrics & Gynaecology, 24*(3), 289–302. doi:10.1016/j.bpobgyn.2009.11.003

Suresh, M. S., Segal, B. S., Preston, R. L., Fernando, C., & Mason, L. (2013). *Shnider & Levinson's anesthesia for obstetrics.* (5th ed.). Philadelphia, PA: Lippincott, Williams, & Wilkins.

Vanita, A., Kajal, J., Babita, G., Jaswinder, K., & Saurabh, D. (2011). Best neonatal outcome following emergency cesarean delivery in nonreassuring fetal heart rate: General or a low-dose spinal anesthesia. *Journal of Obstetric Anaesthesia and Critical Care, 1*(2), 67–72.

Wilson, B. A., Shannon, M. T., & Shields, K. L. (Eds.). (2013). *Pearson's nurse's drug guide: 2012.* Upper Saddle River, NJ: Prentice Hall.

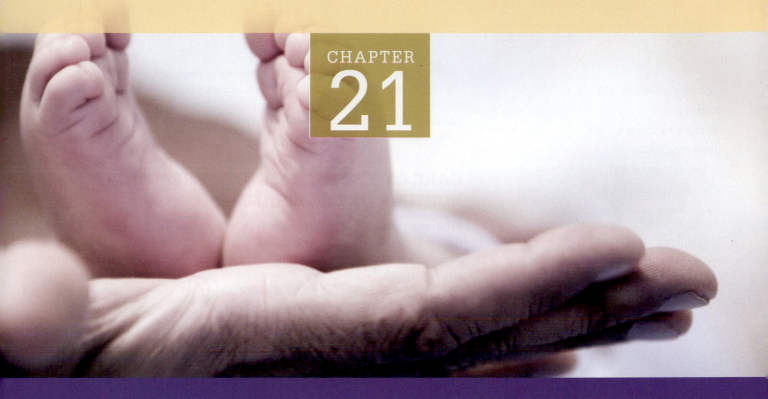

21

Childbirth at Risk: Prelabor Complications

When I learned that we were going to have twins I was stunned. How would we ever manage? Our daughters were born 2 weeks early but both weighed over 5 pounds and did well. The early days were far from easy, especially breastfeeding. I was always tired and it seemed that at least one of the girls was always awake. But they shared a room and after a while they got on the same schedule. That made things easier. They are 2 years old now and such amazing little people. Marcel and I feel that we are blessed with double joy! —Monique, 31

Ryan McVay/Getty Images

LEARNING OUTCOMES

21.1   Explain the possible causes, risk factors, and clinical therapy for premature rupture of the membranes or preterm labor in determining the nursing management of the woman and her fetus/newborn.

21.2   Compare placenta previa and abruptio placentae, including implications for the mother and fetus, as well as nursing care.

21.3   Explain cervical insufficiency and describe its clinical therapy.

21.4   Explain the maternal and fetal/neonatal implications and the clinical therapy in determining the nursing management of the woman with multiple gestation.

21.5   Compare the identification, maternal and fetal/neonatal implications, clinical therapy, and nursing management of the woman with hydramnios and oligohydramnios.

441

After the first trimester, the majority of pregnancies progress smoothly to term. In some cases, however, complications can occur before the onset of labor that significantly impact the outcome of pregnancy. This chapter presents content related to the most common of these conditions. Labor-related complications are discussed in Chapter 22 🔗.

CARE OF THE WOMAN WITH PREMATURE RUPTURE OF MEMBRANES

Premature rupture of membranes (PROM) is spontaneous rupture of the membranes before the onset of labor. PROM affects approximately 8% to 10% of all pregnancies. *Preterm PROM (PPROM)*, which affects approximately 2% to 4% of all pregnancies, is the rupture of membranes occurring before 37 weeks' gestation (Di Renzo, Roura, Facchinetti, et al., 2011). Although the exact cause is unknown, PPROM and PROM are associated with:

- Infection
- Previous history of PPROM/PROM
- Hydramnios
- Multiple pregnancy
- Urinary tract infection (UTI)
- Amniocentesis
- Placenta previa
- Abruptio placentae
- Trauma
- Cervical insufficiency (incompetent cervix)
- History of laser conization or LEEP procedure
- Bleeding during pregnancy
- Maternal genital tract anomalies

Maternal risk is related to infection, specifically *chorioamnionitis* (intra-amniotic infection resulting from bacterial invasion before birth) and *endometritis* (postpartum infection of the endometrium). In addition, abruptio placentae occurs more frequently in women with PROM. Other rare complications include retained placenta and hemorrhage, maternal sepsis, and maternal death.

Fetal/neonatal implications include:

- Risk of respiratory distress syndrome (with PPROM)
- Fetal sepsis caused by ascending pathogens
- Malpresentation
- Prolapse of the umbilical cord
- Nonreassuring fetal heart rate tracings
- Compression of the umbilical cord related to oligohydramnios
- Premature birth
- Increased perinatal morbidity and mortality

PROM that occurs at term is associated with favorable outcomes. Gestations from 32 to 36 weeks generally have favorable outcomes although there may be some complications caused by prematurity. In general, infants born before 32 weeks have some complications, including respiratory distress syndrome (RDS), necrotizing enterocolitis, intraventricular hemorrhage, and sepsis. The earlier the gestational age, the greater the likelihood of infant complications (Hanna & Kiefer, 2012).

Clinical Therapy

A sterile speculum examination is done to detect the presence of amniotic fluid in the vagina. If fluid is not obviously pooling, information can be gained by using Nitrazine paper, which turns deep blue when amniotic fluid is present. Because certain bacterial pathogens can also result in a positive Nitrazine test, a microscopic examination (ferning test) should be used to confirm a rupture. It is considered a definitive test. Digital examination increases the risk of infection and is not recommended until a management plan has been determined.

Fetal well-being is assessed through a fetal heart rate (FHR) tracing or biophysical profile (BPP). In addition, the gestational age of the fetus is calculated to develop a management plan. The gestational age of the fetus and the presence or absence of infection determine the direction of treatment for PROM. If maternal signs and symptoms of infection are evident, antibiotic therapy (usually by intravenous infusion) is begun immediately, and the fetus is born vaginally or by cesarean regardless of the gestational age. Prophylactic antibiotics are often administered for the first 48 hours while awaiting culture results. Upon admission to the nursery, the newborn is assessed for sepsis and placed on antibiotics. (Chapter 28 🔗 provides further information about the newborn with sepsis.)

Management of PPROM in the absence of infection and gestation of less than 37 weeks is usually conservative. The woman is hospitalized on bed rest. On admission, complete blood cell count (CBC), C-reactive protein, and urinalysis are obtained, as are cultures, including chlamydia, gonorrhea, and Group B streptococcus. An ultrasound is done to determine gestational age, amniotic fluid level, and fetal well-being. Continuous electronic fetal monitoring may be ordered at the beginning of treatment but usually is discontinued after a few hours, unless the fetus is estimated to be very low birth weight (VLBW) or if the tracing is of concern. Regular nonstress tests (NSTs) or biophysical profiles are used to monitor fetal well-being. (These tests are discussed in Chapter 14 🔗.) Maternal blood pressure, pulse, temperature, and FHR are assessed every 4 hours. Regular laboratory evaluations are done to detect maternal infection. Vaginal exams are avoided to decrease the chance of infection. As the gestation approaches 34 weeks, fetal lung maturity studies are indicated (see Chapter 14 🔗).

Maternal corticosteroid administration promotes fetal lung maturity and helps to prevent respiratory distress syndrome and other complications. Currently a single course of corticosteroids is recommended (see *Drug Guide: Betamethasone*). Repeat courses of corticosteroids should not be routinely used because they have not been shown to improve neonatal outcomes and are associated with an increased incidence of chorioamnionitis (Gyamfi-Bannerman et al., 2012). Research has not yet determined whether a repeat dose at 30 to 32 weeks may help

stimulate alveoli that were not formed when the initial dose was given (Gyamfi-Bannerman et al., 2012). Administration of corticosteroids to late preterm infants has not been shown to produce clinical benefits (Gyamfi-Bannerman et al., 2012).

NURSING MANAGEMENT *For the Woman with Premature Rupture of Membranes*

Nursing Assessment and Diagnosis

Perform a careful assessment that includes the following:

- Determine the duration of the rupture of the membranes.
- Ask the woman when her membranes ruptured and when labor began.
- Determine gestational age to prepare for the possibility of a preterm birth.
- Observe the mother for signs and symptoms of infection, especially by reviewing her white blood cell (WBC) count, temperature, pulse rate, and the character of her amniotic fluid.
- Assess for maternal fever and hydration status.
- Assess the coping abilities of the woman and her partner, specifically if a preterm birth is anticipated.
- Determine if the woman and her partner have attended childbirth education classes.

Nursing diagnoses that may apply to a woman with PROM include the following (NANDA-I © 2012):

- *Infection, Risk for,* related to premature rupture of membranes
- *Gas Exchange, Impaired,* in the fetus related to compression of the umbilical cord secondary to prolapse of the cord
- *Coping, Ineffective,* related to unknown outcome of the pregnancy

Planning and Implementation

Nursing actions should focus on the woman, her partner, and the fetus:

- Monitor for and report signs of infection to the certified nurse-midwife or physician.
- Evaluate uterine activity and fetal response to the labor, but vaginal exams are not done unless absolutely necessary because this increases the risk of infection.
- Encourage the woman to rest on her side to promote optimal uteroplacental perfusion. Use comfort measures to help promote rest and relaxation.
- Ensure that hydration is maintained, particularly if the woman's temperature is elevated.

Education is another important aspect of nursing care. The woman and her partner, if he is involved, need to understand the implications of PROM and all treatment methods. It is important to address side effects and alternative treatments. The couple needs to know that although the membranes are ruptured, amniotic fluid continues to be produced.

Health Promotion Reducing Risk of Infection During Pregnancy

Pregnant women should avoid all individuals with a history of recent infection, rash-like illness, fever, or unknown illnesses to reduce their risk of acquiring infection during pregnancy.

Drug Guide Betamethasone (Celestone Soluspan)

Overview of Maternal–Fetal Action

Studies have provided ample evidence that glucocorticoids such as betamethasone are capable of inducing pulmonary maturation and decreasing the incidence of respiratory distress syndrome in preterm infants. The mechanism by which corticosteroids accelerate fetal lung maturity is unclear, but it is related to the stimulation of enzyme activity by the drug. The enzyme is required for biosynthesis of surfactant by the type II pneumocytes. Surfactant is of major importance to the proper functioning of the lung in that it decreases the surface tension of the alveoli. Glucocorticoids also increase the rate of glycogen depletion, which leads to thinning of the interalveolar septa and increases the size of the alveoli. The thinning of the epithelium brings the capillaries into closer proximity with the air spaces and improves oxygen exchange.

Route, Dosage, Frequency

Prenatal maternal intramuscular injections of 12 mg of betamethasone are given once a day for 2 days. Dexamethasone has also been given in doses of 6 mg every 12 hours for 4 doses (Desai & Tank, 2012). To obtain maximum results, birth should be delayed for at least 24 hours after completing the first round of treatment.

Repeat courses of corticosteroids should not be used routinely (Desai & Tank, 2012). There is some controversy with administering corticosteroids when membranes are ruptured, fueled by concerns that this could mask infection. Because the onset of infection with ruptured membranes warrants immediate birth, the concern is that sepsis could unknowingly occur.

Contraindications

Inability to delay birth
Adequate L/S ratio
Presence of a condition that necessitates immediate birth (e.g., maternal bleeding)
Presence of maternal infection, diabetes mellitus (relative contraindication)
Gestational age greater than 34 completed weeks

Maternal Side Effects

Increased risk for infection has not been supported in large studies. There may, however, be some increase in the incidence of infection in women with premature rupture of the membranes. Maternal hyperglycemia may occur during corticosteroid administration. Women with insulin-dependent diabetes may require insulin infusions for several days to prevent ketoacidosis. Corticosteroids may increase the risk of pulmonary edema, especially when used concurrently with tocolytics (Wilson, Shannon, & Shields, 2013).

Effects on Fetus/Newborn

Lowered cortisol levels at birth, but rebound occurs by 2 hours of age
Hypoglycemia
Increased risk of neonatal sepsis

Animal studies have shown serious fetal side effects such as reduced head circumference and decreased placental weight. An overall reduction in fetal weight, particularly in female subjects, has also been reported in animal studies. Human studies have not shown these effects, however (Miller et al., 2012).

Nursing Considerations

- Assess for presence of contraindications.
- Provide education regarding possible side effects.
- Administer betamethasone deep into gluteal muscle, avoiding injection into deltoid (high incidence of local atrophy). (Dexamethasone may be administered IM or IV.)
- If membranes are ruptured, temperature monitoring is warranted every 2 hours or more frequently if temperature instability is concerning.
- Periodically evaluate BP, pulse, weight, and edema.
- Assess lab data for electrolytes and blood glucose.
- Although concomitant use of betamethasone and tocolytic agents has been implicated in increased risk of pulmonary edema, the betamethasone has little mineral corticoid activity; therefore, it probably does not add significantly to the salt and water retention effects of beta-adrenergic agonists. Other causes of noncardiogenic pulmonary edema should also be investigated if pulmonary edema develops during administration of betamethasone to a woman in preterm labor.

Providing psychologic support for the couple is critical:

- Help reduce anxiety by listening empathetically, relaying accurate information, and providing explanations of procedures.
- Prepare the couple for a cesarean birth, a preterm newborn, and the possibility of fetal or newborn demise as may be necessary.
- Initiate consultation with the neonatologist or pediatric provider to give the woman and her partner an opportunity to ask questions if a preterm birth is anticipated.

Evaluation

Expected outcomes of nursing care include the following:

- The woman's risk of infection and of cord prolapse decrease.
- The couple is able to discuss the implications of PROM and all treatments and alternative treatments.

Teaching Highlights Explaining Amniotic Membranes

To help a laboring woman and her family understand how the amniotic membranes provide protection, use a color chart that shows a side view of the fetus in the uterus with the membranes intact. Ask the couple to visualize what would happen if the membranes rupture. They will be able to see that pathogens have direct access to the uterus, increasing the risk of infection. They will also see that, when the membranes rupture and the fluid escapes, the cord could "wash out" with the fluid and become trapped between the pelvis and fetal head, causing cord compression.

- The couple verbalizes understanding that they did not cause the event.
- The pregnancy is maintained without trauma to the mother or fetus.

CARE OF THE WOMAN AT RISK BECAUSE OF PRETERM LABOR

Labor that occurs between 20 and 36 completed weeks of pregnancy is called **preterm labor (PTL)**. Prematurity continues to be the number one perinatal and neonatal problem in the United States, with 12.8% of all live births occurring prematurely (Martin, 2011). Often PTL is related to multiple risk factors; only rarely is there a single cause. Table 21–1 presents a list of risk factors for spontaneous preterm labor.

Maternal implications of PTL include psychologic stress related to the baby's condition and physiologic stress related to medical treatment for preterm labor.

Fetal/neonatal implications include increased morbidity and mortality, especially caused by respiratory distress syndrome (RDS), increased risk of trauma during birth, and

Health Promotion   Reduction of Preterm Births

Healthy People 2020 goals include the reduction of preterm births and the reduction of low birth weight (LBW) and very low birth weight (VLBW) infants. Most LBW and VLBW infants are premature and have been delivered prior to the completion of 37 gestational weeks (U.S. Department of Health and Human Services, 2011).

maturational deficiencies (fat storage, heat regulation, immaturity of organ systems).

Clinical Therapy

Women who are at risk for PTL are taught to recognize its symptoms and, if any symptoms are present, to notify their physician/certified nurse-midwife (CNM) immediately. Prompt diagnosis

Table 21–1	Risk Factors for Spontaneous Preterm Labor
Multiple gestation	Cervical shortening/1 cm
DES exposure	Uterine irritability
Known cervical insufficiency	Age (less than 17 or over 35 years)
Hydramnios	Low socioeconomic status
Uterine anomaly	Cigarettes—more than 10/day
Cervix dilated/1 cm at 32 weeks	Substance abuse
Second-trimester abortion	Low maternal weight
Fetal abnormality	Poor weight gain
Febrile illness	More than two first-trimester abortions
Bleeding after 12 weeks	Nonwhite race
History of pyelonephritis or other maternal infection	Cervical cerclage in situ
Diabetes	In vitro fertilization (singleton or multiple gestation)
Previous preterm birth	Sexually transmitted infection (STI) (trichomoniasis, chlamydia)
Previous preterm labor with term birth	Anemia
Abdominal surgery during second or third trimester	Abdominal trauma
History of cone biopsy	Foreign body (e.g., IUD)
Uteroplacental ischemia	*Bacterial vaginosis, E. coli* (ascending intrauterine infection)
Stress	Periodontal disease
Inadequate or no prenatal care	Domestic violence
Lack of social support	Long work hours with prolonged standing
Hypertension (preeclampsia, gestational hypertension, chronic hypertension)	Clotting disorders
Obesity	Interval of less than 6 to 9 months between pregnancies

Evidence-Based Practice Risk Factors for Preterm Births

Clinical Question
What comorbid conditions are risk factors for preterm births?

The Evidence
Understanding the risk factors for preterm births can help the nurse target interventions aimed at preventing this complication. A population-based study focused on identifying rates, associated characteristics, and comorbid conditions of women who had a birth between 34 and 37 weeks' gestation, as compared to women who carried their babies full term. The study included more than 23,000 women; this large sample size and population-based design forms strong evidence for practice. The variables associated with preterm birth were race/ethnicity (African American was highest), age less than 17 or more than 35 years, gestational hypertension, eclampsia, chronic hypertension, and diabetes (Carter, Fowler, Holden, et al., 2011). Some risk factors are modifiable by early counseling and/or lifestyle modification, particularly smoking and those that lead to hypertension and diabetes (Tepper et al., 2012). Improved management of comorbid conditions can result in lower rates of preterm births.

Best Practice
Risk factors for preterm birth should be assessed at each prenatal visit. Counseling and lifestyle modification should be instituted early in the pregnancy to minimize the risk of comorbid conditions that can lead to preterm birth. Managing these conditions carefully during the pregnancy can result in lower preterm birth rates.

Clinical Reasoning
What specific nursing assessments can help detect risk factors for preterm birth? What interventions can help reduce the incidence of comorbid conditions that lead to preterm birth?

---

is necessary to stop preterm labor before it progresses to the point where intervention is ineffective.

Prompt diagnosis of PTL is often difficult because many of the symptoms are common in normal pregnancy. The strongest predictors of preterm birth include the following (Ross, 2011):

- Cervicovaginal fibronectin
- Abnormal cervical length on ultrasound
- History of previous preterm birth
- Presence of infection

Fetal fibronectin (fFN) is a protein normally found in the fetal membranes and decidua. It is in the cervicovaginal fluid in early pregnancy but is not usually present in significant quantities between 22 and 37 weeks' gestation (Ross, 2011). A positive fFN test (fFN found in the cervicovaginal fluid) during this time puts the woman at increased risk for preterm birth. Conversely, a negative fFN in a woman with preterm contractions is associated with a very low risk of birth within 7 to 14 days (Ross, 2011). The test is over 99% accurate for predicting no preterm birth within 7 days. The procedure for collecting a sample is similar to that of the Pap smear; results can be available within 1 hour.

The length of the cervix can be measured fairly reliably after 16 weeks' gestation using an ultrasound probe inserted into the vagina. A cervix that is shorter than expected may help a physician to identify a woman at increased risk for PTL. In such cases, research indicates that vaginal progesterone gel can be used prophylactically to increase gestational age (Ross, 2011). Some clinicians consider that a shorter-than-anticipated cervix reveals the need for a cerclage to prevent preterm birth because of incompetent cervix. However, opinion varies as to the value of cerclage as compared with expectant management (Ross, 2011).

Diagnosis of preterm labor is confirmed if the pregnancy is between 20 and 37 weeks, there are documented uterine contractions (four in 20 minutes or eight in 1 hour), and documented cervical change or cervical dilatation of greater than 1 cm (0.4 in.) or cervical effacement of 80% or more.

SAFETY ALERT!
Because of the risk of adverse maternal and fetal outcomes, labor is not interrupted if one or more of the following conditions are present: severe preeclampsia or eclampsia, chorioamnionitis, hemorrhage, maternal cardiac disease, poorly controlled diabetes mellitus or thyrotoxicosis, severe abruptio placentae, fetal anomalies incompatible with life, fetal death, nonreassuring fetal status, or fetal maturity.

Tocolysis is the use of medications in an attempt to stop labor. Drugs currently used as tocolytics include the β-adrenergic agonists (also called β-mimetics), cyclooxygenase (prostaglandin synthetase) inhibitors, and calcium channel blockers such as nifedipine (Procardia). The β-mimetics terbutaline sulfate (Brethine) and magnesium sulfate were once the most widely used tocolytics but are now commonly being replaced with calcium channel blockers, such as nifedipine (Procardia). Although tocolytic drugs suppress uterine contractions and allow pregnancy to continue, they may cause maternal side effects; the most serious is maternal pulmonary edema. While reducing the dose and duration of therapy sometimes reduces the side effects, long-term use of Brethine is no longer considered the standard of care. Because of risk of maternal morbidity related to pulmonary edema, other medications are commonly used for long-term management.

The selection of magnesium sulfate, calcium channel blockers, or β-mimetics also depends on the experience of the healthcare providers. Although some practitioners use a cocktail approach, using various drugs concurrently, there are no established guidelines or procedures for combination use. Detailed

Health Promotion Risk Factors for Preterm Labor

Women should discontinue all use of alcohol, tobacco, and drugs. They are risk factors for preterm labor and birth.

research trials that examine the effectiveness of a multiphar-macologic approach are needed. Some drugs should not be concurrently used, such as magnesium sulfate and nifedipine (Procardia). For magnesium sulfate, the recommended loading dose is 4 g IV in 100 mL of IV fluid using an infusion pump over 30 minutes, followed by a maintenance dose of 1 to 4 g/hr titrated to response and side effects (Ross, 2011). The therapy is continued for 12 hours after uterine contractions have stopped.

Side effects with the loading dose may include:

- Flushing; feeling warm
- Headache
- Nystagmus
- Nausea
- Dizziness
- Lethargy; sluggishness
- Pulmonary edema

Fetal side effects may include hypotonia and lethargy that persists for 1 or 2 days following birth. Respiratory depression in the newborn can also occur (Ross, 2011). See *Drug Guide: Magnesium Sulfate*.

One calcium channel blocker, nifedipine (Procardia), is be-coming increasingly popular in treating preterm labor because it is easily administered orally or sublingually and has few serious maternal side effects. It decreases smooth muscle contractions by blocking the slow calcium channels at the cell surface. The most common side effects are related to arterial vasodilation and include hypotension, tachycardia, facial flushing, and headache. Nifedipine may be coadministered with the β-mimetics.

SAFETY ALERT!
Nifedipine should *not* be used with magnesium because both drugs block calcium and simultaneous administration has been implicated in serious maternal side effects related to low calcium levels.

Prostaglandin synthesis inhibitors (PSIs) such as indometha-cin (Indocin) have been used for tocolysis in selected instances. Although this medication has been highly effective in delaying birth, potential fetal side effects, such as constriction of the ductus arteriosus, necrotizing enterocolitis (NEC), and intraventricular hemorrhage (IVH), have made it an uncommon treatment mo-dality. Indocin should never be administered after 32 gestational weeks due to its potential to cause heart defects (Stuebe, 2012).

Progesterone supplementation is another form of treatment that has been an effective management tool in reducing preterm births in women with a history of preterm births at less than 34 gestational weeks. Use of progesterone is considered appro-priate to use in singleton pregnancies when there is a past history of PROM or PTL in a previous pregnancy and may be considered in women with a shortened cervical length. It is not routinely administered to women who are asymptomatic with a multiple gestation (American College of Obstetricians and Gynecolo-gists [ACOG], 2008b). The use of hydroxyprogesterone caproate (Makena) injection was approved by the Food and Drug Admin-istration (FDA) in 2011 as a weekly injection, beginning between 16 and 21 weeks. It is used to prevent preterm labor in women with a history of at least one preterm birth. Makena is not indi-cated for women with a multiple gestation (FDA, 2011).

The use of magnesium sulfate treatment has been used for neuroprotection in women with very preterm infants and has been found to offer protection against the development of cere-bral palsy although additional studies are needed. When magne-sium sulfate is given, it should be administered following strict hospital policy because it warrants intensive maternal and fetal monitoring (ACOG, 2010).

Corticosteroids (typically betamethasone or dexametha-sone) should be administered antenatally to any women at risk for preterm birth because of their beneficial effect on preventing neonatal respiratory distress syndrome (RDS), intraventricular hemorrhage (IVH), necrotizing enterocolitis (NEC), and neo-natal mortality (Ross, 2011). Women who are candidates for tocolysis are candidates for antenatal corticosteroids, regardless of fetal gender, race, or availability of surfactant therapy for the newborn, especially between 24 and 34 weeks' gestation (see *Drug Guide: Betamethasone* on page 444). Betamethasone is primarily used and should be administered in 2 intramuscular doses. When dexamethasone is used, 4 doses are given.

NURSING MANAGEMENT *For the Woman with Preterm Labor*

Nursing Assessment and Diagnosis

During the antepartum period, identify the woman at risk for preterm labor by noting the presence of risk factors. During the intrapartum period, assess the progress of labor and the physi-ologic impact of labor on the mother and fetus.

Nursing diagnoses that may apply to the woman with preterm labor include the following (NANDA-I © 2012):

- *Fear* related to risk of early labor and birth
- *Coping, Ineffective,* related to need for constant attention to pregnancy
- *Pain, Acute,* related to uterine contractions

Planning and Implementation
Community-Based Nursing Care

Once the woman at risk for preterm labor has been identified, she needs to be taught about the importance of recognizing the onset of labor (see *Teaching Highlights: Preterm Labor*).

Teaching Highlights Preterm Labor

- Describe the dangers of preterm labor, especially the risk of prematurity in the infant, and all the potential problems.
- Explain that many of the early symptoms of labor, such as backache and increased bloody show, may be subtle initially.
- Summarize self-care measures (see Table 21–2) the woman can take to prevent preterm labor.
- Teach the woman how to palpate for uterine contractions. Demonstrate and ask for a return demonstration.

Drug Guide Magnesium Sulfate

Pregnancy Risk Category: B

Overview of Obstetric Action

Magnesium sulfate acts as a central nervous system (CNS) depressant by decreasing the quantity of acetylcholine released by motor nerve impulses and thereby blocking neuromuscular transmission. This action reduces the possibility of convulsion, which is why magnesium sulfate is used in the treatment of preeclampsia. Because magnesium sulfate secondarily relaxes smooth muscle, it may cause transient blood pressure readings, although it is not considered an antihypertensive. Magnesium sulfate may also decrease the frequency and intensity of uterine contractions; as a result it is also used as a tocolytic in the treatment of preterm labor.

Route, Dosage, Frequency

Magnesium sulfate is generally given intravenously to control dosage more accurately and prevent overdosage. The intravenous route allows for immediate onset of action. It must be given by infusion pump for accurate dosage.

For Treatment of Preterm Labor

Loading dose: 4 to 8 g magnesium sulfate in lactated Ringer's solution administered over a 20- to 60-minute period.

Maintenance dose: 2 to 4 g/hr via infusion pump (Wilson et al., 2013)

For Treatment of Preeclampsia

Loading dose: 4 to 6 g magnesium sulfate administered over a 20- to 30-minute period.

Maintenance dose: 2 to 3 g/hr via infusion pump (Wilson et al., 2013)

Note: Magnesium sulfate is excreted via the kidneys. Because women in preterm labor typically have normal renal function, they generally require higher levels of magnesium to achieve a therapeutic range than women who have preeclampsia and may have compromised renal function. Maintenance dose may need to be adjusted based on serum magnesium levels.

Maternal Contraindications

Diagnosed maternal myasthenia gravis is the only absolute contraindication to the administration of magnesium sulfate. A history of myocardial damage or heart block is a relative contraindication to use of the drug because of the effects on nerve transmission and muscle contractility. Extreme care is necessary in administration to women with impaired renal function because the drug is eliminated by the kidneys, and toxic magnesium levels may develop quickly.

Maternal Side Effects

Most maternal side effects are dose related. Lethargy and weakness related to neuromuscular blockade are common. Sweating, a feeling of warmth, flushing, and nasal congestion may be related to peripheral vasodilation. Other common side effects include nausea and vomiting, constipation, visual blurring, headache, and slurred speech. Signs of developing toxicity include depression or absence of reflexes, oliguria, confusion, respiratory depression, circulatory collapse, and respiratory paralysis. Rapid administration of large doses may cause cardiac arrest. If any of these occur, the drip should be stopped immediately.

Effects on Fetus/Newborn

The drug readily crosses the placenta. Some authorities suggest that transient decrease in FHR variability may occur; others report that no change occurred. In general, magnesium sulfate therapy does not pose a risk to the fetus. Occasionally, the newborn may demonstrate neurologic depression or respiratory depression, loss of reflexes, and muscle weakness. Ill effects in the newborn may actually be related to fetal growth retardation, prematurity, or perinatal asphyxia.

Nursing Considerations

- Monitor the blood pressure every 10 to 15 minutes during administration.
- Monitor maternal serum magnesium levels as ordered (usually every 6 to 8 hours). Therapeutic levels are in the range of 4 to 8 mg/dL. Reflexes often disappear at serum magnesium levels of 9 to 13 mg/dL; respiratory depression occurs at levels of 14 mg/dL; cardiac arrest occurs at levels above 30 mg/L (Wilson et al., 2013).
- Monitor respirations closely. If the rate is less than 12 per minute, magnesium toxicity may be developing, and further assessments are indicated. Many protocols require stopping the medication if the respiratory rate falls below 12 per minute.
- Assess knee jerk (patellar tendon reflex) for evidence of diminished or absent reflexes. Loss of reflexes is often the first sign of developing toxicity. Also note marked lethargy or decreased level of consciousness and hypotension.
- Determine urinary output. Output less than 30 mL/hr may result in the accumulation of toxic levels of magnesium.
- If the respirations or urinary output fall below specified levels or if the reflexes are diminished or absent, no further magnesium should be administered until these factors return to normal. It is important to obtain a baseline of reflexes so that if a change has occurred it can be appropriately detected. Use of both the popliteal and brachial reflexes are used to assess reflex status.
- The antagonist of magnesium sulfate is calcium. Consequently, an ampule of calcium gluconate should be available at the bedside. The usual dose is 1 g given IV over a period of about 3 minutes.
- Monitor fetal heart tones continuously with IV administration.
- Continue magnesium sulfate infusion for approximately 24 hours after birth as prophylaxis against postpartum seizures if given for preeclampsia.
- If the mother has received magnesium sulfate close to birth, the newborn should be closely observed for signs of magnesium toxicity for 24 to 48 hours.
- The antidote for magnesium sulfate is calcium gluconate. Calcium gluconate should always be on hand in case the magnesium levels get too high.

Note: Protocols for magnesium sulfate administration may vary somewhat according to agency policy. Consequently, individuals are referred to their own agency protocols for specific guidelines.

Periodic home visits by a home care nurse are also a common part of care. During these visits it is important to complete physical assessments similar to those done in the hospital and assess the woman's emotional state. Provide information about support groups and other community resources for women at risk for preterm birth.

Teaching the woman to be aware of the signs and symptoms of preterm labor is a primary objective. She should be alert for the following:

- Uterine contractions that occur every 10 minutes or less, with or without pain
- Mild menstrual-like cramps felt low in the abdomen
- Constant or intermittent feelings of pelvic pressure that feel like the baby pressing down
- Rupture of membranes
- Constant or intermittent low, dull backache
- A change in the vaginal discharge (an increase in amount, a change to more clear and watery, or a pinkish tinge)
- Abdominal cramping with or without diarrhea

Teach the woman to evaluate contraction activity once or twice a day. She does so by lying down tilted to one side with a pillow behind her back for support. The woman places her fingertips on the fundus of the uterus, which is above the umbilicus (navel). She checks for contractions (hardening or tightening in the uterus) for about 1 hour. It is important for the pregnant woman to know that uterine contractions occur occasionally throughout the pregnancy. If they occur every 10 minutes for 1 hour, however, the cervix could begin to dilate, and labor could ensue.

Ensure that the woman knows when to report signs and symptoms. If contractions occur every 10 minutes (or more frequently) for 1 hour, if any of the other signs and symptoms are present for 1 hour, or if clear fluid begins leaking from the vagina, the woman should telephone her physician or certified nurse-midwife, clinic, or hospital birthing unit and make arrangements to be checked for ongoing labor. Caregivers need to be aware that the woman's call must be taken seriously. When a woman is at risk for preterm labor, she may have many episodes of contractions and other signs or symptoms. If she is treated positively, she will feel freer to report problems as they arise.

Preventive self-care measures are also important. The nurse has a vital role in communicating the self-care measures described in Table 21–2.

Hospital-Based Nursing Care

Supportive nursing care is important to the woman in preterm labor during hospitalization. This care consists of promoting bed rest, monitoring vital signs (especially blood pressure and respirations), measuring intake and output, and continuous monitoring of fetal heart rate (FHR) and uterine contractions. Place the woman on her left side to facilitate maternal–fetal circulation. Keep vaginal examinations to a minimum. If medications are being used, administer them and monitor the mother and fetus for any adverse effects.

Table 21–2	Self-Care Measures to Prevent Preterm Labor

- Rest two or three times a day lying on your left side.
- Drink 2 to 3 quarts of water or fluid each day. Avoid caffeine drinks. Filling a quart container and drinking from it will eliminate the need to keep track of numerous glasses of fluid.
- Empty your bladder at least every 2 hours during waking hours.
- Avoid lifting heavy objects. If small children are in the home, work out alternatives for picking them up, such as sitting on a chair and having them climb on your lap.
- Avoid prenatal breast preparation such as nipple rolling or rubbing nipples with a towel. This is not meant to discourage breastfeeding but to avoid the potential increase in uterine irritability.
- Pace necessary activities to avoid overexertion.
- Curtail or eliminate sexual activity that involves nipple stimulation or leads to orgasm.
- Find pleasurable ways to help compensate for limitations of activities and boost the spirits.
- Try to focus on 1 day or 1 week at a time rather than on longer periods of time.
- If on bed rest, get dressed each day and rest on a couch rather than becoming isolated in the bedroom.

Source: Prepared in consultation with the Prematurity Prevention Program at the University of Washington Medical Center.

Whether preterm labor is arrested or proceeds, the woman and her partner, if involved, experience intense psychologic stress. The primary aim of the nurse is to decrease the anxiety level associated with the risk of having a preterm newborn by providing emotional support. It is important to recognize the stress of prolonged bed rest and lack of sexual contact and to help the couple find satisfactory ways of dealing with those stresses. With empathetic communication, it is possible to assist the woman and her partner to express their feelings, which commonly include guilt and anxiety, thereby helping them identify and implement coping mechanisms. Keep them informed about the labor progress, the treatment regimen, and the status of the fetus. In the event of imminent vaginal or cesarean birth, the woman or couple should be offered brief but ongoing explanations to prepare them for the actual birth process and the events following the birth. Arrange for consultations with the neonatologist or pediatrician to assist the woman and her partner in anticipating potential neonatal complications and risks for the newborn.

Evaluation

Expected outcomes of nursing care include the following:

- The woman is able to discuss the cause, identification, and treatment of preterm labor.
- The woman states that she feels comfortable in her ability to cope with her situation and has resources available to her.
- The woman can describe appropriate self-care measures and can identify characteristics that need to be reported to her caregiver.
- The woman successfully gives birth to a healthy infant.

CARE OF THE WOMAN AT RISK BECAUSE OF BLEEDING DURING PREGNANCY

Bleeding during pregnancy always requires assessment. The most common causes of bleeding during the first and second trimesters, namely spontaneous abortion, ectopic pregnancy, gestational trophoblastic disease, and incompetent cervix, are addressed in Chapter 16 🔴. The two most clinically significant causes of bleeding in the second half of pregnancy, placenta previa and abruptio placentae, are discussed here. Other placental problems are addressed in Chapter 22 🔴.

Placenta Previa

In **placenta previa**, the placenta is implanted in the lower uterine segment rather than the upper portion of the uterus. This implantation may be on a portion of the lower segment or over the internal cervical os. As the lower uterine segment contracts and dilates in the later weeks of pregnancy, the placental villi are torn from the uterine wall, exposing the uterine sinuses at the placental site. Bleeding begins, but because its amount depends on the number of sinuses exposed, initially it may be either scanty or profuse. Placenta previa is categorized (Figure 21–1 🔴) as being (Cunningham et al., 2010):

- *Low lying*: The placenta is implanted in the lower uterine segment in proximity to but not covering the os.
- *Partial*: The internal os is partially covered.
- *Marginal*: The edge of the placenta is covered.
- *Complete*: The internal os is completely covered.

The cause of placenta previa is unknown. Statistically it occurs in 0.3% to 2% of all women (Marrinan, 2011). Women of African descent and women who have undergone a prior

cesarean birth are at higher risk for placenta previa. Other risk factors include high gravidity, high parity, advanced maternal age, previous miscarriage, previous induced abortion, cigarette smoking, and male fetus (Marrinan, 2011).

Fetal/Neonatal Implications

The prognosis for the fetus depends on the extent of placenta previa. In cases of a marginal previa or a low-lying placenta, the woman may be allowed to labor. Changes in the fetal heart rate (FHR) and meconium staining of the amniotic fluid may be apparent. In a profuse bleeding episode, the fetus is compromised and suffers some hypoxia. FHR monitoring is imperative when the woman is admitted, particularly if a vaginal birth is anticipated, because the presenting part of the fetus may obstruct the flow of blood from the placenta or umbilical cord. If nonreassuring fetal status occurs, cesarean birth is indicated. Women who are diagnosed with a complete or partial previa will undergo a cesarean birth because the risk of intrapartum hemorrhage is high. After birth, blood sampling should be done to determine whether the intrauterine bleeding episodes of the woman have caused anemia in the newborn.

Clinical Therapy

The goal of medical care is to identify the cause of bleeding and to provide treatment that will ensure birth of a mature newborn. Indirect diagnosis is made by localizing the placenta through tests that require no vaginal examination, such as a transabdominal ultrasound scan. Until placenta previa is ruled out, vaginal examinations should never be performed on a woman with bleeding because the examiner's fingers could perforate the placenta if cervical dilatation has occurred. Once placenta previa is ruled out, a vaginal examination can be performed with a speculum to determine the cause of bleeding (such as cervical lesions).

The differential diagnosis of placental or cervical bleeding takes careful consideration. Partial separation of the placenta

A   B   C

🔴 **Figure 21–1** Classification of placenta previa. *A,* Low-lying placental implantation. *B,* Partial placenta previa. *C,* Complete placenta previa.

may also present with painless bleeding, and true placenta previa may not demonstrate overt bleeding until labor begins, thus confusing the diagnosis.

Care of the woman with painless late-gestational bleeding depends on (1) the week of gestation during which the first bleeding episode occurs and (2) the amount of bleeding. If the pregnancy is less than 37 weeks' gestation, expectant management is used to delay birth until about 37 weeks' gestation to allow the fetus time to mature. Expectant management involves the following:

1. Providing bed rest with bathroom privileges as long as the woman is not bleeding

2. Performing no vaginal exams

3. Monitoring blood loss, pain, and uterine contractility

4. Evaluating FHR with an external fetal monitor

5. Monitoring maternal vital signs

6. Performing a complete laboratory evaluation: hemoglobin, hematocrit, Rh factor, and urinalysis

7. Providing intravenous fluid (lactated Ringer's solution)

8. Having two units of cross-matched blood available for transfusion

If frequent, recurrent, or profuse bleeding persists, or if fetal well-being appears threatened, a cesarean birth may be needed. See Table 21–3 for assessment and management of placenta previa.

NURSING MANAGEMENT *For the Woman with Placenta Previa*

Nursing Assessment and Diagnosis

Assessment of the woman with placenta previa must be ongoing to prevent or treat complications that are potentially lethal to the mother and fetus. Painless, bright-red vaginal bleeding is the most accurate diagnostic sign of placenta previa. If this sign develops during the last 3 months of pregnancy, placenta previa should always be considered until ruled out by ultrasound examination. The first bleeding episode is generally scanty. If no vaginal examinations are performed, it often subsides spontaneously. However, each subsequent hemorrhage is more profuse.

The uterus remains soft; if labor begins, it relaxes fully between contractions. The FHR usually remains stable unless profuse hemorrhage and maternal shock occur. As a result of the placement of the placenta, the fetal presenting part is often unengaged, and transverse lie is common.

It is important to assess blood loss, pain, and uterine contractility both subjectively and objectively. Maternal vital signs and the results of blood and urine tests provide additional data about the woman's condition. Evaluate the FHR with continuous external fetal monitoring. Observe and verify the family's ability to cope with the anxiety associated with an unknown outcome.

Nursing diagnoses that may apply include the following (NANDA-I © 2012):

- *Fluid Volume: Deficient,* related to hypovolemia secondary to excessive blood loss

Table 21–3	Assessment and Management of Placenta Previa
Gestation Less Than 37 Weeks	
Assessment	**Management/Action**
Bleeding stopped No uterine contractions No abdominal pain NST reactive	Bed rest Vital signs every 4 hours Provide IV fluids Type and cross-match blood Monitor patient closely
Assessment	**Management/Action**
Bleeding begins again *or* Labor has begun *or* Maternal vital signs decline *or* Fetal status is nonreassuring	Cesarean birth
Assessment	**Management/Action**
Complete previa	Cesarean birth
Gestation More Than 37 Weeks	
Assessment	**Management/Action**

Bleeding minimal or stopped
Reassuring fetal status
	Induction of labor possible if:
	  Low-lying or marginal
	    previa
	  Cervix is ripe
	  Cephalic presentation
	  Fetal head down in pelvis

Assessment	**Management/Action**
Bleeding continues *or* Complete previa	Cesarean birth

Source: Data from Zuspan, F. P., Quilligan, E. J., Blumenfield, M., Kim, M. H., & Evans, C. B. (1998). *Handbook of obstetrics, gynecology, and primary care.* Philadelphia, PA: Elsevier Mosby.

- *Gas Exchange, Impaired,* of the fetus related to decreased blood volume and maternal hypotension

- *Anxiety* related to concern for own personal status and the baby's safety

Planning and Implementation

Monitor the woman and her fetus to determine the status of the bleeding and the responses of the mother and baby. Do the following tasks:

- Take vital signs.

- Record intake and output.

- Perform ongoing continuous fetal monitoring.

Clinical Tip

The amount of bleeding from the vagina is not a reliable guide to the degree of placental separation.

- Perform ongoing continuous uterine activity monitoring with external tocodynamometer.
- Prepare a whole-blood setup to be ready for intravenous infusion.
- Establish a patent intravenous line before caregivers undertake any invasive procedures.
- Monitor maternal vital signs every 15 minutes in the absence of hemorrhage and every 5 minutes with active hemorrhage.

Provision of emotional support for the family is an important nursing care goal. During active bleeding, the assessments and management are directed toward physical support. However, emotional aspects need to be addressed simultaneously. Explain the assessments and treatment measures needed. Provide time for questions, and act as an advocate in obtaining information for the family. Emotional support can also be offered by staying with the family and using touch.

Promotion of neonatal physiologic adaptation is another important nursing responsibility. Check the newborn's hemoglobin, cell volume, and erythrocyte count immediately and then monitor them closely. The newborn may require oxygen, administration of blood, and admission into a special-care nursery.

Evaluation

Anticipated outcomes of nursing care include the following:

- The cause of hemorrhage is recognized promptly and corrective measures are taken.
- The woman's vital signs remain in the normal range.

- Any other complications are recognized and treated early.
- The family understands what has happened and the implications and associated problems of placenta previa.
- The woman and her baby have a safe labor and birth.

Abruptio Placentae

Abruptio placentae is the premature separation of a normally implanted placenta from the uterine wall. Premature separation, the leading cause of perinatal mortality, is considered a catastrophic event because of the severity of the resulting hemorrhage. The incidence of abruptio placentae is 0.5% to 1.0% of all pregnancies, but it accounts for 10% to 15% of all perinatal deaths (Deering, 2011).

The cause of abruptio placentae is largely unknown. Risk factors associated with placental abruption include maternal age over 35 or under 20 years, increased parity, cigarette smoking, alcohol use, cocaine abuse, trauma, retroplacental fibromyoma, post-amniocentesis complication, maternal hypertension, rapid uterine decompression associated with hydramnios and multiple gestation, preterm premature rupture of membranes (PPROM), uterine malformations or fibroids, placental anomalies, short umbilical cord, subchorionic hematoma, elevated second-trimester maternal serum alpha-fetoprotein, previous abruption, and inherited thrombophilia (Deering, 2011).

Abruptio placentae is subdivided into three types (Figure 21–2 ●):

- *Marginal.* The placenta separates at its edges, the blood passes between the fetal membranes and the uterine wall, and the blood escapes vaginally (also called marginal sinus rupture).
- *Central.* The placenta separates centrally, and the blood is trapped between the placenta and the uterine wall. Entrapment of the blood results in concealed bleeding.
- *Complete.* Massive vaginal bleeding is seen in the presence of total separation.

A   B   C

● **Figure 21–2** Abruptio placentae. *A,* Marginal abruption with external hemorrhage. *B,* Central abruption with concealed hemorrhage. *C,* Complete separation.

Abruptio placentae may also be graded according to the severity of clinical and laboratory findings as follows (Deering, 2011):

Grade 1 (Mild): Mild separation with slight vaginal bleeding. Fetal heart rate (FHR) pattern and maternal blood pressure unaffected. Accounts for 40% of abruptions.

Grade 2 (Moderate): Partial abruption with moderate bleeding. Significant uterine irritability is present. Maternal pulse may be elevated although blood pressure is stable. Signs of fetal compromise evident in FHR. Accounts for 45% of abruptions.

Grade 3 (Severe): Large or complete separation with moderate to severe bleeding. Maternal shock and painful uterine contractions present. Fetal death common. Accounts for about 15% of abruptions.

The signs and symptoms of placental abruption are listed in Table 21–4. In severe cases of central abruptio placentae, the blood invades the myometrial tissues between the muscle fibers. This occurrence accounts for the uterine irritability that is a significant sign of abruptio placentae. If hemorrhage continues, eventually the uterus turns entirely blue because the muscle fibers are filled with blood. After birth the uterus contracts poorly. This condition is known as a *Couvelaire uterus* and frequently necessitates hysterectomy.

Maternal Implications

As a result of the damage to the uterine wall and the retroplacental clotting with central abruption, large amounts of thromboplastin are released into the maternal blood supply. This thromboplastin in turn triggers the development of disseminated intravascular coagulation (DIC) and resultant hypofibrinogenemia. Fibrinogen levels, which are ordinarily elevated in pregnancy, may drop in minutes to the point at which blood will no longer coagulate.

Maternal mortality is now uncommon, although maternal morbidity still occurs (Cunningham et al., 2010). Postpartum problems depend in large part on the severity of the intrapartum bleeding, coagulation defects (DIC), hypofibrinogenemia, and time between separation and birth. Moderate to severe hemorrhage results in hemorrhagic shock, which may prove fatal to the mother if it is not rapidly reversed. In the postpartum period, women with this disorder are at risk for hemorrhage and renal failure caused by shock, vascular spasm, intravascular clotting, or a combination of these factors.

Fetal/Neonatal Implications

Perinatal mortality associated with abruptio placentae is about 25% (Cunningham et al., 2010). In severe cases, in which most of the placenta has separated, the infant mortality rate is near 100%. In less severe separation, fetal outcome depends on the level of maturity and the length of time to birth. The most serious complications in the newborn arise from preterm labor,

Table 21–4	Differential Signs and Symptoms of Placenta Previa and Abruptio Placentae	
	Placenta Previa	**Abruptio Placentae**
Onset	Quiet and sneaky	Sudden and stormy
Bleeding	External	External or concealed
Color of blood	Bright red	Dark venous
Anemia	Equal to blood loss	Greater than apparent blood loss
Shock	Equal to blood loss	Greater than apparent blood loss
Toxemia	Absent	May be present
Pain	Only labor	Usually severe and steady
Uterine tenderness	Absent	Present
Uterine tone	Soft and relaxed	Firm to stony hard
Uterine contour	Normal	May enlarge and change shape
Fetal heart tones	Usually present	Present or absent
Engagement	Absent	May be present
Presentation	May be abnormal	No relationship

Source: Oxorn, H. (1986). *Human labor and birth* (5th ed., p. 507). Norwalk, CT: Appleton & Lange.

anemia, and hypoxia. If fetal hypoxia progresses unchecked, irreversible brain damage or fetal demise may result. Thorough assessment and prompt action on the part of the healthcare team can improve both fetal and maternal outcomes.

Clinical Therapy

Disseminated intravascular coagulation (DIC) is a complex pathologic activation of coagulation (blood clotting) mechanisms that can sometimes occur as a complication in pregnancy. In DIC, small clots are formed within blood vessels that consume coagulation proteins and platelets. When this pathologic process occurs, abnormal coagulation and abnormal bleeding result in various systems, including in the skin (e.g., where a needle puncture occurred), gastrointestinal, and respiratory systems. Incisions may also bleed. This cascade of events leads to microclots that disrupt normal blood flow to major organs and can lead to organ failure. DIC is extremely serious and accounts for 25% of maternal deaths (Ramin & Ramin, 2012).

Because of the risk of DIC, evaluating the results of coagulation tests is imperative. In DIC, fibrinogen levels and platelet counts usually decrease; prothrombin times and partial thromboplastin times are normal to prolonged. If the values are not markedly abnormal, serial testing may be helpful in establishing an abnormal trend indicative of coagulopathy. Another test determines levels of fibrin-degradation products; these values rise with DIC.

After establishing the diagnosis, immediate priorities are maintaining the cardiovascular status of the mother and developing a plan for the birth of the fetus. The birth method selected depends on the condition of the woman and fetus and the speed at which the birth will occur; in many circumstances, cesarean birth will be the safest option.

If the separation is mild and the pregnancy is late preterm, labor may be induced and the fetus born vaginally with as little trauma as possible. If rupture of membranes and oxytocin infusion by pump do not initiate labor, a cesarean birth is required. A long delay would raise the risk of increased hemorrhage, with resulting hypofibrinogenemia. Supportive actions to decrease the risk of DIC include typing and cross-matching for blood transfusions (at least three units), evaluating the clotting mechanism, and providing intravenous fluids.

In cases of moderate to severe placental separation, a cesarean birth is done after treatment of hypofibrinogenemia by intravenous infusion of cryoprecipitate or fresh-frozen plasma. Vaginal birth is impossible with a Couvelaire uterus, because the uterus would not contract properly in labor, and a hysterectomy is often needed.

The hypovolemia that accompanies severe abruptio placentae is life threatening and must be combated with whole blood. If the fetus is alive but experiencing stress, emergency cesarean birth is the method of choice. With a stillborn fetus, vaginal birth is preferable if bleeding has stabilized, unless maternal shock from hemorrhage is uncontrollable. Intravenous fluids are administered. Central venous pressure (CVP) monitoring may be needed to evaluate intravenous fluid replacement. An absolute level is not as important as the response to fluid replacement. CVP is evaluated hourly, and the results are communicated to the physician. Elevations of CVP may indicate fluid overload and pulmonary edema. Laboratory testing is ordered to provide ongoing data regarding hemoglobin, hematocrit, and coagulation status. The hematocrit is maintained at 30% through the administration of packed red blood cells or whole blood (Cunningham et al., 2010). Measures are taken to stimulate labor to effect a vaginal birth, if possible. An amniotomy may be performed, and oxytocin is given. Progressive dilatation and effacement usually occur.

Nursing Management. Electronic monitoring of the uterine contractions and resting tone between contractions provides information about the labor pattern and effectiveness of the oxytocin induction. Because uterine resting tone is frequently increased with abruptio placentae, it must be evaluated frequently for further increase. Abdominal girth measurements may be ordered hourly and are obtained by placing a tape measure around the maternal abdomen at the level of the umbilicus. Another method of evaluating uterine size, which increases as more bleeding occurs at the site of abruption, involves placing a mark at the top of the uterine fundus; the distance from the symphysis pubis to the mark may then be measured hourly. Overdistention of the uterus can lead to a ruptured uterus, another life-threatening complication. See *Nursing Care Plan: Hemorrhage in the Third Trimester.*

CARE OF THE WOMAN WITH CERVICAL INSUFFICIENCY

Cervical insufficiency (formerly called *incompetent cervix*) is painless dilatation of the cervix without contractions due to a structural or functional defect of the cervix. The woman is usually unaware of contractions and presents with advanced effacement and dilatation and, possibly, bulging membranes.

The origin of cervical insufficiency is multifactorial. Factors that may contribute to the tendency for the cervix to dilate prematurely can be divided into three categories (Johnson & Iams, 2009):

1. ***Congenital factors.*** May be found in women exposed to diethylstilbestrol (DES) or those with a bicornuate uterus.

2. ***Acquired factors.*** May be related to inflammation, infection, subclinical uterine activity, cervical trauma, cone biopsy, late second-trimester elective abortions, or increased uterine volume (as with a multiple gestation). Loop electrosurgical excision procedure (LEEP) of the cervix has been found to significantly increase the risk of preterm births in both singleton and twin gestations (Noehr, Jensen, Frederiksen, et al., 2009).

3. ***Biochemical (hormonal) factors.*** The hormone relaxin may be an endocrine cause of cervical incompetence.

A woman's obstetric history may give her healthcare provider an indication of increased risk for incompetent cervix. Factors include multiple gestations, repetitive second-trimester losses, previous preterm birth, progressively earlier births with

Nursing Care Plan Hemorrhage in the Third Trimester

Intervention	Rationale	Expected Outcome

1. Nursing Diagnosis: *Fluid Volume, Deficient, Risk for,* related to excessive vascular loss during pregnancy (NANDA-I © 2012)

NIC Primary Intervention:
Fluid management: Promotion of fluid balance and prevention of complications resulting from abnormal or undesired fluid levels

NOC Suggested Outcome:
Fluid balance: Balance of water in the intracellular and extracellular compartments of the body

Goal: The woman will not experience significant fluid volume deficit during the third trimester of pregnancy.

Intervention	Rationale	Expected Outcome
▪ Monitor vital signs (i.e., temperature: normal range is 96.8–100.4°F; pulse: normal is 60–100; respirations: normal is 12–20; blood pressure: normal is 120/80; central venous pressure: normal is 5–10 mm H_2O). Compare present blood pressure with woman's baseline blood pressure. Note pulse pressure.	▪ Any deviations in a woman's baseline vital signs could indicate intravascular fluctuations.	▪ Woman will show signs of adequate fluid volume during pregnancy as evidenced by vital signs within normal limits, capillary refill in less than 3 seconds, adequate sensorium, and urine output greater than 30 mL/hr.
▪ Weigh pads and chux. If the woman has bathroom privileges, instruct her on initiating pad counts. Teach woman how to weigh pads and chux, with each gram = to approximately 1 mL of blood loss.	▪ The combination of weighing and counting pads and chux assists medical personnel in determining the woman's blood loss.	
▪ Report amount of blood loss within a specific period of time (e.g., 50 mL of bright-red blood on pad in 20 minutes).		
▪ Monitor urinary output hourly and measure urine specific gravity (normal: 1.010–1.025).	▪ A decrease in urinary output (less than 30 mL/hr) and an increase in specific gravity suggest dehydration and a need for an increase in fluid intake.	
▪ Palpate bilateral peripheral pulses (normal: equal and strong) and note capillary refill (normal: less than 3 seconds). Also, assess skin color and temperature (normal: pink, warm, dry, and intact).	▪ Helps determine signs of circulatory loss or hypovolemic shock that include weak pulses, capillary refill greater than 3 seconds, skin color that is cyanotic or pallor, and skin temperature that is cool and clammy.	
▪ Assess mental status at frequent intervals.	▪ Excessive blood loss can lead to changes in mentation.	
▪ Assess woman for signs and symptoms of disseminated intravascular coagulation.	▪ Provides vital information on maternal status.	
▪ Instruct the woman on importance of strict bed rest and avoidance of any sexual activity that involves nipple stimulation or that might lead to orgasm.	▪ Bleeding may cease with limited activity. Pressure on the abdomen and orgasms can stimulate uterine activity, thereby causing bleeding. Nipple stimulation may result in uterine contractions, as can orgasm.	
▪ Monitor fetal status and uterine activity by continuous fetal monitoring.	▪ May determine origin of bleeding and fetal well-being.	

(continued)

Nursing Care Plan   Hemorrhage in the Third Trimester—continued

Intervention	Rationale	Expected Outcome
Collaborative:		
■ Collect and review blood work: complete blood count (CBC), type and cross-match, Rh titer, fibrinogen levels, platelet count, activated partial thromboplastin time (APTT), prothrombin time (PT), and hCG levels.	■ Determines blood loss and need for intervention if blood work is abnormal.	
■ Administer appropriate isotonic IV solutions and blood products (e.g., plasma expanders, whole blood, serum albumin, or packed red blood cells) as ordered by physician.	■ Reverses shock symptoms by increasing blood volume.	
■ Insert Foley catheter.	■ Close monitoring of urinary output will aid in determining adequate renal perfusion.	

2. Nursing Diagnosis: *Tissue Perfusion, Peripheral (uteroplacental), Risk for Ineffective,* related to hypovolemia secondary to excessive maternal blood loss (NANDA-I © 2012)

NIC Primary Intervention:		**NOC Suggested Outcome:**
Electronic fetal monitoring: Electronic evaluation of fetal heart rate response to movement, external stimuli, or uterine contractions during antepartum testing		*Circulation status:* Extent to which blood flows unobstructed, unidirectionally, and at an appropriate pressure through large vessels of the systemic and pulmonary circuits
Goal: The fetus will have no evidence of hypoxia during pregnancy.		
■ Assess maternal vital signs.	■ Closely monitoring maternal physiologic status and circulatory status will assist in determining if an episode of bleeding has occurred and allow for interventions to protect maternal and fetal well-being.	
■ Monitor fetal heart tones continuously, assessing for variability, accelerations, and decelerations, and record.	■ Continuous electronic fetal monitoring will aid in detecting signs of fetal hypoxia and allow time for appropriate intervention.	■ Fetus will demonstrate adequate tissue perfusion as evidenced by fetal heart tones that remain within 110–160 beats/min, long-term variability and short-term variability present, positive periodic changes (no variable or late decelerations), and fetal scalp blood pH greater than 7.25.
■ Encourage woman to adhere to a strict lateral-lying bed rest regimen.	■ Promotes good placental/fetal oxygen exchange because pressure on the inferior vena cava is relieved.	
■ Assess fundal height.	■ Determines an approximate gestational age.	
■ Assess labor progression by determining cervical dilatation and effacement if contractions are present.	■ This provides information on maternal labor status.	
Collaborative:		
■ Perform scalp stimulation to assess fetal accelerations.	■ FHR acceleration is considered 15 beats above the baseline lasting for 15 seconds and is indicative of fetal well-being.	
■ Assess amniotic fluid for meconium.	■ Impaired gas exchange relaxes fetal intestinal motility, causing expulsion of meconium into amniotic fluid.	
■ Assist physician during ultrasonography and amniocentesis for lecithin/sphingomyelin (LS) ratio sample.	■ Determines viability and alerts appropriate medical personnel of fetal age if birth is imminent.	

Nursing Care Plan Hemorrhage in the Third Trimester—continued

Intervention	Rationale	Expected Outcome
3. Nursing Diagnosis: *Anxiety* related to personal and fetal well-being secondary to third-trimester hemorrhage (NANDA-I © 2012)		
NIC Primary Intervention: *Anxiety reduction:* Minimizing apprehension, dread, foreboding, or uneasiness related to an unidentified source of anticipated danger		**NOC Suggested Outcome:** *Anxiety control:* Ability to eliminate or reduce disabling feelings of alarm aroused by an identifiable source
Goal: The woman will verbalize a decrease in anxiety.		
■ Maintain frequent contact with the woman and family members.	■ Establishes trust with the woman and her family members, so the patient will not feel alone or abandoned.	■ Woman will actively seek information about diagnosis and prognosis.
■ Provide woman with accurate, reliable information concerning diagnosis and prognosis.	■ Anxiety will lessen when the woman is informed of health status and is allowed to make decisions based on present situation.	■ Woman and her family members will develop appropriate coping strategies that decrease fear and anxiety.
■ Allow woman and family members to verbalize origin of anxiety.	■ Recognizing the origin of anxiety gives the woman and her family the appropriate tool to begin the process of developing coping strategies.	
■ Explain all procedures in an easy-to-understand, nonthreatening manner, and allow woman and family members to ask questions.	■ Accurate information prepares the woman and family members for the impending procedures, thereby reducing anxiety and fear of the unknown.	

each subsequent pregnancy, short labors, previous elective abortion or cervical manipulation, DES exposure, or other uterine anomaly. These women will benefit from close surveillance of cervical length with transvaginal ultrasound beginning between 16 and 24 weeks' gestation. Cervical effacement occurs from the internal os out and can be seen on ultrasound as "funneling." Alteration is apparent in a transvaginal scan when fundal pressure is applied or the woman assumes a standing position. In addition, women at risk for cervical insufficiency need to be informed early in pregnancy of warning signs of impending birth, such as lower back pain, pelvic pressure, and changes in vaginal discharge.

A number of contemporary studies have concluded that endovaginal ultrasound measurements of cervical length between 15 and 28 weeks' gestation identify groups at risk for preterm birth. However, the placement of a cervical cerclage (see the following discussion) does not substantially reduce the risk of prematurity (Johnson & Iams, 2009). This has led to a reconsideration of both medical and surgical treatment options for women with a history of midtrimester losses. Medical therapies used are serial cervical ultrasound assessments, bed rest, progesterone supplementation, antibiotics, and anti-inflammatory drugs (Cunningham et al., 2010).

Cerclage Procedures

A **cerclage** is a surgical procedure in which a stitch is placed in the cervix to prevent a spontaneous abortion or premature birth (*Encyclopedia of Surgery*, 2010). See Figure 21–3 ●. Surgical options include the various types of cerclage procedures. An elective cervical cerclage may be placed late in the first trimester or early in the second trimester with an 80% to 90% success rate

● **Figure 21–3** A cerclage, or purse-string suture, is inserted in the cervix to prevent preterm cervical dilatation and pregnancy loss. After placement, the string is tightened and secured anteriorly.

in preventing fetal loss and premature labor and birth (*Encyclopedia of Surgery*, 2010). A cerclage placed for emergent reasons, when dilatation and effacement have already occurred, is successful in 40% to 60% of cases (*Encyclopedia of Surgery*, 2010).

An abdominal cerclage approach may be required for women with a congenitally short or amputated cervix, cervical defects, a cervix previously scarred, or unhealed lacerations or subacute cervicitis (ACOG, 2008a; Cunningham et al., 2010).

In cases in which cervical dilatation is discovered unexpectedly, an attempt may be made to "rescue" the pregnancy by placing a cerclage after cervical dilatation is advanced. In some instances, decompression of a bulging amniotic sac must be accomplished immediately before the cerclage placement. In this situation, a preoperative evaluation for infection, ruptured membranes, and uterine activity may be prudent. Tocolytics (drugs that stop labor), broad-spectrum antibiotics, and anti-inflammatory agents are given perioperatively and for ongoing treatment. Exposure of the amniotic membranes increases the chance of cerclage failure when compared with an elective placement of a cerclage.

An uncomplicated elective cerclage may be done on an outpatient basis or the woman may be hospitalized and discharged after 24 to 48 hours. An emergency cerclage, however, requires hospitalization for 5 to 7 days or longer. After 37 completed weeks of gestation, the suture may be cut and vaginal birth permitted, or the suture may be left in place and a cesarean birth performed to avoid repeating the procedure in subsequent pregnancies.

CARE OF THE WOMAN WITH MULTIPLE GESTATION

In part because of advances in infertility treatments, the incidence of twins in the United States has increased by 65% since 1980 (Blackburn, 2013). In 2004, the rate of twins was 32.2 per 1000 births. Multifetal births account for only 3% of all births in the United States (Blackburn, 2013). The incidence of spontaneous twins varies but is highest among African Americans, women of greater age and parity, women with a family history of fraternal twins, and women who are tall and overweight. The incidence is low in the Asian and Hispanic populations (Blackburn, 2013). The physiology of multiple gestation is discussed in Chapter 4 🔗.

Twins that occur from two separate ova are called dizygotic (two zygotes), or fraternal, twins. The fetuses may be the same sex or different sexes and are no more closely related genetically than any other siblings. In contrast, 33% of twins are monozygotic, or identical, twins; they develop from one fertilized ovum. They are genetically identical and always the same sex (Blackburn, 2013).

During the prenatal period, visualization of two gestational sacs at 5 to 6 weeks, fundal height greater than expected for the length of gestation, and auscultation of heart rates that differ by at least 10 beats per minute are the most likely clues to multiple-gestation pregnancies. In addition, the alpha-fetoprotein level on the quadruple screen is usually elevated and many women experience severe nausea and vomiting (caused by elevated levels of the human chorionic gonadotropin [hCG] hormone) (Blackburn, 2013).

Maternal Implications

During her pregnancy, the woman may experience physical discomfort such as shortness of breath, dyspnea on exertion, backaches and musculoskeletal disorders, and pedal edema. Other associated problems include (Blackburn, 2013):

- Urinary tract infections
- Threatened abortion
- Anemia
- Gestational hypertension
- Preeclampsia
- Preterm labor and birth
- Premature rupture of membranes
- Thromboembolism
- Placenta previa
- Placenta abruption
- Placenta disorders

Complications during labor include abnormal fetal presentations, uterine dysfunction, prolapsed cord, and hemorrhage at birth or shortly after (Blackburn, 2013).

Fetal/Neonatal Implications

The perinatal mortality rate is approximately 3 times greater for twins than for a single fetus, although the mortality rate for triplets and higher-order multiple births is 4 times higher (Blackburn, 2013). The perinatal mortality rate for monoamniotic siblings has been estimated to be as high as 10% to 32% (Blackburn, 2013). Fetal problems include decreased intrauterine growth rate for each fetus, increased incidence of fetal anomalies, increased risk of prematurity and its associated problems, abnormal presentations, increase in cord accidents, and an increase in cerebral palsy (Blackburn, 2013). Twins are more likely to have long-term disabilities when compared with children who were singleton births. Primiparous women who are pregnant with twins have higher rates of complications and prematurity than multiparous women (Blackburn, 2013). Multifetal pregnancies that are conceived spontaneously have better outcomes than those achieved with assisted reproductive technology. Even singleton births achieved with assisted technology have a higher incidence of adverse outcomes, specifically increased incidences of infants with cerebral palsy (Blackburn, 2013).

Clinical Therapy

Once the presence of twins has been detected, preventing and treating problems that infringe on the development and birth of normal fetuses is the most significant clinical goal. Prenatal visits are more frequent for women with twins than for those with one fetus. Women with multiple-gestation pregnancies need to understand the nutritional implications of multiple fetuses, the assessment of fetal activity, the signs of preterm labor, and the danger signs of pregnancy.

If the initial ultrasound scan performed at 18 to 20 weeks' gestation is normal and no risk factors are identified, serial ultrasounds performed every 3 to 4 weeks are used to assess the growth of each fetus. If the pregnancy has identified risks, including monochorionic diamniotic placentation, ultrasounds are performed every 2 to 3 weeks to detect possible twin-to-twin transfusion syndrome (Cunningham et al., 2010).

A systematic review of studies of hospitalization and bed rest for multiple pregnancy showed insufficient evidence to support routine bed rest (Cunningham et al., 2010). More recent strategies include work leave, lifestyle modifications, and avoidance of sexual activity, although well-designed controlled studies supporting the use of these interventions is lacking in the current literature.

Third-trimester testing usually begins at 32 to 34 weeks' gestation and may include a nonstress test (NST) or biophysical profile (BPP). A reactive NST is associated with good fetal outcome if birth occurs within 1 week of the testing. The NST is done every 3 to 7 days until birth or until results become nonreactive. The BPP is also accurate in assessing fetal status with twin pregnancies. A biophysical profile of 8 or better for each fetus is considered reassuring, and weekly or biweekly BPPs and NSTs continue until birth.

Intrapartum management requires careful attention to maternal and fetal status. The mother should have an IV with a large-bore needle in place. Anesthesia and cross-matched blood should be readily available. The twins are monitored by continuous dual electronic fetal monitoring.

The decision about method of birth, which depends on a variety of factors, may not be made until labor occurs. The presence of maternal complications such as placenta previa, abruptio placentae, or severe preeclampsia usually indicates the need for cesarean birth. Fetal factors such as severe intrauterine growth restriction (IUGR), preterm birth, fetal anomalies, nonreassuring fetal status, and unfavorable fetal position or presentation also require cesarean birth.

Any combination of presentations and positions can occur with multiple births. Figure 21–4 ● shows some possible presentations of twins. When the presenting fetus is in a nonvertex position, cesarean birth is indicated.

Nursing Management

Community-Based Nursing Care.   During pregnancy the woman may need counseling about diet and daily activities. Help her plan meals to meet her increased needs. Nutritional requirements vary

● **Figure 21–4** Twins may be in any of these presentations while in utero.

somewhat based on the mother's prepregnancy weight and the estimated weight of the twins. A daily intake of 3500 kcal (minimum) and 175 g protein is recommended for a woman with normal-weight twins, although an intake of 4000 kcal and 200 g of protein is recommended if the twins are underweight. A prenatal vitamin and 1 mg of folic acid should also be taken daily. A total weight gain of 40 to 45 lb, with a 24-lb gain by 24 weeks, is recommended for women with multiple-gestation pregnancy (Cunningham et al., 2010).

Counseling about daily activities may include encouraging the woman to plan frequent rest periods during the day. The rest period is most effective if the woman rests in a side-lying position (which increases uteroplacental blood flow) and elevates her lower legs and feet to reduce edema. Back discomfort may be relieved by pelvic rocking, maintaining good posture, consistent use of a pregnancy belt to support the abdomen and lower back, and using good body mechanics when lifting objects and moving about.

Hospital-Based Nursing Care.   During labor, the fetal heart rates (FHRs) of the siblings are monitored continuously by an electronic fetal monitor (EFM). Electronic monitoring equipment now makes it possible to monitor the fetuses simultaneously. They are monitored throughout labor and vaginal birth or up to the time of abdominal incision if a cesarean is done. Most multiple gestations are now delivered via cesarean birth.

After birth, prepare to receive two or more newborns instead of one. This means duplicating everything, including resuscitation equipment, radiant warmers, and newborn identification papers and bracelets. Additional staff members should be available for newborn resuscitation, monitoring, and newborn care. Special precautions should be taken to ensure correct identification of the newborns. The first born is usually tagged Baby A; the second, Baby B; and so on.

CARE OF THE WOMAN WITH ABNORMAL AMNIOTIC FLUID VOLUME

Amniotic fluid serves many important functions during pregnancy. However, some pregnancies are complicated by either an excessive amount of amniotic fluid or a reduced amount of fluid.

Hydramnios

Hydramnios (also called *polyhydramnios*), a situation in which there is more than 2000 mL of amniotic fluid, occurs in about 1% of all pregnancies (Cunningham et al., 2010). The exact cause of hydramnios is unknown; however, it often occurs in cases of major congenital anomalies.

During the second half of a normal pregnancy, the fetus begins to swallow and inspire amniotic fluid and to urinate, which contributes to the amount of amniotic fluid present. In cases of hydramnios, no pathology has been found in the amniotic epithelium. However, hydramnios is associated with fetal malformations that affect the fetal swallowing mechanism and neurologic disorders in which the fetal meninges are exposed in the amniotic

cavity. This condition is also found in cases of anencephaly, in which the fetus is thought to urinate excessively because of overstimulation of the cerebrospinal centers. When monozygotic twins manifest hydramnios, it is because the twin with the increased blood volume urinates excessively. Because the weight of the placenta has been found to be increased in some cases of hydramnios, increased functioning of the placental tissue may be a factor.

There are two types of hydramnios: chronic and acute. In the chronic type, the fluid volume gradually increases and is a problem of the third trimester. Most cases are of this variety. In acute cases, the volume increases rapidly over a period of a few days. The acute type is usually diagnosed between 20 and 24 weeks' gestation.

Maternal Implications

When the amount of amniotic fluid is over 3000 mL, the woman experiences shortness of breath and edema in the lower extremities from compression of the vena cava. Milder forms of hydramnios occur more frequently and are associated with minimal symptoms. Hydramnios is associated with maternal disorders such as diabetes and Rh sensitization and with multiple-gestation pregnancies. It can also occur as a result of infections such as syphilis, toxoplasmosis, cytomegalovirus, herpes, and rubella.

If the amniotic fluid is removed rapidly before birth, abruptio placentae can result from too sudden a change in the size of the uterus. Because of overdistention of uterine muscles, uterine dysfunction can occur in the intrapartum period, and the incidence of postpartum hemorrhage increases.

Fetal/Neonatal Implications

Fetal malformations and preterm birth are common with hydramnios; thus, the perinatal mortality rate is fairly high. Prolapsed cord can occur when the membranes rupture, creating a further complication for the fetus. The incidence of malpresentations also increases. In addition, the incidence of preterm labor and cesarean birth is significantly increased in pregnancies complicated by hydramnios.

Clinical Therapy

Hydramnios is managed with supportive treatment unless the intensity of the woman's distress and symptoms dictates otherwise. If the accumulation of amniotic fluid is severe enough to cause maternal dyspnea and pain, hospitalization and removal of the excessive fluid are required. Fluid can be removed vaginally or by amniocentesis. The dangers of performing the technique vaginally are prolapsed cord and the inability to remove the fluid slowly. If amniocentesis is performed, it should be done with the aid of sonography to prevent inadvertent damage to the fetus and placenta. In addition, the fluid should be removed slowly to prevent abruption.

Nursing Management.   Hydramnios should be suspected when the fundal height increases out of proportion to the gestational age. As the amount of fluid increases, it may be difficult to palpate the fetus and auscultate the FHR. In more severe cases, the maternal abdomen appears extremely tense and tight on inspection. On sonography, large spaces can be identified between the fetus and the uterine wall.

When amniocentesis is performed, it is vital to maintain sterile technique to prevent infection. Offer support to the woman and her partner by explaining the procedure to them.

If the fetus has been diagnosed with a congenital defect in utero or is born with a defect, the family needs psychologic support. Often the nurse collaborates with social services to offer the family this additional help.

Oligohydramnios

Oligohydramnios is defined as a less-than-normal amount of amniotic fluid (approximately 500 mL is considered normal). This condition affects 1% to 3% of all pregnancies (Zheng, 2012). Oligohydramnios is diagnosed when the largest vertical pocket of amniotic fluid visible on ultrasound examination is 5 cm (2 in.) or less (Cunningham et al., 2010).

The exact cause of this condition is unknown. It is found in cases of postmaturity; maternal hypertensive disorders, with intrauterine growth restriction (IUGR) secondary to placental insufficiency; and in fetal conditions associated with major renal malformations, including renal aplasia with dysplastic kidneys and obstructive lesions of the lower urinary tract. If oligohydramnios occurs in the first part of pregnancy, there is a danger of fetal adhesions (one part of the fetus may adhere to another part).

Maternal Implications

When oligohydramnios exists, labor can be dysfunctional, and progress is slow. The woman should be monitored for hypertensive disorders.

Fetal/Neonatal Implications

During the gestational period, fetal skin and skeletal abnormalities may occur because fetal movement is impaired as a result of reduced amniotic fluid volume. Because there is less fluid available for the fetus to use during fetal breathing movements, pulmonary hypoplasia may develop. During the labor and birth, oligohydramnios reduces the cushioning effect for the umbilical cord, and cord compression is more likely to occur. Decreased amniotic fluid also contributes to fetal head compression.

Clinical Therapy

During the antepartum period oligohydramnios may be suspected when the uterus does not increase in size according to the dates, the fetus is easily palpated and outlined by the examiner, and the fetus is not ballottable. The fetus can be assessed by biophysical profiles, nonstress tests, and serial ultrasounds. As soon as the fetus is term, induction is typically scheduled because the fetus is at an increased risk for intrauterine fetal demise. During labor, the fetus is monitored by continuous EFM to detect cord compression, which is indicated by variable decelerations. Some clinicians advocate the use of an *amnioinfusion* (a transcervical instillation of 250 mL of warmed sterile saline, followed by a continuous infusion rate of 100 to 200 mL/hr) after membranes have ruptured to decrease the frequency and severity of variable decelerations in the FHR during labor. The fluid is administered in a blood warmer to maintain a constant temperature. It is imperative to monitor for expulsion of the fluid to prevent overdistention of the uterus. The infusion of saline provides more fluid for the umbilical cord to float in and thereby lessens or prevents cord compression. See Chapter 23 ⊘ for more information about amnioinfusion.

Nursing Management. Continuous electronic fetal monitoring is an important part of the assessment during the labor and birth. Evaluate the EFM tracing for the presence of variable decelerations or other nonreassuring signs (such as increasing or decreasing baseline, decreased variability, presence of late decelerations). If variable decelerations are noted, the woman's position can be changed (to relieve pressure on the umbilical cord), and the physician/CNM is notified. If the tracing is not reassuring, a cesarean birth is performed. After the birth, the newborn is evaluated for signs of congenital anomalies, pulmonary hypoplasia, and postmaturity.

Critical Concept Review

LEARNING OUTCOME 21.1: Explain the possible causes, risk factors, and clinical therapy for premature rupture of the membranes or preterm labor in determining the nursing management of the woman and her fetus/newborn.

1. PROM:
   - Although the exact cause is unknown, PPROM is associated with infection, multiple pregnancy, bleeding during pregnancy, trauma, and a variety of other factors.
   - PROM nursing care focuses on prevention of infection such as limiting vaginal exams and changing the bed pads frequently.
   - The fetus is monitored carefully.

2. Preterm labor:
   - Nursing care during preterm labor focuses on administration of tocolytics and monitoring for progression of labor.

LEARNING OUTCOME 21.2: Compare placenta previa and abruptio placentae, including implications for the mother and fetus, as well as nursing care.

1. Abruptio placentae:
   - Condition in which the placenta prematurely separates from the uterine wall.
   - May result in severe hemorrhage.
   - May cause death to mother, fetus, or both.
   - May lead to clotting disorders in the mother.
   - Nursing care involves frequent assessment of uterine tone and measurement of abdominal girth.

2. Placenta previa:
   - Condition in which the placenta implants in the lower segment of the uterus. It may partially or completely cover the cervical os.
   - Bleeding occurs as the cervix begins to dilate. Bleeding may be mild to severe, depending on how much of the placenta covers the cervical os.
   - Fetus may develop hypoxia, anemia, or both from bleeding episode.
   - Nursing care involves assessing blood loss, pain, and uterine contractions.
   - The nurse should NEVER perform a vaginal examination if placenta previa is suspected.

LEARNING OUTCOME 21.3: Explain cervical insufficiency and describe its clinical therapy.

1. Cervical insufficiency (also called incompetent cervix) is the premature dilatation of the cervix; it is the most common cause of second-trimester abortion.

2. It is treated surgically with a cerclage, which involves placing a suture in the cervix to keep it from opening.

LEARNING OUTCOME 21.4: Explain the maternal and fetal/neonatal implications and the clinical therapy in determining the nursing management of the woman with multiple gestation.

1. Care of the woman with more than one fetus includes:
   - Frequent assessment of the fetal heart tones of each fetus.
   - Education of the mother about signs and symptoms of preterm labor.
   - Encouraging the mother to rest frequently.
   - Prior to birth, preparation of equipment needed to care for each individual newborn.

LEARNING OUTCOME 21.5: Compare the identification, maternal and fetal/neonatal implications, clinical therapy, and nursing management of the woman with hydramnios and oligohydramnios.

1. Hydramnios:
   - In this condition, the woman has greater than 2000 mL of amniotic fluid.
   - Associated with fetal swallowing and neurologic disorders.
   - Also associated with maternal gestational diabetes, Rh disorders, and multiple-gestation pregnancies.
   - Woman may experience shortness of breath and lower extremity edema.
   - Amniocentesis may be performed to remove some of the excess fluid.
   - The nurse monitors the mother for complications of the amniocentesis and supports the family if fetal disorders are the cause of the excess fluid.

2. Oligohydramnios:
   - In this condition the amount of amniotic fluid is reduced and concentrated.
   - Often found with some renal fetal disorders, fetal postmaturity, and placental insufficiency.
   - May cause fetal respiratory and skeletal abnormalities.
   - May cause prolonged labor.
   - Amnioinfusion may be used during labor to help to cushion the fetus and umbilical cord.
   - The nurse must continuously monitor the labor pattern for any sign of nonreassuring fetal status.

Clinical Reasoning in Action

Monique Waleski, a 34-year-old G1P0000, at 32 weeks' gestation, contacts her physician's office because she has been experiencing labor contractions that have gradually increased in frequency. She reports that she has been having about eight contractions an hour for the past 2 hours. She is instructed to meet her doctor at the birthing unit for further evaluation.

At the birthing unit a vaginal examination reveals that Monique's cervix is dilated 3 cm and 80% effaced. Contractions continue to occur every 7 to 8 minutes. Her fFN test is positive. She is diagnosed with preterm labor. You position her on her left side and start an IV infusion.

Her physician tells Monique that she wants to begin tocolysis using magnesium sulfate and then prescribes 2 doses of betamethasone. You explain to Monique and her partner that you will be giving her the magnesium sulfate by infusion pump and the betamethasone by IM injection once a day today and tomorrow. She asks you about the two medications including their specific purposes.

1. Explain the concept of tocolysis and the purpose of magnesium sulfate.
2. Describe the concept of a loading dose and maintenance dose.
3. How will you know if Monique is developing toxic levels of magnesium?
4. Describe the role of corticosteroids used during preterm labor.
5. Create a concept map for Monique's care based on her diagnosis of preterm labor. Monique will be receiving magnesium sulfate and betamethasone for her treatment regimen, which should be considered when constructing the concept map.

See www.nursing.pearsonhighered.com for possible responses and an interactive template for a concept map.

References

American College of Obstetricians and Gynecologists (ACOG). (2008a). *Cervical insufficiency* (Practice Bulletin No. 48, issued 2003, reaffirmed 2008). Washington, DC: Author.

American College of Obstetricians and Gynecologists (ACOG). (2008b). *Use of progesterone to reduce preterm birth* (ACOG Committee Opinion No. 419). Washington, DC: Author.

American College of Obstetricians and Gynecologists (ACOG). (2010). *Magnesium sulfate before anticipated preterm birth for neuroprotection* (ACOG Committee Opinion No. 455). Washington, DC: Author.

Blackburn, S. T. (2013). *Maternal, fetal, and neonatal physiology: A clinical perspective* (4th ed.). Philadelphia, PA: Saunders.

Carter, M., Fowler, S., Holden, A., Xenakis, E., & Dudley, D. (2011). The late preterm birth rate and its association with comorbidities in a population-based study. *American Journal of Perinatology, 28*(9), 703–707.

Cunningham, F. G., Leveno, K. J., Bloom, S. L., Hauth, J. C., Rouse, D. J., & Spong, C. Y. (2010). *Williams obstetrics* (23rd ed.). New York, NY: McGraw-Hill Medical.

Deering, S. H. (2011). Abruptio placentae. *eMedicine.* Retrieved from http://emedicine.medscape.com/article/252810-overview#a0101

Desai, S. V., & Tank, P. (2012). *Handbook on preterm prelabor rupture of membranes in a low resource setting.* New Delhi, India: Jaypee Brothers Medical Publishing.

Di Renzo, G. C., Roura, L. C., Facchinetti, F., & European Association of Perinatal Medicine–Study Group on "Preterm Birth." (2011). Guidelines for the management of spontaneous preterm labor: Identification of spontaneous preterm labor, diagnosis of preterm premature rupture of membranes, and preventive tools for preterm birth. *Journal of Maternal Fetal & Neonatal Medicine, 24*(5), 659–667. doi:10.3109/14767058.2011.553694

Encyclopedia of Surgery. (2010). Cervical cerclage. Retrieved from http://www.surgeryencyclopedia.com/Ce-Fi/Cervical-Cerclage.html

Food and Drug Administration (FDA). (2011). *FDA approves drug to reduce risk of preterm birth in at-risk pregnant women.* Retrieved from http://www.fda.gov/NewsEvents/Newsroom/PressAnnouncements/ucm242234.htm?sms_ss=email&at_xt=4d50034cbfa7fa33%2C0

Gyamfi-Bannerman, C., Gilbert, S., Landon, M. B., Spong, C. Y., Rouse, D. J., Varner, M. W., . . . Mercer, B. M.; for the Eunice Kennedy Shriver National Institute of Child Health and Human Development (NICHD) Maternal-Fetal Medicine Units (MFMU) Network. (2012). Effect of antenatal corticosteroids on respiratory morbidity in singletons after late-preterm birth. *Obstetrics & Gynecology, 119*(3), 555–559. doi:10.1097/AOG.0b013e31824758f6

Hanna, N., & Kiefer, D. (2012). A translational view of biomarkers in preterm labor. *American Journal of Reproductive Immunology, 67*(4), 268–272. doi:10.1111/j.1600-0897.2012.01112.x

Johnson, J. R., & Iams, J. D. (2009). *Cervical insufficiency.* Retrieved from http://www.UpToDate.com

Marrinan, G. (2011). Placenta previa imaging. *eMedicine.* Retrieved from http://emedicine.medscape.com/article/404639-overview

Martin, J. A. (2011). Preterm births: United States: 2007. *Morbidity & Mortality Weekly Report (MMWR), 60*(01), 78–79.

Miller, S. L., Sutherland, A. E., Supramaniam, V. G., Walker, D. W., Jenkin, G., & Wallace, E. M. (2012, January 6). Antenatal glucocorticoids reduce growth in appropriately grown and growth-restricted ovine fetuses in a sex-specific manner. *Reproduction, Fertility and Development.* Retrieved from http://dx.doi.org/10.1071/RD11143

Noehr, B., Jensen, A., Frederiksen, K., Tabor, A., & Kjaer, S. K. (2009). Loop electrosurgical excision of the cervix and subsequent risk for spontaneous preterm delivery: A population-based study of singleton deliveries during a 9-year period. *American Journal of Obstetrics & Gynecology, 201*(1), 33.e1–33.e6. Retrieved from http://www.sciencedirect.com

Oxorn, H. (1986). *Human labor and birth* (5th ed., p. 507). Norwalk, CT: Appleton & Lange.

Ramin, S., & Ramkin, K. (2012). *Disseminated intravascular coagulation during pregnancy.* Retrieved from http://www.uptodate.com/contents/disseminated-intravascular-coagulation-during-pregnancy

Ross, M. G. (2011). Preterm labor. *eMedicine.* Retrieved from http://emedicine.medscape.com/article/260998-overview

Stuebe, M. (2012). *Treatment of preterm labor: NSAIDs indomethacin.* Retrieved from http://www.healthline.com/health/pregnancy/preterm-labor-nsaids-indomethacin

Tepper, N., Farr, S., Cohen, B., Nannini, A., Zhang, Z., Anderson, J., . . . Macaluso, M. (2012). Singleton preterm birth: Risk factors and association with assisted reproductive technology. *Maternal & Child Health Journal, 16*(4), 807–813.

U.S. Department of Health and Human Services. (2011). *Healthy People 2020: Improving the health of Americans.* Retrieved from www.healthypeople.gov

Wilson, B. A., Shannon, M. A., & Shields, K. (2013). *Pearson's nurse's drug guide: 2013.* Upper Saddle River, NJ: Prentice Hall.

Zheng, T. (2012). *Comprehensive handbook of obstetrics and gynecology* (2nd ed.). Phoenix, AZ: Phoenix Medical Press.

Zuspan, F. P., Quilligan, E. J., Blumenfield, M., Kim, M. H., & Evans, C. B. (1998). *Handbook of obstetrics, gynecology, and primary care.* Philadelphia, PA: Elsevier Mosby.

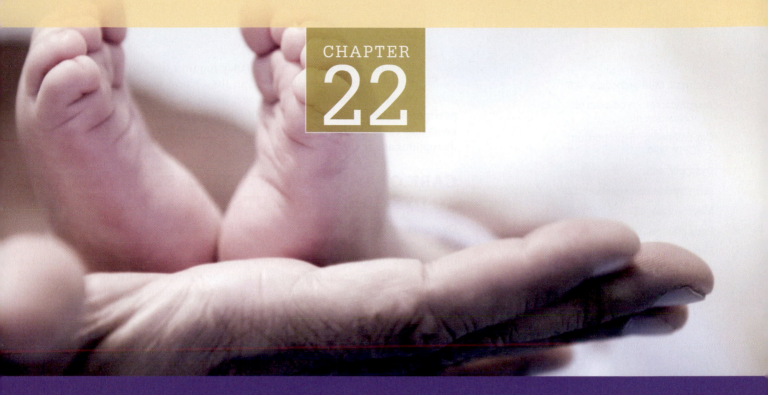

Childbirth at Risk: Labor-Related Complications

We arrived at the birthing unit with such wonderful plans for the birth of our first baby. I was able to do my breathing with the assistance of my husband and the nurse. Then suddenly my baby's heart rate dropped. It lasted for about 20 seconds but it felt like a lifetime. The nurse helped me to my side, and just stayed with us while we waited and watched the fetal monitor. There were no further problems, but I will never forget that moment. —Yolanda, 26

© ArenaCreative/Fotolia.com

LEARNING OUTCOMES

22.1 Compare tachysystolic and hypotonic labor patterns, including the risks, clinical therapy, and nursing management.

22.2 Describe the risks and clinical therapy in determining the nursing management of postterm pregnancy on the childbearing family.

22.3 Relate the various types of fetal malposition and malpresentation to the nursing management for each.

22.4 Explain the identification, risks, and clinical therapy in determining the nursing management of the woman and fetus at risk for fetal macrosomia.

22.5 Relate the maternal implications, clinical therapy, prenatal history, and conditions that may be associated with nonreassuring fetal status to the nursing management of the mother and fetus.

22.6 Describe the nursing management of the mother and fetus with a prolapsed umbilical cord.

22.7 Summarize the identification, maternal and fetal/neonatal implications, clinical therapy, and nursing management of the woman with amniotic fluid embolism (anaphylactoid syndrome of pregnancy).

22.8 Explain the types, maternal and fetal/neonatal implications, and clinical therapy in determining the nursing management of the woman with cephalopelvic disproportion.

22.9 Identify common complications of the third and fourth stages of labor.

22.10 Explain the etiology, diagnosis, and phases of grief in determining the nursing management of the family experiencing perinatal loss.

Successful completion of a pregnancy requires the harmonious functioning of the critical factors discussed in the *Critical Factors in Labor* section in Chapter 17 🔗: the birth passage, the fetus, the relationship between the passage and the fetus, and the forces of labor. Disruptions in any of these components may cause dystocia (abnormal or difficult labor). The most common of these disruptions are discussed in this chapter.

CARE OF THE WOMAN WITH DYSTOCIA RELATED TO DYSFUNCTIONAL UTERINE CONTRACTIONS

Dystocia, or difficult labor, may be caused by a wide variety of problems, the most common of which is dysfunctional (or uncoordinated) uterine contractions. These uncoordinated contractions result in a prolonged labor. Contractions that result in a more normal progression of labor tend to be moderate to strong when palpated and occur regularly (two to four contractions in 10 minutes in early labor and four to five per 10 minutes in later phases). Dysfunctional contractions are typically irregular in strength, timing, or both. These irregular uterine contractions often arrest cervical dilatation.

Tachysystolic Labor Patterns

A normal contraction pattern is shown in Figure 22–1A ●. A tachysystolic labor pattern refers to more than five contractions in 10 minutes, averaged over a 30-minute window. The term is specifically connected with the contraction pattern and does not differ with the presence of fetal heart rate (FHR) decelerations. The presence

A

B

C

● **Figure 22–1** Comparison of labor patterns. *A,* Normal uterine contraction pattern. In this example, contraction frequency is every 3 minutes; duration is 60 seconds. The baseline resting tone is below 10 mm Hg. *B,* Tachysystolic uterine contraction pattern. Note that the contraction frequency is every 1.5 minutes, duration is 90 seconds. The baseline resting tone is 10 mm Hg. *C,* Hypotonic uterine contraction pattern. In this example, the contraction frequency is every 7 minutes (with some uterine activity between contractions), duration is 50 seconds, and intensity increases approximately 25 mm Hg during contractions.

A

B

● **Figure 22–2** Effects of labor on the fetal head. *A,* Caput succedaneum formation. The presenting portion of the scalp area is encircled by the cervix during labor, causing swelling of the soft tissue. *B,* Molding of the fetal head in cephalic presentations: (1) occiput anterior, (2) occiput posterior, (3) brow, (4) face.

or absence of FHR decelerations should be documented. This pattern can be associated with both spontaneous and induced or augmented labors.

Risks of Tachysystolic Labor

Maternal risks of tachysystolic labor include the following:

- Increased discomfort due to uterine muscle cell anoxia
- Fatigue as the pattern continues
- Stress on coping abilities
- Dehydration and increased incidence of infection if labor is prolonged

    Fetal/neonatal risks include the following:

- Nonreassuring fetal status because contractions and increased uterine tone interfere with the uteroplacental exchange of gases and nutrients
- Prolonged pressure on the fetal head, which may result in cephalohematoma, caput succedaneum, or excessive molding (Figure 22–2)

Clinical Therapy

Management of tachysystolic labor may include bed rest and sedation to promote relaxation and reduce pain. Often pharmacologic intervention to promote sedation will stop these contractions. If the tachysystolic pattern continues and develops

● Clinical Tip

To determine whether the fetal heart rate (FHR) is reassuring, look for the following: baseline FHR of 110 to 160 beats/min, presence of variability, and spontaneous accelerations.

into a prolonged latent phase, oxytocin (Pitocin) infusion or amniotomy may be considered (see *Care of the Woman During Labor Induction* in Chapter 23 ⊘). These methods are instituted only after cephalopelvic disproportion (CPD) and fetal malpresentation have been ruled out. If the maternal pelvic diameters are less than average, or if the fetus is particularly large or is in a malpresentation or malposition, CPD is said to be present. In such cases, labor is not stimulated because vaginal birth is not possible. Instead a cesarean birth will be performed.

NURSING MANAGEMENT *For the Woman Experiencing Tachysystolic Labor*

Nursing Assessment and Diagnosis

As part of the labor assessment, evaluate the relationship between the intensity of the pain being experienced and the degree to which the cervix is dilating and effacing. Also note whether anxiety is negatively affecting labor progress. Evidence of increasing frustration and discouragement on the part of the mother and her partner may indicate the need to provide some additional information or assurance. Monitor the fetus closely for signs of nonreassuring fetal status.

Nursing diagnoses that may apply to the woman in tachysystolic labor include the following (NANDA-I © 2012):

- *Fatigue* related to inability to relax and rest secondary to a tachysystolic labor pattern
- *Coping, Ineffective,* related to ineffectiveness of breathing techniques to relieve discomfort
- *Anxiety* related to slow labor progress

Planning and Implementation

A key nursing responsibility is to provide comfort and support to the laboring woman and her partner. The woman experiencing a tachysystolic labor pattern will probably be very uncomfortable because of the increased force of contractions. Her anxiety level and that of her partner may be high. Work to reduce the woman's discomfort and promote a more effective labor pattern.

Suggest supportive measures such as a change of position: left lateral side-lying, high Fowler's, or on her knees in the bed with her arms up around the top of the bed while it is in a high-Fowler's position, rocking in a rocking chair, sitting up, and walking. It may be helpful to offer soothing measures such as a quiet environment, use of music the woman finds calming, back rubs, Therapeutic Touch, and visualization, as well as comfort measures such as mouth care, change of linens, effleurage, and relaxation exercises. The use of tub baths or a warm shower can help promote comfort and uterine relaxation. If sedation is ordered, ensure that the environment is conducive to relaxation. The labor partner may also need assistance in helping the woman cope. A calm, understanding approach offers the woman and her partner further support. Providing information about the cause of the tachysystolic labor pattern and assuring the woman that she is not overreacting to the situation are important nursing actions.

Patient education is key for the woman experiencing tachysystolic labor. She needs information about the dysfunctional labor pattern and the possible implications for her and her baby. Information will help relieve anxiety and thereby increase relaxation and comfort. Explain treatment options and offer opportunities to ask questions.

Evaluation

Expected outcomes of nursing care include the following:

- The woman has increased comfort and decreased anxiety.
- The woman and her partner are able to cope with the labor.
- The woman experiences a more effective labor pattern.

Hypotonic Labor Patterns

A hypotonic labor pattern usually develops in the active phase of labor, after labor has been well established. Hypotonic labor is characterized by fewer than two to three contractions in a 10-minute period (see Figure 22–1C). Hypotonic labor may occur when the uterus is overstretched from a twin gestation, or

---

Clinical Reasoning   Fetal Heart Rate Tracing

A fetal heart rate (FHR) tracing demonstrates the following: baseline heart rate of 140 with variability of 6 to 10 beats/min. When you compare the FHR with the uterine contractions, you note that there is a slowing of the FHR at the time of the contraction and that the FHR tracing looks like the contraction curve, but it is upside down. Based on this tracing, what would you do?
See www.nursing.pearsonhighered.com for possible responses.

---

in the presence of a large fetus, hydramnios, or grand multiparity. Bladder or bowel distention and cephalopelvic disproportion (CPD) may also be associated with this pattern.

Risks of Hypotonic Labor

Maternal implications of hypotonic labor patterns include the following risks:

- Maternal exhaustion
- Stress on coping abilities
- Postpartum hemorrhage from insufficient uterine contractions following birth
- Intrauterine infection if labor is prolonged

  Fetal/neonatal implications include the following:

- Nonreassuring fetal status due to prolonged labor pattern
- Fetal sepsis from pathogens that ascend from the birth canal in the presence of ruptured membranes

Clinical Therapy

The goals of clinical therapy are to improve the quality of the uterine contractions and to ensure a safe outcome for the woman and her baby. Uterine contractions can be stimulated in several ways, including the use of Pitocin, amniotomy, or stimulation of the nipples, which causes the release of oxytocin. Before initiating treatment for hypotonic labor, the physician or certified nurse-midwife (CNM) validates the adequacy of pelvic measurements and completes tests to establish gestational age if fetal maturity is in question. After CPD, fetal malpresentation, and fetal immaturity have been ruled out, Pitocin may be given intravenously (IV) via an infusion pump to improve the quality of uterine contractions. Intravenous fluid is useful to maintain adequate hydration and prevent maternal exhaustion. Amniotomy may be used to stimulate the labor process. The application of an electric breast pump or manual stimulation of the nipples may help strengthen uterine contractions, and is an excellent starting point for women who want an unmedicated birth.

Some physicians support the use of *active management of labor* (AMOL), a process whereby labor is managed from the beginning with amniotomy, timed cervical examinations are performed, and augmentation of labor with IV administration of Pitocin is begun if a specified level of progress is not met. Supporters of AMOL contend that it is a preventive treatment that reduces the chance for protracted labor and decreases the cesarean birth rate. Opponents argue that the use of AMOL increases the incidence of infection (because of frequent vaginal examinations), necessitates the use of additional interventions, and increases the incidence of instrument-assisted births (Simkin, 2011).

An improvement in the quality of uterine contractions is demonstrated by noticeable progress in the labor. If the labor pattern does not become effective or if other complications develop, further interventions, including cesarean birth, may be necessary.

NURSING MANAGEMENT *For the Woman Experiencing Hypotonic Labor*

Nursing Assessment and Diagnosis

Assessment of contractions (for frequency, intensity, and duration), maternal vital signs, and FHR provides data to evaluate maternal–fetal status. Also be alert for signs and symptoms of infection and dehydration. Because of the stress associated with a prolonged labor, observe the woman and her partner's success in implementing coping mechanisms.

Nursing diagnoses that may apply to the woman in hypotonic labor include the following (NANDA-I © 2012):

- *Pain, Acute,* related to uterine contractions secondary to dysfunctional labor
- *Coping, Ineffective,* related to unanticipated discomfort and slow progress in labor
- *Fatigue* related to prolonged labor and discomfort

Planning and Implementation

Nursing measures to promote maternal–fetal physical well-being include frequent monitoring of contractions, maternal vital signs, and FHR. If amniotic membranes are ruptured, assess for the presence of meconium, which makes close observation of fetal status more critical because it often indicates that the fetus is experiencing some form of stress. An intake and output record provides a way of determining maternal hydration or dehydration. Encourage the woman to void every 2 hours, and check her bladder for distention. Because labor may be prolonged, continue to monitor the woman for signs of infection (elevated temperature, chills, foul-smelling amniotic fluid, and fetal tachycardia). Vaginal examinations should be kept to a minimum to decrease the risk of introducing an infection.

Women experiencing a hypotonic labor pattern require emotional support. Help the couple cope with the frustration of a lengthy labor process. Combine a warm, caring approach with techniques to reduce anxiety and discomfort.

The teaching plan needs to include information about the dysfunctional labor process and implications for the mother and baby. Disadvantages of and alternatives to treatment also need to be discussed and understood.

Evaluation

Expected outcomes of nursing care include the following:

- The woman maintains comfort during labor.
- The woman understands the type of labor pattern that is occurring and the treatment plan.

CARE OF THE WOMAN WITH POSTTERM PREGNANCY

A **postterm pregnancy** is one that extends more than 294 days or 42 weeks past the first day of the last menstrual period (LMP). It is distinct from a *postdate* pregnancy, which means that the pregnancy has gone beyond the estimated date of birth (EDB) at 40 weeks. The incidence of postdate pregnancy ranges from 7% to 12% but only 4% of pregnancies last longer than 43 weeks (Caughley, 2011). The cause of true postterm pregnancy is unknown, but it seems to occur more frequently in primigravidas, women with a history of prolonged pregnancy, and in the presence of fetal anencephaly or placental sulfatase deficiency (Caughley, 2011). Women who have experienced a previous postterm pregnancy have a 30% to 40% incidence of postterm pregnancy in subsequent pregnancies (Caughley, 2011).

Risks of Prolonged Pregnancy

Maternal risks associated with prolonged pregnancy include the following (Caughley, 2011):

- Probable labor induction
- Increased risk for large-for-gestational-age (LGA) infant and resultant perineal trauma
- Increased incidence of forceps-assisted, vacuum-assisted, or cesarean birth
- Increased psychologic stress as the due date passes and concern for the baby increases
- Increased risk of infection

    Fetal risks include the following (Caughley, 2011):

- Decreased perfusion from the placenta
- Oligohydramnios (decreased amount of amniotic fluid), which increases the risk of cord compression
- Meconium aspiration (aspiration of meconium-stained amniotic fluid by the fetus at the time of birth), which is more likely if oligohydramnios and thick meconium are present
- Low 5-minute Apgar score

Some fetuses continue to grow beyond the 42nd week of pregnancy and can be excessively large at birth (macrosomia). In other cases the intrauterine environment becomes unfavorable for growth, uteroplacental insufficiency occurs, and at birth the infant has lost muscle mass and subcutaneous fat. This is known as *dysmaturity syndrome*. The macrosomic fetus is at risk for birth trauma, whereas the small-for-gestational-age (SGA) fetus is at risk for nonreassuring fetal status during labor because there is often associated oligohydramnios (Caughley, 2011).

Clinical Therapy

In managing prolonged pregnancy, some caregivers prefer induction at 41 weeks; others advocate expectant management by doing a nonstress test (NST) and biophysical profile (BPP) (especially the amniotic fluid volume portion of the BPP—the

Evidence-Based Practice Induction Versus Expectant Management for Postterm Pregnancy

Clinical Question

What are the risks and benefits of induction versus expectant management for postterm pregnancy?

The Evidence

A postterm pregnancy is one that exceeds 42 completed weeks as dated by ultrasonography. The World Association of Perinatal Medicine charged 12 recognized obstetric experts with evaluating the research regarding the risks, benefits, and management of postterm pregnancy. More than 100 research studies were evaluated by systematic review and meta-analysis to develop practice guidelines for the management of postterm pregnancy. These types of research aggregates by internationally recognized panels form the strongest level of evidence. Early ultrasound evaluation significantly reduces the number of pregnancies diagnosed as postterm; it appears that many pregnancies diagnosed as postterm are actually misdated. Although postterm pregnancies do exhibit higher complication rates, when other sources of maternal and fetal complications are controlled (e.g., intrauterine growth restriction), the extended pregnancy does not appear to be the primary contributor to complications. In the absence of clear maternal or fetal complications, there is little evidence that routine induction before a 42-week gestational age improves outcomes. It does not appear that either induction or expectant management changes the rate of cesarean birth. In cases where induction is preferred, cervical ripening should be used, particularly in nulliparous women (Mandruzzato et al., 2010).

Best Practice

If careful assessment has excluded associated risk factors, mothers whose pregnancies have passed 40 weeks should be provided information about the risks and benefits of both induction and expectant management. It is appropriate for these women to make an informed decision in consultation with their perinatal provider about which management approach to take.

Clinical Reasoning

What are some complications of pregnancy that might require induction in the postterm pregnancy? What are the elements of a teaching plan that can help women make an informed decision about the management approach they want to use?

---

amniotic fluid index) two to three times a week to evaluate fetal well-being (Caughley, 2011). If the fetal assessment tests indicate a problem, interventions are begun to accomplish the birth.

NURSING MANAGEMENT *For the Woman with Postterm Pregnancy*

Nursing Assessment and Diagnosis

When the woman is admitted into the birthing area, ongoing assessments of fetal well-being begin as soon as the postterm condition has been verified. Identify reassuring FHR characteristics and evaluate for the presence of nonreassuring patterns, such as nonperiodic variable decelerations (which may indicate cord compression or oligohydramnios), so that corrective actions can be taken. When the amniotic membranes rupture, assess the fluid for meconium. In addition, assess the woman's knowledge about the condition, implications for her baby, risks, and possible interventions.

Nursing diagnoses that may apply to the woman with postterm pregnancy include the following (NANDA-I © 2012):

- *Fear* related to the unknown outcome for the baby
- *Coping, Ineffective,* related to anxiety about the status of the baby

Planning and Implementation
Community-Based Nursing Care

If the woman has not been assessing fetal movement every day, teach her how to do so. It is vital to stress the importance of identifying inadequate fetal movement and immediately contacting her healthcare provider. (See *Fetal Activity Monitoring* in Chapter 14 for further discussion of techniques to detect fetal movement.)

Patient education about the postterm pregnancy is another important nursing responsibility. Address the implications and associated risks for the baby, as well as possible treatment plans. The woman and her partner need opportunities to ask questions and clarify information.

Hospital-Based Nursing Care

Promoting fetal well-being requires careful assessment of the response of the fetus during labor. If oligohydramnios exists, obtain a continuous FHR tracing and evaluate it frequently. Variable decelerations are often associated with oligohydramnios because the decreased amount of fluid may allow compression of the umbilical cord. If the fetus is macrosomic, carefully assess labor progress (contraction characteristics, progressive cervical dilatation, and fetal descent).

Emotional support is a key nursing intervention for women with pregnancies that extend past the due date. Women experiencing postterm pregnancy frequently feel increased stress and anxiety and have difficulty coping. Encouragement, support, and recognition of the woman's anxiety are helpful strategies.

Evaluation

Expected outcomes of nursing care include the following:

- The woman has knowledge about the postterm pregnancy.
- The woman and her partner feel supported and able to cope with the postterm pregnancy.
- Fetal status is maintained, any abnormalities are quickly identified, and supportive measures are initiated.

CARE OF THE WOMAN AND FETUS AT RISK BECAUSE OF FETAL MALPOSITION

Persistent occiput posterior (POP) position is the most common fetal malposition and occurs when the fetus does not rotate but is born in the occiput posterior (OP) position. (See Figure 17–9 on page 360 🔗 to review fetal presentations.) This position may be normal in women with small pelvises. It may also be related to poor contractions, abnormal flexion of the head, inadequate maternal pushing efforts usually related to epidural anesthesia, or a large fetus. Labor may be prolonged; however, most POP fetuses are born without the aid of forceps.

Risks of Fetal Malposition

Maternal risks related to the POP position include the following:

- Risk of third- or fourth-degree perineal lacerations during birth
- Risk of extension of a midline episiotomy

Fetal implications do not include an increased mortality risk unless labor is prolonged or additional interventions such as forceps-assisted, vacuum-assisted, or cesarean birth are required.

Clinical Therapy

Clinical treatment focuses on close monitoring of maternal and fetal status and labor progress to determine whether vaginal or cesarean birth is the safer method. A cesarean birth is chosen if maternal or fetal problems make a vaginal birth unwise or if cephalopelvic disproportion (CPD) is present. The majority of POP fetuses are born vaginally, either spontaneously or with the assistance of forceps. The forceps can be used to assist in the birth of the fetus while it is still in the occiput posterior position or to rotate the occiput to an anterior position (called Scanzoni's maneuver). (See Chapter 23 🔗 for further discussion of forceps.)

NURSING MANAGEMENT *For the Laboring Woman with the Fetus in Persistent Occiput Posterior Position*

Nursing Assessment and Diagnosis

Signs and symptoms of a POP position include complaints of intense back pain by the laboring woman, a dysfunctional labor pattern, hypotonic labor (the fetal head does not put adequate pressure on the cervix), arrest of dilatation, or arrest of fetal descent. The back pain is caused by the fetal occiput compressing the sacral nerves. Further assessment may reveal a depression in the maternal abdomen above the symphysis. FHR is typically heard far laterally on the abdomen. On vaginal examination the physician/CNM finds the wide, diamond-shaped anterior fontanelle in the anterior portion of the pelvis. This fontanelle may be difficult to feel because of molding of the fetal head.

Nursing diagnoses that may apply to women with POP-positioned fetuses include the following (NANDA-I © 2012):

- *Pain, Acute,* related to back discomfort secondary to the OP position
- *Coping, Ineffective,* related to unanticipated discomfort and slow progress in labor

Planning and Implementation

Changing maternal posture has been used for many years to enhance rotation of OP or occiput transverse (OT) to occiput anterior (OA). A number of position changes may be tried. For instance, the woman may be asked to lie on one side and then asked to move to the other side as the fetus begins to rotate. This side-lying position may promote rotation; it also enables the support person to apply counterpressure on the sacral area to decrease discomfort. A knee–chest position provides a downward slant to the vaginal canal, directing the fetal head downward on descent. A hands-and-knees position is often effective in rotating the fetus. In addition to maintaining a hands-and-knees position on the bed, the woman may try pelvic rocking, and the support person may firmly stroke the abdomen. The stroking begins over the fetal back and swings around to the other side of the abdomen. After the fetus has rotated, the woman lies in a Sims' position on the side opposite the fetal back.

Evaluation

Expected outcomes of nursing care include the following:

- The woman's discomfort is decreased.
- The coping abilities of the woman and her partner are strengthened.

CARE OF THE WOMAN AND FETUS AT RISK BECAUSE OF FETAL MALPRESENTATION

In a normal presentation, the occiput is the presenting part (Figure 22–3A ●). *Fetal malpresentations* include brow, face, breech, shoulder (transverse lie), and compound presentation.

Brow Presentation

In a *brow presentation*, the forehead of the fetus becomes the presenting part. In the *sinciput (military) presentation*, the fetal head is between flexion and extension (Figure 22–3B), whereas in the *occipitomental presentation*, the fetal head enters the birth canal with the widest diameter of the head (approximately 13.5 cm) foremost (Figure 22–3C).

The brow presentation occurs more often in multiparas than in nulliparas and is thought to be due to lax abdominal and pelvic musculature. Many brow presentations spontaneously convert to face or occipital presentations. Brow presentations are the least common types of abnormal presentations.

Risks of Brow Presentation

Maternal implications of brow presentation include increased risk of the following:

- Longer labor due to ineffective contractions and slow or arrested fetal descent
- Cesarean birth if brow presentation persists

Fetal/neonatal risks include increased mortality because of cerebral and neck compression and damage to the trachea and

● **Figure 22–3** Types of cephalic presentations. *A,* The occiput is the presenting part because the head is flexed and the fetal chin is against the chest. The largest anteroposterior (AP) diameter that presents and passes through the pelvis is approximately 9.5 cm. *B,* Sinciput (military) presentation. The head is neither flexed nor extended. The presenting AP diameter is approximately 12.5 cm. *C,* Brow (occipitomental) presentation. The largest diameter of the fetal head (approximately 13.5 cm) presents in this situation. *D,* Face presentation. The AP diameter is 9.5 cm.

larynx. In addition, facial edema, bruising, and exaggerated molding of the newborn's head may be observed.

Clinical Therapy

If a brow presentation fails to convert to occipital or face presentation, cesarean birth is indicated in most cases (Gupta, 2011). If a vaginal birth is attempted, the woman is closely monitored for cephalopelvic disproportion (CPD), facial edema, and nonreassuring fetal status. Attempts to convert brow presentations manually or through the use of forceps or vacuum are contraindicated, as is the use of oxytocin. The use of oxytocin can result in dystocia. Scalp electrodes should not be placed when the fetus is in a brow presentation (Gupta, 2011).

NURSING MANAGEMENT *For the Laboring Woman with the Fetus in Brow Presentation*

Nursing Assessment and Diagnosis

A brow presentation can be detected on vaginal examination by palpation of the diamond-shaped anterior fontanelle on one side and orbital ridges and root of the nose on the other side.

Nursing diagnoses that may apply to a woman with a brow presentation include the following (NANDA-I © 2012):

■ *Knowledge*, *Deficient,* related to lack of information about the possible maternal–fetal effects of brow presentation

■ *Injury, Risk for,* to the fetus related to pressure on fetal structures secondary to brow presentation

■ *Fear* related to sudden need for cesarean birth if conversion does not occur

Planning and Implementation

Closely observe the woman for labor problems and the fetus for signs of hypoxia as evidenced by late decelerations and bradycardia. Provide emotional support to the family. Explain the fetal position to the woman and her support person or interpret what the physician or CNM has told them. Stay close at hand to reassure the couple, inform them of any changes, and assist them with labor-coping techniques. In face and brow presentations, the newborn's face may be edematous. The couple may need help in beginning the attachment process because of the newborn's facial appearance. After the infant is inspected for any abnormalities, the pediatrician and nurse can assure the couple that the facial edema is only temporary and will subside in 3 or 4 days and that the molding will be much less visible in a few days (even though completion of the process takes several weeks).

Evaluation

Expected outcomes of nursing care include the following:

- The woman and her partner understand the implications and associated problems of brow presentation.

- The mother and her baby have a safe labor and birth.

Face Presentation

In a face presentation, the face of the fetus is the presenting part (Figure 22–3D and Figure 22–4 ●). The fetal head is hyperextended even more than in the brow presentation. Face presentation occurs most frequently in multiparas, in preterm birth, and in the presence of anencephaly. The incidence of face presentation is about 1 in 600 births.

A

B

● **Figure 22–4** Mechanism of birth in face (mentoanterior) position. *A,* The submentobregmatic diameter at the outlet. *B,* The fetal head is born by the movement of flexion.

Risks of Face Presentation

Maternal risks related to face presentation include the following:

- Increased risk of CPD and prolonged labor
- Increased risk of infection (with prolonged labor)
- Cesarean birth if fetal chin is posterior (mentum posterior)

  Fetal/neonatal risks include the following:

- Cephalohematoma
- Edema of the face and throat if the fetal chin is anterior (mentum anterior)
- Pronounced molding of the head
- Nonreassuring fetal status

Clinical Therapy

A vaginal birth may be anticipated if no CPD is present, the chin (mentum) is anterior, the labor pattern is effective, and the fetal status is reassuring. Many mentum posterior presentations spontaneously convert to anterior in the late stages of labor. If the mentum remains posterior, a vaginal birth is not possible and a cesarean birth is necessary (Figure 22–5 ●).

NURSING MANAGEMENT *For the Laboring Woman with the Fetus in Face Presentation*

Nursing Assessment and Diagnosis

When performing Leopold's maneuvers, the back of the fetus is difficult to outline with a face presentation, and a deep furrow can be palpated between the hard occiput and the fetal back (Figure 22–6 ●). Fetal heart tones are audible on the side where the fetal feet are palpated. It may be difficult to determine by vaginal examination whether a breech or face is presenting, especially if facial edema is already present. During the vaginal examination, palpation of the saddle of the nose and the gums should be attempted. When assessing engagement, remember that the face has to be deep within the pelvis before the biparietal diameters have entered the inlet.

Nursing diagnoses that may apply to the woman with a fetus in face presentation include the following (NANDA-I © 2012):

- *Fear* related to unknown outcome of the labor and a possible instrument-assisted or cesarean birth
- *Injury, Risk for,* to the newborn's face related to edema secondary to the birth process

Planning and Implementation

Nursing interventions are the same as those indicated for the brow presentation.

Evaluation

Expected outcomes of nursing care include the following:

- The woman and her partner understand the implications and associated problems of face presentation.
- The mother and her baby have a safe labor and birth.

● **Figure 22–5** Face presentation. Mechanism of birth in mentoposterior position. Fetal head is unable to extend farther. The face becomes impacted.

A

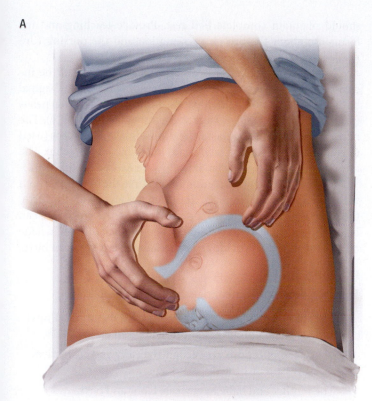

- Increased risk of cervical cord injuries caused by hyperextension of the fetal head during vaginal birth
- Increased risk of asphyxia and nonreassuring fetal status
- Increased risk of birth trauma (especially of the head) during either vaginal or cesarean breech birth

Clinical Therapy

Current clinical therapy is directed toward converting the breech presentation to a cephalic presentation prior to the beginning of labor. Some physicians attempt an external cephalic version (ECV) at 36 to 38 weeks' gestation as long as the woman is not in labor. (See Chapter 23 for discussion of external version.) The American College of Obstetricians and Gynecologists (2010) recommends a planned cesarean birth for the fetus in a breech presentation because of the significant increase in complications associated with breech vaginal births.

B

● **Figure 22–6** Face presentation. **A,** Palpation of the maternal abdomen with the fetus in right mentum posterior (RMP) position. **B,** Vaginal examination may permit palpation of facial features of the fetus.

Breech Presentation

In a breech presentation the fetal head is not the presenting part but rather is found in the fundus of the uterus. The exact cause of breech presentation (Figure 22–7 ●) is unknown. This malpresentation occurs in about 3% to 4% of labors and is frequently associated with preterm birth, placenta previa, hydramnios, multiple gestation, uterine anomalies (such as bicornuate uterus), and fetal anomalies (especially anencephaly and hydrocephaly) (Cunningham et al., 2010).

Risks of Breech Presentation

The maternal implication of breech presentation is a likelihood of cesarean birth. Fetal/neonatal implications include the following (Cunningham et al., 2010):

- Higher perinatal morbidity and mortality rates
- Increased risk of prolapsed cord, especially in incomplete breeches, because space is available between the cervix and presenting part

● **Figure 22–7** Breech presentation. **A,** Frank breech. **B,** Incomplete (footling) breech. **C,** Complete breech in left sacral anterior (LSA) position. **D,** On vaginal examination the nurse may feel the anal sphincter. The tissue of the fetal buttocks feels soft.

> ### Complementary Care Moxibustion to Promote Version in Breech Presentations
>
> Traditional Chinese medicine uses the herb mugwort in the form of moxa to promote version in a breech presentation. Moxa is a system of treatment, often combined with acupuncture, in which an herb is dried, rolled into cones (like incense cones), and placed on certain meridian points of the body. The moxa is then lit and allowed to burn close to the skin, hence the "bustion" component of the name. The heat and pungency of mugwort stimulate the point, and it is believed that the energy moves through the body and increases fetal activity.
>
> The meridian point that is used in moxibustion to promote version in breech presentation is acupoint BL 67, located beside the outer corner of the fifth toenail. Treatment may take from 7 days to 2 weeks. There is limited evidence suggesting that moxibustion is an effective modality in managing breech presentations; however, when combined with acupuncture and postural techniques (knee–chest position), the incidence of version increases (Coyle, Smith, & Peat, 2012).

NURSING MANAGEMENT *For the Laboring Woman with the Fetus in Breech Presentation*

Nursing Assessment and Diagnosis

Frequently it is the nurse who first recognizes a breech presentation. On palpation the firm fetal head is felt in the uterine fundus and the wider sacrum in the lower part of the abdomen. If the sacrum has not descended, ballottement causes the entire fetal body to move. Furthermore, fetal heart rate (FHR) is usually auscultated above the umbilicus. Passage of meconium into the amniotic fluid due to compression of the fetus's intestinal tract is common.

If membranes are ruptured, be particularly alert for a prolapsed umbilical cord, especially in footling breeches, because there is space between the cervix and presenting part through which the cord can slip. If the infant is small and the membranes rupture, the danger is even greater. The risk of a prolapsed umbilical cord is one reason any woman with ruptured membranes should not ambulate until a full assessment, including vaginal examination, has been performed.

Nursing diagnoses that may apply to a woman with a breech presentation include the following (NANDA-I © 2012):

- *Gas Exchange, Impaired,* in the fetus related to interruption in umbilical blood flow secondary to compression of the cord
- *Knowledge, Deficient,* related to lack of information about the implications and associated complications of breech presentation for the mother and fetus

Planning and Implementation

During labor, promote maternal–fetal physical well-being by frequently assessing fetal and maternal status. Because the fetus is at increased risk for prolapse of the cord, agency protocols may call for continuous fetal monitoring. If the head is not completely engaged, continuous monitoring is warranted and the woman should maintain complete bed rest. Provide teaching and information about the breech presentation and the nursing care needed.

Most physicians perform cesarean births because of the increased fetal risks associated with breech vaginal birth. Vaginal birth is more common in multiparous women with a proven pelvis (prior birth of a normal or large size fetus without difficulty). The nurse assists with the vaginal birth by including Piper forceps (used to guide the after-coming fetal head) in the birth table setup. The nurse may assist the physician if forceps are needed for the birth.

Vaginal breech births commonly occur in the operating room with a "double setup" in place. If difficulties arise with the birth, the room is already prepared for a cesarean so the procedure can be performed quickly. If the family and physician/CNM decide on a cesarean birth, provide assistance as with any cesarean birth.

Evaluation

Expected outcomes of nursing care include the following:

- The woman and her partner understand the implications and associated problems of breech presentation.
- Major complications are recognized early and corrective measures are instituted.
- The mother and baby have a safe labor and birth.

Transverse Lie (Shoulder Presentation) of a Single Fetus

A transverse lie occurs in approximately 1 in 300 term births (Cunningham et al., 2010). Maternal conditions associated with a transverse lie are grand multiparity with relaxed uterine muscles, preterm fetus, abnormal uterus, excessive amniotic fluid, placenta previa, and contracted pelvis (Figure 22–8 ●).

Clinical Therapy

The management of shoulder presentation depends on the gestational age. If discovered before term, the management is expectant (watchful), because some fetuses may change presentation without intervention. When a shoulder presentation is still evident at 37 completed weeks of gestation, an external cephalic version (ECV) attempt (followed, if successful, by induction of labor) is recommended, because the associated risk of prolapsed cord is significant. Intrapartum ECV is often successful in early labor and can reduce the need for cesarean birth. If it is unsuccessful, cesarean birth is indicated.

Nursing Management

The nurse can identify a transverse lie by inspection and palpation of the abdomen, by auscultation of the FHR, and by vaginal examination. On inspection the woman's abdomen appears widest from side to side as a result of the long axis of the infant's body lying parallel to the ground and across the mother's uterus.

On palpation no fetal part is felt in the fundal portion of the uterus or above the symphysis. The head may be palpated on one side and the breech on the other. Fetal heart rate is usually auscultated just below the midline of the umbilicus. If a presenting part is palpated on vaginal examination, it is the ridged thorax or possibly an arm compressed against the chest.

Scapula
Ribs
Humerus
Acromion process

B

● **Figure 22–8** Transverse lie. *A,* Shoulder presentation. *B,* On vaginal examination the nurse may feel the acromion process as the fetal presenting part.

Assist in the interpretation of the fetal presentation and provide information and support to the couple. Assess maternal and fetal status frequently, and prepare the woman for a cesarean birth (see Chapter 23 🔗).

Compound Presentation

A compound presentation is one in which there are two presenting parts, such as the occiput and fetal hand or the complete breech and fetal hand. Most compound presentations resolve themselves spontaneously, but others require additional manipulation at birth.

CARE OF THE WOMAN AND FETUS AT RISK FOR MACROSOMIA

Fetal **macrosomia** is defined as a birth weight of more than 4500 g (Cunningham et al., 2010). (*Note:* Some sources say 4000 g.) The condition is more common with prepregnancy maternal obesity, excessive maternal weight gain, maternal diabetes, prior history of macrosomia, a male fetus, grand multiparity, prolonged gestation, and in women of Hispanic ethnic background (Jazayeri, 2010). Macrosomia is also more common in fetuses who have erythroblastosis fetalis (Cunningham et al., 2010).

Risks of Macrosomia

Maternal implications of macrosomia include increased risk of the following:

- CPD
- Dysfunctional labor and prolonged labor

- Soft-tissue laceration during vaginal birth
- Postpartum hemorrhage

Fetal/neonatal implications include increased risk of the following:

- Meconium aspiration
- Asphyxia
- Shoulder dystocia, in which, after birth of the head, the anterior shoulder fails to deliver either spontaneously or with gentle traction (unresolved shoulder dystocia can lead to fetal death)
- Upper brachial plexus injury and fractured clavicles
- Hypoglycemia, polycythemia, and hyperbilirubinemia

Clinical Therapy

The occurrence of maternal and fetal problems associated with excessively large infants may be lessened somewhat by identifying macrosomia before the onset of labor. If a large fetus is suspected, the maternal pelvis should be evaluated carefully. Fetal size can be estimated by palpating the crown-to-rump length of the fetus in utero and by ultrasound or x-ray pelvimetry. Studies indicate that palpation and ultrasound provide equally effective assessments of fetal weight. When the uterus appears excessively large, hydramnios, an oversized fetus, or multiple gestation must be considered as the possible cause.

When fetal weight is estimated to be 4500 g or more, a cesarean birth is usually planned. The best method of birth for an estimated fetal weight of 4000 to 4500 g is debatable. The discussion centers primarily on the incidence of shoulder dystocia during vaginal birth and the difficulty in accurately estimating the fetal weight. Unexpected shoulder dystocia during vaginal birth can be a grave problem. Shoulder dystocia is marked by the presence of "turtle sign," in which the fetal head emerges and then quickly retracts as the shoulder becomes wedged beneath the pubic bone. As an emergency measure, the physician/CNM may ask the nurse to assist the woman into the McRoberts maneuver (sharp flexion of the thighs toward the hips and abdomen) or to apply gentle suprapubic pressure in an attempt to aid in the birth of the fetal shoulders. Fundal pressure should never be used because it can further wedge the anterior shoulder under the symphysis pubis.

Nursing Management

Assist in identifying women who are at risk for carrying a large fetus and those who exhibit signs of macrosomia. Because these women are prime candidates for dystocia and its complications, frequently assess the fetal heart rate (FHR) for indications of nonreassuring fetal status and evaluate the rates of cervical dilatation and fetal descent.

Apply the fetal monitor for continuous fetal evaluation. Early decelerations (caused by fetal head compression) could mean size disproportion at the bony inlet. Report any sign of labor dysfunction or nonreassuring fetal status to the physician/CNM immediately. Lack of fetal descent is another indicator that should alert the nurse to the possibility that the infant is too large for a vaginal birth.

Provide support for the laboring woman and her partner and information about the implications of macrosomia and possible associated problems. During the birth, continue to provide support and encouragement to the woman or the couple.

Inspect macrosomic newborns after birth for cephalohematoma, Erb's palsy, and fractured clavicles, and inform the nursery staff of any problems so that the newborn can be closely monitored for cerebral, neurologic, and motor problems.

In a woman with a macrosomic fetus, the uterus has been stretched farther than it would have been with an average-sized fetus. Blood glucose monitoring of the fetus is recommended since macrosomia is often associated with gestational diabetes. The overstretching may lead to contractile problems during labor or after birth. After birth the overstretched uterus may not contract well (uterine atony) and will feel boggy (soft). In this case, uterine hemorrhage is likely. The fundus of the uterus is massaged to stimulate contraction; IV or IM Pitocin may be needed. Monitor maternal vital signs closely for deviations suggestive of shock.

CARE OF THE WOMAN AND FETUS IN THE PRESENCE OF NONREASSURING FETAL STATUS

When the oxygen supply is insufficient to meet the physiologic needs of the fetus, a nonreassuring fetal status may result. This status may be transient or chronic, and may be prompted by a variety of factors. The most common are cord compression and uteroplacental insufficiency, possibly caused by preexisting maternal or fetal disease or placental abnormalities. If the resulting hypoxia persists and metabolic acidosis occurs, the situation could cause permanent damage to or be life threatening for the fetus.

Maternal Implications

Indications of nonreassuring fetal status greatly increase the psychologic stress of a laboring woman and her family members. Professional staff members may become so involved in assessing fetal status and initiating corrective measures that they fail to provide the woman and her partner with explanations and emotional support. It is imperative to offer both. In many instances, if birth is not imminent, the woman must undergo cesarean birth. This method of birth may be a source of fear and frustration, too, if the couple prepared for a shared vaginal birth experience.

Clinical Therapy

The most common initial signs of nonreassuring fetal status are variations from the normal heart rate pattern and decreased fetal movement. Meconium-stained amniotic fluid and the presence of ominous fetal heart rate (FHR) patterns such as persistent late decelerations (regardless of the depth of deceleration), persistent and severe variable decelerations (especially if the return to baseline is prolonged), and prolonged decelerations are signs of nonreassuring fetal status. When these patterns are detected, **intrauterine resuscitation** (corrective measures used to optimize

the oxygen exchange within the maternal–fetal circulation) should be started without delay.

Treatment of maternal hypotension involves having the woman turn to a left lateral position (right lateral may also be tried), beginning an IV infusion or increasing the flow rate if an infusion is already in place, or, if cord prolapse is suspected, having the woman assume a knee–chest position. Position changes that result in an increase in the fetal heart rate should be maintained. Perform a vaginal examination to attempt to detect a prolapsed cord. Decrease uterine activity by discontinuing IV Pitocin administration or administering a tocolytic agent (such as terbutaline) to decrease contraction frequency and intensity. Administer oxygen to the woman via facial mask.

Caregivers can obtain additional information about the condition of the fetus by fetal scalp blood sampling, fetal scalp stimulation, or fetal acoustic stimulation (see *Fetal Acoustic and Vibroacoustic Stimulation Tests* in Chapter 14 🔗). See Table 22–1 for management of nonreassuring fetal status.

Nursing Management

Review the woman's prenatal history and note the presence of any conditions (such as preeclampsia, diabetes, renal disease, or intrauterine growth restriction [IUGR]) that may be associated with decreased uteroplacental–fetal blood flow. When the membranes rupture, assess the FHR immediately and note the characteristics of the amniotic fluid. As labor progresses, be especially

Table 22–1	Management of Nonreassuring Fetal Status

- Recognize pattern changes that are indicative of nonreassuring fetal status such as:
  - Deep, repetitive variable decelerations
  - Prolonged decelerations
  - Ongoing late decelerations

- Begin intrauterine resuscitation measures:
  - Change maternal position.
  - Correct maternal hypotension.
  - Discontinue Pitocin.
  - Administer medications, such as terbutaline, to decrease uterine activity.
  - Increase intravenous fluid rate or begin IV immediately if not already established.
  - Assess for prolapsed cord via vaginal examination.

- If abnormal patterns resolve, continue with continuous electronic fetal monitoring.

- If abnormal patterns do not resolve and vaginal birth is imminent, proceed with vaginal birth as quickly as possible.

- If birth not imminent and bradycardia persists, or if a scalp pH level is less than 7.20, a cesarean birth is indicated.

- If these tests are reassuring, cautious assessments can continue every 15 minutes until birth occurs.

- If testing becomes nonreassuring, a cesarean should be performed.

alert to suspicious changes in the FHR. At all times, encourage and support maternal positioning that maximizes uteroplacental–fetal blood flow.

CARE OF THE WOMAN AND FETUS WITH A PROLAPSED UMBILICAL CORD

A **prolapsed umbilical cord** results when the umbilical cord precedes the fetal presenting part. When this occurs, pressure is placed on the umbilical cord as it is trapped between the presenting part and the maternal pelvis. Consequently the vessels carrying blood to and from the fetus are compressed (Figure 22–9 ●). Prolapse of the cord may occur with rupture of the membranes if the presenting part is not well engaged in the pelvis.

Risks of Prolapsed Umbilical Cord

Although a prolapsed cord does not directly precipitate physical alterations in the woman, her immediate concern for the baby creates enormous stress. The woman may need to deal with some unusual interventions, a cesarean birth, and, in some circumstances, the death of her baby.

For the fetus, compression of the cord results in decreased blood flow and leads to nonreassuring fetal status. If labor is under way, the cord is compressed further with each contraction. If the pressure on the cord is not relieved, the fetus will die.

Clinical Therapy

Preventing prolapse of the cord is the preferred medical approach. A laboring woman with a confirmed rupture of membranes will be kept horizontal, usually in bed, until the fetal head is well engaged and the risk of a prolapse is significantly decreased. If a prolapse occurs, relieving the compression on the cord is critical to fetal outcome. The medical and nursing team must work together to facilitate birth.

Bed rest is indicated for all laboring women with a history of ruptured membranes, until engagement with no cord prolapse

has been documented. Furthermore, with spontaneous rupture of membranes or amniotomy, the fetal heart rate (FHR) should be auscultated for at least a full minute and at the beginning and end of contractions for several contractions. If fetal bradycardia is detected on auscultation, perform a vaginal examination to rule out cord prolapse. In the presence of cord prolapse, electronic monitor tracings show severe, moderate, or prolonged variable decelerations with baseline bradycardia.

If a loop of cord is discovered, the examiner's gloved fingers must remain in the vagina to provide firm pressure on the fetal head (to relieve compression) until the physician/CNM arrives. This is a lifesaving measure. Give the mother oxygen via face mask, and monitor the FHR to determine whether the cord compression is adequately relieved.

The force of gravity can be employed to relieve umbilical cord compression. The nurse can instruct the woman to assume the knee–chest position or can adjust the bed to the Trendelenburg position, and transport the woman to the delivery or operating room in this position (Figure 22–10 ●). The cord may be occultly prolapsed with an actual loop extending into the vagina or lying alongside the presenting part. It may be pulsating strongly or so weakly that it is difficult to determine upon palpation of the cord whether the fetus is alive.

Nursing Management

Because there are few outward signs of cord prolapse, each pregnant woman is advised to call her physician/CNM when the membranes rupture and to go to the office, clinic, or birthing facility. Perform a sterile vaginal examination to determine if there is danger of cord prolapse. If the presenting part is well engaged, the risk of cord prolapse is minimal, and the woman may ambulate as desired. If the presenting part is not well engaged, bed rest is recommended to prevent cord prolapse.

Because cord prolapse can be associated with fetal death, some physicians/CNMs insist that bed rest be maintained after rupture of membranes regardless of fetal engagement. This can lead to conflict if the laboring woman and her partner do not hold the same opinions. Ease this situation by helping the physician/CNM and the couple communicate.

During labor any alteration of the FHR or the presence of meconium in the amniotic fluid indicates the need to assess for cord prolapse. Vaginal birth is possible with prolapsed cord if the cervix is completely dilated and pelvic measurements are adequate. If these conditions are not present, cesarean birth

● **Figure 22–9** Prolapse of the umbilical cord.

● **Figure 22–10** Knee–chest position is used to relieve cord compression during cord prolapse emergency.

is the method of choice. (See Skill 3–9 in the *Clinical Skills Manual* SKILLS.)

CARE OF THE WOMAN AND FETUS AT RISK DUE TO ANAPHYLACTOID SYNDROME OF PREGNANCY

In the presence of a small tear in the amnion or chorion high in the uterus, a small amount of amniotic fluid may leak into the chorionic plate and enter the maternal system as an **amniotic fluid embolism**, a condition called **anaphylactoid syndrome of pregnancy**. The fluid can also enter at areas of placental separation or cervical tears. Under pressure from the contracting uterus, the fluid is driven into the maternal circulation and then the maternal lungs. The more debris in the amniotic fluid (such as meconium), the greater the maternal problems. This condition, although rare, can be catastrophic. Risk factors associated with it include a tumultuous labor, placental abruption, trauma, induction of labor, eclampsia, operative vaginal birth, cesarean birth, and multiple gestation, among other things (Blackburn, 2013).

Maternal Implications

The woman with an amniotic fluid embolism experiences sudden onset of respiratory distress, circulatory collapse, acute hemorrhage, and cor pulmonale (failure of the right ventricle) as the embolism blocks the vessels of the lungs. She exhibits dyspnea and cyanosis leading to hemorrhagic shock and coma and may develop seizures. Birth must be facilitated immediately to obtain a live fetus.

Clinical Therapy

Any woman exhibiting chest pain, dyspnea, cyanosis, frothy sputum, tachycardia, hypotension, and massive hemorrhage requires the cooperation of every member of the health team if her life is to be saved. Medical interventions are supportive. Recovery is contingent on return of the mother's cardiovascular and respiratory stability. If necessary, a cesarean birth is performed.

Nursing Management

In the absence of the physician/CNM, the nurse administers oxygen under positive pressure until medical help arrives. An intravenous line is quickly established. If respiratory and cardiac arrest occur, initiate cardiopulmonary resuscitation (CPR) immediately.

Ready the equipment necessary for blood transfusion and for the insertion of the CVP line. As the blood volume is replaced, using fresh whole blood to provide clotting factors, the CVP must be monitored frequently. In the presence of cor pulmonale, fluid overload could easily occur.

CARE OF THE WOMAN WITH CEPHALOPELVIC DISPROPORTION

The birth passage includes the maternal bony pelvis, beginning at the pelvic inlet and ending at the pelvic outlet, and the maternal soft tissues within these anatomic areas. A contracture

(narrowed diameter) in any of the described areas can result in **cephalopelvic disproportion (CPD)** if the fetus is larger than the pelvic diameters. Abnormal fetal presentations and positions occur in CPD as the fetus moves to accommodate its passage through the maternal pelvis.

The gynecoid and anthropoid pelvic types are usually adequate for vertex birth, but the android and platypelloid types are predisposed to CPD. Certain combinations of types also can result in pelvic diameters inadequate for vertex birth. (See Chapter 17 🔗 for a description of pelvic types and their implications for childbirth.)

Types of Contractures

The pelvic inlet is contracted if the shortest anterior-posterior diameter is less than 10 cm or the greatest transverse diameter is less than 12 cm. The anterior-posterior diameter may be approximated by measuring the diagonal conjugate, which in the contracted inlet is less than 11.5 cm. Clinical and x-ray pelvimetry are used to determine the smallest anterior-posterior diameter through which the fetal head must pass.

The treatment goal is to allow the natural forces of labor to push the biparietal diameter of the fetal head beyond the potential interspinous obstruction. Although forceps may be used, they cause difficulty because pulling on the head destroys flexion, and the space is further diminished. A bulging perineum and crowning indicate that the obstruction has been passed.

An interischial tuberous diameter of less than 8 cm constitutes an outlet contracture. Outlet and midpelvic contractures frequently occur simultaneously. Whether vaginal birth can occur depends on the woman's interischial tuberous diameters and the fetal posteriosagittal diameter.

Risks of Cephalopelvic Disproportion

When CPD is present, the mother experiences prolonged labor. Membrane rupture can result from the force of the unequally distributed contractions being exerted on the fetal membranes. In obstructed labor, in which the fetus cannot descend, uterine rupture can occur. With delayed descent, necrosis of maternal soft tissues can result from pressure exerted by the fetal head. Eventually necrosis can cause fistulas from the vagina to other nearby structures. Difficult, forceps-assisted births can also result in damage to maternal soft tissue.

If the membranes rupture and the fetal head has not entered the inlet, there is a danger of cord prolapse. Excessive molding of the fetal head can result. Traumatic, forceps-assisted birth can damage the fetal skull and central nervous system.

Clinical Therapy

Fetopelvic relationships can be assessed by comparing pelvic measurements obtained by a manual examination before labor and by computed tomography (CT). An estimated weight of the fetus is obtained by ultrasound measurements.

When the pelvic diameters are borderline or questionable, a *trial of labor* (TOL) may be advised. In this process the woman continues to labor, and careful, frequent assessments of cervical dilatation and fetal descent are made. As long as there is continued progress, the TOL continues. If progress ceases, the decision for a cesarean birth is made.

Nursing Management

The adequacy of the maternal pelvis for a vaginal birth should be assessed both during and before labor. During the intrapartum assessment, the size of the fetus and its presentation, position, and lie must also be considered. (See Chapter 18 🔴 for intrapartum assessment techniques.)

The nurse should suspect CPD when labor is prolonged, cervical dilatation and effacement are slow, and engagement of the presenting part is delayed. The couple may need support in coping with the stresses of this complicated labor. Keep the couple informed of what is happening and explain the procedures being used. This knowledge reassures the couple that measures are being taken to resolve the problem.

Nursing actions during the TOL are similar to care during any labor except that cervical dilatation and fetal descent are assessed more frequently. Both contractions and the fetus should be monitored continuously. Report any signs of nonreassuring fetal status to the physician/CNM immediately.

The mother may be positioned in a variety of ways to increase the pelvic diameters. Sitting or squatting increases the outlet diameters and may be effective when there is failure of, or slow, fetal descent. Changing from one side to the other or maintaining a hands-and-knees position may assist the fetus in the occiput posterior position to change to an occiput anterior position. The mother may instinctively want to assume one of these positions. If not, the nurse can encourage a change of position.

CARE OF THE WOMAN WITH A COMPLICATION OF THE THIRD OR FOURTH STAGE OF LABOR

Common complications of the third and fourth stages of labor include retained placenta, lacerations, and placenta accreta.

Retained Placenta

Retention of the placenta beyond 30 minutes after birth is termed **retained placenta**. It occurs in 1 in 100 to 1 in 200 vaginal births (Benirschke, Burton, & Baergen, 2012). Bleeding as a result of a retained placenta can be excessive. If placenta expulsion does not occur, the physician/CNM attempts to remove the placenta manually. In women who do not have an epidural in place, intravenous sedation may be required because of the discomfort caused by the procedure. Failure to retrieve the placenta via manual removal usually necessitates surgical removal by curettage. If the woman does not have an epidural in place, the procedure can be performed under general anesthesia. Retained placenta may be a symptom of an accreta, increta, or percreta (to be discussed shortly).

Lacerations

Lacerations of the cervix or vagina may be indicated when bright-red vaginal bleeding persists in the presence of a well-contracted uterus. The incidence of lacerations is higher when the childbearing woman is young or a nullipara, has an epidural, has forceps-assisted birth and an episiotomy, and has not done perineal massage or preparation during pregnancy. Vaginal and perineal lacerations are often categorized in terms of degree, as follows:

- First-degree laceration is limited to the fourchette, perineal skin, and vaginal mucous membrane.

- Second-degree laceration involves the perineal skin, vaginal mucous membrane, underlying fascia, and muscles of the perineal body; it may extend upward on one or both sides of the vagina.

- Third-degree laceration extends through the perineal skin, vaginal mucous membranes, and perineal body and involves the anal sphincter; it may extend up the anterior wall of the rectum.

- Fourth-degree laceration is the same as third-degree but extends through the rectal mucosa to the lumen of the rectum; it may be called a third-degree laceration with a rectal wall extension.

Placenta Accreta

The chorionic villi attach directly to the myometrium of the uterus in *placenta accreta*. Two other types of placental adherence are *placenta increta*, in which the myometrium is invaded, and *placenta percreta*, in which the myometrium is penetrated. The adherence itself may be total, partial, or focal, depending on the amount of placental involvement. The incidence of placenta accreta is 1 in 533 births (Oyelese & Canterino, 2011). It is the most common type, accounting for almost three-fourths of adherent placentas.

The primary complication with placenta accreta is maternal hemorrhage and failure of the placenta to separate following birth of the infant. An abdominal hysterectomy may be necessary, depending on the amount and depth of involvement.

CARE OF THE WOMAN AND FETUS WITH PLACENTAL PROBLEMS

The most common types of placental problems—placenta previa and abruptio placentae—are discussed in Chapter 21 🔴. Other problems of the placenta are presented in Table 22–2.

CARE OF THE FAMILY EXPERIENCING PERINATAL LOSS

Perinatal loss is death of a fetus or infant from the time of conception through the end of the newborn period 28 days after birth. Spontaneous abortion (miscarriage) in the antepartum period is discussed in Chapter 16 🔴; this section discusses intrauterine fetal death (IUFD) after 20 weeks' gestation, often referred to as *stillbirth* or *fetal demise*.

Common Causes of Perinatal Loss

Antepartum fetal deaths, although infrequent, account for about half of all perinatal mortality in the United States. About 70% to 90%

Table 22–2   Placental and Umbilical Cord Variations

Placental Variation	Maternal Implications	Fetal/Neonatal Implications	
SUCCENTURIATE PLACENTA			
One or more accessory lobes of fetal villi will develop on the placenta.	Postpartum hemorrhage from retained lobe	None, as long as all parts of the placenta remain attached until after birth of the fetus	
CIRCUMVALLATE PLACENTA			
A double fold of chorion and amnion form a ring around the umbilical cord, on the fetal side of the placenta.	Increased incidence of late abortion, antepartum hemorrhage, and preterm labor	Intrauterine growth restriction, prematurity, fetal death	
BATTLEDORE PLACENTA			
The umbilical cord is inserted at or near the placental margin.	Increased incidence of preterm labor and bleeding	Prematurity, nonreassuring fetal status	
VELAMENTOUS INSERTION OF THE UMBILICAL CORD			
The vessels of the umbilical cord divide some distance from the placenta in the placental membranes.	Hemorrhage if one of the vessels is torn	Nonreassuring fetal status, hemorrhage	

of all stillbirths occur before the onset of labor, with more than half occurring between 20 and 28 weeks' gestation (Flenady et al., 2011). The cause may be unknown, or it may be related to fetal factors such as chromosomal disorders, birth defects, exposure to teratogens, infections, or complications of multiple gestation or fetal growth restriction; maternal factors such as chronic hypertension, preeclampsia or eclampsia, diabetes, advanced maternal age, Rh incompatibility, uterine rupture, or ascending maternal infection; or placental factors such as placenta previa, abruptio placentae, or a cord accident. In 25% of fetal deaths, the cause remains unknown even after autopsy (Flenady et al., 2011).

Perinatal loss in industrialized countries has declined in recent years as early diagnosis of congenital anomalies and advances in genetic testing techniques have increased the use of elective termination. Fetal death occurs more frequently in monochorionic twins and in pregnancies conceived by assisted reproductive technologies (Tsoumpou et al., 2011). Certain genetic testing procedures such as amniocentesis and chorionic villus sampling (CVS) can actually cause fetal loss.

In industrialized countries, maternal obesity, advanced maternal age, maternal smoking, primiparity, small-for-gestational-age (SGA) fetuses, abruptions, maternal hypertension, and diabetes are the most common etiologies of stillbirth (Flenady et al., 2011). In developing countries, infection plays a significant role in fetal deaths. Ascending bacterial organisms include *Escherichia coli*, Group B streptococci, and *Ureaplasma urealyticum*. These infections can occur either before or after the membranes have ruptured, resulting in fetal demise. Viral causes of fetal demise include parvovirus and coxsackievirus. *Toxoplasma gondii, Listeria monocytogenes,* and the organisms that cause leptospirosis, Q fever, and Lyme disease have also been identified as causative factors for stillbirth. Untreated syphilis is associated with a high stillborn rate as are malaria infections when contracted for the first time by the mother during pregnancy (Flenady et al., 2011). These infections carry a much higher morbidity and mortality rate in developing countries.

Certain maternal conditions can also be associated with higher rates of fetal death. Past maternal exposure to certain bacterial and viral antigens can produce an autoimmune response that can result in fetal death (Blackburn, 2013). Women with acquired and immune thrombophilia have higher rates of miscarriage and fetal demise than those without hematologic alterations (Helgadottir, Skjeldestad, Jacobsen, et al., 2011).

Maternal Physiologic Implications

Prolonged retention of the dead fetus may lead to the development of disseminated intravascular coagulation (DIC), also called consumption coagulopathy, in the mother. After the release of thromboplastin from the degenerating fetal tissues into the maternal bloodstream, the extrinsic clotting system is activated, triggering the formation of multiple tiny blood clots. Fibrinogen and factors V and VII are subsequently depleted, and the woman begins to display symptoms of DIC. Fibrinogen levels begin a linear descent 3 to 4 weeks after the death of the fetus and continue to decrease in the absence of appropriate medical intervention.

Besides DIC, other adverse outcomes can occur if the onset of labor and subsequent birth are delayed. Women with prolonged retention of a dead fetus are more prone to infection. A resulting infection can cause endometritis or sepsis. The longer the pregnancy continues, the higher the incidence of maternal infection.

Although immediate induction is routinely performed, there may be situations in which induction is delayed, such as maternal refusal or the presence of a multiple gestation. In these cases, fibrinogen levels are monitored weekly or biweekly to recognize and prevent progressive coagulopathy from occurring (Hanan, Al-Kadri, & Tamim, 2012).

Clinical Therapy

When fetal death has occurred, abdominal x-ray examination may reveal Spalding's sign, an overriding of the fetal cranial bones. In addition, maternal estriol levels fall. Diagnosis of IUFD is confirmed by absence of heart action on ultrasound. Without medical intervention, most women have spontaneous labor within 2 weeks of fetal death. The once common practice of waiting for the onset of labor has largely been abandoned in recent years since the risks of complications increase with delaying the birth. Prompt birth also increases the ability to identify the cause of death.

In modern practice, most women with a diagnosed fetal demise are given the option of waiting a few days or scheduling an induction procedure immediately. Most women will elect for an induction within a day or two of the final diagnosis. The mode of induction is dependent on the gestational age of the fetus, the readiness of the cervix, and previous mode of birth. In women who have had a previous cesarean birth, a repeat cesarean may be performed since the use of Pitocin or prostaglandin agents can increase the risk of a uterine rupture.

Women with an unfavorable cervix may be given vaginal prostaglandin agents, misoprostol, or laminaria tents. *Laminaria tents*, made from dried seaweed, work by drawing water out of the cervical tissue, allowing the cervix to soften and dilate. They are commonly used to dilate the cervix in preterm gestations when induction is warranted.

Women less than 28 weeks' gestation are typically given prostaglandin E$_2$ (PGE$_2$) vaginal suppositories every 4 to 6 hours or oral or vaginal misoprostol every 4 to 6 hours until spontaneous labor occurs (Spong & Dudley, 2011). Because PGE$_2$ suppositories can cause severe vomiting and diarrhea, women are commonly pretreated with antiemetic and antidiarrheal preparations to prevent or lessen these unpleasant side effects (Spong & Dudley, 2011).

Postbirth Evaluation

Identifying the causative factor of fetal loss assists many families in progressing through the grieving process. Information obtained from a postmortem examination or postmortem studies can provide vital information related to the cause of the fetal death, the possibility for reoccurrence, and closure for the couple. The types of studies and tests performed depend on the parents' past history, medical history, and preferences for the depth of testing desired. Chromosome studies should be considered if the couple has a history of other second- or third-trimester losses or if either parent has a suspected balanced translocation or mosaic chromosomal pattern (Spong & Dudley, 2011).

If an intra-amniotic infection is the suspected cause, cultures of both the placenta and the fetus should be obtained. If specific infections are being considered, both IgM and IgG antibodies should be drawn to determine if an acute infectious process has occurred.

All stillborn infants should have a careful visual inspection at the time of birth for obvious defects or abnormalities. The placenta and membranes should also be closely examined, and the placenta should be sent to pathology for further testing. The umbilical cord should be inspected for true knots, a velamentous insertion, lack of Wharton's jelly, or a short cord to determine if a cord accident was the cause. If a specific cause is suspected, blood tests and x-rays can be performed. An autopsy is the best mechanism to determine the cause of death; however, in the event that the parents decline an autopsy, magnetic resonance imaging (MRI) can also provide detailed information (Spong & Dudley, 2011).

Most practitioners perform a CBC and antibody screen upon admission. Because diabetes is a causative factor, a random or postpartum glucose level can be obtained to rule out this cause. Additional maternal factors that can also be evaluated are listed in Table 22–3.

Phases of Grief

Grief is an individual's total response to a loss, including physical symptoms, thoughts, feelings, functional limitations, and spiritual reactions. It may be manifested by certain behaviors and rituals of *mourning*, such as weeping or visiting a gravesite, which help the person experience, accept, and adjust to the loss. The period of adjustment to loss is known as *bereavement*. (*Note:* Grief as it relates to the birth of an at-risk newborn is discussed in Chapter 31 .)

The behaviors that couples exhibit while mourning may be associated with the five stages of grieving described in *On Death and Dying* (Kubler-Ross, 1969). Often the first stage is *denial* of the death of the fetus. Even when the initial healthcare provider suspects fetal demise, the couple is hoping that a second opinion may be different. Some couples may not be convinced of the death until they see and hold the stillborn infant after birth. The second stage is *anger,* resulting from feelings of loss, loneliness, and perhaps guilt. The anger may be projected at significant others and healthcare team members, or it may be absent when the death is sudden and unexpected. The mother may attempt to identify a specific event that caused the death and may blame herself. *Bargaining,* the third stage, may or may not be present, depending on the couple's preparation for the death of the fetus. If the death is unanticipated, the couple may not have time for bargaining. When the death is expected, such as in the case of a known lethal congenital anomaly, bargaining is more commonly seen. It is marked by the couple making mental trade-offs in exchange for the fetus being healthy. In the fourth stage, *depression* is evidenced by preoccupation, weeping, and withdrawal. Changing hormonal levels in the first 24 to 48 hours after birth may compound the depression and associated grief.

The final stage, *acceptance,* surfaces when resolution occurs. This stage is highly individualized and may take months to years to complete.

Maternal Death

Maternal death is defined by the World Health Organization (WHO) as "the death of a woman while pregnant or within 42 days of termination of pregnancy, irrespective of the duration and the site of the pregnancy, from any cause related to or aggravated by the pregnancy or its management, but not from accidental or incidental causes" (2012). The most common causes of maternal death are hemorrhage, hypertensive disorders, embolism, infection, and preexisting chronic conditions, such as diabetes and cardiovascular disease. Obesity is also becoming a significant factor in maternal deaths because of the medical conditions that result (Joint Commission, 2010). The national maternal mortality rate was 13.2 deaths per 100,000 live births (Heron et al., 2009). A recent number of reports indicate that maternal mortality may be rising in the United States, although there has been a change in the classification system that may have resulted in the identification of more deaths as pregnancy related (WHO, 2012). The numbers of maternal deaths are certainly not decreasing, however, and the death of even one mother on a perinatal unit can be a devastating experience for all involved.

For the husband, or father of the child, the death of his partner is shocking (even if she had previous medical problems) and traumatic. There is an even deeper shock presenting here, in that the

Table 22–3	Tests to Determine Cause of Fetal Loss
Fetal Testing	**Maternal Testing**
Fetal blood tests and x-rays	Diabetes testing
Autopsy or MRI	CBC with platelet count
Placental studies	Kleihauer-Betke test
Chromosomal studies (if indicated)	Abnormal antibody testing (lupus anticoagulant, anticardiolipin antibodies)
	TSH levels
	Infectious disease testing (rubella, syphilis, malaria, toxoplasmosis, cytomegalovirus)
	Hereditary thrombophilia testing
	Toxicology testing

Clinical Tip

No matter who you are or how much nursing experience you have, when an expectant family is in pain because of their loss, it can be difficult to know the right thing to say. A good start is to say "I'm so sorry, I don't know what to say." The nurse can play a therapeutic role by sitting quietly with the mother, holding her hand, and speaking of the beauty of the baby's fingers, toes, and hair, and other specific characteristics of the baby.

death is surrounding an expectedly joyous event, a birth. The grieving process is complicated by a number of factors (such as possibly caring for the newborn infant while grieving his partner) and too comprehensive a topic for this text. What is important for nurses caring for the father and/or other family members is to recognize that initial grief reactions may be extremely intense. As long as no one is violating the foundational principles of grief reaction (i.e., not hurting themselves, others, or personal property), the father and family should be fully supported through this initial time with all support available to them and the facility in which the nurse is practicing. Interactions should be brief and direct, such as offering tissues and straightforward condolences (i.e. "I'm so sorry this is happening to you"). As with all losses, it is important to resist offering explanations or platitudes. There are no adequate explanations and platitudes are not helpful and, in most cases, prove harmful.

For the staff, a maternal death on the perinatal unit can be traumatic as well. When a death occurs on any unit, there are individual as well as group reactions to the event (Garko, 2007). The individual nurses involved may experience feelings of shock, sadness, anger, guilt, and other grief-associated reactions. The unit as a whole may experience feelings of inadequacy, anger, guilt, confusion, and depression. For the nurses directly involved, the father and family must still be cared for and for everyone on the unit, nursing care continues.

It is important for management in these situations to step in and provide an opportunity for the staff to express their feelings in a safe environment. Intervention for the staff could include professional debriefing or, where professional assistance is not available, simply calling a staff meeting to allow the nurses to work through some of the emotions while supporting one another (Dietz, 2009; Garko, 2007). The most important thing for the nurse to remember is to take care of his or her own grief reactions and allow time for personal healing. Focusing on the positive aspects of the situation where they exist (such as personal kindness shown to the mother before the death, or to the family in the aftermath) is an important step in the healing process as well as reflecting objectively on those things out of one's personal control (the mother's underlying medical issues or unforeseen complications). The idea, as with the loss of an infant, is to eventually memorialize the event with a balanced perspective, recognizing where personal effectiveness as well as limitations exists and learning to live with them, both personally and professionally.

NURSING MANAGEMENT *For the Family Experiencing Perinatal Death*

Nursing Assessment and Diagnosis

Cessation of fetal movement reported by the mother to the nurse is frequently the first indication of fetal death. It is followed by a gradual decrease in the signs and symptoms of pregnancy. Fetal heart tones are absent, and fetal movement is no longer palpable. Once fetal demise has been established, assess the family members' ability to adapt to their loss. Open communication between the mother, her partner, and the healthcare team members contributes to a realistic understanding of the medical condition and its associated treatments. Discuss prior experiences the family has had with loss and what they feel were their perceived coping abilities at that time. Identifying the family's social supports and resources is also important.

Perinatal loss may also occur in the intrapartum period as a result of an intrapartum complication, such as an unresolved shoulder dystocia, prolapsed umbilical cord, abruptio placentae, or other complication. In such emergency situations, healthcare team members often focus on the physical needs of the mother and an attempt to save the fetus's life. Commonly, the family is not informed that a perinatal death has occurred until the infant is born. Thus, the parents are faced with the sudden and completely unanticipated death of their infant. The most common reaction is protest or disbelief.

Although the physician/CNM informs the family of the death, the nurse continues one-on-one care with the family, providing both physical and emotional support throughout this crucial period. Assist the family members in the grief process and explore their immediate wishes for viewing and holding their deceased child.

Nursing diagnoses that may apply include the following (NANDA-I © 2012):

- *Grieving* related to imminent loss of a child
- *Coping: Family, Compromised,* related to the death of a child/unresolved feelings regarding perinatal loss
- *Hopelessness* related to sudden, unexpected fetal loss
- *Spiritual Distress*, *Risk for,* related to intense suffering secondary to unexpected fetal loss

Planning and Implementation

Most facilities have an established protocol to follow in the event of perinatal death. The protocol typically provides a holistic focus for family-centered nursing care. It is important for the entire healthcare team to be notified so collaborative care can be initiated. When fetal death has been confirmed before admission, the entire staff on the unit is informed so they can avoid making inappropriate remarks. Many facilities have a symbol, such as a card with a leaf, heart, or cluster of flowers, that is placed on the mother's door so all staff members are aware of the loss (Figure 22–11 ●).

Preparing the Family for the Birth

On arrival at the facility, the couple with a known or suspected fetal demise should immediately be placed in a private room. When possible the woman should be in a room that is farthest away from other laboring women. Take care not to leave the

● **Figure 22–11** Door card.

Source: ©Share Pregnancy & Infant Loss Support, Inc. www.nationalshare.org.

couple in the waiting room with other expectant parents or visitors waiting for news from other women in labor.

The couple should be allowed to remain together as much as they wish. Provide privacy as needed and maintain a supportive environment. Give the couple complete information about what to expect and what will happen. Encourage and answer questions. Stay with the couple so they do not feel alone and isolated; however, continuously assess cues from the couple that they want to be alone. Some couples may want outside support, such as family members or friends, to be present during the labor. Facilitate the couple's wishes.

When possible the same nurse should provide care for the couple so a therapeutic relationship can be established. As the relationship develops, provide solace by listening to the couple without offering commentary. Also provide ongoing opportunities for the couple to ask questions. It is not uncommon for the family to ask the same questions repeatedly as part of the initial grief process. Provide clear explanations and straightforward answers.

Consider cultural factors in providing care. Although not everyone from a given culture responds to loss in the same way, responses to fetal death are often influenced by cultural and personal beliefs. Similarly, responses to loss may be influenced by spiritual beliefs. In considering religious practices, it is prudent simply to ask the family how they can best be helped to meet their religious needs. Some families may desire to see a spiritual adviser. If so, offer to contact the hospital chaplain or another cleric for them. It is important to let the family process their own beliefs and feelings about the meaning, purpose, and significance of the life and death of their infant.

If a grief counselor is available, arrange an initial interaction with the couple if they are willing. A social worker is commonly involved. Coordinate members of the collaborative care team so a comprehensive plan of care can be initiated.

Explain details of the plan of care and allow the family to ask questions and make decisions for their labor and birth preferences. Review the availability of anesthesia and analgesia. The woman typically can have pain medication whenever she desires. Facilitate the participation of the woman and her partner in the labor and birth process.

Remember that, in contrast to a typical birth experience, the birth of a stillborn infant marks both the beginning and the end. It is imperative that the couple and family have all wishes and preferences respected. However, the family may have difficulty making decisions during this period. Assist the couple to explore their feelings and help them to make decisions about who is present and what rituals will occur during and following the birth. Examples of birth preferences include the following:

- Use of music, dimmed lighting, or other environmental preferences
- Laboring or birthing in a specific position
- Having the infant placed on the mother's chest immediately after birth
- Allowing the father to cut the umbilical cord
- Presence of other family members or friends at the birth

> ### Developing Cultural Competence
> **Grief Responses and Interactions**
>
> - Cultures that are stoic in nature can be difficult to assist. Stoicism may stem from family or cultural background, shock, or denial. It is important to ascertain the underlying reason so that appropriate interventions, where warranted, can occur.
> - In male-dominant cultures, mothers experiencing perinatal loss may tend to focus on their "failure" as a woman to successfully reproduce. Reassure these women (while respecting cultural beliefs) that nothing they did or did not do affected the outcome. A reiteration of known medical causes may be helpful.
> - In cultures in which the extended family is the couple's main source of support, it is important to allow as much interaction with family members as possible. In cultures where privacy is valued above all, help the family limit visitors if that is their preference.
> - Avoidance is not therapeutic. If you are not certain what the family needs, simply ask them how you can help to accommodate their wishes. Families appreciate an honest and caring attitude.

Sometimes couples worry that others may view their preferences as "strange" or "wrong." Reassure the family that it is their experience and that there are no right or wrong feelings or wishes.

The couple may have waves of overwhelming grief, disbelief, or sadness. Encourage the couple to experience the grief that they feel. It is not uncommon for one partner to attempt to put on a "brave front," feeling that by showing grief he or she will make the other partner feel worse. It is also not uncommon for partners to have intense feelings that they are unable to share. Encourage partners to express their emotions freely to the extent they are able. Help them understand that they may each experience different feelings.

Supporting the Family in Viewing the Stillborn Infant

Advocates of seeing the stillborn infant believe that viewing assists in dispelling denial and enables the couple to progress to the next step in the grieving process. If they choose to see their stillborn infant, prepare the couple for what they will see by saying "She is going to feel cold," "He is going to be blue," or other appropriate statements. If the parents have shared with you the name they had chosen for their baby, use that name in discussing the baby, for example, "Jessie's face is bruised." Another common practice is to wrap the infant in a blanket or apply a hat to cover birth defects. This allows the parents an opportunity to view the infant before seeing the birth defect. Most parents will eventually remove the covering to inspect the infant; however, applying a covering allows them time to adjust to the appearance at their own pace.

Some families will hold their infant for a short time before returning him or her to the nurse, whereas others will wish to spend a great deal of time with their infant. Allow the infant to remain with the family for as long as the family desires. Some parents may elect to bathe or dress their stillborn baby; support them in their choice. Some couples may want other family members, friends, or their other children to see the infant. Act as an advocate to ensure that the family's wishes are respected.

Providing Discharge Care

Most facilities prepare a remembrance box or package for the family to take home. This typically consists of a photograph taken of the infant or the family, a card with the baby's footprints, a crib card, identification band, a lock of hair, and possibly a blanket or clothing worn by the infant. In the event that the couple declines the package, it is common for the hospital to retain these items for a specific period in case they change their minds.

After the birth, give the option of an early discharge (as early as 6 to 8 hours after the birth) to the couple. Facility protocol will dictate where mothers are transferred after a perinatal loss. Some hospitals have the women remain on the birthing unit; others give the mother the option of choosing a postpartum room or one on a medical unit. If the mother is transferred to a postpartum room, select a room for her that is far away from other rooms and the newborn nursery. It is imperative that all staff members, as well as student nurses, be notified of the mother's status.

Include information on the grief process in discharge information (Figure 22–12 ●). Prepare the couple to return home by stressing that others may not know what to say, and that even loved ones may make inappropriate comments because they do not know how to respond to grief and loss. This can prepare the couple for the reactions of others. If there are siblings, each will usually progress through age-appropriate grieving. Provide the parents with information about normal mourning reactions, both psychologic and physiologic.

When caring for a family suffering from a perinatal loss, it is important to remember that the nurse experiences many of the same grief reactions as the parents of a stillborn infant. It is important to have colleagues and family members available for counseling and support.

Facilitating the Family's Grief Work

The parents of a stillborn infant suffer a devastating experience that precipitates an intense emotional trauma. During pregnancy the couple has already begun the attachment process, which now must be ended through the grieving process. Facilitating the family's grief work is thus a critical nursing intervention—one that requires skill, sensitivity, and compassion.

Following discharge, some families may need closure of the intrapartum event in order to continue their grief work. A consultation can be scheduled with the practitioner who cared for them during the pregnancy and birth. Families may also wish to read the results of tests performed during the intrapartum period and the autopsy report. Provide a copy of the medical record to the couple and encourage them to ask questions, express their feelings, and ask for clarification.

Families are routinely referred for counseling services after a perinatal loss has occurred. A counselor who specializes in perinatal issues can provide expertise and assist the couple in their grieving. Partners should be allowed to verbalize fears and concerns about future pregnancies. When appropriate, also provide referrals to genetic counselors, religious support persons, and social service agencies.

Besides referral information, the woman should receive scheduled, follow-up phone calls to assess the family's functioning and their progress with grief work. Use these follow-up phone calls to provide pertinent information and identify additional resources for the family.

As the grief process ensues, encourage families to implement cultural, religious, or social customs that will assist them in grieving and mourning. Advise the family that certain upcoming milestones, such as holidays, future birthdays, baby showers, Mother's Day, Father's Day, and other social events may trigger their grief. The family can better cope with these events if they are adequately prepared.

Referring the Family to Community Services

Although most facilities have an established protocol for families experiencing perinatal loss, more comprehensive intervention programs are being established in communities to assist these families. Community support groups that focus on perinatal loss can provide an important support network and resources. Specialized groups, such as those focused on early pregnancy loss, stillbirth, and perinatal loss associated with specific congenital anomalies, allow families the opportunity to interact with peers who have lost infants under similar circumstances. Provide the group name, contact person (if possible), and phone number. Various books written by mothers who have lost children are available in bookstores and are valuable resources for grieving parents.

Internet technology has allowed large numbers of individuals to share resources and information and to participate in online support groups. Internet resources can be effective for all families and may be the only resources available for families in rural, underserved areas.

Specialized community outreach programs are another resource that can provide assistance to grieving families; some provide early counseling to parents whose fetus has a known lethal congenital anomaly. In perinatal hospice programs, parents

● **Figure 22–12** Bereavement literature.

Source: Share Pregnancy & Infant Loss, Inc.

are given the opportunity to explore options, such as elective termination or waiting for the onset of spontaneous labor or a medically indicated induced labor. For families wishing to continue their pregnancies, the program typically assigns a multidisciplinary team who provides compassionate care, ongoing counseling, referral to support groups, and spiritual guidance (Ramer-Chrastek & Thygesen, 2005).

Care of the Couple Who Has Experienced Loss in a Previous Pregnancy

Couples who have had previous perinatal loss typically enter a subsequent pregnancy with conflicting feelings and may experience ambivalence, fear, and anxiety. Many times, their past experience is relived when another pregnancy occurs. Some couples conceive soon after a loss, while others wait years. Some couples enter a subsequent pregnancy with grief work largely completed while others are still experiencing unresolved grief.

The nurse caring for a couple who has had a previous loss needs to be kind, compassionate, and patient. Couples need specific information and clear explanations of all prenatal information. Make referrals to genetic counselors when appropriate. Some couples may wish to have a consultation with a perinatologist. If unresolved grief issues are present or the family experiences extreme anxiety, counseling may be beneficial.

Interventions to decrease anxiety can help the couple tremendously. At the first visit, an early ultrasound can be performed to verify the presence of the fetal heart. In early pregnancy, women may be fearful when first-trimester pregnancy symptoms begin to resolve. It may be helpful for these women to come in for weekly visits for a period of time simply to hear the fetal heartbeat. This intervention may continue to be helpful until the woman begins to feel fetal movement. Throughout the pregnancy, the office or clinic nurse can play a key role by providing reassurance and answering questions that the woman may have.

Women with a previous loss typically receive additional antepartum testing throughout the pregnancy. Ultrasounds can be used to provide reassurance and assess fetal growth and development, placental functioning, and cord variations. Nonstress testing and biophysical profiles can be performed weekly after 32 weeks to ensure fetal well-being. Fetal kick counts should be initiated at 28 weeks and continue until the birth occurs. Women with a previous loss should give birth at their expected date of birth or when the pregnancy is at term and should not go over their due date, since placental functioning can decline in postdate pregnancies.

Evaluation

Expected outcomes of nursing care for the family experiencing perinatal loss include the following:

- Family members express their feelings about the death of their baby.
- Family members participate in the decision making regarding preferences for the labor, birth, and the immediate postpartum period.
- Family members participate in the decision of whether to see their baby and other decisions about the baby.
- The family has resources available for continued support.
- Family members know the community resources available and have names and phone numbers to use if they choose.
- The family is moving into and through the grieving process.

Critical Concept Review

LEARNING OUTCOME 22.1: Compare tachysystolic and hypotonic labor patterns, including the risks, clinical therapy, and nursing management.

1. Tachysystolic labor patterns:
   - Characterized by increased frequency but decreased effectiveness of contraction in effacing and dilating the cervix. Usually leads to a prolonged latent phase.
   - May cause mother to become fatigued and have difficulty coping with stress of labor.
   - Pattern may cause prolonged pressure on the fetal head.
   - Clinical therapy may involve sedation, pain medication, and bed rest. Pitocin may be given only if CPD and fetal malpresentation are ruled out.
   - Nursing management includes decreasing environmental stimuli, decreasing anxiety, and promoting comfort.

2. Hypotonic labor patterns:
   - Characterized by less than two or three contractions in a 10-minute period during the active phase of labor.
   - Mother may experience fatigue and coping difficulties.
   - Mother is at risk for intrauterine infection and postpartum hemorrhage.
   - Fetus is at risk for sepsis.
   - Clinical therapy includes assessment of adequacy of pelvic measurement and fetal maturity; the use of Pitocin or nipple stimulation once CPD and fetal malpresentation are ruled out.
   - Nursing management includes close monitoring for signs and symptoms of infection and dehydration, and keeping vaginal exams to a minimum.

LEARNING OUTCOME 22.2: Describe the risks and clinical therapy in determining the nursing management of postterm pregnancy on the childbearing family.

1. Postterm pregnancy may result in an increased possibility of:
   - Probable labor induction.
   - Forceps or vacuum-assisted or cesarean birth.
   - Decreased perfusion to the placenta.
   - Decreased amount of amniotic fluid and possible cord compression.
   - Increased possibility of meconium aspiration.
   - Increased risk for macrosomia or a loss of fat and muscle mass resulting in small-for-gestational age (SGA).

LEARNING OUTCOME 22.3: Relate the various types of fetal malposition and malpresentation to the nursing management for each.

1. Occiput posterior position:
   - Baby is face up instead of face down as it enters the vagina.
   - May prolong labor.
   - Baby is usually able to be born vaginally but may need forceps assistance to turn baby.
2. Brow presentation:
   - Forehead of the fetus becomes the presenting part.
   - May cause labor to be prolonged.
   - Cesarean birth necessary if brow presentation persists.

3. Face presentation:
   - Face of the fetus is the presenting part.
   - Vaginal birth may be possible, but cesarean birth remains a significant possibility.
4. Breech presentation:
   - Fetal buttocks or foot/feet are the presenting part.
   - Ninety percent of breech presentations result in cesarean birth.
5. Transverse lie:
   - Fetal shoulder is the presenting part.
   - Fetus must be born by cesarean.

LEARNING OUTCOME 22.4: Explain the identification, risks, and clinical therapy in determining the nursing management of the woman and fetus at risk for fetal macrosomia.

1. Identification of fetal macrosomia is conducted through:
   - Palpation of fetus in utero.
   - Ultrasound of fetus.
   - X-ray pelvimetry.
2. Management of fetal macrosomia involves the following:
   - Cesarean birth performed if fetus is greater than 4500 g.
   - Continuous fetal monitoring if labor is allowed to progress.
   - Notification of physician for early decelerations, labor dysfunction, or nonreassuring fetal status.

3. Care of newborn with macrosomia requires:
   - Assessment of newborn for cephalohematoma, Erb's palsy, and fractured clavicles.
4. Care of the mother after birth of newborn with macrosomia requires:
   - Fundal massage to prevent maternal hemorrhage from overstretched uterus.
   - Close monitoring of vital signs.

LEARNING OUTCOME 22.5: Relate the maternal implications, clinical therapy, prenatal history, and conditions that may be associated with nonreassuring fetal status to the nursing management of the mother and fetus.

1. Nursing actions (intrauterine resuscitation) include:
   - Turn the woman to left lateral position to treat hypotension.
   - Begin or increase IV flow rate.
   - Perform vaginal exam to check for cord prolapse.
   - Have woman assume knee–chest position if cord prolapse is suspected.
   - Discontinue Pitocin or administer a tocolytic agent to decrease contraction frequency and intensity.
   - Administer oxygen.
   - Notify physician.
   - Obtain additional information about fetus by fetal scalp blood sampling or fetal acoustical stimulation.

LEARNING OUTCOME 22.6: Describe the nursing management of the mother and fetus with a prolapsed umbilical cord.

1. Umbilical cord precedes fetal presenting part, placing pressure on cord and diminishing blood flow to the fetus.
2. Bed rest is recommended if engagement has not occurred and membranes have ruptured.
3. Assess for nonreassuring fetal status.

LEARNING OUTCOME 22.7: Summarize the identification, maternal and fetal/neonatal implications, clinical therapy, and nursing management of the woman with amniotic fluid embolism (anaphylactoid syndrome of pregnancy).

1. Amniotic fluid embolism:
   - Caused by a small tear in the chorion or amnion high in the uterus, which may allow amniotic fluid to enter the maternal circulatory system.
   - Usually occurs during or after birth.
   - The woman experiences sudden symptoms of respiratory distress leading to severe hemorrhage.
   - This disorder is life threatening, so medical management and nursing care are aimed at delivering lifesaving treatments such as CPR and transfusion until the woman is stabilized.

LEARNING OUTCOME 22.8: Explain the types, maternal and fetal/neonatal implications, and clinical therapy in determining the nursing management of the woman with cephalopelvic disproportion.

1. Labor is usually prolonged in the presence of CPD.
2. Vaginal birth may be possible depending on the type of CPD.
3. Woman may increase pelvic diameter during labor by squatting, sitting, rolling from side to side, or maintaining a knee–chest position.
4. CPD may make cesarean birth the only available method of birth.

LEARNING OUTCOME 22.9: Identify common complications of the third and fourth stages of labor.

1. The most common complications are:
   - Retained placenta:
     - If not expelled, the placenta must be manually removed from the uterus.
   - Lacerations:
     - Suspected when there is bright-red bleeding in the presence of a contracted uterus.
     - Usually repaired immediately after birth of child.
   - Placenta accreta:
     - In this condition, the chorionic villi attach directly to the myometrium of the uterus.
     - May result in maternal hemorrhage and failure of the placenta to separate from the uterus.
     - May result in the need for hysterectomy at time of birth.

LEARNING OUTCOME 22.10: Explain the etiology, diagnosis, and phases of grief in determining the nursing management of the family experiencing perinatal loss.

1. Perinatal loss results from three factors:
   - Fetal factors: The fetus has or develops a disorder that is incompatible with life.
   - Maternal factors: The mother has a disorder such as diabetes or preeclampsia that creates a hostile environment for the fetus.
   - Placental or other factors: Certain conditions such as abruptio placentae or cord accident cut off blood supply to the fetus, leading to death.
2. Diagnosis may be made when the mother notices lack of movement in the fetus or at a regularly scheduled physician's visit when a fetal heart tone cannot be found.

3. Nursing care involves supporting the family through the grief work:
   - Assist the family through the labor and birth.
   - Provide for the woman's physical needs after the birth.
   - Encourage family members to express and share their thoughts and feelings about the loss.
   - Give the family an opportunity to view, hold, and name the infant.
   - Prepare items for the family to keep to remember the infant.
   - Provide opportunities for religious or spiritual counseling and cultural practices.
   - Visit or phone the family after discharge to assist in closure.
   - Make referrals to appropriate perinatal loss counseling services if indicated.

Clinical Reasoning in Action

June Dice, a 25-year-old G3P1011, is admitted to you in labor and delivery at 38 weeks with a moderate amount of dark red vaginal bleeding. June's prenatal history is significant for late prenatal care (20 weeks' gestation by ultrasound) and cocaine abuse. An ultrasound is done upon admission that demonstrates a marginal placenta abruption. You place June on the fetal monitor and observe a fetal heart rate baseline of 146 to 155 with accelerations to 166 with fetal movement. There are occasional mild variable decelerations with a quick return to baseline. Contraction pattern is interpreted as an irritable uterus. An intravenous infusion with Ringer's lactate is started with a #18 intracath. June's vital signs are within normal limits. Her hematocrit is 29%. You assist the physician with a vaginal exam to rupture membranes and insert a fetal scalp electrode and intrauterine pressure catheter. A small amount of light yellow-green amniotic fluid is observed. The exam shows June is 4 cm dilated, 50% effaced, vertex at −1 station. You follow protocol and start an oxytocin induction/augmentation. June is asking why oxytocin is needed.

1. Explain the goal of labor induction/augmentation in response to June's question.
2. Explain potential risk factors associated with oxytocin induction of labor.
3. You observe a nonreassuring fetal heart rate of 144 to 150 beats/min with decreased variability, and persistent late decelerations with each contraction. What interventions would you immediately take?
4. What supportive actions are taken to decrease the risk of hypofibrinogenemia?
5. What complications might be present in the newborn at birth?
6. Create a concept map for June's care based on the presence of marginal placenta abruption, history of cocaine abuse, maternal anemia, and presence of meconium-stained amniotic fluid. June is also undergoing Pitocin augmentation, which should be incorporated into the concept map as well.

See www.nursing.pearsonhighered.com for possible responses and an interactive template for a concept map.

References

American College of Obstetricians and Gynecologists. (2010). *Mode of term singleton breech delivery* (ACOG Committee Opinion No. 340). Washington, DC: Author.

Benirschke, K., Burton, G., & Baergen, R. (2012). Involution of implantation site: Retained placenta. *Pathology of the Human Placenta*, 241–248. doi:10.1007/978-3-642-23941-0_10

Blackburn, S. T. (2013). *Maternal, fetal, & neonatal physiology: A clinical perspective* (4th ed.). St. Louis, MO: Saunders.

Caughley, A. B. (2011). Postterm pregnancy. *eMedicine.* Retrieved from http://emedicine.medscape.com/article/261369-overview#aw2aab6b6

Coyle, M. E., Smith, C. A., & Peat, B. (2012). Cephalic version by moxibustion for breech presentation. *Cochrane Database of Systematic Reviews,* Issue 5. Art. No.: CD003928. doi:10.1002/14651858.CD003928.pub3

Cunningham, F. G., Leveno, K. J., Bloom, S. L., Hauth, J. C., Rouse, D. J., & Spong, C. Y. (2010).

Williams' obstetrics (23rd ed.). New York, NY: McGraw-Hill Medical.

Dietz, D. (2009). Debriefing to help perinatal nurses cope with a maternal loss. *Maternal Child Health, 34*(4), 243–248. doi:10.1097/01.NMC.0000357917.41100.c5

Flenady, V., Koopmans, L., Middleton, P., Frøen, J. F., Smith, G. C., Gibbons, K., . . . Ezzeti, M. (2011). Major risk factors for stillbirth in high-income countries: A systematic review and meta-analysis.

The Lancet, 377(9774), 1331–1340. doi:10.1016/S0140-6736(10)62233-7

Garko, C. (2007). Painful lessons: When a mother dies, staff must grieve—and then learn. *Nursing for Women's Health, 11*(4), 357–361.

Gupta, S. (2011). *A comprehensive textbook of obstetrics and gynecology.* New Delhi, India: Jaypee Brothers Publishing.

Hanan, M., Al-Kadri, F., & Tamim, H. (2012). Factors contributing to intra-uterine fetal death. *Archives of Gynecology and Obstetrics.* doi:10.1007/s00404-012-2426-z

Helgadottir, L. B., Skjeldestad, F. E., Jacobsen, A. F., Sandset, P. M., & Jacobsen, E. M. (2011). The association of inherited thrombophilia and intrauterine fetal death: A case-control study. *Blood Coagulation & Fibrinolysis, 22*(8), 651–656.

Heron, M. P., Hoyert, D. L., Murphy, S. L., Xu, J., Kochanek, K. D., & Tejada-Vera, B. (2009). Deaths: Final data for 2006. *National Vital Statistics Report,* 57(14). Retrieved from www.cdc.gov/nchs/data/nvsr/nvsr57/nvsr57_14.pdf

Jazayeri, A. (2010). Macrosomia. *eMedicine.* Retrieved from http://emedicine.medscape.com/article/262679-overview

Joint Commission. (2010). Preventing maternal death. *Sentinel Event Alert,* (44). Retrieved from http://www.jointcommission.org/SentinelEvents/SentinelEventAlert/sea_44.htm

Kubler-Ross, E. (1969). *On death and dying.* New York, NY: Macmillan.

Mandruzzato, G., Alfirevic, A., Chervenak, F., Gruenebaum, A., Heimstad, R., Heinonen, S., . . . Thilaganathan, B. (2010). Guidelines for the management of postterm pregnancy. *Journal of Perinatal Medicine, 38*(2010), 111–119.

Oyelese, Y., & Canterino, J. C. (2011). Placenta previa and placenta accrete. *Bleeding During Pregnancy* (Part 3), 135–150. doi:10.1007/978-1-4419-9810-1_8

Ramer-Chrastek, J., & Thygesen, N. V. (2005). A perinatal hospice for an unborn child with a life-limiting condition. *International Journal of Palliative Nursing, 11*(6), 274–276.

Simkin, P. (2011). *The labor progress handbook: Early interventions to prevent and treat dystocia.* London, UK: Wiley Publications.

Spong, C., & Dudley, D. J. (2011). Medical management including delivery. In *Stillbirth: Prediction, prevention and management.* Oxford, UK: Wiley-Blackwell. doi:10.1002/9781444398038.ch14

Tsoumpou, I., Mohamed, A. M., Tower, C., Roberts, S. A., & Nardo, L. C., (2011). Failed IVF cycles and the risk of subsequent preeclampsia or fetal growth restriction: A case-control exploratory study. *Fertility and Sterility, 95*(3), 973–978. doi:10.1016/j.fertnstert.2010.07.1053

World Health Organization. (2012). *Maternal mortality.* Retrieved from http://www.who.int/mediacentre/factsheets/fs348/en/index.html

Birth-Related Procedures

With our first baby, all of a sudden I had to have a cesarean. Everything happened so fast but our son was OK, and that's all that mattered. With our second baby, I wanted to try a vaginal birth. Even though I wanted to, I was afraid. I don't know what I would have done without my nurse. She stayed with me the whole time and kept giving me support. She explained what was happening and gave encouragement. I felt safe. I had a beautiful baby girl after 8 hours of labor. —Marianne, 22

Larry D. Gordon/Getty Images

LEARNING OUTCOMES

23.1 Explain the methods, purpose, and contraindications of external and podalic versions that determine nursing management.

23.2 Describe the use of amniotomy in the nursing management of the woman and fetus.

23.3 Compare the methods for inducing labor, explaining their advantages and disadvantages in determining the nursing management of women during labor induction.

23.4 Describe the measures to prevent episiotomy, the types of episiotomy performed, and the associated nursing management.

23.5 Explain the indications and maternal and neonatal risks that impact nursing management during forceps-assisted birth.

23.6 Describe the use of and risk of vacuum extraction to assist birth.

23.7 Explain the indications for cesarean birth, impact on the family unit, preparation and teaching needs, and associated nursing management.

23.8 Examine the risks, guidelines, and nursing management of the woman undergoing trial of labor after cesarean.

Most births occur without the need for operative obstetric intervention. In some instances, however, procedures are necessary to maintain the safety of the woman and the fetus. The most common of these procedures are version, amniotomy, amnioinfusion, cervical ripening, induction of labor, episiotomy, forceps- or vacuum-assisted birth, cesarean birth, and vaginal birth following a previous cesarean birth.

Generally, women are aware of the possible need for an obstetric procedure during their labor and birth. However, some women expect to have a "natural" experience and feel disappointed, angry, or even guilty when an unanticipated procedure is needed. This conflict between expectation and the need for intervention presents a challenge to maternity nurses. The nurse provides information regarding any procedure to help the woman and her partner understand what is proposed, the anticipated benefits and possible risks, and any alternatives.

CARE OF THE WOMAN DURING VERSION

Version, or turning the fetus, is a procedure used to change the fetal presentation by abdominal or intrauterine manipulation. The most common type of version is **external cephalic version (ECV)**, in which the fetus is changed from a breech to a cephalic presentation by external manipulation of the maternal abdomen (Figure 23–1 ●). A less common type of version, called **podalic version**, is used only with the second fetus during a vaginal twin birth and only if the twin does not descend readily or if the heart rate is nonreassuring. The use of podalic versions is declining as more women with a second twin in a non-vertex presentation are counseled to undergo a cesarean birth (Webster & Loughley, 2011). The success rates of ECV in singleton pregnancies averages approximately 50% with ranges from 35% to 86% (Ehrenberg-Buchner, 2011).

Criteria for External Cephalic Version

If breech or shoulder presentation (transverse lie) is detected in the later weeks of pregnancy, an external cephalic version may be attempted. Before the ECV is begun, an ultrasound is used to locate the placenta and to confirm fetal presentation.

The following criteria should be met before performing external version:

- The pregnancy is at 36 or more weeks of gestation. A version may result in complications that require immediate birth by cesarean (Ehrenberg-Buchner, 2011).
- A nonstress test (NST), obtained immediately before performing the version, is reactive. A reactive NST indicates fetal well-being.
- The fetal breech is not engaged. Once the presenting part is engaged, it is difficult—if not impossible—to do a version.

Contraindications for External Version

Contraindications include the following:

- Maternal problems, such as uterine anomalies, uncontrolled preeclampsia, or third-trimester bleeding
- Complications of pregnancy, such as rupture of membranes, oligohydramnios, hydramnios, or placenta previa or vasa previa
- Previous cesarean birth or other significant uterine surgery
- Multiple gestations
- Nonreassuring fetal heart rate (FHR) or other evidence of uteroplacental insufficiency
- Fetal abnormalities, such as intrauterine growth restriction (IUGR) or nuchal cord

Before the external version procedure begins, an intravenous line may be established to administer medications in case of difficulty. The woman may receive

● **Figure 23–1** External (or cephalic) version of the fetus. A new technique involves applying pressure to the fetal head and buttocks so that the fetus completes a "backward flip" or "forward roll."

terbutaline subcutaneously to relax the uterus. Some physicians may also order regional anesthesia for the procedure. Both tocolytics and regional anesthesia have been associated with higher success rates and fewer cesarean births (Goetzinger, Harper, Tuuli, et al., 2011). Ultrasound is frequently used to provide information about the fetal position. The version is discontinued in the presence of severe maternal pain or significant fetal bradycardia or decelerations.

Nursing Management

On admission, begin a thorough assessment by verifying that there are no contraindications to the version procedure. Obtain maternal vital signs and a reactive NST. This initial assessment period provides an ideal time for educating the woman and her partner and for addressing their concerns. They can be encouraged to express their understanding and expectations of the procedure. At the same time, the possibility of failure of the ECV and slight risk of cesarean birth if the FHR becomes nonreassuring can be discussed. Explain what will occur in either of these circumstances to better prepare the woman and her partner if intervention becomes necessary. Although the physician is ultimately responsible for obtaining informed consent, it is also the nurse's role to ensure that the woman understands the procedure and has the opportunity to ask questions and voice her concerns or fears.

SAFETY ALERT!

External cephalic version is considered a safe procedure but should be performed only when there is the ability to provide a cesarean delivery if necessary (Goetzinger et al., 2011).

 Clinical Tip

Because the ECV procedure can be uncomfortable, encourage the woman to take slow, deep breaths. Using distraction and speaking in a calm, reassuring voice can help decrease fear and anxiety.

Place an intravenous (IV) line before beginning the procedure to maintain IV access in case of a complication. Throughout the procedure, continue to monitor maternal blood pressure, pulse, and comfort level frequently (because the mother may experience pain during the procedure). Fetal well-being is ascertained before, intermittently during, and for (at least) 30 minutes following the procedure, using electronic fetal monitoring (EFM), ultrasound, or both. Also assess maternal–fetal response to the tocolytic. Provide aftercare instructions, which may include maternal monitoring for contractions and fetal movement (fetal kick counts).

CARE OF THE WOMAN DURING AMNIOTOMY

Amniotomy is the artificial rupture of the amniotic membranes (AROM). It is probably the most common invasive procedure in obstetrics. Because the amniotomy requires that an instrument, called an amnihook, be inserted through the cervix, at least 2 cm (0.8 in.) of cervical dilatation is required. Some clinicians may also perform amniotomy by inserting a fetal scalp electrode on the fetal head as a means to rupture membranes.

SAFETY ALERT!

The fetal head should be engaged prior to rupturing the membranes to prevent a possible prolapsed umbilical cord, a situation in which the umbilical cord slips through the cervical opening ahead of the presenting part. This constitutes an obstetric emergency and can be avoided by using strict criteria before an amniotomy is performed. (For a discussion of umbilical cord prolapse, see Chapter 22 ●).

Amniotomy has been used as a means to shorten labor. A recent study that examined amniotomy and the length of labor did show a reduction in the first stage of labor, which in turn resulted in a shortage of time needed for oxytocin induction, fewer cesarean births, and no increases in maternal fever (Gagnon-Gervais et al., 2012). Amniotomy can also be used at any time during the first stage to augment labor (accelerate the progress). Amniotomy is more effective in multiparous women. This is because the cervix is more pliable. Amniotomy manipulates both hormones and mechanical factors to stimulate labor. Upon rupturing the membranes, natural prostaglandins are released that stimulate uterine contractions. The escape of amniotic fluid allows the presenting part to descend and place direct pressure on the cervix, thus resulting in an acceleration of dilatation.

Amniotomy may also be done during labor to apply an internal fetal heart monitoring electrode to the scalp or to insert an intrauterine pressure catheter. In addition, amniotomy allows assessment of the color and composition of amniotic fluid.

AROM Procedure

While performing a vaginal examination, the physician/certified nurse-midwife (CNM) introduces an amnihook into the vagina and makes a small tear in the amniotic membrane, which allows amniotic fluid to escape.

Nursing Management

Explain the AROM procedure to the woman and then assess fetal presentation, position, and station, because amniotomy is usually delayed until engagement has occurred. Ask the woman to assume a semireclining position and drape her to provide privacy. The fetal heart rate (FHR) is assessed just before and immediately after the amniotomy, and the two FHR assessments are compared. If there are marked changes, check for prolapse of the cord. The amniotic fluid is inspected for amount, color, odor, and the presence of meconium or blood. While wearing disposable gloves, cleanse and dry the woman's perineal area and change the underpads as needed. Because there is now an open pathway for organisms to ascend into the uterus, the number of vaginal exams must be kept to a minimum to reduce the chance of introducing an infection. In addition, monitor the woman's temperature a minimum of every 2 hours. Provide information regarding the expected effects of the amniotomy. It is important for the woman to know that amniotic fluid is constantly produced, because some women may worry that they will experience a "dry birth." See Skill 3–2, Assisting with Amniotomy, in the *Clinical Skills Manual* SKILLS .

CARE OF THE WOMAN DURING AMNIOINFUSION

Amnioinfusion (AI) is a technique by which warmed, sterile normal saline or Ringer's lactate solution is introduced into the uterus through an intrauterine pressure catheter (IUPC). Amnioinfusion can be used intrapartally to increase the volume of fluid in cases of oligohydramnios, in which cord compression causes fetal heart rate (FHR) deceleration and nonreassuring fetal status. It provides an extra cushion of fluid that relieves pressure on the umbilical cord and promotes increased perfusion to the fetus. Amnioinfusion may also be indicated for preterm labor with premature rupture of membranes.

Nursing Management

The nurse is often the first person to detect changes in fetal heart rate associated with cord compression. When cord compression

 Clinical Tip

Before the AROM procedure, place several layers of disposable pads under the woman's buttocks and a folded towel between her legs. The towel readily absorbs the fluid released during the procedure and prevents soiling of the bed linens. After the procedure, remove the towel as well as all layers of absorbent pads that have been soiled. To increase the woman's comfort, place several clean absorbent pads under her buttocks because amniotic fluid will continue to leak from the vagina.

is suspected, the immediate intervention is to assist the laboring woman to another position. If this intervention is not successful in restoring the FHR, an amnioinfusion may be considered.

Help administer the AI, assess the woman's vital signs and contraction status, and monitor the fetal heart rate by continuous electronic fetal monitoring (EFM). It is important to provide ongoing information to the laboring woman and her partner and to answer questions as they arise. Comfort measures and positioning are vital because the woman is now on bed rest. Frequent changing of disposable underpads and perineal care are also needed because of the constant leakage of fluid from the vagina. Ensure that fluids that are infused into the uterus are being adequately expelled. Fluid expulsion is evaluated by counting sanitary pads and visual observation during perineal care.

CARE OF THE WOMAN DURING CERVICAL RIPENING

Cervical ripening is softening and effacing of the cervix. It may be used for the pregnant woman who is at term or late preterm when there is a medical or obstetric indication for induction of labor. In general, cervical ripening agents are used when the cervix is unfavorable for induction. The Bishop score is a scoring system that notes the favorability of the cervix for labor. A score of less than 8 indicates that it is unlikely for labor to occur and therefore the use of a cervical ripening agent is warranted. A score of 8 means that the cervix is favorable for labor and will respond favorably to Pitocin induction. A score above 9 indicates that spontaneous labor will likely result. Pharmacologic methods of cervical ripening include the use of prostaglandin agents (Prepidil, Cervidil) and Cytotec, which is a synthetic PGE_1 analogue. The use of prostaglandin agents became popular when Prepidil gel, which contains 0.5 mg dinoprostone, a prostaglandin E_2 (PGE_2) agent, was first used to induce women with an unfavorable cervix. It is placed either intracervically or intravaginally. Prostaglandin agents placed intravaginally are superior to intracervical placement (American College of Obstetricians and Gynecologists [ACOG], 2009). Most facilities are now using newer agents such as Cervidil or Cytotec (misoprostol) for labor induction.

Dinoprostone (Cervidil)

Cervidil is packaged as a 2-cm (0.8-in.) square vaginal insert that resembles a thin piece of cardboard. It releases 10 mg of dinoprostone at a rate of 0.3 mg/hour over 12 hours. In recent studies, women being induced with Cervidil had less pain than women who had received prostaglandin gel, resulting in improved physical and emotional well-being of the mother (Zanconato et al., 2011).

Cervidil has been associated with cervical ripening, reducing the length of labor, and lowering the requirements for Pitocin during labor induction (ACOG, 2009). Prostaglandin agents are typically used when labor induction is indicated, but not emergent, such as maternal gestational diabetes, postdates, or large-for-gestational-age (LGA) fetuses who warrant birth occurring in the near future. For example, a woman who is over

Clinical Tip

Advise the woman that prostaglandin agents commonly cause uterine stimulation after insertion. Review the signs of labor that warrant further assessment after discharge home. Teach the woman the difference between common reactions to the prostaglandin agents (such as cramping, uterine irritability, and gel leakage) and the true signs of labor (strong regular contractions, rupture of membranes) before she leaves the hospital.

41 weeks of gestation but has a very unfavorable cervix may be given prostaglandin gel to ripen her cervix before a Pitocin induction is scheduled. See *Drug Guide: Dinoprostone (Cervidil) Vaginal Insert* for more information.

Misoprostol (Cytotec)

Misoprostol (Cytotec) is a synthetic PGE_1 analogue that some healthcare agencies use to ripen the cervix and induce labor. It is available as a tablet and can be administered using several routes including the following: oral, vaginal, rectal, sublingual, or buccal. Although the last two routes are effective, they are rarely used. The rectal route is primarily used when attempting to control postpartum hemorrhaging (Mansouri & Alsahly, 2011). While practitioners may opt to administer the medication using different routes, a Cochrane review found that the rectal and vaginal routes are more commonly associated with uterine tachysystolic patterns and that the oral route is just as effective in producing cervical ripening while reducing the duration of Pitocin infusion (Hofmeyr, Gülmezoglu, & Pileggi, 2010). Studies also provide evidence that using dosages of 25 mcg at intervals of 4 hours or more is associated with a lower incidence of tachysystole (Hofmeyr et al., 2010). Although conflicting research findings can be confusing, it is important to note that Cytotec is delivered via various routes and yields successful results.

Since the 1990s, Cytotec has been contraindicated for inducing labor in women who have had a previous cesarean birth or have a scar on their uterus (ACOG, 2009). Although quite rare, Cytotec has also been associated with uterine rupture in women who have no previous scar on their uterus (Hofmeyr et al., 2010). Other risk factors for uterine rupture include a high-dose regimen (100 mcg or higher), advanced gestational age, and five or more previous pregnancies (Hofmeyr et al., 2010). After a careful review of the literature and current studies, ACOG (2009) issued the following recommended guidelines for Cytotec administration:

- Use only during the third trimester for cervical ripening or labor induction.
- One-fourth tablet or 25 mcg should be the initial dosage.

Drug Guide Dinoprostone (Cervidil) Vaginal Insert

Pregnancy Risk Category: C

Overview of Maternal–Fetal Action

Dinoprostone is a naturally occurring form of prostaglandin E_2. Dinoprostone can be used at term to ripen the cervix and can stimulate the smooth muscle of the uterus to enhance uterine contractions. Cervidil is administered by placing the insert into the posterior vagina where the moist environment triggers the release of the dinoprostone as the insert swells.

Route, Dosage, Frequency

Each insert measures 29 mm × 9.5 mm, is 0.8 mm thick, and releases 0.3 mg/hr of dinoprostone. The insert is placed in the posterior fornix of the vagina, and the patient is typically advised to maintain bed rest with bathroom privileges while the insert is in place. The mother is cautioned to avoid removing the insert when toileting and to advise the nurse if the insert becomes dislodged. Continuous electronic monitoring is typically used after administration. Women should be routinely monitored to ensure fetal well-being and to assess for tachysystole contraction patterns. If tachysystole occurs or if active labor ensues, the insert should be promptly removed. The insert may be left in place for up to 12 hours.

Contraindications

- Patient with known sensitivity to prostaglandins
- Presence of nonreassuring fetal status
- Unexplained bleeding during pregnancy
- Strong suspicion of cephalopelvic disproportion
- Patient already receiving Pitocin
- Patient who is not anticipated to be able to give birth vaginally
- Previous cesarean birth, uterine scar, or uterine rupture

Dinoprostone vaginal gel should be used with CAUTION in patients with ruptured membranes, a fetus in breech presentation, presence of glaucoma, or history of asthma (Wilson, Shannon, & Shields, 2013).

Maternal Side Effects

Uterine hyperstimulation with or without nonreassuring fetal status has occurred in a very small number (6.6%) of patients. Other reported maternal side effects include gastrointestinal disturbance (fewer than 1% of patients have experienced fever, nausea, vomiting, diarrhea, or abdominal pain) (Wilson et al., 2013).

Effects on Fetus/Newborn

Nonreassuring fetal heart rate patterns

Nursing Considerations

- Assess for presence of contraindications.
- Monitor maternal vital signs, cervical dilatation, and effacement carefully.
- Monitor fetal status for presence of reassuring fetal heart rate pattern (baseline 110 to 160 beats/min, presence of variability, presence of accelerations with fetal movement, absence of late or variable decelerations).
- Prepare to administer terbutaline if uterine hyperstimulation, sustained uterine contractions, nonreassuring fetal status, or any other adverse reactions occur.

- Recurrent administration should not exceed dosing intervals of more than 3 to 6 hours.
- Pitocin should not be administered less than 4 hours after the last Cytotec dose.
- Continuous fetal and uterine monitoring should be performed in a hospital setting.

Absolute contraindications for the use of Cytotec include the following:

- Presence of uterine contractions 3 times in 10 minutes
- Significant maternal asthma (Hofmeyr et al., 2010)
- History of previous cesarean birth or other uterine scar
- Bleeding during the pregnancy
- Presence of placenta previa
- Fetal tachycardia, nonreassuring fetal heart rate tracing, meconium passage (Hofmeyr et al., 2010)

Nursing Management

Physicians, certified nurse-midwives (CNMs), and birthing room nurses who have had special education and training may administer cervical ripening agents. Provide the woman and her support person(s) information about the procedure, and answer any questions they may have. Assess baseline maternal vital signs, and apply an electronic fetal monitor (EFM). The EFM tracing should indicate minimal or absent uterine activity, a reassuring fetal heart rate (FHR) pattern, and a reactive nonstress test (NST). If uterine contractions are not occurring regularly, the ripening agent is inserted into the vagina. If prescribed, Cytotec is administered every 3 to 6 hours until adequate cervical change occurs (ACOG, 2009). Instruct the woman to lie supine with a right hip wedge for a specified time (usually at least 1 hour). The woman can then assume any comfortable position. As discussed previously, monitor the woman for uterine hyperstimulation and FHR abnormalities (changes in baseline rate, variability, presence of decelerations) for at least 2 hours following insertion. The insert should be removed immediately if uterine hyperstimulation or nonreassuring fetal status occurs. A beta-adrenergic agent should also be administered if hyperstimulation occurs (Forrest Pharmaceuticals, 2013).

CARE OF THE WOMAN DURING LABOR INDUCTION

ACOG defines **labor induction** as the stimulation of uterine contractions before the spontaneous onset of labor, with or without ruptured amniotic membranes, for the purpose of accomplishing birth. Induction may be indicated in the presence of the following (Ehrenthal, Jiang, & Strobino, 2010):

- Diabetes mellitus
- Preeclampsia/eclampsia
- Premature rupture of membranes (PROM) with established fetal maturity
- Chorioamnionitis

- Postterm gestation, especially in association with oligohydramnios
- Intrauterine fetal demise (IUFD)
- Intrauterine fetal growth restriction (IUGR)
- Alloimmunization
- Nonreassuring antepartum testing

Relative indications include chronic hypertension, systemic lupus erythematosus, gestational diabetes, hypercoagulation disorders, cholestasis of pregnancy, polyhydramnios, fetal anomalies requiring specialized neonatal care, logistical factors (risk of rapid birth, distance from hospital, psychologic factors, advanced cervical dilatation), and previous stillbirth (Ehrenthal et al., 2010).

All contraindications to spontaneous labor and vaginal birth are contraindications to the induction of labor. Maternal contraindications include but are not limited to the following (Ehrenthal et al., 2010; Thorpe, 2009):

- Patient refusal
- Placenta previa or vasa previa
- Floating fetal presenting part
- Prior uterine incision that would preclude a trial of labor
- Active genital herpes infection
- Umbilical cord prolapse
- Acute severe nonreassuring fetal status
- Absolute cephalopelvic disproportion

Relative contraindications include cervical carcinoma; malpresentation, such as breech; and funic presentation. A **funic presentation** is when the umbilical cord is interposed between the cervix and the presenting part. It can be located by clinical evaluation or by ultrasound (Ehrenthal et al., 2010; Thorpe, 2009).

Labor Readiness

Before attempting an induction, assess fetal maturity and cervical readiness to ensure that both the woman and fetus are ready for the onset of labor.

Fetal Maturity

The gestational age of the fetus is best evaluated by accurate maternal menstrual dating and early ultrasounds. Amniotic fluid studies also provide valuable information in assessing fetal lung maturity (see Chapter 14 🔗).

Cervical Readiness

The findings on vaginal examination help determine whether cervical changes favorable for induction have occurred. Bishop (1964) developed a prelabor scoring system that is helpful in predicting the potential success of induction (Table 23–1). Components evaluated are cervical dilatation, effacement, consistency, and position, as well as the station of the fetal presenting part. A score of 0, 1, 2, or 3 is given to each assessed characteristic. The higher the total score for all the criteria, the more likely it is that labor will occur. The lower the total score, the higher the

Table 23-1	Prelabor Status Evaluation Scoring System			
	Assigned Value			
Factor	**0**	**1**	**2**	**3**
Cervical dilatation	Closed	1 to 2 cm	3 to 4 cm	5 cm or more
Cervical effacement	0% to 30%	40% to 50%	60% to 70%	80% or more
Fetal station	−3	−2	−1, 0	+1, or lower
Cervical consistency	Firm	Moderate	Soft	
Cervical position	Posterior	Midposition	Anterior	

Source: Data from Bishop, E. H. (1964). Pelvic scoring for elective inductions. *Obstetrics & Gynecology, 24,* 266.

failure rate. A favorable cervix is the most important criterion for a successful induction (Ehrenthal et al., 2010; Thorpe, 2009). The presence of a cervix that is anterior, soft, 50% effaced, and dilated at least 2 cm (0.8 in.), with the fetal head at 1 to +1 station or lower (Bishop score of 8 or 9), is favorable for successful induction (Teixeira, Lunet, Rodrigues, et al., 2012). If the cervix is unfavorable, a method of cervical ripening may be tried.

Methods of Inducing Labor

When the cervix is favorable, the most frequently used methods of induction are amniotomy (discussed previously), stripping the amniotic membranes, mechanical dilatation with intracervical catheter, intravenous Pitocin infusion, and complementary methods.

Stripping the Membranes

A nonpharmacologic method of induction frequently used by physicians/CNMs is stripping (or sweeping) the amniotic membranes. The practitioner inserts a gloved finger into the internal os and rotates it 360 degrees twice, separating the amniotic membranes that are lying against the lower uterine segment. This is thought to release prostaglandins that stimulate uterine contractions. The procedure is usually uncomfortable and can result in cramping, uterine contractions, and vaginal bleeding.

Mechanical Dilatation with Intracervical Catheter

An intracervical catheter is sometimes used to facilitate mechanical dilatation of the cervix when the cervix is unfavorable or a low Bishop score has been established. When first used in obstetrics, Foley catheters were placed within the cervix and the balloon was inflated to facilitate mechanical dilatation of the cervix. This method has been shown to be effective in stretching the cervix without increasing the incidence of infection and without causing fetal tachysystole, which can occur with the use of prostaglandin agents (Fox et al., 2011). The disadvantages include difficulty with placement and failure to maintain placement. Women are limited in their ability to ambulate postinsertion because of the risk of displacement. Mechanical dilatation is sometimes performed with weighted, double-ballooned catheters, which have been shown to decrease the first stage of

labor (Lutgendorf, Johnson, Terpstra, et al., 2012). Some practitioners may also combine intracervical balloon dilatation with prostaglandin agents to shorten the first stage of labor (Kehl et al., 2011).

Pitocin Infusion

Administration of Pitocin is effective for initiating uterine contractions to induce labor and may also be used to enhance ineffective contractions (labor augmentation). A primary line of 1000 mL of electrolyte solution (e.g., lactated Ringer's solution) is started intravenously. Ten units of Pitocin are added to a secondary line of intravenous (IV) fluid so the resulting mixture will contain 10 milliunits/mL of Pitocin (1 milliunit/min, or 6 mL/hr), and the prescribed dose can be calculated easily. After the primary infusion is started, the Pitocin solution is piggybacked into the primary tubing port closest to the catheter insertion. The infusion is then administered using an infusion pump to control the flow rate precisely. The rate of infusion is based on physician/CNM protocol and careful assessment of the contraction pattern. The goal for induction is to achieve stable contractions every 2 to 3 minutes that last 40 to 60 seconds. The uterus should relax to full baseline resting tone between each contraction. Progress is determined by changes in the effacement and dilatation of the cervix and station of the presenting part.

Pitocin induction is not without some associated risks, including hyperstimulation of the uterus, resulting in uterine contractions that are too frequent or too intense, with an increased resting tone. Hypertonic contractions may lead to decreased placental perfusion and nonreassuring fetal status. Other risks include uterine rupture, water intoxication, fetal hypoxia, and in rare circumstances fetal death (Wilson et al., 2013).

Complementary Methods

Although not frequently presented in medical (allopathic) or nursing texts, a variety of more natural, noninvasive methods of inducing labor can be effective. These methods include sexual intercourse; self or partner nipple or breast stimulation; the use of herbs, castor oil, or enemas; and acupuncture. Many CNMs and their patients desire a less medical approach to birth and want to use natural methods when possible. The cautions and contraindications for these natural methods are the same as those for medical induction of labor. It is also important to understand that some of them may not have undergone scientific research as rigorous as that used for pharmacologic agents.

Sexual intercourse is a logical method of inducing cervical ripening and uterine contractions; female orgasm stimulates contractions, and male ejaculate is a rich source of prostaglandins. Penetration during intercourse can also stimulate the lower uterine segment and cause uterine contractions. In addition, breast and nipple stimulation, which are often part of lovemaking, cause the production of endogenous oxytocin, which in turn stimulates the uterus to contract (Chaudhry, Fischer, & Schaffir, 2011).

Herbal preparations and other homeopathic solutions have not been scientifically studied to the same extent as other natural methods. The caregiver needs a thorough personal knowledge or ongoing consultation with a homeopathic physician to safely recommend the use of these approaches during late pregnancy. Some herbal products, such as blue cohosh, have been found to cause complications and should not be routinely recommended during pregnancy (Hall, McKenna, & Griffiths, 2011).

Although ingesting castor oil has been used for many years, it has not been well studied as a method of labor induction. The mechanism of action is not understood. A Cochrane review found that no clinical effectiveness could be established and that all women who ingested castor oil experienced nausea, indicating that such recommendations lack evidence-based guidelines and should not be routinely recommended (Dowswell, Kelly, Livio, et al., 2010).

Acupuncture and acupressure have been used for centuries in Eastern medicine as a means for inducing labor or preventing postdate pregnancies although the number of carefully researched studies in this area is limited. Women who receive acupressure and acupuncture are less likely to need labor induction than women who do not receive these therapies (Smith & Crowther, 2009).

Nursing Management.   Aspects to address during patient teaching about induction of labor include the purpose, the procedure itself, nursing care that will be provided, assessments, comfort measures, and a review of breathing techniques that may be used during labor. Regardless of the induction method used, close observation and accurate, ongoing assessments are mandatory to provide safe, optimal care for both woman and fetus. A qualified clinician should be readily accessible to manage any complications that may occur.

As contractions are established, perform vaginal examinations to evaluate cervical dilatation, effacement, and station. The frequency of vaginal examinations primarily depends on the woman's parity, comfort level, and strength of her contractions. If evaluating the need for analgesia, perform a vaginal examination to avoid giving the medication too early and increasing the risk of prolonging labor. This examination also helps identify advanced dilatation and imminent birth.

Pitocin induction protocols recommend obtaining baseline data (maternal temperature, pulse, respirations, blood pressure), a 20- to 30-minute electronic fetal monitor (EFM) recording demonstrating a reassuring fetal heart rate (FHR), a reactive nonstress test (NST), and the contraction status before starting an induction. Use a fetal monitor to provide continuous data.

Clinical Reasoning   Determining Infusion Rate

You are a birthing center nurse caring for Wendy Johnson, G2P1, during a Pitocin infusion to induce her labor. Wendy has been receiving the medication via infusion pump for 4 hours and currently is receiving 6 milliunits/min (36 mL/hr). You have just completed your assessments and found the following: BP 120/80, pulse 80, respirations 16; contractions every 3 minutes lasting 60 seconds and of strong intensity; the FHR baseline is 144 to 150 with average variability; and cervical dilatation is 6 cm (2.4 in.). Will you continue the same infusion rate, increase the rate, or decrease the rate?

See www.nursing.pearsonhighered.com for possible responses.

 Evidence-Based Practice   Risks Associated with Elective Induction of Labor

Clinical Question

What are the risks associated with elective induction of labor?

The Evidence

Elective induction of labor is at an all-time high in the United States despite the known risks. Two cross-sectional retrospective studies compared mothers who elected induction for nonmedical reasons with mothers who did not. More than 63,000 women were represented by these studies. Cross-sectional studies with these large sample sizes form the strongest level of evidence. Women who had nonmedical, elective inductions had nearly twice as many cesarean births as women who did not (Wilson, Effken, & Butler, 2010). Length of stay was longer for these mothers, even after controlling for the effects of a surgical birth. Rates of other complications, for both mother and baby, were also higher with elective induction; these rates were highest for nulliparous women. The most serious risks were maternal hemorrhage and the need for neonatal resuscitation. There were no identified improvements in maternal or neonatal outcomes with elective induction of labor (Vardo, Thornburg, Glantz, et al., 2011).

Best Practice

Elective induction for nonmedical reasons is contrary to a focus on patient safety for both mother and baby. Mothers who are considering elective induction should be educated about the risks for themselves and their babies, and should be encouraged to consider the increased risk of cesarean birth when discussing this possibility.

Clinical Reasoning

What are the reasons that mothers may consider an elective induction for nonmedical reasons? How can the nurse help the mother determine alternative ways to address these needs?

Before each increase of the Pitocin infusion rate, assess the following:

- Maternal blood pressure, pulse, respirations, temperature, and pain level
- Contraction status including frequency, duration, intensity, and resting tone

- FHR baseline, variability, and reactivity, noting the presence of accelerations, any decelerations, or bradycardia

For additional information about nursing interventions during use of Pitocin, see *Drug Guide: Oxytocin (Pitocin)* and *Nursing Care Plan: The Induction of Labor.*

 ## Drug Guide Oxytocin (Pitocin)

Overview of Obstetric Action

Oxytocin (Pitocin) exerts a selective stimulatory effect on the smooth muscle of the uterus and blood vessels. Oxytocin affects the myometrial cells of the uterus by increasing the excitability of the muscle cell, increasing the strength of the muscle contraction, and supporting propagation of the contraction (movement of the contraction from one myometrial cell to the next). Its effect on the uterine contraction depends on the dosage used and on the excitability of the myometrial cells. During the first half of gestation, there is little excitability of the myometrium, and the uterus is fairly resistant to the effects of oxytocin. However, from midgestation on, the uterus responds increasingly to exogenous intravenous oxytocin. Cautious use of diluted oxytocin administered intravenously at term results in a slow rise of uterine activity.

The circulatory half-life of oxytocin is 3 to 5 minutes. It takes approximately 40 minutes for a particular dose of oxytocin to reach a steady-state plasma concentration (Wilson et al., 2013).

The effects of oxytocin on the cardiovascular system can be pronounced. Blood pressure initially may decrease, but after prolonged administration may increase by 30% above the baseline. Cardiac output and stroke volume increase. With doses of 20 milliunits/min or above, oxytocin exerts an antidiuretic effect, decreasing free water exchange in the kidney and markedly decreasing urine output.

Oxytocin is used to induce labor at term and to augment uterine contractions in the first and second stages of labor. Oxytocin may also be used immediately after birth to stimulate uterine contraction and thereby control uterine atony.

Route, Dosage, Frequency
For Induction of Labor or Augmentation of Labor

- Start with primary IV tubing and piggyback secondary IV with 10 units of Pitocin (1 mL) to 1000 mL of intravenous solution. (The resulting concentration is 10 milliunits oxytocin per 1 mL of intravenous fluid.) Oxytocin is infused using an infusion pump.
- Using an infusion pump, administer IV, starting at 0.5–1 milliunit/min and increase by 1–2 milliunits/min every 40–60 minutes. Alternatively, start at 1–2 milliunits/min and increase by 1 milliunit/min every 15 minutes until an adequate contraction pattern (every 2–3 minutes and lasting 40–60 seconds) is achieved.
- Provide continuous monitoring of the fetus and uterine contractions, and ensure that vital signs, including maternal blood pressure, heart rate, and oxygen saturation, are being assessed every 15 minutes.
- In some settings or in a situation when limited fluids may be administered, a more concentrated solution may be used. When 10 units Pitocin are added to 500 mL IV solution, the resulting concentration

is 1 milliunit/min = 3 mL/hr. If 10 units Pitocin are added to 250 mL IV solution, the concentration is 1 milliunit/min = 1.5 mL/hr.

SAFETY ALERT!

It is imperative for the nurse to know the concentration of Pitocin in milliunits per minute to prevent accidental overdosage, which can result in tachysystolic labor patterns, nonreassuring fetal status, and fetal bradycardia.

For Administration After Expulsion of Placenta

- One dose of 10 units of Pitocin (1 mL) is given intramuscularly or added to IV fluids for continuous infusion.
- Assess maternal blood pressure, pulse, and uterine resting tone before each increase in oxytocin infusion rate.
- Record all assessments and IV rate on patient's chart. Record oxytocin infusion rate in milliunits per minute and milliliters per hour (e.g., 0.5 milliunits/min [3 mL/hr]).
- Record all patient activities and procedures.
- Apply nursing comfort measures.
- If bleeding is well controlled, often oxytocin is discontinued after the initial postpartum infusion.

Maternal Contraindications

- Severe preeclampsia/eclampsia
- Predisposition to uterine rupture (in nullipara over 35 years of age, multigravida 4 or more, overdistention of the uterus, previous major surgery of the cervix or uterus)
- Cephalopelvic disproportion
- Malpresentation or malposition of the fetus, cord prolapse
- More than one previous cesarean birth
- Preterm infant
- Rigid, unripe cervix; total placenta previa
- Presence of nonreassuring fetal status

Maternal Side Effects

Hyperstimulation of the uterus results in hypercontractility, which in turn may cause the following:

- Abruptio placentae
- Impaired uterine blood flow, leading to fetal hypoxia
- Rapid labor and birth, leading to lacerations of cervix, vagina, or perineum; uterine atony; fetal trauma
- Uterine rupture
- Water intoxication (nausea, vomiting, hypotension, tachycardia, cardiac arrhythmia) if oxytocin is given in electrolyte-free solution or at a rate exceeding 20 milliunits/min; hypotension with rapid IV bolus administration postpartum

(continued)

Effect on Fetus/Newborn

- Fetal effects are primarily associated with the presence of hyper-contractility of the maternal uterus. Hypercontractility decreases the oxygen supply to the fetus, which is reflected by irregularities or decrease in fetal heart rate (FHR), as well as hypoxia
- Hyperbilirubinemia (Wilson et al., 2013)
- Trauma from rapid birth
- Hypoxia as an effect of maternal hypotension

Nursing Considerations

- Explain induction or augmentation procedure to patient.
- Apply fetal monitor, and obtain 15- to 20-minute tracing and non-stress test (NST) to assess FHR before starting IV oxytocin.
- For induction or augmentation of labor, start with primary IV, and piggyback secondary IV with oxytocin and infusion pump. Pitocin can never be run without an infusion pump and must always be run using a secondary line.
- Ensure continuous fetal and contraction monitoring. Telemetry units can be worn for ambulation or use of bath tubs.
- The maximum rate is 40 milliunits/min (ACOG, 2009). Not all protocols recommend a maximum dose. When indicated, the maximum dose is generally between 16 and 40 milliunits/min. Decrease oxytocin by similar increments once labor has progressed to 5–6 cm dilatation. Protocols may vary from one agency to another.

0.5 milliunit/min = 3 mL/hr	8 milliunits/min = 48 mL/hr
1.0 milliunit/min = 6 mL/hr	10 milliunits/min = 60 mL/hr
1.5 milliunits/min = 9 mL/hr	12 milliunits/min = 72 mL/hr
2 milliunits/min = 12 mL/hr	15 milliunits/min = 90 mL/hr
4 milliunits/min = 24 mL/hr	18 milliunits/min = 108 mL/hr
6 milliunits/min = 36 mL/hr	20 milliunits/min = 120 mL/hr

- Maternal vital signs, including blood pressure, heart rate, and oxygen saturation, are monitored every 15 minutes.
- Assess FHR; frequency, duration, and intensity of uterine contractions; and presence of decelerations, accelerations, and uterine resting tone every 15 minutes and before each increase in the oxytocin infusion rate.
- Record patient activities (such as change of position, vomiting), procedures done (amniotomy, sterile vaginal examination), and administration of analgesic agents to allow for interpretation and evaluation of tracing.
- Assess cervical dilatation as needed.
- Discontinue IV oxytocin infusion and infuse primary solution when (1) nonreassuring fetal status is noted (bradycardia, late or variable decelerations); (2) uterine contractions are more frequent than every 2 minutes; (3) duration of contractions exceeds more than 60 seconds; or (4) insufficient relaxation of the uterus between contractions or a steady increase in resting tone is noted (ACOG, 2009). In addition to discontinuing IV oxytocin infusion, turn patient to side, and if nonreassuring fetal status is present, administer oxygen by tight face mask at 7–10 L/min; notify physician/CNM.
- Maintain intake and output record.

SAFETY ALERT!

Women receiving Pitocin warrant ongoing assessment every 15 minutes and need closer ongoing observation when Pitocin levels are increased. If the nurse cannot adequately monitor the woman immediately following a dosage increase, it is advisable to wait to increase the medication until careful monitoring capabilities are available.

 Nursing Care Plan The Induction of Labor

Intervention	Rationale	Expected Outcome
1. Nursing Diagnosis: *Injury, Risk for,* related to hypersystole of uterus caused by induction of labor (NANDA-I © 2012)		
NIC Priority Intervention: Health education		NOC Suggested Outcome: Maternal status: Intrapartum; patient will remain free from injury

Goal: The woman will experience progression of labor without difficulty or complications.

Obtain a baseline for maternal blood pressure, pulse, respirations, temperature, and pain level.	Pitocin induction can affect the cardiovascular system. Blood pressure may initially be decreased. If the induction is prolonged, the blood pressure may increase by 30%. Respirations can become elevated because of pain sensation, anxiety, or physiologic causes. Temperature is obtained to monitor for infection. The pain level is assessed continuously to determine if pain medication is warranted or changes in vital signs are caused by maternal discomfort.	
Place patient on external fetal monitor for 20 minutes to obtain a baseline for fetal heart rate (FHR) and variability.	Assesses for fetal well-being. Normal FHR ranges from 110 to 160 beats/min. Variability measuring three to five fluctuations in 1 minute is documented as average. Continuous electronic fetal monitoring (EFM) is performed during a Pitocin induction.	

Nursing Care Plan   The Induction of Labor—continued

Intervention	Rationale	Expected Outcome
■ Perform nonstress test.	■ A nonstress test is performed to assess the fetal heart rate in response to fetal movement. Accelerations of fetal heart rate with fetal movement may indicate the fetus has adequate oxygenation and an intact central nervous system. A reactive nonstress test indicates there were at least two accelerations of 15 beats/min above baseline, lasting 15 seconds in a 20-minute period.	
■ Insert IV line and begin primary infusion with 1000 mL of electrolyte solution.	■ An electrolyte solution such as lactated Ringer's is used for the primary solution. A primary IV allows continuous intravenous access and fluid infusion in the event the Pitocin drip needs to be discontinued.	
■ Piggyback Pitocin solution into primary IV tubing, via pump, in the port closest to the IV insertion site.	■ Pitocin is mixed in 1000 mL of an electrolyte solution (usually 5% dextrose in lactated Ringer's solution) and piggybacked to main IV line. A pump is used to ensure dosage accuracy.	
■ Begin Pitocin infusion per agency protocol.	■ The rate to be used is determined by physician/CNM orders or agency protocol.	■ Contractions will increase in frequency, duration, and intensity. An increase in cervical dilatation, effacement, and intensity will be achieved. The uterus will maintain adequate resting tone (remain soft) between contractions.
■ Monitor infusion pump and connections.	■ This ensures adequate dosing. Early identification of problems with the infusion site, the piggyback connection, or flow rate will minimize effects on uterine contractions and FHR. If a problem is found, correct and restart infusion at the beginning dose.	
■ Monitor and evaluate maternal blood pressure and pulse before each increase in the Pitocin infusion rate.	■ Prolonged inductions may increase the blood pressure by 30%. The Pitocin infusion rate should not be advanced if maternal hypertension or hypotension is present or if there are any radical changes in pulse rate.	
■ Evaluate urine output.	■ Dosages of Pitocin above 20 milliunits/min have an antidiuretic effect. This level decreases free water exchange in the kidneys, therefore markedly decreasing urine output.	
■ Evaluate and document fetal heart rate before each increase in Pitocin infusion rate.	■ During Pitocin infusion, fetal heart rate should range between 110 and 160 beats/min. Hypersystole of the maternal uterus may cause nonreassuring fetal status. Fetal bradycardia may occur along with a decrease in variability, leading to fetal hypoxia. Fetal tachycardia may also occur. If persistent fetal bradycardia or fetal tachycardia occurs, the Pitocin is discontinued.	

(continued)

Nursing Care Plan   The Induction of Labor—continued

Intervention	Rationale	Expected Outcome
■ Evaluate and document contraction pattern before each increase of the Pitocin infusion rate.	■ Contractions every 2 to 3 minutes, lasting 40 to 60 seconds with moderate intensity, are considered adequate. Cervical dilatation progresses an average of 1.2 to 1.5 cm/hr (0.5 to 0.6 in./hr) during the active phase of labor.	
■ Increase Pitocin infusion dosage until adequate contractions are achieved or the maximum dose per agency protocol is reached.	■ Pitocin may be increased every 20 to 40 minutes until an adequate contraction pattern is achieved.	
■ Evaluate contraction frequency, duration, and intensity before increasing the infusion rate. Discontinue Pitocin infusion and infuse primary solution if signs of hypersystole of the uterus are detected.	■ Signs of hypersystole include contraction frequency less than 2 minutes, duration exceeding 60 seconds, and increased resting tone. Hypersystole of the uterus puts the patient at risk for abruptio placentae and uterine rupture.	
■ Initiate treatment measures to reverse the effects of Pitocin infusion if fetal tachycardia or bradycardia occurs.	■ When the FHR falls outside the normal range (110 to 160 beats/min), treatment measures should be initiated. To reverse the effects of Pitocin, immediately discontinue Pitocin, infuse primary solution, administer oxygen by tight face mask at 7 to 10 L/min, place patient in side-lying position, and notify physician/CNM.	

CARE OF THE WOMAN DURING AN EPISIOTOMY

An **episiotomy** is a surgical incision of the perineal body to enlarge the outlet. It is the second-most-common procedure in maternal–child care and has long been thought to minimize the risk of lacerations of the perineum and the overstretching of perineal tissues. However, episiotomy may actually increase the risk of fourth-degree perineal lacerations (ACOG, 2011). Though very common, the routine use of episiotomy has been seriously questioned for several years. Research suggests that (1) rather than protecting the perineum from lacerations, the presence of an episiotomy makes it more likely that the woman will have anal sphincter tears and (2) perineal lacerations heal more quickly than deep perineal tears (ACOG, 2011). In clinical practice, research has shown that the incidence of major perineal trauma (extension to or through the anal sphincter) is more likely to happen if a midline episiotomy is done (ACOG, 2011). Women with previous episiotomies were more likely to have a repeat episiotomy or a spontaneous laceration when compared with those women who had a spontaneous laceration without the use of episiotomy during their first pregnancies (Lurie, Kedar, Boaz, et al., 2012). Additional complications associated with episiotomy are blood loss, infection, pain, and perineal discomfort that may continue for days or weeks past birth, including painful intercourse (Lurie et al., 2012).

Factors That Predispose Women to Episiotomy

Overall factors that place a woman at increased risk for episiotomy are primigravid status, large or macrosomic fetus, occiput-posterior position, use of forceps or vacuum extractor, and shoulder dystocia. Other factors that may be mitigated by nurses and physicians/CNMs include the following:

■ Use of lithotomy and other recumbent positions (cause excessive and uneven stretching of the perineum)

■ Encouraging or requiring sustained breath holding during second-stage pushing (causes excessive and rapid perineal stretching, can adversely affect blood flow in mother and fetus, and requires woman to be responsive to caregiver directions rather than to her own urges to push spontaneously)

■ Arbitrary time limit placed by the physician/CNM on the length of the second stage

Preventive Measures

These general tips help reduce the incidence of routine episiotomies:

■ Perineal massage during pregnancy for nulliparous women

■ Natural pushing during labor, and avoiding the lithotomy position or pulling back on legs (which tightens the perineum)

- Side-lying position for pushing, which helps slow birth and diminish tears
- Warm or hot compresses on the perineum and firm counterpressure
- Encouraging a gradual expulsion of the infant at the time of birth by encouraging the mother to "push, take a breath, push, take a breath" thereby easing the infant out slowly
- Avoiding immediate pushing after epidural placement

Episiotomy Procedure

The two types of episiotomy in current practice are midline and mediolateral (Figure 23–2). Just before birth, when approximately 3 to 4 cm (1.2 to 1.6 in.) of the fetal head is visible during a contraction, the episiotomy is performed using sharp scissors with rounded points. The midline incision begins at the bottom center of the perineal body and extends straight down the midline to the fibers of the rectal sphincter. The mediolateral incision begins in the midline of the posterior fourchette and extends at a 45-degree angle downward to the right or left. The mediolateral episiotomy is seldom used and is typically reserved for severe cases when a large incision is made in emergent situations, such as a prolapsed umbilical cord or undiagnosed breech birth.

The episiotomy is usually performed with regional or local anesthesia but may be done without anesthesia in emergency situations. It is generally proposed that as crowning occurs, the

Clinical Tip

Although it is no longer recommended, some practitioners continue to routinely perform episiotomy. Therefore, nurses should provide information about episiotomy and encourage women to talk to their practitioner about the incidence of its use within the practice. Encourage women who are opposed to an episiotomy to discuss their objection to the procedure with their healthcare provider at a prenatal visit before the onset of labor. Advise women that episiotomies are sometimes indicated, such as in cases of severe fetal nonreassuring status, macrosomia, instrument-assisted births, or an unresolving shoulder dystocia.

distention of the tissues causes numbing. Repair of the episiotomy (episiorrhaphy) and any lacerations is completed either during the period between birth of the newborn and expulsion of the placenta or after expulsion of the placenta. Adequate anesthesia must be given for the repair. Many practitioners prefer to wait until the placenta has been delivered in case complications occur and manual exploration of the uterus is indicated.

Nursing Management

The woman needs to be supported during the episiotomy and the repair because she may feel some pressure or pulling or tugging sensations. If anesthesia is inadequate, she may feel pain. Placing

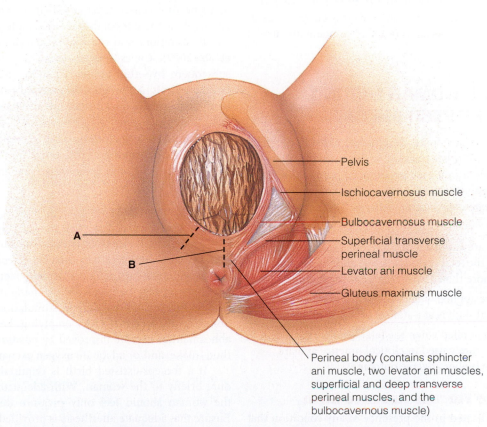

Pelvis

Ischiocavernosus muscle

Bulbocavernosus muscle

Superficial transverse perineal muscle

Levator ani muscle

Gluteus maximus muscle

Perineal body (contains sphincter ani muscle, two levator ani muscles, superficial and deep transverse perineal muscles, and the bulbocavernous muscle)

● **Figure 23–2** The two common types of episiotomies are midline and mediolateral. *A,* Right mediolateral. *B,* Midline.

a hand on the woman's shoulder and talking with her can provide comfort and distraction from the repair process. If the woman is having more discomfort than she can handle, act as an advocate in communicating the woman's needs to the physician/CNM. At all times the woman needs to be the one who decides whether the amount of discomfort she is experiencing is tolerable. She should never be told, "This doesn't hurt." She is the person experiencing the discomfort, and her evaluation needs to be respected.

Record the type of episiotomy on the birth record. Include this information in a report to subsequent caregivers so that adequate assessments can be made and relief measures can be instituted.

Comfort measures may begin immediately after birth with the application of an ice pack to the perineum. For optimal effect the ice pack should be applied for 20 to 30 minutes and removed for at least 20 minutes before being reapplied. Assess the perineal tissues frequently to prevent injury from the ice pack. Inspect the episiotomy site every 15 minutes during the first hour after the birth for redness, swelling, tenderness, bruising, and hematomas. To adequately assess the episiotomy site, have the woman roll onto her side with the head of the bed in the lowered position. Lift the woman's top leg and inspect the suture line carefully. Instruct the mother in postpartum care, such as perineal hygiene, self-care, and comfort measures. (See further discussion on nursing care after episiotomy in Chapter 30 🌐.)

It is important to recognize that perineal pain continues for a period of time, and it may be significant. Do not discount this pain. Women who experience prolonged perineal pain tend to have problems with breastfeeding and depression and are reluctant to reestablish sexual activity.

Nursing advocacy is needed to promote selective rather than routine episiotomy. It is imperative to stay current regarding new information and research in order to maintain current practice standards.

CARE OF THE WOMAN DURING FORCEPS-ASSISTED BIRTH

Forceps are surgical instruments designed to assist in the birth of a fetus by providing either traction or the means to rotate the fetal head to an occiput-anterior position. In medical literature and practice, **forceps-assisted birth** is also known as *instrumental delivery* or *operative vaginal delivery*. Three categories of forceps application exist:

1. Outlet forceps are applied when the fetal skull has reached the perineum, the fetal scalp is visible, and the sagittal suture is not more than 45 degrees from the midline.
2. Low forceps are applied when the leading edge (presenting part) of the fetal skull is at a station of +2 or more.
3. Midforceps are applied when the fetal head is engaged. Midforceps are rarely used in clinical practice and are associated with higher adverse outcomes.

Indications for Forceps-Assisted Birth

Forceps may be indicated in the presence of any condition that threatens the mother or fetus and that can be relieved by birth.

Conditions that put the woman at risk include heart disease, pulmonary edema, infection, and exhaustion. Fetal conditions include premature placental separation and nonreassuring fetal status. Forceps may be used to shorten the second stage of labor and assist the woman's pushing effort. They may also be used when regional anesthesia has affected the woman's motor innervation and she cannot push effectively.

Before forceps are used, the following conditions must be met (Al-Suhel, Gill, Robson, et al., 2009):

- The cervix must be completely dilated and the exact position and station of the fetal head known.
- Membranes must be ruptured to allow a firm grasp on the fetal head, which must be engaged and in vertex or face presentation.
- The type of pelvis should be known, because certain pelvic types do not permit rotation.
- The maternal bladder should be empty and adequate anesthesia given.
- No degree of cephalopelvic disproportion can be present.
- The operator must have the knowledge to perform the procedure.
- Maternal anesthesia is available.
- Adequate staff is available with the ability to perform a cesarean birth if indicated.
- Maternal consent has been obtained.

Neonatal and Maternal Risks

Some newborns may develop a small area of ecchymosis and/or edema along the sides of the face as a result of forceps application. Facial lacerations and brachial plexus can also occur (Al-Suhel et al., 2009). Caput succedaneum or cephalhematoma (with subsequent hyperbilirubinemia) may occur, as may transient facial paralysis. Although rare, cerebral hemorrhages, fractures, brain damage, and fetal death have also been reported (Al-Suhel et al., 2009).

Maternal risks include possible lacerations of the birth canal; extensions of a midline episiotomy into the anus; increased bleeding, bruising, and perineal edema; and anal incontinence (Al-Suhel et al., 2009).

Nursing Management

Using ongoing assessment, note the variables that are associated with an increased rate of instrument-assisted or operative birth. Nursing care measures can then be directed toward variables that may reduce the incidence of these factors. For example, labor dystocia may be corrected by changing maternal position, ambulation, use of breast/nipple stimulation or an electric breast pump, and frequent bladder emptying. Fetal heart rate (FHR) abnormalities may be improved by position changes, increased fluid intake, and/or adequate oxygen exchange.

If a forceps-assisted birth is required, explain the procedure briefly to the woman. With adequate regional anesthesia the woman should feel only pressure during the procedure. Ensure that adequate anesthesia is provided by alerting the physician if the woman experiences discomfort or pain. Encourage the woman to use breathing techniques that help prevent her from pushing during application of the forceps (Figure 23–3 ●). Monitor contractions and advise the physician when one is present. With each contraction the physician provides traction on the forceps as the woman pushes. Reinforce to the woman that she needs to push while traction is being applied, explaining that the combined efforts help with expulsion of the fetus. It is not uncommon to observe mild fetal bradycardia as traction is being applied to the forceps. This bradycardia results from head compression and is transient.

● **Figure 23–3** Application of forceps in occiput-anterior (OA) position. *A,* The left blade is inserted along the left side wall of the pelvis over the parietal bone. *B,* The right blade is inserted along the right side wall of the pelvis over the parietal bone. *C,* With correct placement of the blades, the handles lock easily. During uterine contractions, traction is applied to the forceps in a downward and outward direction to follow the birth canal.

Immediately following birth, assess the newborn for facial edema, bruising, caput succedaneum, cephalhematoma, and any signs of cerebral edema. In the fourth stage, assess the woman for perineal swelling, bruising, hematoma, excessive bleeding, and hemorrhage. In the postpartum period it is important to assess for signs of infection if lacerations occurred during the procedure. Provide an opportunity for the woman to ask questions and reiterate explanations as needed.

CARE OF THE WOMAN DURING VACUUM-ASSISTED BIRTH

Vacuum-assisted birth is an obstetric procedure used to facilitate the birth of a fetus by applying suction to the fetal head. The vacuum extractor is composed of a soft suction cup attached to a suction bottle (pump) by tubing. The suction cup, which comes in various sizes, is placed against the fetal occiput, and the pump is used to create negative pressure (suction) inside the cup. Traction is applied in coordination with uterine contractions, descent occurs, and the fetal head is born (Figure 23–4 ●). General recommendations include that there should be progressive descent with the first two pulls and that the procedure should be limited to prevent cephalhematomas, brain injury, and fetal death (Edgar, Baskett, Young, et al., 2012).

Two types of vacuums are available. The Mityvac® is used in settings where a sterile instrument is not required. The nurse typically holds the pump and operates it while the physician applies the vacuum to the fetal head and exerts traction. The Kiwi vacuum can be used in both sterile and nonsterile settings and is much smaller in size. The Kiwi is also associated with a lower incidence of cephalhematoma and caput. The availability and use of vacuums may be dependent on what the facility has in stock and physician preference.

Nursing Management

Keep the woman and her partner informed about what is happening during the procedure. If adequate regional anesthesia has been administered, the woman feels only pressure during the procedure. Assess fetal heart rate (FHR) by continuous electronic fetal monitoring (EFM). During the vacuum procedure, a slow incremental increase in vacuum pressure is recommended before applying traction, starting at a negative pressure and increasing gradually at 0.2 kg/cm^2 every 2 minutes to achieve a pressure of approximately 0.8 kg/cm^2 (alternatively expressed as 500–600 mm Hg, 500–600 torr, 23.6 in Hg, or 11.6 lb/in.^{2}) (Ali & Norwitz, 2009). The maximum allowable time should not exceed 8 to 10 minutes (Ali & Norwitz, 2009). Frequent pop-offs are associated with failure and a higher rate of complications and warrant reconsideration about continuing with the attempt.

Assessment of the newborn should include inspection and continued observation for cephalhematomas, intracerebral hemorrhage, and retinal hemorrhages (Edgar et al., 2012). Because infants born via vacuum are at increased risk for jaundice, carefully assess the infant's skin color. Finally, reassure the parents that the caput (chignon) on the baby's head will disappear within 2 to 3 days.

A

B

C

● **Figure 23–4** Vacuum extractor traction. *A,* The cup is placed on the fetal occiput, creating suction. Traction is applied in a downward and outward direction. *B,* Traction continues in a downward direction as the fetal head begins to emerge from the vagina. *C,* Traction is maintained to lift the fetal head out of the vagina.

Vacuum Extraction

Video

CARE OF THE FAMILY DURING CESAREAN BIRTH

Cesarean birth, the birth of the infant through an abdominal and uterine incision, is one of the oldest surgical procedures known. Until the 20th century cesarean procedures were primarily used in an attempt to save the fetus of a dying woman. As the maternal and perinatal morbidity and mortality rates associated with cesarean birth steadily decreased throughout the 20th century, the proportion of cesarean births increased. Beginning in the early 1970s the cesarean birth rate rose steadily for almost two decades. In 1989, however, in an effort to control healthcare costs, the number of cesarean births began to decline. In 2010, the rate of cesarean births performed in the United States was 32.8% (Centers for Disease Control and Prevention, 2012). Canada's cesarean section rate is also at an all-time high at 26% (Women's Health Data Directory, 2012).

Cesarean birth rates differ dramatically around the globe. It is estimated that more than 18.5 million cesarean births are performed annually (World Health Organization [WHO], 2011). Cesarean birth is the least common in the Sub-Saharan African countries with rates averaging 0.3%. In these areas, however, many women do not have access to cesarean births, which leads to the world's highest maternal and infant morbidity (WHO, 2011). The cesarean birth rate in East Asia, the Caribbean, and Latin America continues to rise. Brazil (45.9%) and the Dominican Republic (41.9%) have the highest cesarean birth rates in the world (WHO, 2011). Other countries with cesarean rates over 30% include China, United States, Mexico, Argentina, Italy, Australia, Chile, Paraguay, Cuba, Portugal, Uruguay, Iran, and South Korea (WHO, 2011). Countries with low cesarean birth rates include Iceland (15.6%), Qatar (15.9%), Belgium (15.9%), Poland (16.1%), and Finland (16.3%) (WHO, 2011). Overall, the incidence of cesarean birth has continued to increase around the world.

The increasing rate in the United States is linked to a rise in repeat cesarean births fueled by concerns regarding the risk of uterine rupture with a vaginal birth after a previous cesarean birth. There is also an increase in requests from women for cesarean births so that they can avoid the pain of labor and vaginal birth. The trend increased further when some medical literature stated that vaginal births could result in pelvic floor damage during the birth process, although the majority of pelvic floor injuries are associated with operative vaginal births (Handa et al., 2011). There is also an emerging trend to "schedule" birth into busy routines to meet specific needs of the parents, such as coordinating work projects, arranging for babysitting of older children, or arranging for relatives who live in other geographic locations to travel to be present for the birth itself.

During the past few years, there has been a rise in the number of nulliparous women requesting cesarean births. This trend has led to further increases in the cesarean birth rate. Although cesarean birth on request is associated with a reduction in maternal hemorrhage risk, it is also associated with increases in neonatal respiratory problems, longer hospitalizations, and an increase in complications in subsequent pregnancies, including placenta implantation problems and uterine rupture (Demers, 2011).

Therefore, cesarean birth without medical indications should not be recommended for women desiring several children, for women less than 39 gestational weeks, or when pregnancy dating is unknown or may be inaccurate. It should also not be motivated by the lack of anesthesia availability in an institution (Demers, 2011). In some developing countries, such as Nigeria, cesarean by request is viewed as a guarantee that a woman will deliver a live infant and will avoid labor pains (Okonkwo, Ojengbede, Morhason-Bello, et al., 2012).

Many other factors have contributed to the rise in the cesarean birth rate and need to be considered in any discussion about decreasing the rate. These factors include an increased use of epidural anesthesia, maternal age over 35, failed inductions, decline in vaginal breech deliveries, decreases in operative vaginal deliveries, increased repeat cesarean rates, reduced vaginal birth after cesarean birth rates, increased physician scheduling of cesarean births for personal convenience, policy statements from professional organizations encouraging cesarean birth, political pressure from malpractice insurance carriers who attempt to dictate practice standards, and fear of litigation (Demers, 2011).

Indications

Commonly accepted indications for cesarean birth include complete placenta previa, cephalopelvic disproportion, placental abruption, active genital herpes, umbilical cord prolapse, failure to progress in labor, nonreassuring fetal status, previous classical incision on the uterus (either previous cesarean birth or myomectomy), more than one previous cesarean birth, benign and malignant tumors that obstruct the birth canal, and cervical cerclage.

Certain maternal medical conditions are contraindications to a vaginal birth and warrant a cesarean birth. These include cardiac disorders; severe maternal respiratory disease; central nervous system disorders that increase intracranial pressure; mechanical vaginal obstruction, such as an ovarian mass or lower uterine segment fibroids; HIV infection in the mother; and severe mental illness that results in an altered state of consciousness (Society for Maternal–Fetal Medicine, 2012). Other indications that are now commonly associated with cesarean birth include breech presentation, previous cesarean birth, major congenital anomalies, and severe Rh alloimmunization. Note, however, that in some of these circumstances, the infants may be able to be delivered vaginally.

Maternal Mortality and Morbidity

Cesarean births have a higher maternal mortality rate than vaginal births. For every 100,000 who give birth via a successful trial of labor after cesarean (TOLAC), 4 maternal deaths will occur compared to 13 deaths that will occur as a result of an elective repeat cesarean delivery (ERCD) (National Institutes of Health Consensus Development Conference Panel, 2010). Perinatal morbidity is often associated with infection, hypertensive disorders, reaction to anesthesia, blood clots, and bleeding problems (Goldenberg, McClure, & Kamath, 2012).

In addition to the complications associated with cesarean birth, there are also risks that increase maternal mortality and morbidity in subsequent pregnancies. Women who have

Video | Cesarean Birth

previously given birth via cesarean have a 1% risk of uterine rupture in subsequent pregnancies (ACOG, 2009). Women who have had a previous cesarean birth have an increased risk of bleeding problems in future pregnancies. The risk of placenta previa in subsequent pregnancies is 8.7 per 1000 (Gurol-Urganci et al., 2011), and the risk of abruptio placentae is 12 per 1000 (Oyelese & Canterino, 2011). There is also an increase in fetal demise and in neonatal respiratory distress and the need for oxygen administration in fetuses whose mothers have previously given birth via cesarean (Oyelese & Canterino, 2011).

Skin Incisions

The skin incision for a cesarean birth is either transverse (Pfannenstiel) or vertical and is not indicative of the type of incision made into the uterus. The transverse incision (Figure 23–5 ●) is made across the lowest and narrowest part of the abdomen. Because the incision is made just below the pubic hairline, it is almost invisible after healing. The limitation of this type of skin incision is that it does not allow for extension of the incision if needed. This incision is used when time permits (e.g., with failure to progress and stable fetal and maternal status), because it usually requires more time to make and repair.

The vertical incision, which is rarely used in current obstetric practice, is made between the navel and the symphysis pubis. This type of incision is quicker and is therefore preferred in cases of nonreassuring fetal status when rapid birth is indicated, with preterm or macrosomic infants, or when the woman is significantly obese (Cunningham et al., 2010). Time factors, patient preference, previous vertical skin incision, or physician preference determines the type of skin incision.

Uterine Incisions

The type of uterine incision depends on the need for the cesarean. The choice of incision affects the woman's opportunity for a subsequent vaginal birth and her risks of a ruptured uterine scar with a subsequent pregnancy.

The two major locations of uterine incisions are in the lower uterine segment and in the upper segment of the uterine corpus.

● **Figure 23–5** Transverse skin incision for a cesarean birth.
Source: Courtesy of Wilson Garcia and The Valley Hospital, Ridgewood, NJ.

> ### Developing Cultural Competence
> **Translating Operative Reports**
>
> Women from other countries who have had a previous cesarean birth typically have a vertical skin incision; however, the skin incision does not provide data on the type of uterine incision that was performed. Obtain an operative report if possible. Operative reports in other languages need to be translated by personnel familiar with medical terminology. If an operative report cannot be obtained, which is common, provide the woman with a thorough explanation regarding the need for a repeat cesarean.

The most common lower uterine segment incision is a transverse incision (Figure 23–6 ●). Another incision, the classic vertical incision, which is made into the upper uterine segment, was the method of choice for many years but is almost never performed in modern obstetrics. More blood loss results, and it is more difficult to repair. Most important, it carries an increased risk of uterine rupture with subsequent pregnancy, labor, and birth because the upper uterine segment is the most contractile portion of the uterus.

See Table 23–2 for the advantages and disadvantages of the three types of uterine incisions.

Analgesia and Anesthesia

There is no perfect anesthesia for cesarean birth. Each has its advantages, disadvantages, possible risks, and side effects. Goals for analgesia and anesthesia administration include safety, comfort, and emotional satisfaction for the patient. (For a discussion of analgesia and anesthesia, see Chapter 20 ●.)

NURSING MANAGEMENT *For the Woman Undergoing a Cesarean Birth*

Preparation for Cesarean Birth

Because one of every four births is a cesarean, preparation for this possibility should be an integral part of all prenatal education. Pregnant women and their partners should be encouraged to discuss the possibility of a cesarean birth with their physician/CNM and at the same time discuss their specific needs and desires under those circumstances. Their preferences may include the following:

- Participating in the choice of anesthetic
- Father or significant other being present during the procedures and/or birth
- Father or significant other being present in the recovery or postpartum room
- Video recording and/or taking pictures of the birth as allowed by facility
- Delayed instillation of eye drops to promote eye contact between parent and infant in the first hours after birth

Fallopian tube

Ovary

Site of incision

Bladder

Vagina

A

B

C

● **Figure 23–6** Uterine incisions for a cesarean birth. **A,** This transverse incision in the lower uterine segment is called a Kerr incision. **B,** The Sellheim incision is a vertical incision in the lower uterine segment. **C,** This view illustrates the classic uterine incision that is done in the body (corpus) of the uterus. The classic incision was commonly done in the past and is associated with increased risk of uterine rupture in subsequent pregnancies and labor.

- Physical contact or holding the infant while in the operating and/or recovery room (by the father if the mother cannot hold the newborn)
- Breastfeeding in the recovery area within the first hour of birth

Information that couples need about cesarean birth includes the following:

- What preparatory procedures to expect
- Description or viewing of the birthing room
- Types of anesthesia for birth and analgesia available postpartum
- Sensations that may be experienced
- Roles of significant others
- Interaction with newborn
- Immediate recovery phase
- Postpartum phase

Preparing the woman and her family for birth involves more than the procedures of establishing an intravenous line, instilling a urinary indwelling catheter, and performing an abdominal prep. As discussed previously, good communication skills are essential for preparing the woman and her support person. Use therapeutic touch and direct eye contact (if culturally acceptable and possible) to assist the woman in maintaining a sense of control and to lessen anxiety.

If the cesarean birth is scheduled and not an emergency, there is ample time for preoperative teaching. Relay this information in a birth-oriented rather than surgery-oriented context. This provides an opportunity for the woman to express her concerns, ask questions, and develop a relationship with you.

In preparation for surgery, the woman is given nothing by mouth. To reduce the likelihood of serious pulmonary damage if gastric contents are aspirated, antacids may be administered

Table 23–2	Types of Uterine Incisions for Cesarean Birth

Lower Uterine Segment Transverse Incision (Kerr) (Most Commonly Used)

Advantages	*Disadvantages*
Less blood loss because it is the thinnest part of the uterus	Takes longer to make a transverse incision and complete the repair
Easier to repair	Size of incision is limited because of the presence of major vessels on either side of the uterus
Requires minimal dissection of the bladder from underlying myometrium	
Less chance of adherence of bowel or omentum to the incision line	Can extend laterally into the uterine vessels
Area is less likely to rupture during subsequent pregnancies	Incision may stretch and become a thin sheath, causing problems in subsequent labors

Lower Uterine Segment Vertical Incision (Sellheim)

Advantages	*Disadvantages*
Preferred for:	Incision may extend into the cervix
Multiple gestation	Extensive dissection of the bladder
Placenta previa	Controlling bleeding and closure can be difficult
Nonreassuring fetal status	Carries a high risk of rupture with subsequent labor
Abnormal presentation	Future births need to be cesarean
Preterm and macrosomic fetuses	

Upper Uterine Segment Vertical Incision (Classic)

Advantages	*Disadvantages*
None; now used infrequently	Heavy blood loss
	Difficult to repair
	Increased risk of uterine rupture with subsequent pregnancy

Source: Data from Cunningham, F. G., Leveno, K. J., Bloom, S. L., Hauth, J. C., Gilstrap, L. C., & Wenstrom, K. D. (2010). *Williams obstetrics* (23rd ed.). New York, NY:McGraw-Hill Medical.

Clinical Tip

Women undergoing elective cesarean birth can be taught many aspects of postoperative teaching before their birth experience. Important components of patient education that can be emphasized before birth include dealing with postoperative discomfort, splinting the incision to decrease pain, frequent deep breathing and coughing, and the importance of early ambulation. Women who receive this information before the birth are more apt to remember it when it is reviewed in the early postpartum period.

within 30 minutes of surgery. If epidural anesthesia is used, you may assist with the procedure, monitor the woman's blood pressure and response, and continue electronic fetal monitoring (EFM). Perform an abdominal and perineal prep, insert an indwelling catheter to prevent bladder distention, and start an intravenous line with a large-bore needle to permit blood administration if it becomes necessary. Order preoperative medication, notify the pediatrician, and prepare to receive the new baby. Ensure that the infant warmer is working and that resuscitation equipment is available.

Assist in positioning the woman on the operating table. Fetal heart rate (FHR) is assessed before surgery and during preparation because fetal hypoxia can result from the supine position. The operating room table is adjusted so it slants slightly to one side or a hip wedge (folded blanket or towels) is placed under the woman's right hip to tip the uterus slightly and reduce compression of blood vessels. The uterus should be displaced 15 degrees from the midline. This helps relieve the pressure of the heavy uterus on the vena cava and lessens the incidence of vena cava compression and maternal supine hypotension. The suction should be in working order and the urine collection bag should be positioned under the operating table to obtain proper drainage. Auscultation or EFM of the fetal heart rate is continued until immediately before the procedure. A last-minute check is done to ensure that the fetal scalp electrode has been removed if the fetus was internally monitored.

Continue to provide reassurance and describe the various procedures being performed along with their rationales to ease anxiety and give the woman a sense of control.

Preparation for Elective Birth After Cesarean Birth

When a couple is anticipating an elective birth after cesarean (EBAC), they have a general understanding of what will occur, which can help them make informed choices about their birth experience. Couples who have had previous negative experiences need an opportunity to describe what they felt.

Encourage them to identify what they would like to do differently and to list options that would make the experience more positive. Those who have already had positive experiences need reassurance that their needs and desires will be met in a similar manner and should be allowed to discuss any fears or anxieties. For women who previously labored and then had an unexpected cesarean birth, the experience may be perceived as negative. Positive aspects that can be emphasized include participation in selecting the birth date, lack of fatigue related to labor, ability to prepare and make arrangements for other children, and ability for other family members or friends to be present at the hospital during or immediately after birth if desired by the couple.

Preparation for Emergency Cesarean Birth

When the need for a cesarean birth emerges suddenly, the period preceding surgery must be used to its greatest advantage. It is imperative that caregivers use their most effective communication skills in supporting the couple. Describe what the couple may anticipate during the next few hours. Asking the couple "What questions or concerns do you have about the decision?" gives them an opportunity for clarification. Prepare the woman in stages, giving her information and the rationales for interventions before beginning any procedure. It is essential to tell the woman (1) what is going to happen, (2) why it is being done, and (3) what sensations she may experience. This allows the woman to be informed and to consent to the procedure, which gives her a sense of control and reduces her feelings of helplessness.

Supporting the Father or Partner

Every effort should be made to include the father or partner in the birth experience. When attending the cesarean birth, the partner wears protective coverings similar to those worn by others in the operating suite. A stool can be placed beside the woman's head so that the partner can sit nearby to provide physical touch, visual contact, and verbal reassurance.

To promote the participation of the father/partner who chooses not to be in the operating suite, you can do the following:

1. Allow the father to be nearby, where he can hear the newborn's first cry.

2. Allow the father to hold the newborn near the head of the mother to facilitate early parental bonding.

3. Encourage the father to carry or accompany the infant to the nursery for the initial assessment.

4. Involve the father in postpartum care in the recovery room.

Some facilities have policies that prohibit a support person from being in the operating room if the woman requires general anesthesia or if an emergency birth is being performed. In these situations, the support person should receive a thorough explanation of what is happening and why, be advised when the staff will return to provide information, know the expected length of time for the procedure, and be reassured that the mother is receiving the care she and the baby need. Because this exclusion is stressful for family members, staff should try to provide information as soon as possible after providing emergency care to the mother. Having another staff member check in on the family and provide updates and reassurance often helps decrease the family's anxiety.

Immediate Postnatal Recovery Period

After birth assess the Apgar score and complete the same initial assessment and identification procedures used for vaginal births. Infant identification bands must be placed on the infant and the mother (as well as the father or support person, if present) before removing the infant from the operating room. Every effort should be made to assist the parents in bonding with their infant. If the mother is awake, one of her arms can be freed to enable her to touch and stroke the infant. The newborn may be placed on the mother's chest or held in an *en face* position. If physical contact is not possible, provide a running narrative so the mother knows what is happening with her baby. Assist the anesthesiologist or nurse anesthetist with raising the mother's head so she can see her infant immediately after birth. The parents can be encouraged to talk to the baby, and the father can hold the baby until she or he is taken to the nursery.

Assess the mother's vital signs every 5 minutes until they are stable, then every 15 minutes for 2 hours, then every 4 hours until she is discharged to the postpartum unit. Remain with the woman until she is stable.

Evaluate the dressing and perineal pad every 15 minutes for at least an hour. The fundus should be gently palpated to determine whether it is remaining firm; it may be palpated by placing a hand to support the incision. Intravenous Pitocin is usually administered to promote the contractility of the uterine musculature. If the woman has been under general anesthesia, she should be positioned on her side to facilitate drainage of secretions, turned, and assisted with coughing and deep breathing every 2 hours for at least 24 hours. If she has received a spinal or epidural anesthetic, the level of anesthesia is checked every 15 minutes until full sensation has returned. It is important to monitor intake and output and to observe the urine for a bloody tinge, which could mean surgical trauma to the bladder. The physician prescribes medication to relieve the mother's pain and nausea, and it is administered as needed.

 Clinical Tip

Promote bonding by allowing the mother to hold or nurse the infant during this time period. If the infant has been moved to a separate area, such as the nursery, encourage maternal participation by allowing the support person to visit the infant and report back to the mother. The support person can take digital pictures or bring back the blanket that was used to wrap up the baby immediately after the birth. Offering frequent updates such as "Your baby's doing just fine" provide reassurance to the mother if separation is needed.

CARE OF THE WOMAN UNDERGOING TRIAL OF LABOR AFTER CESAREAN (TOLAC) AND VAGINAL BIRTH AFTER CESAREAN (VBAC)

In the late 1990s there was an increasing trend to have a trial of labor and attempt **vaginal birth after cesarean (VBAC)**, now also known as a **trial of labor after cesarean (TOLAC)**, in cases of nonrecurring indications for a cesarean (such as umbilical cord prolapse, breech, placenta previa, or nonreassuring fetal status). This trend was influenced by consumer demand and studies that supported VBAC as a viable alternative to repeat cesarean.

In current practice, TOLAC should be performed in facilities where there is immediate access to perform an emergency cesarean birth if medically indicated. This requires in-house anesthesia and in-house, round-the-clock obstetric services. In facilities that cannot meet these criteria, the availability of TOLAC may be limited and require women who desire a TOLAC to travel to larger hospital facilities.

Between 1970 and 2007, media reports identifying risks of VBAC have introduced extensive debate regarding its safety. At the same time, trends in counseling women to have an elective repeat cesarean birth are driving cesarean births to an all-time high in the United States. Although TOLAC is associated with a higher risk of uterine rupture, the overall maternal mortality rates are higher for women undergoing an elective repeat cesarean delivery (ERCD), which prompted revision of protocols to determine which groups of women could safely have a TOLAC.

The ACOG (2010) guidelines update states that the following aspects are encouraging when considering a TOLAC:

- A woman with one or two previous cesarean births and a low transverse uterine incision
- A clinically adequate pelvis based on clinical pelvimetry or prior vaginal birth
- A woman with one previous cesarean birth with an undocumented uterine scar unless there is a high suspicion there was a classical incision performed previously
- Absence of other uterine scars or history of previous uterine rupture

The most common risks associated with failed TOLAC births are maternal hemorrhage, infection, operative injury, thromboembolism, hysterectomy, and death (ACOG, 2010). Complications associated with uterine rupture include hemorrhage, uterine scar separation or uterine rupture, hysterectomy, surgical injuries, infant death, and neurologic complications (see Chapter 21 🔗). The incidence of uterine rupture is 0.5% to 0.9% of all trials of labors when the mother has had a previous cesarean birth. The incidence of uterine rupture is directly correlated with the type of uterine incision the woman has obtained in a previous birth. Low transverse incisions have the lowest risk, whereas classical and vertical incisions carry a higher risk

of uterine rupture (ACOG, 2010). Women who go into spontaneous labor have a much lower incidence of uterine rupture (0.4%) compared with women who undergo Pitocin induction (0.9% to 1.1%) (ACOG, 2010). Prostaglandin agents should not be used in women attempting a TOLAC because of the increased risk of uterine rupture. The incidence of uterine rupture in women who receive a prostaglandin agent is as high as 1.4 per 100 (ACOG, 2010).

Conservative policies, such as awaiting spontaneous labor, avoiding prostaglandin agents, and avoiding elective inductions, can assist in reducing the incidence of uterine rupture. Women with an unfavorable cervix who are in need of an induction for medical indications may be treated with a transcervical catheter to initiate mechanical dilatation; however, research findings are inconsistent, with one study finding a slightly higher incidence of uterine rupture compared to spontaneous labor (ACOG, 2010).

Women who have a successful TOLAC have lower incidences of infection, less blood loss, fewer blood transfusions, and shorter hospital stays. Healthcare costs are considerably lower for women who have a TOLAC than for those who have a repeat cesarean birth (ACOG, 2010). After a woman had one successful VBAC, the risks of neonatal and maternal complications were low in subsequent attempts. In general, 60% to 80% of women who undergo a TOLAC have a successful VBAC.

Research shows a close correlation between maternal weight and success for TOLAC (O'Dwyer et al., 2011). In one study that examined obese and morbidly obese women, the TOLAC success rate was only 2.3% although the neonatal death rate rose significantly as a mother's body mass index (BMI) rose (Belogolovkin et al., 2012). Although ACOG does not provide specific guidelines on obesity as a contraindication to TOLAC, all factors should be presented to the woman so she can make an informed choice related to her intended birth options.

Nursing Management

The nursing care of a woman undergoing TOLAC varies according to institutional protocols. Generally, a saline lock is inserted for IV access if needed or an intravenous infusion of fluids is started, continuous electronic fetal monitoring (EFM) is used, and clear fluids may be taken. A woman at higher risk may require additional precautionary measures, such as internal monitoring after the membranes have ruptured. Take care to ensure that the woman and her partner feel safe but not unduly restricted by the TOLAC status. When available, telemetry monitors can be utilized so mothers can ambulate within the hallways and take tub baths and showers.

Supportive and comfort measures are very important. The woman may be excited about this opportunity to experience labor and vaginal birth, or she may be hesitant and frightened about the possibility of complications. The presence of the nurse is important in providing information and encouragement for the laboring woman and her partner.

Critical Concept Review

LEARNING OUTCOME 23.1: Explain the methods, purpose, and contraindications of external and podalic versions that determine nursing management.

1. An external version (cephalic version) may be done after 36 weeks' gestation to change a breech presentation to a cephalic presentation.
   - Physician applies external manipulation to the maternal abdomen.
   - Fetal part must not be engaged.
   - NST performed to establish fetal well-being.
   - Tocolytic given during procedure to relax uterus.

2. Podalic version is used to turn a second twin during a vaginal birth.
   - Used only if second fetus does not descend readily and heartbeat is not reassuring.
   - Physician reaches into uterus and grabs feet of fetus and pulls them down through cervix.
   - A tocolytic is given to relax uterus.
   - An epidural may be given to reduce discomfort during the procedure and increase success rates.

LEARNING OUTCOME 23.2: Describe the use of amniotomy in the nursing management of the woman and fetus.

1. An amniotomy (artificial rupture of the amniotic membranes) is used for several reasons:
   - To induce labor.
   - To accelerate labor.
   - To apply an internal fetal monitor or insert an intrauterine pressure catheter.

2. Risks include prolapsed cord and infection.

LEARNING OUTCOME 23.3: Compare the methods for inducing labor, explaining their advantages and disadvantages in determining the nursing management of women during labor induction.

1. Cervical ripening:
   - May hasten the beginning of labor or shorten the course of labor.
   - May cause hyperstimulation of the uterus.
2. Stripping the membranes:
   - May not induce labor; if labor is initiated, it typically begins within 48 hours.
   - May cause bleeding.

3. Mechanical dilatation of the cervix:
   - Is used to stretch the cervix and shorten the first stage of labor without causing hypersystole.
   - Can be used with weighted catheter or in combination with prostaglandin agents.
4. Pitocin infusion:
   - Is usually effective at producing contractions.
   - May cause hyperstimulation of uterus.

LEARNING OUTCOME 23.4: Describe the measures to prevent episiotomy, the types of episiotomy performed, and the associated nursing management.

1. Preventive measures:
   - Perineal massage during pregnancy.
   - Natural pushing during labor.
   - Side-lying position for pushing; avoid lithotomy position or pulling back on legs.
   - Avoid immediate pushing after epidural placement.
   - Encourage a gradual expulsion of the infant by doing controlled breathing pattern.

2. Two types of episiotomy are used:
   - Midline.
   - Mediolateral.
3. During the episiotomy the nurse supports the woman, explaining the procedure.
4. After the birth:
   - Place an ice pack to the perineum.
   - Inspect the perineum frequently.
   - Instruct the woman in perineal hygiene, self-care, and comfort measures.

LEARNING OUTCOME 23.5: Explain the indications and maternal and neonatal risks that impact nursing management during forceps-assisted birth.

Indications:
1. To shorten the second stage of labor.
   - Used in the presence of nonreassuring fetal status and premature placental separation.
2. To assist woman's pushing effort.
   - Used in the presence of maternal exhaustion, or when regional anesthesia impairs woman's ability to push effectively.

Maternal and neonatal risks:
1. Newborn bruising, facial edema, facial lacerations, cephalhematoma, and transient facial paralysis.
2. Woman may experience vaginal lacerations, increased bleeding, bruising, and perineal edema.

LEARNING OUTCOME 23.6: Describe the use and risk of vacuum extraction to assist birth.

1. Vacuum extractor assists birth by applying suction to the fetal head.
   - May cause cephalhematoma.
   - Increases risk for jaundice.

LEARNING OUTCOME 23.7: Explain the indications for cesarean birth, impact on the family unit, preparation and teaching needs, and associated nursing management.

1. Most common indications for cesarean birth are:
   - Nonreassuring fetal status.
   - Lack of labor progression.
   - Maternal infection.
   - Pelvic size disproportion.
   - Placenta previa.
   - Previous cesarean birth.
2. Couples should be encouraged to participate in as many choices as possible concerning the surgical birth.
3. Preparation for cesarean birth requires:
   - Establishing IV lines.
   - Placing an indwelling catheter.
   - Performing an abdominal prep.

4. Teaching needs include:
   - What to expect before, during, and after birth.
   - Role of significant others.
   - Interaction with newborn.
5. Associated nursing care:
   - Routine postpartum care including fundal checks.
   - Care of incision.
   - Monitoring intake and output.
   - Assessment of respiratory system and returning bowel sounds.
   - Assessment of maternal pain level and provision of pain relief.

LEARNING OUTCOME 23.8: Examine the risks, guidelines, and nursing management of the woman undergoing trial of labor after cesarean.

1. Most common risks are:
   - Hemorrhage.
   - Uterine rupture.
   - Infant death.

2. Nursing care:
   - Continuous EFM.
   - Internal monitoring.
   - IV fluid.
3. Prostaglandin agent induction should be avoided if possible.

Clinical Reasoning in Action

Betsy Jones, a 28-year-old G1P0 at 39 weeks' gestation, and her husband present to you in the labor suite for an external cephalic version procedure by her obstetrician. You introduce yourself and review her prenatal record for any significant risk factors or contraindications to the version procedure. Her prenatal chart is significant in that the fetus has been in a persistent frank breech position. You encourage Betsy and her husband to express their understanding and expectations of the procedure. You discuss certain criteria to be met prior to the procedure and obtain vital signs as follows: T 98.8°F, P 88, R 14, BP 110/80, urine screening negative for sugar, albumin, and ketones. You place Betsy on the external electronic fetal monitor, which demonstrates a fetal heart rate baseline of 140 to 152 with long-term variability.

There are no contractions observed by the monitor or Betsy. After explaining how to record fetal movement on the monitor, you proceed with an NST.

1. Explain the contraindications to the version procedure.
2. Discuss the criteria that should be met prior to performing external version.
3. How would you explain to Betsy and her husband what to expect during the version procedure?
4. What support would you give Betsy during the procedure?
5. Explain postversion discharge teaching.
6. Create a concept map for Betsy's care based on the need for an external cephalic version based on the diagnosis of frank breech presentation.

See www.nursing.pearsonhighered.com for possible responses and an interactive template for a concept map.

References

Ali, U. A., & Norwitz, E. R. (2009). Vacuum-assisted vaginal delivery. *Reviews in Obstetrics & Gynecology, 2*(1), 5–17.

Al-Suhel, R., Gill, S., Robson, S., & Shadbolt, B. (2009). Kjelland's forceps in the new millennium. Maternal and neonatal outcomes of attempted rotational forceps delivery. *Australian and New Zealand Journal of Obstetrics and Gynaecology, 49*, 510–514. doi:10.1111/j.1479-828X.2009.01060.x

American College of Obstetricians and Gynecologists (ACOG). (2009). *Induction of labor* (ACOG Practice Bulletin No. 107). Washington, DC: Author.

American College of Obstetricians and Gynecologists (ACOG). (2010). *Vaginal birth after previous cesarean delivery* (Practice Bulletin No. 115). Washington, DC: Author.

American College of Obstetricians and Gynecologists (ACOG). (2011). *Episiotomy* (ACOG Practice Bulletin No. 71). Washington, DC: Author.

Belogolovkin, V., Crisan, L., Lynch, O., Weldeselasse, H., August, E. M., Alio, A. P., & Salihu, H. M. (2012). Neonatal outcomes of successful VBAC among obese and super-obese mothers. *Journal of Maternal–Fetal and Neonatal Medicine, 25*(6), 714–718. doi:10.3109/14767058.2011.596594

Bishop, E. H. (1964). Pelvic scoring for elective inductions. *Obstetrics and Gynecology, 24*, 266.

Centers for Disease Control and Prevention. (2012). *Birth trends.* Retrieved from http://www.cdc.gov/nchs/births.htm

Chaudhry, Z., Fischer, J., & Schaffir, J. (2011). Women's use of nonprescribed methods to induce labor: A brief report. *Birth, 38*, 168–171. doi:10.1111/j.1523-536X.2010.00465.x

Cunningham, F. G., Leveno, K. J., Bloom, S. L., Hauth, J. C., Gilstrap, L. C., & Wenstrom, K. D. (2010). *Williams obstetrics* (23rd ed.). New York, NY: McGraw-Hill Medical.

Demers, A. (2011). Should patients be entitled to cesarean section on demand? No. *Canadian Family Physician, 57*(11), 1247–1248.

Dowswell, T., Kelly, A. J., Livio, S., Norman, J. E., & Alfirevic, Z. (2010). Different methods for the induction of labour in outpatient settings. *Cochrane Database of Systematic Reviews 2010*, Issue 8. Art. No.: CD007701. doi:10.1002/14651858.CD007701 .pub2

Edgar, D. C., Baskett, T. F., Young, D. C., & O'Connell, T. M. (2012). Neonatal outcome following failed Kiwi OmniCup vacuum extraction. *Journal of Obstetrics & Gynaecology in Canada, 34*(7), 620–625.

Ehrenberg-Buchner, S. (2011). External cephalic version. *Medscape.* Retrieved from http://medicine.medscape .com/article/1848353-overview

Ehrenthal, D. B., Jiang, X., & Strobino, D. M. (2010). Labor induction and the risk of a cesarean delivery among nulliparous women at term. *Obstetrics & Gynecology, 116*(1), 35–42.

Forrest Pharmaceuticals. (2013). *Cervidil dinoprostone 10 mg vaginal insert.* St. Louis, MO: Author.

Fox, N., Saltzman, D., Roman, A., Klauser, C., Moshier, E., & Rebarber, A. (2011). Intravaginal misoprostol versus Foley catheter for labour induction: A meta-analysis. *BJOG: An International Journal of Obstetrics & Gynaecology, 118*, 647–654. doi:10.1111/j.1471-0528.2011.02905.x

Gagnon-Gervais, K., Bujold, E., Iglesias, M., Duperron, L., Masse, A., Mayrand, M., . . . Audibert, F. (2012). Early versus late amniotomy for labour induction: A randomized controlled trial. *Journal of Maternal–Fetal and Neonatal Medicine, 25*(11), 2326–2329. doi:10. 3109/14767058.2012.695819

Goetzinger, K. R., Harper, L. M., Tuuli, M. G., Macones, G. A., & Colditz, G. A. (2011). Effect of regional anesthesia on the success rate of external cephalic version: A systematic review and meta-analysis. *Obstetrics & Gynecology, 118*(5),1137–1144. doi:10.1097/AOG.0b013e3182324583

Goldenberg, R. L., McClure, E. M., & Kamath, B. D. (2012). Intrapartum perinatal mortality. *Indian Pediatrics, 49*(3),187–190. doi:10.1007/ s13312-012-0050-4

Gurol-Urganci, I., Cromwell, D. A., Edozien, L. C., Smith, G. C. S., Onwere, C., Mahmood, T. A., . . . van der Meulen, J. H. (2011). Risk of placenta previa in second birth after first birth cesarean section: A population-based study and meta-analysis. *BMC Pregnancy and Childbirth, 11*, 95. doi:10.1186/1471-2393-11-95

Hall, H. G., McKenna, L. G., & Griffiths, D. (2011). Complementary and alternative medicine for induction of labour. *Women and Birth, 25*(3), 142–148. doi:10.1016/j.wombi.2011.03.006

Handa, V. L., Blomquist, J. L., Knoepp, L. R., Hoskey, K. A., McDermott, K. C., & Muñoz, A. (2011). Pelvic floor disorders 5–10 years after vaginal or cesarean childbirth. *Obstetrics & Gynecology, 118*(4),777–784. doi:10.1097/AOG.0b013e3182267f2f

Hofmeyr, G. J., Gülmezoglu, A. M., & Pileggi, C. (2010). Vaginal misoprostol for cervical ripening and induction of labour. *Cochrane Database of Systematic Reviews 2010*, Issue 10. Art. No.: CD000941. doi:10.1002/14651858.CD000941.pub2

Kehl, S., Ehard, A., Berlit, S., Spaich, S., Sütterlin, M., & Siemer, J. (2011). Combination of misoprostol and mechanical dilation for induction of labour: A randomized controlled trial. *European Journal of Obstetrics & Gynecology and Reproductive Biology, 159*(2), 315–319. doi.org/10.1016/j.ejogrb.2011.09.010

Lurie, S., Kedar, D., Boaz, M., Golan, A., & Sadan, O. (2012). Need for episiotomy in a subsequent delivery following previous delivery with episiotomy. *Archives of Gynecology and Obstetrics.* doi:10.1007/ s00404-012-2551-8

Lutgendorf, M. A., Johnson, A., Terpstra, E. R., Snider, T. C., & Magann, E. F. (2012). Extra-amniotic balloon for preinduction cervical ripening: a randomized comparison of weighted traction versus unweighted. *Journal of Maternal–Fetal and Neonatal Medicine, 25*(6), 581–586. doi:10.3109/14767058.2011 .587063

Mansouri, H. A., & Alsahly, N. (2011). Rectal versus oral misoprostol for active management of third stage of labor: A randomized controlled trial. *Archives of Gynecology and Obstetrics, 283*(5), 935–939. doi:10.1007/s00404-010-1466-5

National Institutes of Health Consensus Development Conference Panel. (2010). National Institutes of Health Consensus Development conference statement: Vaginal birth after cesarean: New insights. March 8–10, 2010. *Obstetrics & Gynecology, 115*(6), 1279.

O'Dwyer, V., Fattah, C., Farah, N., Hogan, J., Kennelly, M. M., & Turner, M. J. (2011). Vaginal birth after caesarean section (VBAC) and maternal obesity. *Archives of Diseases in Child Fetal Neonatal Education, 96*, Fa82. doi:10.1136/archdischild.2011.300162.24

Okonkwo, N. S., Ojengbede, O. A., Morhason-Bello, I. O., & Adedokun, B. O. (2012). Maternal demand for cesarean section: Perception and willingness to request by Nigerian antenatal patients. *International Journal of Women's Health, 4*, 141–148. doi:10.2147/IJWH.S10325

Oyelese, Y., & Canterino, J. C. (2011). Placenta previa and placenta accreta. *Bleeding During Pregnancy, 3*, 135–150. doi:10.1007/978-1-4419-9810-1_8

Smith, C. A., & Crowther, C. A. (2009). Acupuncture for induction of labour. *Cochrane Database of Systematic Reviews 2009*, Issue 1. Art. No.: CD002962. doi:10.1002/14651858.CD002962.pub2

Society for Maternal–Fetal Medicine. (2012). *High-risk pregnancy care, research, and education for over 35 years.* Retrieved from https://www.smfm.org/ attachedfiles/SMFMMonograph3.1.pdf

Teixeira, C., Lunet, N., Rodrigues, T., & Barros, H. (2012). The Bishop Score as a determinant of labour induction success: A systematic review and meta-analysis. *Archives of Gynecology and Obstetrics, 286*(3), 739–753. doi:10.1007/s00404-012-2341-3

Thorpe, J. M. (2009). Clinical aspects of normal and abnormal labor. In R. K. Creasy, R. Resnik, & J. D. Iams (Eds.), *Obstetrics: Normal and problem pregnancies* (6th ed., pp. 691–724). Philadelphia, PA: Saunders.

Vardo, J., Thornburg, L., Glantz, J., & Christopher, J. (2011). Maternal and neonatal morbidity among nulliparous women undergoing elective induction of labor. *Journal of Reproductive Medicine, 56*(1–2), 25–30.

Webster, S. N. E., & Loughley, A. D. (2011). Internal podalic version with breech extraction. *The Obstetrician & Gynaecologist, 13*(1), 7–14. doi:10.1576/ toag.13.1.7.27635

Wilson, B., Effken, J., & Butler, R. (2010). The relationship between cesarean section and labor induction. *Journal of Nursing Scholarship, 42*(2), 130–138.

Wilson, B. A., Shannon, M. T., & Shields, K. M. (Eds.). (2013). *Nursing drug guide: 2012.* Upper Saddle River, NJ: Pearson.

Women's Health Data Directory. (2012). *Cesarean section.* Retrieved from http://www.womenshealthdata. ca/category.aspx?catid=108&rt=3

World Health Organization (WHO). (2011). *The global numbers and costs of additionally needed and unnecessary caesarean sections performed per year: Overuse as a barrier to universal coverage* (World Health Report, Background Paper No. 30). Retrieved from http://www.who.int/healthsystems/topics/ financing/healthreport/30C-sectioncosts.pdf

Zanconato, G., Bergamini, V., Mantovani, E., Carlin, R., Bortolami, O., & Franchi, M. (2011). Induction of labor and pain: A randomized trial between two vaginal preparations of dinoprostone in nulliparous women with an unfavorable cervix. *Journal of Maternal–Fetal and Neonatal Medicine, 24*(5), 728–731. doi:10.310 9/14767058.2011.557108

CHAPTER
24

The Physiologic Responses of the Newborn to Birth

I remember clearly when they held him up for us to see and my husband and I cried and laughed and it was so amazing. He was 9 1/2 pounds and was so beautiful. Even though my labor was long, his Apgars were high, and he didn't even cry—not until we dressed him, anyway. —Crystal, 26

Scott T. Baxter/Getty Images

LEARNING OUTCOMES

24.1 Explain the respiratory and cardiovascular changes that occur during the newborn's transition to extrauterine life and during stabilization in determining the nursing care of the newborn.

24.2 Compare the factors that modify the newborn's blood values to the corresponding results.

24.3 Relate the process of thermogenesis in the newborn and the major mechanisms of heat loss to the challenge of maintaining newborn thermal stability.

24.4 Explain the steps involved in conjugation and excretion of bilirubin in the newborn.

24.5 Identify the reasons a newborn may develop jaundice and nursing interventions to decrease the probability of jaundice.

24.6 Delineate the functional abilities of the newborn's gastrointestinal tract and liver.

24.7 Relate the development of the newborn's kidneys to the newborn's ability to maintain fluid and electrolyte balance.

24.8 Describe basic newborn immunologic responses.

24.9 Explain the physiologic and behavioral characteristics of newborn neurologic function, patterns of behavior during the periods of reactivity, and possible nursing interventions.

24.10 Describe the normal sensory-perceptual abilities and behavioral states seen in the newborn period and the associated nursing care.

519

The newborn period is the time from birth through the 28th day of life. During this period, the newborn adjusts from intrauterine to extrauterine life. The nurse needs to be knowledgeable about a newborn's normal physiologic and behavioral adaptations and to recognize alterations from normal.

The first few hours of life, in which the newborn stabilizes respiratory and circulatory functions, are called **neonatal transition**. All other newborn body systems change their level of functioning and become established over a longer period of time during the neonatal period.

RESPIRATORY ADAPTATIONS

To begin life as a separate being, the baby must immediately establish respiratory functioning and ventilation. Adequate gas exchange in conjunction with marked circulatory changes are radical and rapid changes crucial to successful transition to extrauterine life.

Intrauterine Factors Supporting Respiratory Function

Even before the significant respiratory events occur at birth, certain intrauterine factors also enhance the newborn's ability to breathe. Adequate fetal lung development allows the newborn to expand the lungs and exchange oxygen and carbon dioxide gases. Even before birth the fetus practices breathing movements, which allow the newborn to breathe immediately after birth.

Fetal Lung Development

The respiratory system is in an ongoing state of development during fetal life, and lung development continues into early childhood. During the first 20 weeks' gestation, development is limited to the differentiation of pulmonary, vascular, and lymphatic structures. From 20 to 28 weeks, alveolar ducts begin to appear, followed by primitive alveoli. During this time, the alveolar epithelial cells begin to differentiate into type I cells (structures necessary for gas exchange) and type II cells (structures that provide for the synthesis and storage of surfactant). **Surfactant**, a lipoprotein that coats the inner surfaces of the alveoli, is composed of surface-active phospholipids (lecithin and sphingomyelin), which are critical for alveolar stability. At 28 to 32 weeks' gestation, the number of type II cells increases further, and surfactant is produced by a more stable cellular pathway. Surfactant peaks at about 35 weeks' gestation and remains high until term, paralleling late fetal lung development. At this time, the lungs are structurally developed enough to permit maintenance of lung expansion and adequate exchange of gases, although a fetus born at this gestation may need intensive care to survive.

Clinically, the peak production of lecithin—one component of surfactant—corresponds closely to the marked decrease in the incidence of respiratory distress syndrome for babies born after 35 weeks' gestation. Production of sphingomyelin (the other component of surfactant) remains constant during gestation. The newborn born before the lecithin/sphingomyelin (L/S) ratio is 2:1 will have varying degrees of respiratory distress. (See discussion of L/S ratio and respiratory distress syndrome in Chapter 29 ✐.)

Fetal Breathing Movements

The newborn's ability to breathe air immediately after birth appears to result from fetal breathing movements (FBM), the intrauterine practice respiratory movements that begin around the 17th to 20th week of gestation. In this respect, breathing can be seen as a continuation of an intrauterine process; the lungs convert from a fluid-filled organ to a gas-filled organ capable of gas exchange.

These breathing movements are essential for developing the chest wall muscles and the diaphragm and, to a lesser extent, for regulating lung fluid volume and resultant lung growth.

Initiation of Breathing

To maintain life, the lungs must function immediately after birth. Two radical changes must take place for the lungs to function:

1. Pulmonary ventilation must be established through lung expansion following birth.

2. A marked increase in the pulmonary circulation must occur.

The first breath of life in response to mechanical and reabsorptive, chemical, thermal, and sensory changes associated with birth initiates the serial opening of the alveoli. So begins the transition from a fluid-filled environment to an air-breathing, independent, extrauterine life. Figure 24–1 • summarizes the initiation of respiration.

Mechanical and Reabsorptive Processes

During the latter half of gestation, the fetal lungs continuously produce fluid. This fluid expands the lungs almost completely, filling the air spaces. Some of the lung fluid moves up into the trachea and into the amniotic fluid and is then swallowed by the fetus.

In preparation for birth, lung fluid production normally decreases and fetal breathing movement decreases 24 to 36 hours before the onset of true labor. However, approximately 80 to 100 mL of lung fluid remains in the respiratory passages of a normal full-term fetus at the time of birth. Excess fluid must be removed from the alveolar spaces after birth for effective gas exchange to occur.

As the fetus experiences labor there is a fetal gasp and active exhalation that initiates the removal of fluid from the lungs. Also during labor a glucocorticoids and catecholamine surge promotes fluid clearance from the lungs. During the vaginal birthing process, a *thoracic squeeze* occurs and squeezes a small amount of fluid out of the lungs. The significance of the thoracic squeeze appears minimal, and the process of labor is primarily responsible for the initial movement of lung fluid out of the lungs (Blackburn, 2013; Cloherty, Eichenwald, Hansen, et al., 2012). If the baby doesn't experience labor (e.g., the mother has a planned cesarean section), then the infant has an increased chance of getting transient tachypnea (see Chapter 28 🔗).

After this first inspiration, the newborn exhales, with crying, against a partially closed glottis, creating positive intrathoracic pressure. The high positive intrathoracic pressure distributes the inspired air throughout the alveoli and begins to establish *functional residual capacity* (FRC), the air left in the lungs at the end of a normal expiration. The higher intrathoracic pressure also increases absorption of fluid via the capillaries and lymphatic system. The negative intrathoracic pressure created when the diaphragm moves down with inspiration causes lung fluid to flow from the alveoli across the alveolar membranes into the pulmonary interstitial tissue.

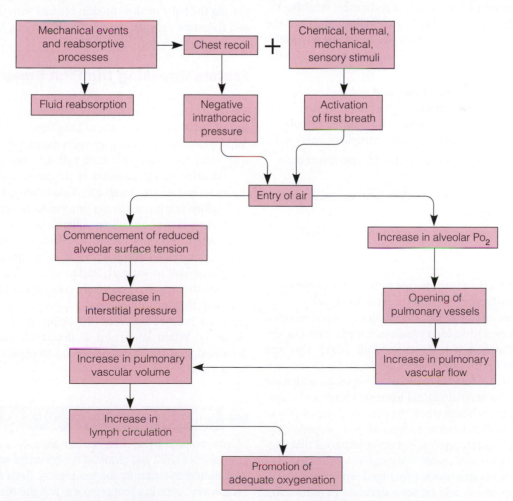

• **Figure 24–1** Initiation of respiration in the newborn.

At birth the alveolar epithelium is temporarily more permeable. This, combined with decreased cellular resistance at the onset of breathing, may facilitate passive liquid absorption. With each succeeding breath, the lungs continue to expand, stretching the alveolar walls and increasing the alveolar volume. Protein molecules are too large to pass through capillary walls. The presence of more protein molecules in the pulmonary capillaries than in the interstitial tissue creates oncotic pressure. This pressure draws the interstitial fluid into the capillaries and lymphatic tissue to balance the concentration of protein. Lung expansion helps the remaining lung fluid move into the interstitial tissue. As pulmonary vascular resistance decreases, pulmonary blood flow increases, and more interstitial fluid is absorbed into the bloodstream. In the healthy term newborn, lung fluid moves rapidly into the interstitial tissue but may take several hours to move into the lymph and blood vessels (see Skill 5–1, Performing Nasal Pharyngeal Suctioning, in the *Clinical Skills Manual* SKILLS).

Newborns may have problems clearing the fluid from their lungs and beginning respiration for a variety of reasons:

- The lymphatic system may be underdeveloped, thus decreasing the rate at which the fluid is absorbed from the lungs.
- Complications that occur before or during labor and birth can interfere with adequate lung expansion and cause failure to decrease pulmonary vascular resistance, resulting in decreased pulmonary blood flow. Excess fluid must exit the alveoli, and pulmonary blood flow must increase to match ventilation with perfusion. These complications include the following:
  - Inadequate compression of the chest wall in very small newborns (small for gestational age [SGA] or very low birth weight [VLBW]) because of immature muscular development that causes an overly compliant chest wall
  - Absence of chest wall compression in a newborn born by cesarean birth
  - Respiratory depression secondary to maternal analgesia or anesthesia agents
  - Aspiration of amniotic fluid, meconium, or blood

Chemical Stimuli

An important chemical stimulator that contributes to the onset of breathing is transitory asphyxia of the fetus and newborn. The first breath is an inspiratory gasp, the result of central nervous system (CNS) reaction to sudden pressure, temperature change, and other external stimuli (Cheffer & Rannalli, 2011). This first breath is triggered by the slight elevation in pCO_2 (hypercapnia) and decrease in pH (acidosis) and pO_2 (hypoxia), which are the natural result of a normal vaginal labor and birth and cessation of placental gas exchange when the cord is clamped. These stressors, present in all newborns to some degree, stimulate the aortic and carotid chemoreceptors, initiating impulses that trigger the medulla's respiratory center. Although this brief period of asphyxia is a significant stimulator, prolonged asphyxia is abnormal, depresses respiration, and causes a decrease in pulmonary blood flow. Another chemical factor involves hormonal changes during the labor and delivery process. The levels of prostaglandin, a hormone that suppresses respiration, fall with the clamping of the umbilical cord, thus increasing the infant's respiratory drive (Blackburn, 2013).

Thermal Stimuli

A significant decrease in environmental temperature after birth, 37°C to 21°C–23.9°C (98.6°F to 70°F–75°F), results in sudden chilling of the moist newborn (Blackburn, 2013). The cold stimulates skin nerve endings, and the newborn responds with rhythmic respirations. Normal temperature changes that occur at birth are apparently within acceptable physiologic limits. Excessive cooling may result in profound depression and evidence of cold stress (see Chapter 28 🔗 for discussion of cold stress).

Sensory Stimuli

During intrauterine life, the fetus is in a dark, sound-dampened, fluid-filled environment and is nearly weightless. As the fetus moves from a familiar, comfortable, quiet environment to one of sensory abundance, a number of physical and sensory influences help respiration begin and be sustained after birth. They include the numerous tactile, auditory, and visual stimuli of birth and the normal handling after delivery. Joint movement also results in enhanced proprioceptor stimulation to the respiratory center to sustain respirations. Thoroughly drying the newborn and placing the baby in skin-to-skin contact with the mother's chest and abdomen provide ample stimulation in a far more comforting way and also decrease heat loss.

Factors Opposing the First Breath

Three major factors may oppose the initiation of respiratory activity: (1) the contracting force between alveoli—called *alveolar surface tension*; (2) viscosity of lung fluid within the respiratory tract, which is influenced by surfactant levels; and (3) the ease with which the lung is able to fill with air—called *lung compliance*.

Alveolar surface tension is the contracting force between the moist surfaces of the alveoli. This tension, which is necessary for healthy respiratory function, would nevertheless cause the small airways and alveoli to collapse between each inspiration if surfactant were not present. Surfactant is important because it reduces surface tension of the fluid lining the alveoli, permitting the alveoli to expand. Surfactant stabilizes the alveoli and prevents them from completely collapsing during each expiration and thus promotes lung expansion. Similarly, surfactant promotes lung compliance, the ability of the lung to fill with air easily. When surfactant is decreased, compliance is also decreased, and the pressure needed to expand the alveoli with air increases.

> ## Clinical Tip
>
> Gentle, thorough drying of the newborn and skin-to-skin contact with the mother's chest and abdomen is emphasized when using external stimulation means for the first breaths. These methods provide ample stimulation in a comforting way and also decrease heat loss.

Resistive forces of the fluid-filled lung, combined with the small radii of the airways, necessitate pressures of 30 to 40 cm (11.8 to 15.7 in.) of water to open the lung initially (Niermeyer & Clarke, 2011).

The first breath usually establishes FRC that is 30% to 40% of the fully expanded lung volume. This FRC allows alveolar sacs to remain partially expanded on expiration, decreasing the need for continuous high pressures for each of the following breaths. Subsequent breaths require only 6 to 8 cm H$_2$O pressure to open alveoli during inspiration. Therefore, the first breath of life is usually the most difficult.

Cardiopulmonary Physiology

The onset of respiration stimulates changes in the cardiovascular system necessary for successful transition to extrauterine life, hence the term **cardiopulmonary adaptation**. As air enters the lungs, pO$_2$ rises in the alveoli, which stimulates the relaxation of the pulmonary arteries and triggers a decrease in pulmonary vascular resistance. As pulmonary vascular resistance decreases, the vascular flow in the lung increases rapidly and achieves 100% normal flow at 24 hours of life. This delivery of greater blood volume to the lungs contributes to the conversion from fetal circulation to newborn circulation.

After pulmonary circulation is established, blood is distributed throughout the lungs, although the alveoli may or may not be fully open. For adequate oxygenation to occur, the heart must deliver sufficient blood to functional, open alveoli. Shunting of blood is common in the early newborn period. Bidirectional blood flow, or right-to-left shunting through the ductus arteriosus, may divert a significant amount of blood away from the lungs, depending on the pressure changes of respiration, crying, and the cardiac cycle. This shunting in the newborn period is also responsible for the unstable transitional period in cardiopulmonary function.

Oxygen Transport

The transportation of oxygen to the peripheral tissues depends on the type of hemoglobin in the red blood cells. In the fetus and newborn, a variety of hemoglobins exist, the most significant being fetal hemoglobin (HbF) and adult hemoglobin (HbA). Approximately 70% to 90% of the hemoglobin in the fetus and newborn is of the fetal variety. The greatest difference between HbF and HbA relates to the transport of and release of oxygen to the tissues.

Because HbF has a greater affinity for oxygen than does HbA, the oxygen saturation in the newborn's blood is greater than in the adult's, but the amount of oxygen released to the tissues is less. Because of this high concentration of oxygen in the blood with HbF, hypoxia in the newborn is particularly difficult to recognize. Clinical manifestations of cyanosis do not appear until low blood levels of oxygen are present.

Maintaining Respiratory Function

The lung's ability to maintain oxygenation and ventilation (the exchange of oxygen and carbon dioxide) is influenced by such factors as lung compliance and airway resistance. Lung compliance is influenced by the elastic recoil of the lung tissue and

anatomic differences in the newborn. The newborn has a relatively large heart and mediastinal structures that reduce available lung space. Also, the newborn chest is equipped with weak intercostal muscles and a rigid rib cage with horizontal ribs and a high diaphragm, which restricts the space available for lung expansion. The large abdomen further encroaches on the high diaphragm to decrease lung space. Another factor that limits ventilation is airway resistance, which depends on the radii, length, and number of airways. Airway resistance is increased in the newborn when compared with adults.

Characteristics of Newborn Respiration

The normal newborn respiratory rate is 30 to 60 breaths per minute. Initial respirations may be largely diaphragmatic, shallow, and irregular in depth and rhythm. The abdomen's movements are synchronous with the chest movements. When the breathing pattern is characterized by pauses lasting 5 to 15 seconds, **periodic breathing** is occurring. Periodic breathing is rarely associated with differences in skin color or heart rate changes, and it has no prognostic significance. Tactile or other sensory stimulation increases the inspired oxygen and converts periodic breathing patterns to normal breathing patterns during neonatal transition. With deep sleep, the pattern is reasonably regular. Periodic breathing occurs with rapid-eye-movement (REM) sleep, and grossly irregular breathing is evident with motor activity, sucking, and crying. Cessation of breathing lasting more than 20 seconds is defined as *apnea* and is abnormal in term newborns. Apnea may or may not be associated with changes in skin color or heart rate (drop below 100 beats per minute). Apnea always needs to be further evaluated.

Newborns tend to be obligatory nose breathers because the nasal route is the primary route of air entry. This is because of the high position of the epiglottis and the position of the soft palate (Blackburn, 2013). Newborns need to breathe through their noses in order to feed without choking. Although many term newborns can breathe orally, with nasal occlusion, nasal obstructions can cause respiratory distress. Therefore, it is important to keep the nose and throat clear. Immediately after birth, and for about the next 2 hours, respiratory rates of 60 to 70 breaths per minute are normal. Some cyanosis and acrocyanosis are normal for several hours; thereafter, the infant's color improves steadily. If respirations drop below 30 or exceed 60 per minute when the infant is at rest, or if retractions, cyanosis, or nasal flaring and expiratory grunting occur, the clinician should be notified. Any increased use of the intercostal muscles (retractions) may indicate respiratory distress. (See Chapter 28 🔗 and Table 28–1 🔗 on page 673 for signs of respiratory distress.) Some institutions do pulse oximetry, which should be greater than 95% in term newborns. But it takes about 8 minutes on average for pulse oxygen saturations to rise above 90% (Raab & Kelly, 2013).

CARDIOVASCULAR ADAPTATIONS

As described earlier, the onset of respiration triggers increased blood flow to the lungs after birth. This greater blood volume contributes to the conversion from fetal circulation to neonatal circulation.

Fetal-Newborn Transitional Physiology

During fetal life, blood with the higher oxygen content is diverted to the heart and brain. Blood in the descending aorta is less oxygenated and supplies the kidney and intestinal tract before it is returned to the placenta. Limited amounts of blood, pumped from the right ventricle toward the lungs, enter the pulmonary vessels. In the fetus, increased pulmonary resistance forces most of this blood through the ductus arteriosus into the descending aorta (Table 24–1).

Marked changes occur in the cardiovascular system at birth. Expansion of the lungs with the first breath decreases pulmonary vascular resistance and increases pulmonary blood flow. Pressure in the left atrium increases as blood returns from the pulmonary veins. Pressure in the right atrium drops, and systemic vascular resistance increases as umbilical venous blood flow is halted when the cord is clamped. These physiologic mechanisms mark the transition from fetal to neonatal circulation and show the interplay of cardiovascular and respiratory systems (Figure 24–2 ●).

Five major areas of change occur in cardiopulmonary adaptation (Figure 24–3 ●):

1. *Increased aortic pressure and decreased venous pressure.*
   Clamping of the umbilical cord eliminates the placental vascular bed and reduces the intravascular space. Consequently, aortic (systemic) blood pressure increases. At the same time, blood return via the inferior vena cava decreases, resulting in a decreased right atrial pressure and a small decrease in pressure within the venous circulation.

Table 24–1	Fetal and Neonatal Circulation	
System	**Fetal**	**Neonatal**
Pulmonary blood vessels	Constricted, with very little blood flow; lungs not expanded	Vasodilation and increased blood flow; lungs expanded; increased oxygen stimulates vasodilation.
Systemic blood vessels	Dilated, with low resistance; blood mostly in placenta	Arterial pressure rises because of loss of placenta; increased systemic blood volume and resistance.
Ductus arteriosus	Large, with no tone; blood flow from pulmonary artery to aorta	Reversal of blood flow; now from aorta to pulmonary artery because of increased left atrial pressure. Ductus is sensitive to increased oxygen and body chemicals and begins to constrict.
Foramen ovale	Patent, with increased blood flow from right atrium to left atrium	Increased pressure in left atrium attempts to reverse blood flow and shuts one-way valve.

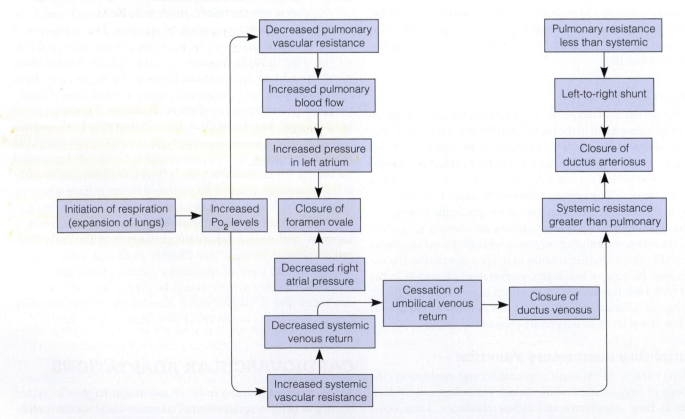

● **Figure 24–2** Transitional circulation: Conversion from fetal to neonatal circulation.

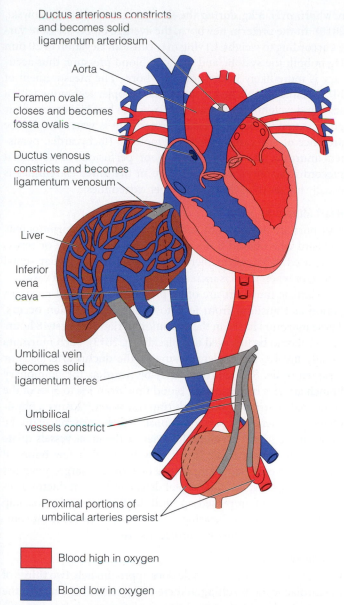

Ductus arteriosus constricts
and becomes solid
ligamentum arteriosum

Aorta

Foramen ovale
closes and becomes
fossa ovalis

Ductus venosus
constricts and becomes
ligamentum venosum

Liver

Inferior
vena
cava

Umbilical vein
becomes solid
ligamentum teres

Umbilical
vessels constrict

Proximal portions of
umbilical arteries persist

■ Blood high in oxygen

■ Blood low in oxygen

● **Figure 24–3** Major changes that need to occur in the newborn's circulatory system to complete the transition to neonatal circulation.

Source: Reprinted with permission from Hole, J. W. (1993). *Human anatomy and physiology* (6th ed.). Dubuque, IA: W. C. Brown. All rights reserved.

2. *Increased systemic pressure and decreased pulmonary artery pressure.* With the loss of the low-resistance placenta, systemic resistance pressure increases, resulting in greater systemic pressure. At the same time, lung expansion increases pulmonary blood flow, and the increased blood pO_2 associated with initiation of respirations dilates pulmonary blood vessels. The combination of vasodilation and increased pulmonary blood flow decreases pulmonary artery resistance. As the pulmonary vascular beds open, the systemic vascular pressure increases, enhancing perfusion of the other body systems.

3. *Closure of the foramen ovale.* Closure of the foramen ovale is a function of changing atrial pressures. In utero, pressure is greater in the right atrium, and the foramen ovale

is open after birth. Decreased pulmonary resistance and increased pulmonary blood flow increase the pulmonary venous return into the left atrium, thereby increasing left atrial pressure slightly. The decreased pulmonary vascular resistance and the decreased umbilical venous return to the right atrium also decrease right atrial pressure. The pressure gradients across the atria are now reversed, with the left atrial pressure now greater, and the foramen ovale is functionally closed 1 to 2 hours after birth. However, a slight right-to-left shunting may occur in the early newborn period. Any increase in pulmonary resistance or right atrial pressure, such as occurs with crying, acidosis, or cold stress, may cause the foramen ovale to reopen, resulting in a temporary right-to-left shunt. Anatomic closure occurs within 30 months (Blackburn, 2013).

4. *Closure of the ductus arteriosus.* Initial elevation of the systemic vascular pressure above the pulmonary vascular pressure increases pulmonary blood flow by reversing the flow through the ductus arteriosus. Blood now flows from the aorta into the pulmonary artery. Furthermore, although the presence of oxygen causes the pulmonary arterioles to dilate, an increase in blood pO_2 triggers the opposite response in the ductus arteriosus—it constricts.

In utero, the placenta provides prostaglandin E_2 (PGE_2), which causes ductus vasodilation. With the loss of the placenta and increased pulmonary blood flow, PGE_2 levels drop, leaving the active constriction by PO_2 unopposed. If the lungs fail to expand or if PO_2 levels drop, the ductus remains patent. Functional closure starts by 10 to 15 hours after birth, and fibrosis of the ductus occurs within 4 weeks after birth (Blackburn, 2013).

5. *Closure of the ductus venosus.* Although the mechanism initiating closure of the ductus venosus is not known, it appears to be related to mechanical pressure changes after severing of the cord, redistribution of blood, and cardiac output. Closure of the bypass forces perfusion of the liver. Fibrosis of the ductus venosus occurs within 2 months. Figure 24–3 depicts the changes in blood flow and oxygenation as the fetal cardiopulmonary circulation changes to neonatal circulation.

Characteristics of Cardiac Function

Evaluation of the newborn's heart rate, blood pressure, heart murmurs, and cardiac workload provides data for evaluating cardiac function.

Heart Rate

Shortly after the first cry and the start of changes in cardiopulmonary circulation, the newborn heart rate can accelerate to 180 beats per minute. The average resting heart rate in the first week of life is 110 to 160 beats per minute in a healthy, full-term newborn but may vary significantly during deep sleep or active awake states. In the full-term newborn, the heart rate may drop to 80 to 100 beats per minute during deep sleep (Furdon & Benjamin, 2010).

Apical pulse rates should be obtained by auscultation for a full minute, preferably when the newborn is asleep (Figure 24–4 ●).

● **Figure 24–4** Apical pulse rates should be obtained by auscultation for a full minute, preferably when the newborn is asleep.

Source: Courtesy of Wilson Garcia.

The heart rate should be evaluated for abnormal rhythms or beats. Peripheral pulses of all extremities should also be evaluated to detect any inequalities or unusual characteristics. While radial pulses are readily found, peripheral pedal pulses may be difficult to palpate in the newborn. Additionally, brachial and femoral pulses are usually easily palpated in the well newborn.

Blood Pressure

Blood pressure (BP) tends to be highest immediately after birth and then descends to its lowest level at about 3 hours of age. By days 4 to 6, the blood pressure rises and plateaus at a level approximately the same as the initial level. Blood pressure is sensitive to the changes in blood volume that occur in the transition to newborn circulation (Figure 24–5 ●). Peripheral perfusion pressure is a particularly sensitive indicator of the newborn's ability to compensate for alterations in blood volume before changes in blood pressure. Capillary refill should be less than 2 to 3 seconds when the skin is blanched.

Blood pressure values during the first 12 hours of life vary with the birth weight and gestational age. The average mean blood pressure is 42 to 60 mm Hg in the full-term, resting

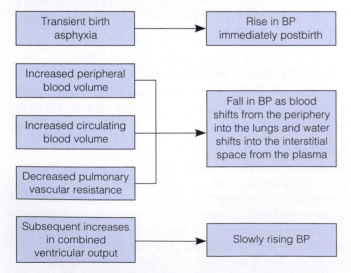

● **Figure 24–5** Response of blood pressure (BP) to neonatal changes in blood volume.

newborn over 3 kg during the first 12 hours of life (Sadowski, 2010). In the preterm newborn, the average blood pressure varies according to weight. Crying may cause an elevation of 20 mm Hg in both the systolic and diastolic blood pressure; thus accuracy is more likely in the quiet newborn. The measurement of BP is best accomplished by using the Doppler technique with a size- and weight-appropriate cuff over the brachial artery. Four point extremity blood pressure assessment is warranted in the presence of any cardiovascular symptoms (tachycardia, persistent murmur, abnormal pulses, poor perfusion, or abnormal precordial activity). Blood pressure in the lower extremities is usually higher than that in the upper extremities.

Heart Murmurs

Murmurs are produced by turbulent blood flow. Murmurs may be heard when blood flows across an abnormal valve or across a stenosed valve, when there is an atrial or ventricular septal defect, or when there is increased flow across a normal valve.

Cardiac murmurs are often present in the initial newborn period as transition from fetal to neonatal circulation occurs. These murmurs heard in the transition period (the first 48 hours of life) should be followed up (Blackburn, 2013). Such murmurs usually involve incomplete closure of the ductus arteriosus or foramen ovale. Soft murmurs may be heard as the pulmonary branch arteries increase their blood flow from 7% to 50% of the combined ventricular output during transition, causing a physiologic peripheral pulmonary stenosis. Clicks may normally be heard at the lower left sternal border as the great vessels dilate to accommodate systolic blood flow in the first few hours of life. Because of the current practice of early discharge, murmurs associated with ventricular septal defect and patent ductus arteriosus are not often picked up until the first well-baby checkup at 4 to 6 weeks of age. Hearing a murmur is often the most common means of recognizing cardiac disease.

Cardiac Workload

Before birth, the right ventricle does approximately two thirds of the cardiac work, resulting in increased size and thickness of the right ventricle at birth. After birth, the left ventricle has a significantly greater increase in volume load than the right ventricle, and it needs to progressively increase in size and thickness. This may explain why right-sided heart defects are better tolerated than left-sided ones and why left-sided heart defects rapidly become symptomatic after birth.

HEMATOPOIETIC SYSTEM

In the first days of life, hematocrit may rise 1 to 2 g/dL above fetal levels as a result of placental transfusion, low oral fluid intake, and diminished extracellular fluid volume. By 1 week postnatally, peripheral hemoglobin is comparable to fetal blood counts. The hemoglobin level declines progressively over the first 2 months of life. This initial decline in hemoglobin creates a phenomenon known as **physiologic anemia of infancy**. The newborn usually tolerates this physiologic state without any clinical difficulties. Hemoglobin values fall, mainly from a decrease in red cell mass rather than from the dilutional effect of increasing plasma volume. The fact that red cell survival is lower in newborns than in adults, and that red cell production is less, also contributes to this anemia. Neonatal red blood cells (RBCs) have a life span of 60 to 80 days, approximately two thirds the life span of adult RBCs (Luchtman-Jones & Wilson, 2011). Erythropoiesis resumes normally when levels of erythropoietin rise in response to low hemoglobin levels and tissue oxygen needs (Cloherty et al., 2012). Once erythropoiesis resumes, iron stores will be used to produce new RBCs. Most infants require supplemental iron to maintain adequate iron stores.

Leukocytosis is a normal finding, because the stress of birth stimulates increased production of neutrophils during the first few days of life. Neutrophils then decrease to 35% of the total leukocyte count by 2 weeks of age. Lymphocytes play a role in antibody formation and eventually become the predominant type of leukocyte and the total white blood cell count falls.

Blood volume is approximately 85 mL/kg of body weight for a term infant (Luchtman-Jones & Wilson, 2011). For example, a 3.6 kg (8 lb) newborn has a blood volume of 306 mL. Blood volume varies based on the amount of placental transfusion received during the delivery of the placenta, as well as other factors, including the following:

1. *Delayed cord clamping and the normal shift of plasma to the extravascular spaces.* Newborn hemoglobin and hematocrit values are higher when a placental transfusion occurs after birth. Placental vessels contain about 75 to 125 mL of blood at term, most of which can be transfused into the newborn by holding the newborn below the level of the placenta and delaying clamping of the cord. Blood volume increases by 10% with delayed cord clamping (Luchtman-Jones & Wilson, 2011). The increase is reflected by a rise in hemoglobin level and an increase in the hematocrit. For greatest accuracy, the initial hemoglobin and hematocrit levels should be measured in the cord blood, although this is not a routine practice. In term newborns a delay in clamping the umbilical cord appears to offer protection from anemia without harmful effects. In preterm or small-for-gestational-age (SGA) newborns a delay in cord clamping may have risks. It can speed and worsen symptoms of hyperbilirubinemia and cause hypervolemia.

2. *Gestational age.* There appears to be a positive association between gestational age, RBC numbers, and hemoglobin concentration.

3. *Prenatal and/or perinatal hemorrhage.* Significant prenatal or perinatal bleeding decreases the hematocrit level and causes hypovolemia.

4. *The site of the blood sample.* Hemoglobin and hematocrit levels are significantly higher in capillary blood than in venous blood. Sluggish peripheral blood flow creates RBC stasis, thereby increasing RBC concentration in the capillaries. Consequently, blood samples taken from venous blood sites are more accurate than those from capillary sites.

The concentration of serum electrolytes in the blood indicates the fluid and electrolyte status of the newborn. See Table 24–2 for normal term newborn electrolyte and blood values.

Table 24–2	Normal Term Newborn Cord Blood Values
Laboratory Data	**Normal Range**
Hemoglobin	14–20 g/dL
Hematocrit	43%–63%
WBC	10,000–30,000/mm^3
WBC differential	
Neutrophils	40%–80%
Lymphocytes	20%–40%
Monocytes	3%–10%
Platelets	150,000–350,000/mm^3
Reticulocytes	3%–7%
Blood volume	82.3 mL/kg (third day after early cord clamping), 92.6 mL/kg (third day after delayed cord clamping)
Sodium	129–144 mEq/L
Potassium	3.4–9.9 mEq/L
Chloride	103–111 mEq/L
Bicarbonate	18–23 mEq/L
Carbon dioxide	13–29 mmol/L
Calcium	8.2–111 mg/dL
Glucose	45–96 mg/dL
Total protein	4.8–7.3 g/dL

Source: Adapted from Fanaroff, A. A., & Martin, R. J. (Eds.). (2011). *Neonatal-perinatal medicine* (9th ed.). St. Louis, MO: Mosby.

TEMPERATURE REGULATION

Temperature regulation is the maintenance of thermal balance by the loss of heat to the environment at a rate equal to heat production. Newborns are *homeothermic;* they attempt to stabilize their internal (core) body temperatures within a narrow range in spite of significant temperature variations in their environment.

Thermoregulation in the newborn is closely related to the rate of metabolism and oxygen consumption. Within a specific environmental temperature range, called the **neutral thermal environment (NTE)** zone, the rates of oxygen consumption and metabolism are minimal, and internal body temperature is maintained because of thermal balance (Blackburn, 2013). For an *unclothed, full-term newborn,* the NTE is an ambient environmental temperature range of 32°C to 33.5°C (89.6°F to 92.3°F) within 50% relative humidity; for a *clothed, full-term newborn,* the NTE is 24°C to 27°C (75.2°F to 80.6°F) and can be adjusted according to the needs of individual infants (Blackburn, 2013). Thus, the normal newborn requires higher environmental temperatures to maintain a thermoneutral environment. Several newborn characteristics affect the establishment of thermal stability:

- The newborn has less subcutaneous fat than an adult and a thin epidermis.
- Blood vessels in the newborn are closer to the skin than those of an adult. Therefore, the circulating blood is influenced by changes in environmental temperature and in turn influences the hypothalamic temperature-regulating center.
- The flexed posture of the term newborn decreases the surface area exposed to the environment, thereby reducing heat loss.

A table listing neutral thermal environmental temperatures gives a recommended temperature range depending on the weight and age of the infant (see Skill 5–3, Thermoregulation of the Newborn, in the *Clinical Skills Manual* SKILLS). Generally speaking, the smaller infants in each weight group will require a temperature in the higher portion of the temperature range. Within each time range, the younger the infant, the higher the temperature required. For example, the preterm or small-for-gestational-age (SGA) newborn has less adipose tissue and is hypoflexed, and therefore requires higher environmental temperatures to achieve a neutral thermal environment. Larger, well-insulated newborns may be able to cope with lower environmental temperatures. If the environmental temperature falls below the lower limits of the NTE, the newborn responds with increased oxygen consumption and metabolism, which results in greater heat production. Prolonged exposure to the cold may result in depleted glycogen stores and acidosis. Oxygen consumption also increases if the environmental temperature is above the NTE.

Heat Loss

A newborn is at a distinct disadvantage in maintaining a normal temperature. With a large body surface in relation to mass and a limited amount of insulating subcutaneous fat, the full-term newborn loses about four times the heat of an adult. The newborn's poor thermal stability is primarily because of excessive heat loss rather than impaired heat production. Because of the risk of hypothermia and possible cold stress, minimizing heat loss in the newborn after birth is essential (see Chapters 19 🔗 and 26 🔗 for nursing management).

Two major routes of heat loss are from the internal core of the body to the body surface and from the external surface to the environment. Usually the core temperature is higher than the skin temperature, resulting in continuous transfer or conduction of heat to the surface. The greater the difference in temperature between core and skin, the more rapidly heat transfers. The transfer is accomplished through an increase in oxygen consumption, depletion of glycogen stores, and metabolization of brown fat. Heat loss from the body surface to the environment takes place in four ways—by convection, radiation, evaporation, and conduction (Figure 24–6 ●).

- **Convection** is the loss of heat from the warm body surface to the cooler air currents. Air-conditioned rooms, air currents with a temperature below the infant's skin

A. Convection

B. Radiation

C. Evaporation

D. Conduction

● **Figure 24–6** Methods of heat loss. *A,* Convection. *B,* Radiation. *C,* Evaporation. *D,* Conduction. The distribution of brown adipose tissue (brown fat) in the newborn is shown in the shaded areas.

temperature, oxygen by mask, and removal from an incubator for procedures increase convective heat loss in the newborn. The amount of heat transferred depends on the velocity of the moving air, the temperature difference between the air and the infant's skin, and the proportion of body surface area exposed.

- **Radiation** losses occur when heat transfers from the heated body surface to cooler surfaces and objects not in direct contact with the body. The walls of a room or of an incubator are potential causes of heat loss by radiation, even if the ambient temperature of the incubator is within the thermal neutral range for that infant. Placing cold objects (such as ice for blood gases) onto the incubator or near the infant in the radiant warmer will increase radiant losses.

- **Evaporation** is the loss of heat incurred when water is converted to a vapor. The newborn is particularly prone to lose heat by evaporation immediately after birth (when the baby is wet with amniotic fluid) and during baths; thus, drying the newborn is critical. Evaporation accounts for 25% of heat loss immediately after delivery (Blackburn, 2013). Evaporation also occurs from expired air from the respiratory tract. Radiant warming beds and bank phototherapy lights accentuate evaporative loss.

- **Conduction** is the loss of heat to a cooler surface by direct skin contact. Chilled hands, cool scales, cold examination tables, and cold stethoscopes can cause loss of heat by conduction. Even if objects are warmed to the incubator temperature, the temperature difference between the infant's core temperature and the ambient temperature may be significant. This difference results in heat transfer.

Once the infant has been dried after birth, the highest losses of heat generally result from radiation and convection. The newborn can respond to the cooler environmental temperature with adequate peripheral vasoconstriction, but this mechanism is not entirely effective because of the minimal amount of fat insulation present, the large body surface, and ongoing thermal conduction. Because of these factors, minimizing the baby's heat loss and preventing hypothermia are imperative. (See Chapter 28 🔗 for nursing measures to prevent hypothermia.)

Most hospitalized infants are weighed daily. Placing unclothed infants on a cold scale can induce heat loss. A safer and more developmentally beneficial way to weigh an infant is by doing a "swaddled weight." Place blankets, diaper, hat, and infant

clothing on the scale before calibrating the scale to zero. Then you will be able to dress and swaddle the infant for weighing and the scale will reflect only the infant's weight.

Heat Production (Thermogenesis)

When exposed to a cool environment, the newborn requires additional heat. The newborn has several physiologic mechanisms that increase heat production, or *thermogenesis*. These mechanisms include increased basal metabolic rate, muscular activity, and chemical thermogenesis (also called *nonshivering thermogenesis [NST]*).

Nonshivering thermogenesis is an important mechanism of heat production unique to the newborn. It occurs when skin receptors perceive a drop in the environmental temperature and, in response, transmit sensations to stimulate the sympathetic nervous system. NST uses the newborn's stores of **brown adipose tissue (BAT)** (also called brown fat) to provide heat. It increases in the fetus at about 25 to 26 weeks' gestation and continues to increase until 3 to 5 weeks after the birth of a term infant, unless the fat is depleted by cold stress (Blackburn, 2013). Brown fat is deposited in the midscapular area, around the neck, and in the axillas, with deeper placement around the trachea, esophagus, abdominal aorta, kidneys, and adrenal glands (see Figure 24–6). BAT receives its name from the dark color caused by its enriched blood supply, dense cellular content, and abundant nerve endings. These characteristics of brown fat cells promote rapid metabolism, heat generation, and heat transfer to the peripheral circulation. The large numbers of brown fat cells increase the speed with which triglycerides are metabolized to produce heat.

Shivering, a form of muscular activity common in the cold adult, is rarely seen in the newborn. If the newborn shivers, it means the newborn's metabolic rate has already doubled. The extra muscular activity does little to produce needed heat.

Thermographic studies of newborns exposed to cold show an increase in the skin heat produced over the newborn's brown fat deposits between 1 and 14 days of age. However, if the brown fat supply has been depleted, the metabolic response to cold is limited or lacking. An increase in basal metabolism as a result of hypothermia results in an increase in oxygen consumption. A decrease in the environmental temperature of 2°C, from 33°C to 31°C, is a drop sufficient to double the oxygen consumption of a term newborn. Keeping the normal newborn warm promotes normal oxygen requirements, whereas chilling can cause the newborn to show signs of respiratory distress.

When exposed to cold, the normal term newborn is usually able to cope with the increase in oxygen requirements, but the preterm newborn may be unable to increase ventilation to the necessary level of oxygen consumption. (See Chapter 28 🔗 for a discussion of

Clinical Tip

Bath time is when many newborns experience cold stress. To minimize the risk, always bathe infants in a warm room, gather all supplies prior to beginning the bath, and pre-warm soaps or shampoos. Dry infants with warmed blankets and dress immediately. The infant's head accounts for a large portion of body surface area and has great capacity for heat loss, so placing a hat on the infant is an effective way to minimize heat loss. Placing the infant skin to skin with the mother after bathing is a good way to help rewarm and maintain body temperature.

Developing Cultural Competence
Newborn Baths in Jordan

In Jordan, the birth of a male infant is a much celebrated event. The newborn is bathed daily during the first week of life. During the final bath, salt is added to the water to help the newborn's skin adjust to the external environment and protect it from changes in the weather.

cold stress.) Because oxidation of fatty acids depends on the availability of oxygen, glucose, and adenosine triphosphate (ATP), the newborn's ability to generate heat can be altered by pathologic events such as hypoxia, acidosis, and hypoglycemia or by medication that blocks the release of norepinephrine. The effect of certain drugs such as meperidine (Demerol) may also prevent metabolism of brown fat. Newborn hypothermia prolongs as well as potentiates the effects of many analgesic and anesthetic drugs in the newborn.

Response to Heat

Sweating is the term newborn's usual initial response to hyperthermia. The newborn sweat glands have limited function until after the fourth week of extrauterine life; heat is lost through peripheral vasodilation and evaporation of insensible water loss. The term infant will be flaccid and assume a position of extension to facilitate heat loss (Blackburn, 2013). Oxygen consumption and metabolic rate also increase in response to hyperthermia. Severe hyperthermia can lead to death or to gross brain damage if the baby survives.

HEPATIC ADAPTATIONS

In the newborn, the liver is frequently palpable 2 to 3 cm below the right costal margin at the midclavicular line (Gardner & Goldson, 2011). It is relatively large and occupies about 40% of the abdominal cavity. The newborn liver plays a significant role in iron storage, carbohydrate metabolism, conjugation of bilirubin, and coagulation.

Iron Storage and RBC Production

As red blood cells (RBCs) are destroyed after birth, the iron is stored in the liver until needed for new RBC production. Newborn iron stores are determined by total body hemoglobin content and length of gestation. The term newborn has about 270 mg of iron at birth, and about 140 to 170 mg of this amount is in the hemoglobin. If the mother's iron intake has been adequate, enough iron will be stored to last until the infant is about 5 months of age. See Chapter 33 🔗 for discussion of iron supplementation after 6 months of age.

Carbohydrate Metabolism

At term, the newborn's cord blood glucose level is 15 mg/dL lower than the maternal blood glucose level. Newborn carbohydrate reserves are relatively low. One third of this reserve is in the form of liver glycogen. Newborn glycogen stores are twice those of the adult. The newborn enters an energy crunch at the time of birth, with the removal of the maternal glucose supply and the increased energy expenditure associated with the birth process and extrauterine life. Fuel sources are consumed at a faster rate because of the work of breathing, loss of heat when exposed to cold, activity, and activation of muscle tone. Glucose is the main source of energy in the first 4 to 6 hours after birth. During the first 2 hours of life, the serum blood glucose level declines, then rises, and finally reaches a steady state by 3 hours after birth (Cloherty et al., 2012).

The nurse may assess the glucose level on admission if risk factors are present or per agency protocol (see *Care of the Newborn with Hypoglycemia* in Chapter 28 🔗). As stores of liver and muscle glycogen and blood glucose decrease, the newborn compensates by changing from a predominantly carbohydrate

metabolism to fat metabolism. Energy can be derived from fat and protein, as well as from carbohydrates. The amount and availability of each of these "fuel substrates" depend on the ability of immature metabolic pathways (which lack specific enzymes or hormones) to function in the first few days of life.

Conjugation of Bilirubin

Conjugation, or the changing of bilirubin into an excretable form, is the conversion of the yellow lipid-soluble pigment (unconjugated, indirect) into water-soluble pigment (excretable, direct). Unconjugated bilirubin is fat soluble, has a propensity for fatty tissues, is not in an excretable form, and is a potential toxin. **Total bilirubin** is the sum of conjugated (direct) and unconjugated (indirect) bilirubin.

Fetal unconjugated bilirubin crosses the placenta to be excreted, so the fetus does not need to conjugate bilirubin. Total bilirubin at birth is usually less than 3 mg/dL unless an abnormal hemolytic process has been present in utero. After birth the newborn's liver must begin to conjugate bilirubin. This produces a normal rise in serum bilirubin levels in the first few days of life.

The bilirubin formed after RBCs are destroyed is transported in the blood bound to albumin. The bilirubin is transferred into the hepatocytes and bound to intracellular proteins. These proteins determine the amount of bilirubin held in a liver cell for processing and consequently determine the amount of bilirubin uptake into the liver. The activity of uridine-diphosphoglucuronosyl transferase (UDPGT) enzyme results in the attachment of unconjugated bilirubin to glucuronic acid (product of liver glycogen), producing conjugated (direct) bilirubin. Direct bilirubin is excreted into the tiny bile ducts, then into the common duct and duodenum. The conjugated bilirubin then progresses down the intestines, where bacteria transform it into urobilinogen (urine bilirubin) and stercobilinogen. Stercobilinogen is not reabsorbed but is excreted as a yellow-brown pigment in the stools.

Even after the bilirubin has been conjugated and bound, it can be changed back to unconjugated bilirubin via the enterohepatic circulation. In the intestines β-D-glucuronidase enzyme acts to split off (deconjugate) the bilirubin from glucuronic acid if it has not first been acted on by gut bacteria to produce urobilinogen; the free bilirubin is reabsorbed through the intestinal wall and brought back to the liver via portal vein circulation. This recycling of the bilirubin and decreased ability to clear bilirubin from the system are prevalent in babies with very high β-D-glucuronidase activity levels, those who are exclusively breastfed, and those with delayed bacterial colonization of the gut (such as with the use of antibiotics) and further increases the newborn's susceptibility to jaundice (Figure 24–7 ●).

The newborn liver has relatively less glucuronyl transferase activity in the first few weeks of life than an adult liver. This reduction in hepatic activity, along with a relatively large bilirubin load, decreases the liver's ability to conjugate bilirubin and increases susceptibility to jaundice.

Physiologic Jaundice

Physiologic jaundice is caused by accelerated destruction of fetal RBCs, impaired conjugation of bilirubin, and increased bilirubin reabsorption from the intestinal tract. This condition does

Other sources

| Catabolism of RBC | Ineffective erythropoiesis | } Bone marrow |
| | Tissue heme Heme proteins | } Liver |

75% Heme   25% Heme

Biliverdin

Heme oxygenase
Biliverdin reductase
} Reticuloendothelial system

Unconjugated bilirubin
+
Serum albumin
} Circulation

Intracellular proteins

Smooth endoplasmic reticulum

Uridine diphospho-glucuronosyl transferase (UDPGT)
} Hepatic system

Bilirubin glucuronides

Enterohepatic circulation of bilirubin

Kidney

β-D-Glucuronidase

Bacterial flora

Bilirubin
} Gastrointestinal system

Urobilinogen

Fecal bilirubin (stercobilinogen)

Urine bilirubin

● **Figure 24–7** Conjugation of bilirubin in newborns.

not have a pathologic basis but is a normal biologic response of the newborn.

Maisels describes five factors—several of which can also be related to pathologic events—that may interact to create physiologic jaundice (Cloherty et al., 2012).

1. *Increased amounts of bilirubin delivered to the liver.* The increased blood volume because of delayed cord clamping combined with faster RBC destruction in the newborn leads to an increased bilirubin level in the blood. A proportionately larger amount of nonerythrocyte bilirubin forms in the newborn. Therefore, newborns have two to three times greater production or breakdown of

bilirubin than do adults. The use of forceps or vacuum extraction, which sometimes causes facial bruising or cephalhematoma (entrapped hemorrhage), can increase the amount of bilirubin to be handled by the liver.

2. *Defective hepatic uptake of bilirubin from the plasma.* If the newborn does not ingest adequate calories, the formation of hepatic binding proteins diminishes, resulting in higher bilirubin levels.

3. *Defective conjugation of the bilirubin.* Decreased uridine-diphosphoglucuronosyl activity as in hypothyroidism or inadequate caloric intake causes the intracellular binding proteins to remain saturated and results in greater

unconjugated bilirubin levels in the blood. The fatty acids in breast milk are thought to compete with bilirubin for albumin-binding sites and therefore impede bilirubin processing.

4. *Defect in bilirubin excretion.* A congenital infection may cause impaired excretion of conjugated bilirubin. Delay in introduction of bacterial flora and decreased intestinal motility can also delay excretion and increase enterohepatic circulation of bilirubin.

5. *Increased reabsorption of bilirubin from the intestine.* Reduced bowel motility, intestinal obstruction, or delayed passage of meconium increases the circulation of bilirubin in the enterohepatic pathway, thereby resulting in higher bilirubin values.

Approximately 50% to 60% of full-term and 80% of preterm newborns exhibit physiologic jaundice on about the second or third day after birth (Blackburn, 2013). The characteristic yellow color results from increased levels of unconjugated (indirect) bilirubin, which are a normal product of RBC breakdown and reflect the body's temporary inability to eliminate bilirubin. Serum levels of bilirubin are about 4 to 6 mg/dL before the yellow coloration of the skin and sclera appears. *The signs of physiologic jaundice appear after the first 24 hours postnatally.* This time frame differentiates physiologic jaundice from pathologic jaundice (see Chapter 28 for further discussion), which is clinically seen at birth or within the first 24 hours of postnatal life. Major risk factors for developing severe hyperbilirubinemia in late preterm and term infants place the total serum levels in the high-risk zone on the bilirubin nomogram.

There is no consistent definition of neonatal hyperbilirubinemia; what is considered to be in that range varies with population characteristics and postbirth age (Blackburn, 2013). Peak bilirubin levels are reached between days 3 and 5 in the full-term infant and between days 5 and 7 in the preterm infant. These values are established for European and American Caucasian newborns. Chinese, Japanese, Korean, and Native American newborns have considerably higher bilirubin levels that are not as apparent and that persist for longer periods with no apparent ill effects (Blackburn, 2013).

The nursery or postpartum environment, including lighting, may hinder the early detection of the degree and type of jaundice. Pink walls and artificial lights mask the beginning of jaundice in newborns but daylight can help to recognize jaundice early as it eliminates distortions from artificial light.

If jaundice is suspected, the nurse can assess the newborn's coloring by pressing the skin, on the forehead or nose, with a finger. As blanching occurs, the nurse can observe the icterus (yellow coloring). The newborn develops jaundice in cephalocaudal progression, meaning that jaundice is first seen in the face and then travels down the trunk.

SAFETY ALERT!

Universal screening for hyperbilirubinemia and not visual inspection alone is necessary to identify elevated bilirubin levels in newborns. (AWHONN, Clinical Position Statement, 2005, reaffirmed 2009).

Several newborn care procedures will decrease the probability of high bilirubin levels.

- Maintain the newborn's skin temperature at 36.5°C (97.8°F) or above; cold stress results in acidosis. Acidosis decreases available serum albumin-binding sites, weakens albumin-binding powers, and causes elevated unconjugated bilirubin levels.

- Monitor stool for amount and characteristics. Bilirubin is eliminated in the feces; inadequate stooling may result in reabsorption and recycling of bilirubin. Early breastfeeding should be encouraged because the laxative effect of colostrum increases excretion of meconium and transitional stool.

- Encourage early feedings to promote intestinal elimination and bacterial colonization and provide caloric intake necessary for hepatic binding proteins to form.

If jaundice becomes apparent, nursing care is directed toward keeping the newborn well hydrated and promoting intestinal elimination. (For specific nursing management and therapies, see *Nursing Care Plan: The Newborn with Hyperbilirubinemia* on page 689 in Chapter 28.)

Physiologic jaundice may upset parents; provide emotional support and thorough explanation of the condition. If the baby is placed under phototherapy, a few additional days of hospitalization may be required, which may also upset parents. Encourage them to meet the emotional needs of their newborn by continuing to feed, hold, and caress the infant. If the mother is discharged, encourage the parents to return for feedings and to telephone or visit when possible. In many instances, the mother, especially if she is breastfeeding, may elect to remain hospitalized with her newborn; the nurse should support this decision. If insurance limitations make this unrealistic, it may be possible to find an empty room for the discharged mother and her family to use while visiting the newborn. As an alternative to continued hospitalization, the newborn may be treated with home phototherapy. (See *Phototherapy* in Chapter 28 for more information.)

Breastfeeding Jaundice and Breast Milk Jaundice

Breastfeeding is implicated in prolonged jaundice in some newborns. *Breastfeeding jaundice* occurs in the first days of life in breastfed newborns. It appears to be associated with poor feeding practices and not with any abnormality in milk composition

---

Developing Cultural Competence
Interpreting Illness Through Cultural Beliefs

Cultural beliefs lead mothers to interpret illness within their cultural framework, especially when left without clear and understood explanations (Lauderdale, 2012). For example, some Latina women believe that showing strong maternal emotions during pregnancy and during breastfeeding can be detrimental. They blame jaundice in their newborn on *bili* associated with anger. Such maternal reactions can be lessened by careful explanations to the mothers about the diagnosis, prognosis, duration, and management options for jaundice, and possibility for recurrence.

(McGrath & Hardy, 2011). Prevention of early breastfeeding jaundice includes encouraging frequent (every 2 to 3 hours) breastfeeding, avoiding supplementation, and accessing maternal lactation counseling.

In *breast milk jaundice*, the bilirubin level begins to rise after the first week of life, when physiologic jaundice is waning after the mother's milk has come in. The level peaks at 5 to 10 mg/dL at 2 to 3 weeks of age and declines over the first several months of life (McGrath & Hardy, 2011).

In contrast to breastfeeding jaundice, breast milk jaundice is related to milk composition promoting increased bilirubin reabsorption from the intestine. Some women's breast milk contains several times the normal concentration of certain free fatty acids. These free fatty acids may compete with bilirubin for binding sites on albumin and inhibit the conjugation of bilirubin or increase lipase activity, which disrupts the RBC membrane. Increased lipase activity enhances absorption of bile across the gastrointestinal tract membrane, thereby increasing the entero-hepatic circulation of bilirubin. The exact mechanism of true breast milk jaundice is unknown but it is thought to be due to unidentified factors in breast milk interfering with bilirubin metabolism (Cloherty et al., 2012).

Newborns with breastfeeding jaundice appear well, and at present development of kernicterus (toxic levels of bilirubin in the brain) has not been documented. Temporary cessation of breastfeeding may be advised if bilirubin reaches presumed toxic levels of approximately 20 mg/dL or if the interruption is necessary to establish the cause of the hyper-bilirubinemia. Most physicians believe that breastfeeding may be resumed once other causes of jaundice have been ruled out and as long as serum bilirubin levels remain below 20 mg/dL. In cases of breast milk jaundice, within 24 to 36 hours after breastfeeding is discontinued, the newborn's serum bilirubin levels begin to fall dramatically. With resumption of breastfeeding, the bilirubin concentration may have a slight rise of 2 to 3 mg/dL, with a subsequent decline (Table 24–3).

Coagulation

The liver plays an important part in blood coagulation during fetal life and continues this function following birth. Coagulation factors II, VII, IX, and X (synthesized in the liver) are activated under the influence of vitamin K and therefore are considered vitamin K dependent. The absence of normal flora needed to synthesize vitamin K in the newborn gut results in low levels of vitamin K and creates a transient blood coagulation alteration between the second and fifth day of life. From a low point at about 2 to 3 days after birth, these coagulation factors rise slowly, but they do not approach adult levels until 9 months of age or later (Manco-Johnson, Rodden, & Hays, 2011). Other coagulation

Table 24–3 Factors in Physiologic, Breast Milk, and Breastfeeding Jaundice

PHYSIOLOGIC JAUNDICE

- Physiologic jaundice occurs after the first 24 hours of life.
- During the first week of life, bilirubin should not exceed 13 mg/dL. Some pediatricians allow levels up to 15 mg/dL.
- Bilirubin levels peak at 3 to 5 days in term infants.

BREAST MILK JAUNDICE

- Bilirubin levels begin to rise after the first week of life when mature breast milk comes in.
- A peak of 5 to 10 mg/dL is reached at 2 to 3 weeks of age.
- It may be necessary to interrupt breastfeeding for a short period when bilirubin reaches 20 mg/dL.

BREASTFEEDING JAUNDICE

- Bilirubin levels rise after the first 24 hours of age.
- Levels peak on the third or fourth day of life and decline through the first month to normal levels.
- The incidence can be decreased by increasing the number of breastfeeding episodes to 8 to 12 in 24 hours.

factors with low umbilical cord blood levels are XI, XII, and XIII. Fibrinogen and factors V and VII are near adult.

Although newborn bleeding problems are rare, an injection of vitamin K (AquaMEPHYTON) is given prophylactically on the day of birth to combat potential clinical bleeding problems. (Chapter 26 ● discusses administration of vitamin K to newborns, and Chapter 28 ● discusses hemorrhagic disease of the newborn in greater depth.)

Platelet counts at birth are in the same range as for older children, but newborns may manifest mild transient difficulty in platelet aggregation functioning. This platelet problem is accentuated by phototherapy. Prenatal maternal therapy with phenytoin sodium (Dilantin) or phenobarbital also causes abnormal clotting studies and newborn bleeding in the first 24 hours after birth. Infants born to mothers receiving warfarin (Coumadin) compounds may bleed, because these agents cross the placenta and accentuate existing vitamin K-dependent factor deficiencies. Transient neonatal thrombocytopenia may occur in infants born to mothers with severe hypertension or HELLP syndrome (*h*emolysis, *e*levated *l*iver enzymes, and *l*ow *p*latelet count) and in infants born to mothers who have idiopathic isoimmune thrombocytopenic purpura.

GASTROINTESTINAL ADAPTATIONS

By 36 to 38 weeks' gestation, the gastrointestinal system is adequately mature, with enzymatic activity and the ability to transport nutrients.

Digestion and Absorption

The full-term newborn has sufficient intestinal and pancreatic enzymes to digest most simple carbohydrates, proteins, and fats. The carbohydrates requiring digestion in the newborn are

Clinical Tip

Encourage and support mothers who desire to breastfeed their infants. Assist and instruct them on how to pump and express milk during the interrupted breastfeeding period. Reassure them that nothing is wrong with their milk or mothering abilities.

usually disaccharides (lactose, maltose, sucrose), which are split into monosaccharides (galactose, fructose, and glucose) by the enzymes of the intestinal mucosa. Lactose is the primary carbohydrate in the breastfeeding newborn and is generally easily digested and well absorbed. The only enzyme lacking is pancreatic amylase, which remains relatively deficient during the first few months of life. Newborns have trouble digesting starches (changing more complex carbohydrates into maltose) so they should not eat solids until after the first 6 months of life.

Although proteins require more digestion than carbohydrates, they are well digested and absorbed from the newborn intestine. The newborn digests and absorbs fats less efficiently because of the minimal activity of the pancreatic enzyme lipase. The newborn excretes about 10% to 20% of the dietary fat intake, compared with 10% for the adult. The newborn absorbs the fat in breast milk more completely than the fat in cows' milk, because breast milk consists of more medium-chain triglycerides and contains lipase. (See Chapter 33 🔗 for further discussion of newborn nutrition.)

By birth, the newborn has experienced swallowing, gastric emptying, and intestinal propulsion. In utero, fetal swallowing is accompanied by gastric emptying and peristalsis of the fetal intestinal tract. By the end of gestation, peristalsis becomes much more active in preparation for extrauterine life. Fetal peristalsis is also stimulated by hypoxia, causing the expulsion of meconium into the amniotic fluid in postterm fetuses.

Air enters the stomach immediately after birth. The small intestine is filled with air within 2 to 12 hours and the large bowel within 24 hours. The salivary glands are immature at birth, and the newborn produces little saliva until about 3 months of age. The newborn's stomach can hold 50 to 60 mL. It empties intermittently, starting within a few minutes of the beginning of a feeding and ending 2 to 4 hours after feeding. Bowel sounds are present within the first 30 to 60 minutes of birth, and the newborn can successfully feed during this time. The newborn's gastric pH becomes less acidic about a week after birth and remains less acidic than that of adults for the next 2 to 3 months.

The cardiac sphincter is immature, as is neural control of the stomach, so some regurgitation may be noted in the newborn period. Regurgitation of the first few feedings during the first day or two of life can usually be lessened by avoiding overfeeding and by burping the newborn well during and after the feeding.

When no other signs and symptoms are evident, vomiting is limited and ceases within the first few days of life. Continuous vomiting or regurgitation should be observed closely. If the newborn has swallowed bloody or purulent amniotic fluid, lavage of the stomach may be indicated in the term newborn to relieve the problem. Bilious vomiting is abnormal and must be evaluated thoroughly because it might represent a condition that warrants prompt surgical intervention.

Adequate digestion and absorption are essential for newborn growth and development. If optimal nutritional support is available, postnatal growth should parallel intrauterine growth; that is, after 30 weeks' gestation, the fetus gains 30 g per day and adds 1.2 cm (0.5 in.) to body length daily. To gain weight at the intrauterine rate, the term newborn requires 120 cal/kg/day. After birth, caloric intake is often insufficient for weight gain until the newborn is 5 to 10 days old. During this time, there

may be a weight loss of 5% to 10% in term newborns. A shift of intracellular water to extracellular space and insensible water loss accounts for the weight loss; thus, failure to lose weight when caloric intake is inadequate may indicate fluid retention.

Elimination

Term newborns usually pass meconium within 8 to 24 hours of life and almost always within 48 hours. **Meconium** is formed in utero from the amniotic fluid and its constituents, intestinal secretions, and shed mucosal cells. It is recognized by its thick, tarry black or dark green appearance. Transitional (thin brown to green) stools consisting of part meconium and part fecal material are passed for the next day or two, and then the stools become entirely fecal. Generally the stools of a breastfed newborn are pale yellow (but may be pasty green); they are more liquid and more frequent than those of formula-fed newborns, whose stools are paler and often the consistency of peanut butter (see Figure 26–23 🔗 on page 607). Frequency of bowel movement varies but ranges from one every 2 to 3 days to as many as 10 daily. Totally breastfed infants often progress to stools that occur every 5 to 7 days. Mothers should be counseled that the newborn is not constipated as long as the bowel movement remains soft. Table 24–4 summarizes the newborn's physiologic adaptation to extrauterine life.

Clinical Reasoning Newborn Weight Loss

Jonathon Sykes is a 5-day-old term male infant who has returned to the hospital for a lactation visit. Jonathon's birth weight was 3260 grams (7 pounds, 3 ounces) and his current weight is 2963 grams (6 pounds, 8 1/2 ounces). The lactation nurse is worried about this weight loss and shares her concerns with Jonathon's mother. What would you tell Jonathon's mother about his weight loss since birth? What are other questions you might ask Jonathon's mother about his daily habits? Based on his birth weight, what is the appropriate number of kilocalories that Jonathon needs to grow?
See www.nursing.pearsonhighered.com for possible responses.

Table 24–4	Physiologic Adaptations to Extrauterine Life

- Periodic breathing may be present.

- Desired axillary temperature of 36.5°C to 37.5°C (97.7°F to 99.5°F) stabilizes 4 to 6 hours after birth for term infant (Cloherty et al., 2012).

- Desired blood glucose level reaches 60 to 70 mg/dL by third postnatal day.

- Stools progress from (for detailed discussion see Chapter 26 🔗):
  - Meconium (thick, tarry, black; meconium plug may be expelled)
  - Transitional stools (thin, brown to green)
  - Breastfed infants (yellow-gold, soft or mushy)
  - Formula-fed infants (pale yellow, formed, and pasty)

URINARY TRACT ADAPTATIONS

Kidney Development and Function

Certain physiologic features of the newborn's kidneys influence the newborn's ability to handle body fluids and excrete urine.

1. The term newborn's kidneys have a full complement of functioning nephrons by 34 to 36 weeks' gestation.

2. The glomerular filtration rate of the newborn's kidney is low compared with the adult rate. Because of this physiologic decrease in kidney glomerular filtration, the newborn's kidney is unable to dispose of water rapidly when necessary.

3. The juxtamedullary portion of the nephron has limited capacity to reabsorb HCO_3^1 and H^1 and concentrate urine (reabsorb water back into the blood). The limitation of tubular reabsorption can lead to inappropriate loss of substances present in the glomerular filtrate, such as amino acids, bicarbonate, glucose, sodium, chloride, phosphate, and urea.

The ability to concentrate urine fully is attained by 3 months of age. Feeding practices have limited effect on urine concentration.

Because the newborn has difficulty concentrating urine, the effect of excessive insensible water loss or restricted fluid intake is unpredictable. The newborn kidney is also limited in its dilutional capabilities. The concentrating and dilutional abilities of the kidneys are an important consideration in monitoring fluid therapy to prevent dehydration or overhydration.

Characteristics of Newborn Urinary Function

Many newborns void immediately after birth, and the voiding frequently goes unnoticed. Among normal newborns, 90% void by 24 hours after birth and 99% void by 48 hours after birth (Cloherty et al., 2012). A newborn who has not voided by 48 hours should be assessed for adequacy of fluid intake, bladder distention, restlessness, and symptoms of pain. The appropriate clinical personnel should be notified if indicated.

The initial bladder volume is 6 to 44 mL of urine. Unless edema is present, normal urinary output is often limited, and the voidings are scanty until fluid intake increases. (The fluid of edema is eliminated by the kidneys, so infants with edema have a much higher urinary output.) The first 2 days postnatally, the newborn voids two to six times daily, with a urine output of 15 mL/kg/day. The newborn subsequently voids 5 to 25 times every 24 hours, with a volume of 25 mL/kg/day. Observation and documentation of adequate output is necessary given the large number of term infants who have early hospital discharge.

Following the first voiding, the newborn's urine frequently appears cloudy (because of mucus content) and has a high specific gravity, which decreases as fluid intake increases. Occasionally pink stains ("brick dust spots") appear on the diaper. These are caused by urates and are innocuous. Blood may occasionally be observed on the diapers of female newborns. This *pseudomenstruation* is related to the withdrawal of maternal hormones. Males may have bloody spotting from a circumcision if

Table 24–5	Newborn Urinalysis Values
Protein less than 5 to 10 mg/dL	
WBC less than 2 to 3/hpf	
RBC 0	
Casts 0	
Bacteria 0	
Color pale yellow	

performed. In the absence of apparent causes for bleeding, the clinician should be notified. During early infancy, normal urine is straw colored and almost odorless, although odor occurs when certain drugs are given, metabolic disorders exist, or infection is present. Table 24–5 contains urinalysis values for the normal newborn.

IMMUNOLOGIC ADAPTATIONS

The newborn's immune system is not fully activated until sometime after birth. Limitations in the newborn's inflammatory response result in failure to recognize, localize, and destroy invasive bacteria. Thus, the signs and symptoms of infection are often subtle and nonspecific in the newborn. The newborn also has a poor hypothalamic response to pyrogens; therefore, fever is not a reliable indicator of infection. In the neonatal period, hypothermia is a more reliable sign of infection.

Of the three major types of immunoglobulins that are primarily involved in immunity—IgG, IgA, and IgM—only IgG crosses the placenta. The pregnant woman forms antibodies in response to illness or immunization. This process is called **active acquired immunity**. When IgG antibodies are transferred to the fetus in utero, **passive acquired immunity** results, because the fetus does not produce the antibodies itself. IgG antibodies are very active against bacterial toxins.

Because the maternal IgG is transferred primarily during the third trimester, preterm newborns (especially those born before 34 weeks' gestation) may be more susceptible to infection. In general, newborns have immunity to tetanus, diphtheria, smallpox, measles, mumps, poliomyelitis, and a variety of other bacterial and viral diseases. The period of resistance varies: Immunity against common viral infections such as measles may last 4 to 8 months, whereas immunity to certain bacteria may disappear within 4 to 8 weeks.

Although newborn infants are more vulnerable to infection, the normal newborn does produce antibodies in response to an antigen but not as effectively as an older child does. It is customary to begin the majority of routine immunizations at 2 months of age so that the infant can develop active acquired immunity. Some immunizations for specific viruses (such as hepatitis B) are even given in the first day after birth. (See discussion of newborn immunization in Chapter 26 🔗.)

IgM antibodies are produced in response to blood group antigens, gram-negative enteric organisms, and some viruses in the expectant mother. Because IgM does not normally cross the placenta, most or all of it is produced by the fetus beginning at 10 to 15 weeks' gestation. Elevated levels of IgM at birth may indicate placental leaks or, more commonly, antigenic stimulation in utero. Consequently elevations suggest that the newborn was exposed to an intrauterine infection such as syphilis or TORCH syndrome (toxoplasmosis, rubella, cytomegalovirus, herpesvirus hominis type 2 infection). (For further discussion, see Chapter 16 🔗.) The lack of available maternal IgM in the newborn also accounts for the susceptibility to gram-negative enteric organisms such as *Escherichia coli*.

IgA immunoglobulins appear to provide protection mainly on secreting surfaces such as the respiratory tract, gastrointestinal tract, and eyes. Serum IgA does not cross the placenta and is not normally produced by the fetus in utero. Unlike the other immunoglobulins, IgA is not affected by gastric action. Colostrum, the forerunner of breast milk, is very high in the secretory form of IgA. Consequently it may be of significance in providing some passive immunity to the infant of a breastfeeding mother. Newborns begin to produce secretory IgA in their intestinal mucosa about 4 weeks after birth.

NEUROLOGIC AND SENSORY-PERCEPTUAL FUNCTIONING

The newborn's brain is about one quarter the size of an adult's, and myelination of nerve fibers is incomplete. Unlike the cardiovascular and respiratory systems, which undergo tremendous changes at birth, the nervous system is minimally influenced by the actual birth process. Because many biochemical and histologic changes have yet to occur in the newborn's brain, the postnatal period is considered a time of risk with regard to the development of the brain and nervous system. For neurologic development—including development of intellect—to proceed, the brain and other nervous system structures must mature in an orderly, unhampered fashion. (For discussion of cranial nerves, see Chapter 25 🔗.)

Intrauterine Environment Influence on Newborn Behavior

Newborns respond to and interact with the environment in a predictable pattern of behavior that is somewhat shaped by their intrauterine experience. This intrauterine experience is affected by intrinsic factors such as maternal nutrition and external factors such as the mother's physical environment. Depending on the newborn's temperament, neonatal behavioral responses to different stresses vary. Some newborns react quietly to stimulation, others become overreactive and tense, and some may exhibit a combination of the two.

Factors such as exposure to intense auditory stimuli in utero can eventually be manifested in the behavior of the newborn. For example, the fetal heart rate (FHR) initially increases when the pregnant woman is exposed to auditory stimuli, but repetition of the stimuli leads to decreased FHR. Thus, the newborn who was exposed to intense noise during fetal life is significantly less reactive to loud sounds postnatally.

Characteristics of Newborn Neurologic Function

Normal newborns are usually in a position of partially flexed extremities with the legs near the abdomen. When awake, the newborn may exhibit purposeless, uncoordinated bilateral movements of the extremities. The organization and quality of the newborn's motor activity are influenced by a number of factors, including the following (Brazelton & Nugent, 2011):

- Sleep-alert states
- Presence of environmental stimuli, such as heat, light, cold, and noise
- Conditions causing a chemical imbalance, such as hypoglycemia
- Hydration status
- State of health
- Recovery from the stress of labor and birth

The newborn's body growth progresses in a cephalocaudal (head-to-toe), proximal-distal fashion. The newborn is somewhat hypertonic; that is, there is resistance to extending the elbow and knee joints. Muscle tone should be symmetric. Diminished muscle tone and flaccidity may indicate neurologic dysfunction.

Specific symmetric deep tendon reflexes can be elicited in the newborn. The knee-jerk reflex is brisk; a normal ankle clonus may involve three to four beats. Plantar flexion is present. Other reflexes, including the Moro, grasping, Babinski, rooting, and sucking reflexes, are characteristic of neurologic integrity. (For discussion of reflexes see Chapter 25 🔗.) Complex behavioral patterns reflect the newborn's neurologic maturation and integration. A newborn who can bring a hand to the mouth may be demonstrating motor coordination as well as a self-quieting technique, thus increasing the complexity of the behavioral response. **Self-quieting ability** is the ability of newborns to use their own resources to quiet and comfort themselves.

Newborns also possess complex, organized defensive motor patterns. **Habituation** is the newborn's ability to process and respond to complex stimulation. For example, when a bright light is flashed into the newborn's eyes, the initial response is blinking, constriction of the pupil, and perhaps a slight startle reaction. However, with repeated stimulation, the newborn's responses gradually diminish and disappear. The capacity to ignore repetitious disturbing stimuli is a defense mechanism readily allowing the newborn to shut out overwhelming and disturbing stimuli. Sensory abilities include visual, auditory, olfactory, taste, and tactile capacities.

Periods of Reactivity

The newborn usually shows a predictable pattern of behavior during the first several hours after birth, characterized by two **periods of reactivity** separated by a sleep phase.

First Period of Reactivity

The first period of reactivity lasts approximately 30 minutes after birth. During this period the newborn is awake and active and may appear hungry and have a strong sucking reflex. This is the natural and best opportunity to initiate breastfeeding if the mother has chosen it. Bursts of random, diffuse movements alternating with relative immobility may occur. Respirations are rapid, as high as 80 breaths per minute, and there may be retraction of the chest, transient flaring of the nares, and grunting. The heart rate is rapid, and the rhythm may be irregular. Bowel sounds are usually absent.

Period of Inactivity to Sleep Phase

After approximately half an hour the newborn's activity gradually diminishes, and the heart rate and respirations decrease as the newborn enters the sleep phase. The sleep phase may last from a few minutes to 2 to 4 hours. During this period, the newborn will be difficult to awaken and will show no interest in sucking. Bowel sounds become audible, and cardiac and respiratory rates return to baseline values.

Second Period of Reactivity

During the second period of reactivity, the newborn is again awake and alert. This period lasts 4 to 6 hours in the normal newborn. Physiologic responses are variable during this stage. The heart and respiratory rates increase; however, the nurse must be alert for apneic periods, which may cause a drop in the heart rate and oxygen level (desaturation). The newborn is stimulated to continue breathing during such times. The newborn may develop rapid color changes and become mildly cyanotic or mottled during these fluctuations. Production of respiratory and gastric mucus increases, and the newborn responds by gagging, choking, and regurgitating.

SAFETY ALERT!

Because infants are often unable to handle oral secretions effectively enough to protect their airway, parents must be instructed in the proper use of the bulb syringe. The bulb syringe used correctly creates mild suction for removal of oral and nasal secretions. Overuse or vigorous use of the bulb syringe causes unnecessary trauma and inflammation of the small nasal airways resulting in swelling and partial airway obstruction. See Skill 5–1, Performing Nasal Pharyngeal Suctioning, in the *Clinical Skills Manual* SKILLS .

Continued close observation and intervention may be required to maintain a clear airway during this period of reactivity. The gastrointestinal tract becomes more active. The newborn often passes the first meconium stool and may also have an initial voiding. The newborn will indicate readiness for feeding by such behaviors as sucking, rooting, and swallowing. If feeding was not initiated in the first period of reactivity, it is done at this time. (See Chapter 26 ✏ for further discussion of this first feeding.)

Behavioral States of the Newborn

The behavior of the newborn can be divided into two categories, the sleep state and the alert state (Gardner & Goldson, 2011). These postnatal behavioral states are similar to those that have been identified during pregnancy. Subcategories are identified under each major category.

Sleep States

The sleep states are as follows:

1. *Deep or quiet sleep.* Deep or quiet sleep is characterized by closed eyes with no eye movements; regular, even breathing; and jerky motions or startles at regular intervals. Behavioral responses to external stimuli are likely to be delayed. Startles are rapidly suppressed, and changes in state are not likely to occur. Heart rate may range from 100 to 120 beats per minute.

2. *Active or light sleep (rapid eye movement [REM] sleep).* The baby has irregular respirations; eyes closed, with REM; irregular sucking motions; minimal activity; and irregular but smooth movement of the extremities. Environmental and internal stimuli may initiate a startle reaction and a change of state.

Newborn sleep cycles have been recognized and defined according to duration. The length of the sleep cycle depends on the age of the newborn. At term, REM active sleep and quiet sleep occur in intervals of 50 to 60 minutes (Gardner & Goldson, 2011). About 45% to 50% of the newborn's total sleep is active sleep, 35% to 45% is quiet sleep, and 10% is transitional between these two periods. Growth hormone secretion depends on regular sleep patterns. Any disturbance of the sleep-wake cycle can result in irregular spikes of growth hormone. REM sleep stimulates the highest peaks of growth hormone and the growth of the neural system. Over time, the newborn's sleep-wake patterns become diurnal; that is, the newborn sleeps at night and stays awake during the day. (See *Assessment of Neurologic Status* in Chapter 25 ✏ for a short discussion of Brazelton's assessment of newborn states.)

Alert States

In the first 30 to 60 minutes after birth, many newborns display a quiet alert state, characteristic of the first period of reactivity (Figure 24–8 ●). Nurses should use these alert states to encourage

● **Figure 24–8** Mother and newborn gaze at each other. This quiet alert state is the optimum state for interaction between baby and parents.
Source: Superstock Royalty Free.

bonding and breastfeeding. These periods of alertness tend to be short the first 2 days after birth to allow the baby to recover from the birth process. Subsequent alert states are of choice or of necessity (Gardner & Goldson, 2011). Increasing choice of wakefulness by the newborn indicates a maturing capacity to achieve and maintain consciousness. Heat, cold, and hunger are but a few of the stimuli that can cause wakefulness by necessity. Once the disturbing stimuli are removed, the newborn tends to fall back asleep.

The following are subcategories of the alert state (Gardner & Goldson, 2011).

1. *Drowsy or semidozing.* The behaviors common to the drowsy state are open or closed eyes; fluttering eyelids; semidozing appearance; and slow, regular movements of the extremities. Mild startles may be noted from time to time. Although the reaction to a sensory stimulus is delayed, a change of state often results.

2. *Quiet alert.* In the wide-awake state, the newborn is alert and follows and fixates on attractive objects, faces, or auditory stimuli. Motor activity is minimal, and the response to external stimuli is delayed.

3. *Active alert.* In the active alert awake state the newborn's eyes are open and motor activity is quite intense, with thrusting movements of the extremities. Environmental stimuli increase startles or motor activity, but individual reactions are difficult to distinguish because of the generally high activity level.

4. *Crying.* Intense crying is accompanied by jerky motor movements. Crying serves several purposes for the newborn. It may be a distraction from disturbing stimuli such as hunger and pain. Fussiness often allows the newborn to discharge energy and reorganize behavior. Most important, crying elicits an appropriate response of help from the parents.

Sensory Capacities of the Newborn

Visual Capacity

Orientation is the newborn's ability to be alert to, to follow, and to fixate on appealing and attractive complex visual stimuli. The newborn prefers the human face and eyes and bright shiny objects. As the face or object comes into the line of vision, the newborn responds with bright, wide eyes, still limbs, and fixed staring. This intense visual involvement may last several minutes, during which time the newborn is able to follow the stimulus from side to side. The newborn uses this sensory capacity to become familiar with family, friends, and surroundings.

Auditory Capacity

The newborn responds to auditory stimulation with a definite, organized behavior repertoire. The stimulus used to assess auditory response should be selected to match the state of the newborn. A rattle is appropriate for light sleep, a voice for an awake state, and a clap for deep sleep. As the newborn hears the sound, the cardiac rate rises, and a minimal startle reflex may be seen. If the sound is appealing, the newborn will become alert and search for the site of the auditory stimulus. Newborns prefer the sound of the human voice to nonhuman sounds and have very acute hearing immediately after birth (Cheffer & Rannalli, 2011). The newborn's hearing should be evaluated prior to discharge.

Olfactory Capacity

Newborns can select their mother by smell and are apparently able to select people by smell (Cheffer & Rannalli, 2011). Newborns are able to distinguish their mothers' breast pads from those of other mothers at just 1 week postnatally and will preferentially turn toward the mother's odor.

Taste and Sucking

The newborn responds differently to varying tastes. They can distinguish between sweet and sour at 3 days of age (Cheffer & Rannalli, 2011). Sugar, for example, increases sucking. Newborns fed with a rubber nipple versus the breast also show sucking pattern variations. While breastfeeding, the newborn sucks in bursts, with frequent regular pauses. The bottle-fed newborn tends to suck at a regular rate, with infrequent pauses.

When awake and hungry, the newborn displays rapid searching motions in response to the rooting reflex. Once feeding begins, the newborn establishes a sucking pattern according to the method of feeding. Finger sucking is seen in utero as well as after birth. The newborn frequently uses nonnutritive sucking as a self-quieting activity, which assists in the development of self-regulation. For bottle-fed infants, there is no reason to discourage nonnutritive sucking with a pacifier. Pacifiers should be offered to breastfed infants only after breastfeeding is well established. If the pacifier is offered too soon, a phenomenon called "nipple confusion" may occur in which the breastfed infant has difficulty learning to suck from the breast and will nurse less (see *Supplementary Formula-Feeding for Breastfed Infants* in Chapter 26 🔗).

Tactile Capacity

The newborn is very sensitive to being touched, cuddled, and held. Often a mother's first response to an upset or crying newborn is touching or holding. Swaddling, placing a hand on the abdomen, or holding the arms to prevent a startle reflex are other methods of soothing the newborn. The quieted newborn is then able to attend to and interact with the environment. Touch is also used to rouse a drowsy infant, making him or her more alert for feeding.

> ## Teaching Highlights Newborn Crying
>
> While the mother and infant are in the hospital, the nurse has a perfect opportunity to teach parents techniques to deal with infant crying and fussiness. It is important for parents and caregivers to know that for the first several months crying is the only means of communication available to the newborn and usually signifies unmet needs.

Critical Concept Review

LEARNING OUTCOME 24.1: Explain the respiratory and cardiovascular changes that occur during the newborn's transition to extrauterine life and during stabilization in determining the nursing care of the newborn.

1. Newborn respiration is initiated primarily by chemical, mechanical, and reabsorptive processes associated with thermal and sensory stimulation.
2. Onset of respirations stimulates cardiovascular changes:
   - Air enters the lungs; oxygen content rises in alveoli and stimulates relaxation of pulmonary arteries.

- This leads to a decrease in pulmonary vascular resistance, which allows complete vascular flow to the lungs.
- With increased oxygenated pulmonary blood flow and loss of the placenta, systemic blood flow increases and the foramen ovale and ductus arteriosus begin to close.

LEARNING OUTCOME 24.2: Compare the factors that modify the newborn's blood values to the corresponding results.

1. Newborn blood values are affected by:
   - Site of the blood sample: venous versus capillary
   - Gestational age

- Prenatal and/or perinatal hemorrhage
- Timing of the clamping of the umbilical cord

LEARNING OUTCOME 24.3: Relate the process of thermogenesis in the newborn and the major mechanisms of heat loss to the challenge of maintaining newborn thermal stability.

1. Thermogenesis is achieved by:
   - Increased basal metabolic rate
   - Muscular activity
   - Nonshivering thermogenesis
   - Metabolizing of brown adipose fat

2. Heat loss is created by:
   - Evaporation (infant is wet from amniotic fluid and/or bath)
   - Convection
   - Radiation
   - Conduction

LEARNING OUTCOME 24.4: Explain the steps involved in the conjugation and excretion of bilirubin in the newborn.

1. Unconjugated bilirubin is a by-product of the destruction of red blood cells.
2. Bilirubin is bound to albumin. It is transferred into liver cells and bound to intracellular proteins. These proteins determine the amount of bilirubin uptake into the liver.

3. The uridine-diphosphoglucuronosyl transferase (UDPGT) enzyme causes unconjugated bilirubin to attach to glucuronic acid, producing conjugated bilirubin. This is excreted into bile ducts, then into the common duct, and into the duodenum.
4. In the intestines, bacteria transform the conjugated bilirubin into urobilinogen (urine bilirubin) and stercobilinogen, which is excreted as a pigment in the stools.

LEARNING OUTCOME 24.5: Identify the reasons a newborn may develop jaundice and nursing interventions to decrease the probability of jaundice.

1. A newborn may develop jaundice because of:
   - Accelerated destruction of fetal RBCs
   - Impaired conjugation of bilirubin
   - Increased bilirubin reabsorption from the intestinal tract

2. Early nursing interventions to decrease jaundice are:
   - Maintain the newborn's skin temperature.
   - Monitor stool for amount and characteristics for excretion of meconium.
   - Encourage early feedings to promote intestinal elimination.

LEARNING OUTCOME 24.6: Delineate the functional abilities of the newborn's gastrointestinal tract and liver.

1. At birth the newborn is able to digest most simple carbohydrates, proteins, and fats. They have trouble digesting starches.
2. The newborn usually passes meconium within 24–48 hours after birth and begins to have normal bowel movements.

3. The newborn liver is slightly less active than the adult liver, which is indicative in the liver's decreased ability to conjugate all of the bilirubin produced by the destruction of fetal RBCs.
4. The liver plays a crucial role in iron storage, carbohydrate metabolism, and coagulation.

LEARNING OUTCOME 24.7: Relate the development of the newborn's kidneys to the newborn's ability to maintain fluid and electrolyte balance.

1. The following characteristics of a newborn's kidneys cause difficulty in maintaining fluid and electrolyte balance:
   - Decreased rate of glomerular flow and limited excretion of solutes

   - Limited tubular reabsorptions
   - Limited ability to concentrate urine
2. Most newborns void within 48 hours of birth.

LEARNING OUTCOME 24.8: Describe basic newborn immunologic responses.

1. The newborn is unable to recognize, localize, and destroy invasive bacteria.
2. The newborn has passive acquired immunity from the mother, lasting from 4 weeks to 8 months.

3. The newborn begins to produce own immunity at about 4 weeks of age.

LEARNING OUTCOME 24.9: Explain the physiologic and behavioral characteristics of newborn neurologic function, patterns of behavior during the periods of reactivity, and possible nursing interventions.

1. Neurologic responses:
   - Newborn interacts with environment
   - Presence of synchronized motor activity
   - Well-developed sensory capacities
2. Periods of reactivity:
   - First period of reactivity (lasts 30 minutes after birth):
     - The newborn is awake and active, appears hungry, and has a strong suck.
     - The nurse should help the mother to initiate breastfeeding.
     - Vital signs are elevated at this time.
   - Period of inactivity to sleep (30 minutes to 4 hours after birth):
   - The newborn is difficult to awaken.
   - Vital signs return to normal.
   - Second period of reactivity (lasts 4–6 hours after period of inactivity):
     - The newborn is awake and alert.

- Vital signs are variable and the nurse must observe the newborn closely during this time for periods of apnea, gagging, and regurgitation.
- The newborn often passes meconium stool.
- The newborn shows a readiness to feed.

3. Behavioral states:
   - Sleep state:
   - Deep or quiet sleep: closed eyes with no eye movement
   - Light sleep (active rapid eye movements)
   - Alert state:
     - Subcategories include: drowsy or semidozing, quiet alert, active alert, and crying.
     - The mother and nurse should use this time to facilitate feedings.

LEARNING OUTCOME 24.10: Describe the normal sensory-perceptual abilities and behavioral states seen in the newborn period and the associated nursing care.

1. The normal sensory-perceptual abilities of the newborn are:
   - Visual:
     - The newborn is able to be alert to, follow, and fixate on complex visual stimuli for short periods of time.
   - Auditory:
     - The newborn is able to be alert to and search for an appealing auditory stimulus.
   - Olfactory:
     - The newborn is able to select people by smell.

- Taste and sucking:
  - The newborn is able to respond selectively to different tastes.
- Tactile:
  - The newborn is very sensitive to being touched, cuddled, and held.
  - The newborn is able to attend to and interact with the environment.

2. Some of the behavioral capabilities of the newborn that assist in adaptation to extrauterine life include self-quieting ability and habituation.

Clinical Reasoning in Action

Sandra Dee, a 21-year-old, G1, P0000, at 36 weeks' gestation, has been in labor for the last 12 hours and is fully dilated with caput visible on the perineum. The fetal heart rate is 148 to 152 with early deceleration down to 142 with contraction and pushing. Her contractions are 4 to 5 minutes apart of good quality. Sandra's mother and sister are present for the birth. Her prenatal record shows no significant pregnancy problems or complications, and her vital signs have been stable within normal limits. Sandra has received 2 doses of Stadol for a total of 2 mg IV for pain relief during her labor. The last dose was given 2 hours ago. You assist with the vaginal birth of a live baby without an episiotomy. You observe the sex and time as the midwife places the infant girl on the mother's abdomen, suctions out the baby's mouth and nose, and proceeds to clamp the cord. You dry and stimulate the infant

to breathe, remove the wet blanket and replace it with a dry one, and place the infant skin to skin on the mother's chest. You assess the need for infant resuscitation. The baby has a lusty cry spontaneously less than 30 seconds after birth. You palpate the cord, obtaining a heart rate of 120, and observe that the baby's chest and face are pink, and the legs and arms are flexed with open fist.

1. Explain the changes that must occur in the infant's cardiopulmonary system at birth.
2. What criteria do you look for when you assess the newborn for adequate cardiopulmonary adaptation at birth?
3. What steps do you take to maintain a neutral thermal environment at birth?
4. Sandra plans to breastfeed. When would you initiate the first feeding?
5. Discuss nursing actions that can decrease the probability of high bilirubin levels in the newborn.

See www.nursing.pearsonhighered.com for possible responses.

References

Association of Women's Health, Obstetric and Neonatal Nurses (AWHONN). (2005, reaffirmed 2009). *Clinical position statement: Universal screening for hyperbilirubinemia* [Position statement]. Washington, DC: Author.

Blackburn, S. T. (2013). *Maternal, fetal, & neonatal physiology: A clinical perspective* (4th ed.). St. Louis, MO: Saunders.

Brazelton, T. B., & Nugent, J. K. (2011). *The neonatal behavioral assessment scale* (4th ed.). London, England: MacKeith.

Cheffer, N. D., & Rannalli, D. A. (2011). Transitional care of the newborn. In S. Mattson & J. E. Smith (Eds.), *Core curriculum for maternal-newborn nursing* (4th ed., pp. 345–361). St. Louis, MO: Saunders.

Cloherty, J. R., Eichenwald, E. C., Hansen, A. R., & Stark, A. R. (2012). *Manual of neonatal care* (7th ed.). Philadelphia, PA: Lippincott Williams & Wilkins.

Furdon, S. A., & Benjamin, K. (2010). Physical assessment. In M. T. Verklan & M. Walden (Eds.), *Core curriculum for neonatal intensive care nursing* (4th ed., pp. 121–155). St. Louis, MO: Saunders.

Gardner, S. L., & Goldson, E. (2011). The neonate and the environment: Impact on development. In S. L. Gardner, B. S. Carter, M. Enzman-Hines, & J. A. Hernandez (Eds.), *Merenstein & Gardner's handbook of neonatal intensive care* (7th ed., pp. 270–331). St. Louis, MO: Mosby.

Lauderdale, J. (2012). Transcultural perspectives in childbearing. In M. M. Andrews & J. S. Boyle (Eds.), *Transcultural concepts in nursing care* (6th ed., pp. 91–122). Philadelphia, PA: Wolters Kluwer/Lippincott Williams & Wilkins.

Luchtman-Jones, L., & Wilson, D. B. (2011). The blood and hematopoietic system. In R. J. Martin, A. A. Fanaroff, & M. C. Walsh (Eds.), *Fanaroff & Martin's Neonatal-perinatal medicine* (9th ed., pp. 1308–1373). St. Louis, MO: Elsevier-Mosby.

Manco-Johnson, M., Rodden, D. J., & Hays, T. (2011). Newborn hematology. In S. L. Gardner, B. S. Carter, M. Enzman-Hines, & J. A. Hernandez (Eds.), *Merenstein & Gardner's handbook of neonatal intensive care* (7th ed., pp. 503–530). St. Louis, MO: Mosby.

McGrath, J. M., & Hardy, W. (2011). The infant at risk. In S. Mattson & J. E. Smith (Eds.), *Core curriculum for maternal-newborn nursing* (4th ed., pp. 362–414). St. Louis, MO: Saunders.

Niermeyer, S., & Clarke, S. (2011). Delivery room care. In S. L. Gardner, B. S. Carter, M. Enzman-Hines, & J. A. Hernandez (Eds.), *Merenstein & Gardner's handbook of neonatal intensive care* (7th ed., pp. 52–77). St. Louis, MO: Mosby.

Raab, E. L., & Kelly, L. K. (2013). Normal newborn assessment & care. In A. H. Decherney, L. Nathan, N. Laufer, & A. S. Roman (Eds.), *Current diagnosis & treatment: Obstetrics & gynecology* (11th ed., pp. 181–189). New York, NY: McGraw-Hill.

Sadowski, S. L. (2010). Cardiovascular disorders. In M. T. Verklan & M. Walden (Eds.), *Core curriculum for neonatal intensive care nursing* (4th ed., pp. 534–588). St. Louis, MO: Saunders.

Nursing Assessment of the Newborn

Like most parents, when I held my son for the first time, I checked that all his fingers and toes were present. Then he looked at me with wide, bright, serious eyes and began my introduction to his unique personality. —Leah, 23

Radius Images/Alamy

LEARNING OUTCOMES

25.1 Describe the physical and neuromuscular maturity characteristics assessed to determine the gestational age of the newborn.

25.2 Summarize the components of a systematic physical assessment of the newborn.

25.3 Describe the normal physical characteristics and normal variations of the newborn and compare abnormal findings to possible causes and nursing responses.

25.4 Describe the components of a neurologic assessment and the neurologic/neuromuscular characteristics of the newborn and the reflexes that may be present at birth.

25.5 Compare the components of the newborn behavioral assessment with the normal behavioral characteristics and normal variations of the newborn.

25.6 Correlate findings in a newborn behavioral assessment to nursing responses and to teach and involve parents in the care of their newborn.

Newborns communicate their needs primarily by behavior. Because nurses are the most consistent professional observers of the newborn, they can translate this behavior into information about a newborn's condition and respond with appropriate nursing interventions. This chapter focuses on the assessment of the newborn and the interpretation of these findings.

Newborn assessment is a continuous process designed to evaluate development and adjustments to extrauterine life. In the birth setting, the Apgar scoring procedure and careful observation form the basis of assessment and are correlated with information such as the following:

- Maternal prenatal history
- Birthing history
- Maternal analgesia and anesthesia
- Complications of labor or birth
- Treatment instituted immediately after birth, in conjunction with determination of clinical gestational age
- Consideration of the classification of newborns by weight and gestational age and by neonatal mortality risk
- Physical examination of the newborn

The nurse incorporates data from these sources with the assessment findings during the first 1 to 4 hours after birth to formulate a plan for nursing intervention.

The various newborn assessments and the data obtained from them are valuable only to the degree to which they are shared with the parents. The parents must be included in the assessment process from the moment of their child's birth. The *Apgar* score and its meaning should be explained immediately to the family (see Chapter 19 🔵 for a discussion of the Apgar score). As soon as possible, the parents should take part in the physical and behavioral assessments as well.

The nurse encourages the parents to identify the unique behavioral characteristics of their newborn and to learn nurturing activities. Attachment is promoted when parents have an opportunity to explore their newborn in private and identify individual physical and behavioral characteristics. The nurse's supportive responses to parents' questions and observations are essential throughout the assessment process. The newborn physical examination is the beginning of newborn health surveillance and health education for the newborn's family that continues into the community setting.

TIMING OF NEWBORN ASSESSMENTS

During the first 24 hours of life, the newborn makes the critical transition from intrauterine to extrauterine life. The risk of mortality and morbidity is statistically high during this period. Assessment of the newborn is essential to ensure that the transition proceeds successfully.

There are major time frames for assessments of newborns while they are in the birth facility.

- Delivery room disposition. The first assessment is done in the birthing area immediately after birth to determine the need for resuscitation or other interventions. The stable newborn should stay with the family after birth to initiate early attachment. The newborn with complications is usually taken to the special nursery for further evaluation and intervention.
- Nursery or couplet care admission examination. A second assessment may be done by the nursery nurse as part of routine admission procedures. During this assessment, the nurse carries out a brief physical examination to estimate gestational age and evaluate the newborn's adaptation to extrauterine life. No later than 2 hours after birth, the admitting nursery nurse should evaluate

the newborn's status and any problems that place the newborn at risk (Gleason & Devaskar, 2012).

- Before discharge examination. A certified nurse-midwife (CNM), physician, or nurse practitioner will carry out an exam similar to the well-baby admission exam. This includes a behavioral assessment and additional information from the baby's stay in the birthing unit to assess if the infant is ready for routine care at home. A complete physical examination is done to detect any emerging or potential problems. When the birthing center stay is short, a combination admission-discharge exam is appropriate.

This chapter presents the procedures for estimating gestational age and performing the complete physical examination and behavioral assessment. Chapter 19 🕐 discusses the immediate postbirth assessment. Chapter 26 🕐 describes the brief assessment performed during the first 4 hours of life.

ESTIMATION OF GESTATIONAL AGE

The nurse must establish the newborn's gestational age in the first 4 hours after birth so that careful attention can be given to age-related problems. Traditionally, a newborn's gestational age was determined from the date of the pregnant woman's last menstrual period. However, this method was accurate only 75% to 85% of the time. Because of the problems that develop with the preterm newborn or the newborn whose weight is inappropriate for gestational age, a more accurate system was developed to postnatally evaluate the newborn. Once learned, the procedure can be done in a few minutes.

SAFETY ALERT!

It is essential that the nurse wear gloves when assessing the newborn in these early hours after birth and before the first bath until amniotic fluid, as well as vaginal and bloody secretions on the skin, are removed.

Clinical **gestational age assessment tools** have two components: (1) external physical characteristics and (2) neurologic or neuromuscular development. Physical characteristics generally include the following:

- Sole creases
- Amount of breast tissue
- Amount of lanugo
- Cartilaginous development of the ear
- Testicular descent and scrotal rugae in the male
- Labial development in the female

These objective clinical criteria are not influenced by labor and birth and do not change significantly within the first 12 hours after birth.

The neurologic examination facilitates assessment of functional or physiologic maturation in addition to physical development. A variety of factors can affect the newborn's nervous system, which is unstable during the first 24 hours of life;

neurologic evaluation findings based on reflexes or assessments dependent on the higher brain centers may not be reliable. If the neurologic findings drastically deviate from the gestational age derived by evaluation of external characteristics, a second assessment is done in 24 hours.

The neurologic assessment components (excluding reflexes) can aid in assessing the gestational age of newborns of less than 34 weeks' gestation. Between 26 and 34 weeks, neurologic changes are significant, whereas significant physical changes are less evident. Ballard, Khoury, Wedig, et al. (1991) developed the *estimation of gestational age by maturity rating*, a simplified version of the well-researched *Dubowitz tool*. The Ballard tool omits some of the neuromuscular tone assessments, which are difficult to assess in very ill newborns or those on respirators, and leg recoil. In the Ballard tool, each physical and neuromuscular finding is given a value, and the total score is matched to a gestational age. The maximum score on the Ballard tool is 50, which corresponds to a gestational age of 44 weeks.

For example, on completion of a gestational assessment of a 1-hour-old newborn, the nurse gives a score of 3 to all the physical characteristics, for a total of 18, and gives a score of 3 to all neuromuscular assessments, for a total of 18. The physical characteristics score of 18 is added to the neurologic score of 18 for a total score of 36, which correlates with 38+ weeks' gestation. Because all newborns vary slightly in the development of physical characteristics and maturation of neurologic function, scores usually vary instead of all being 3.

Postnatal gestational age assessment tools can overestimate preterm newborns of less than 28 weeks' gestational age and underestimate postterm or more than 43 weeks' gestation. Ballard et al. (1991) in the **New Ballard Score (NBS)** added criteria for more accurate assessment of the gestational age of newborns between 20 and 28 weeks' gestation and less than 1500 g. They suggest that the assessments should be made within 12 hours of birth to optimize accuracy, especially in infants of less than 26 weeks' gestational age. Also the Ballard assessment may be overstimulating to infants of less than 27 weeks' gestation (Gardner & Hernandez, 2011). Some maternal conditions, such as preeclampsia, diabetes, and maternal analgesia and anesthesia, may affect certain gestational assessment components and warrant further evaluation. Maternal diabetes, although it appears to accelerate fetal physical growth, seems to retard maturation. Maternal hypertension states, which retard fetal physical growth, seem to speed maturation.

Newborns of women with preeclampsia on magnesium sulfate may have a poor correlation with the neuromuscular criteria involving active muscle tone and edema. Maternal analgesia and anesthesia may cause respiratory depression in the baby. Babies with respiratory distress syndrome (RDS) tend to be flaccid and edematous and to assume a "froglike" posture (see Chapter 29 🕐 for a discussion of RDS). These characteristics affect the scoring of the neuromuscular components of the assessment tool used. The NBS gestational age assessment tool will be used throughout the chapter to demonstrate the assessment of the physical and neuromuscular criteria associated with gestational age.

A

B

C

● **Figure 25–1** Resting posture. *A,* Infant exhibits beginning of flexion of the thigh. The gestational age is approximately 31 weeks. Note the extension of the upper extremities. Score 1 or 2. *B,* Infant exhibits stronger flexion of the arms, hips, and thighs. The gestational age is approximately 35 weeks. Score 3. *C,* The full-term infant exhibits hypertonic flexion of all extremities. Score 4.

Source: George Dodson/Lightworks Studio/Pearson Education.

Assessment of Physical Maturity Characteristics

The nurse first evaluates observable characteristics without disturbing the baby. Selected physical characteristics are presented here in the order in which they might be most effectively evaluated:

1. *Resting posture,* although a neuromuscular component, should be assessed as the baby lies undisturbed on a flat surface (Figure 25–1 ●).

2. *Skin* in the preterm newborn appears thin and transparent, with veins prominent over the abdomen early in gestation. As the newborn approaches term, the skin appears opaque because of increased subcutaneous tissue. Disappearance of the protective vernix caseosa promotes skin desquamation; this is commonly seen in postmature infants (infants of more than 42 weeks' gestational age) and those showing signs of placental insufficiency.

3. *Lanugo,* a fine hair covering, decreases as gestational age increases. The amount of **lanugo** is greatest at 28 to 30 weeks and then disappears, first from the face and then from the trunk and extremities. It is most abundant over the back (particularly between the scapulae), although it will be noted over the face, legs, and arms (Figure 25–2 ●).

4. *Sole (plantar) creases* are reliable indicators of gestational age in the first 12 hours of life. Later the skin of the foot begins drying, and superficial creases appear. Development of plantar creases begins at the top (anterior) portion of the sole and, as gestation progresses, proceeds to the heel (Figure 25–3 ●). Peeling may also occur. Plantar creases

● **Figure 25–2** Lanugo.

Source: Courtesy of Jo Engle, RN, MSN, NNP-BC and Vanessa Howell, RN, MSN.

vary with race. In newborns of African descent, plantar creases may be less developed at term.

5. The nurse inspects the *areola* and gently palpates the *breast bud tissue* by applying the forefinger and middle finger to the breast area and measuring the tissue between them in centimeters or millimeters (Figure 25–4 ●). At term gestation, the tissue measures between 0.5 and 1 cm (5 and 10 mm). During the assessment, the nipple should not be grasped firmly because skin and subcutaneous tissue will prevent accurate estimation of size. The nurse must do this procedure gently to avoid causing trauma to the breast tissue.

As gestation progresses, the breast bud tissue mass and areola enlarge. However, a large breast tissue mass

A B C

● **Figure 25–3** Sole creases. *A,* Infant has a few sole creases on the anterior portion of the foot. Note the slick heel. Score 2. The gestational age is approximately 35 weeks. *B,* Infant has a deeper network of sole creases on the anterior two thirds of the sole. Note the slick heel. Score 3. The gestational age is approximately 37 weeks. *C,* The full-term infant has deep sole creases down to and including the heel as the skin loses fluid and dries after birth. Score 4. Sole (plantar) creases can be seen even in preterm infants.

Source: George Dodson/Lightworks Studio/Pearson Education.

can occur as a result of specific conditions other than advanced gestational age or the effects of maternal hormones on the baby. In the large-for-gestational-age (LGA) infant, a diabetic mother's accelerated development of breast tissue is a reflection of subcutaneous fat deposits. Small-for-gestational-age (SGA) (head sparing) term or postterm newborns may have used subcutaneous fat (which would have been deposited as breast tissue) to survive in utero; as a result, their lack of breast tissue may indicate a gestational

age of 34 to 35 weeks, even though other factors indicate a term or postterm newborn (Cloherty, Eichenwald, Hansen, et al., 2012).

6. *Ear form and cartilage distribution* develop with gestational age. The cartilage gives the ear its shape and substance (Figure 25–5 ●). In a newborn of less than 34 weeks' gestation, the ear is relatively shapeless and flat; it has little cartilage, so the ear folds over on itself and remains folded. By approximately 36 weeks' gestation, some cartilage and

A B

● **Figure 25–4** Breast tissue. *A,* Newborn has a visible raised area greater than 0.75 cm (0.3 in.) diameter. Score 3. The gestational age is 38 weeks. *B,* Gently compress the tissue between the middle and index fingers and measure the tissue in centimeters or millimeters. Absence of or decreased breast tissue often indicates a premature or small-for-gestational-age (SGA) newborn.

Source: George Dodson/Lightworks Studio/Pearson Education.

A   B   C

● **Figure 25–5** Ear form and cartilage. *A,* The ear of the infant at approximately 36 weeks' gestation shows incurving of the upper two thirds of the pinna. Score 2. *B,* Infant at term shows well-defined incurving of the entire pinna. Score 3. *C,* The pinna is folded toward the face and released. If the auricle stays in the position in which it is pressed or returns slowly to its original position, it usually means the gestational age is less than 38 weeks.

Source: A & B. George Dodson/Lightworks Studio/Pearson Education. C. Courtesy of Jo Engle, RN, MSN, NNP-BC and Vanessa Howell, RN, MSN.

incurving of the upper pinna are present, and the pinna springs back slowly when folded. (The nurse tests this response by holding the top and bottom of the pinna together with the forefinger and thumb and then releasing them or by folding the pinna of the ear forward against the side of the head, releasing it, and observing the response.) By term, the newborn's pinna is firm, stands away from the head, and springs back quickly from the folding.

7. *Male genitals* are evaluated for size of the scrotal sac, presence of rugae (wrinkles and ridges in the scrotum), and descent of the testes (Figure 25–6 ●). Before 36 weeks, the scrotum has few rugae, and the testes are palpable in the inguinal canal. By 36 to 38 weeks, the testes are in the upper scrotum, and rugae have developed over the anterior portion of the scrotum. By term, the testes are generally in

the lower scrotum, which is pendulous and covered with rugae.

8. The appearance of the *female genitals* depends in part on subcutaneous fat deposition and therefore relates to fetal nutritional status (Figure 25–7 ●). The clitoris varies in size, and occasionally is so swollen that it is difficult to identify the sex of the newborn. This swelling may be caused by adrenogenital syndrome, which causes the adrenals to secrete excessive amounts of androgen and other hormones. At 30 to 32 weeks' gestation, the clitoris is prominent, and the labia majora are small and widely separated. As gestational age increases, the labia majora increase in size. At 36 to 40 weeks, they nearly cover the clitoris. At 40 weeks and beyond, the labia majora cover the labia minora and clitoris.

A   B

● **Figure 25–6** Male genitals. *A,* Preterm newborn's testes are not within the scrotum. The scrotal surface has few rugae. Score 2. *B,* Term newborn's testes are generally fully descended. The entire surface of the scrotum is covered by rugae. Score 3.

Source: George Dodson/Lightworks Studio/Pearson Education.

A   B   C

● **Figure 25–7** Female genitals. *A,* Infant has a prominent clitoris. The labia majora are widely separated, and the labia minora, viewed laterally, would protrude beyond the labia majora. Score 1. The gestational age is 30 to 36 weeks. *B,* The clitoris is still visible. The labia minora are now covered by the larger labia majora. Score 2. The gestational age is 36 to 40 weeks. *C,* The term infant has well-developed, large labia majora that cover both the clitoris and labia minora. Score 3. The labia minora is often dark in some ethnic and racial groups of infants.

Source: A & B. George Dodson/Lightworks Studio/Pearson Education. *C.* Courtesy of Christine Mescolotto.

Other physical characteristics assessed by some gestational age scoring tools include the following:

1. *Vernix* covers the preterm newborn. The postterm newborn has no vernix. After noting vernix distribution, the birthing area nurse (wearing gloves) dries the newborn to prevent evaporative heat loss, thus disturbing the vernix and potentially altering this gestational age criterion. The birthing area nurse must communicate to the neonatal nurse the amount of vernix and the areas of vernix coverage.

2. *Hair* of the preterm newborn has the consistency of matted wool or fur and lies in bunches rather than in the silky, single strands of the term newborn's hair.

3. *Skull firmness* increases as the fetus matures. In a term newborn the bones are hard, and the sutures are not easily displaced. The nurse should not attempt to displace the sutures forcibly.

4. *Nails* appear and cover the nail bed at about 20 weeks' gestation. Nails extending beyond the fingertips may indicate a postterm newborn.

Assessment of Neuromuscular Maturity Characteristics

The central nervous system of the fetus matures at a fairly constant rate. Tests have been designed to evaluate neurologic status as manifested by development of neuromuscular tone. One significant neuromuscular change is that muscle tone progresses from extensor tone to flexor tone and from the lower to the upper extremities as the neurologic system matures in a *caudocephalad* (tail-to-head) progression. The neuromuscular evaluation requires more manipulation and disturbances than the physical evaluation of the newborn. The neuromuscular evaluation is best performed when the infant has stabilized.

1. The *square window sign* is elicited by gently flexing the newborn's hand toward the ventral forearm until resistance is felt. The angle formed at the wrist is measured (Figure 25–8 ●).

2. *Recoil* is a test of flexion development. Because flexion first develops in the lower extremities, recoil is first tested in the legs. Place the newborn on its back on a flat surface. With a hand on the newborn's knees, the nurse places the baby's legs in flexion, then extends them parallel to each other and flat on the surface. The response to this maneuver is recoil of the newborn's legs. According to gestational age, they may not move or they may return slowly or quickly to the flexed position. Preterm infants have less muscle tone than term infants, so preterm infants have less recoil.

    Test arm recoil by flexion at the elbow and extension of the arms at the newborn's side. While the baby is in the supine position, the nurse completely flexes both elbows, holds them in this position for 5 seconds, extends the arms at the baby's side, and releases them. On release, the elbows of a full-term newborn form an angle of less than 90 degrees and rapidly recoil back to a flexed position. The elbows of a preterm newborn have slower recoil time and form an angle greater than 90 degrees. Arm recoil is also slower in healthy but fatigued newborns after birth; therefore, arm recoil is best elicited after the first hour of birth, when the baby has had time to recover from the stress of the birth. The deep sleep state also decreases the arm recoil response. Assessment of arm recoil should be bilateral to rule out brachial palsy.

3. The *popliteal angle* (degree of knee flexion) is determined with the newborn flat on its back. The thigh is flexed on the abdomen and chest, and the nurse places the index finger of the other hand behind the newborn's ankle to extend the lower leg until resistance is met. The angle formed is then measured. Results vary from no resistance in the

A   B   C

● **Figure 25–8** Square window sign. **A,** This angle is 90 degrees and suggests an immature newborn of 28 to 32 weeks' gestation. Score 0. **B,** A 30- to 40-degree angle is commonly found in newborns from 38 to 40 weeks' gestation. Score 2 to 3. **C,** A 0- to 15-degree angle occurs in newborns from 40 to 42 weeks' gestation. Score 4.

Source: A & B. George Dodson/Lightworks Studio/Pearson Education. C. Courtesy of Jo Engle, RN, MSN, NNP-BC and Vanessa Howell, RN, MSN.

very immature newborn to an 80-degree angle in the term newborn.

4. The *scarf sign* is elicited by placing the newborn supine and drawing an arm across the chest toward the newborn's opposite shoulder until resistance is met. The location of the elbow is then noted in relation to the midline of the chest (Figure 25–9 ●). A preterm infant's elbow will cross the midline of the chest, whereas a full-term infant's elbow will not cross midline.

5. The *heel-to-ear extension* is performed by placing the newborn in a supine position and then gently drawing the foot toward the ear on the same side until resistance is felt. The nurse should allow the knee to bend during the test. It is important to hold the buttocks down to keep from rolling the baby. Both the proximity of foot to ear and the degree of knee extension are assessed. A preterm, immature newborn's leg will remain straight and the foot will go to the ear or beyond (Figure 25–10 ●). With advancing gestational age, the newborn demonstrates increasing resistance to this maneuver. Maneuvers involving the lower extremities of newborns who had frank breech presentations should be delayed to allow for resolution of leg positioning.

6. *Ankle dorsiflexion* is determined by flexing the ankle on the shin. The nurse uses a thumb to push on the sole of the newborn's foot while the fingers support the back of the leg. Then the angle formed by the foot and the interior leg is measured (Figure 25–11 ●). Intrauterine position and congenital deformities can influence this sign.

A   B   C

● **Figure 25–9** Scarf sign. **A,** No resistance is noted until after 30 weeks' gestation. The elbow can be readily moved past the midline. Score 1. **B,** The elbow is at midline at 36 to 40 weeks' gestation. Score 2. **C,** Beyond 40 weeks' gestation, the elbow will not reach the midline. Score 4.

Source: A & B. George Dodson/Lightworks Studio/Pearson Education. C. Courtesy of Jo Engle, RN, MSN, NNP-BC and Vanessa Howell, RN, MSN.

● **Figure 25–10** Heel to ear. No resistance. Leg fully extended. Score 0.

Source: George Dodson/Lightworks Studio/Pearson Education.

7. *Head lag* (neck flexor) is measured by pulling the newborn to a sitting position and noting the degree of head lag. Total lag is common in newborns up to 34 weeks' gestation. Full-term newborns can support their heads momentarily.

8. *Ventral suspension* (horizontal position) is evaluated by holding the newborn prone on the nurse's hand. The

A

B

● **Figure 25–11** Ankle dorsiflexion. *A,* A 45-degree angle indicates 32 to 36 weeks' gestation. A 20-degree angle indicates 36 to 40 weeks' gestation. Score 2 to 3. *B,* A 15- to 0-degree angle is common at 40 weeks' or more gestational age. Score 4.

Source: George Dodson/Lightworks Studio/Pearson Education.

position of the head and back and the degree of flexion in the arms and legs are noted. Some flexion of arms and legs indicates 36 to 38 weeks' gestation; fully flexed extremities, with head and back even, are characteristic of a term newborn.

9. *Major reflexes* such as *sucking, rooting, grasping, Moro, tonic neck,* and others are evaluated during the newborn exam. These reflexes are discussed later in the chapter.

A supplementary method for estimating gestational age (done by the physician or nurse practitioner) is to view the vascular network of the cornea with an ophthalmoscope. The nurse may need to delay administration of prophylactic eye ointment in preterm infants until after this vascular eye exam is done. The amount of vascularity present over the surface of the lens assists in identifying infants of 27 through 34 weeks' gestational age.

When the gestational age determination and birth weight are considered together, the newborn can be identified as one whose growth is:

■ *Small for gestational age (SGA)* (below the 10th percentile)

■ *Appropriate for gestational age (AGA)* (between the 10th and 90th percentile)

■ *Large for gestational age (LGA)* (above the 90th percentile)

This determination (Figure 25–12 ●) enables the nurse to anticipate possible physiologic problems. This information is used in conjunction with a complete physical examination to establish a plan of care appropriate for the individual newborn. For example, an SGA or LGA newborn often requires frequent

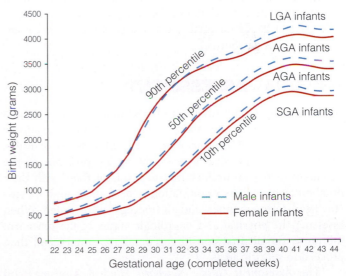

● **Figure 25–12** Select reference percentiles for birth weight at each gestational age from 22 to 44 completed weeks for male and female singleton infants: 10th, 50th, and 90th percentiles. Data from 3,423,215 male and 3,267,502 female infants in the 1999–2000 U. S. Natality datasets.

Source: Oken, E., Kleinman, K. P., Rich-Edwards, J., & Gillman, M. W. (2003). A nearly continuous measure of birth weight for gestational age using a United States national reference. *BMC Pediatrics, 3,* 6. Retrieved from http://www.biomedcentral.com/1471-2431/3/6 © 2003 Oken et al.; licensee BioMed Central Ltd. This is an open access article: verbatim copying and redistribution of this article are permitted in all media for any purpose, provided this notice is preserved along with the article's original URL.

Clinical Reasoning Determining Gestational Age

A nurse has completed the gestational assessment on newborn Travis Bell who weighs 3000 g and is 48 cm long with a head circumference of 33 cm. His Apgar scores were 8 at 1 minute and 9 at 5 minutes. Other assessment data include skin dry and cracking with pale areas and rare veins, no lanugo, sole creases covering the entire sole, raised areola 3 mm, well-curved pinna soft with ready recoil, and testes descended with moderate rugae. Reflex data include square window at 0 degree, arm recoil 100 degree, popliteal angle 100 degree, scarf sign yield elbow will not reach midline, heel to ear 90 degree, and posture fully flexed. The parents express concerns over his small size.

What are the newborn's physical maturity score and neuromuscular maturity score?

Interpret the newborn's combined scores of neuromuscular and physical maturity.

Determine if the newborn is small for gestational age (SGA), appropriate for gestational age (AGA), or large for gestational age (LGA).

What should the nurse tell the parents regarding their concern over his small size?

See www.nursing.pearsonhighered.com for possible responses.

glucose monitoring and early feedings. (See Chapter 28 🔗 for a more complete discussion of these categories and the potential problems associated with them.)

The nurse also plots the gestational age against the newborn's length, head circumference, and weight on the appropriate growth chart to determine if these measurements fall within the average range—the 10th to 90th percentile for the corresponding gestational age. These correlations further document the level of maturity and appropriate category for the newborn. (See Chapter 27 🔗 for further discussion of the various gestational age SGA newborns.)

PHYSICAL ASSESSMENT

After the initial determination of gestational age and related potential problems, the nurse carries out a more extensive physical assessment in a warm, well-lit area that is free of drafts. Completing the physical assessment in the presence of the parents provides an opportunity to acquaint them with their unique newborn. The examination is performed in a systematic, head-to-toe manner, and all findings are recorded. When assessing the physical and neurologic status of the newborn, the nurse should first consider general appearance and then proceed to specific areas.

The *Assessment Guide: Newborn Physical Assessment* on pages 571–580 outlines how to systematically assess the newborn. Normal findings, alterations, and related causes are presented and correlated with suggested nursing responses. The findings are typical for a full-term newborn.

General Appearance

The newborn's head is disproportionately large for its body. The neck looks short because the chin rests on the chest. Newborns

have a prominent abdomen, sloping shoulders, narrow hips, and rounded chests. The center of the baby's body is the umbilicus rather than the symphysis pubis as in the adult. The body appears long and the extremities short.

Newborns tend to stay in a flexed position similar to the one maintained in utero and will offer resistance when the extremities are straightened. This flexed position contributes to the short appearance of the extremities. The hands are tightly clenched. After a breech birth, the feet are usually dorsiflexed, and it may take several weeks for the infant to assume the typical newborn posture.

Weight and Measurements

The normal full-term Caucasian newborn has an average birth weight of 3405 g (7 lb, 8 oz). Newborns of African, Asian, or Mexican American descent are usually somewhat smaller at term. Other factors that influence weight are age, size, and health of the mother (smoking and malnutrition decrease birth weight). After the first week, and for the first 6 months, the newborn's weight increases about 198 g (7 oz) weekly.

Approximately 70% to 75% of the newborn's body weight is water. During the initial newborn period (the first 3 or 4 days), term newborns have a physiologic weight loss of about 5% to 10% because of fluid shifts. This weight loss may reach 15% for preterm newborns. Large babies also tend to lose more weight because of greater fluid loss in proportion to birth weight. If weight loss is greater than 10%, clinical reappraisal is indicated. Factors contributing to weight loss include insufficient fluid intake resulting from delayed breastfeeding or a slow adjustment to the formula, increased volume of meconium excreted, urination, and dehydration or consistent chilling (because of nonshivering thermogenesis).

The length of the normal newborn is difficult to measure because the legs are flexed and tensed. To measure length, the nurse should place newborns flat on their backs with their legs extended as much as possible (Figure 25–13 ●). The average length is 50 cm (20 in.), and the range is 46 to 56 cm (18 to 22 in.).

● **Figure 25–13** Measuring the length of the newborn.
Source: Courtesy of Vanessa Howell, RNC, MSN.

A   B

● **Figure 25–14** *A,* Measuring the head circumference of the newborn. *B,* Measuring the chest circumference of the newborn.
Source: Courtesy of Vanessa Howell, RNC, MSN.

The newborn will grow approximately 2.5 cm (1 in.) a month for the next 6 months. This is the period of most rapid growth.

At birth the newborn's head is one fourth the size of an adult's head. The circumference (biparietal diameter) of the newborn's head is 32 to 37 cm (12.5 to 14.5 in.). For accurate measurement, the nurse places the tape over the most prominent part of the occiput and brings it just above the eyebrows (Figure 25–14*A* ●). The circumference of the newborn's head is approximately 2 cm (0.8 in.) greater than the circumference of the newborn's chest at birth, and will remain in this proportion for the next few months. (Factors that alter this measurement are discussed in the section titled "Head" later in this chapter.) It is best to take another head circumference on the second day if the newborn experienced significant head molding or developed a caput from the birth process.

The average circumference of the chest is 32 cm (12.5 in.) and ranges from 30 to 35 cm (12 to 14 in.). Chest measurements are taken with the tape measure placed at the lower edge of the scapulae and brought around anteriorly, directly over the nipple line (Figure 25–14*B* ●). The abdominal circumference, or girth, may also be measured at this time, by placing the tape around the newborn's abdomen at the level of the umbilicus, with the bottom edge of the tape at the top edge of the umbilicus (Table 25–1).

Temperature

Initial assessment of the newborn's temperature is critical. In utero, the temperature of the fetus is about the same as, or slightly higher than, the expectant mother's. When babies enter the outside world, their temperature can suddenly drop as a result of exposure to cold drafts and the skin's heat loss mechanisms.

If no heat conservation measures are started, the normal term newborn's deep body temperature falls 0.1°C (0.2°F) per minute; skin temperature drops 0.3°C (0.5°F) per minute. Skin temperature markedly decreases within 10 minutes after exposure to room air. The temperature should stabilize within 8 to 12 hours. Temperature is monitored at least every 30 minutes until the newborn's status has remained stable for 2 hours (American Academy of Pediatrics [AAP] Committee on Fetus and Newborn & American College of Obstetricians and Gynecologists [ACOG], 2012).

Thereafter, the nurse should assess temperature at least once every 8 hours, or according to institutional policy. In infants who have been exposed to group B hemolytic streptococcus, more frequent temperature monitoring may be required (see Chapter 24 ✪ for a discussion of the physiology of temperature regulation).

Table 25–1	Newborn Measurements			
Measurement		**Average**	**Range**	**Growth**
Weight (Weight is influenced by a variety of factors, and maternal age and size. Physiologic weight loss 5% to 10% for term newborns, up to 15% for preterm newborns.)		3405 g (7 lb, 8 oz)	2500–4000 g (5 lb, 8 oz–8 lb, 13 oz)	198 g (7 oz) per week for first 6 mo
Length		50 cm (20 in.)	46–56 cm (18–22 in.)	2.5 cm (1 in.) per month for first 6 mo
Head circumference (Approximately 2 cm larger than chest circumference)		33–35 cm (13–14 in.)	32–37 cm (12.5–14.5 in.)	
Chest circumference		32 cm (12.5 in.)	30–35 cm (12–14 in.)	

● **Figure 25–15** Axillary temperature measurement. The thermometer should remain in place for 3 minutes. The newborn's arm should be tightly but gently pressed against the thermometer and the newborn's side, as illustrated.

Source: Courtesy of Jo Engle, RN, MSN, NNP-BC and Vanessa Howell, RN, MSN.

Temperature can be assessed by the axillary skin method, a continuous skin probe, or may be via the rectal route. Axillary temperature reflects body (core) temperature and the body's compensatory response to the thermal environment. In preterm and term newborns, there is less than 0.1°C (0.2°F) difference between temperatures at the two sites and the axillary method is preferred. Axillary temperature ranges from 36.4°C to 37.2°C (97.5°F to 99°F) (Figure 25–15 ●).

Skin temperature is measured most accurately by means of continuous skin probe, especially for small newborns or newborns maintained in incubators or under radiant warmers. Normal skin temperature is 36°C to 36.5°C (96.8°F to 97.7°F). Continuous assessment of skin temperature allows time for initiation of interventions before a more serious fall in core temperature occurs (Figure 25–16 ●).

● **Figure 25–16** Temperature monitoring for the newborn. A skin thermal sensor is placed on the newborn's abdomen, upper thigh, or arm and secured with porous tape or a foil-covered foam pad.

Source: © Tom McCarthy/Photoedit.

Rectal temperature is assumed to be the closest approximation to core temperature, but the accuracy of this method depends on the depth to which the thermometer is inserted. Normal rectal temperature is 36.6°C to 37.2°C (97.8°F to 99°F). The rectal route is *not* recommended as a routine method, if done with a digital or electronic thermometer (American Academy of Pediatrics, 2011).

Temperature instability, a deviation of more than 1°C (2°F) from one reading to the next, or a subnormal temperature may indicate an infection. In contrast to an elevated temperature in older children, an increased temperature in a newborn may indicate a reaction to too many coverings, too hot a room, or dehydration. Dehydration, which tends to increase body temperature, occurs in newborns whose feedings have been delayed for any reason. Newborns may respond to overheating (a temperature greater than 37.5°C [99.5°F]) by increased restlessness and eventually by perspiration after 35 to 40 minutes of exposure (Blackburn, 2013). The perspiration appears initially on the head and face and then on the chest. Many newborns initially cannot perspire, so they increase their respiratory and heart rates, which increases oxygen consumption. Whether the initial temperature is elevated or subnormal the newborn must have a stable temperature per agency protocol prior to leaving the nursery.

Skin Characteristics

Although the newborn's skin color varies with genetic background, all healthy newborns have a pink tinge to their skin. The ruddy hue results from increased red blood cell concentrations in the blood vessels and limited subcutaneous fat deposits.

Skin pigmentation is slight in the newborn period, so color changes may be seen even in darker skinned babies. Caucasian newborns often have a pink-tinged or ruddy skin tone a few hours after birth, and African American newborns may have a reddish brown to pale pink with yellow or red tinge skin color. Hispanic and Asian newborns range from a pink or rosy red to olive or yellow skin tone (Cloherty et al., 2012). Skin pigmentation deepens over time; therefore, variations in skin color indicating illness are more difficult to evaluate in African American and Asian newborns (Cloherty et al., 2012). A newborn who is cyanotic at rest and pink only with crying may have *choanal atresia* (congenital blockage of the passageway between the nose and pharynx). If crying increases the cyanosis, heart or lung problems should be suspected. Very pale newborns may be anemic or have hypovolemia (low blood pressure) and should be evaluated for these problems.

Developing Cultural Competence
Keeping Newborns Warm

In the Latino culture and others, parents may be overly concerned about keeping their newborn baby warm. Parents should be informed that overdressing babies while they are sleeping is related to a higher risk of sudden infant death syndrome (SIDS) and that bundling them excessively can be uncomfortable and lead to heat rash.

● **Figure 25–17** Acrocyanosis.

● **Figure 25–18** Erythema toxicum on leg.

Acrocyanosis (bluish discoloration of the hands and feet) may be present in the first 2 to 6 hours after birth but can be normal for up to 24 hours (Figure 25–17 ●). This condition is caused by poor peripheral circulation, which results in vasomotor instability and capillary stasis, especially when the baby is exposed to cold. Therefore, blue hands and nails are a poor indicator of decreased oxygenation in a newborn. If the central circulation is adequate, the blood supply should return quickly (2 to 3 seconds) to the extremity after the skin is blanched with a finger. The nurse assesses the face and mucous membranes for pinkness that reflects adequate oxygenation. Further oxygenation assessment is needed if there are signs of respiratory distress. Pulse oximetry can be obtained.

Mottling (lacy pattern of dilated blood vessels under the skin) occurs as a result of general circulation fluctuations. It may last several hours to several weeks or may come and go periodically. Mottling may be related to chilling or prolonged apnea, sepsis, or hypothyroidism.

Harlequin sign (clown) color change is occasionally noted: A deep red color develops over one side of the newborn's body while the other side remains pale, so that the skin resembles a clown's suit. This color change results from a vasomotor disturbance in which blood vessels on one side dilate while the vessels on the other side constrict (Lomax, 2011). It usually lasts from 1 to 20 minutes. Affected newborns may have single or multiple episodes, but they are transient and clinically insignificant. The nurse should document each occurrence.

Jaundice (yellowish discoloration of skin and mucous membranes) is first detectable on the face (where skin overlies cartilage) and the mucous membranes of the mouth and has a head-to-toe progression (Cloherty et al., 2012). Jaundice advances from head to toe and regresses in the opposite direction. Evaluation and determination of the cause of jaundice must be initiated immediately to prevent possibly serious sequelae. Any jaundice noted before a newborn is 24 hours of age should be reported to the physician or neonatal nurse practitioner. Breastfeeding is a possible cause of late onset jaundice. (For discussion of various types of jaundice see Chapter 24 🔗, and for detailed discussion of causes and treatment for jaundice see Chapter 29 🔗.)

Erythema toxicum is an eruption of lesions in the area surrounding a hair follicle that are firm, vary in size from 1 to 3 mm, and consist of a white or pale yellow papule or pustule with an erythematous base. It is often called "newborn rash" or "flea bite" dermatitis. The rash may appear suddenly, usually over the trunk and diaper area, and is frequently widespread (Figure 25–18 ●). The lesions do not appear on the palms of the hands or the soles of the feet. The peak incidence is at 24 to 48 hours of life. The condition rarely presents at birth or after 5 days of life. The cause is unknown, and no treatment is necessary. Some clinicians believe it may be caused by irritation from clothing. The lesions disappear in a few hours or days. If a maculopapular rash appears, a smear of the aspirated papule will show numerous eosinophils on staining; no bacteria will be cultured.

Milia, which are exposed sebaceous glands, appear as raised white spots on the face, especially across the nose (Figure 25–19 ●). No treatment is necessary, because they will clear spontaneously within the first month. Infants of African heritage have a similar condition called transient neonatal pustular melanosis.

Skin turgor is assessed to determine hydration status, the need to initiate early feedings, and the presence of any infectious processes. The usual place to assess skin turgor is over the abdomen, forearm, or thigh. Skin should be elastic and should return rapidly to its original shape.

● **Figure 25–19** Facial milia over bridge of nose.
Source: © Jack Sullivan/Alamy.

Vernix caseosa, a whitish, cheeselike substance, covers the fetus while in utero and lubricates the skin of the newborn. The skin of the term or postterm newborn has less vernix and is frequently dry. Peeling is common, especially on the hands and feet, in the postterm infant.

Forceps marks may be present after a vaginal birth. The newborn may have reddened areas over the cheeks and jaws. It is important to reassure the parents that these marks will disappear, usually within 1 or 2 days. Transient facial paralysis resulting from the forceps pressure is a rare complication. Vacuum extractor suction marks (abrasions or ecchymosis) on the vertex of the scalp may be seen when vacuum extractors are used to assist with the birth (Gleason & Devaskar, 2012).

Sucking blisters (vesicles or bullae) may appear on the lips, fingers, or hands of newborns as a result of vigorous sucking, either in utero or after birth. These sucking blisters (Figure 25–20 ●) may be intact or ruptured and require no treatment.

Birthmarks

Telangiectatic nevi (stork bites) appear as pale pink or red spots and are frequently found on the eyelids, nose, lower occipital bone, and nape of the neck (Figure 25–21 ●). These lesions are common in newborns with light complexions and are more noticeable during periods of crying. These areas have no clinical significance and usually fade by the second birthday.

Mongolian blue spots are macular areas of bluish black or gray-blue pigmentation on the dorsal area and the buttocks (Figure 25–22 ●). They are common in newborns of Asian, Hispanic, and African descent and other dark-skin races and can be seen in 1% to 9% of Caucasians. They gradually fade during

● **Figure 25–21** Stork bites over left eyelid and near right eyebrow.
Source: Courtesy of Anne Garcia.

the first or second year of life. They may be mistaken for bruises and should be documented in the newborn's chart.

Nevus flammeus (port-wine stain) is a capillary angioma directly below the epidermis. It is a nonelevated, sharply demarcated, red-to-purple area of dense capillaries (Figure 25–23 ●). In infants of African descent, it may appear as a purple-black stain. The size and shape vary, but it commonly appears on the face. It does not grow in size, does not fade with time, and does not blanch as a rule. The birthmark may be concealed by using an opaque cosmetic cream. If convulsions and other neurologic problems accompany the nevus flammeus, the clinical picture is suggestive of *Sturge-Weber syndrome,* with involvement of the fifth cranial nerve (the ophthalmic branch of the trigeminal nerve).

Nevus vasculosus (strawberry mark) is a capillary hemangioma. It consists of newly formed and enlarged capillaries in the dermal and subdermal layers. It is a raised, clearly delineated,

● **Figure 25–20** Sucking blister in middle of upper lip.
Source: Courtesy of Jo Engle, RN, MSN, NNP-BC and Vanessa Howell, RN, MSN.

● **Figure 25–22** Mongolian blue spots.

● **Figure 25–23** Port-wine stain over temple area.
Source: Courtesy of Alyssa Torres.

● **Figure 25–24** Overlapped cranial bones produce a visible ridge in a premature newborn. Easily visible overlapping does not occur often in term infants.
Source: Courtesy of Jo Engle, RN, MSN, NNP-BC and Vanessa Howell, RN, MSN.

dark red, rough-surfaced birthmark commonly found in the head region. Such marks usually grow (often rapidly) starting during the second or third week of life and may not reach their fullest size until about 6 months (Cloherty et al., 2012). They begin to shrink and start to resolve spontaneously several weeks to months after they reach peak growth. A pale purple or gray spot on the surface of the hemangioma signals the start of resolution. The best cosmetic effect is achieved when the lesions are allowed to resolve spontaneously.

Head

The newborn's head is large (approximately one fourth of the body size), with soft, pliable cranial skull bones. The head may appear asymmetric in the newborn of a vertex birth. This asymmetry, called **molding**, is caused by the overriding of the cranial bones during labor and birth (Figure 25–24 ●). The degree of molding varies with the amount and length of pressure exerted on the head. Within a few days after birth, the overriding usually diminishes and the suture lines become palpable; therefore, a second measurement is indicated a few days after birth. Any extreme differences in head size may indicate microcephaly (abnormally small head) or hydrocephalus (an abnormal buildup of fluid in

Clinical Tip

Birthmarks are frequently a cause of concern for parents. The mother may be especially anxious, fearing that she is to blame ("Is my baby 'marked' because of something I did?"). Guilt feelings are common in the presence of misconceptions about the cause. Birthmarks should be identified and explained to the parents. By providing appropriate information about the cause and course of birthmarks, the nurse frequently relieves the fears and anxieties of the family. The nurse should note any bruises, abrasions, or birthmarks seen on admission to the nursery.

the brain) and can result in an enlarged head. Variations in the shape, size, or appearance of the head measurements may be caused by *craniosynostosis* (premature closure of the cranial sutures), which will need to be corrected through surgery to allow brain growth, and *plagiocephaly* (asymmetry caused by pressure on the fetal head during gestation) (Lomax, 2011).

Two *fontanels* ("soft spots") may be palpated on the newborn's head. Fontanels, which are openings at the juncture of the cranial bones, can be measured with the fingers. Accurate measurement necessitates that the examiner's finger be measured in centimeters. The assessment should be carried out with the newborn in a sitting position and not crying. The *diamond-shaped anterior fontanel* is approximately 3 to 4 cm long by 2 to 3 cm wide. It is located at the juncture of the frontal and parietal bones. The *posterior fontanel*, smaller and triangular, is formed by the parietal bones and the occipital bone and is 0.5 by 1 cm. Because of molding, the fontanels are smaller immediately after birth than several days later. The anterior fontanel closes within 18 months, whereas the posterior fontanel closes within 8 to 12 weeks.

The fontanels are a useful indicator of the newborn's condition. The anterior fontanel may swell when the newborn cries or passes a stool or may pulsate with the heartbeat, which is normal. The sutures between the cranial bones should be palpated for the amount of overlapping. In newborns whose growth has been restricted the sutures may be wider than normal, and the fontanels may also be larger because of impaired growth of the cranial bones. In addition to inspecting the newborn's head for degree of molding and size, the nurse should evaluate it for soft-tissue edema and bruising.

Cephalohematoma

Cephalohematoma is a collection of blood resulting from ruptured blood vessels between the surface of a cranial bone (usually parietal) and the periosteal membrane (Figure 25–25 ●). The scalp in these areas feels loose and slightly edematous. These areas emerge as defined hematomas between the first and second day. Although external pressure may cause the mass to fluctuate, it does not increase in size when the newborn cries. Cephalohematomas may be unilateral or bilateral and do not cross suture lines. They are relatively common in vertex births and may disappear within 2 weeks to 3 months. They may be associated with physiologic jaundice, because extra red blood cells are being destroyed within the cephalohematoma. A large cephalohematoma can lead to anemia and hypotension.

Caput Succedaneum

Caput succedaneum is a localized, easily identifiable, soft area of the scalp, generally resulting from a long and difficult labor or vacuum extraction (Figure 25–26 ●). The sustained pressure of the presenting part against the cervix results in compression of local blood vessels, and venous return is slowed. Slowed venous return causes an increase in tissue fluids, an edematous swelling, and occasional bleeding under the periosteum. The caput may vary from a small area to a severely elongated head. The fluid in the caput is reabsorbed within 12 hours to a few days after birth. Caputs resulting from vacuum extractors are sharply outlined, circular areas up to 2 cm (0.8 in.) thick. They disappear more slowly than naturally occurring edema. See Table 25–2.

Hair

The term newborn's hair is smooth with texture variations depending on ethnic background. Scalp hair is usually high over the eyebrows. Assessment of the newborn's hair characteristics such as color, quantity, texture, hairlines, direction of growth,

Scalp
Sagittal suture
Periosteum
Blood
Skull bone

A

Sagittal suture
Serum
Periosteum
Skull bone

A

B

● **Figure 25–25** Cephalohematoma is a collection of blood between the surface of a cranial bone and the periosteal membrane. This is a cephalohematoma over the right parietal bone.
Source: Courtesy of Jo Engle, RN, MSN, NNP-BC and Vanessa Howell, RN, MSN.

B

● **Figure 25–26** Caput succedaneum is a collection of fluid (serum) under the scalp.

Table 25–2	Comparison of Cephalohematoma and Caput Succedaneum	
Cephalohematoma	**Caput Succedaneum**	
Collection of blood between cranial (usually parietal) bone and periosteal membrane	Collection of fluid, edematous swelling of the scalp	
Caused by subperiosteal hemorrhage	Caused by pressure of the fetal head against the cervix during labor, which decreases blood flow to the area and results in edema	
Does not cross suture lines	Crosses suture lines	
Appears on first and second day, increases in size for 2–3 days	Present at birth or shortly thereafter, does not increase in size	
Disappears after 2–3 weeks or may take months	Reabsorbed within 12 hours or a few days after birth	

● **Figure 25–27** Facial paralysis. Paralysis of the right side of the face from injury to the right facial nerve.
Source: © Wellcome Image Library/Custom Medical Stock Photo.

and hair whorls can identify genetic, metabolic, and neurologic disorders (Lomax, 2011). For example, coarse, brittle, and dry hair may indicate hypothyroidism.

Face

The newborn's face is well designed to help the newborn suckle. Sucking (fat) pads are located in the cheeks, and a labial tubercle (sucking callus) is frequently found in the center of the upper lip. The chin is recessed, and the nose is flattened. The lips are sensitive to touch, and the sucking reflex is easily initiated. Symmetry of the eyes, nose, and ears is evaluated. See *Assessment Guide: Newborn Physical Assessment* on pages 571–580 for deviations in symmetry and variations in size, shape, and spacing of facial features. Facial movement symmetry should be assessed to determine the presence of facial palsy. Facial paralysis appears when the newborn cries; the affected side is immobile, and the palpebral (eyelid) fissure widens (Figure 25–27 ●). Paralysis may result from forceps-assisted birth or pressure on the facial nerve from the maternal pelvis during birth. Facial paralysis usually disappears within a few days to 3 weeks, although in some cases it may be permanent.

Eyes

The eyes of the newborn of northern European descent are a blue-gray or slate blue-gray color. Dark-skin newborns tend to have dark eyes at birth. Scleral color tends to be bluish white because of its relative thinness. A blue sclera is associated with osteogenesis imperfecta. The infant's eye color is usually established at approximately 3 months, although it may change any time up to 1 year.

The eyes should be checked for size, equality of pupil size, reaction of pupils to light, blink reflex to light, and edema and inflammation of the eyelids. The eyelids are usually edematous during the first few days of life because of the pressure associated with birth.

Erythromycin and tetracycline (in some agencies) are used prophylactically instead of silver nitrate and usually do not cause chemical irritation of the eye (see Chapter 26 ⊘). The instillation of silver nitrate drops in the newborn's eyes may cause edema, and **chemical conjunctivitis** may appear a few hours after instillation, but it disappears in 1 to 2 days (Cloherty et al., 2012). If infectious conjunctivitis exists, the newborn has the same purulent (greenish yellow) discharge exudate as in chemical conjunctivitis, but it is caused by gonococcus, *Chlamydia*, staphylococci, or a variety of gram-negative bacteria. It requires treatment with ophthalmic antibiotics. Onset is usually after the second day. Edema of the orbits or eyelids may persist for several days, until the newborn's kidneys can eliminate the fluid.

Small **subconjunctival hemorrhages** appear in about 10% of newborns and are commonly found on the sclera. These hemorrhages are caused by the changes in vascular tension or ocular pressure during birth. They will remain for a few weeks and are of no pathologic significance. Parents need reassurance that the newborn is not bleeding from within the eye and that vision will not be impaired.

The newborn may demonstrate transient strabismus caused by poor neuromuscular control of eye muscles (Figure 25–28 ●). It gradually regresses in 3 to 4 months. The "doll's eye" phenomenon is also present for about 10 days after birth. As the newborn's head position is changed to the left and then to the right, the eyes move to the opposite direction. "Doll's eye" results from underdeveloped integration of head-eye coordination.

The nurse should observe the newborn's pupils for opacities or whiteness and for the absence of a normal red retinal reflex. Red retinal reflex is a red-orange flash of color observed when an ophthalmoscope light reflects off the retina. In a newborn with dark skin color, the retina may appear paler or more grayish.

● **Figure 25–28** Transient strabismus in the newborn may be due to poor neuromuscular control.

Source: Biophoto Associates/Photo Researchers, Inc.

The color of the red reflex can also be abnormal with retinoblastoma. Absence of red reflex occurs with cataracts. Congenital cataracts should be suspected in newborns of mothers with a history of rubella, cytomegalic inclusion disease, or syphilis. Brushfield spots (black or white spots on the periphery of the iris) can be associated with trisomy 21 (Gleason & Devaskar, 2012).

The cry of the newborn is commonly tearless because the lacrimal structures are immature at birth and are not usually fully functional until the second month of life. However, some babies produce tears during the newborn period.

Poor oculomotor coordination and absence of accommodation limit visual abilities, but newborns have peripheral vision, can fixate on objects near (20.3 to 25.4 cm [8 to 10 in.]) and in front of their face for short periods, can accommodate to large objects (7.6 cm [3 in.] tall by 7.6 cm [3 in.] wide), and can seek out high-contrast geometric shapes. Newborns can perceive faces, shapes, and colors and begin to show visual preferences early. Newborns generally blink in response to bright lights, to a tap on the bridge of the nose (glabellar reflex), or to a light touch on the eyelids. Pupillary light reflex is also present. Examination of the eye is best accomplished by rocking the newborn from an upright position to the horizontal a few times or by other methods, such as diminishing overhead lights, which elicit an opened-eye response.

Nose

The newborn's nose is small and narrow. Infants are characteristically nose breathers for the first few months of life and generally remove obstructions by sneezing. Nasal patency is ensured if the newborn breathes easily with the mouth closed. If respiratory difficulty occurs, the nurse checks for choanal atresia (congenital blockage of the passageway between the nose and pharynx) and observes the newborn feeding since they are obligatory nose breathers.

The newborn has the ability to smell after the nasal passages are cleared of amniotic fluid and mucus. Newborns demonstrate this ability by the search for milk. Newborns turn their heads toward a milk source, whether bottle or breast. Newborns react to strong odors, such as alcohol, by turning their heads away or blinking.

Mouth

The lips of the newborn should be pink, and a touch on the lips should produce sucking motions. Saliva is normally scant. The taste buds develop before birth, and the newborn can easily discriminate between sweet and bitter flavors.

The easiest way to examine the mouth completely is to stimulate infants to cry such as by gently depressing the tongue, thereby causing them to open the mouth fully. It is extremely important to examine the entire mouth to check for a cleft palate, which can be present even in the absence of a cleft lip. The examiner moves an unpowdered, gloved index finger along the hard and soft palate to feel for any openings (Figure 25–29 ●). Occasionally, an examination of the gums will reveal *precocious teeth* over the area where the lower central incisor will erupt. If they appear loose, they should be removed to prevent aspiration. Gray-white lesions (inclusion cysts) on the gums may be confused with teeth. On the hard palate and gum margins, **Epstein pearls**, small glistening white specks (keratin-containing cysts) that feel hard to the touch, are often present. They usually disappear in a few weeks and are of no significance. **Thrush** may appear as white patches that look like milk curds adhering to the mucous membranes, and bleeding may occur when patches are removed. Thrush is caused by *Candida albicans,* often acquired from an infected vaginal tract during birth, antibiotic use, or poor hand washing when the mother handles her newborn. Thrush is treated with a preparation of nystatin (Mycostatin).

A newborn who is tongue-tied has a ridge of frenulum tissue attached to the underside of the tongue at varying lengths from its base, causing a heart shape at the tip of the tongue. Cutting the ridge of tissue is not currently recommended. This ridge

● **Figure 25–29** The nurse inserts a gloved index finger into the newborn's mouth and feels for any openings along the hard and soft palates. *Note:* Gloves or a finger cot are always worn to examine the palate.

Source: Courtesy of Vanessa Howell, RNC, MSN.

does not usually affect speech or eating, but cutting creates an entry for infection.

Transient nerve paralysis resulting from birth trauma may be manifested by asymmetric mouth movements when the newborn cries or by difficulty with sucking and feeding.

Ears

The ears of the newborn are soft and pliable and should recoil readily when folded and released. In the normal newborn, the top of the ear (pinna) should be parallel to the outer and inner canthus of the eye. The ears should be inspected for shape, size, firmness of cartilage, and position. *Low-set ears* are characteristic of many syndromes and may indicate chromosomal abnormalities (especially trisomies 13 and 18), intellectual disability, and internal organ abnormalities, especially bilateral renal agenesis as a result of embryologic developmental deviations (Figure 25–30 ●). *Preauricular skin tags* may be present just in front of the ear. Visualization of the tympanic membrane is not usually done soon after birth because blood and vernix block the ear canal.

Following the first cry, the newborn's hearing becomes acute as mucus from the middle ears is absorbed, the eustachian tubes become aerated, and the tympanic membranes become visible. The newborn's hearing initially can be evaluated by noting the baby's response to loud or moderately loud noises that are not accompanied by vibrations. The sleeping newborn should stir or awaken in response to nearby sounds. (This is not a very accurate test, but it may alert the examiner to a possible problem.) The newborn can discriminate the individual characteristics of the human voice and is especially sensitive to sound levels within the normal conversational range. The newborn in a noisy nursery may habituate to the sounds and not stir unless the sound is sudden or much louder than usual.

The AAP has endorsed universal newborn hearing screening (UNHS) before discharge from the birthing unit as the standard of care (AAP & ACOG, 2012). See Chapter 26 ℰ for discussion of newborn hearing screening.

Neck

A short neck, creased with skin folds, is characteristic of the normal newborn. Because muscle tone is not well developed, the neck cannot support the full weight of the head, which rotates freely.

 Clinical Tip

Measuring weight and height often aggravate newborns and may alter their vital signs. For better accuracy, take the newborn's vital signs before weighing and measuring.

The head lags considerably when the newborn is pulled from a supine to a sitting position, but the prone newborn is able to raise the head slightly. The neck is palpated for masses and the presence of lymph nodes and is inspected for webbing. Adequacy of range of motion and neck muscle function is determined by moving the head while supporting the newborn to prevent injury. Injury to the sternocleidomastoid muscle (congenital torticollis) must be considered in the presence of neck rigidity.

The nurse evaluates the clavicles for evidence of fractures, which occasionally occur during difficult births or in newborns with broad shoulders. The normal clavicle is straight. If fractured, a lump and a grating sensation (crepitus) during movements may be palpated along the course of the side of the break. The nurse also elicits the Moro reflex (page 568) to evaluate bilateral equal movement of the arms. If the clavicle is fractured, the response will be demonstrated only on the unaffected side.

Chest

The thorax is cylindric and symmetric at birth, and the ribs are flexible. The general appearance of the chest should be assessed. A protrusion at the lower end of the sternum, called the xiphoid cartilage, is frequently seen. It is under the skin and will become less apparent after several weeks as adipose tissue accumulates.

Engorged breasts occur frequently in both male and female newborns. This condition, which occurs by the third day, is a result of maternal hormonal influences and may last up to 2 weeks (Figure 25–31 ●). A whitish secretion from the nipples may also be noted. The newborn's breast should not be massaged or squeezed, because this may cause a breast abscess. Supernumerary nipples are occasionally noted below and medial to the true nipples. These harmless pink or brown (in dark-skin newborns) spots vary in

● **Figure 25–30** The position of the external ear may be assessed by drawing a line across the inner and outer canthus of the eye to the insertion of the ear. *A*, Normal position. *B*, True low-set position.

● **Figure 25–31** Breast hypertrophy.

Clinical Tip

Vital sign assessments are most accurate if the newborn is at rest, so measure pulse and respirations first if the baby is quiet. To soothe a crying baby, try placing your moistened gloved finger in the baby's mouth, and then complete your assessment while the baby suckles.

size and do not contain glandular tissue. Accessory nipples can be differentiated from pigmented nevi (moles) by placing the fingertips alongside the accessory nipple and pulling the adjacent tissue laterally. The accessory nipple will appear dimpled.

Cry

The newborn's cry should be strong, lusty, and of medium pitch. A high-pitched, shrill cry is abnormal and may indicate neurologic disorders or hypoglycemia. Periods of crying usually vary in length after consoling measures are used. Babies' cries are an important method of communication and alert caregivers to changes in their condition and needs (see Chapter 31 🌐).

Respiration

Normal breathing for a term newborn is 30 to 60 respirations per minute and is predominantly diaphragmatic, with associated rising and falling of the abdomen during inspiration and expiration. The nurse should note any signs of respiratory distress, nasal flaring, intercostal or xiphoid retraction, expiratory grunt or sigh, seesaw respirations, or tachypnea (greater than 60 breaths per minute). Hyperextension (chest appears high) or hypoextension (chest appears low) of the anteroposterior diameter of the chest should also be noted. Both the anterior and posterior chest are auscultated. Some breath sounds are heard best when the newborn is crying, but localizing and identifying breath sounds is difficult in the newborn. Upper airway noises and bowel sounds can be heard over the chest wall, making auscultation difficult. Because sounds may be transmitted from the unaffected lung to the affected lung, the absence of breath sounds may not be diagnosed. Air entry may be noisy in the first couple of hours until lung fluid resolves, especially after cesarean births. Brief periods of periodic breathing occur, but no color or heart rate changes occur in healthy, term newborns. Sepsis should be suspected in full-term newborns experiencing apneic episodes.

Heart

Heart rates can be as rapid as 180 beats per minute (beats/min) in newborns and fluctuate a great deal, especially if the baby moves or is startled. The normal range is 110 to 160 beats/min. The heart is examined for rate and rhythm, position of the apical impulse, and heart sound intensity. Dysrhythmias should be evaluated by the physician.

The pulse rate is variable and is influenced by physical activity, crying, state of wakefulness, and body temperature. Auscultation is performed over the entire heart region (precordium), below the left axilla, and below the scapula. *Apical pulse rates are obtained by auscultation for a full minute, preferably when the newborn is asleep.*

The placement of the heart in the chest should be determined when the newborn is in a quiet state. The heart is relatively large at birth and is located mid to left chest and high in the chest, with its apex somewhere between the fourth and fifth intercostal space.

A shift of heart tones in the mediastinal area to either side may indicate pneumothorax, dextrocardia (heart placement on the right side of the chest), or a diaphragmatic hernia. The experienced nurse can detect these and many other problems early with a stethoscope. Auscultate heart sounds using both the bell and diaphragm of the stethoscope. Normally, the heartbeat has a "toc tic" sound. A slur or slushing sound (usually after the first sound) may indicate a *murmur.* Although 90% of all murmurs are transient and are considered normal, they should be monitored closely by a physician. Many murmurs are secondary to closing of patent ductus arteriosus or patent foramen ovale, which should close 1 to 2 days after birth. (See Chapters 27 🌐 and 48 🌐 for discussions of congenital heart defects in the infant and child.)

Peripheral pulses (brachial, femoral, pedal) are also evaluated to detect any lags or unusual characteristics. Brachial pulses are palpated bilaterally for equality and compared with the femoral pulses. Femoral pulses are palpated by applying gentle pressure with the middle finger over the femoral canal (Figure 25–32 ●). Decreased or absent femoral pulses may indicate coarctation of the aorta or hypovolemia and require additional evaluation. A wide difference in blood pressure between the upper and lower extremities also indicates coarctation of the aorta.

The measurement of blood pressure is best accomplished by using a noninvasive blood pressure device (Figure 25–33 ●). If a blood pressure cuff is used, the newborn's extremities must be immobilized during the assessment, and the cuff should cover two thirds of the upper arm or upper leg. Movement, crying, and inappropriate cuff size can give inaccurate measurements of the blood pressure.

Blood pressure may not be measured routinely on healthy newborns, but it is essential for newborns who are having distress, are premature, or are suspected of having a critical cardiac anomaly, renal disease, or clinical signs of hypotension (Lomax, 2011). Infants who have birth asphyxia and are on ventilators have significantly lower systolic and diastolic blood pressures than healthy infants. If a cardiac anomaly is suspected, blood pressure is measured in all four extremities (Table 25–3). At birth, systolic values usually range from 70 to 50 mm Hg and diastolic values from 45 to 30 mm Hg. By the tenth day of life, blood pressure rises to 90/50 mm Hg.

Clinical Tip

If possible, obtain blood pressure measurement during quiet sleep or sleep state. Place the cuff on the infant's arm or leg and give the infant time to quiet. Obtain an average of two to three measurements when making clinical decisions. Follow mean blood pressure to monitor changes, as it is less likely to be erroneous. Noninvasive blood pressure may overestimate blood pressure in very-low-birth-weight infants.

A   **B**

● **Figure 25–32** *A,* Bilaterally palpate the femoral arteries for rate and intensity of the pulses. Press fingertip gently at the groin as shown. *B,* Compare the femoral pulses to the brachial pulses by palpating the pulses simultaneously for comparison of rate and intensity.

● **Figure 25–33** Blood pressure measurement using the Dinamap and Doppler devices. The cuff can be applied to either the newborn's upper arm or the thigh.

Source: Courtesy of Vanessa Howell, RNC, MSN.

Table 25–3	Newborn Vital Signs
PULSE	
110–160 beats/min During sleep as low as 80 beats/min; if crying, up to 180 beats/min (Lomax, 2011) Apical pulse counted for 1 full minute	
RESPIRATIONS	
30–60 respirations/minute Predominantly diaphragmatic but synchronous with abdominal movements Respirations counted for 1 full minute	
BLOOD PRESSURE	
70–50/45–30 mm Hg at birth 90/50 mm Hg at day 10	
TEMPERATURE	
Normal range: 36.5°C to 37.5°C (97.7°F to 99.4°F) Axillary: 36.4°C to 37.2°C (97.5°F to 99°F) Skin: 36°C to 36.5°C (96.8°F to 97.7°F) Rectal: 36.6°C to 37.2°C (97.8°F to 99°F)	

Abdomen

The nurse can learn a great deal about the newborn's abdomen without disturbing the infant. The abdomen should be cylindric, protrude slightly, and move with respiration. A certain amount of laxness of the abdominal muscles is normal. A scaphoid (hollow-shaped) appearance suggests the absence of abdominal contents, often seen in diaphragmatic hernias. No cyanosis should be present, and few if any blood vessels should be apparent to the eye. There should be no gross distention or bulging. The more distended the abdomen, the tighter the skin becomes, with engorged vessels appearing. Distention is the first sign of many gastrointestinal abnormalities.

Before palpation of the abdomen, the nurse should auscultate for the presence or absence of bowel sounds in all four quadrants. Bowel sounds may be present by 1 hour after birth. Palpation can cause a transient decrease in bowel sounds intensity.

Abdominal palpation should be done systematically. The nurse palpates each of the four abdominal quadrants and moves in a clockwise direction until all four quadrants have been palpated for softness, tenderness, and the presence of masses. The nurse should place one hand under the back for support during palpation.

Umbilical Cord

Initially the umbilical cord is white and gelatinous in appearance, with the two umbilical arteries and one umbilical vein readily apparent. Because a single umbilical artery is frequently associated with congenital anomalies, the nurse should count the vessels during the newborn assessment. The cord begins drying within 1 or 2 hours of birth and is shriveled and blackened by the second or third day. (Care of the umbilical cord is discussed in Chapter 26 🔗.)

Cord bleeding is abnormal and may result from tension on the cord or clamp. Foul-smelling drainage is also abnormal and is generally caused by infection, which requires immediate treatment to prevent septicemia. Serous or serosanguineous drainage that continues after the cord falls off may indicate a granuloma. If the newborn has a patent urachus (abnormal connection between the umbilicus and bladder), moistness or draining urine may be apparent at the base of the cord. Another umbilical cord anomaly that can occur is umbilical cord hernia and associated patent omphalomesenteric duct (Figure 25–34 ●). Umbilical hernias are more common in infants of African American descent than in Caucasian infants (Gleason & Devaskar, 2012). Umbilical hernias usually close spontaneously by 2 years of age.

Genitals

Female Infants

Examine the labia majora, labia minora, and clitoris and note the size of each as appropriate for gestational age. A vaginal tag or hymenal tag is often evident and will usually disappear in a few weeks. During the first week of life, the female newborn may have a vaginal discharge composed of thick, whitish mucus. This discharge, which can become tinged with blood, is called **pseudomenstruation** and is caused by the withdrawal

> ### Developing Cultural Competence
> **Native Americans and Umbilical Cord Care**
>
> In the Woodland Indian tribe, upon birth, the umbilical cord is tied and a small piece is saved. This section of the umbilical cord is sewn into a deerskin diamond-shaped pocket. The pocket is hung over the infant's crib to provide protection for the infant.

● **Figure 25–34** Umbilical hernia.
Source: George Dodson/Lightworks Studio/Pearson Education.

of maternal hormones. *Smegma,* a white, cheeselike substance, is often present between the labia. Do not remove it because it may traumatize tender tissue.

Male Infants

The nurse inspects the penis to determine whether the urinary orifice is correctly positioned. *Hypospadias* occurs when the urinary meatus is located on the ventral surface of the penis, whereas in *epispadias,* the meatus is on the dorsal surface of the glans. Hypospadias occurs most commonly among people of Western European descent. *Phimosis* is a condition in which the opening of the foreskin (prepuce) is small and the foreskin cannot be pulled back over the glans at all. This condition may interfere with urination, so the adequacy of the urinary stream should be evaluated.

The scrotum is inspected for size and symmetry. Scrotal color variations are especially prominent in African American, Indian, and Hispanic newborns (Cloherty et al., 2012). The scrotum should be palpated to verify the presence of both testes and to rule out *cryptorchidism* (failure of testes to descend). The testes are palpated separately between the thumb and forefinger, with the thumb and forefinger of the other hand placed together over the inguinal canal. Scrotal edema and discoloration are common in breech births. *Hydrocele* (a collection of fluid surrounding the testes in the scrotum) is common in newborns and should be identified. It usually resolves without intervention. The presence of a discolored or dusky scrotum and solid testis should raise the suspicion of testicular torsion which should be reported immediately.

Anus

The anal area is inspected to verify that it is patent and has no fissure. Imperforate anus and rectal atresia may be ruled out by observation. Digital examination, if necessary, is done by a physician or nurse practitioner. The nurse also notes the passage of the first meconium stool. Atresia of the gastrointestinal tract or meconium ileus with resultant obstruction must be considered if the newborn does not pass meconium in the first 24 hours of life.

Extremities

Extremities are examined for gross deformities, extra digits or webbing, clubfoot, and range of motion. Normal newborn extremities appear short, are generally flexible, and move symmetrically.

Arms and Hands

Nails extend beyond the fingertips in term newborns. The nurse should count fingers and toes. *Polydactyly* is the presence of extra digits on either the hands or the feet. *Syndactyly* refers to fusion (webbing) of fingers or toes, which can be hereditary or associated with trisomy 21 (Down syndrome). The hands are inspected for normal palmar creases. A single palmar crease is frequently present in children with trisomy 21.

Brachial palsy, paralysis of portions of the arm, results from trauma to the brachial plexus during a difficult birth. It occurs commonly when strong traction is exerted on the head of the newborn in an attempt to deliver a shoulder lodged behind the symphysis pubis in the presence of shoulder dystocia. Brachial palsy may also occur during a breech birth if an arm becomes trapped over the head and traction is exerted.

The portion of the arm affected is determined by the nerves damaged. **Erb-Duchenne paralysis (Erb's palsy)** involves damage to the upper arm (fifth and sixth cervical nerves) and is the most common type. Injury to the eighth cervical and first thoracic nerve roots and the *lower portion* of the plexus produces the relatively rare lower arm injury. The *whole-arm type* results from damage to the entire plexus.

With Erb-Duchenne paralysis the newborn's arm lies limply at the side. The elbow is held in extension, with the forearm pronated. The newborn is unable to elevate the arm, and the Moro reflex cannot be elicited on the affected side (Figure 25–35 ●). Lower arm injury causes paralysis of the hand and wrist; complete paralysis of the limb occurs with the whole-arm type.

The degree of nerve damage, which results from the trauma and hemorrhage within the nerve sheath, determines recovery. Complete recovery occurs within a few months with minimal trauma. Moderate trauma may result in partial paralysis. Recovery is unlikely with severe trauma, and muscle wasting may develop.

Legs and Feet

The legs of the newborn should be of equal length, with symmetric skin folds. However, they may assume a fetal posture, similar to the position in utero, and it may take several days for the legs and feet to relax into a normal position. The nurse should assess for asymmetry of inner thigh folds, limited hip abduction, and Allis sign (an indication of fracture in the neck of the femur in which a finger easily sinks into the relaxed fascia between the great trochanter and the iliac crest). To further evaluate hip dislocation or hip instability, the Ortolani and Barlow maneuvers are performed. The nurse (or more commonly, the physician or nurse practitioner) performs the **Barlow maneuver** (Figure 25–36*B* ●) to rule out the possibility of developmental dysplastic hip, also called congenital hip dysplasia (hip dislocatability). The examiner grasps and adducts the infant's thigh and applies gentle downward pressure. Dislocation can be felt as the femoral head slips out of the acetabulum.

The **Ortolani maneuver** (Figure 25–36*D* ●) should be performed with the newborn relaxed and quiet on a firm surface. With hips and knees flexed at a 90-degree angle, the experienced nurse grasps the infant's thigh with the middle finger over the greater trochanter and lifts the thigh to bring the femoral head from its posterior position toward the acetabulum. With gentle abduction of the thigh, the femoral head is returned to the acetabulum and the examiner feels a sense of reduction or a "clunk" as the femoral head returns, confirming the diagnosis of an unstable or dislocatable hip.

Examine the feet for evidence of a talipes deformity (clubfoot). Intrauterine position frequently causes the feet to appear to turn inward (Figure 25–37 ●); this is termed a *"positional" clubfoot*. If the feet can easily be returned to the midline by manipulation, no treatment is indicated and the nurse teaches range of motion exercises to the family. Further evaluation is indicated when the foot will not turn to a midline position or align readily. This is considered the most severe type of "true clubfoot," or talipes equinovarus.

Back

With the newborn prone, examine the back. The spine should appear straight and flat, because the lumbar and sacral curves do not develop until the newborn begins to sit. The base of the spine is examined for a dermal sinus. A nevus pilosus ("hairy nerve") is occasionally found at the base of the spine in newborns. It is significant because it is frequently associated with spina bifida. A pilonidal dimple should be examined to ascertain that there is no connection to the spinal canal.

Assessment of Neurologic Status

The neurologic examination should begin with a period of observation, noting the general physical characteristics and behaviors of the newborn. Important behaviors to assess are the *state of alertness, resting posture, cry,* and *quality of muscle tone and motor activity.*

The usual position of the newborn is with partially flexed extremities, with the legs abducted to the abdomen. When awake, the newborn may exhibit purposeless, uncoordinated bilateral movements of the extremities. If these movements are absent, minimal, or obviously asymmetric, neurologic dysfunction should be suspected. Eye movements are observable during the first few days of life. An alert newborn is able to fixate on faces and brightly colored objects. Shining a bright light in the newborn's eyes elicits the blinking response.

Evaluate muscle tone by moving various parts of the body while the head of the newborn is in a neutral position. The newborn is somewhat hypertonic; that is, there should be resistance to extending the elbow and knee joints. Muscle tone should be

 Clinical Tip

Always examine more closely any infant who is reluctant to move an extremity. Fractures are often asymptomatic in the newborn. Paralytic injuries are characterized by immobility of an extremity.

● **Figure 25–36** *A,* The asymmetry of gluteal and thigh fat folds seen in infant with left developmental dysplasia of the hip. *B,* The Barlow (dislocation) maneuver. Baby's thigh is grasped and adducted (placed together) with gentle downward pressure. *C,* Dislocation is palpable as the femoral head slips out of the acetabulum. *D,* The Ortolani maneuver puts downward pressure on the hip and then inward rotation. If the hip is dislocated, this maneuver will force the femoral head back into the acetabular rim with a noticeable "clunk."

Head of femur

Acetabulum

Greater
trochanter

● **Figure 25–37** *A,* Bilateral talipes equinovarus (clubfoot). *B,* To determine the presence of clubfoot, the nurse moves the foot to the midline. Resistance indicates true clubfoot.

symmetric. Diminished muscle tone and flaccidity require further evaluation.

Jitteriness (tremor-like movements) in the full-term newborn must be evaluated to differentiate the tremors from seizures. Tremors may also be related to hypoglycemia, hypocalcemia, or substance withdrawal. Environmental stimuli may initiate tremors. Jitteriness may be distinguished from tonic-clonic seizure activity because it usually can be stopped by the infant's sucking on the extremity or by the nurse holding or flexing the involved extremity. A fine jumping of the muscle is likely to be a central nervous system (CNS) disorder and requires further evaluation. Newborn seizures may consist of no more than chewing or swallowing movements, deviations of the eyes, rigidity, or flaccidity because of CNS immaturity. In contrast to tremors, seizures are not usually initiated by stimuli, and cannot be stopped by holding.

Specific deep tendon reflexes can be elicited in the newborn but have limited value unless they are obviously asymmetric.

The knee jerk is typically brisk; a normal ankle clonus may involve three or four beats. Plantar flexion is present.

The immature CNS of the newborn is characterized by a variety of reflexes. Because the newborn's movements are uncoordinated, methods of communication are limited, and control of body functions is restricted, the reflexes serve a variety of purposes. Some aid in feeding (rooting, sucking) and may not be very active if the infant has eaten recently, and some stimulate human interaction (grasping). In addition, newborns can blink, gag, yawn, cough, sneeze, and draw back from pain (protective reflexes). They can even move a little on their own. When placed on their stomachs, they push up and try to crawl (prone crawl). Absence or a variance in the response requires motor function by a specialist. Absence of the *plantar grasp* and *Galant (truncal) incurvation* reflexes requires neurologic evaluation. The most common reflexes found in the normal newborn are shown in Table 25–4.

Table 25–4	Common Newborn Reflexes

Tonic neck reflex (fencer position). Elicited when the newborn is supine and the head is turned to one side. In response, the extremities on the same side straighten, whereas on the opposite side they flex. This reflex may not be seen during the early newborn period, but once it appears it persists until about the third month.

Tonic neck reflex.
Source: George Dodson/Lightworks Studio/Pearson Education.

Palmar grasping reflex. Elicited by stimulating the newborn's palm with a finger or object; the newborn grasps and holds the object or finger firmly enough to be lifted momentarily from the crib.

Palmar grasping reflex.

(continued)

| Table 25–4 | Common Newborn Reflexes—continued |

Moro reflex. Elicited when the newborn is startled by a loud noise or lifted slightly above the crib and then suddenly lowered. In response, the newborn straightens arms and hands outward while the knees flex. Slowly the arms return to the chest, as in an embrace. The fingers spread, forming a C, and the newborn may cry. This reflex may persist until about 6 months of age.

Moro reflex.
Source: George Dodson/Lightworks Studio/Pearson Education.

Rooting reflex. Elicited when the side of the newborn's mouth or cheek is touched. In response, the newborn turns toward that side and opens the lips to suck (if not fed recently).

Rooting reflex.
Source: George Dodson/Lightworks Studio/Pearson Education.

Stepping reflex. When held upright with one foot touching a flat surface, the newborn puts one foot in front of the other and "walks." This reflex is more pronounced at birth and is lost in 4 to 8 weeks.

The stepping reflex disappears between 4 and 8 weeks of age.

| **Table 25–4** | Common Newborn Reflexes—continued |

Sucking reflex. Elicited when an object is placed in the newborn's mouth or anything touches the lips. Newborns suck even while sleeping; this is called nonnutritive sucking, and it can have a quieting effect on the baby. Disappears by 12 months.

Sucking reflex.

The nurse uses the following steps to assess CNS integration:

1. Insert a gloved finger into the newborn's mouth to elicit a sucking reflex.

2. As soon as the newborn is sucking vigorously, assess hearing and vision responses by noting changes in sucking in the presence of a light, a rattle, and a voice.

3. The newborn should respond to such stimuli with a brief cessation of sucking, followed by continuous sucking with repetitious stimulation.

This CNS integration exam demonstrates auditory and visual integrity as well as the capability of complex behavioral interactions. As healthcare providers carry out the newborn physical and neurologic assessment, they are always on the alert to recognize possible alterations and possible injuries related to the birth process that require further investigation and intervention. (See Table 25–5 for potential types of birth trauma.)

The Brazelton Neonatal Behavioral Assessment Scale

The **Brazelton Neonatal Behavioral Assessment Scale** attempts to identify the newborn's repertoire of behavioral responses to the environment and also documents the newborn's neurologic adequacy and capabilities. (For complete discussion of all test items and maneuvers, see Brazelton & Nugent, 2011.) It provides a way for the nurse, in conjunction with the parents (primary caregivers), to identify and understand the individual newborn's states and capabilities. Families learn which responses, interventions, or activities best meet the special needs of their newborn, and this understanding fosters positive attachment experiences.

Because the first few days after birth are a period of behavioral disorganization, the complete assessment should be done on the third day after birth. The nurse should make every effort to elicit the best response. This may be accomplished by

| **Table 25–5** | Potential Types of Birth Trauma |

Classification	Examples*
Soft-tissue injuries	Lacerations, abrasions, bruising, fat necrosis
Skull injuries	Cephalohematoma, *fractures
Scalp laceration/abscess	Fetal scalp electrode
Intracranial hemorrhage	Subdural, subarachnoid
Eye injuries	*Subconjunctival and retinal hemorrhages
Bone fractures	Clavicle, *facial bones, humerus, femur
Nasal injuries	Dislocation, *fractures
Dislocations	Hips
Cranial nerve injuries	Facial nerve, *brachial plexus, *phrenic nerve, recurrent laryngeal nerve (vocal cord paralysis), Horner syndrome

*Most common birth injuries seen in newborns.

Clinical Reasoning Newborn Behavior

Maria Reyes, a 19-year-old G2 (now P2) mother, delivered a 40-week-old female newborn 24 hours ago. The newborn exam was normal. Mrs. Reyes asks about the newborn's exam. She says she has noticed that the baby cries more than her first child did and seems to require holding for longer periods of time after feeding before "quieting down." She is concerned that she is doing something wrong and wants to know when her newborn will start to act like her first baby. What should you discuss with her about newborn behavior?
See www.nursing.pearsonhighered.com for possible responses.

repeating tests at different times or by testing during situations that facilitate the best possible response, such as when the parents are holding, cuddling, rocking, or singing to their baby.

The behavioral assessment of the newborn should be carried out initially in a quiet, dimly lighted room, if possible. The nurse first determines the newborn's state of consciousness, because scoring and introduction of the test items are correlated with the sleep or waking state. The newborn's state depends on physiologic variables, such as the amount of time from the last feeding, positioning, environmental temperature, health status, presence of such external stimuli as noises and bright lights, and the wake-sleep cycle of the infant. An important characteristic of the newborn period is the pattern of states, as well as the transitions from one state to another. The pattern of states is a predictor of the newborn's receptivity and ability to respond to stimuli in a cognitive manner. Babies learn best in a quiet, alert state and in an environment that is supportive and protective and that provides appropriate stimuli.

Observe the newborn's sleep-wake patterns (as discussed in Chapter 24 🔴), including the rapidity with which the newborn moves from one state to another, the ability to be consoled, and the ability to diminish the impact of disturbing stimuli. The following questions may provide the nurse with a framework for assessment:

- Does the newborn's response style and ability to adapt to stimuli indicate a need for parental interventions that will alert the newborn to the environment so that he or she can grow socially and cognitively?

- Are parental interventions necessary to lessen the outside stimuli, as in the case of the baby who responds to sensory input with intensity?

- Can the baby control the amount of sensory input that he or she must deal with?

The behaviors, and the sleep-wake states in which they are assessed, are categorized as follows:

- *Habituation.* The nurse assesses the newborn's ability to diminish or shut down innate responses to specific repeated stimuli, such as a rattle, bell, light, or pinprick.

- *Orientation to inanimate and animate visual and auditory assessment stimuli.* The nurse observes how often and where the newborn attends to auditory and visual stimuli. Orientation to the environment is determined by an ability to respond to clues given by others and by a natural ability to fix on and follow a visual object horizontally and vertically. This capacity and parental appreciation of it are important for positive communication between infant and parents; the parents' visual (*en face*) and auditory (soft, continuous voice) presence stimulates their newborn to orient to them. Inability or lack of response may indicate visual or auditory problems. It is important for parents to know that their newborn can turn to voices soon after birth or by 3 days of age and can become alert at different times with a varying degree of intensity in response to sounds.

- *Motor activity.* Several components are evaluated. Motor tone of the newborn is assessed in the most characteristic state of responsiveness. This summary assessment includes

overall use of tone as the newborn responds to being handled—whether during spontaneous activity, prone placement, or horizontal holding—and overall assessment of body tone as the newborn reacts to all stimuli.

- *Variations.* Frequency of alert states, state changes, color changes (throughout all states as examination progresses), activity, and peaks of excitement are assessed.

- *Self-quieting activity.* This assessment is based on how often, how quickly, and how effectively newborns can use their resources to quiet and console themselves when upset or distressed. Considered in this assessment are such self-consolatory activities as putting hand to mouth, sucking on a fist or the tongue, and attuning to an object or sound (Figure 25–38 🔴). The newborn's need for outside consolation must also be considered (e.g., seeing a face; being rocked, held, or dressed; using a pacifier; being swaddled).

    Newborns who are neurologically impaired are unable to use self-quieting activities and require more frequent comforting from caregivers when stimulated. For example, drug-positive newborns often exhibit abnormal sleep and feeding patterns and irritability. Swaddling newborns is a way to provide comfort and security. Swaddling also helps the newborn organize and control body movements and behaviors. Blanket swaddling should be loose and should allow the infant easy hand to mouth access to promote self-soothing abilities. Tight swaddling, "straitjacket" techniques with arms at sides, is not comforting and may further agitate the infant.

- *Cuddliness or social behaviors.* This area encompasses the newborn's need for, and response to, being held. Also considered is how often the newborn smiles. These behaviors influence the parents' self-esteem and feelings of acceptance or rejection. Cuddling also appears to be an indicator of personality. Cuddlers appear to enjoy, accept, and seek physical contact; are easier to placate; sleep more; and form

🔴 **Figure 25–38** The newborn can bring hand to mouth as a self-soothing activity.

Source: George Dodson/Lightworks Studio/Pearson Education.

earlier and more intense attachments. Noncuddlers are active and restless, have accelerated motor development, and are intolerant of physical restraint. Smiling, even as a grimace reflex, greatly influences parent-newborn feedback. Parents identify this response as positive.

Newborn Physical Assessment Guide

Review the Newborn Physical Assessment Guide for systematically assessing the newborn. Normal findings, alterations, and related causes are presented and correlated with suggested nursing responses. The findings are typical for a full-term newborn.

Assessment Guide · Newborn Physical Assessment

Physical Assessment/Normal Findings	Alterations and Possible Causes*	Nursing Responses to Data†
Vital Signs		
Blood pressure (BP): At birth: 70–50/45–30 mm Hg Day 10: 90/50 mm Hg (may be unable to measure diastolic pressure with standard sphygmomanometer)	Low BP (hypovolemia, shock)	Monitor BP in all cases of distress, prematurity, or suspected anomaly. Low BP: Refer to physician immediately so measures to improve circulation are begun.
Pulse: 110–160 beats/min (if asleep, as low as 80 beats/min; if crying, up to 180 beats/min)	Weak pulse (decreased cardiac output) Bradycardia (severe asphyxia) Tachycardia (over 160 beats/min at rest) (infection, CNS problems, arrhythmia, stress, hypovolemia)	Assess skin perfusion by blanching (capillary refill test—normal 2–3 sec). Carry out neurologic and thermoregulation assessments.
Respirations: 30–60 breaths/min Synchronization of chest and abdominal movements Diaphragmatic and abdominal breathing	Tachypnea (pneumonia, respiratory distress syndrome [RDS]) Rapid, shallow breathing (hypermagnesemia caused by large doses given to mothers with preeclampsia) Respirations below 30 breaths/min (maternal anesthesia or analgesia)	Identify sleep-wake state; correlate with respiratory pattern. Evaluate for all signs of respiratory distress; report findings to physician.
Transient tachypnea	Expiratory grunting, subcostal and substernal retractions; flaring of nares (respiratory distress); apnea (cold stress, respiratory disorder)	Evaluate for cold stress. Report findings to physician/neonatal nurse practitioner.
Crying: Strong and lusty Moderate tone and pitch Cries vary in length from 3–7 min after consoling measures are used	High-pitched, shrill (neurologic disorder, hypoglycemia) Weak or absent (CNS disorder, laryngeal problem) Inconsolable crying (GI discomforts, feeding intolerances)	Discuss newborn's use of cry for communication. Assess and record abnormal cries. Reduce environmental noises.
Temperature: Axilla 36.4°C–37.2°C (97.5°F–99°F) Heavier newborns tend to have higher body temperatures	Elevated temperature (room too warm, too much clothing or covers, dehydration, sepsis, brain damage) Subnormal temperature (brainstem involvement, cold, sepsis) Swings of more than 2°F from one reading to next or subnormal temperature (infection)	Notify physician of elevation or drop. Counsel parents on possible causes of elevated or low temperatures, appropriate home care measures, and when to call physician. Teach parents how to take rectal and/or axillary temperature; assess parents' information regarding use of thermometer; provide teaching as needed.
Weight: 2500–4000 g (5 lb, 8 oz–8 lb, 13 oz)	Less than 2748 g (less than 6 lb) = SGA or preterm infant Greater than 4050 g (greater than 9 lb) = LGA or infant of diabetic mother	Plot weight and gestational age on growth chart to identify high-risk infants. Ascertain body build of parents. Counsel parents regarding appropriate caloric intake.
Within first 3–4 days, normal weight loss of 5–10% Large babies tend to lose more because of greater fluid loss in proportion to birth weight except infants of diabetic mothers	Loss greater than 15% (low fluid intake, loss of meconium and urine, feeding difficulties, diabetes insipidus)	Notify physician of net losses or gains. Calculate fluid intake and losses from all sources (insensible water loss, radiant warmers, and phototherapy lights).

*Possible causes of alterations are identified in parentheses.

†This column provides guidelines for further assessment and initial nursing interventions.

(continued)

Assessment Guide Newborn Physical Assessment—continued

Physical Assessment/Normal Findings	Alterations and Possible Causes*	Nursing Responses to Data†
Length: 46–56 cm (18–22 in.) Grows 10 cm (3 in.) during first 3 months	Less than 45 cm (congenital dwarf) Short/long bones proximally (achondroplasia) Short/long bones distally (Ellis-van Creveld syndrome)	Assess for other signs of dwarfism. Determine other signs of skeletal system adequacy. Plot progress at subsequent well-baby visits.
Posture Body usually flexed, hands may be tightly clenched, neck appears short as chin rests on chest In breech presentations feet are usually dorsiflexed	Only extension noted, inability to move from midline (trauma, hypoxia, immaturity) Constant motion (maternal caffeine intake or drug withdrawal)	Record spontaneity of motor activity and symmetry of movements. If parents express concern about newborn's movement patterns, reassure and evaluate further if appropriate.
Skin *Color:* Color consistent with genetic background Newborns of European descent: pink-tinged or ruddy color over face, trunk, extremities Newborns of African descent: reddish brown to pale pink with yellow or red tinge Newborns of Asian, Native American, Hispanic descent: pink or rosy red to yellow, olive tinge	Pallor of face, conjunctiva (anemia, hypothermia, anoxia) Beefy red (hypoglycemia, immature vasomotor reflexes, polycythemia)	Discuss with parents common skin color variations to allay fears. Document extent and time of occurrence of color change.
Common variations: acrocyanosis, circumoral cyanosis, Mongolian spots, or harlequin color change	Meconium staining (nonreassuring fetal status) Jaundice (hemolytic reaction from blood incompatibility within first 24 hours, sepsis)	Obtain Hgb and hematocrit values, obtain bilirubin levels. Assess for respiratory difficulty. Differentiate between physiologic and pathologic jaundice.
Mottled when undressed	Cyanosis (choanal atresia, CNS damage or trauma, respiratory or cardiac problem, cold stress)	Assess degree of (central or peripheral) cyanosis and possible causes; refer to physician.
Minor bruising: over buttocks in breech presentation and over eyes and forehead in facial presentations		Discuss with parents cause and course of minor bruising related to labor and birth.
Texture: Smooth, soft, flexible, may have dry, peeling hands and feet	Generalized cracked or peeling skin (SGA or postterm; blood incompatibility; metabolic, kidney dysfunction) Seborrheic dermatitis (cradle cap) Absence of vernix (postmature)\ Yellow vernix (meconium staining)	Report to physician. Instruct parents to shampoo the scalp and anterior fontanel areas daily with soap; rinse well; avoid use of oil.
Turgor: Elastic, returns to normal shape after pinching	Maintains tent shape (dehydration)	Assess for other signs and symptoms of dehydration.
Pigmentation: Clear; milia across bridge of nose, forehead, or chin will disappear within a few weeks Café-au-lait spots (one or two)	Six or more (neurologic disorder such as von Recklinghausen disease, cutaneous neurofibromatosis)	Advise parents not to pinch or prick these pimplelike areas. If there are six or more café-au-lait spots, refer for genetic and neurologic consult.
Mongolian spots common over dorsal area and buttocks in dark-skin infants		Assure parents of normalcy of this pigmentation; it will fade in first year or two.
Erythema toxicum	Impetigo (group A β-hemolytic streptococcus or *Staphylococcus aureus* infection)	If impetigo occurs, instruct parents about hand washing and linen precautions during home care.
Telangiectatic nevi	Hemangiomas: Nevus flammeus (port-wine stain) Nevus vascularis (strawberry hemangioma) Cavernous hemangiomas	Collaborate with physician. Counsel parents about birthmark's progression to allay misconceptions. Record size and shape of hemangiomas. Refer for follow-up at well-baby clinic.

*Possible causes of alterations are identified in parentheses.

†This column provides guidelines for further assessment and initial nursing interventions.

Assessment Guide Newborn Physical Assessment—continued

Physical Assessment/Normal Findings	Alterations and Possible Causes*	Nursing Responses to Data†
Rashes	Rashes (infection)	Assess location and type of rash (macular, papular, vesicular). Obtain history of onset, prenatal history, and related signs and symptoms.
Petechiae of head or neck (breech presentation, cord around neck)	Generalized petechiae (clotting abnormalities)	Determine cause; advise parents if further health care is needed.
Head		
General appearance, size, movement Round, symmetric, and moves easily from left to right and up and down; soft and pliable	Asymmetric, flattened occiput on either side of the head (plagiocephaly) Head held at angle (torticollis)	Instruct parents to change infant's positions frequently when awake. When awake, needs to spend "tummy time." Infants should be placed supine for sleep per "back to sleep" guidelines.
	Unable to move head side to side (neurologic trauma)	Determine adequacy of all neurologic signs.
Circumference 32–37 cm (12.5–14.5 in.); 2 cm greater than chest circumference; head one fourth of body size	Extreme differences in size may be microencephaly (Cornelia de Lange syndrome, cytomegalic inclusion disease [CID], rubella, toxoplasmosis, chromosome abnormalities), hydrocephalus (meningomyelocele, achondroplasia), anencephaly (neural tube defect) Head is 3 cm or more larger than chest circumference (preterm, hydrocephalus)	Measure circumference from occiput to frontal area using metal or paper tape. Measure chest circumference using metal or paper tape and compare to head circumference. Record measurements on growth chart. Reevaluate at well-baby visits.
Common variations: Molding: Breech and cesarean newborns' heads are round and well shaped	Cephalohematoma (trauma during birth, may persist up to 3 months) Caput succedaneum (long labor and birth; disappears in 1 week)	Evaluate neurologic response. Observe for hyperbilirubinemia. Check Hct. Reassure parents regarding common manifestations caused by birth process and when they should disappear.
Fontanels: Palpation of juncture of cranial bones Anterior fontanel: 3–4 cm long by 2–3 cm wide, diamond shaped Posterior fontanel: 1–2 cm at birth, triangle shaped Slight pulsation Moderate bulging noted with crying, stooling, or pulsations with heartbeat	Overlapping of anterior fontanel (malnourished or preterm newborn) Premature closure of sutures (craniosynostosis) Late closure (hydrocephalus) Moderate to severe pulsation (vascular problems) Constant bulging (increased intracranial pressure, meningitis) Sunken (dehydration)	Discuss normal closure times with parents and care of "soft spots" to allay misconceptions. Refer to physician. Observe for signs and symptoms of hydrocephalus. Refer to physician. Evaluate hydration status. Evaluate neurologic status. Report to physician.
Hair		
Texture: Smooth with fine texture variations (Note: Variations depend on ethnic background.)	Coarse, brittle, dry hair (hypothyroidism) White forelock (Waardenburg syndrome)	Instruct parents regarding routine care of hair and scalp.
Distribution: Scalp hair high over eyebrows (Spanish, Mexican hairline begins midforehead and extends down back of neck.)	Low forehead and posterior hairlines may indicate chromosomal disorders	Assess for other signs of chromosomal aberrations. Refer to physician.
Face		
Symmetric movement of all facial features, normal hairline, eyebrows and eyelashes present		Assess and record symmetry of all parts, shape, regularity of features, sameness or differences in features.
Spacing of features: Eyes at same level, nostrils equal size, cheeks full, and sucking pads present	Eyes wide apart—ocular hypertelorism (Apert syndrome, cri du chat, Turner syndrome)	Observe for other signs and symptoms indicative of disease states or chromosomal aberrations.

*Possible causes of alterations are identified in parentheses.

†This column provides guidelines for further assessment and initial nursing interventions.

(continued)

Assessment Guide   Newborn Physical Assessment—continued

Physical Assessment/Normal Findings	Alterations and Possible Causes*	Nursing Responses to Data†
Lips equal on both sides of midline	Abnormal face (Down syndrome, cretinism, gargoylism)	
Chin recedes when compared with other bones of face	Abnormally small jaw—micrognathia (Pierre Robin syndrome, Treacher Collins syndrome)	Maintain airway; do not position supine. Initiate surgical consultation and referral.
Movement: Makes facial grimaces	Inability to suck, grimace, and close eyelids (cranial nerve injury)	Initiate neurologic assessment and consultation.
Symmetric when resting and crying	Asymmetry (paralysis of facial cranial nerve)	Assess and record symmetry of all parts, shape, regularity of features, and sameness or differences in features.

Eyes

Physical Assessment/Normal Findings	Alterations and Possible Causes*	Nursing Responses to Data†
General placement and appearance: Bright and clear; even placement; slight nystagmus (involuntary cyclic eye movements)	Gross nystagmus (damage to third, fourth, and sixth cranial nerves)	
Concomitant strabismus	Constant and fixed strabismus	Reassure parents that strabismus is considered normal up to 6 months.
Move in all directions		
Blue or slate blue-gray	Lack of pigmentation (albinism) Brushfield spots may indicate Down syndrome (a light or white speckling of the outer two thirds of the iris)	Discuss with parents any necessary eye precautions. Assess for other signs of Down syndrome.
Brown color at birth in dark-skin infants		
Eyelids: Position: above pupils but within iris, no drooping	Elevation of (hydrocephalus) or retraction of upper lid (hyperthyroidism)	Discuss with parents that permanent eye color is usually established by 3 months of age.
	"Sunset sign" lid elevation and downward gaze (hydrocephalus), ptosis (congenital or paralysis of oculomotor muscle)	Assess for signs of hydrocephalus and hyperthyroidism.
Eyes on parallel plane	Upward slant in non-Asians (Down syndrome)	Evaluate interference with vision in subsequent well-baby visits.
Epicanthal folds in Asians and 20% of newborns of northern European descent	Epicanthal folds (Down syndrome, cri du chat syndrome)	Assess for other signs of Down syndrome.
Movement: Blink reflex in response to light stimulus Eyes open wide in dimly lighted room	Blink absent (CNS injury, cranial nerve damage)	Evaluate neurologic status. Refer to physician.
Inspection: Edematous for first few days of life, resulting from birth; no lumps or redness	Purulent drainage (infection); infectious conjunctivitis (gonococcus, chlamydia, staphylococcus, or gram-negative organisms) Marginal blepharitis (lid edges red, crusted, scaly)	Initiate good hand washing. Refer to physician. Evaluate infant for seborrheic dermatitis; scales can be removed easily.
Cornea: Clear Corneal reflex present	Ulceration (herpes infection); large cornea or corneas of unequal size (congenital glaucoma) Clouding, opacity of lens (cataract)	Refer to ophthalmologist. Assess for other manifestations of congenital herpes; institute nursing care measures.
Sclera: May appear bluish in newborn, then white; slightly brownish color frequent in newborns of African descent	True blue sclera (osteogenesis imperfecta)	Refer to physician.

*Possible causes of alterations are identified in parentheses.

†This column provides guidelines for further assessment and initial nursing interventions.

Assessment Guide Newborn Physical Assessment—continued

Physical Assessment/Normal Findings	Alterations and Possible Causes*	Nursing Responses to Data†
Pupils: Pupils equal in size, round, and react to light by accommodation	Anisocoria—unequal pupils (CNS damage) Dilation or constriction (intracranial) damage, retinoblastoma, glaucoma; pupils nonreactive to light or accommodation (brain injury)	Refer for neurologic examination.
Slight nystagmus in newborn who has not learned to focus Pupil light reflex demonstrated at birth or by 3 weeks of age	Nystagmus (labyrinthine disturbance, CNS disorder)	
Conjunctiva: Chemical conjunctivitis Subconjunctival hemorrhage	Pale color (anemia)	Obtain hematocrit and hemoglobin. Reassure parents that chemical conjunctivitis will subside in 1–2 days and subconjunctival hemorrhage disappears in a few weeks.
Palpebral conjunctiva (red but not hyperemic)	Inflammation or edema (infection, blocked tear duct)	
Vision: 20/200 Tracks moving object to midline Fixed focus on objects at a distance of about 10–20 in.; may be difficult to evaluate in newborn Prefers faces, geometric designs, and black and white to colors	Cataracts (congenital infection)	Record any questions about visual acuity, and initiate follow-up evaluation at first well-baby checkup.
Lashes and lacrimal glands: Presence of lashes (lashes may be absent in preterm newborns)	No lashes on inner two thirds of lid (Treacher Collins syndrome); bushy lashes (Hurler syndrome); long lashes (Cornelia de Lange syndrome)	
Cry commonly tearless	Excessive tearing (plugged lacrimal duct, natal narcotic withdrawal), glaucoma	Demonstrate to parents how to milk blocked tear duct. Refer to ophthalmologist if tearing is excessive before third month of life.
Nose		
Appearance of external nasal aspects: May appear flattened as a result of birth process	Continued flat or broad bridge of nose (Down syndrome)	Arrange consultation with specialist.
Small and narrow in midline, even placement in relationship to eyes and mouth	Low bridge of nose, beaklike nose (Apert syndrome, Treacher Collins syndrome) Upturned (Cornelia de Lange syndrome)	Initiate evaluation of chromosomal abnormalities.
Patent nares bilaterally (nose breathers)	Blockage of nares (mucus and/or secretions), choanal atresia	Inspect for obstruction of nares.
Sneezing common to clear nasal passages	Flaring nares (respiratory distress)	Maintain oral airway until surgical correction is made.
Responds to odors, may smell breast milk	No response to stimulating odors	Inspect for obstruction of nares.
Mouth		
Function of facial, hypoglossal, glossopharyngeal, and vagus nerves: Symmetry of movement and strength	Mouth draws to one side (transient seventh cranial nerve paralysis caused by pressure in utero or trauma during birth, congenital paralysis) Fishlike shape (Treacher Collins syndrome)	Initiate neurologic consultation. Administer artificial tears if eye on affected side of face is unable to close.
Presence of gag, swallowing, coordinated with sucking reflexes; Adequate salivation	Suppressed or absent reflexes	Evaluate other neurologic functions of these nerves.
	*Possible causes of alterations are identified in parentheses.	†This column provides guidelines for further assessment and initial nursing interventions.

(continued)

Assessment Guide   Newborn Physical Assessment—continued

Physical Assessment/Normal Findings	Alterations and Possible Causes*	Nursing Responses to Data†
Palate (soft and hard): Hard palate dome-shaped Uvula midline with symmetric movement of soft palate	High-steepled palate (Treacher Collins syndrome), bifid uvula (congenital anomaly)	Assess for other congenital anomalies.
Palate intact, sucks well when stimulated	Clefts in either hard or soft palate (polygenic disorder)	Initiate a surgical consultation referral.
Epithelial (Epstein) pearls appear on mucosa		Assure parents that these are normal and will disappear at 2 or 3 months of age.
Esophagus patent, some drooling common in newborn	Excessive drooling or bubbling (esophageal atresia)	Test for patency of esophagus.
Tongue: Free moving in all directions, midline	Tongue-tied Lack of movement or asymmetric movement (neurologic damage) Fasciculations (fine tremors) Spinal muscular atrophy	Further assess neurologic functions. Test reflex elevation of tongue when depressed with tongue blade.
Pink color, smooth to rough texture, noncoated	Deviations from midline (cranial nerve damage) White cheesy coating (thrush) Tongue has deep ridges	Check for signs of weakness or deviation. Differentiate between thrush and milk curds by wiping patches: if white patches don't come off easily, it is thrush. Reassure parents that tongue pattern may change from day to day.
Tongue proportional to mouth	Large tongue with short frenulum (cretinism, Down syndrome, other syndromes)	Evaluate in well-baby clinic to assess development delays. Initiate referrals.
Ears		
External ear: Without lesions, cysts, or nodules	Nodules, cysts, or sinus tracts in front of ear Adherent earlobes Low-set ears (genetic anomaly or syndrome) Preauricular skin tags	Evaluate characteristics of lesions. Counsel parents to clean external ear with washcloth only; discourage use of cotton-tip applicators. Refer to physician for ligation.
Hearing: Eustachian tubes are cleared with first cry	Presence of one or more risk factors	Assess history of risk factors for hearing loss.
Attends to sounds; sudden or loud noise elicits Moro reflex	No response to sound stimuli (deafness)	Test for Moro reflex.
Neck		
Appearance: Short, straight, creased with skin folds	Abnormally short neck (Turner syndrome) Arching or inability to flex neck (meningitis, congenital anomaly)	Report findings to physician.
Posterior neck lacks loose extra folds of skin	Webbing of neck (Turner syndrome, Down syndrome, trisomy 18)	Assess for other signs of these syndromes.
Clavicles: Straight and intact	Knot or lump on clavicle (fracture during difficult birth)	Obtain detailed labor and birth history; apply figure-8 bandage. Consider oral analgesics.
Moro reflex elicitable	Unilateral Moro reflex response on unaffected side (fracture of clavicle, brachial palsy, Erb-Duchenne paralysis)	Collaborate with physician.
Symmetric shoulders	Hypoplasia	

*Possible causes of alterations are identified in parentheses.

†This column provides guidelines for further assessment and initial nursing interventions.

Assessment Guide   Newborn Physical Assessment—continued

Physical Assessment/Normal Findings	Alterations and Possible Causes*	Nursing Responses to Data†
Chest		
Appearance and size: Circumference: 32.5 cm (12.8 in.), 1–2 cm (0.4–0.8 in.) less than head Wider than it is long Normal shape without depressed or prominent sternum Lower end of sternum (xiphoid cartilage) may be protruding; is less apparent after several weeks Sternum 8 cm (3.1 in.) long	Funnel chest (congenital or associated with Marfan syndrome) Continued protrusion of xiphoid cartilage (Marfan syndrome, "pigeon chest") Barrel chest	Measure at level of nipples after exhalation. Determine adequacy of other respiratory and circulatory signs. Assess for other signs and symptoms of various syndromes.
Expansion and retraction: Bilateral expansion	Unequal chest expansion (pneumonia, pneumothorax, respiratory distress)	Assess respiratory effort regularity, flaring of nares, difficulty on both inspiration and expiration.
No intercostal, subcostal, or supracostal retractions	Retractions (respiratory distress) Seesaw respirations (respiratory distress)	
Auscultation: Breath sounds are louder in infants than adults due to less subcutaneous tissue to muffle transmission	Decreased breath sounds (decreased respiratory activity, atelectasis, pneumothorax)	Obtain transillumination. Record findings and consult physician. Perform assessment and report to physician any positive findings.
Chest and axillae clear on crying	Increased breath sounds (resolving pneumonia or in cesarean births)	
Bronchial breath sounds (heard where trachea and bronchi closest to chest wall, above sternum and between scapulae): Bronchial sounds bilaterally Air entry clear Rales may indicate normal newborn atelectasis Cough reflex absent at birth, appears in 2 or more days	Adventitious or abnormal sounds (respiratory disease or distress)	Evaluate color for pallor or cyanosis. Report to physician.
Breasts: Flat with symmetric nipples Breast tissue diameter 5 cm (2 in.) or more at term Distance between nipples 8 cm (3.1 in.) Breast engorgement occurs on third day of life; liquid discharge may be expressed in term newborns	Lack of breast tissue (preterm or SGA) Discharge Enlargement Breast abscesses Supernumerary nipples Dark-colored nipples	Evaluate for infection. Reassure parents of normality of breast engorgement. No intervention is necessary.
Heart		
Auscultation: Location: lies horizontally, with left border extending to left of midclavicle Regular rhythm and rate Determination of point of maximal impulse (PMI)	Arrhythmia (anoxia), tachycardia, bradycardia Malpositioning (enlargement, abnormal placement, pneumothorax, dextrocardia, diaphragmatic hernia)	Refer all arrhythmia and gallop rhythms. Initiate cardiac evaluation.
Functional murmurs No thrills	Location of murmurs (possible congenital cardiac anomaly)	Evaluate murmur: location, timing, and duration; observe for accompanying cardiac pathology symptoms; ascertain family history.
Horizontal groove at diaphragm shows flaring of rib cage to mild degree	Marked rib flaring (vitamin D deficiency) Inadequacy of respiratory movement	Initiate cardiopulmonary evaluation; assess pulses and blood pressures in all four extremities for equality and quality.

*Possible causes of alterations are identified in parentheses.

†This column provides guidelines for further assessment and initial nursing interventions.

(continued)

Assessment Guide   Newborn Physical Assessment—continued

Physical Assessment/Normal Findings	Alterations and Possible Causes*	Nursing Responses to Data†
Abdomen		
Appearance: Cylindric with some protrusion, appears large in relation to pelvis, some laxness of abdominal muscles No cyanosis, few vessels seen Diastasis recti—common in infants of African descent	Distention, shiny abdomen with engorged vessels (gastrointestinal abnormalities, infection, congenital megacolon) Scaphoid abdominal appearance (diaphragmatic hernia) Increased or decreased peristalsis (duodenal stenosis, small bowel obstruction) Localized flank bulging (enlarged kidneys, ascites, or absent abdominal muscles)	Examine abdomen thoroughly for mass or organomegaly. Measure abdominal girth. Report deviations of abdominal size. Assess other signs and symptoms of obstruction. Refer to physician.
Umbilicus: No protrusion of umbilicus (protrusion of umbilicus common in infants of African descent) Bluish white color Cutis navel (umbilical cord projects), granulation tissue present in navel	Umbilical hernia Patent urachus (congenital malformation) Omphalocele (covered defect) Gastroschisis (uncovered defect) Redness or exudate around cord (infection) Yellow discoloration (hemolytic disease, meconium staining)	Measure umbilical hernia by palpating the opening and record; it should close by 1 year of age; if not, refer to physician. Cover omphalocele and gastroschisis with sterile, moist dressing or plastic sterile bag. Instruct parents on cord care and hygiene.
Two arteries and one vein apparent Begins drying 1–2 hours after birth No bleeding	Single umbilical artery (congenital anomalies) Discharge or oozing of blood from the cord	Refer anomalies to physician.
Auscultation of all four quadrants:	Bowel sounds in chest (diaphragmatic hernia)	Collaborate with physician.
Soft bowel sounds heard shortly after birth every 10–30 seconds	Absence of bowel sounds Hyperperistalsis (intestinal obstruction)	Assess for other signs of dehydration or infection.
Femoral pulses: Palpable, equal bilateral	Absent or diminished femoral pulses (coarctation of aorta)	Monitor blood pressure in upper and lower extremities.
Inguinal area: No bulges along inguinal area No inguinal lymph nodes felt	Inguinal hernia	Initiate referral. Continue follow-up in well-baby clinic.
Bladder: Percusses 1–4 cm (0.4–1.6 in.) above symphysis Should void within 24 hours after birth; if not, at time of birth Urine—inoffensive, mild odor	Failure to void within 24–48 hours after birth Exposure of bladder mucosa (exstrophy of bladder) Foul odor (infection)	Check whether baby voided at birth. Obtain urine specimen if infection is suspected. Consult with clinician.
Genitals Gender clearly delineated	Ambiguous genitals	Refer for genetic consultation.
Male *Penis:* Slender in appearance, about 2.5 cm (1 in.) long, 1 cm (0.4 in.) wide at birth. Normal urinary orifice, urethral meatus at tip of penis	Micropenis (congenital anomaly) Meatal atresia Hypospadias, epispadias	Observe and record first voiding. Collaborate with physician in presence of abnormality. Delay circumcision.
Noninflamed urethral opening	Urethritis (infection)	Palpate for enlarged inguinal lymph nodes and record painful urination.
Foreskin adheres to glans	Ulceration of meatal opening (infection, inflammation)	Evaluate whether ulcer is because of diaper rash; counsel regarding care.
Uncircumcised foreskin tight for 2–3 months	Phimosis—if still tight after 3 months	Instruct parents on how to care for uncircumcised penis.
Circumcised		Teach parents how to care for circumcision.
Erectile tissue present		

*Possible causes of alterations are identified in parentheses.

†This column provides guidelines for further assessment and initial nursing interventions.

Physical Assessment/Normal Findings	Alterations and Possible Causes*	Nursing Responses to Data†
Scrotum: Skin loose and hanging or tight and small; extensive rugae and normal size. Normal skin color Scrotal discoloration common in breech	Large scrotum containing fluid (hydrocele) Minimal rugae, small scrotum Red, shiny scrotal skin (orchitis)	Shine a light through scrotum (transilluminate) to verify diagnosis. Assess for prematurity.
Testes: Descended by birth; not consistently found in scrotum	Undescended testes (cryptorchidism)	If testes cannot be felt in scrotum, gently palpate femoral, inguinal, perineal, and abdominal areas for presence.
Testes size 1.5–2 cm (0.6–0.8 in.) at birth	Enlarged testes (tumor) Small testes (Klinefelter syndrome or adrenal hyperplasia)	Refer and collaborate with physician for further diagnostic studies.

Female

Mons: Normal skin color, area pigmented in dark-skin infants Labia majora cover labia minora in term and postterm newborns; symmetric size appropriate for gestational age	Hematoma, lesions (trauma) Labia minora prominent	Evaluate for recent trauma. Assess for prematurity.
Clitoris: Normally large in newborn Edema and bruising in breech birth	Hypertrophy (hermaphroditism)	Refer for genetic workup.
Vagina: Urinary meatus and vaginal orifice visible (0.5 cm [0.2 in.] circumference) Vaginal tag or hymenal tag disappears in a few weeks	Inflammation; erythema and discharge (urethritis) Congenital absence of vagina	Collect urine specimen for laboratory examination. Refer to physician.
Discharge; smegma under labia	Foul-smelling discharge (infection)	Collect data and further evaluate reason for discharge.
Bloody or mucoid discharge	Excessive vaginal bleeding (blood coagulation defect)	

Buttocks and Anus

Buttocks symmetric	Pilonidal dimple	Examine for possible sinus. Instruct parents about cleansing this area.
Anus patent and passage of meconium within 24–48 hours after birth	Imperforate anus, rectal atresia (congenital gastrointestinal defect)	Evaluate extent of problems. Initiate surgical consultation. Perform digital examination to ascertain patency if patency uncertain.
No fissures, tears, or skin tags	Fissures	

Extremities and Trunk

Short and generally flexed, extremities move symmetrically through range of motion but lack full extension	Unilateral or absence of movement (spinal cord involvement) Fetal position continued or limp (anoxia)	Review birth record to assess possible cause.
All joints move spontaneously; good muscle tone, of flexor type, birth to 2 months	Spasticity when infant begins using extensors (cerebral palsy)	Collaborate with physician.
Arms: Equal in length Bilateral movement Flexed when quiet	Brachial palsy (difficult birth) Erb-Duchenne paralysis Muscle weakness, fractured clavicle Absence of limb or change of size (phocomelia, amelia)	Report to clinician.
Hands: Normal number of fingers	Polydactyly (Ellis-van Creveld syndrome) Syndactyly—one limb (developmental anomaly) Syndactyly—both limbs (genetic component)	Report to clinician.

*Possible causes of alterations are identified in parentheses.

†This column provides guidelines for further assessment and initial nursing interventions.

(continued)

Assessment Guide Newborn Physical Assessment—continued

Physical Assessment/Normal Findings	Alterations and Possible Causes*	Nursing Responses to Data†
Normal palmar crease	Single palmar crease (Down syndrome)	Refer for genetic workup.
Normal size hands	Short fingers and broad hand (Hurler syndrome)	
Nails present and extend beyond fingertips in term newborn	Cyanosis and clubbing (cardiac anomalies) Nails long or yellow stained (postterm)	Evaluate for history of distress in utero. Carry out cardiac and respiratory assessments. Check pulse oximetry.
Spine: C-shaped spine Flat and straight when prone Slight lumbar lordosis Easily flexed and intact when palpated At least half of back devoid of lanugo Full-term infant in ventral suspension should hold head at 45-degree angle, back straight	Spina bifida occulta (nevus pilosus) Dermal sinus Myelomeningocele Head lag, limp, floppy trunk (neurologic problems)	Evaluate extent of neurologic damage; initiate care of spinal opening. Elicit reflex to assess degree of involvement.
Hips: No sign of instability	Sensation of abnormal movement, jerk, or snap of hip dislocation	Physician or nurse practitioner examines all newborn infants for dislocated hip before discharge from birthing center.
Hips abduct to more than 60 degrees	Limited abduction (developmental dysplasia of hip)	If this is suspected, refer to orthopedist for further evaluation. Reassess at well-baby visits.
Inguinal and buttock skin creases: Symmetric inguinal and buttock creases	Asymmetry (dislocated hips)	Refer to orthopedist for evaluation. Counsel parents regarding symptoms of concern, and discuss therapy.
Legs: Legs equal in length Legs shorter than arms at birth	Shortened leg (dislocated hips) Lack of leg movement (fractures, spinal defects)	Refer to orthopedist for evaluation. Counsel parents regarding symptoms of concern, and discuss therapy.
Feet: Foot is in straight line Positional clubfoot—based on position in utero	Talipes equinovarus (true clubfoot)	Discuss differences between positional and true clubfoot with parents. Teach parents passive manipulation of foot.
Fat pads and creases on soles of feet	Incomplete sole creases in first 24 hours of life (premature)	Refer to orthopedist if not corrected by 3 months of age.
Talipes planus (flat feet) normal under 3 years of age		Reassure parents that flat feet are normal in infants.
Neuromuscular		
Motor function: Symmetric movement and strength in all extremities	Limp, flaccid, or hypertonic (CNS disorders, infection, dehydration, fracture)	Appraise newborn's posture and motor functions by observing activities and motor characteristics.
May be jerky or have brief twitchings	Tremors (hypoglycemia, hypocalcemia, infection, neurologic damage)	Evaluate for electrolyte imbalance, hypoglycemia, and neurologic functioning.
Head lag not over 45 degrees	Delayed or abnormal development (preterm, neurologic involvement)	
Neck control adequate to maintain head erect briefly	Asymmetry of tone or strength (neurologic damage)	Refer for genetic evaluation.

*Possible causes of alterations are identified in parentheses.

†This column provides guidelines for further assessment and initial nursing interventions.

Critical Concept Review

LEARNING OUTCOME 25.1: Describe the physical and neuromuscular maturity characteristics assessed to determine the gestational age of the newborn.

1. The common physical characteristics included in the gestational age assessment are:
   - Skin
   - Lanugo
   - Plantar (sole) creases
   - Breast tissue and size
   - Ear form and cartilage
   - Genitalia
2. The neuromuscular components of gestational age scoring tools are:
   - Posture
   - Square window

   - Popliteal angle
   - Arm recoil
   - Heel-to-toe extension
   - Scarf sign

3. By assessing the physical and neuromuscular components specified in a gestational age tool, the nurse determines the gestational age of the newborn and identifies the newborn as SGA, AGA, or LGA and prioritizes individual needs.

LEARNING OUTCOME 25.2: Summarize the components of a systematic physical assessment of the newborn.

1. Basis for complete newborn assessment includes:
   - Perinatal history
   - Determination of gestational age
   - Physical assessment
   - Behavioral assessment
2. Components of a complete newborn physical assessment include:
   - Vital signs
   - Weight, length, and head circumference
   - Skin appearance and presence of birthmarks
   - Examination of the head for size, appearance, symmetry, presence, and status of fontanels

   - Hair appearance
   - Appearance, condition, and symmetry of face, eyes, and ears
   - Appearance and condition of nose and mouth
   - Appearance of chest and auscultation of lungs and heart
   - Appearance of abdomen and presence of bowel sounds
   - Inspection of umbilical stump for two arteries and one vein
   - Appearance of appropriate genitalia
   - Condition and patency of anus
   - Position and condition of extremities, trunk, and spine

LEARNING OUTCOME 25.3: Describe the normal physical characteristics and normal variations of the newborn and compare abnormal findings to possible causes and nursing responses.

1. Normal ranges for newborn vital signs include:
   - Heart rate, 110 to 160 beats/min
   - Respirations, 30 to 60 respirations per minute
   - Axillary temperature, 36.4°C to 37.2°C (97.5°F to 99°F); skin temperature, 36°C to 36.5°C (96.8°F to 97.7°F); rectal temperature, 36.6°C to 37.2°C (97.8°F to 99°F)
   - Blood pressure at birth, 70–50/45–30 mm Hg
2. Normal newborn measurements include:
   - Weight range, 2500 to 4000 g (5 lb, 8 oz to 8 lb, 13 oz), with weight dependent on maternal size and age
   - Length range, 46 to 56 cm (18 to 22 in.)
   - Head circumference range, 32 to 37 cm (12.5 to 14.5 in.)— approximately 2 cm larger than the chest circumference.
3. The newborn infant should have a head that appears large for its body.

4. The normal newborn has a prominent abdomen, sloping shoulders, narrow hips, and rounded chest. The body appears long and the extremities short.
5. Newborns tend to stay in a flexed position and will resist straightening of the extremities. Hands remain clenched.
6. The nurse should be knowledgeable about variations that are indicative of normal newborn responses as well as those that indicate a need for further investigation.
7. See the newborn physical assessment guide for possible causes of abnormal findings and possible nursing responses.
8. An important role of the nurse during the physical assessment of the newborn is to teach parents about their newborn and involve them in their baby's care.

LEARNING OUTCOME 25.4: Describe the components of a neurologic assessment and the neurologic/neuromuscular characteristics of the newborn and the reflexes that may be present at birth.

1. Neurologic assessment characteristics are:
   - State of alertness
   - Resting position
   - Muscle tone
   - Cry
   - Motor activity
2. Neuromuscular assessment characteristics are:
   - Symmetric movements and strength of all extremities
   - Head lag less than 45 degrees
   - Ability to hold head erect briefly

3. Normal reflexes
   - Blink
   - Pupillary reflex
   - Moro
   - Rooting and sucking
   - Palmar grasp
   - Stepping
   - Tonic neck

LEARNING OUTCOME 25.5: Compare the components of the newborn behavioral assessment with the normal behavioral characteristics and normal variations of the newborn.

1. Components of Brazelton Neonatal Behavioral Assessment include:
   - Newborn state changes
   - Temperament
   - Individual behavioral patterns
2. The categories of the newborn behavioral characteristics are:
   - Habituation
   - Orientation to inanimate and animate visual and auditory assessment stimuli
   - Motor activity
   - Variations. Frequency of alert states, state changes, color changes, activity, and peaks of activity
   - Self-quieting activity
   - Cuddliness or social behavior

LEARNING OUTCOME 25.6: Correlate findings in a newborn behavioral assessment to nursing responses and to teach and involve parents in the care of their newborn.

1. Behaviorally, the infant will sleep the majority of the time and wake for feeding. The infant should be easily consoled when upset.
2. An important role of the nurse during the behavioral assessment of the newborn is to teach parents about their newborn and involve them in their baby's care. This involvement facilitates the parents' identification of their newborn's uniqueness, allays their concerns, and fosters positive attachment experiences.

Clinical Reasoning in Action

Susan Pine, a 21-year-old G2, now P1011, delivers a 39 2/7-weeks' gestation female newborn. The vaginal birth is assisted with a vacuum extractor. The prenatal record is significant for an increase of maternal blood pressure to 140/90 on the day of birth. Susan is treated with magnesium sulfate during her labor and has an epidural analgesia for the pain of labor. The baby's Apgar is 8 and 9 at 1 and 5 minutes, and she has been admitted to the newborn nursery. The newborn's admission exam is normal except for a 2-cm round caput succedaneum. Now, 8 hours later, the baby's condition is stable and she needs to be bottle-fed. You take her to her mother's room where you observe that Susan does not reach out to take her from you. She seems unsure when handling her baby. Susan asks you about the swelling on her baby's head and wonders if it will ever go away.

1. How would you explain the cause of Susan's baby's caput succedaneum?
2. Compare the difference between a cephalohematoma and caput succedaneum.
3. Explore with Susan her baby's reflexes and state of alertness.
4. Susan asks you how she will know what her baby needs. How would you respond?
5. Develop a concept map to meet the potential needs of a baby who has a cephalohematoma.

See www.nursing.pearsonhighered.com for possible responses and an interactive template for a concept map.

References

American Academy of Pediatrics. (2011). *How to take a child's temperature.* Retrieved from http://www.healthychildren.org/English/health-issues/conditions/fever

American Academy of Pediatrics (AAP) Committee on Fetus and Newborn & American College of Obstetricians and Gynecologists (ACOG) Committee on Obstetrics. (2012). *Guidelines for perinatal care* (7th ed.). Evanston, IL: Author.

Ballard, J. L., Khoury, J. C., Wedig, K., Wang, L., Eilers-Walsman, B. L., & Lipp, R. (1991). New Ballard score, expanded to include extremely premature infants. *Journal of Pediatrics, 119*(3), 417–423.

Blackburn, S. T. (2013). *Maternal, fetal, neonatal physiology: A clinical perspective* (4th ed.). London, England: MacKeith.

Brazelton, T. B., & Nugent, J. K. (2011). *The neonatal behavioral assessment scale* (4th ed.). London, England: MacKeith.

Cloherty, J. P., Eichenwald, E. C., Hansen, A. R., & Stark, A. R. (2012). *Manual of neonatal care* (7th ed.). Philadelphia, PA: Lippincott Williams & Wilkins.

Gardner, S. L., & Hernandez, J. A. (2011). Initial nursery care. In S. L. Gardner, B. S. Carter, M. Enzman-Hines, & J. A. Hernandez (Eds.), *Merenstein & Gardner's handbook of neonatal intensive care* (7th ed., pp. 78–112). St. Louis, MO: Mosby.

Gleason, C. A., & Devaskar, S. U. (2012). *Avery's diseases of the newborn* (9th ed.). St. Louis, MO: Elsevier/Saunders.

Lomax, A. (2011). *Examination of the newborn: An evidence-based guide.* Chichester, UK: Blackwell Publishing.

The Normal Newborn: Needs, Care, and Feeding

When our daughter was laid in my arms right after birth she was so delicate. I had not dared to hope that we would be blessed with a girl because there were so few girls in my husband's family. Our 2-year-old niece was the first girl in 107 years, so I had pretty much decided that another boy would be just fine. But here she was, right here in my arms. —Catherine, 32

LEARNING OUTCOMES

26.1 Summarize essential information to be obtained about a newborn's birth experience and immediate postnatal period.

26.2 Explain how the physiologic and behavioral responses of the newborn during the first 4 hours after birth (admission and transitional period) determine the nursing care of the newborn.

26.3 Explain the advantages and disadvantages of breastfeeding and formula-feeding in determining the nursing care of both mother/family and newborn.

26.4 Formulate guidelines for helping both breast- and formula-feeding mothers to feed their newborns successfully in hospital and community-based settings.

26.5 Identify activities that should be included in a daily care plan for a normal newborn.

26.6 Describe the common concerns of families regarding their newborn.

26.7 Identify opportunities to individualize parent teaching and enhance each parent's abilities and confidence while providing infant care in the birthing unit.

26.8 Explain the influence of cultural values on infant care, especially feeding practices.

At the moment of birth, numerous physiologic adaptations begin to take place in the newborn's body. Because of these dramatic changes, newborns require close observation to determine how smoothly they are making the transition to extrauterine life. Newborns also require specific care that enhances their chances of making the transition successfully.

The two broad goals of nursing care during this period are (1) to promote the physical well-being of the newborn, and (2) to support the establishment of a well-functioning family unit. To meet the first goal, the nurse provides comprehensive care to the newborn in the mother-baby unit. To meet the second goal, the nurse teaches family members how to care for their new baby and supports their efforts so that they feel confident and competent. Thus, the nurse must be knowledgeable about necessary family adjustments as well as the healthcare needs of the newborn. It is important that the family return home confident, knowing that they have the support, information, and skills to care for their newborn. Equally important is the need for each member of the family to begin a unique relationship with the newborn. The cultural and social expectations of individual families and communities affect the ways in which normal newborn care is carried out.

The previous two chapters presented an informational database of the physiologic and behavioral changes occurring in the newborn and the pertinent nursing assessments that are needed. This chapter discusses nursing management while the newborn is in the birthing unit and feeding methods for the full-term, healthy infant.

NURSING CARE DURING ADMISSION AND THE FIRST FOUR HOURS OF LIFE

Immediately after birth, the baby is formally admitted to the healthcare facility.

Nursing Diagnoses

Physiologic alterations of the newborn form the basis of many nursing diagnoses, as does the family members' incorporation of them in caring for their newborn. Nursing diagnoses are based on an analysis of the assessment findings. As discussed in Chapter 24 ⊘, the newborn's physiologic adaptation to extrauterine life occurs rapidly and all body systems are affected. Therefore, many of these nursing diagnoses and associated interventions must be identified and implemented in a very short period.

Nursing diagnoses that may apply to newborns include the following (NANDA-I © 2012):

- *Airway Clearance, Ineffective,* related to presence of mucus and retained lung fluid
- *Body Temperature*, *Imbalanced, Risk for,* related to evaporative, radiant, conductive, and convective heat losses
- *Pain, Acute,* related to heel sticks for glucose or hematocrit tests, vitamin K injection, or hepatitis B immunization

Nursing Plan and Implementation

Initiating Admission Procedures

After birth, the newborn is formally admitted to the healthcare facility. The admission procedures include a review of prenatal and birth information for possible risk factors, a gestational age assessment, and an assessment to ensure that the newborn's adaptation to extrauterine life is proceeding normally. This evaluation of the newborn's status and risk factors must be done no later than 2 hours after birth (American Academy of Pediatrics [AAP] Committee on Fetus and Newborn & American College of Obstetricians and Gynecologists [ACOG] Committee on Obstetrics, 2012).

If the initial assessment indicates that the newborn is not at risk physiologically, the nurse performs many of the routine admission procedures in the presence of the parents in the birthing area. Some care measures indicated by the assessment findings may be performed by the nurse or by the family members under the guidance of the nurse in an effort to educate and support the family. Other interventions may be delayed until the newborn has been transferred to a nursery.

The nurse responsible for the newborn first checks and confirms the newborn's identification with the mother's identification and then obtains and records all significant information. The essential data to be recorded on the newborn's chart are as follows:

1. *Condition of the newborn.* Pertinent information includes the newborn's Apgar scores at 1 and 5 minutes, any resuscitative measures required in the birthing area, physical examination, vital signs, voidings, and passing of meconium. Complications to be noted are excessive mucus, delayed spontaneous respirations or responsiveness, abnormal number of cord vessels, and obvious physical abnormalities.

2. *Labor and birth record.* A copy of the labor and birth record should be placed in the newborn's chart or be accessible on the computer. The record contains the significant data about the birth—for example, duration, course, and status of mother and fetus throughout labor and birth and any analgesia or anesthesia administered to the mother. The nurse notes any variation or difficulties, such as prolonged rupture of membranes, abnormal fetal position, presence or absence of meconium-stained amniotic fluid, signs of nonreassuring fetal heart rate during labor, nuchal cord (cord around the newborn's neck at birth), precipitous birth, use of forceps or vacuum extraction assisted device, maternal analgesics and anesthesia received within 1 hour before birth, and administration of antibiotics during labor.

3. *Antepartum history.* Any maternal problems that may have compromised the fetus in utero, such as preeclampsia, spotting, illness, recent infections (evidence of chorioamnionitis), blood type, rubella status, serology results, hepatitis B screen results, colonization with group B streptococci, or a history of maternal substance abuse, are of immediate concern in newborn assessment. The chart should also include information about maternal age, estimated date of birth (EDB), previous pregnancies, and presence of any congenital anomalies. An HIV serology test should be encouraged and performed according to state law (AAP & ACOG, 2012).

4. *Parent–newborn interaction information.* The nurse notes parents' interactions with their newborn and their desires regarding care, such as rooming in, circumcision, and the type of feeding. Information about other children in the home, available support systems, interactional patterns within each family unit, situations that compromise lactation (breast surgery, previous lactation failure), and any high-risk circumstances (adolescent mother, domestic violence, history of child abuse) helps in providing comprehensive care (AAP & ACOG, 2012).

● **Figure 26–1** Weighing of newborn: The scale is cleaned and balanced before each weighing, with the protective pad in place.
Source: George Dodson, Lightworks Studio/Pearson Education.

As part of the admission procedure, the nurse weighs the newborn in both grams and pounds. In the United States, parents understand weight best when it is stated in pounds and ounces (Figure 26–1 ●). The nurse cleans, covers, and sets the scale to zero each time a newborn is weighed to prevent cross-infection. Since the nurse needs to remove all clothing and blankets for accurate weight, it best to do the weighing under a warmer light to avoid heat loss from conduction.

The nurse then measures the newborn, recording the measurements in both centimeters and inches. The three routine measurements are length, head circumference, and chest circumference. In some facilities, abdominal girth may also be measured (see Table 25–1: Newborn Measurements 🔗 on page 553). Rapidly assess the baby's color, muscle tone, alertness, and general state. Remember that the first period of reactivity may have concluded, and the baby may be in the sleep-inactive phase, which makes the infant hard to arouse. Do basic assessments for estimating gestational age and complete the physical assessment (see *Assessment Guide: Newborn Physical Assessment* beginning on page 571 in Chapter 25 🔗).

In addition to obtaining vital signs, perform a hematocrit and blood glucose evaluation on at-risk newborns or as clinically indicated (such as for small-for-gestational-age [SGA] or large-for-gestational-age [LGA] infants, or if the newborn is jittery). These procedures may be done on admission or within the first 2 hours after birth (AAP & ACOG, 2012). (See Skill 10–1: Performing a Capillary Puncture, in the *Clinical Skills Manual* SKILLS .)

Maintaining a Clear Airway and Stable Vital Signs

Free flow oxygen should be readily available. The nurse positions the newborn on his or her back (or side, if the infant has copious secretions). If necessary, the nurse should use a bulb syringe or DeLee wall suction (see Chapter 19 and Figure 19–7 🔗 on page 417 and Skill 5–1 in the *Clinical Skills Manual* SKILLS) to remove mucus from the stomach to help prevent possible aspiration. When possible, this procedure should be delayed for 10 to 15 minutes after birth, reducing the potential for severe vasovagal reflex apnea.

In the absence of any newborn distress, continue with the admission by taking the newborn's vital signs (see Table 25–3: Newborn Vital Signs on page 563). The initial temperature is taken by the axillary method. A wider range of normal exists for axillary temperature, specifically 36.4°C to 37.2°C (97.5°F to 99°F).

Once the initial temperature is taken, the nurse monitors the core temperature either by obtaining axillary temperatures at intervals or by placing a skin sensor on the newborn for continuous reading. The usual skin sensor placement site is the newborn's abdomen, but placement on the upper thigh or arm can give a reading closely correlated with the mean body temperature. The vital signs for a healthy term newborn should be monitored at least every 30 minutes until the newborn's condition has remained stable for 2 hours (AAP & ACOG, 2012). The newborn's respirations may be irregular yet still be normal. Brief periods of apnea, lasting only 5 to 10 seconds with no color or heart rate changes, are considered normal. The normal pulse range is 110 to 160 beats per minute (beats/min), and the normal respiratory range is 30 to 60 respirations per minute.

Maintaining a Neutral Thermal Environment

A neutral thermal environment is essential to minimize the newborn's need for increased oxygen consumption and use of calories to maintain body heat in the optimal range of 36.4°C to 37.2°C (97.5°F to 99°F). If the newborn becomes hypothermic, the body's response can lead to metabolic acidosis, hypoxia, and shock.

A neutral thermal environment is best achieved by performing the newborn assessment and interventions with the newborn unclothed and under a radiant warmer. The radiant warmer's thermostat is controlled by the thermal skin sensor taped to the newborn's abdomen, upper thigh, or arm (see Figure 25–16 on page 554). The sensor indicates when the newborn's temperature exceeds or falls below the acceptable temperature range. The nurse should be aware that leaning over the newborn may block the radiant heat waves from reaching the newborn (Blackburn, 2013).

In light of early discharge practices (12 to 48 hours), healthy term infants can be safely bathed immediately after the admission assessment is completed. The baby is bathed while still under the radiant warmer; bathing may be done in the parents' room and by the parents. Bathing the newborn offers an excellent opportunity for teaching and welcoming parents' involvement in the care of their newborn. If there is any doubt regarding the infant's condition, a sponge bath may be given when the baby's temperature is normal and vital signs are stable (about 2 to 4 hours after birth), when the baby's condition dictates, or when the parents wish to give the first bath. The nurse rechecks the newborn's temperature after the bath and, if it is stable, dresses him or her in a shirt, diaper, and cap; wraps the baby; and places the newborn in an open crib at room temperature. If the newborn's axillary temperature is below 36.5°C (97.7°F), the nurse returns the newborn to the radiant warmer. The rewarming process should be gradual to prevent hyperthermia. (See Chapter 25 for information about temperature assessment and instability and Table 26–1.)

Table 26–1	Maintenance of Stable Newborn Temperature

Take action to help the newborn maintain a stable temperature:

- Keep the newborn's clothing and bedding dry.
- Double-wrap the newborn and put a stocking cap on him or her.
- Use the radiant warmer during procedures.
- Reduce the newborn's exposure to drafts.
- Warm objects that will be in contact with the newborn (e.g., stethoscope, blankets).
- Encourage the mother to snuggle with the newborn under blankets or to breastfeed the newborn with hat and light cover on.

Clinical Tip

A cap can be fashioned from a piece of stockinette to help reduce heat loss from the head.

Preventing Vitamin K Deficiency Bleeding

A prophylactic injection of vitamin K_1 (AquaMEPHYTON) is recommended to prevent hemorrhage, which can occur because of low prothrombin levels in the first few days of life (see *Drug Guide: Vitamin K_1 Phytonadione [AquaMEPHYTON]*). The potential for hemorrhage is considered to result from the absence of gut bacterial flora, which influences the production of vitamin K_1 in the newborn (see *Coagulation* in Chapter 24 for further discussion). Current recommendations underscore the need for treatment in infants who are exclusively breastfed (Blackburn, 2013).

The vitamin K_1 injection is given intramuscularly in the middle third of the vastus lateralis muscle, located in the lateral aspect of the thigh (Figure 26–2 ●). Before injecting, the nurse must thoroughly clean the newborn's skin site for the injection with a small alcohol swab. The nurse uses a 25-gauge, 5/8-in. needle for the injection. An alternative site is the rectus femoris muscle in the anterior aspect of the thigh. However, this site is near the sciatic nerve and femoral artery; therefore, injections here should be done with caution (Figure 26–3 ●).

Preventing Eye Infection

The nurse is also responsible for giving the legally required prophylactic eye treatment for *Neisseria gonorrhoeae*, which may have infected the newborn of an infected mother during the birth process. A variety of topical agents appear to be equally effective. Ophthalmic ointments that are used include 0.5% erythromycin (Ilotycin Ophthalmic) (see *Drug Guide: Erythromycin Ophthalmic Ointment [Ilotycin Ophthalmic]* on page 588), 1% tetracycline, or per agency protocol. All are also effective against chlamydia, which has a higher incidence rate than gonorrhea.

Successful eye prophylaxis requires that the medication be instilled into the lower conjunctival sac of each eye (Figure 26–4 ●). The nurse massages the eyelid gently to distribute the ointment. Instillation may be delayed up to 1 hour after birth to allow eye contact during parent–newborn bonding.

Eye prophylaxis medications can cause chemical conjunctivitis, which gives the newborn some discomfort and may

● **Figure 26–2** Procedure for vitamin K injection. Cleanse area thoroughly with alcohol swab and allow skin to dry. Bunch the tissue of the upper outer thigh (vastus lateralis muscle) and quickly insert a 25-gauge, 5/8-in. needle at a 90-degree angle to the thigh. Aspirate, then slowly inject the solution to distribute the medication evenly and minimize the baby's discomfort. Remove the needle and gently massage the site with an alcohol swab.

Source: © Marlon Lopez/Shutterstock.

Greater trochanter
Sciatic nerve
Femoral and deep femoral artery
Femoral and deep femoral vein
Rectus femoris muscle
Vastus lateralis muscle
Patella

● **Figure 26–3** Injection sites. The middle third of the vastus lateralis muscle is the preferred site for intramuscular injection in the newborn. The middle third of the rectus femoris is an alternative site, but its proximity to major vessels and the sciatic nerve requires caution in using this site for injection.

interfere with the ability to focus on the parents' faces. The resulting edema, inflammation, and discharge may cause concern if the parents have not been informed that the side effects will clear in 24 to 48 hours and that this prophylactic eye treatment is necessary for the newborn's well-being.

Early Assessment of Neonatal Distress

During the first 24 hours of life, the nurse should be constantly alert for signs of distress. If the newborn is with the parents during this period, the nurse must take extra care to teach them how to maintain their newborn's temperature, recognize the hallmarks of newborn distress, and respond immediately to signs of

respiratory problems. The parents learn to observe the newborn for changes in color or activity, grunting or "sighing" sounds with breathing, rapid breathing with chest retractions, or facial grimacing. Their interventions include nasal and oral suctioning with a bulb syringe, positioning, and vigorous fingertip stroking of the newborn's spine to stimulate respiratory activity if necessary. The nurse must be available immediately if the newborn develops distress (Table 26–2).

Drug Guide Vitamin K₁ Phytonadione (AquaMEPHYTON)

Pregnancy Risk Category: C

Overview of Neonatal Action

Phytonadione is used in prophylaxis and treatment of vitamin K deficiency bleeding (VKDB), formerly known as hemorrhagic disease of the newborn. It promotes liver formation of the clotting factors II, VII, IX, and X. At birth, the newborn does not have the bacteria in the colon that are necessary for synthesizing fat-soluble vitamin K₁. Therefore, the newborn may have decreased levels of prothrombin during the first 5 to 8 days of life, reflected by a prolongation of prothrombin time.

Route, Dosage, Frequency

Intramuscular injection is given in the vastus lateralis thigh muscle. A one-time-only prophylactic dose of 0.5 to 1 mg is given intramuscularly within 1 hour of birth or may be delayed until after the first breastfeeding in the delivery/birthing area (Wilson, Shannon, & Shields, 2013).

If the mother received anticoagulants during pregnancy, an additional dose may be ordered by the physician and is given 6 to 8 hours after the first injection.

Neonatal Side Effects

Pain and edema may occur at the injection site. Allergic reactions, such as rash and urticaria, may also occur.

Nursing Considerations

- Protect drug from light.
- Give vitamin K₁ before circumcision procedure.
- Observe for signs of local inflammation.
- Observe for bleeding (usually occurs on second or third day). Bleeding may be seen as generalized ecchymoses or bleeding from umbilical cord, circumcision site, nose, or gastrointestinal tract. Results of serial prothrombin time (PT) and international normalized ratio (INR) should be assessed.
- Observe for jaundice and kernicterus, especially in preterm infants.

● **Figure 26–4** Ophthalmic ointment. Retract the lower eyelid outward to instill a 1/4-in. (1 cm) long strand of ointment from a single-dose tube along the lower conjunctival surface. Make sure that the tip of the tube does not touch the eye.

Table 26–2	Signs of Newborn Distress

- Increased respiratory rate (more than 60/minute) or difficult respirations
- Sternal retractions
- Nasal flaring
- Grunting
- Excessive mucus
- Facial grimacing
- Cyanosis (central: skin, lips, tongue)
- Abdominal distention or mass
- Vomiting of bile-stained material
- Absence of meconium elimination within 24 hours of birth
- Absence of urine elimination within 24 hours of birth
- Jaundice of the skin within 24 hours of birth or because of a hemolytic process
- Temperature instability (hypothermia or hyperthermia)
- Jitteriness or glucose less than 40 mg%

Source: Adapted from Tappero, E. P., & Honeyfield, M. E. (2009). *Physical assessment of the newborn* (3rd ed.). Petaluma, CA: NICU Inc.

A common cause of neonatal distress is early-onset group B streptococcal (GBS) disease. Infected mothers transmit GBS infection to their infants during labor and birth; thus it is recommended that at-risk mothers receive intrapartum antimicrobial prophylaxis (IAP) for GBS disease. All infants of mothers identified as at risk should be assessed and observed for signs and symptoms of sepsis (see Chapter 16 🔗 for discussion of maternal care).

Facilitating Early Parent–Newborn Attachment

To facilitate **parent–newborn attachment**, eye-to-eye contact between the parents and their newborn is extremely important during the early hours after birth when the newborn is in the first period of reactivity. The newborn is alert during this time,

---

Clinical Reasoning Early Respiratory Efforts

You overhear Mr. Johannson speaking to his mother on the phone. He is telling her about the "cute little noises" his 30-minute-old baby makes. The infant is in the room with the mother. What is your best course of action?
See www.nursing.pearsonhighered.com for possible responses.

Drug Guide Erythromycin Ophthalmic Ointment (Ilotycin Ophthalmic)

Pregnancy Risk Category: B

Overview of Neonatal Action

Erythromycin (Ilotycin Ophthalmic) is used as prophylactic treatment of ophthalmia neonatorum, which is caused by the bacteria *Neisseria gonorrhoeae*. Preventive treatment of gonorrhea in the newborn is required by law. Erythromycin is also effective against ophthalmic chlamydial infections. It is either bacteriostatic or bactericidal, depending on the organisms involved and the concentration of drug.

Route, Dosage, Frequency

Ophthalmic ointment (0.5%) is instilled as a narrow ribbon or strand, 1 cm long, along the lower conjunctival surface of each eye, starting at the inner canthus. It is instilled only once in each eye (AAP & ACOG, 2012). The ointment may be administered in the birthing area or, alternatively, later in the nursery so that eye contact between infant and parent is facilitated and the bonding process immediately after birth is not interrupted. After administration, gently close the eye and manipulate to ensure the spread of ointment (Wilson et al., 2013).

Neonatal Side Effects

Sensitivity reaction may occur; the ointment may interfere with the ability to focus and may cause edema and inflammation. Side effects usually disappear in 24 to 48 hours.

Nursing Considerations

- Wash hands immediately before instillation to prevent introduction of bacteria.
- Do not irrigate the eyes after instillation. Use a new tube or single-use container for ophthalmic ointment administration shortly after birth. May wipe away excess after 1 minute.
- Observe for hypersensitivity.
- Teach parents about the need for eye prophylaxis. Educate them regarding side effects and signs that need to be reported to the healthcare provider.

Activity

Care Plan: Infant Care During Transition

the eyes are wide open, and the baby often makes direct eye contact with human faces within optimal range for visual acuity (7 to 8 in.). It is theorized that this eye contact is an important foundation in establishing attachment in human relationships (Klaus & Klaus, 1985). Consequently, administration of the prophylactic eye medication is often delayed, but no more than 1 hour, to provide an opportunity for a period of eye contact between parents and their newborn, thus facilitating the attachment process (AAP & ACOG, 2012). Parents who cannot be with their newborns in this first period because of maternal or infant distress may need reassurance that the bonding process can proceed normally as soon as both mother and baby are stable.

Another situation that can facilitate attachment is the interactive bath. While bathing their newborn for the first time, parents attend closely to their baby's behavior. In this way, the newborn becomes an active participant and parents are drawn into an interaction with their newborn. The nurse can interpret the infant's behavior, model ways to respond to the behavior, and support parental strategies for doing so.

Evaluation

When evaluating the nursing care provided during the period immediately after birth, the nurse may anticipate the following outcomes:

- The newborn's adaptation to extrauterine life is successful as demonstrated by all vitals within acceptable parameters.
- The newborn's physiologic and psychologic integrity is supported.
- Positive interactions between parent and infant will be supported.

NURSING CARE OF THE NEWBORN FOLLOWING TRANSITION

Once a healthy newborn has demonstrated successful adaptation to extrauterine life, he or she needs appropriate observations for the first 6 to 12 hours after birth and the remainder of the stay in the birthing facility.

Nursing Diagnoses

Examples of nursing diagnoses that may apply during daily care of the newborn include the following (NANDA-I © 2012):

- *Breathing Pattern, Ineffective,* related to periodic breathing
- *Nutrition, Imbalanced: Less than Body Requirements,* related to limited nutritional and fluid intake and increased caloric expenditure
- *Urinary Elimination, Impaired,* related to meatal edema secondary to circumcision
- *Infection, Risk for,* related to umbilical cord healing, circumcision site, immature immune system, or potential birth trauma (forceps or vacuum extraction birth)

Clinical Reasoning **Newborn Breathing Difficulties**

Aisha Khan gave birth to a healthy girl 2 hours ago; she calls you to her room. She sounds frightened and says her baby cannot breathe. You find Aisha cradling her newborn in her arms. The baby is mildly cyanotic, is waving her arms, and has mucus coming from her nose and mouth. What would you do?
See www.nursing.pearsonhigher.com for possible responses.

- *Knowledge, Readiness for Enhanced,* related to information about basic newborn care, male circumcision, and breastfeeding and/or formula-feeding
- *Family Processes, Readiness for Enhanced,* related to integration of newborn into family or demands of newborn care and feeding

Nursing Plan and Implementation
Maintaining Cardiopulmonary Function

Assess vital signs every 6 to 8 hours or more, depending on the newborn's status. The newborn should be placed on the back (supine) for sleeping. A bulb syringe is kept within easy reach should the newborn need oral-nasal suctioning. If the newborn has respiratory difficulty, the nurse clears the airway. Vigorous fingertip stroking of the baby's spine will frequently stimulate respiratory activity. A cardiorespiratory monitor can be used on newborns that are not being observed at all times and are at risk for decreased respiratory or cardiac function. Indicators of risk are pallor, cyanosis, ruddy color, apnea, and other signs of instability. Changes in skin color may indicate the need for closer assessment of temperature, cardiopulmonary status, hematocrit, glucose, and bilirubin levels.

Maintaining a Neutral Thermal Environment

Make every effort to maintain the newborn's temperature within the normal range by continuing interventions started in the first 4-hour period. A newborn whose temperature falls below optimal level uses calories to maintain body heat rather than for growth. Chilling also decreases the affinity of serum albumin for bilirubin, thereby increasing the likelihood of newborn jaundice. In addition, it increases oxygen use and may cause respiratory distress. An overheated newborn will increase activity and respiratory rate in an attempt to cool the body. Both measures deplete caloric reserves, and the increased respiratory rate leads to increased insensible fluid loss (Blackburn, 2013).

Clinical Reasoning **Maintaining the Newborn's Temperature**

John Fredricks, the father of a newborn less than a day old, has the infant lying on its back with only a diaper. When you suggest that the baby may need more covering, he responds: "He doesn't like all that stuff on. After all, he's been naked until now."
   What actions and teaching are appropriate in this situation?
See www.nursing.pearsonhigered.com for possible responses.

Promoting Adequate Hydration and Nutritional Status

Record caloric and fluid intake and enhance adequate hydration by maintaining a neutral thermal environment and offering early and frequent feedings. Early feedings promote gastric emptying and increase peristalsis, thereby decreasing the potential for hyperbilirubinemia by decreasing the amount of time fecal material is in contact with enzyme β-glucuronidase in the small intestine. This enzyme frees the bilirubin from the feces, allowing it to be reabsorbed into the vascular system. The nurse records voiding and stooling patterns. The first voiding should occur within 24 hours and the first passage of stool within 48 hours. When they do not occur, the nurse continues the normal observation routine while assessing for abdominal distention, bowel sounds, hydration, fluid intake, and temperature stability.

The newborn is weighed at the same time each day for accurate comparisons and must be kept warm during the weighing. A weight loss of up to 10% for term newborns is considered within normal limits during the first week of life (Cloherty, Eichenwald, Hansen, et al., 2012). This weight loss is the result of limited intake, loss of excess extracellular fluid, and passage of meconium. Parents should be told about the expected weight loss, the reason for it, and the expectations for regaining the birth weight. Birth weight is usually regained by 2 weeks if feedings are adequate.

Excessive handling can cause an increase in the newborn's metabolic rate and caloric use and cause fatigue. The nurse should be alert to the newborn's subtle cues of fatigue, including a decrease in muscle tension and activity in the extremities and neck, as well as loss of eye contact, which may be manifested by fluttering or closure of the eyelids. The nurse quickly ceases stimulation when signs of fatigue appear. The nurse should demonstrate to parents the need to be aware of newborn cues and to wait for periods of alertness for contact and stimulation. Assess the woman's comfort and latching-on techniques if she is breastfeeding, or assess the bottle-feeding techniques. Breastfeeding and formula-feeding the newborn are discussed in detail later in this chapter.

Promoting Skin Integrity

Newborn skin care, including bathing, is important for the health and appearance of the individual newborn and for infection control within the nursery. Ongoing skin care involves cleansing the buttock and perianal areas with fresh water and cotton or a mild soap and water with diaper changes. If commercial baby wipes are used, those without alcohol should be selected. Perfumed and latex-free wipes are also available.

The umbilical cord is assessed for signs of bleeding or infection. Removal of the cord clamp within 24 to 48 hours of birth reduces the chance of tension injury to the area. Keeping the umbilical stump clean and dry can reduce the chance for infection (Figure 26–5 ●). See Skill 5–4 in the *Clinical Skills Manual* SKILLS .

Many types of routine cord care are practiced, including the use of air-drying, triple dye, an antimicrobial agent such as bacitracin, or application of 70% alcohol to the cord stump. These practices are largely based on tradition rather than evidence-based findings. The skin absorption and toxicity of triple-dye agents in newborns have not been carefully studied. No single method of umbilical cord care has been proven to be superior in preventing umbilical cord colonization and infection (omphalitis) (Cloherty et al., 2012). The use of air-drying results in umbilical cords

● **Figure 26–5** Routine umbilical cord care. The umbilical cord base is carefully cleansed.

Source: George Dodson, Lightworks Studio/Pearson Education.

separating more quickly than those treated with alcohol (Cloherty et al., 2012). Folding the diaper down to avoid covering the cord stump can prevent contamination of the area and promote drying. The nurse is responsible for cord care per agency policy. The cord should look dark and dry up before falling off (Figure 26–6 ●). It is also the nurse's responsibility to instruct parents in caring for the cord and observing for signs and symptoms of infection after discharge, such as foul smell, redness and greenish yellow drainage, localized heat and tenderness, or bright red bleeding or if the area remains unhealed 2 to 3 days after the cord stump has sloughed off.

Promoting Safety

Safety of the newborn is paramount. It is essential that the nurse and other caregivers verify the identity of the newborn by comparing the numbers and names on the identification bracelets of mother and newborn before giving a newborn to a parent (AAP & ACOG, 2012). An additional form of identification band has a built-in sensor unit that sounds an alarm if the newborn is

● **Figure 26–6** The umbilical cord looks dark and dries up prior to falling off.

Source: Courtesy of Anna Garcia.

transported beyond set birthing unit boundaries. Individual birthing units should practice safety measures to prevent infant abduction and provide information to parents regarding their role in this area and in general newborn safety measures. Parental measures to prevent abduction and provide for safety include the following:

Security

- Check that identification bands are in place as they care for their newborn. If bands are missing, parents should ask that they be replaced immediately.

- Allow only people with proper birthing unit picture identification to bring the baby or remove the baby from the room. If parents do not know the staff person, they should call the nurse for assistance.

- Report the presence of any suspicious people on the birthing unit.

Safety

- Never leave the newborn alone in the room. If they walk in the halls or take a shower, parents should have a family member watch the newborn or return the newborn to the nursery.

- A parent who feels weak, faint, or unsteady should not lift the newborn. Instead, the parent should call for assistance.

- Always keep an eye and hand on the newborn when he or she is out of the crib.

- Protect newborns from infection even though they do possess some immunity. Parents should ask visitors to leave if they have any of the following: cold, diarrhea, discharge from sores, or a contagious disease.

Preventing Complications

Newborns are at continued risk for the complications of hemorrhage, late-onset cardiac symptoms, and infection. Pallor may be an early sign of hemorrhage and must be reported to the physician. The newborn is placed on a cardiorespiratory monitor to permit continuous assessment. Several newborn conditions put newborns at risk for hemorrhage. Cyanosis that is not relieved by oxygen administration requires emergency intervention, may indicate a congenital cardiac condition or shock, and requires ongoing assessment.

Infection in the nursery is best prevented by requiring that all personnel who have direct contact with newborns scrub for 2 to 3 minutes from the fingertips up to and including the elbows at the beginning of each shift. The hands must also be washed with soap and rubbed vigorously for 15 seconds before and after contact with every newborn and after touching any soiled surface such as the floor or one's hair or face. Parents are instructed to practice good hand washing and/or use of an antiseptic hand cleaner before touching the newborn. They are also instructed that anyone holding the baby should practice good hand washing, even after the family returns home. In some clinical settings family members are asked to wear gowns (preferably disposable) over their street clothes during their contact with infants. These are good opportunities for the nurse to reinforce the efficacy of hand washing in preventing the spread of infection.

Jaundice occurs in most newborn infants. Most jaundice is benign, but because of the potential toxicity of bilirubin, newborn infants must be monitored to identify those who might develop severe hyperbilirubinemia and, in rare cases, acute bilirubin encephalopathy or kernicterus (see Chapter 28 🔗 for more detailed discussion) (AAP & ACOG, 2012). Current recommendations include obtaining a total serum bilirubin level in any infant that is visibly jaundiced in the first 24 hours of life, and obtaining either a serum or transcutaneous bilirubin level before discharge. Nomograms for evaluating risk factors based on bilirubin levels and age of infant are available (see Chapter 24 🔗).

Circumcision

Circumcision was originally a religious rite practiced by Jews and Muslims. Many parents choose circumcision because they want their male child to have a physical appearance similar to that of his father or the majority of other children or they may feel that it is expected by society. Another commonly cited reason for circumcising newborn males is to prevent the need for anesthesia, hospitalization, pain, and trauma if the procedure is needed later in life (Healthy Children, 2013a). To ensure informed consent, parents should be advised during the prenatal period about possible long-term medical effects of circumcision and noncircumcision.

Circumcision is a surgical procedure in which the prepuce, an epithelial layer covering the penis, is separated from the glans penis and excised. This permits exposure of the glans for easier cleaning. As in the past, recommendations regarding circumcision have varied. The 2005 AAP policy statement reaffirmed that it does not recommend *routine* circumcision but acknowledges that medical indications for circumcision still exist (Cloherty et al., 2012). The policy recommends that acceptable methods of analgesia (dorsal penile nerve block [DPNB], subcutaneous ring block, and eutectic mixture of local anesthetics [EMLA] cream) be used during circumcision to decrease procedural pain (Cloherty et al., 2012). The DPNB and subcutaneous ring block are the most effective options.

Circumcision *should not be performed* if the newborn is premature or compromised, has a known bleeding problem, or is born with a genitourinary defect such as hypospadias or epispadias, which may necessitate the use of the foreskin in future surgical repairs.

Nursing Management. A well-informed nurse can allay parents' anxiety by sharing information and allowing them to express their concerns. In order for parents to make a truly informed decision, they must be knowledgeable about the potential risks and outcomes of circumcision. Hemorrhage, infection, difficulty in voiding, separation of the edges of the circumcision, discomfort, and restlessness are early potential problems (Cloherty et al., 2012).

The parents of an uncircumcised male infant require information from the nurse about good hygienic practices. Tell them that the foreskin and glans are two similar layers of cells that separate from each other. The separation process begins prenatally and is normally completed between 3 to 5 years of age. In the process of separation, sterile sloughed cells build up between the layers. This buildup looks similar to the smegma secreted after puberty, and it is harmless. Occasionally during the daily bath, the parent can gently test for retraction. If retraction has occurred, daily gentle washing of the glans with soap and water is sufficient to maintain adequate cleanliness. The parents should teach the child to incorporate this practice into his daily self-care activities. Most uncircumcised males have no difficulty doing so.

If circumcision is desired, the procedure is performed when the newborn is well stabilized and has received his initial physical examination by a healthcare provider. Before a circumcision, ensure that the physician has explained the procedure, determine whether the parents have any further questions about the procedure, and verify that the circumcision permit is signed. As with any surgical procedure, the infant's identification band should be checked to verify his identity before the procedure begins. Gather the equipment and prepare the newborn by removing the diaper and placing him on a padded circumcision board or some other type of restraint, but restraining only the legs. These restraint measures along with the application of warm blankets to the upper body increase infant comfort during the procedure. In Jewish circumcision ceremonies, the infant is held by the father or godfather and given wine before the procedure.

A variety of devices (Gomco clamp, Plastibell, Mogen clamp) are used for circumcision (Figures 26–7 ● and 26–8 ●), and all

produce minimal bleeding. Therefore, make special note of infants with a family history of bleeding disorders or with mothers who took anticoagulants, including aspirin, prenatally. During the procedure, assess the newborn's response. One important consideration is pain experienced by the newborn. A DPNB or ring block using 1% lidocaine without epinephrine or similar anesthetic significantly minimizes the pain and shifts in behavioral patterns such as crying, irritability, and erratic sleep cycles associated with circumcision. Other studies are investigating the use of topical anesthetic applied 60 to 90 minutes before prepuce removal and the use of sucrose pacifiers before and during the procedure. Studies indicate that a combination of methods is most effective in reducing pain during circumcision.

During the procedure, provide comfort measures such as swaddling, lightly stroking the newborn's head, providing a

Slit here

A

B

● **Figure 26–7** Circumcision using the Yellen or Gomco clamp. **A,** The prepuce is drawn over the cone and **B,** the clamp is applied. Pressure is maintained for 3 to 4 minutes, and then excess prepuce is cut away.

A

B

● **Figure 26–8** Circumcision using the Plastibell. **A,** The bell is fitted over the glans. A suture is tied around the bell's rim and the excess prepuce is cut away. The plastic rim remains in place for 3 to 4 days until healing occurs. The bell may be allowed to fall off; it is removed if still in place after 8 days. **B,** Plastibell.

Source: B, Courtesy of Jo Engle, RN, MSN, NNP-BC, and Vanessa Howell, RN, MSN.

Health Promotion Newborn Circumcision Care

Teach family members how to assess for unusual bleeding, how to respond if it is present, and how to care for the newly circumcised penis. Parents of newborns circumcised with a method other than Plastibell should receive the following information:

- Clean with warm water with each diaper change.
- Apply petroleum ointment for the next few diaper changes to help prevent further bleeding and to protect the healing tissue afterward (Figure 26–9 ●).
- If bleeding does occur, apply light pressure with a sterile gauze pad to stop the bleeding within a short time. If this is not effective, contact the physician immediately, or take the newborn to the healthcare provider.
- The glans normally has granulation tissue (a yellowish film) on it during healing. Continued application of a petroleum ointment (or ointment suggested by the healthcare provider) can help protect the granulation tissue that forms as the glans heals.
- Report to the care provider any signs or symptoms of infection, such as increasing swelling, pus drainage, and cessation of urination.
- When diapering, ensure that the diaper is not too loose to cause rubbing with movement, or too tight to cause pain.
- If the infant's care provider recommends oral analgesics, follow instructions for proper measuring and administration.

● **Figure 26–9** Following circumcision, petroleum ointment may be applied to the site for the next few diaper changes.

Source: George Dodson, Lightworks Studio/Pearson Education.

---

pacifier for nonnutritive sucking, and talking to him. Following the circumcision, the infant should be held and comforted by a family member or the nurse. Be alert to any behavioral cues that these measures are overstimulating the newborn instead of comforting him. Such cues include turning away of the head, increased generalized body movement, skin color changes, hyperalertness, and hiccoughing. See Skill 5–5 in the *Clinical Skills Manual* SKILLS .

Ideally, assess the circumcision every 30 minutes for at least 2 hours following the procedure. It is important to observe the first voiding after a circumcision to evaluate for urinary obstruction related to penile injury or edema.

If the Plastibell is used, provide information to the parents about normal appearance and how to observe for infection. Inform them that the Plastibell should fall off within 8 days. If it remains on after 8 days, they should consult with the newborn's physician. Though no ointments or creams should be used while the bell remains, application of petroleum ointment may protect granulation tissue afterward.

Enhancing Parent–Newborn Attachment

The nurse encourages parent–newborn attachment by involving all family members with the new member of the family. (For specific interventions see Chapter 19 ● and Chapter 30 ● and *Teaching Highlights: What Parents Need to Know About Enhancing Attachment.*) Infant massage is a common childcare practice in many parts of the world, especially Africa and Asia, and has recently gained attention in the United States. Parents can be taught to use infant massage as a method to facilitate the bonding process and to reduce the stress and pain associated with teething, constipation, inoculations, and colic. Infant massage not only

Developing Cultural Competence
Infant Naming in Kenya

In Kenya, the naming of a child is an important event. Names are commonly selected to mirror important or current events. For example, an infant who is born while traveling may be given a name that means "wanderer" or "traveler." Other names may be chosen after a relative who is among the "living-dead" (deceased). It is believed that this results in a partial reincarnation of that relative, especially if the child has characteristics in common with that individual. It is also believed there is a connection between newborns and the spirit world.

induces relaxation for the infant but also provides a calming and "feel-good" interaction for the parents that fosters the development of warm, positive relationships.

The nurse can discuss waking activities such as talking with the newborn while making eye contact, holding the newborn in an upright position (sitting or standing), gently bending the newborn back and forth while grasping under the knees and supporting the head and back with the other hand, or gently rubbing the newborn's hands and feet. Quieting activities may include swaddling or bundling the baby to increase a sense of security; using slow, calming movements; and talking softly, singing, or humming to the newborn.

Caring for newborns in the birthing setting and fostering parent–infant attachment means that the nurse will have contact with patients from a wide variety of racial, religious, and cultural backgrounds. Though it may not be possible to be conversant with all cultures, the nurse can demonstrate cultural competence with both colleagues and patients. The nurse must be sensitive

Teaching Highlights **What Parents Need to Know About Enhancing Attachment**

- Information on the periods of reactivity, expected newborn responses, and normal newborn physical characteristics.
- The gradual developmental nature of the bonding process and the reciprocal interactive nature of the process.
- The infant's capabilities for interaction such as nonverbal communication abilities. Nonverbal communications include movement, gaze, touch, facial expressions, and vocalizations—including crying. Eye contact is considered one of the cardinal factors in developing infant–parent attachment and will be integrated with touching and vocal behaviors.
- Touching, including stroking, patting, massaging, and kissing, will progress to interactive touch between parent and infant; parents need to assimilate these and other comforting behaviors (talking, singing, swaddling, rocking) into daily routines with their baby.
- The infant's behaviors will change as the infant matures, and it is important for parents to be consistent in response to their infant's cues and needs.
- Information about pamphlets, videos, and support groups in the community.

to the cultural beliefs and values of the family and be aware of cultural variations in newborn care such as naming the newborn, giving compliments about the newborn, and using good luck charms (see *Developing Cultural Competence: Examples of Cultural Beliefs and Practices Regarding Baby Care*).

Evaluation

When evaluating the nursing care provided during the newborn period, the nurse may anticipate the following outcomes:

- The baby's physiologic and psychologic integrity is supported by maintaining stable vital signs and interactions based on normal newborn behaviors.
- The newborn feeding pattern will be satisfactorily established.
- The parents express understanding of the bonding process and display attachment behaviors.

INFANT FEEDING

Early nutrition has a significant impact on the present and future health and well-being of the infant because this is a period of rapid growth and brain development. Good nutrition fosters physical growth and helps maintain a healthy immune

Developing Cultural Competence **Examples of Cultural Beliefs and Practices Regarding Baby Care***

Umbilical Cord

- People of Latin American or Filipino cultural background may use an abdominal binder or bellyband to protect against dirt, injury, and umbilical hernia. They may also apply oils to the stump of the cord or tape metal to the umbilicus to ward off evil spirits (D'Avanzo & Geissler, 2008).
- People of northern European ancestry may expect a sterile cutting of the cord at birth. They may allow the stump to air-dry and discard the cord once it falls off.
- Some Latin American parents cauterize the stump with a hot flame, hot coal, or the like (WHO, 1999).
- In Kenya, women may express colostrum onto the cord stump (WHO, 1999).
- In Ecuador, the cord stump is left long in girls to prevent a small uterus and problems with childbirth (WHO, 1999).

Parent–Infant Contact

- People of Asian ancestry may pick up the baby as soon as it cries, or they may carry the baby at all times.
- Several native North American nations' people, notably the Navajos, may use cradle boards, so the infant can be with family even during work and feel secure (Woodring & Andrews, 2012).
- The Muslim father traditionally calls praise to Allah in the newborn's right ear and cleans the infant after birth.

Circumcision

- People of Muslim and Jewish ancestry practice circumcision as a religious ritual.

- Many natives of Africa and Australia practice circumcision as a puberty rite.
- Native Americans and people of Asian and Latin American cultures rarely perform circumcision (Lipson & Dibble, 2008).
- According to 2006 global estimates, about 30% of males are circumcised (WHO, 2008).

Health and Illness

- Some people from Latin American cultural backgrounds may believe that touching the face or head of an infant when admiring it will ward off the "evil eye." They may also neglect to cut the baby's nails to avoid nearsightedness and instead put mittens on the baby's hands to prevent scratching. They also may believe that fat babies are healthy (Woodring & Andrews, 2012).
- Some people of Asian heritage may not allow anyone to touch the baby's head without asking permission.
- Some Orthodox Jews believe that saying the baby's name before the formal naming ceremony will harm the baby.
- Asians and Haitians may delay naming their infants until after confinement month (D'Avanzo & Geissler, 2008).
- Some people of Vietnamese ancestry believe that cutting a baby's hair or nails will cause illness.

**Note:* The information is meant only to provide examples of the behaviors that may be found within certain cultures. Not all members of a culture practice the behaviors described.

system. In addition, infant feeding is an important component of newborn socialization that promotes cognitive and emotional development.

The newborn's diet must supply all the nutrients required by the body in the proper quantities to meet the newborn's rapid rate of physical and neurologic growth and development. A newborn's diet should provide adequate hydration and sufficient calories and must include protein, carbohydrates, fat, vitamins, and minerals. Exclusive breast milk and/or iron-fortified 20-calorie/ounce formula are sufficient as sole sources of nutrition to meet the dietary needs of the newborn from birth up to 6 months of age. Complementary solid foods are introduced in the second half of the first year, and the infant continues to receive breast milk and/or formula until at least 12 months of age (American Academy of Pediatrics Section on Breastfeeding, 2012). See Chapter 33 *⊘* for a discussion of infant nutrition.

CHOICE OF FEEDING: BREAST VERSUS FORMULA

Feeding their newborn is an exciting, satisfying, but often worrisome task for parents. Meeting this essential need of their new child helps parents strengthen their attachment to their child and fosters their self-images as nurturers and providers, yet carries great responsibility. Whether a woman chooses to breastfeed or formula-feed, she can adequately meet her infant's needs. As questions about feeding arise, the nurse works with the woman to help her develop skill in her chosen method. In every interaction, it is the nurse's responsibility to support the parents and promote the family's sense of confidence.

The mother usually decides to breastfeed or formula-feed by the sixth month of pregnancy and often even before conception. However, she may not make her final decision until admission to the birth center. The decision is often influenced by relatives, especially the baby's father and maternal grandmother (Association of Women's Health, Obstetric and Neonatal Nurses [AWHONN], 2007), by friends, and by social customs rather than being based on knowledge about the nutritional and psychologic needs of the mother and her newborn.

Once the parents have made an informed choice of feeding method, the nurse's primary responsibilities are to support the family's decision and to help the family achieve a positive result. No woman should be made to feel either inadequate or superior because of her choice in feeding. There are advantages and disadvantages to breastfeeding and bottle-feeding, but positive bonds in parent–child relationships can be developed with either method.

BREASTFEEDING

Breast Milk Production

The female breast is divided into 15 to 20 lobes, separated from one another by fat and connective tissue, and interspersed with blood vessels, lymphatic vessels, and nerves. These lobes are subdivided into connected lobules composed of small units

called alveoli where milk is synthesized by the alveolar secretory epithelium. The lobules have a system of lactiferous ducts that join larger ducts and eventually open onto the nipple surface (Riordan & Wambach, 2010). Mothers are often surprised to see milk coming out of multiple nipple pores when they express their milk. See Figure 26–10 *●* to view the anatomy of the breast.

Physiologic and Endocrine Control of Lactogenesis

During pregnancy, increased levels of estrogen stimulate breast duct proliferation and development, and elevated progesterone levels promote the development of lobules and alveoli in preparation for lactation. Prolactin levels rise from approximately 10 ng/mL prepregnancy to 200 ng/mL at term. However, lactation is suppressed during pregnancy by elevated progesterone levels secreted by the placenta. Once the placenta is expelled

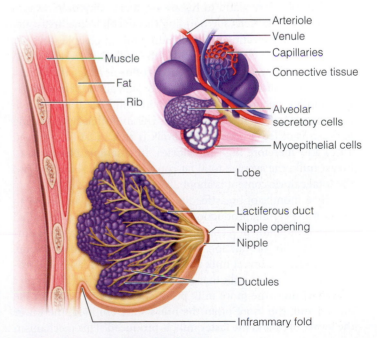

● **Figure 26–10** Anatomy of the breast.

at birth, progesterone levels fall and the inhibition is removed, triggering milk production. This occurs whether the mother has breast stimulation or not. However, if by the third or fourth day breast stimulation is not occurring, prolactin levels begin to drop.

Initially, lactation is under endocrine control. The hormone **prolactin** is released from the anterior pituitary in response to breast stimulation from suckling or the use of a breast pump. Prolactin levels double each time the infant suckles at the breast, regardless of the age of the infant or duration of lactation. Prolactin stimulates the milk-secreting cells in the alveoli to produce milk, then rapidly drops back to baseline. If more than approximately 3 hours occur between stimulation, prolactin levels begin to drop below baseline. To reverse the overall decline in prolactin level, the mother can be encouraged to stimulate her breasts more frequently (e.g., every 1.5 to 2 hours). Mothers should be strongly encouraged to stimulate their breasts frequently if their infants are not effective feeders or if they are separated from their infants. Prolactin receptors are established during the first 2 weeks postpartum in response to frequency of breast stimulation (Human Milk Banking Association of North America [HMBANA], 2011). Inadequate development of prolactin receptors during this time is likely to negatively impact the mother's long-term milk volume. By 2 weeks postpartum, prolactin levels will be back to prepregnancy levels and milk production will cease if stimulation of the breasts by breastfeeding or pumping does not occur (Lawrence & Lawrence, 2011).

The milk that flows from the breast at the start of a feeding or pumping session is called **foremilk**. The foremilk is watery milk high in protein and low in fat (1% to 2%). This milk has trickled down from the alveoli between feedings to fill the lactiferous ducts. It is low-fat milk because the fat globules made in the alveoli stick to each other and to the walls of the alveoli and do not trickle down.

In addition to prolactin release, stretching of the nipple and compression of the areola signal the hypothalamus to trigger the posterior pituitary gland to release oxytocin. **Oxytocin** acts on the myoepithelial cells surrounding the alveoli in the breast tissue to contract, ejecting milk, including the fat globules present, into the ducts. This process is called the *milk ejection reflex*, better known in lay terms as the **letdown reflex** or *letdown response*. The average initial letdown response occurs about 2 minutes after an infant begins to suckle, and there will be 4 to 10 letdown responses during a feeding session. The milk that flows during letdown is called hindmilk. **Hindmilk** is rich in fat (can exceed 10%) and therefore high in calories. In a sample of expressed breast milk, the average total fat concentration is about 4% and the total caloric content is about 20 calories/ounce.

By 6 months of breastfeeding, prolactin levels are only 5 to 10 ng/mL, yet milk production continues. A whey protein called feedback inhibitor of lactation (FIL) has been identified as influencing milk production through a negative feedback loop. FIL is present in breast milk and functions to decrease milk production. The more milk that remains in the breast for a longer period of time, the more milk production is decreased. On the other hand, the more often the breasts are emptied, the lower the level of FIL and the faster milk is produced. This mechanism of regulating milk at the local level is called autocrine control.

This process is key to understanding how a mother maintains or loses her milk supply (Blackburn, 2013).

A number of factors can delay or impair lactogenesis. Maternal factors include cesarean birth, primiparity, long duration of stage 1 or stage 2 of labor, postpartum hemorrhage, type 1 diabetes, untreated hypothyroidism, obesity, polycystic ovary syndrome, retained placenta fragments, vitamin B_6 deficiency, history of previous breast surgery, insufficient glandular breast tissue, and significant stress (Riordan & Wambach, 2010). Other factors that can interfere with breastfeeding include smoking and use of alcohol, as well as some prescription and over-the-counter medications (e.g., antihistamines, combined birth control pills).

Stages of Human Milk

During the establishment of lactation there are three stages of human milk: colostrum, transitional milk, and mature milk.

Colostrum is the initial milk that begins to be secreted during midpregnancy and is immediately available to the baby at birth. Colostrum is a thick, creamy yellowish fluid with concentrated amounts of protein, fat-soluble vitamins, and minerals, and it has lower amounts of fat and lactose compared with mature milk. It also contains antioxidants and high levels of lactoferrin and secretory IgA. It promotes the establishment of *Lactobacillus bifidus* flora in the digestive tract, which helps to protect the infant from disease and illness. Colostrum also has a laxative effect on the infant, which helps the baby pass meconium stools, which in turn helps decrease hyperbilirubinemia. Although the volume of colostrum is small, it encourages the newborn to nurse frequently, helping to stimulate milk production. No supplementation with other fluids is necessary unless there is a medical condition.

The onset of copious milk secretion begins between 32 and 96 hours postpartum. For most women this is observed on day 3. Laypeople refer to this as the milk "coming in," and it is called **transitional milk**. Transitional milk has qualities intermediate to colostrum and mature milk but may look indistinguishable from colostrum. It is still light yellow in color but is more copious than colostrum and contains more fat, lactose, water-soluble vitamins, and calories. See Figure 26–11 ● to view a picture of transitional milk. By day 5, most mothers are producing about 16 oz/day (Riordan & Wambach, 2010).

Mature milk is white or slightly blue-tinged in color. It is present by 2 weeks postpartum and continues thereafter until lactation ceases. Mature milk contains about 13% solids (carbohydrates, proteins, and fats) and 87% water. Although mature human milk appears similar to skim cow's milk and may cause mothers to question whether their milk is "rich enough," mothers should be reassured that this is the normal appearance of mature human milk and that it provides the infant with all the necessary nutrients. Although gradual changes in composition do occur continuously over periods of weeks to accommodate the needs of the growing newborn, in general the composition of mature milk is fairly consistent with the exception of the fat content as noted previously. Milk production continues to increase slowly over the first month. By 6 months postpartum a mother produces about 27 oz (800 mL) per day (Blackburn, 2013).

Immunologic Advantages

The immunologic advantages of breast milk include varying degrees of protection from respiratory tract and gastrointestinal tract infections, necrotizing enterocolitis, urinary tract infections, otitis media, bacterial meningitis, bacteremia, and allergies (AWHONN, 2007). Transplacental passage of maternal immunoglobulin gradually diminishes over the first 6 months of life until the infant can begin to produce his or her own immunoglobulins. Human milk-derived immunologic protection helps supplement this protection.

Secretory IgA, an immunoglobulin present in colostrum and breast milk, has antiviral, antibacterial, and antigenic-inhibiting properties, specifically across mucosal surfaces such as the intestinal tract. Secretory IgA plays a role in decreasing the permeability of the small intestine to help prevent large protein molecules from triggering an allergic response. Other constituents of colostrum and breast milk that act to inhibit the growth of bacteria or viruses are *Lactobacillus bifidus,* lysozymes, lactoperoxidase, lactoferrin, transferrin, and various immunoglobulins.

All babies should receive vaccination following a schedule as recommended by the Centers for Disease Control and Prevention (CDC, 2013). The current vaccination schedule can be viewed online at the CDC website for Breastfeeding Resources (CDC, 2013). (See Chapter 44 🔗 for discussion of immunizations.) Mothers may worry that their antibodies will inactivate the live poliovirus. But breastfeeding does not adversely affect immunization and is not a contraindication for any vaccine. Some mothers also wonder if it is safe for them to receive vaccinations while breastfeeding. Mothers should be reassured that most vaccines can safely be taken during the lactation period.

Psychosocial Benefits of Breastfeeding

The psychosocial advantages of breastfeeding include increased self-esteem, enhanced bonding, and a decrease in stress for the mother and infant.

A mother's self-esteem is increased in knowing that she has provided the perfect food for her baby and provided protection with her own antibodies. For many mothers breastfeeding takes effort, understanding, and an emotional commitment to endure the demands of this lifestyle choice. The mother's sense of accomplishment in being able to satisfy her baby's needs for nourishment and comfort can be a tremendous source of personal satisfaction. Also breastfeeding can provide the infant with a fresh, clean, naturally warm source of nutrition. Women who breastfeed, by its nature, have close contact with their infants. Newborns are very responsive to touch, and it is vital for the infant's emotional well-being. The tactile stimulation associated with breastfeeding can communicate warmth, closeness, comfort, and the opportunity to learn each other's behavioral cues and needs. From the release of prolactin and oxytocin while breastfeeding, mothers may feel more affectionate toward their newborns, have improved letdown response, and breastfeed more frequently and for longer periods of time (AWHONN, 2007). See Table 26–3 for a comparison of breastfeeding and formula-feeding.

● **Figure 26–11** Transitional human milk.
Source: Courtesy of Brigitte Hall, RNC, MSN, IBCLC.

Advantages of Breast Milk

In their breastfeeding policy statement, the American Academy of Pediatrics recommends exclusive breastfeeding as the preferred feeding for all infants, with a few exceptions, for the first 6 months and continued breastfeeding during the introduction of solids until the infant is 12 months old or older, as desired. There is overwhelming scientific evidence that shows that breastfeeding provides newborns and infants with specific nutritional, immunologic, and psychosocial advantages over formula-feeding (AAP & ACOG, 2012).

Nutritional Advantages

Human milk provides optimum nutrition for the human infant because it is species specific. The macronutrients such as protein, fat, and carbohydrates (lactose) are synthesized by the mother in the alveoli of the breasts by specialized secretory cells. Micronutrient elements such as vitamins and minerals derive from the circulating maternal plasma. There are more than 200 distinct components in breast milk, with more remaining to be identified (Lawrence & Lawrence, 2011).

Additional health advantages for breastfed infants include reduced risk of developing type 1 or type 2 diabetes mellitus, lymphoma, leukemia, Hodgkin disease, obesity, hypercholesterolemia, and asthma. The mother who breastfeeds has health advantages such as burning additional calories making milk (quicker return to prepregnancy weight), has a decreased risk of developing breast cancer and ovarian cancer, and may have a decreased risk of developing postmenopausal osteoporosis (AWHONN, 2007).

Table 26–3   Comparison of Breastfeeding and Formula-Feeding

Breastfeeding	Formula-Feeding (Iron-Enriched)
INFANT NUTRITION	

Breastfeeding	Formula-Feeding (Iron-Enriched)
■ An ideal balance of nutrients, efficiently absorbed. High bioavailability of iron leaves lower iron for bacterial growth and cell injury. ■ Higher levels of essential fatty acids, lactose, cystine, and cholesterol, necessary for brain and nerve growth. ■ Composition varies according to gestational age and stage of lactation, meeting changing nutritional needs. ■ Long-term decreased incidence of diabetes, cancer, obesity, and asthma. ■ Contains unsaturated fats. ■ Infants determine the volume of milk consumed. ■ Frequency of feeding is determined by infant cues. May feed more frequently as milk digests faster.	■ Derived from bovine milk and/or plant sources. Lower bioavailability of nutrients requires higher concentrations in milk. Additives may cause intolerance. ■ Still missing numerous ingredients. Formulas do not contain cholesterol. Soy and hydrolysate formulas do not contain lactose. DHA and ARA now added. ■ Nutritional value not varied. Nutritional adequacy depends on proper preparation/dilution. ■ Contains saturated fats. ■ Parents or healthcare provider determines the volume consumed. Overfeeding may occur if caregiver is determined that baby empty bottle. ■ Frequency of feeding is determined by infant's cues. May feed less frequently as milk digestion is slower.

IMMUNOLOGIC PROPERTIES

Breastfeeding	Formula-Feeding (Iron-Enriched)
■ Contains immunoglobulins, enzymes, and leukocytes that protect against pathogens. Nutrients promote growth of *Lactobacillus*, protective bacteria. Lower rates of urinary tract infections, otitis media, and other infectious diseases. ■ Anti-infective properties present in the milk permit longer storage duration. ■ Breast milk is hypoallergenic, with minimal risk of protein allergy/intolerance.	■ No anti-infective properties. Formula is linked to an increased incidence of gastrointestinal and respiratory tract infections. ■ Potential for bacterial contamination exists during preparation and storage. ■ Cow's milk protein allergy is relatively common.

MATERNAL HEALTH

Breastfeeding	Formula-Feeding (Iron-Enriched)
■ Faster return to prepregnancy weight. ■ Breastfeeding associated with lower risk of breast and ovarian cancer. ■ Concerns over breastfeeding and medications.	■ Provides infant nutrition when breast milk is not available because of maternal illness, medication/drug use, or lactation failure (breast surgery, endocrine disease).

PSYCHOSOCIAL ASPECTS

Breastfeeding	Formula-Feeding (Iron-Enriched)
■ Skin-to-skin contact enhances bonding. ■ Hormones of lactation promote maternal feelings and sense of well-being. ■ Some mothers may feel ashamed or embarrassed because of the value system of modern society. ■ Leaking of breast milk. ■ Breastfeeding after returning to work may be difficult.	■ Both parents can participate in positive parent–infant interaction during feeding. ■ Father can assume feeding responsibilities.

COST

Breastfeeding	Formula-Feeding (Iron-Enriched)
■ Healthy diet for mother. ■ Savings for infant medical costs: approximately $400 average in first year of life. ■ Ancillary costs: nursing pads, nursing bras. ■ A breast pump may be needed. ■ Refrigeration is necessary for storing expressed milk.	■ Formula cost per year: $1200 for standard formula, $2500 for hypoallergenic formulas. ■ Ancillary costs: bottles or bottle liners, nipples, cleaning costs. ■ Refrigeration is needed if preparing more than one bottle at a time.

CONVENIENCE

Breastfeeding	Formula-Feeding (Iron-Enriched)
■ Milk is always the perfect temperature. No preparation time is needed. ■ The mother must be available to feed or will need to provide expressed milk to be given in her absence. ■ If she misses a feeding, the mother must express milk to maintain lactation. ■ The mother may experience breast tenderness and engorgement in the early days of lactation. ■ Limited birth control options and vaginal dryness.	■ Formula must be purchased commercially. ■ Preparation is time consuming. Less convenient for traveling or for night feedings. ■ Mother need not be present—anyone can feed the infant

Potential Contraindications

There are some instances when breastfeeding is or may be contraindicated:

- Mother is HIV-positive or has AIDS, is counseled against breastfeeding except in countries where the risk of neonatal death from diarrhea and other disease (excluding AIDS) is high (AAP & ACOG, 2012).

- Mother has active, untreated tuberculosis; has varicella; is HTLV1–positive (human T-cell leukemia virus type 1); or has another illness, on a case-by-case basis.

- Mother has active herpes on her breast—the infant may still feed on the unaffected side only until the lesion has healed.

- Mother uses illicit drugs (e.g., cocaine, heroin) or is an alcoholic.

- Mother smokes posing health risks to herself and potential secondhand exposure risks to her baby. Research shows that smoking by breastfeeding mothers can significantly alter infants' sleep-wake cycles, causing infants to sleep less, and also affects milk flavor. Maternal smoking can result in breast milk concentrations of nicotine of 1.5 to 3 times the maternal plasma concentration. However, babies who receive breast milk from mothers who smoke are healthier than babies who receive formula and live in a household with smokers. Mothers who smoke cigarettes can breast-feed. To minimize effects on the baby, mothers should time their smoking to immediately *after* breastfeeding and should not smoke in the same room as the infant (AAP & ACOG, 2012).

- Mother takes specific medications (e.g., radioactive iso-topes, antimetabolites, chemotherapy drugs, and a few others). A mother with a diagnosis of breast cancer should not breastfeed so that she can begin treatment immediately.

- Infant has galactosemia.

Postpartum maternal concerns about breastfeeding are discussed in Chapter 30 🔗.

Potential Problems in Breastfeeding

Because mothers are discharged from the birthing unit before breastfeeding is well established, they are frequently alone when they encounter changes in the breastfeeding process. Many women stop nursing if the situations they encounter seem to pose problems. Nurses can offer anticipatory guidance regarding common breastfeeding phenomena and provide resources for the woman's use after discharge. (See Chapter 30 🔗 for a detailed discussion of self-care measures the nurse can suggest to a woman with a breastfeeding problem after discharge from the birthing unit.)

Timing of Newborn Feedings

The timing of newborn feedings is ideally determined by physiologic and behavioral cues rather than a set schedule.

Initiating the First Feeding

The timing of the first feeding varies depending on whether the newborn is to be breastfed or formula-fed and whether there were any complications during pregnancy or birth, such as maternal diabetes or intrauterine growth restriction (IUGR). Mothers who choose to breastfeed their newborns should be encouraged to put the baby to the breast during the first period of reactivity. This practice should be encouraged because successful, long-term breastfeeding during infancy appears to be related to beginning breastfeedings in the first few hours of life. Sleep-wake states affect feeding behavior and need to be considered when evaluating the newborn's sucking ability.

Formula-fed newborns usually begin the first feedings by 5 hours of age, during the second period of reactivity when they awaken and appear hungry. Observing the earlier, more subtle cues that the newborn is ready to nurse provides an opportunity for the nurse to teach the parents to recognize these cues and respond before the newborn is frustrated and crying.

The nurse should assess for active bowel sounds, absence of abdominal distention, and a lusty cry that quiets and is replaced with rooting and sucking behaviors when a stimulus is placed near the lips. These signs indicate that the newborn is hungry and physically ready to tolerate the initial feeding.

If there are no complications at the birth and the mother is not overly sedated, the infant may be placed on the mother's chest after birth. This skin-to-skin contact after birth helps the baby maintain body temperature, helps with self-regulation, increases maternal oxytocin levels, helps the mother to notice subtle feeding cues, and promotes bonding (Figure 26–12 ●).

Throughout the first 2 hours after birth, but especially during the first hour of life, the infant is usually alert and ready to breastfeed. This first feeding should not be forced. Some babies are content just licking the nipple or nuzzling up against the breast initially. Early breastfeeding can enhance maternal–infant bonding and facilitate release of oxytocin, which helps contract the uterus, expelling the placenta and decreasing the risk of post-partum hemorrhage.

● **Figure 26–12** Mother and infant skin-to-skin.
Source: Courtesy of Brigitte Hall, RNC, MSN, IBCLC.

Activity

Case Study: Breastfeeding Patient

Early feedings benefit the newborn because they enhance maternal–infant attachment; stimulate peristalsis, helping to eliminate the by-products of bilirubin conjugation (which decreases the risk of jaundice); help prevent hypoglycemia; promote the passage of meconium; provide the immunologic protection of colostrum; and begin to stimulate further maternal milk production, helping prevent later feeding difficulties.

If the mother plans to bottle-feed, she and her newborn can still enjoy skin-to-skin contact initially. Formula-feedings are not typically initiated in the birthing room. Bottle-fed newborns are offered formula as soon as they show an interest or feeding cues, or per agency policy. For both breastfed and formula-fed infants, early feeding enhances maternal–infant attachment and stimulates peristalsis, helping to eliminate the by-products of bilirubin conjugation (which decreases the risk of jaundice).

Assessment of the newborn's physiologic status is a primary and ongoing concern to the nurse throughout the first feeding. Extreme fatigue coupled with tachypnea, dusky color, and diaphoresis while feeding is most likely symptomatic for respiratory and/or cardiac problems or, rarely, esophageal anomalies (see Chapter 27 🔗). Findings associated with esophageal anomalies include maternal polyhydramnios and increased oral mucus in the infant. Although the nurse is always on the alert for any complications, keep in mind that it is not unusual for healthy newborns to regurgitate a small amount of mucus, fluid, or milk shortly after feeding, or to develop hiccups. Most babies have "wet burps" at some point and virtually all have some degree of reflux. Holding the baby upright on the parent's chest for 15 to 20 minutes after a feeding and not placing the baby in a car seat or swing (which increases abdominal pressure) for that time can help decrease the incidence of reflux. Once the newborn is tolerating feeding, the infant's normal position after feeding is on his or her back.

Establishing a Feeding Pattern

An "on-demand" feeding program facilitates each baby's own rhythm and helps a new mother establish lactation. Unrestricted feedings are best accomplished by hospitals that provide mother-baby rooming-in practices on a 24-hour basis. When the father is able to room in with the mother and new baby, it allows both parents to participate and learn how to care for their infant; this has been shown to be important in the development of the family relationship. Having the father room in also allows the mother with a cesarean delivery to keep her baby at the bedside. When mothers and babies are not separated after birth, mothers and fathers are better able to respond to their babies' needs more quickly than the nursery staff may be able to, resulting in less infant crying, natural feeding intervals, and an adequate number of feedings in a 24-hour period.

Following the initial alert period (approximately the first 2 hours after birth), the newborn typically falls into a deep sleep for several hours. Mothers should be encouraged to rest during this time too. When the newborn awakens, he or she will likely want to nurse frequently, alternating between relatively short periods of light sleep and quiet wakefulness. As wakefulness and interest in nursing increase, the infant will often cluster 5 to 10 feeding episodes over 2 to 3 hours (Riordan & Wambach, 2010). The mother may misinterpret "cluster feedings" in the first few days of life to mean that her infant is not satisfied because she is not producing enough milk. The nurse should take this opportunity to reinforce the mother's perception that the infant wants additional milk, but point out that cluster feeding is a normal and necessary pattern to stimulate the mother's milk production. Formula supplementation is not indicated and will actually delay milk production.

Some healthy infants are uninterested in nursing and just want to sleep for the first few days after birth. This pattern is noted in babies whose mothers have had a difficult labor, a prolonged pushing stage during delivery, or medication (especially multiple dosing) for labor pain or for a cesarean birth.

Late-preterm infants (infants born between 35 weeks' but less than 38 weeks' gestation) also tend to be very sleepy for the first few days, much more so than full-term infants. In addition, male infants who have undergone a circumcision procedure often become very sleepy after surgery. These sleepy babies are at risk of losing an excessive amount of weight, becoming dehydrated, and developing exaggerated jaundice in just a few days after birth. In addition, the mother may develop pathologic engorgement if her baby does not wake up to breastfeed frequently and effectively during this time.

Complementary Care Herbs for Breastfeeding

Galactogogues are commonly used to increase a mother's milk production when her supply is decreased, to assist in reestablishing a milk supply after weaning, and to assist in initiating lactation such as when an adoptive mother desires to nurse her infant. They include fenugreek, goat's rue, milk thistle, anise, basil, blessed thistle, fennel seeds, and marshmallow (Academy of Breastfeeding Medicine [ABM], 2011).

Most mothers taking galactogogues notice an increase in their milk supply within 1 to 3 days. A mother should be counseled that taking a galactogogue alone will not solve her low milk supply problem. She must also increase the frequency of breastfeeding (or pumping with a good quality breast pump) to have the best results. Ideally, the mother should stimulate her breasts 8 to 12 times a day, especially while lactation is getting reestablished. She also needs to balance the demands in her life and try to get rest when she can and lessen her stress. (Stress has a negative impact on a mother's milk supply.) She must also continue to drink to quench her thirst and eat a healthy diet, which includes receiving a minimum of 1800 calories per day. These behaviors will also help to increase her milk supply.

Herbal galactogogues can be consumed as a tea, or can be taken as capsules or as a tincture added to liquid to drink. Fenugreek is probably the most well-known herbal galactogogue among lactation consultants in the United States. Mothers with diabetes, asthma, or allergies to peanuts, soy, chickpeas, or garbanzo beans, or who are taking warfarin sodium (Coumadin) should consult with their healthcare provider before taking this herb (Academy of Breastfeeding Medicine [ABM], 2011). Other herbs thought to increase milk supply include alfalfa, dandelion, fennel, horsetail, red raspberry, caraway, and anise. Women with lupus should read labels to avoid preparations that include alfalfa which can exacerbate their disease.

To avoid these complications, parents can be taught techniques to wake their sleepy baby whenever the infant shows signs of being in the light state-of-sleep cycle. With a little help, the baby may be gently aroused to breastfeed. One method is to remove the baby's blanket and clothing so that the infant is wearing only a diaper and T-shirt. Babies feed better when they are not bundled, and they can actually achieve a better attachment without the bulk of extra clothing and blankets in the way. If the room is too cool for the newborn to feed in just a diaper and T-shirt, have the mother apply a blanket over the top of her baby *after* the baby has attached to the breast. Another technique is to undo and check the baby's diaper. Sitting the baby in a burping position and gently "walking" fingers along the back will usually arouse the baby. Parents should also be encouraged to talk or sing to their baby while trying these techniques to further arouse their baby from sleep.

If the newborn falls asleep after the first few suckles, encourage the mother to use tactile stimulation while the newborn is still attached to the breast. The mother can also be encouraged to use breast compression or breast massage while the infant is breastfeeding to keep milk trickling into the infant's mouth until the infant stimulates the mother to release her milk. If this is not sufficient to keep the baby actively feeding, suggest that the mother remove the baby from the breast momentarily and try to burp the infant. The infant may not actually burp but the burping technique may help wake the infant.

An infant's feeding pattern may change again when the mother's breasts become fuller. Mothers' breasts begin to look and feel noticeably heavier between the second and fourth day postpartum. When milk production has noticeably increased, the "cluster feeding" pattern ceases until the infant has the first growth spurt at about 2 weeks of age. Now an infant generally feeds every 1 ½ to 3 hours around the clock, about 8 to 12 feedings per day. Feeding intervals are counted from the time of the start of one feeding to the start of the next feeding. During this engorgement phase of lactation some infants may struggle initially with latch-on, especially if the mother allows greater than 3 hours to lapse between feedings. If the newborn is not breastfeeding often or effectively enough to soften the breasts, then the breasts may become quite firm and the mother's nipple may become less pliable and this can lead to a shallow latch attachment and sore nipples. If this occurs, the mother can try to express some milk to soften her areola before latching her infant. When her baby breastfeeds on this fuller than usual breast, it is not uncommon for the infant to only want to feed on just the one side. This feeding pattern usually does not last long either. Within days the infant will be back to feeding at both breasts again.

Formula-fed newborns generally sleep longer at a stretch and awaken to feed every 3 to 4 hours, typically feeding only 6 to 8 times per day. To compensate for sleeping longer between feedings, formula-fed infants feed a larger volume at each feeding. It will be awhile before the baby sleeps through the night.

Regardless of whether a mother is breastfeeding or formula-feeding her infant, many parents are distressed by their infant's erratic feeding pattern. Parents need to be informed about normal infant feeding and sleeping patterns and be aware that these patterns vary among babies and change over days, weeks, and months according to the infant's growth and development. In the beginning, the "average" newborn sleeps a total of 16 hours a day. Infants wake to feed and generally fall back to sleep within an hour.

Satiety behaviors are the same for formula-fed babies as for breastfed babies. These behaviors include longer pauses toward the end of the feeding and noticeable total body relaxation (the baby lies limp with hands down at his side and unclenched). The infant may also release the mother's nipple or the bottle nipple, and may fall asleep. If a baby is satiated and content following feedings, is meeting daily output expectations, and is gaining weight as expected, then feedings are going well.

On the other hand, if a breastfeeding baby awakens shortly after feeding and is exhibiting feeding cues, this baby should be offered the breast again regardless of when he or she was last fed. The newborn may be cluster feeding or may not have fed efficiently at the previous feeding. Pacifier use in response to this early waking is especially inappropriate. The pacifier needlessly postpones the feeding, which is indicated based on hunger cues and can have a negative consequence for the mother's milk supply and the infant's weight. The American Academy of Pediatrics recommends waiting to introduce a pacifier in the breastfeeding newborn until breastfeeding is well established, generally when the infant is 3 to 4 weeks old. A formula-feeding infant can be offered a pacifier any time after birth, which is thought to help reduce the risk for sudden infant death syndrome (SIDS) (AAP, 2013b).

SAFETY ALERT!

Parents should be instructed never to put honey or corn syrup on their infant's pacifier to encourage an infant to accept it. Honey and possibly corn syrup may be contaminated with *Clostridium botulinum*, a bacterium that causes infantile botulism. Botulism is rare, but when it occurs it causes serious illness.

Both breastfed and formula-fed infants experience growth spurts at certain times and require increased feeding. The breastfeeding mother may meet these increased demands by nursing more frequently to increase her milk supply. It takes about 72 hours for the milk supply to increase adequately to meet the new demand. A slight increase in feedings meets the formula-fed infant's needs.

Nourishing her newborn is a major concern of the new mother. Her feelings of success or failure may influence her self-concept as she assumes her maternal role. With proper instruction, support, and encouragement from professionals, breastfeeding becomes a source of pleasure and satisfaction to both the parents and infant.

Cultural Considerations in Infant Feeding

Healthcare professionals can learn about an individual patient's cultural background by engaging in discussions with the patient and asking questions in a sensitive and respectful way. This provides opportunity to validate healthy practices and to exert a positive influence on other matters. An occasion for this kind of dialogue might arise during interactions with a new mother who may have misconceptions about breastfeeding. For example, if a new mother says she heard that getting upset or angry will spoil her milk, you can point out that this belief likely stems from the correct observation that the breastfeeding infant can sense maternal tension (which also may delay letdown) and may therefore act fussy as well, appearing to behave as if he or she were getting "spoiled milk." Then reassure the mother that there is no evidence that the milk composition itself is changed. This will allow you to focus on the real issues of bonding and relaxation technique. Simply understanding what is really going on may help the mother to be more relaxed.

Whenever possible, it is best to have a female, non-family member translator present to interpret for a mother. For Muslim women, it is culturally unacceptable for them to speak about intimate matters in front of their families. Therefore, it would be inappropriate to ask the new mother's husband or her children to be her interpreter. Even among those who speak English, language barriers and miscommunications still exist due in part to words having different meanings to people of different cultures. It is important to give enough explanation to ensure that the mother clearly understands the information provided. These are but a few of the numerous cultural influences related to feeding. (See *Developing Cultural Competence: Breastfeeding in Other Cultures.*) When nurses are faced with an infant care practice different from the ones to which they are accustomed, they need to evaluate the effect of the practice. Different practices are not necessarily inferior. The nurse should intervene only if the practice is actually harmful to the mother or baby.

Breastfeeding Technique

Breastfeeding Positions and Latching On

Breastfeeding is not instinctive, it is learned. It is a natural process, but it takes "know-how." Ideally, each breastfeeding mother should have a breastfeeding evaluation to determine any knowledge deficits, acknowledge any concerns, provide instructions, and assist with breastfeeding.

Positioning. There are many breastfeeding positions, but only the four classic breastfeeding positions will be discussed here: (1) modified cradle position, (2) cradle position, (3) football (or clutch) hold position, and (4) side-lying position (Figures 26–13 ● through 26–16 ●). After a mother has fed using one position, encourage her to try a different position when she offers her second breast. Alternating positions facilitates drainage of the breasts and changes the pressure points on the breast. This will provide some relief to the mother with sore nipples.

Latching On. It is important to have the mother and baby positioned properly in order to achieve an optimal attachment. If, for example, the infant is lying flat on the back (supine position) to feed, then the infant can obtain only a shallow latch (not attached far back onto the areola). The infant's shoulder becomes an obstacle putting distance between the infant's mouth and the mother's breast. Anything that contributes to a shallow latch is going to cause sore nipples and other complications. Nipple trauma, although relatively common, is not normal. (See Chapter 30 ● for a discussion of breastfeeding with inverted or flat nipples.)

The infant needs to attach the lips onto the breast or, more accurately, far back onto the areola, not on the nipple. If the infant attaches just to the nipple, the mother will have sore nipples

and pain may inhibit the letdown reflex. To obtain a deep latch, the mother needs to be taught how to elicit the infant's rooting reflex, stimulating the infant to open the mouth as widely as possible (like a big yawn). Once the infant does this, the mother should quickly but gently draw her baby in toward her. During the first few days of life, the newborn typically only opens the mouth widely for a second or so, and then begins to close the mouth again. If the mother misses her chance to get her baby latched on, she needs to simply start over again.

Figures 26–17 ● through 26–22 ● demonstrate various positions and techniques used in latching on.

Clinical Tip

As you assist new mothers with breastfeeding, it is important to create a relaxed environment and approach to breastfeeding. Encourage the mother to get into a comfortable position, well supported with pillows. Remind her to bring the baby to her breast rather than leaning forward to the baby.

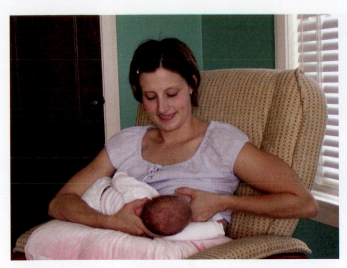

- Have the mother sit comfortably in upright position using good body alignment. Use pillows for support (may use Boppy, body pillow, or standard bed pillows). Lap pillow should help bring the baby up to breast level so the mother does not lean over baby.
- Place the baby on the mother's lap and turn the baby's entire body toward the mother (the baby is in side-lying position). Position the baby's body so that the baby's nose lines up to the nipple. Maintain the baby's body in a horizontal alignment.
- To feed at left breast, the mother supports the baby's head with her right hand at nape of the baby's neck (allow head to slightly lag back); the mother's right thumb by the baby's left ear, and right forefinger near the baby's right ear.
- With the mother's free left hand, she can offer her left breast.

● Figure 26–13 Modified cradle position.
Source: Courtesy of Brigitte Hall, RNC, MSN, IBCLC.

- Have the mother sit comfortably in upright position using good body alignment. Use pillows for support (may use Boppy, body pillow, or standard bed pillows). Lap pillow should help bring the baby up to breast level so the mother does not lean over the baby.
- Place the baby on the mother's lap and turn the baby's entire body toward the mother (the baby is in side-lying position). Position the baby's body so that the baby's nose lines up to the nipple. Maintain the baby's body in a horizontal alignment.
- If feeding from the left breast, have the mother cradle the baby's head near the crook of her left arm while supporting her baby's body with her left forearm.
- With the mother's free right hand, she can offer her left breast.

● Figure 26–14 Cradle position.
Source: Courtesy of Brigitte Hall, RNC, MSN, IBCLC.

- Have the mother sit comfortably and use pillows to raise the baby's body to breast level. If using a Boppy and the Boppy is in "normal" position on the mother's lap, turn it counterclockwise slightly (if feeding at left breast) to provide extended support for the baby's body resting along the mother's left side and near the back of the mother's chair.
- If feeding at left breast, place the baby on the left side of the mother's body, heading the baby into position feet first. The baby's bottom should rest on the pillow near the mother's left elbow.
- Turn the baby slightly on her side so that she faces the breast.
- The mother's left arm clutches the baby's body close to the mother's body. The baby's body should feel securely tucked in under the mother's left arm.
- Have the mother support the baby's head with her left hand. With the mother's free right hand, she can offer her breast. (Good position for the mother with c-section.)

● Figure 26–15 Football hold position.
Source: Courtesy of Brigitte Hall, RNC, MSN, IBCLC.

- Have the mother rest comfortably lying on her side (left side for this demonstration). Use pillows to support the mother's head and back, and provide support for the mother's hips by placing a pillow between her bent knees.
- Place the baby in side-lying position next to the mother's body. The baby's body should face the mother's body. The baby's nose should line up to the mother's nipple. Place a roll behind the baby's back, if desired.
- With the mother's free right hand, she can offer her left breast. After the baby is securely attached, mom can rest her right hand anywhere that is comfortable for her.

● **Figure 26–16** Side-lying position.
Source: Courtesy of Brigitte Hall, RNC, MSN, IBCLC.

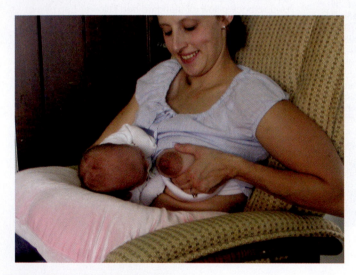

To be ready to draw the baby's mouth onto the mother's breast, as soon as the baby opens her mouth widely enough, the mother needs to have her hand supporting her breast in the ready position. She can use various hand holds, but she needs to keep her fingers well behind the areola. One such hand position is called the "C-hold." In this hold, the thumb is placed on top of the breast near 12:00 position and the other four fingers are placed on the underside of the breast near the 6:00 position (depends on mother's hand size and length of fingers). The key point is to keep the fingers at least 1 1/2 inches back from the base of the nipple as the fingers support the breast. Mothers are not often aware of where they place their fingers especially on the underside of the breast. If the fingers are too far forward (too close to the nipple), then the infant cannot grasp a large amount of areola in her mouth and this results in a "shallow" latch. A shallow latch is associated with nipple pain and ineffective drainage of the breast.
An alternate hand hold not shown is a "U-hold" hand position. The thumb and forefinger are near the 3 and 9 position on the breast again with fingers at least 1 1/2 inches back from the base of the nipple; the body of the hand rests on the lower portion of the breast. Using this hand hold, the mother's arm position is down at her side rather than sticking outward as it is when supporting the breast using the C-hold position.

● **Figure 26–17** C-hold hand position.
Source: Courtesy of Brigitte Hall, RNC, MSN, IBCLC.

Breastfeeding Assessment

During the birthing unit stay, the nurse must carefully monitor the progress of the breastfeeding pair. A systematic assessment of several breastfeeding episodes provides the opportunity to teach the new mother about lactation and the breastfeeding process, provide anticipatory guidance, and evaluate the need for follow-up care after discharge. Criteria for evaluating a breastfeeding session include maternal and infant cues, latch-on, position, let-down, nipple condition, infant response, and maternal response. The literature provides various tools to guide the assessment and documentation of the breastfeeding efforts.

Breastfeeding Efficiency

The mother should be taught to observe the infant for effective breastfeeding. The infant should have a rhythmic suckling pattern (the slight pause between jaw compressions on the breast permits the mouth to fill with milk before swallowing). To note if the jaw compressions are strong enough, the mother should observe or feel if there is movement at the bilateral temporomandibular joints located in front of the infant's ears.

The infant should maintain a rhythmic feeding pattern with only brief pauses (lasting only seconds, not minutes) between spurts of active feeding, with the feeding session typically

The scissor hold is often discouraged because mothers (especially mothers with small hands) have a difficult time keeping their fingers off the areola or at least 1½ inches back from the base of the areola. Here, the mother is able to support her breast well without letting her fingers encroach onto the areola.

The mother should be instructed to gently support the breast and not press too deeply, which can obstruct the flow of milk through the ducts.

● **Figure 26–18** Scissor hold hand position.
Source: Courtesy of Brigitte Hall, RNC, MSN, IBCLC.

Before eliciting the rooting reflex, it is important to have the baby in good alignment. When the infant opens his mouth to latch on, the goal is to achieve a deep, asymmetric latch attachment. The goal is *not* to center the nipple in the baby's mouth. The rationale for this is to optimize oral-motor function. The jaw is a hinge joint. The upper jaw is immobile; the lower jaw compresses the breast. The breast is efficiently drained if more areola is drawn into the baby's mouth from the inferior aspect of the breast and a smaller amount drawn in from the superior aspect of the areola. Aligning the infant to the mother with baby's nose facing mother's nipple permits the jaw to be in a lower position. The next step is to let the infant drop his head back (head in "sniff position"), so that the infant leads into the breast with the chin.

● **Figure 26–19** Nose to nipple.
Source: Courtesy of Brigitte Hall, RNC, MSN, IBCLC.

To trigger the rooting reflex, teach the mother to use her nipple to stroke downward in a vertical motion across the middle of baby's lower lip. Initially, the infant may respond by licking or smacking. This is a normal response to the stimulus. Encourage the mother to keep stimulating the infant's lower lip until the infant finally opens his mouth widely. If the infant is not responding at all, then the infant is probably too sleepy and may need help waking up. After trying wake up techniques, the infant may be ready to try breastfeeding again.

● **Figure 26–20** Initial attempt to elicit the rooting reflex.
Source: Courtesy of Brigitte Hall, RNC, MSN, IBCLC.

Teach the mother to be patient and wait for the infant's mouth to gape open as widely as possible. Here the infant needs to open the mouth even wider before the mother draws her baby toward the breast. The mother should be encouraged to continue stroking the infant's lip until the infant opens the mouth wider.

● **Figure 26–21** Continued attempt to elicit rooting reflex.
Source: Courtesy of Brigitte Hall, RNC, MSN, IBCLC.

Once the baby has latched onto the breast, the mother should check that the baby is latched-on properly. The infant's chin should be embedded into the mother's breast. The infant's nose should be very close but not actually touching the breast. The nose should be centered. If the mother feels a little pinch on her areola, she can slowly release the hand supporting her breast so she can have a free hand to attempt to move her baby's jaw gently downward. To do this maneuver, the mother needs to place the thumb or forefinger of her free hand (the hand that just released the breast) on the baby's lower jaw (there is a horizontal groove to use as leverage—the groove on the baby's chin is parallel with the baby's lips). With gentle downward pressure the mother should feel relief of any persistent tenderness. This procedure opens the jaw wider and it also helps to roll out the infant's lower lip that may have been inadvertently drawn into the baby's mouth. As the baby begins to suckle, there should be no dimpling of the infant's cheeks and no smacking or clicking noises.

● **Figure 26–22** Baby is latched on.
Source: Courtesy of Brigitte Hall, RNC, MSN, IBCLC.

 Clinical Tip

With a sleepy baby, unwrap the baby, encourage lots of skin-to-skin contact between the mother and baby, and have the mother rest with her baby near her breast so that the baby can feel and smell the breast. Encourage the mother to watch for feeding cues, such as hand-to-mouth activity, fluttering eyelids, vocalization (but not necessarily crying), and mouthing activities.

lasting for 10 to 20 minutes on the first breast. The infant may feed only a few minutes on the second breast or not at all, so the mother should alternate the first breast at the next feeding. The mother should visually observe for swallowing and later, as her milk is abundant, she will hear the infant's swallows. Discourage the mother from watching the clock to determine when the infant needs to switch breast sides but rather encourage her to watch the newborn's feeding pattern to note when active feeding ceases. When satiated, the infant will either pull away from the breast or fall asleep. The infant will be extremely relaxed at the end of the feeding and will sleep until the next feeding is due (at least an hour). As the infant matures, the feeding intervals will lengthen.

Another indicator of breastfeeding efficiency is softening of the mother's breasts, although this is not a reliable indicator in the first few days postpartum while breast milk volume is low. Within a week, however, this is a good indicator of milk transfer.

The infant who feeds well will have a characteristic output. See Figure 26–23 ● for breastfeeding intake and output expectations. The infant should also have the characteristic weight loss followed by weight gain pattern discussed earlier in this chapter.

- Infants should breastfeed 8 to 12 times per day and should appear relaxed after feeding.
- Colostrum is all that a newborn needs in the first few days of life in most cases.
- It is normal for an infant to lose up to 7% of birth weight in the first few days; however, up to 10% weight loss is tolerated if the mother's breasts are full, the infant is observed to breastfeed well, and the infant is not dehydrated.
- Infants should gain 10 grams/kg/day after the mother's milk supply is abundant (about day 4 of life).
- Infants should be back to their birth weight by 2 weeks of age.
- Infant's stool should change in color, consistency, and frequency during the first few days of life. The photo images noted below depict stool color progression. Some babies progress faster to yellow milk stools, as early as day 3.

Day 1

Day 2

Day 3

Day 4

Day 5

Minimum Output

On day 1, the infant should produce at least one wet diaper and one meconium stool by 24 hours of age.

Note the pinkish-red "brick dust" appearance on the diaper. The uric acid crystals produced by the kidneys is associated with concentrated urine. A red flag is raised if their presence is continued beyond day 2 or 3 of life.

On day 2, the infant should produce at least two wet diapers and two early transitional stools in a 24-hour period by 48 hours of age.

On day 3, the infant should produce at least three wet diapers and three transitional stools in a 24-hour period by 72 hours of age.

When a mother's milk supply is abundant on day 2, some babies will have transitioned to yellow milk stools as early as day 3.

On day 4, the infant should produce at least four wet diapers and three to four yellow-green transitional stools or yellow milk stools in a 24-hour period by 96 hours of age.

On day 5, the infant should produce at least five wet diapers and three to four yellow milk stools per day; the stools are typically explosive and have a curdy or seedy appearance.

Hereafter, breastfeeding infants will consistently produce at least six well-saturated wet diapers per day. These infants will typically continue to produce at least three to four yellow milk stools daily, but may have up to 10 stools per day until they are about a month old. Infants 4 weeks or older may suddenly decrease their stool frequency, even skipping days.

● **Figure 26–23** Breastfeeding intake and output expectations.
Source: Courtesy of Brigitte Hall, RNC, MSN, IBCLC.

● **Figure 26–24** Hand expression.
Source: Courtesy of Brigitte Hall, RNC, MSN, IBCLC.

In situations where there is a question regarding milk transfer effectiveness, it can be most reliably measured by obtaining pre- and postbreastfeeding weight checks using an accurate infant scale. The difference in prefeed and postfeed weights is the amount of milk (each gram increase reflects 1 mL) transferred to the infant and may be useful in assessing breastfeeding efficiency and maternal milk volume.

Bottle-Feeding Breast Milk

There are a number of reasons for bottle-feeding breast milk. The nurse should evaluate the indications in order to recommend the best technique for the mother and her particular need.

Hand Expression. Some mothers prefer to hand express their milk rather than use a breast pump, and many find that in the immediate postpartum period hand expression of milk may be a more effective method of removing drops of colostrum than using an electric breast pump. Nurses should teach all mothers the skill of hand expressing breast milk, as it is possible the mother will find herself in a situation without a breast pump but needing to relieve herself from engorgement.

To facilitate hand expressing breast milk, the mother should be sure her breasts are clean (avoid using soap on nipples), her hands are washed, and she has taken a few minutes to relax and gently massage her breasts before beginning. She should be sitting up straight or leaning slightly forward (a pillow behind the back is helpful), because gravity aids in the flow of milk. The mother should then use the Marmet Technique of hand expression described in the following steps:

1. The mother will position her thumb at the 12:00 position on the top edge of the areola (about 1 to 1½ inches back from the tip of her nipple) and her forefinger and middle fingerpads at the 6:00 position on the bottom edge of the areola (about 1 to 1½ inches from the tip of her nipple). If positioned correctly, a line between the thumb and fingers will cross the nipple (see Figure 26–24 ●).

2. Next the mother will stretch her areola back toward her chest wall without lifting her fingers off her breast.

3. Now she should roll her thumb and fingers simultaneously forward. This action compresses the ducts beneath the areola and stimulates the breast to empty both manually and by triggering the letdown reflex.

4. The mother should repeat the sequence multiple times to completely drain her breasts. She should try to maintain a steady rhythm, cycling 45 to 60 times/minute. It is also more effective if the mother repositions her fingers to other positions on the same breast (3:00 and 9:00, 1:00 and 7:00, etc.) when the milk flow slows.

The mother should take care not to traumatize her breasts or nipples. Hand expression should not be painful. Most mothers will need assistance in learning this technique initially. Reassure the mother that this skill is learned; with practice, she can become an expert at hand expression.

Breast Pump. Although hand expression can be efficient, many mothers will choose to use a mechanical breast pump to express their milk. Not all breast pumps are of the same quality, even within the same category (see Figures 26–25 ●, 26–26 ●,

● **Figure 26–25** Manual breast pump.
Source: Courtesy of Brigitte Hall, RNC, MSN, IBCLC.

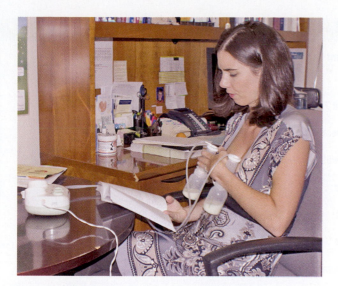

● **Figure 26–26** Individual double electric breast pump.
Source: Courtesy of Brigitte Hall, RNC, MSN, IBCLC.

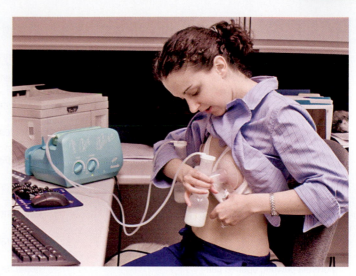

● **Figure 26–27** Hospital-grade multiuser breast pump.
Source: Courtesy of Brigitte Hall, RNC, MSN, IBCLC.

and 26–27 ● and Table 26–4). Pumps generally cycle from low to high suction at a frequency similar to that of a breastfeeding infant (about 45 to 60 cycles per minute). However, differences in the quality of the pump motor or the presence or absence of controls over suction pressure mean that some pumps will generate inadequate pressure or cycle too slowly to be effective, whereas others may exert too high a suction that can cause injury. Breast flange size, proper fit, and comfort are other variables to consider. Some good quality pumps have multiple flange sizes available to accommodate the various nipple sizes of mothers. Excessive rubbing of the mother's nipple in the flange tunnel can cause discomfort and result in a decreased volume expressed. The nurse should refer the mother to a lactation consultant or other person knowledgeable regarding different breast pumps.

Storing Human Breast Milk.   There are different guidelines for storage of expressed breast milk (EBM) depending on whether the infant is a healthy full-term infant or a premature or sick

Table 26–4	Types of Breast Pumps and Indications for Use			
Indication	Manual Breast Pump (Figure 26–25)	Small Battery/Electric Breast Pump	Individual Double Electric Breast Pump (Figure 26–26)	Hospital-Grade Multiuser Double Electric Breast Pump (Figure 26–27)
A missed feeding	■	◊		
An evening out	■	◊		
Working part-time	■	◊		
Convenience—occasional use	■	◊		
Working full-time			*	*
Premature/hospitalized infant				*
Low milk supply				*
Sore nipples/engorgement			*	*
Latch-on problems/infection			■	*
Drawing out flattish nipples	■	◊	*	*

■ Good ◊ Better * Best

Source: Adapted from the *Medela Breastfeeding Information Guide Tips and Products.* (2002). Table: Which Breastpump Is Best for You? (p. 3). Medela, Inc.

Table 26–5	Storage Guidelines for Breast Milk and Formula	
Milk	**Environment**	**Time Until Discard**
Breast milk or formula, opened/reconstituted	Being fed	Finish feed within 1 hour
Breast milk or formula, opened/reconstituted	Environment 79 degrees	1 hour
Breast milk or formula, opened/reconstituted	Room temperature	4 hours
Breast milk or formula, opened/reconstituted	Cooler pack/59 degrees	24 hours
Thawed breast milk	Refrigerator	24 hours
Formula, opened/reconstituted	Refrigerator	24 to 48 hours (see label)
Fresh breast milk	Refrigerator	8 days
Formula powder, opened can	Room temperature	1 month
Fresh breast milk	Freezer	3 months
Formula/powder in sealed container	Avoid excessive heat	Printed expiration date
Thawed breast milk	Freezer	Do not refreeze
Formula	Freezer	Do not freeze

Sources: Adapted from Human Milk Banking Association of North America (HMBANA). (2011). *Best practice for expressing, storing and handling human milk in hospitals, homes and child care settings.* Raleigh, NC: Author; Mead-Johnson Nutritionals. (2012). *Pediatric products handbook.* New York, NY: Bristol-Myers Squibb Company. http://www.meadjohnson.com; and Ross Products Division. (2010). *Pediatric nutritionals product guide.* Columbus, OH: Abbott Laboratories. http://www.abbottnutrition.com

infant in the hospital. The guidelines in Table 26–5 (which also includes storage guidelines for formula) are intended as a resource for the mother of a healthy, full-term infant.

Supplementary Formula-Feeding for Breastfed Infants

Supplementary formula-feedings for the breastfeeding infant after birth are not routinely recommended. Supplementation should only be given when medically indicated (ABM, 2009). Routine supplements are unnecessary in the early days after birth, and bottle-feeding may cause the infant to develop an incorrect sucking pattern or may cause the infant to refuse the breast altogether (Riordan & Wambach, 2010). Early supplementation with formula may contribute to a delay in early maternal milk production, may result in maternal engorgement after the mother's milk production has increased, and may possibly sensitize an at-risk infant for milk-protein allergy. These types of problems have been implicated in early breastfeeding terminations (Mercer, Teasley, Hopkinson, et al., 2010).

"Nipple confusion" or "nipple preference" can cause some babies to develop an incorrect sucking technique, or to simply refuse to breastfeed again. This potential problem occurs because the techniques for breastfeeding and formula-feeding are different. In breastfeeding, the infant has to open the mouth very wide to latch on. To transfer milk the baby has to extend the tongue forward, cupping the nipple and drawing the mother's nipple deep into the mouth until the teat reaches the "comfort zone" near the junction of the infant's hard and soft palate. After the infant creates suction from the tongue and cheeks and seals the latch with the lips, then the infant rhythmically compresses the breast with his or her jaw while the tongue moves in an undulating motion to move fluid toward the pharynx before swallowing, in coordination with breathing. On average, it takes a couple of minutes before the breastfeeding mother's milk flow increases during letdown. With bottle-feeding, the infant keeps the tongue retracted and uses the tip of the tongue to block the flow of milk, which otherwise drips continuously by gravity even when suction is not applied. The bottle-feeding baby merely needs to create suction with the mouth on the bottle nipple and the fluid easily flows.

At times there are valid medical indications for supplementation of the breastfeeding infant. These include delayed lactogenesis; unavailability of the mother because of severe illness or separation; primary lactation failure; hypoglycemia; significant dehydration; weight loss of 8% to 10% with exclusive breastfeeding; delayed passage of stool (presence of meconium on day 5); hyperbilirubinemia related to poor intake, prematurity, or low birth weight; and refusal of or ineffective breastfeeding.

When supplementation is indicated, the first choice is to use the mother's own milk (fresh, previously expressed, or frozen/thawed). If maternal breast milk is not available, pasteurized donor milk is the next choice, and then formula (HMBANA, 2011). The method of supplementation chosen is based on the particular situation, parental preference, and agency policy.

Evidence-Based Practice Risk Factors for Delayed Lactogenesis

Clinical Question

What are the modifiable risk factors for delayed lactogenesis?

The Evidence

Delayed breast milk production (lactogenesis) is a primary cause of lack of success in breastfeeding. When adequate breast milk is not available, excess neonatal weight loss and early weaning may occur. Many causes of lactogenesis are not modifiable but some are. Nutrition experts conducted a retrospective cohort study of 431 women, and a systematic review of 12 studies confirmed the findings. These aggregates of multiple studies form the strongest level of evidence. Women who had the least success persisting in breastfeeding were more likely to be obese, primiparous, and have unsuccessful first

efforts to breastfeed in the immediate postpartum period (Bojcicki, 2011; Nommsen-Rivers, Chantry, Peerson, et al., 2010).

Best Practice

Helping potential parents modify risk factors such as obesity before conception will have a host of benefits, including earlier onset of lactogenesis. Other modifiable risk factors include lack of success in the early postpartum period; spending enough time with these mothers to ensure their first breastfeeding efforts are successful will set the stage for persistence.

Clinical Reasoning

How can the nurse assist the new mother in achieving success in the first breastfeeding attempts?

Promotion of Successful Infant Breastfeeding

With the trend toward earlier discharge from the birthing center, there is limited time for inpatient education. Teaching moments, when they occur, may not be optimal because of the distraction of visitors and the mother's being sleep deprived, uncomfortable, or under the effects of an analgesic. It is important that parents receive verbal and written instructions and community resource information to which they can later refer. (See Chapter 30 🌱 for a complete discussion of self-care measures the nurse can suggest to a woman with a breastfeeding problem after discharge from the birthing center.)

To promote a supportive hospital environment for breastfeeding, the Baby-Friendly Hospital Initiative recognizes hospitals and birthing centers that offer optimal lactation services and comply with the 10 steps outlined in Table 26–6. Baby-Friendly status

is not easy to achieve. One obstacle to achieving Baby-Friendly status, among many, is having to agree not to accept free or low-cost formula. Currently there are approximately 159 hospitals in the United States with Baby-Friendly designation as of January 2013 according to an update on the Baby-Friendly Hospital Initiative USA website (BFHI USA, 2013).

FORMULA-FEEDING

With more attention placed on promoting and assisting breastfeeding mothers, the teaching needs of the mother who is formula-feeding may inadvertently get overlooked. Nurses may assume that families can simply follow the formula preparation instructions on the side of the formula containers. Parents need teaching, counseling, and support. Parents need to learn about the feeding pattern for a formula-feeding infant, the intake and output expectations, the recommended type of formula for their infant, how to prepare and store formula, what equipment they will need, feeding technique, and safety precautions. (See Table 26–3 on page 598.)

Formula-Feeding Guidelines and Technique

Commercial formulas are available in three forms: powder, concentrate, and ready-to-feed. There are situations in which one formula may be better to use than another, but in general, convenience and cost usually influence the parents' decision.

- *Powdered formula* is the least expensive type of formula. This formula can be made up one bottle at a time, or multiple bottles can be prepared, but they must be used within 24 to 48 hours. Standard powdered formula is made by adding one level scoop of powdered formula to 60 mL of water. Powdered formulas are not sterile. Powdered formula is made from pasteurized liquid that is then freeze-spray dried into a powder; contamination with microorganisms can occur in the final stages of production. Preparation of any infant formula, but especially powdered formulas, requires careful handling to avoid contamination with microorganisms.

Table 26–6	Baby-Friendly Requirements

BABY-FRIENDLY 10 STEPS TO SUCCESSFUL BREASTFEEDING

- Have a written breastfeeding policy that is routinely communicated to all healthcare staff.
- Train all healthcare staff in skills necessary to implement this policy.
- Inform all pregnant women about the benefits and management of breastfeeding.
- Help mothers initiate breastfeeding within one hour of birth.
- Show mothers how to breastfeed and maintain lactation, even if they should be separated from their infants.
- Give newborn infants no food or drink other than breast milk, unless medically indicated.
- Practice rooming in—that is, allow mothers and infants to remain together 24 hours a day.
- Encourage breastfeeding on demand.
- Give no artificial teats or pacifiers (also called dummies or soothers) to breastfeeding infants.
- Foster the establishment of breastfeeding support groups and refer mothers to them on discharge from the hospital or clinic.

Source: World Health Organization/United Nations Children's Emergency Fund (WHO/UNICEF). (2010). *U.S. committee for UNICEF interim program in the United States to promote the Baby-Friendly ten steps to successful breastfeeding.* Washington, DC: Government Printing Office.

■ *Formula concentrate* is more expensive than powder but is not as expensive as ready-to-feed formula. Formula concentrate is commercially sterile. This formula must be diluted with an equal part of water. By adding boiled water that has been cooled, sterility can be maintained.

■ *Ready-to-feed* formula is the easiest to use because it does not require any mixing; however, this convenience comes at a cost—it is the most expensive formula. It is indicated for use when adequate water is not available, when the infant is immunocompromised and requires commercially sterile (pasteurized) formula, when an inexperienced baby-sitter will be feeding the infant, and for convenience.

Whatever the type of formula chosen, the nurse should underscore the importance of proper preparation and prompt refrigeration. Parents will need to be briefed on safety precautions during formula preparation. A primary concern is proper mixing to reconstitute formula. Parents need clear instructions to avoid unintentional harm to their infant. Parents should be instructed to follow the directions on the formula can label precisely as written. They should know that adding too much water during preparation dilutes the nutrients and caloric density. This contributes to undernourishment, insufficient weight gain, and possibly water intoxication, which can cause hyponatremia and seizures. Not adding enough water concentrates nutrients and calories and can tax an infant's immature kidneys and digestive system as well as cause dehydration. See Table 26–5 for storage guidelines for formula.

Some recommended sanitary precautions and additional safety precautions are listed here:

■ Check the expiration date on the formula container.

■ Ensure good hand washing before preparing formula; never dip into the can without clean hands.

■ Clean bottles, nipples, rings, disks, and bottle caps.
   a. Washing in a dishwasher when available (small items and heat-sensitive items on top rack secured in a basket), or
   b. Boiling briefly (1 to 2 minutes) in a pot of water, or
   c. Cleaning using a microwave sterilization kit, or
   d. Cleaning using very warm soapy water and a nipple and bottle brush.

■ Inspect and replace bottle nipples as soon as they show wear; worn nipples can break apart and can become a choking hazard.

■ Wash the top of the formula container before piercing the lid.

■ Shake the liquid formulas well before pouring off the desired amount.

■ Shake prepared milk that has been sitting in the refrigerator before feeding.

■ Allow tap water to run for 1 minute before obtaining water to use for mixing—this helps clear any lead standing in the pipes. Also, always use cold tap water, as warm water tends to contain higher levels of lead as well.

■ Use only the scoop supplied in the can of formula when formula preparation instructions call for a "scoop" of powdered formula. A scoop should not be "packed" and should be leveled off (e.g., with the back of a knife).

■ Do not add anything else to the bottle, except under direction of the baby's healthcare provider.

■ Milk in a bottle should be warmed by placing the bottle in a bowl of warm tap water for no longer than 15 minutes. Do not fill the bowl with water higher than the rim of the bottle. (Babies can take cold formula but most young infants will prefer it warm.)

■ Allow freshly prepared (unused) formula to sit out at room temperature for no longer than 2 hours; use an insulated pack to transport formula. Milk left over in the bottle after a feeding should be discarded.

■ In warm weather, transport reconstituted formula or concentrate from an open can in an insulated pack with frozen gel packs.

■ Travel with water and formula separated—carry premeasured water bottles and bottles with premeasured amounts of powdered formula, or carry premeasured commercially prepared formula packets, or have the can of formula available.

■ Holding the infant during feeding (even when the infant can hold the bottle) promotes bonding and prevents supine feedings.

■ Do not allow the infant to formula-feed in a supine position because this increases the risk of otitis media and dental caries in the older infant.

■ Never prop a bottle—this is a choking hazard.

■ Allow infants to take what they want AND to stop when they want. Overfeeding can lead to obesity.

Parents also need guidance about what kind of water to use to reconstitute formula (see Table 26–7 to review types of water sources) and should discuss with their infant's healthcare provider whether to boil the water before use. If boiling is used, parents need to be instructed to heat the water until it reaches a rolling boil, to continue to let the water boil for 1 to 2 minutes, and, most importantly, to allow the water to cool before using it to reconstitute the formula. Parents should also be instructed not to let the water boil down to a low level in the pan because this can cause minerals in the water to become concentrated.

Use of distilled bottle water and filtered tap water raises concerns with regard to fluoride. The American Academy of Pediatrics recommends that no fluoride supplements be given to an infant before 6 months of age (AAP & ACOG, 2012). Parents should be encouraged to read the labels on bottled water to see if fluoride has been added and to determine if the water source is suitable depending on the infant's age (Table 26–7).

Parents often have questions about the kind of bottles and nipples to purchase. Many newly designed bottles are marketed to lessen air intake while an infant feeds. There is not a particular bottle design that is best for all babies. A key point to emphasize to the families is feeding technique. Parents should try to avoid situations in which an infant is crying for a prolonged time. Crying results in increased ingestion of air even before the infant

Table 26–7	Water Sources
Type	**Description**
Distilled water	Minerals and most other impurities have been removed. It will not contain any fluoride. An acceptable water source for reconstituting formula.
Filtered tap water	Some minerals and impurities removed during filtration, including fluoride. This is an acceptable water source for reconstituting formula.
Natural mineral water	Comes from protected groundwater and by law cannot be treated. Naturally contains high levels of minerals and sodium and so is not suitable for infants or for reconstituting formula.
Spring water	Comes from a single nonpolluted groundwater source, but unlike natural mineral water, it can be further treated. Because there is no regulation requiring the mineral content to be printed on the bottle label, it is best to avoid this water source for reconstituting formula.
Tap water	Water from the municipal water supply, and regulated by drinking water regulations. It is treated and considered safe for use in reconstituting formula.
Well water	Needs to be tested before use. Higher risk of nitrate poisoning. Untested water is not recommended for use in reconstituting formula.

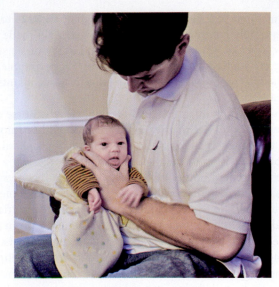

● **Figure 26–28** Burping baby sitting up on lap.
Source: Courtesy of Brigitte Hall, RNC, MSN, IBCLC.

● **Figure 26–29** Burping baby over the shoulder.
Source: Courtesy of Brigitte Hall, RNC, MSN, IBCLC.

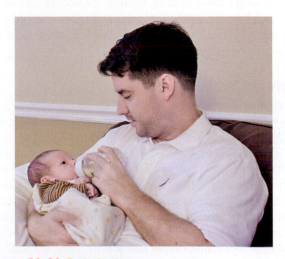

● **Figure 26–30** Bottle-feeding.
Source: Courtesy of Brigitte Hall, RNC, MSN, IBCLC.

has started feeding. Infants who are very hungry also gulp more air. For these situations, instruct the parents to burp their infant frequently to prevent the infant from having a large emesis (Figure 26–28 ● and Figure 26–29 ●). The parent may even want to attempt to pat the baby's back briefly before starting the feeding to calm a crying infant and possibly burp as well. Another tip to avoid excessive ingestion of air is to have the parent hold the infant cradled in his or her arms while bottle-feeding, and tilting the bottle at a 45-degree angle in order for fluid to cover the nipple. This prevents the infant from sucking in air and swallowing it. The vented bottle design eliminates the negative effects of a vacuum and channels air through an internal vent system above the milk avoiding air bubbles in the milk. See Figure 26–30 ● to view an infant bottle-feeding.

Parents will want to consider a slow-flow nipple for all newborns and for older breastfeeding babies learning to formula-feed—over time the infant will graduate to medium-flow and high-flow nipples. Nipples come in different shapes. Generally, nipple shape plays a greater importance for breastfeeding babies receiving expressed breast milk or supplemental formula in a bottle. Breastfed babies transition best going from breast to bottle and back to breast again when using a bottle nipple that has a relatively wide base (to help maintain a wide open latch) and a medium to long nipple length. Another variable to consider is nipple construction. Nipples are generally made from either rubber or silicone. Families with a history of sensitivity to latex are advised to use silicone nipples. Silicone nipples also have less of an odor, which may be an issue for some infants who are breastfed.

To know if an infant is bottle-feeding well, the nurse needs to observe a bottle-feeding session. Parents should be informed that if the infant is sucking effectively, the parents should observe bubbles rising in the fluid of standard bottles. (If a family is using vented bottles or bottles with liners that retract as fluid is removed, bubbles will not be detected.) No bubbles will be observed if the parent unintentionally places the bottle nipple under the infant's tongue, preventing the infant from sucking effectively. Some infants, especially premature infants, raise the tongue to the roof of the mouth and so it is sometimes a challenge to place the nipple on top of the tongue. Infants who persistently leak milk from the side of the mouth may be getting fluid too quickly. The nurse could suggest using a slower flowing nipple. If symptoms persist, the infant should have an oral evaluation. The infant could have a short lingual frenulum (tongue-tied) and not be able to properly cup the tongue under the nipple and channel fluid to the back of the throat, or may have an oral-motor dysfunction and need speech therapy or occupational therapy evaluation.

There has been a growing concern regarding specific chemicals used in the manufacture of plastic baby bottles, the material used in lining formula cans, and soft plastics such as bisphenol-A (BPA) that could leach from polycarbonate plastic used in the manufacture of some baby bottles and transfer into the baby's milk.

SAFETY ALERT!

Parents need to be instructed to read product labels to see if the merchandise they are purchasing is free of these potentially harmful chemicals. If product labels do not explicitly state that they are free of these chemicals, then it cannot be assumed they are BPA-free, PVC-free, lead-free, and phthalates-free.

If parents cannot afford to purchase new BPA-free bottles, then encourage them to limit heating the bottles (avoid using the dishwasher and bottle warmers) and throw out old bottles with scratches. The harmful chemicals are leached most when the plastic is heated or damaged.

Involving Fathers

Our traditional view of the family following the birth of a child places most of the attention on the mother and newborn, oftentimes leaving the father out. Nurses need to recognize this and make every effort to speak to both parents when entering the patient's room. Fathers play a vital role in the family by providing support to the mother and care for their newborn. If a mother has chosen not to breastfeed, the father can be involved with bottle-feedings from the start. However, if the mother is breastfeeding, it is important to ask the father to wait to introduce a bottle until the mother's milk supply and breastfeeding are well established. The father can be encouraged to assist with breastfeeding in the meantime. He can help the mother get in position and

● **Figure 26–31** Father and infant skin-to-skin.
Source: Courtesy of Brigitte Hall, RNC, MSN, IBCLC.

help tweak the baby's latch if the mother complains of any discomfort. The father can also massage the mother's breasts during breastfeeding to help stimulate the sleepy baby to feed better and to relieve any engorgement.

The father can help with other aspects too. He can help burp the baby, change diapers, and bathe and comfort the baby. The father can also provide skin-to-skin contact that enhances bonding, provides comfort to the newborn, and calms the baby down before offering the breast. One strategy is to have the father hold the baby vertically on his chest and let the baby suck on a clean finger for a minute or so (see Figure 26–31 ●). These are just a few ways to involve the father after the birth of the baby. These interactions promote father–mother–infant bonding and are important for paternal role development.

NURSING MANAGEMENT IN PREPARATION FOR DISCHARGE

Although the adjustment to parenting is a normal process, going home presents a critical transition for the family. The parents become the primary caregivers for the newborn and must provide a nurturing environment in which the emotional and physical needs of the newborn can be met. Nursing interventions focus on promoting health and preventing possible problems.

Nursing Assessment and Diagnosis

When preparing for discharge, assess whether parents have realistic expectations of the newborn's behavior and the depth of their knowledge in caring for their newborn.

Nursing diagnoses that may apply to the newborn's family include the following (NANDA-I © 2012):

- *Parenting, Readiness for Enhanced,* related to appropriate behavioral expectations for the newborn
- *Family Processes, Readiness for Enhanced,* related to integration of newborn into family unit or demands of newborn care and feeding.

Planning and Implementation

Parent Teaching

To meet the parent's need for information, the nurse who is responsible for the care of the mother and newborn should assume the primary responsibility for parent education. Nearly every contact with the parents presents an opportunity for sharing information that can facilitate their sense of competence in newborn care. The nurse also needs to recognize and respect the many good ways of providing safe care. Unless their care methods are harmful to the newborn, the parents' methods of giving care should be reinforced rather than contradicted.

The information that follows is provided to increase the nurse's knowledge of newborn care and can also be used to meet parents' needs for information. If they are new parents, the sensitive nurse gently teaches them by example and provides instructions geared to their needs and previous knowledge about the various aspects of newborn care.

The nurse observes how parents interact with their newborn during feeding and caregiving activities. Even during a short stay (48 hours or less), there are opportunities for the nurse to provide information and observe whether the parents are comfortable with changing the diapers of, wrapping, handling, and feeding their newborn (Figure 26–32 ●). Do both parents get involved in the newborn's care? Is the mother depending on someone else to help her at home? Does the mother give reasons (e.g., "I'm too tired," "My stitches hurt," or "I'll learn later") for not wanting to be involved in her baby's care? As the family provides care, the nurse can enhance parental confidence by giving them positive feedback. If the parents encounter problems, the nurse can express confidence in their abilities to master the new skill or information, suggest alternatives, and serve as a role model. All these factors need to be considered when evaluating the educational needs of the parents. Providing mother-baby care and home care instruction on the night shift assists with education needs for early discharge parents.

One-to-one teaching while the nurse is in the mother's room is the most effective educational method rated as such

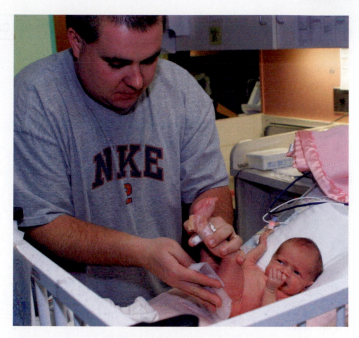

● **Figure 26–32** A father demonstrates competence and confidence in diapering his newborn daughter.
Source: George Dodson/Lightworks Studio/Pearson Education.

by both first-time and experienced postpartum parents. With shorter stays, most teaching unfortunately tends to focus on infant feeding and immediate physical care needs of the mother, with limited anticipatory guidance provided in other areas. To address this deficit, see *Teaching Highlights: What to Tell Parents About Infant Care*, which includes a broad range of information important to share with new parents.

General Instructions for Newborn Care

One of the first concerns of anyone who has not had the experience of picking up a baby is how to do it correctly. The newborn is easily picked up by sliding one hand under the neck and shoulders and the other hand under the buttocks or between the newborn's legs and then gently lifting upward. This technique provides security and support for the head (which the newborn is unable to support until 3 or 4 months of age).

The nurse can be an excellent role model for families in the area of safety. Safety topics include proper positioning of the newborn on the back to sleep and correct use of the bulb syringe. The baby should never be left alone anywhere but in the crib. The mother is reminded that while she and her newborn are together in the birthing unit, she should never leave her baby alone for security reasons and because newborns spit up frequently the first day or two after birth. Other newborn safety measures are discussed in detail in Chapter 30 ✇.

Demonstrating a bath (see Chapter 30 ✇), cord care, and temperature assessment is the best way for the nurse to provide information on these topics to parents. See Table 26–1 on page 586.

The nurse demonstrates and reviews the taking of axillary or tympanic temperatures and discourages the use of mercury thermometers. It is important that families understand the differences and know how to select a thermometer. The newborn's

Clinical Tip

For patients who are hearing impaired, videotapes with information in both spoken and signed formats are most helpful. Birthing centers should have handouts available for families who do not speak English and either birthing center interpreters (not family members) or language interpreter phones.

Teaching Highlights What to Tell Parents About Infant Care

Immediate Safety Measures for the Newborn
- Watch for excessive mucus: use a bulb syringe to remove mucus.
- Have baby sleep on his or her back in a crib or in someone's arms.

Voiding and Stool Characteristics and Patterns
- Urine is straw to amber color without foul smell. Small amounts of uric acid crystals are normal in first days of life (may be mistaken by parents as blood in diaper because of reddish "brick dust" appearance).
- At least 6 to 10 wet diapers a day after the first few days of life.
- Normal progression of stool changes: (1) meconium (thick, tarry, dark green); (2) transitional stools (thin, brown to green); (3a) breastfed infant: yellow gold, soft or mushy stools; (3b) formula-fed infant: pale yellow, formed and pasty stools.
- Only one to two stools a day for formula-fed baby.
- Six to 10 small, loose yellow stools per day or only one stool every few days after breastfeeding is well established (after about 1 month).

Cord Care
- Wash hands with clean water before and after care.
- Keep the cord dry and exposed to air or loosely covered with clean clothes. (If cultural custom demands binding of the abdomen, a sanitary method such as the use of a clean piece of gauze can be recommended.)
- Clean the cord and skin around the base with a cotton swab or cotton ball. Clean two to three times a day or with each diaper change. Touching the cord, applying unclean substances to it, and applying bandages should be avoided.
- Do not give tub baths until the cord falls off in 7 to 14 days.
- Fold diapers below the umbilical cord to air-dry the cord (contact with wet or soiled diapers slows the drying process and increases the possibility of infection).
- Check the cord each day for any odor, oozing of greenish yellow material, or reddened areas around the cord. Expect tenderness around the cord and darkening and shriveling of the cord. Report to the healthcare provider any signs of infection.
- Normal changes in cord: The cord should look dark and dry up before falling off. A small drop of blood may present when the cord falls off.
- Never pull the cord or attempt to loosen it.

Care Required for Circumcision and Uncircumcised Infants
Circumcision Care
- Squeeze water over the circumcision site once a day.
- Rinse the area off with warm water and pat dry.

- Apply a small amount of petroleum jelly (unless a Plastibell is in place) with each diaper change.
- Fasten a diaper over the penis snugly enough so that it does not move and rub the tender glans.
- Because the glans is sensitive, avoid placing baby on the stomach for the first day after the procedure.
- Check for any foul-smelling drainage or bleeding at least once a day.
- Let the Plastibell fall off by itself (about 8 days after circumcision). It should not be pulled off.
- Light, sticky, yellow drainage (part of healing process) may form over the head of the penis.

Uncircumcised Care
- Clean the uncircumcised penis with water during diaper changes and with bath.
- Do not force the foreskin back over the penis; foreskin will retract normally over time (may take 3 to 5 years).

Techniques for Waking and Quieting Newborns
Waking Baby
- Loosen clothing, change diaper.
- Hand-express milk onto baby's lips.
- Talk with baby while making eye contact.
- Hold baby in upright position (sitting or standing).
- Have baby do sit-ups (gently and rhythmically bend baby back and forth while grasping the baby under his or her knees and supporting baby's head and back with your other hand).
- Play patty-cake with baby.
- Stimulate the rooting reflex (brush one cheek with a hand or nipple).
- Increase skin contact (gently rub hands and feet).

Quieting Baby
- Check for a soiled diaper.
- Hold swaddled baby upright against midchest, supporting the bottom and back of head. Baby can hear heartbeat, feel warmth, and hear your softly spoken words or calming sounds.
- Use slow, calming movements with baby.
- Softly talk, sing, or hum to baby.

Signs of Illness
See Table 26–8: When Parents Should Call Their Healthcare Provider on page 620.

---

temperature needs to be taken only when signs of illness are present. Parents are advised to call their physician or pediatric nurse practitioner immediately if they observe any signs of illness.

Nasal and Oral Suctioning

Most newborns are obligatory nose breathers for the first months of life. They generally maintain air passage patency by coughing or sneezing. During the first few days of life, however, the newborn has increased mucus, and gentle suctioning with a bulb syringe may be indicated but only in cases of obvious obstruction.

The newborn's mouth should be suctioned first so that there is nothing to aspirate if the newborn gasps when the nose is suctioned (AAP & ACOG, 2012). The nurse can demonstrate the use of the bulb syringe in the mouth and nose and have the parents do a return demonstration. The parents should repeat this demonstration of suctioning and cleansing the bulb before discharge so they feel confident in performing the procedure. Care should be taken to apply only gentle suction to prevent nasal bleeding.

To suction the newborn, the bulb syringe is compressed before the tip is placed in the nostril. The nurse or parent must

● **Figure 26–33** Nasal and oral suctioning. The bulb is compressed, the tip is placed in either the mouth or the nose, and the bulb is released.

 Clinical Tip

Remember that left-handed people tend to hold the baby over their right shoulder, and right-handed people do the opposite. This keeps the dominant hand free. However, most health personnel wear their nametags on the left side. To avoid scratching the baby's face, wear your nametag on the same side as your dominant hand.

take care not to occlude the passageway. The bulb is permitted to reexpand slowly by releasing the compression on the bulb (Figure 26–33 ●). The bulb syringe is removed from the nostril, and drainage is then compressed out of the bulb and onto a tissue. The bulb syringe may also be used in the mouth if the newborn is spitting up and unable to handle the excess secretions. The bulb is compressed, the tip of the bulb syringe is placed about 1 inch to one side of the newborn's mouth, and compression is released. This draws up the excess secretions. The procedure is repeated on the other side of the mouth. The roof of the mouth and the back of the throat are avoided because suction in these areas might stimulate the gag reflex. The bulb syringe should be washed in warm, soapy water and rinsed in warm water daily and as needed after use. Rinsing with a half-strength white vinegar solution followed by clear water may help to extend the useful life of the bulb syringe by inhibiting bacterial growth. A bulb syringe should always be kept near the newborn. New parents and nurses who are inexperienced with babies may fear that the baby will choke and are relieved to know how to take action if such an event occurs. They should be advised to turn the newborn's head to the side or hold the newborn with the head down as soon as there is any indication of gagging or vomiting and to use the bulb syringe as needed. See Skill 5–1 in the *Clinical Skills Manual* SKILLS .

Some infants may have transient edema of the nasal mucosa following suctioning of the airway after birth. The nurse can demonstrate the use of normal saline to loosen secretions, and instruct parents in the gentle and moderate use of the bulb syringe to avoid further irritation of the mucous membranes. If parents will be using humidifiers at home, they should be instructed to follow the manufacturer's cleaning instructions carefully so that molds, spores, and bacteria from a dirty humidifier do not enter the baby's environment.

Sleep and Activity

The National Institute of Child Health and Human Development and the American Academy of Pediatrics recommend that healthy term infants be placed on their backs to sleep. Parents are taught the importance of following "Back to Sleep Guidelines" to reduce the incidence of sudden infant death syndrome (SIDS) (American Academy of Pediatrics [AAP], 2013b). Though infants may need to be placed on their sides initially because of copious or thick secretions, placing them on their backs in the newborn period serves to educate parents regarding infant positioning. Studies indicate that parents position their babies in the same positions they observe in the hospital setting, so nurses must demonstrate this behavior to reduce the risk of SIDS. If exceptions are warranted, these should be explained to families so they do not misinterpret what they observe. The placement of babies in a prone position during supervised wakeful play sessions or "tummy time" should be encouraged as well (AAP, 2013c). Parents are also encouraged to hold their babies and not allow them to remain in infant carriers for prolonged periods of time.

Perhaps nothing is more individual to each baby than the sleep-activity cycle. It is important for the nurse to recognize the individual variations of each newborn and to assist parents as they develop sensitivity to their infant's communication signals and rhythms of activity and sleep. See Chapter 24 🔗 for a more detailed discussion of sleep-wake activity.

Car Safety Considerations

Half of the children killed or injured in automobile accidents could have been protected by the use of federally approved car seats. Newborns must go home from the birthing unit in a car seat adapted to fit them (Figure 26–34 ●). Babies should never be placed in the front seat of a car equipped with a passenger-side airbag. The car seat should be positioned to face the rear of the car until the baby is 2 years old, or until they reach maximum height and weight for their seat (AAP, 2013a). Nurses need to ensure that all parents are knowledgeable about the benefits of child safety seat use and proper installation. Nurses can encourage parents to have their infant safety seats checked by local groups trained specifically for that purpose. The Seat Check Initiative provides locations and information about child safety seats.

Newborn Screening and Immunization Programs

Before the newborn and mother are discharged from the birthing unit, the nurse informs the parents about the **newborn screening tests** and tells them when to return to the birthing center or clinic if further tests are needed.

Several disorders that can be identified from a few drops of blood obtained by a heelstick are cystic fibrosis, galactosemia, congenital adrenal hyperplasia, congenital hypothyroidism, maple syrup urine disease, phenylketonuria (PKU), sickle cell trait, biotinidase deficiency, and hemoglobinopathies

● **Figure 26–34** An infant car restraint such as this one should be used from birth to about 24 months of age.

Source: George Dodson/Lightworks Studio/Pearson Education.

● **Figure 26–35** Newborn hearing screen.

Source: Courtesy of Jo Engle, RN, MSN, NNP-BC and Vanessa Howell, RN, MSN.

(Cloherty et al., 2012). The Health Resources and Services Administration (HRSA) recommends that states test for a core panel of 29 treatable congenital conditions including hearing loss in the newborn (Genetics Home Reference, 2013). Phenylketonuria and congenital hypothyroidism are the only tests that are performed in all 50 states and the District of Columbia. Early newborn discharge puts infants at risk for delayed or even missed diagnosis of PKU and congenital hypothyroidism because the likelihood of detecting PKU increases as the infant grows older; the infant must be at least 24 hours old for a valid test. A second test is required in most states, usually between 1 week and 1 month of age, to minimize the chance of a positive child going undetected. PKU and other inborn errors of metabolism are discussed further in Chapter 54 🔗.

Hearing loss is found in 1 to 3 per 1000 infants in the normal newborn population (Healthy Children, 2013b). The recommended initial newborn hearing screening should be accomplished before discharge from the birthing unit with appropriate follow-up if the newborn fails to pass the initial screen in all hospitals providing obstetric services. (For further discussion, see Chapter 25 🔗.) According to the National Center for Hearing Assessment and Management, 97% of all infants obtain hearing screening in the United States. Sometimes infants fail to pass these tests for reasons other than hearing loss. Amniotic fluid in the ear canals is a frequent cause of suboptimal test results. In these cases, infants are retested in a week or two. The current goal is to screen all infants by 1 month of age, confirm hearing loss with audiologic examination by 3 months of age, and treat with comprehensive early intervention services before 6 months of age (CDC, 2012). Typically, screening programs use a two-stage screening approach (otoacoustic emissions [OAE]

repeated twice, OAE followed by auditory brainstem response [ABR], or automated ABR repeated twice). Families need to be educated about appropriate interpretation of screening test results and appropriate steps for follow-up (Figure 26–35 ●).

Immunization programs against the hepatitis B virus during the newborn period and infancy are in place in many states, at least 20 countries, and high-incidence areas such as American Samoa. Universal vaccination of infants is recommended. See *Drug Guide: Hepatitis B Vaccine (Engerix-B, Recombivax HB)*. Parents need to be advised whether their birthing center provides newborn hepatitis vaccination so that an adequate follow-up program can be set in motion.

The nurse should teach the family all necessary caregiving methods before discharge. A checklist may be helpful to determine whether the teaching has been completed and to verify the parents' knowledge on leaving the birthing unit (Figure 26–36 ●). The nurse needs to review all areas for understanding or answer outstanding questions with the mother and father, without rushing, and take time to resolve all queries. Any concerns of the parents or nurse are noted.

Community-Based Nursing Care

The nurse discusses with parents ways to meet their newborn's needs, ensure safety, and appreciate the newborn's unique characteristics and behaviors. By assisting parents in establishing links with their community-based healthcare provider, the nurse can get the new family off to a good start. Parents also need to know the signs of illness, how to reach the pediatrician or after-hours clinic, and the importance of follow-up after discharge (Table 26–8). Parents should also check with their clinician for advice about over-the-counter medications to be kept in the medicine cabinet.

The family should have the care provider's phone number, address, and any specific instructions. Having the birthing unit or nursery phone number is also reassuring to a newborn's family. They are encouraged to call with questions. Follow-up

FOR NURSES ONLY

NURSERY TEACHING CHECKLIST

Please read the *Mother/Baby* information booklet given to you after birth. After reading it, please go through the following list and check whether you understand each topic or need to know more.

		I know this already	Doesn't apply to me	I need to know more	Taught/reviewed/demonstrated
Baby Care	What to do if baby is choking or gagging				
	Safety				
	How to do skin care/cord care				
	How to take care of the circumcision or genital area				
	How to know if my baby is sick and what to do				
	What is jaundice and how to detect it				
	Use of thermometer				
	Use of bulb syringe				
	How and when to burp baby				
	Newborn behavior: crying/comforting				
	How to position baby after feeding				
	What does demand scheduling mean				
Breastfeeding	I attended breastfeeding class/watched breastfeeding video	YES ☐	NO ☐		
	How to position baby for feeding				
	How to get baby to latch on to my nipple properly				
	When and how long to breastfeed				
	Removal of baby from my nipple				
	What is the supply and demand concept				
	What is the let-down reflex				
	When does breast milk come in				
	Supplementing				
	Proper diet for breastfeeding mothers				
	Prevention and comfort measures for sore nipples				
	Prevention and comfort measures for engorgement				
	When and how to use a breast pump				
	How to express milk by hand				
	How to go back to work and continue to breastfeed				
Bottle-Feeding	How to feed my baby a bottle				
	Reasons for NOT propping bottles				
	How to clean nipple/bottle				
	How to mix formula				
	What formula should my baby drink				
Safety	**Use of infant car seat**				
	Back to Sleep				
	Shaken Baby Syndrome				

Other information:

_____

_____

_____

_____

I have received and understand the instructions given on the above topics.

_____   _____
MOTHER'S SIGNATURE   DATE

Videos viewed/ Literature given:

_____

Language Spoken by Mother:

☐ English ☐ Spanish ☐ Other _____

Interpreter Used? ☐ Yes ☐ No ☐ Family Interprets

Nurse's Signature(s):

_____

_____

● **Figure 26–36** Nursery teaching checklist. An infant teaching checklist is completed by the time of discharge.

Source: Adapted from Presbyterian/St. Luke's Medical Center, Denver, CO.

Drug Guide Hepatitis B Vaccine (Engerix-B, Recombivax HB)

Overview of Neonatal Action

Recombinant hepatitis B vaccine is used as a prophylactic treatment against all subtypes of hepatitis B virus. It provides passive immunization for newborns of HBsAg-negative and HBsAg-positive mothers. Hepatitis B can be transmitted across the placenta, but most newborns are infected during birth.

The vaccine is produced from baker's yeast and plasmid containing the HBsAg gene.

Hepatitis B (thimerosal-free) vaccine contains more than 95% HBsAg protein and is an inactivated (noninfective) product.

Infants of HBsAg-positive mothers should concurrently receive 0.5 mL of hepatitis B immunoglobulin (HBIG) prophylaxis at separate injection sites (CDC, 2013; Wilson et al., 2013).

Route, Dosage, Frequency

The first dose of 0.5 mL (10 mcg) is given intramuscularly into the anterolateral thigh within 12 hours of birth for infants born to HBsAg-positive mothers. The second dose of vaccine is given at least 1 month after the first dose and followed by a final dose at least 4 months after the first dose and at least 3 months after the second dose, but not before 6 months of age (CDC, 2013).

Infants born to HBsAg-negative mothers receive their first dose of vaccine at birth, the second dose at 1 to 2 months, and the third dose at 6 to 18 months (AAP & ACOG, 2012).

Infants whose mother's HBsAg status is unknown should receive the same doses of vaccine as infants born to HBsAg-positive mothers.

Neonatal Side Effects

The only common side effect is soreness at the injection site. Occasionally, there is erythema, swelling, warmth, and induration at the injection site, irritability, or a low-grade fever (37.7°C [99.8°F]).

Nursing Considerations

Delay administration during active infection, as the vaccine will not prevent infection during its incubation period.

- The vaccine should be used as supplied. Do not dilute. Shake well.
- Do not inject intravenously or intradermally.
- Monitor for adverse reactions. Monitor temperature closely.
- Have epinephrine available to treat possible allergic reactions.
- Responsiveness to the vaccine is age dependent. Preterm infants weighing less than 1000 g have lower seroconversion rates. Consider delaying the first dose until the infant is term postconceptual age (PCA) or use a 4-dose schedule.

Table 26–8	When Parents Should Call Their Healthcare Provider

Temperature above 38°C (100.4°F) axillary or below 36.6°C (97.8°F) axillary

Continual rise in temperature

More than one episode of forceful vomiting or frequent vomiting over a 6-hour period

Refusal of two feedings in a row

Lethargy (listlessness), difficulty in awakening baby

Cyanosis (bluish discoloration of skin) with or without a feeding

Absence of breathing longer than 20 seconds

Inconsolable infant (quieting techniques are not effective) or continuous high-pitched cry

Discharge or bleeding from umbilical cord, circumcision, or any opening (except vaginal mucus or pseudomenstruation)

Two consecutive green, watery stools or black stools or increased frequency of stools

No wet diapers for 18 to 24 hours or fewer than six to eight wet diapers per day after 4 days of age

Development of eye drainage

calls lend added support by providing another opportunity for parents to have their questions answered.

Some institutions have initiated postpartum and/or newborn follow-up home visits especially for infants discharged before 48 hours after birth. The follow-up infant examination should be within 48 hours of discharge when the family is unable to visit their primary care physician within that time period. The home visit focuses on normal newborn care, assessment for hyperbilirubinemia (jaundice), extreme weight loss, feeding problems, and knowledge related to newborn care and feeding within the family unit.

Routine well-baby visits should be scheduled with the clinic, pediatric nurse practitioner, or physician. Regardless of the type of follow-up services available in the community, the nurse contributes to the newborn's health by stressing the importance of routine care and by helping families who have no follow-up plans to connect to local resources for care. (For a detailed discussion of home care, see Chapter 30 ⊘.)

Evaluation

When evaluating the nursing care provided in preparation for discharge, the nurse may anticipate the following outcomes:

- The parents demonstrate safe techniques in caring for their newborn.
- Parents verbalize developmentally appropriate behavioral expectations of their newborn and knowledge of community-based newborn follow-up care.

Critical Concept Review

LEARNING OUTCOME 26.1: Summarize essential information to be obtained about a newborn's birth experience and immediate postnatal period.

Information is gathered from these sources:

1. Condition of the newborn:
   - Apgar scores.
   - Any resuscitation effort.
   - Vital signs.
   - Voiding.
   - Passage of meconium.
2. Labor and birth record:
   - Length and course of labor.
   - Type of delivery.
   - Conditions at delivery.
   - Medications given during labor.

3. Antepartum record:
   - Infections during pregnancy.
   - EDB.
   - Previous pregnancies.
   - Any congenital anomalies.
   - HIV test result.
4. Parent–newborn interaction information:
   - Type of infant feeding desired.
   - Desire for circumcision if infant is male.
   - Support system available.
   - Whether rooming in is desired.

LEARNING OUTCOME 26.2: Explain how the physiologic and behavioral responses of the newborn during the first 4 hours after birth (admission and transitional period) determine the nursing care of the newborn.

1. Maintaining a clear airway and stable vital signs:
   - The infant's cardiovascular and respiratory systems are changing rapidly.
   - The infant is dried and stimulated to breathe.
   - Free flow oxygen is available if needed, to assist the infant's transition.
   - Apgar score and vital signs are used to assess the infant's transition.
2. Maintaining a neutral thermal environment:
   - The infant is stressed by the change from the warm, moist environment of the uterus to the dry, drafty environment of the birthing room and nursery.
   - A neutral thermal environment is needed to prevent the need for increased oxygen and calories.
   - The newborn is dried and placed under a radiant warmer.
   - A cap is placed on the infant's head to prevent heat loss.
   - Temperature is checked frequently and the infant is kept from drafts and open windows.
3. Preventing hemorrhagic disease in the newborn:
   - Newborn lacks intestinal bacterial flora, which is necessary for the production of vitamin K.
   - Prothrombin levels are low during the first few days of life.
   - Vitamin K injection is given IM quickly after birth.
4. Preventing eye infection:
   - Infant may come in contact with infected material during birth.
   - Eye prophylaxis is given to all newborns to prevent serious eye infection.

5. Assessment of neonatal distress:
   - The nurse assesses and teaches parents signs and symptoms of respiratory distress such as tachypnea, grunting, retractions, or change in color.
   - Parents are taught to use the bulb syringe and proper positioning to prevent respiratory problems.
6. Expected periods of reactivity:
   - The infant is usually alert for the first hour after birth.
   - The nurse should encourage eye-to-eye contact between the infant and parents.
   - The nurse should initiate first feedings if the infant is stable.
7. Nursing interventions during the first 4 hours after birth include:
   - Monitor vital signs: every hour, four times daily.
   - Assess and monitor skin color, including acrocyanosis.
   - Assess condition of cord (note number and type of vessels).
   - Assess weight, length, and head circumference.
   - Determine gestational age classification.
   - Assess for the presence of any anomalies.
   - Identify infant and initiate security system.
   - Check for expected reflexes.
   - Assess ability to suck and swallow.
   - Bathe infant when temperature is stable.
   - Assist mother to feed as soon as infant is stable.
   - Administer necessary medications.

LEARNING OUTCOME 26.3: Explain the advantages and disadvantages of breastfeeding and formula-feeding in determining the nursing care of both mother/family and newborn.

1. Advantages of breastfeeding:
   - Provides immunologic protection.
   - Infant digests and absorbs components of breast milk easier.
   - Provides most vitamins to infant if mother's diet is adequate.
   - Strengthens the mother–infant attachment.
   - No additional cost.
   - Breast milk requires no preparation.
2. Disadvantages of breastfeeding:
   - Many medications pass through to breast milk.
   - Father is unable to participate equally in actual feeding of infant.
   - Mother may have difficulty being separated from infant.

3. Advantages of bottle-feeding:
   - Provides good nutrition to infant.
   - Father can participate in infant feeding activities.
4. Disadvantages of bottle-feeding:
   - May need to try different formulas before finding one that is well tolerated by the infant.
   - Formula must be purchased and prepared.
   - Proper preparation is necessary for nutritional adequacy.

LEARNING OUTCOME 26.4: Formulate guidelines for helping both breast- and formula-feeding mothers to feed their newborns successfully in hospital and community-based settings.

1. The breastfeeding mother needs to know:
   - How breast milk is produced.
   - How to correctly position and facilitate "latching on" by the infant for feeding.
   - The procedure for feeding the infant.
   - Number of times per day the breastfed infant should be put to the breast.
   - How to express, pump, and store breast milk.
   - How and when to supplement with formula.
   - How to care for the breasts.
   - Medications that pass through breast milk.
   - Support groups for breastfeeding.

2. The bottle-feeding mother needs to know:
   - Types of formula available and how to prepare each type.
   - The procedure for feeding the infant.
   - How to correctly position the infant for bottle-feeding.
   - How to safely store the formula.
   - How to safely care for bottles and nipples.

LEARNING OUTCOME 26.5: Identify activities that should be included in a daily care plan for a normal newborn.

1. Subsequent daily care includes:
   - Monitor vital signs every 6 to 8 hours.
   - Assess weight.
   - Assess overall color.
   - Assess and care for umbilical cord and circumcision, if performed.
   - Assess intake and output.
   - Assess infant's ability to void and stool.
   - Assess nutritional status.
   - Determine if infant is feeding adequately.
   - Swaddle infant to provide for warmth.
   - Initiate necessary immunizations.
   - Initiate newborn screening tests such as hearing test, if applicable.
   - Assess parent attachment.
   - Provide teaching to parents concerning newborn care.

LEARNING OUTCOME 26.6: Describe the common concerns of families regarding their newborn.

Parent concerns and teaching about newborn and infant care include:
1. Immediate health status of the newborn.
2. Measures to ensure infant safety:
   - How to properly use a bulb syringe.
   - Place baby on back to sleep.
   - How to safely position infant in crib.
3. Voiding and stool characteristics and patterns:
   - Normal color of urine and appropriate number of voidings.
   - Color, type, and number of expected stools.
4. How to provide general infant care.
   Cord care:
   - How to keep cord clean and dry.
   - How to keep diapers from irritating cord.
   - Normal changes of cord.
   - Possible cord complications.
   Male genitalia care:
   - Care of circumcision site.
   - Signs and symptoms of complications from circumcision.
   - Care and cleaning of uncircumcised infant.
   How to awaken infant:
   - Dress, undress, or bathe hands and feet of infant.
   - Change diaper.
   - Talk to infant, place in upright position.
   - Increase skin contact.
   How to quiet infant:
   - Move infant slowly and calmly.
   - Burp infant or change soiled diaper.
   - Swaddle infant.
   - Talk to or coo to infant.

Prior to discharge, review with parents about:
1. How to properly feed infant.
   Breastfeeding, if applicable:
   - Position of baby.
   - Supply and demand.
   - Latching on and breaking suction.
   - Supplementing.
   - How to express milk by hand and the use of a breast pump.
   Bottle-feeding, if applicable:
   - Position for feeding and burping the baby.
   - How to prepare formula and how to clean bottles and nipples.
   - Determination of proper formula.
2. General baby care:
   - Safety measures.
   - Skin and cord care.
   - How to detect jaundice.
   - Normal newborn behavior.
   - How to know if infant is sick, take a temperature, and phone number of and when to call infant's healthcare provider.
   - The proper use of car seats.
   - Remaining newborn screenings.
   - Schedule for newborn immunizations.
   - Appointment for infant's next visit with healthcare provider.

LEARNING OUTCOME 26.7: Identify opportunities to individualize parent teaching and enhance each parent's abilities and confidence while providing infant care in the birthing unit.

Individualized parent teaching is best accomplished by:

1. Observation and demonstration of common infant activities such as:
   - Feeding.
   - Bathing.
   - Diaper changing.
   - Cord care.
   - Circumcision care.

2. Videotapes of selected infant care activities.
3. Written handouts of selected infant care activities.
4. Return demonstration of parents completing selected infant care activities.

LEARNING OUTCOME 26.8: Explain the influence of cultural values on infant care, especially feeding practices.

Nurses must:

1. Describe how cultural values influence infant feeding practices.
2. Be sensitive to ethnic backgrounds of minority populations.
3. Understand that the dominant culture in any society defines normal maternal infant feeding interactions.

Clinical Reasoning in Action

Alice Fine, age 32, G1, now P1001, spontaneously delivers a 7.25 pound baby girl over a median episiotomy. The baby's Apgars are 7 and 9 at 1 and 5 minutes. The baby is suctioned, stimulated, and given free flow oxygen at birth. As the nurse on duty, you admit baby Fine to the newborn nursery, place her under a radiant heater, and perform a newborn assessment. You obtain the vital signs of temperature 97°F, heart rate 128, respiration 55. A physical exam demonstrates no abnormalities, and you note that there were no significant problems with the pregnancy, the mother's blood type is A+, and she plans to bottle-feed. You monitor the baby until her vital signs are stable and then take her to the mother's room for her first bottle-feeding at 60 minutes old.

1. How would you review measures to promote the safety of the newborn from abduction?
2. How would you explain the technique to suction the newborn with a bulb syringe?
3. Describe the care of the newborn's cord.
4. How would you review bottle-feeding with the mother?

See www.nursing.pearsonhighered.com for possible responses.

References

Academy of Breastfeeding Medicine (ABM). (2009). Protocol #3: Hospital guidelines for the use of supplementary feedings in the healthy term breastfed neonate, revised 2009. *Breastfeeding Medicine, 4*(3), 175–182. doi:10.1089/bfm.2009.9991

Academy of Breastfeeding Medicine (ABM). (2011). Protocol #9: Use of galactogogues initiating or augmenting the rate of maternal milk secretion. *Breastfeeding Medicine,* http://www.bfmed.org/Resources/Protocols.aspx

American Academy of Pediatrics (AAP). (2013a). *AAP updates recommendation on car seats.* Retrieved from http://www.healthychildren.org

American Academy of Pediatrics (AAP). (2013b). *Reduce the risk of SIDS.* Retrieved from http://www.healthychildren.org/English/ages-stages/sleep/pages/Preventing-SIDS

American Academy of Pediatrics (AAP). (2013c). *Sleep position: Why back is best.* Retrieved from http://www.healthychildren.org/English/ages-stages/baby/sleep/pages/Sleep-Position

American Academy of Pediatrics (AAP) Committee on Fetus and Newborn & American College of Obstetricians and Gynecologists (ACOG) Committee on Obstetrics. (2012). *Guidelines for perinatal care* (7th ed.). Evanston, IL: Author.

American Academy of Pediatrics (AAP) Section on Breastfeeding. (2012). Policy statement: Breastfeeding and the use of human milk. *Pediatrics, 129,* e827–e841.

Association of Women's Health, Obstetric and Neonatal Nurses (AWHONN). (2007). *Breastfeeding support: Prenatal care through the first year. Evidence-based clinical practice guideline* (2nd ed., pp. 1–89). Washington, DC: Author.

Baby-Friendly Hospital Initiative USA (BFHI USA). (2013). *Implementing the UNICEF/WHO baby-friendly hospital initiative in the U.S.* Retrieved from http://www.babyfriendlyusa.org/eng/index.html

Blackburn, S. T. (2013). *Maternal, fetal, & neonatal physiology: A clinical perspective* (4th ed.). St. Louis, MO: Saunders.

Bojcicki, J. (2011). Maternal prepregnancy body mass index and initiation and direction of breastfeeding: A review of the literature. *Journal of Women's Health, 20*(3), 341–347.

Callister, L. C. (2008). Integrating cultural beliefs and practices when caring for childbearing women and families. In K. R. Simpson & P. A. Creehan, *Perinatal nursing* (3rd ed., pp. 29–57). Philadelphia, PA: Lippincott Williams & Wilkins.

Centers for Disease Control and Prevention (CDC). (2012). *Hearing loss in newborn: Screening and diagnosis.* Retrieved from http://www.cdc.gov/Features/NewbornScreening/

Centers for Disease Control and Prevention (CDC) Advisory Committee on Immunization Practices. (2013). *Recommended childhood and adolescent immunization schedule, United States 2013.* Retrieved from http://www.cdc.gov/vaccines/schedules/downloads/child/0-18yrs-schedule.pdf

Cloherty, J. R., Eichenwald, E. C., Hansen, A. R., & Stark, A. R. (2012). *Manual of neonatal care* (7th ed.). Philadelphia, PA: Lippincott Williams & Wilkins.

D'Avanzo, C. E., & Geissler, E. M. (2008). *Pocket guide to cultural assessment* (4th ed.). St. Louis, MO: Mosby.

Genetics Home Reference. (2013). *Newborn screening.* Retrieved from http://www.ghr.nlm.nih.gov/nbs

Healthy Children. (2013a). *Circumcision*. Retrieved from http://www.healthychildren.org/english/ages-stages/baby/prenatal/decisions-to-make/pages/circumcision

Healthy Children. (2013b). *Purpose of newborn hearing screening*. Retrieved from http://www.healthychildren.org/english/ages-stages/baby/pages/purpose-of-newborn-hearing

Human Milk Banking Association of North America (HMBANA). (2011). *Best practice for expressing, storing and handling human milk in hospitals, homes and child care settings* (3rd ed.). Raleigh, NC: Author.

Klaus, M., & Klaus, P. (1985). *The amazing newborn*. Menlo Park, CA: Addison-Wesley.

Lawrence, R. A., & Lawrence, R. M. (2011). *Breastfeeding: A guide for the medical profession* (7th ed.). Philadelphia, PA: Mosby.

Lipson, J. G., & Dibble, S. L. (2008). *Culture & clinical care* (7th ed.). San Francisco, CA: The Regents, University of California.

Mercer, A. M., Teasley, S. L., Hopkinson, J., McPherson, D. M., Simon, S. D., & Hall, R. T. (2010). Evaluation of a breastfeeding assessment score in a diverse population. *Journal of Human Lactation, 26*(1), 42–48.

Nommsen-Rivers, L., Chantry, C., Peerson, J., Cohen, R., & Dewey, K. (2010). Delayed onset of lactogenesis among first-time mothers is related to maternal obesity and factors associated with ineffective breastfeeding. *American Journal of Clinical Nutrition, 92*(3), 574–584.

Ott, B. B., Al-Khadhuri, J., & Al-Junaibi, S. (2003). Preventing ethical dilemmas: Understanding Islamic health care practices. *Pediatric Nursing, 29*(3), 227–230.

Riordan, J., & Wambach, K. (2010). *Breastfeeding and human lactation* (4th ed.). Boston, MA: Jones & Bartlett.

Teh, L. (undated). *No bathing, no visiting, and no drinking water: The confinement of Chinese mothers*. Retrieved from http://www.geocities.com/Wellesley/3321/win14c.htm

United States Breastfeeding Committee. (2011). *Healthy People 2020: Breastfeeding objectives*. Retrieved from http://www.usbreastfeeding.org/Legislation-Policy/FederalPolicies/HealthyPeople2020Breast-feedingObjectives/tabid/120/Default.aspx

Wilson, B. A., Shannon, M. T., & Shields, K. M. (2013). *Prentice Hall nurse's drug guide 2013*. Upper Saddle River, NJ: Pearson Education.

Woodring, B. C., & Andrews, M. M. (2012). Transcultural perspectives in the nursing care of children and adolescents. In M. M. Andrews & J. S. Boyle (Eds.), *Transcultural concepts in nursing care* (6th ed., pp. 123–156). Philadelphia, PA: Lippincott.

World Health Organization (WHO). (1999). *Care of the umbilical cord: A review of the evidence*. Retrieved from http://www.whoint/en/documents/MSM98-4

World Health Organization (WHO). (2008). *Male circumcision information package*. Retrieved from http://www.who.int/hiv/pub/malecircumcision/infopack/en/index.html

Pearson Nursing Student Resources Find additional review materials at: **nursing.pearsonhighered.com**

The Newborn at Risk: Conditions Present at Birth

There is an initial flurry of activity when my baby is taken into the NICU. Now my entire universe, everything that I am, constricts down to focus on our little one. She hardly dents this world, a withery face that shows a kind of infinitely pained acceptance, breath and heartbeat almost nothing, and a pose that moves to rest, resisting nothing. I look at my small daughter with eyes naked with amazement and unsure joy. —Jontelle, 42

Digital Vision/Getty Images

LEARNING OUTCOMES

27.1 Explain the factors present at birth that indicate an at-risk newborn.

27.2 Compare the underlying etiologies of the physiologic complications of small-for-gestational-age (SGA) newborns and preterm appropriate-for-gestational-age (Pr AGA) newborns and the nursing management for each.

27.3 Explain the impact of maternal diabetes mellitus on the newborn.

27.4 Compare the characteristics and potential complications that influence nursing management of the postterm newborn and the newborn with postmaturity syndrome.

27.5 Discuss the physiologic and behavioral characteristics of the preterm newborn that predispose each body system to various complications and that are used in developing a plan of care that includes nutritional management.

27.6 Summarize the nursing assessments of and initial interventions for a newborn with selected congenital anomalies.

27.7 Explain the special care needed by an alcohol- or drug-exposed newborn.

27.8 Relate the consequences of maternal HIV/AIDS to the nursing management of infants at risk for HIV/AIDS in the neonatal period and the issues for their caregivers.

27.9 Identify the physical examination findings during the early newborn period that would make the nurse suspect a congenital cardiac defect or congestive heart failure.

Many levels of nursery care have evolved in response to increasing knowledge about at-risk newborns. Along with the newborn's parents, the nurse is an important caregiver in all these settings. As a member of the collaborative healthcare team, the nurse is a technically competent professional who contributes the high-touch human care necessary in the high-tech perinatal environment.

In addition to the availability of a high level of newborn care, various other factors influence the outcome of at-risk infants, including the following:

- Birth weight
- Gestational age
- Type and length of newborn illness
- Environmental factors
- Maternal factors
- Maternal–infant separation

IDENTIFICATION OF AT-RISK NEWBORNS

An at-risk newborn is one susceptible to illness (morbidity) or even death (mortality) because of dysmaturity, immaturity, physical disorders, or complications during or after birth. In most cases, the infant is the product of a pregnancy involving one or more predictable risk factors, including the following:

- Low socioeconomic level of the mother
- Limited access to health care or no prenatal care
- Exposure to environmental dangers, such as toxic chemicals and illicit drugs
- Preexisting maternal conditions such as heart disease, diabetes, hypertension, hyperthyroidism, and renal disease
- Maternal factors such as age and parity
- Medical conditions related to pregnancy and their associated complications
- Pregnancy complications such as abruptio placentae, oligohydramnios, preterm labor, premature rupture of membranes, preeclampsia

Various risk factors and their specific effects on the pregnancy outcome are listed in Table 10–1 on page 198. Because these factors and the perinatal risks associated with them are known, the birth of at-risk newborns can often be anticipated. The pregnancy can be closely monitored, treatment can be started as necessary, and arrangements can be made for birth to occur at a facility with appropriate resources to care for both mother and baby.

Whether or not prenatal assessment indicates that the fetus is at risk, the course of labor and birth and the infant's ability to withstand the stress of labor cannot be predicted. Thus, the nurse's use of electronic fetal heart monitoring or fetal heart auscultation by Doppler plays a significant role in detecting stress or distress in the fetus. Immediately after birth the Apgar score is a helpful tool for identifying the at-risk newborn, but it is not a definite indication of an acute intrapartum hypoxic event.

The newborn classification and neonatal mortality risk chart is another useful tool for identifying newborns at risk. Before this classification tool was developed, birth weight of less than 2500 g was the sole criterion for determining immaturity. Clinicians then recognized that a newborn could weigh more than 2500 g and still be immature. Conversely, an infant weighing less than 2500 g might be functionally at term or beyond. Thus birth weight and gestational age together are now the criteria used to assess neonatal maturity, morbidity, and mortality risk.

According to the newborn classification and neonatal mortality risk chart, gestation (postmenstrual age) is divided as follows (Gardner & Hernandez, 2011):

- *Preterm:* less than 37 (completed) weeks
- *Late preterm:* 34 to 36 6/7 (completed) weeks
- *Early term:* 37 to 38 6/7 (completed) weeks
- *Term:* 37 to 41 6/7 (completed) weeks
- *Postterm:* greater than 42 weeks

Late preterm is an emerging classification that refers to subgroups of infants between 34 and 36 6/7 weeks' gestation; however, it is not yet used consistently for a single age range (Cloherty, Eichenwald, Hansen, et al., 2012; Glomella, 2013). See Chapter 30 🔗 for a discussion of the long-term needs of late preterm infants. It has been identified that morbidities associated with prematurity continue into early term gestation and are compounded by socioeconomic status (SES) (Ruth, Roos, Hildes-Ripstein, et al., 2013).

Generally newborns are classified as LGA, SGA, or AGA, based on weight and gestational age (Koops, Morgan, & Battaglia, 1982). **Large-for-gestational-age (LGA)** newborns are those who plot above the 90th percentile curve on intrauterine growth curves. Appropriate-for-gestational-age (AGA) newborns are those that plot between the 10th percentile and 90th percentile growth curves. **Small-for-gestational-age (SGA)** newborns are those that plot below the 10th percentile growth curve. See Figure 25–12 🔗 on page 551. A newborn is assigned to a category depending on birth weight, length, occipital-frontal head circumference, and gestational age. For example, a newborn classified as Pr SGA is preterm and small for gestational age. The full-term newborn whose weight is appropriate for gestational age is classified FAGA. It is important to note that intrauterine growth charts are influenced by altitude and the ethnicity of the newborn population used to create the chart. Also, the assigned newborn classification may vary according to the intrauterine growth curve chart used; therefore, the chart used should correlate with the characteristics of the patient population.

Neonatal mortality risk is the infant's chance of death within the newborn period—that is, within the first 28 days of life. Neonatal mortality risk decreases as both gestational age and birth weight increase. Infants who are Pr SGA have the highest neonatal mortality risk. The previously high mortality rates for LGA newborns have decreased at most perinatal centers because of both improved management of diabetes in pregnancy and increased recognition of potential complications of LGA newborns.

Neonatal morbidity can be anticipated based on birth weight and gestational age. The neonatal morbidity by birth weight and gestational age tool assists in determining the needs of particular infants for special observation and care. For example, an infant of 2000 g at 40 weeks' gestation should be carefully assessed for evidence of neonatal distress, hypoglycemia, congenital anomalies, congenital infection, and polycythemia.

Identifying the nursing care needs of the at-risk newborn depends on minute-to-minute observations of the changes in the newborn's physiologic status. The organization of nursing care must be directed toward the following:

- Decreasing physiologically stressful situations
- Observing constantly for subtle signs of change in clinical condition
- Interpreting laboratory data and coordinating interventions
- Conserving the infant's energy for healing and growth
- Providing for developmental stimulation and maintenance of sleep cycles
- Assisting the family in developing attachment behaviors
- Involving the family in planning and providing care

CARE OF THE SMALL-FOR-GESTATIONAL-AGE/INTRAUTERINE GROWTH RESTRICTION NEWBORN

Currently infants are considered small for gestational age (SGA) when they are less than the 10th percentile for birth weight; very small for gestational age is when they are two standard deviations below the population norm or less than the third percentile (Rozance & Rosenberg, 2012) (Figure 27–1 ●). *Note:* An SGA newborn may be preterm, term, or postterm. An undergrown newborn may also be said to have **intrauterine growth restriction (IUGR)**, which describes pregnancy circumstances of advanced gestation and limited fetal growth. This classification of abnormal growth is also enhanced by looking at growth potential by adjusting birth weight reference limits for first-trimester maternal height, birth order, and fetal neonatal sex.

SGA infants are commonly seen with mothers who smoke or have high blood pressure, causing these infants to have an increased incidence of perinatal asphyxia and perinatal mortality when compared with AGA infants (Gleason & Devaskar, 2012). The incidence of polycythemia and hypoglycemia is also higher in this group of infants.

● **Figure 27–1** Thirty-one-week gestational age, 2-day-old baby girl.
Source: Carol Harrigan, RN, MSN, NNP-BC

Factors Contributing to IUGR

IUGR may be caused by maternal, placental, or fetal factors and may not be apparent antenatally. Intrauterine growth is linear (follows expected growth line) in the normal pregnancy from approximately 28 to 38 weeks' gestation. After 38 weeks, growth is variable, depending on the growth potential of the fetus and placental function. The most common causes of growth restriction are as follows:

- *Maternal factors.* Primiparity, grand multiparity, multiple-gestation pregnancy (twins and higher-order multiples), lack of prenatal care, age extremes (<16 years or >40 years), and low socioeconomic status (which can result in inadequate health care, inadequate education, and inadequate living conditions) affect IUGR (Cloherty et al., 2012). Before the third trimester, the nutritional supply to the fetus far exceeds its needs. Only in the third trimester are maternal malnutrition and drug abuse limiting factors in fetal growth.

- *Maternal disease.* Maternal heart disease, substance abuse (drugs, tobacco, alcohol), sickle cell disease, phenylketonuria (PKU), lupus erythematosus, and asymptomatic pyelonephritis are associated with SGA and IUGR. Complications associated with preeclampsia, chronic hypertensive vascular disease, and advanced diabetes mellitus can diminish blood flow to the uterus, thereby decreasing oxygen delivery to the fetus.

- *Environmental factors.* High altitude, exposure to x-rays, excessive exercise, work-related exposure to toxins, hyperthermia, and maternal use of drugs that have teratogenic effects, such as nicotine, alcohol, antimetabolites, anticonvulsants, narcotics, and cocaine, affect fetal growth (Cloherty et al., 2012).

- *Placental factors.* Placental conditions such as small placenta, infarcted areas, abnormal cord insertions, placenta previa, and thrombosis may affect circulation to the fetus, which becomes more deficient with increasing gestational age.

- *Fetal factors.* Congenital infections such as TORCH infections (*t*oxoplasmosis, *o*ther agents, *r*ubella, *c*ytomegalovirus, *h*erpes simplex virus), syphilis congenital malformations, discordant twins, sex of the fetus (females tend to be smaller), chromosomal syndromes (trisomies 13, 18, 21), two-vessel umbilical cord, and inborn errors of metabolism can predispose a fetus to fetal growth disturbances.

Identifying fetuses with IUGR is the first step in detecting common disorders associated with affected newborns. The perinatal history of maternal conditions, early dating of pregnancy by first-trimester ultrasound measurements, antepartum testing (nonstress test, contraction stress test, biophysical profile; for more information on these tests, see Chapter 14 🔴), Doppler velocimetry of placenta, gestational age assessment, and the physical and neurologic assessment of the newborn are important methods (Cloherty et al., 2012).

Clinical Tip

In assessing a growth-restricted infant resulting from unexplained maternal etiology (e.g., hypertension, placental insufficiency), an in utero viral infection may be the cause.

Patterns of IUGR

Intrauterine growth occurs by an increase in both cell number and cell size. If insult occurs early during the critical period of organ development in the fetus, fewer new cells are formed, organs are small, and organ weight is subnormal. In contrast, growth failure that begins later in pregnancy does not affect the total number of cells, only their size. The organs are normal, but their size is diminished. There are two clinical pictures of IUGR newborns:

- *Symmetric (proportional) IUGR* is caused by long-term maternal conditions (such as chronic hypertension, severe malnutrition, chronic intrauterine viral infection, substance abuse [drugs, alcohol, tobacco], anemia) or fetal genetic abnormalities (Gleason & Devaskar, 2012). Symmetric IUGR can be noted by ultrasound in the first half of the second trimester. In symmetric IUGR there is chronic, prolonged restriction of growth in the size of organs, weight, length, and, especially, head circumference.

- *Asymmetric (disproportional) IUGR* is associated with an acute compromise of uteroplacental blood flow. Some associated causes are placental infarcts, preeclampsia, and poor weight gain in pregnancy. The growth restriction is usually not evident before the third trimester because, although weight is decreased, length and head circumference (used as a growth indicator) remain appropriate for that gestational age. After 36 weeks' gestation, the abdominal circumference of a normal fetus becomes larger than the head circumference. In asymmetric IUGR, the head circumference remains larger than the abdominal circumference. Thus measuring only the biparietal diameter on ultrasound will not reveal asymmetric IUGR. An early indicator of asymmetric IUGR is a decrease in the growth rate of the abdominal circumference, reflecting subnormal liver growth, a reduction in glycogen stores, and a scarcity of subcutaneous fat (Gleason & Devaskar, 2012). Birth weight is below the 10th percentile, whereas head circumference and/or length may be between the 10th and 90th percentiles. Asymmetric SGA newborns related to IUGR are particularly at risk for asphyxia, pulmonary hemorrhage, hypocalcemia, and hypoglycemia.

Despite growth restriction, physiologic maturity develops according to gestational age. The SGA/IUGR newborn's chances for survival are better than those of the preterm AGA newborn because of organ maturity, although this newborn still faces many potential difficulties.

Common Complications of the SGA/IUGR Newborn

The complications occurring most frequently in the SGA/IUGR newborn include the following:

- *Fetal hypoxia (impaired oxygenation).* The SGA/IUGR newborn suffers chronically lower-than-normal oxygen levels in utero, which leaves little reserve to withstand the demands of normal labor and birth. Thus intrauterine asphyxia and its potential systemic problems can occur. Cesarean birth may be necessary.

- *Aspiration syndrome.* In utero hypoxia can cause the fetus to gasp during birth, resulting in aspiration of amniotic fluid into the lower airways. It can also lead to relaxation of the anal sphincter and passage of meconium. This may result in aspiration of the meconium in utero or with the first breaths after birth.
- *Hypothermia.* Diminished subcutaneous fat (used for survival in utero), depletion of brown fat in utero, and a large surface area decrease the IUGR newborn's ability to conserve heat. The flexed position assumed by the term SGA newborn diminishes the effect of surface area.
- *Hypoglycemia.* An increase in metabolic rate in response to heat loss and poor hepatic glycogen stores causes hypoglycemia. In addition, the newborn is compromised by inadequate supplies of enzymes to activate gluconeogenesis (conversion of nonglucogen sources such as fatty acids and proteins to glucose).
- *Polycythemia.* The number of red blood cells is increased (central hematocrit > 65%) in the SGA/IUGR newborn. This finding is considered a physiologic response to in utero chronic hypoxic stress. Polycythemia may contribute to hypoglycemia and hyperviscosity.

Newborns who have significant SGA/IUGR tend to have a poor prognosis, especially when born before 37 weeks' gestation. Factors contributing to poor outcome include the following:

- *Congenital malformations.* Congenital malformations occur in 5% of SGA/IUGR infants (Cloherty et al., 2012). The more severe the IUGR, the greater the chance for malformation as a result of impaired mitotic activity and cellular hypoxia.
- *Intrauterine infections.* When fetuses are exposed to intrauterine infections such as rubella and cytomegalovirus, they are profoundly affected by direct invasion of the brain and other vital organs by the offending virus.
- *Continued growth difficulties.* SGA newborns tend to be shorter than newborns of the same gestational age. Asymmetric IUGR infants can be expected to catch up in weight and approach their inherited growth potential when given an optimal environment.
- *Cognitive difficulties.* Often SGA/IUGR newborns can exhibit subsequent learning disabilities. The disabilities are characterized by hyperactivity, short attention span, and poor fine motor coordination (writing and drawing) (Daily, Carter, & Carter, 2011).

Clinical Therapy

The goal of medical therapy for SGA/IUGR infants is early recognition and implementation of the medical management of potential problems.

NURSING MANAGEMENT *For the SGA/IUGR Newborn*

Nursing Assessment and Diagnosis

The nurse is responsible for assessing gestational age and identifying signs of potential complications associated with SGA

infants. All body parts of the symmetric IUGR infant are in proportion (the head does not appear overly large or excessively long in relation to the other body parts), but they are below normal size for the baby's gestational age. These newborns are generally vigorous.

The asymmetric IUGR infant appears long, thin, and emaciated, with loss of subcutaneous fat tissue and muscle mass. The baby may have loose skinfolds; dry, desquamating skin; and a thin and often meconium-stained cord. The head appears relatively large (although it approaches normal size) because the chest size and abdominal girth are decreased. The baby may have a vigorous cry and appear alert and wide-eyed.

Nursing diagnoses that may apply to the SGA newborn include those listed in the *Nursing Care Plan: The Small-for-Gestational-Age Newborn* and the following (NANDA-I © 2012):

- *Hypothermia* related to decreased subcutaneous fat
- *Tissue Integrity, Impaired,* related to increased blood viscosity
- *Parenting, Risk for Impaired,* related to prolonged separation of newborn from parents secondary to illness

Planning and Implementation

Hospital-Based Nursing Care

Hypoglycemia, the most common metabolic complication of IUGR, produces such sequelae as CNS abnormalities and mental retardation (intellectual disability). Conditions such as asphyxia, hyperviscosity, and cold stress may also affect the baby's outcome. Meticulous attention to physiologic parameters is essential for immediate nursing management and reduction of long-term disorders. (See *Nursing Care Plan: The Small-for-Gestational-Age Newborn* on pages 630–632.)

Community-Based Nursing Care

The long-term needs of the SGA/IUGR newborn include careful follow-up evaluation of patterns of growth and possible disabilities that may later interfere with learning or motor functioning. Long-term follow-up care is essential for infants with congenital malformations, congenital infections, and obvious sequelae from physiologic problems. Parents of the SGA/IUGR newborn need support, because a positive atmosphere can enhance the baby's growth potential and the child's ultimate outcome.

Evaluation

Expected outcomes of nursing care include the following:

- The SGA/IUGR newborn is free from respiratory compromise.
- The SGA/IUGR newborn maintains a stable temperature.
- The SGA/IUGR infant is free from hypoglycemic episodes and maintains glucose homeostasis.
- The SGA/IUGR newborn gains weight and takes breast or formula feedings without developing physiologic distress or fatigue.
- The parents verbalize their concerns about their baby's health problems and understand the rationale behind management of their newborn.

Nursing Care Plan The Small-for-Gestational-Age Newborn

Intervention	Rationale	Expected Outcome

1. Nursing Diagnosis: *Gas Exchange, Impaired,* related to amniotic fluid and meconium aspiration (NANDA-I © 2012)

NIC Priority Intervention:
Respiratory monitoring: Collection and analysis of patient data to ensure airway patency and adequate gas exchange

NOC Suggested Outcome:
Respiratory status: Gas exchange: alveolar exchange of CO_2 or O_2 to maintain arterial blood gas concentrations

Goal: The newborn's respirations will be stable and maintained within normal limits.

Intervention	Rationale	Expected Outcome
■ Obtain maternal prenatal, labor, and birth records.	■ Provides information about fetal stress that may have occurred during the prenatal or intrapartum period. In addition, the birth record will provide information concerning infant's respiratory status at birth; for example, the Apgar score.	■ Infant will maintain adequate respiratory gas exchange as evidenced by respirations of 30–60/min with no periods of apnea or evidence of worsening distress.
■ Maintain airway patency through judicious suctioning.	■ Respiratory distress in SGA newborns is due to in utero hypoxia and aspiration of meconium.	
■ Observe for worsening signs of respiratory distress such as generalized cyanosis; worsening retractions, grunting, and nasal flaring, as evidenced by Silverman respiratory index; sustained tachypnea; apnea episodes; inequality of breath sounds; presence of rales and rhonchi.		
■ Monitor and maintain adequate body temperature (36°C±0.2°C [97.7°F±0.5°F]) to avoid increased oxygen consumption.	■ Temperature elevation may cause metabolic rate and oxygen needs to increase when associated with meconium aspiration.	
■ Administer oxygen per order for relief of respiratory distress signs. (See *Care of the Newborn with Respiratory Distress* in Chapter 28 for nursing care and treatment of meconium aspiration, infant resuscitation.)	■ Provides healthcare personnel with cardiac and pulmonary status.	
■ Implement treatment plan for respiratory distress.		
■ Monitor glucose levels.	■ Respiratory distress increases consumption of glucose.	
■ **Collaborative:** Obtain arterial blood gases per physician's orders.		
■ Monitor infant's cardiac status and pulmonary status; pulse oximetry and arterial blood gases (ABGs).	■ Oxygen demands increase with meconium aspiration. Obtaining ABGs will provide medical personnel with baseline information about infant's respiratory status so effective medical interventions can be initiated.	

2. Nursing Diagnosis: *Thermoregulation, Ineffective,* secondary to decreased subcutaneous fat (NANDA-I © 2012)

NIC Priority Intervention:
Temperature regulation: Attaining and/or maintaining body temperature within a normal range

NIC Suggested Outcome:
Temperature regulation: Balance among heat production, heat gain, and heat loss during the neonatal period.

Goal: The infant's temperature will be stable and maintained within normal limits.

Intervention	Rationale	Expected Outcome
■ Provide neutral thermal zone (NTZ) range for infant based on postnatal weight.	■ Neutral thermal environment charts used for preterm infant are not reliable for weight of SGA infant.	■ Infant will not exhibit signs and symptoms of hypothermia as evidenced by axillary temperature maintenance of 36.4°C–37.2°C (97.5°F–99°F) and no signs and symptoms of respiratory distress.

Nursing Care Plan The Small-for-Gestational-Age Newborn—continued

Intervention	Rationale	Expected Outcome
■ Use a skin probe to maintain infant's skin temperature at 36°C–36.5°C (97.5°F–99°F).	■ A neutral thermal environment requires minimal oxygen consumption to maintain a normal core temp.	
■ Obtain axillary temps and compare to registered skin probe temp. If discrepancy exists evaluate potential cause.	■ Discrepancies between axillary and skin probe monitor temp may be due to mechanical causes or the burning of brown fat.	
■ Adjust and monitor incubator or radiant warmer to maintain skin temp.		
■ Minimize heat losses and prevent cold stress by: ■ Warming and humidifying oxygen without blowing over face in order to avoid increasing oxygen consumption. ■ Keeping skin dry, especially immediately following delivery. ■ Keeping isolettes, radiant warmers, and cribs away from windows and cold external walls and out of drafts. ■ Avoiding placing infant on cold surfaces such as metal treatment tables, cold x-ray plates, and scales. ■ Padding cold surfaces with diapers and using radiant warmers during procedures. ■ Warming blood for exchange transfusions.	■ Physical principles of heat loss effects include: ■ Evaporation—lungs and skin when cooling occurs as a result of water evaporation ■ Convection—air currents ■ Conduction—skin contact with cooler object ■ Radiation—loss of warmth to cooler surrounding objects	
■ Observe for signs and symptoms of cold stress: decreased temperature, lethargy, pallor (for further discussion, see Chapter 28).	■ Hypothermia is a potential problem for SGA infant because: 1. SGA infant has decreased stores of brown fat available for thermogenesis, because SGA infant has used these stores in utero for survival. 2. SGA infant has poor insulation due to use of subcutaneous tissues in utero for survival.	

3. Nursing Diagnosis: *Tissue integrity, Impaired,* related to decreased glycogen stores and impaired gluconeogenesis (NANDA-I © 2012)

NIC Priority Intervention:
High-risk infant care: Identification and management of a high-risk infant to promote healthy outcomes for the baby

NOC Suggested Outcome:
Risk control: Actions to eliminate or reduce actual, personal, and modifiable health threats

Goal: The newborn will have a normal blood glucose level.

Intervention	Rationale	Expected Outcome
■ Monitor chemstrip per SGA protocol and report values <45 mg/dL.	■ Combined with depletion of glycogen stores, impaired gluconeogenesis predisposes SGA infants to profound hypoglycemia within first 2 days of life.	■ Fetus will not exhibit signs and symptoms of hypoglycemia as evidenced by a euglycemic state and blood glucose greater than 20 mg/dL.
■ Observe, record, and report signs of hypoglycemia: cyanosis, lethargy, jitteriness, seizure activity, and apnea.	■ Hypoglycemia in SGA infant is indicated by whole blood sugar less than 20 mg/dL.	
■ Initiate feeding schedule for SGA newborns per agency protocol.	■ Frequent monitoring of Dextrostix assists in identifying decreasing glucose levels.	
■ Provide glucose intake either through early enteral feeding (before 4 hr) or by IV per physician's order.	■ Provision of glucose through early feedings (begin before 4 hr of age) assists in maintaining glucose levels.	

See further discussion of hypoglycemia in Chapter 28 .

(continued)

Nursing Care Plan   The Small-for-Gestational-Age Newborn—continued

Intervention	Rationale	Expected Outcome

4. Nursing Diagnosis: *Nutrition, Imbalanced: Less Than Body Requirements,* related to increased metabolic needs in the infant (NANDA-I © 2012)

NIC Priority Intervention: *Newborn monitoring:* Measurement and interpretation of physiologic status of the newborn for the first 24 hr		**NOC Suggested Outcome:** *Nutritional status:* Food and fluid intake: amount of food and fluid taken into the body over a 24-hr period

Goal: The newborn will gain weight and tolerate nipple feedings without tiring.

■ Assess suck, swallow, gag, and cough reflexes.	■ Sterile water may be used to test gag and swallow reflex because it causes fewer pulmonary complications in the presence of gastrointestinal tract abnormalities and/or aspiration of feeding. ■ Prevents feeding problems and assists in determining the best method of feeding for infant.	■ Infant will maintain steady weight gain as evidenced by less than 2%/day weight loss, will tolerate oral feedings, and will have urine output of 1–3 mL/kg/hr.
■ Initiate formula feeding per protocol at 1 hr of age; move early to formula feeding every 2–3 hr.	■ SGA newborns require more calories per kilogram for growth than AGA newborns because of increased metabolic activity and oxygen consumption secondary to increased percentage of body weight made up by visceral organs.	
■ Supplement oral feedings with IV intake per orders. ■ Use concentrated formulas that supply more calories in less volume, such as 22 or 24 cal/oz.	■ Small, frequent feedings of high-caloric formula are used because of limited gastric capacity and decreased gastric emptying.	
■ Promote growth by providing caloric intake of 120–150 cal/kg/day in small amounts.	■ Growth is evaluated by increase in weight (about 20 g/day), length, and other body measurements.	
■ Observe, record, and report signs of respiratory distress or fatigue occurring during feedings.	■ Decrease in exhaustion is an important consideration in feeding SGA infant. ■ Adequate nutritional intake promotes growth and prevents such complications as metabolic catabolism and hypoglycemia.	
■ Supplement gavage or nipple feedings with IV therapy per physician order until oral intake is sufficient to support growth.	■ Gavage feedings require less energy expenditure on the part of the newborn.	
■ Establish a nipple feeding program that is begun slowly and progresses slowly, such as nipple feed once per day, nipple feed once per shift, and then nipple feed every other feeding.		
■ Monitor daily weight with anticipation of small amount of weight loss when nipple feedings start.	■ Nipple feeding, an active rather than passive intake of nutrition, requires energy expenditure and burning of calories by infant.	

CARE OF THE LARGE-FOR-GESTATIONAL-AGE (LGA) NEWBORN

A newborn whose birth weight is at or above the 90th percentile on the intrauterine growth curve (at any week of gestation) is considered large for gestational age (LGA). Some AGA newborns

have been incorrectly categorized as LGA because of miscalculation of the date of conception caused by postconceptual bleeding. Careful gestational age assessment is essential to identify the potential needs and problems of these infants.

The most well-known condition associated with excessive fetal growth is maternal diabetes; however, only a small fraction of large newborns are born to diabetic mothers. The cause of the majority of cases of LGA newborns is unclear, but certain factors or situations have been found to correlate with their birth (Cloherty et al., 2012):

- Genetic predisposition is correlated proportionately to the mother's prepregnancy weight and to weight gain during pregnancy. Large parents tend to have large infants.

- Multiparous women have two to three times the number of LGA infants as primigravidas.

- Male infants are typically larger than female infants.

- Infants with erythroblastosis fetalis, Beckwith-Wiedemann syndrome (a genetic condition associated with omphalocele and neonatal hypoglycemia and hyperinsulinemia), or transposition of the great vessels are usually large.

The increase in the LGA infant's body size is characteristically proportional, although head circumference and body length are in the upper limits of intrauterine growth. The exception to this rule is the infant of the diabetic mother, whose body weight increases while length and head circumference may remain in the normal range. Macrosomic infants have poor motor skills and have difficulty regulating behavioral states. LGA infants tend to be more difficult to arouse to a quiet alert state.

Common Complications of the LGA Newborn

Complications of the LGA newborn can include the following:

- *Birth trauma caused by cephalopelvic disproportion (CPD).* Often LGA newborns have a biparietal diameter greater than 10 cm (4 in.) or are associated with a maternal fundal height measurement greater than 42 cm (16 in.) without the presence of polyhydramnios. Because of their excessive size, there are more breech presentations and shoulder dystocia. These complications may result in asphyxia, fractured clavicles, brachial palsy, facial paralysis, phrenic nerve palsy, depressed skull fractures, cephalohematoma, and intracranial hemorrhage caused by birth trauma.

- *Complications of hypoglycemia, polycythemia, and hyperviscosity.* These disorders are most often seen in infants of diabetic mothers, infants with erythroblastosis fetalis, or infants with Beckwith-Wiedemann syndrome.

Nursing Management

The perinatal history, in conjunction with ultrasonic measurement of fetal skull (biparietal diameter) and gestational age testing, is important in identifying an at-risk LGA newborn. Essential components of the nursing assessment are monitoring vital signs, screening for hypoglycemia and polycythemia, and observing for signs and symptoms related to birth trauma. Address parental concerns about the visual signs of birth trauma and the potential for continuation of the overweight pattern. Help parents learn to arouse and console their newborn and facilitate attachment behaviors. Mothers of LGA infants with facial or head bruising may be reluctant to interact with their newborns because they fear hurting their infants. The nursing care involved in the complications associated with LGA

newborns is similar to the care needed by the infant of a diabetic mother and is discussed in the next section.

CARE OF THE INFANT OF A DIABETIC MOTHER

The **infant of a diabetic mother (IDM)** is considered at risk and requires close observation during the first few hours to the first few days of life. Mothers with severe diabetes or diabetes of long duration associated with vascular complications may give birth to small-for-gestational-age (SGA) infants. The typical IDM, when the diabetes is poorly controlled or gestational, is large for gestational age (LGA). The infant is macrosomic, ruddy in color, and has excessive adipose (fat) tissue (Figure 27–2 ●). The umbilical cord is thick and the placenta is large. There is a higher incidence of macrosomic infants born to certain ethnic groups (Native Americans, Mexican Americans, African Americans, Pacific Islanders).

IDMs have decreased total body water, particularly in the extracellular spaces, and are therefore not edematous. Their excessive weight is because of increased weight of the visceral organs, cardiomegaly (hypertrophy), and increased body fat. The only organ not affected is the brain.

The excessive fetal growth of the IDM is caused by exposure to high levels of maternal glucose, which readily crosses the placenta. The fetus responds to these high glucose levels with increased insulin production and hyperplasia of the pancreatic beta cells. The main action of the insulin is to facilitate the entry of glucose into muscle and fat cells. Once in the cells, glucose is converted to glycogen and stored. Insulin also inhibits the breakdown of fat to free fatty acids, thereby maintaining lipid synthesis; increases the uptake of amino acids; and promotes protein

● **Figure 27–2** Macrosomic infant of a Class B insulin-dependent diabetic mother born at 38 weeks' gestation weighing 3402 grams.

Source: Carol Harrigan, RN, MSN, NNP-BC

synthesis. Insulin is an important regulator of fetal metabolism and has a "growth hormone" effect that results in increased linear growth. Infants of diabetic mothers may be obese as children (Gleason & Devaskar, 2012).

Common Complications of the IDM

Although IDMs are usually large, they have immature physiologic functions and exhibit many of the problems of the preterm (premature) infant. The complications most often seen in an IDM are as follows:

- *Hypoglycemia.* Hypoglycemia is defined as a blood sugar less than 40 mg/dL. Even though the high maternal blood supply is lost, the IDM continues to produce high levels of insulin, which deplete the infant's blood glucose within hours after birth. IDMs also have less ability to release glucagon and catecholamines, which normally stimulate glucagon breakdown and glucose release. The incidence of hypoglycemia in IDMs varies according to the degree of success in controlling the maternal diabetes, the maternal blood sugar level at the time of birth, the length of labor, the class of maternal diabetes, and early versus late feedings of the newborn (Gleason & Devaskar, 2012). Signs and symptoms of hypoglycemia include tremors, cyanosis, apnea, temperature instability, poor feeding, and hypotonia. Seizures may occur in severe cases.

- *Hypocalcemia.* Tremors are the obvious clinical sign of hypocalcemia. They may be caused by the increased incidence of prematurity in IDMs and by the stresses of a difficult pregnancy, labor, and birth. Diabetic women tend to have decreased serum magnesium levels at term secondary to increased urinary calcium excretion, which causes secondary hypoparathyroidism in their infants. Other factors may include vitamin D antagonism, which results from elevated cortisol levels, hypophosphatemia from tissue catabolism, and decreased serum magnesium levels.

- *Hyperbilirubinemia.* This condition may be seen at 48 to 72 hours after birth. It may be caused by slightly decreased extracellular fluid volume, which increases the hematocrit level. This elevation facilitates an increase in red blood cell breakdown, thereby increasing bilirubin levels. The presence of hepatic immaturity may impair bilirubin conjugation. Enclosed hemorrhages resulting from complicated vaginal birth may also cause hyperbilirubinemia.

- *Birth trauma.* Because most IDMs are macrosomic, trauma may occur during labor and birth from shoulder dystocia.

- *Polycythemia.* Fetal hyperglycemia and hyperinsulinism result in increased oxygen consumption, which can lead to fetal hypoxia (Raab & Kelly, 2013). Glycohemoglobin (HbA$_{1c}$) binds to oxygen, decreasing the oxygen available to the fetal tissues. This tissue hypoxia stimulates increased erythropoietin production, which increases both the hematocrit level and the potential for hyperbilirubinemia. See Chapter 15 🔴 for discussion of HbA$_{1c}$.

- *Respiratory distress syndrome (RDS).* This complication occurs especially in newborns of diabetic mothers who are not well controlled (Cloherty et al., 2012). Insulin antagonizes the cortisol-induced stimulation of lecithin synthesis that is necessary for lung maturation. Therefore, IDMs may have less mature lungs than expected for their gestational age. There is also a decrease in the phospholipid phosphatidylglycerol (PG), which stabilizes surfactant. The insufficiency of PG increases the incidence of RDS. Therefore, it is important to test for the presence of PG in the amniotic fluid before birth.

    RDS does not appear to be a problem for infants born of diabetic mothers who have decreased placental perfusion; instead, the stresses of poor uterine blood supply may lead to increased production of steroids, which accelerates lung maturation. IDMs may also have a delay in closure of the ductus arteriosus and decreases in postnatal pulmonary artery pressure (Cloherty et al., 2012).

- *Congenital birth defects.* These may include congenital heart defects (transposition of the great vessels, ventricular septal defect, patent ductus arteriosus), small left colon syndrome, renal anomalies, neural tube defects, and sacral agenesis (caudal regression) (Cloherty et al., 2012). Early close control of maternal glucose levels before and during pregnancy decreases the risk of birth defects. See Chapter 15 🔴 for more information.

Clinical Therapy

Prenatal management is directed toward controlling maternal glucose levels, which minimizes the common complications of IDMs. Because the onset of hypoglycemia occurs between 1 and 3 hours after birth in IDMs (with a spontaneous rise to normal levels by 4 to 6 hours), blood glucose determinations should be done on cord blood or by heelstick hourly during the first 4 hours after birth and then at 4-hour intervals until the risk period (about 48 hours) has passed or per agency protocol.

IDMs whose serum glucose level falls below 40 mg/dL should have early feedings with formula or breast milk (colostrum). If normal glucose levels cannot be maintained with oral feedings, an intravenous (IV) infusion of glucose will be necessary. (See Chapter 28 🔴 for detailed discussion of hypoglycemia in the newborn.)

NURSING MANAGEMENT *For the Infant of a Diabetic Mother (IDM)*

Nursing Assessment and Diagnosis

Do not be lulled into thinking that a big baby is a mature baby. In almost every case, because of the infant's large size, the IDM will appear older than gestational age scoring indicates. Consider both the gestational age and whether the baby is AGA or

 Clinical Tip

When beginning fluids on an IDM, it is sometimes best to start at a higher than normal concentration of dextrose to avoid hypoglycemia episodes.

LGA in planning and providing safe care. In caring for the IDM, assess for signs of respiratory distress, hyperbilirubinemia, birth trauma, and congenital anomalies.

Nursing diagnoses that may apply to IDMs include the following (NANDA-I © 2012):

- *Nutrition, Imbalanced: Less Than Body Requirements,* related to increased glucose metabolism secondary to hyperinsulinemia
- *Gas Exchange, Impaired,* related to respiratory distress secondary to impaired production of surfactant
- *Tissue Integrity, Impaired,* related to poor maternal metabolic control
- *Family Processes, Interrupted,* related to the illness of the baby

Planning and Implementation

Nursing care of the IDM is directed toward early detection and ongoing monitoring of hypoglycemia (by performing glucose tests) and polycythemia (by obtaining central hematocrits), RDS, and hyperbilirubinemia. (These conditions are presented in Chapter 28 .) Assess for signs of birth trauma and congenital anomalies.

Parent teaching is directed toward preventing macrosomia and the resulting fetal/neonatal problems by instituting early and ongoing diabetic control. Advise parents that with early identification and care, most IDMs' neonatal problems have no significant sequelae.

Evaluation

Expected outcomes of nursing care include the following:

- The IDM's respiratory distress and metabolic problems are minimized.
- The parents understand the effects of maternal diabetes on the baby's health and preventive steps they can initiate to decrease its impact on subsequent pregnancies.
- The parents verbalize their concerns about their baby's health problems and understand the rationale behind management of their newborn.

CARE OF THE POSTTERM NEWBORN

The **postterm newborn** is any newborn born after 42 completed weeks of gestation. Postterm or prolonged pregnancy occurs in less than 3% to 14% of all pregnancies (Cloherty et al., 2012). The cause of postterm pregnancy is not completely understood, but several factors are known to be associated with it. (See Chapter 21 for a discussion of maternal factors.) Many pregnancies classified as prolonged are thought to be a result of inaccurate estimates of date of birth (EDB). Postterm pregnancy is more common in Australian, Greek, and Italian ethnic groups.

Most babies born as a result of prolonged pregnancy are of normal size and health; some continue growing and are over 4000 g at birth, which supports the contention that the postterm fetus can remain well nourished. Potential intrapartum problems for these healthy but large fetuses are cephalopelvic disproportion (CPD) and shoulder dystocia. (See Chapter 22 for discussion of the necessary assessments and interventions.)

Common Complications of the Newborn with Postmaturity Syndrome

The term **postmaturity** applies only to the infant who is born after 42 completed weeks of gestation and also demonstrates characteristics of *postmaturity syndrome*. Postterm infants have begun to lose weight but usually have a normal length and head circumference (Cloherty et al., 2012).

The characteristics of postmature newborns are primarily caused by a combination of advanced gestational age, placental aging and decreased placental function, and continued exposure to amniotic fluid. The truly postmature newborn is at high risk for morbidity and has a mortality rate two to three times greater than that of term infants. Although today the percentages are extremely low, the majority of postmature fetal deaths occur during labor, because the fetus uses up necessary body reserves.

The following are common disorders of the postmature newborn:

- Hypoglycemia, from nutritional deprivation and depleted glycogen stores
- Meconium aspiration in response to in utero hypoxia as the stress of labor begins (The presence of oligohydramnios increases the danger of aspirating thick meconium. Severe meconium aspiration syndrome increases the baby's chance of developing persistent pulmonary hypertension, pneumothorax, and pneumonia.)
- Polycythemia caused by increased production of red blood cells (RBCs) in response to hypoxia
- Congenital anomalies of unknown cause
- Seizure activity because of hypoxic insult
- Cold stress because of loss or poor development of subcutaneous fat

Clinical Therapy

The aim of antenatal management is to differentiate the fetus who has postmaturity syndrome from the fetus who at birth is large, well nourished, alert, and tolerating the prolonged (postterm) pregnancy. Antenatal tests that are done to evaluate fetal status and determine obstetric management and their use in postterm pregnancy are discussed in more depth in Chapters 15 and 21 . If the amniotic fluid is meconium stained, an amnioinfusion may be done during labor. This procedure dilutes the meconium by directly infusing either normal saline or Ringer's lactate into the uterus, decreasing the risk of meconium aspiration syndrome. (For detailed discussion of clinical management and care of the newborn at risk for meconium aspiration, see Chapter 28 .)

Hypoglycemia is monitored by serial glucose determinations per agency protocols. The baby may be placed on glucose infusions or given early feedings if respiratory distress is not present, but these measures must be instituted with caution because of the frequency of asphyxia in the first 24 hours. Postmature newborns are often voracious eaters.

For the small-for-gestational-age (SGA) infant who is postmature, peripheral and central hematocrits are tested to determine the presence of polycythemia. Fluid resuscitation can be initiated. In extreme cases a partial exchange transfusion may be necessary to prevent polycythemia and adverse sequelae such as hyperviscosity. Oxygen is provided for respiratory distress. In addition, temperature instability and excessive loss of heat can result from decreased liver glycogen stores. (See Chapter 28 🔗 for thermoregulation techniques.)

NURSING MANAGEMENT *For the Newborn with Postmaturity Syndrome*

Nursing Assessment and Diagnosis

The newborn with postmaturity syndrome appears alert. This wide-eyed, alert appearance is not necessarily a positive sign because it may indicate chronic intrauterine hypoxia. The infant typically has dry, cracking, parchment-like skin without vernix or lanugo (Figure 27–3 ●). Fingernails are long, and scalp hair is profuse. The infant's body appears long and thin. The wasting involves depletion of previously stored subcutaneous tissue, causing the skin to be loose. Fat layers are almost nonexistent.

Postmature newborns frequently have meconium staining, which colors the nails, skin, and umbilical cord. The varying shades (yellow to green) of meconium staining can give some clue as to whether the expulsion of meconium in utero was a recent or chronic problem. Green coloring indicates a more recent event.

Nursing diagnoses that may apply to the postmature newborn include the following (NANDA-I © 2012):

- *Hypothermia* related to decreased liver glycogen and brown fat stores

- *Nutrition, Imbalanced: Less Than Body Requirements,* related to increased use of glucose secondary to in utero stress and decreased placenta perfusion

- *Gas Exchange, Impaired,* related to airway obstruction from meconium aspiration

- *Tissue Perfusion: Peripheral, Ineffective,* related to increased blood viscosity caused by polycythemia

Planning and Implementation

Nursing care of the postmature infant is directed toward early detection and ongoing monitoring of hypothermia (by regulating thermoregulation), hypoglycemia (by performing glucose tests), polycythemia (by obtaining central hematocrits), and meconium aspiration and RDS (by monitoring cardiopulmonary status). (These conditions are discussed in Chapter 28 🔗.)

Encourage parents to express their feelings and fears about the newborn's condition and potential long-term problems. Give careful explanations of procedures, include the parents in the development of care plans for their baby, and encourage follow-up care as needed.

Evaluation

Expected outcomes of nursing care include the following:

- The postterm newborn establishes effective respiratory function.

- The postmature baby is free of metabolic alterations (hypoglycemia) and maintains a stable temperature.

CARE OF THE PRETERM (PREMATURE) NEWBORN

A **preterm infant** is any infant born at 37 or fewer weeks' gestation (Gardner & Hernandez, 2011) (Figure 27–4 ●). With the help of modern technology, infants are surviving at younger gestational ages, but not without significant morbidity. The incidence of all preterm births in the United States is approximately 12.7%.

● **Figure 27–3** Postterm infant demonstrates deep cracking and peeling of skin.
Source: © Wellcome Image Library/Custom Medical Stock Photo.

● **Figure 27–4** A 6-day-old, 27-week gestational age, 960-g preterm infant.
Source: Carol Harrigan, RN, MSN, NNP-BC

African American women are more than three times as likely to have an extremely preterm infant (<28 weeks of gestation) (Cloherty et al., 2012). The rise in multiple birth rates has markedly influenced overall rates of low-birth-weight (LBW) infants. Prematurity and low birth weight are common in single women and adolescents.

The major problem of the preterm newborn is the variable immaturity of all systems. The degree of immaturity depends on the length of gestation. Because of immaturity, the premature newborn is ill equipped to smoothly traverse the complex, interconnected pathways from intrauterine to extrauterine life.

Alteration in Respiratory and Cardiac Physiology

The preterm newborn is at risk for respiratory problems because of the following critical factors in the development of respiratory distress:

1. The preterm infant is unable to produce adequate amounts of surfactant. (See Chapter 24 for a discussion of respiratory adaptation and development.) Inadequate surfactant lessens compliance (ability of the lung to fill with air easily), thereby increasing the inspiratory pressure needed to expand the lungs with air. This progressive atelectasis leads to an inability to develop a functional residual capacity (FRC), causing an ineffective exchange of oxygen and carbon dioxide. As a result, the infant becomes hypoxic, pulmonary blood flow is inefficient, and the preterm newborn's available energy is depleted.

2. The muscular coat of pulmonary blood vessels is incompletely developed. Consequently, the pulmonary arterioles do not constrict as well in response to decreased oxygen levels. This lowered pulmonary vascular resistance leads to left-to-right shunting of blood through the ductus arteriosus, which increases the blood flow back into the lungs.

3. Normally the ductus arteriosus responds to increasing oxygen levels and prostaglandin E levels by vasoconstriction; in the preterm infant, who is more susceptible to hypoxia, the ductus may remain open. A patent ductus increases the blood volume to the lungs, causing pulmonary congestion, increased respiratory effort, carbon dioxide retention, and bounding femoral pulses.

The common complications of the cardiopulmonary system in preterm infants are discussed later in this chapter and in Chapter 28.

Heat loss is a major problem in preterm newborns. Two factors limiting heat production are the decreased availability of glycogen in the liver and the amount of brown fat available for heat production, both of which appear in the third trimester. Because the muscle mass is small in preterm infants, and muscular activity is diminished (they are unable to shiver), heat production is further limited.

Five physiologic and anatomic factors increase heat loss in the preterm infant:

1. The preterm baby has a higher ratio of body surface to body weight. This means that the baby's ability to produce heat (based on body weight) is much less than the potential for losing heat (based on surface area). The loss of heat in a preterm infant weighing 1500 g is five times greater per unit of body weight than in an adult.

2. The preterm baby has very little subcutaneous fat, which is the human body's insulation. Without adequate insulation, heat is easily conducted from the core of the body (warmer temperature) to the surface of the body (cooler temperature). Heat is lost from the body as the blood vessels, which lie close to the skin surface in the preterm infant, transport blood from the body core to the subcutaneous tissues.

3. The preterm baby has thinner, more permeable skin than the term infant. This increased permeability contributes to a greater insensible water loss as well as to heat loss.

4. Flexion of the extremities decreases the amount of surface area exposed to the environment. Extension increases the surface area exposed to the environment and thus increases heat loss. The gestational age of the infant influences the amount of flexion, from completely hypotonic and extended at 28 weeks to strong flexion displayed by 36 weeks.

5. The preterm baby has a decreased ability to vasoconstrict superficial blood vessels and conserve heat in the body core.

In summary, gestational age is directly proportional to the ability to maintain thermoregulation; thus the more preterm the newborn, the less able the infant is to maintain heat balance. Preventing heat loss by providing a neutral thermal environment using a servocontrol skin probe is one of the most important considerations in nursing care management of the preterm infant. Cold stress, with its accompanying severe complications, can be prevented (see *Care of the Newborn with Cold Stress* in Chapter 28).

Alteration in Gastrointestinal Physiology

Maturation of the digestive and absorptive process is more variable, however, and occurs later in gestation. As a result of gastrointestinal (GI) immaturity, the preterm newborn has the following ingestion, digestive, and absorption problems:

- A marked danger of aspiration and its associated complications because of the infant's poorly developed gag reflex, incompetent esophageal cardiac sphincter, and poor sucking and swallowing reflexes.

- Difficulty in meeting high caloric and fluid needs for growth because of small stomach capacity.

- Limited ability to convert certain essential amino acids to nonessential amino acids. Certain amino acids, such as histidine, taurine, and cysteine, are essential to the preterm infant but not to the term infant.

- Inability to handle the increased osmolarity of formula protein because of kidney immaturity. The preterm infant requires a higher concentration of whey protein than of casein.

- Difficulty absorbing saturated fats because of decreased bile salts and pancreatic lipase. Severe illness of the newborn may also prevent intake of adequate nutrients.

- Difficulty with lactose digestion initially because processes may not be fully functional during the first few days of a preterm infant's life. The preterm newborn can digest and absorb most simple sugars.
- Deficiency of calcium and phosphorus may exist because two thirds of these minerals are deposited in the last trimester. Rickets and significant bone demineralization caused by deficiency of calcium and phosphorus, which are deposited primarily in the last trimester, are also problems.
- Increased basal metabolic rate and increased oxygen requirements caused by fatigue associated with sucking.
- Feeding intolerance and necrotizing enterocolitis (NEC) as a result of diminished blood flow and tissue perfusion to the intestinal tract due to a combination of contributing factors including prematurity, formula feeding, bacterial colonization, and hypoxemia/ischemia events.

Alteration in Renal Physiology

Specific characteristics of the preterm infant that pose clinical problems in the management of fluid and electrolyte balance include the following:

- The glomerular filtration rate (GFR) is directly related to lower gestational age and increases steadily after 34 weeks' postconceptual age (PCA). The GFR is also decreased in the presence of diseases or conditions that decrease the renal blood flow and perfusion, such as severe respiratory distress, hypotension, and asphyxia. Anuria and oliguria may also be observed. A low systolic blood pressure can reflect any diseases that decrease cardiac output and affect renal blood flow. Systolic blood pressure varies with gestational age and PCA.

Clinical Tip

A gradual decline in urine may be associated with a drop in the infant's blood pressure.

- The preterm infant's kidneys are limited in their ability to concentrate urine or to excrete excess amounts of fluid. This means that if excess fluid is administered, the infant is at risk for fluid retention and overhydration. If too little is administered, the infant will become dehydrated because of the inability to retain adequate fluid.
- The preterm kidneys begin excreting glucose (glycosuria) at a lower serum glucose level than that of the term infant. Therefore, glycosuria with hyperglycemia can lead to osmotic diuresis and polyuria.
- The kidney's buffering capacity is reduced, predisposing the infant to metabolic acidosis. Bicarbonate is excreted at a lower serum level, and acid is excreted more slowly. Therefore, after periods of hypoxia or insult, the preterm infant's kidneys require a longer time to excrete the lactic acid that accumulates.
- The immaturity of the renal system affects the preterm infant's ability to excrete drugs. Because excretion time

is longer, many drugs are given over longer intervals (e.g., every 24 hours instead of every 12 hours). Urine output must be carefully monitored when the infant is receiving nephrotoxic drugs such as gentamicin and vancomycin. In the event that urine output is poor, drugs can become toxic in the infant much more quickly than in the adult.

Alteration in Immunologic Physiology

The preterm infant has an increased susceptibility to infections acquired in utero that may have precipitated preterm labor and birth. However, all preterm infants have immature specific and nonspecific immunity.

In utero the fetus receives passive immunity against a variety of infections from maternal IgG immunoglobulins, which cross the placenta. Because most of this immunity is acquired in the last trimester of pregnancy, the preterm infant has few antibodies at birth. (See *Care of the Newborn with Infection* in Chapter 28 .)

The other immunoglobulin significant for the preterm infant is secretory IgA, which does not cross the placenta but is found in breast milk. Breast milk's secretory IgA provides immunity to the mucosal surfaces of the GI tract, protecting the newborn from enteric infections such as those caused by *Escherichia coli* and *Shigella*.

Another altered defense against infection in the preterm infant is the skin surface. In very small infants the skin is easily excoriated, and this factor, coupled with many invasive procedures, places the infant at great risk for nosocomial infections. It is vital to use good hand washing techniques in the care of these infants to prevent unnecessary infection.

Alteration in Neurologic Physiology

Because the period of most rapid brain growth and development occurs during the third trimester of pregnancy, the closer to term an infant is born, the better the neurologic prognosis. A common interruption of neurologic development in the preterm infant is caused by intraventricular hemorrhage (IVH) and intracranial hemorrhage (ICH). Hydrocephalus may develop as a consequence of an IVH caused by an obstruction at the cerebral aqueduct (Scher, 2013).

Alteration in Reactivity Periods and Behavioral States

The newborn infant's response to extrauterine life is characterized by two periods of reactivity (see Chapter 24). The preterm infant's periods of reactivity, however, are delayed. In the very ill infant, these periods of reactivity may not be observed at all because the infant may be hypotonic and unreactive for several days

Clinical Tip

The sudden onset of apnea and bradycardia, coupled with metabolic acidosis in an otherwise healthy, growing premature infant, may be suggestive of bacterial sepsis, especially if a central line is present.

Clinical Question
What nonpharmacologic pain management tools are effective for managing preterm neonatal procedural pain?

The Evidence
Nonpharmacologic pain management tools such as nonnutritive sucking and facilitated tucking have been shown to be effective in full-term newborns who must undergo painful procedures, such as heelsticks. *Facilitated tucking* involves a caregiver hand-swaddling an infant by placing a hand on the infant's head and feet while providing flexion and containment. Two groups of obstetric nursing experts applied these interventions to preterm neonates in the NICU. Both utilized randomized control trial designs, which form the strongest level of evidence for practice. Nonnutritive sucking on either a pacifier or glucose water is effective in reducing pain during heelstick. Facilitated

tucking, particularly when done by the parents, is also effective in reducing pain in these babies (Liaw, Wang, Yang, et al., 2012). Of the two procedures, nonnutritive sucking was the most effective in pain control, while tucking was effective in stabilizing the baby during the procedure.

Best Practice
Nonnutritive sucking is an effective pain management tool for preterm infants undergoing painful procedures. Facilitated tucking—particularly if done by the parents—can both manage pain and immobilize the baby for the procedure.

Clinical Reasoning
How can the nurse involve the parents in facilitated tucking during a painful procedure? What other benefits might this involvement generate?

after birth. In general, stable preterm infants do not demonstrate the same behavioral states as term infants. Preterm infants tend to be more disorganized in their sleep–wake cycles and are unable to attend as well to the human face and objects in the environment. Neurologically, their responses (sucking, muscle tone, states of arousal) are weaker than full-term infants' responses.

Management of Nutrition and Fluid Requirements

Early feedings are extremely valuable for the premature infant in maintaining normal metabolism and lowering the possibility of such complications as hypoglycemia, hyperbilirubinemia, hyperkalemia, osteopenia of prematurity, and other digestive system problems.

Nutritional Requirements
Oral (enteral) caloric intake necessary for growth in a healthy preterm newborn is 95 to 130 kcal/kg/day (Blackburn, 2013). In addition to these relatively high caloric needs, the preterm newborn requires more protein than the full-term infant. To meet these needs, many institutions use breast milk or special preterm formulas. Feeding regimens are established based on the infant's weight and estimated stomach capacity. Initial formula feedings are gradually increased as the infant tolerates them. It may be necessary to supplement oral feedings with parenteral fluids to maintain adequate hydration and caloric intake until the baby is on full oral feedings.

In addition to a higher calorie and protein formula, preterm infants should receive supplemental multivitamins, including

vitamins A, D, and E, iron, and trace minerals. A diet high in polyunsaturated fats (which preterm infants tolerate best) increases the requirement for vitamin E. Preterm formulas also need to contain medium-chain triglycerides (MCT) and additional amino acids such as cysteine, as well as calcium, phosphorus, and vitamin D supplements to increase mineralization of bones.

Nutritional intake is considered adequate when there is consistent weight gain of 20 to 30 g/day. Initially, no weight gain may be noted for several days, but total weight loss should not exceed 15% of the total birth weight or more than 1% to 2% per day. Some institutions add the criteria of head circumference growth and increase in body length of 1 cm (0.4 in.) per week, once the newborn is stable.

Methods of Feeding
The preterm infant is fed by various methods depending on the infant's gestational age, health and physical condition, and neurologic status. The three most common oral feeding methods are bottle, breast, and gavage.

Bottle Feeding. Preterm infants who have a coordinated as well as rhythmic suck–swallow–breathing pattern are usually between 35 and 36 weeks' postconceptual age and may be fed by bottle. Oral readiness to feed is best described by the following behaviors: remaining engaged in the feeding, organizing oral–motor functioning, coordinating the suck–swallow–breath skill, and maintaining physiologic stability. Those premature infants who root when their cheek is stroked and actively search for the nipple are neurodevelopmentally ready to initiate oral feeding. To avoid excessive expenditure of energy, a soft, yellow, single-hole nipple is usually used (milk flow is less rapid). The infant is fed in a semisitting position and burped gently after each ½ to 1 oz. The feeding should take no longer than 15 to 20 minutes (nippling requires more energy than other methods). Premature infants who are progressing from gavage feedings to bottle feeding should start with one session of bottle feeding a day and slowly increase the number of times a day a bottle is given until the baby tolerates all feedings from a bottle.

Sucking may be affected by age, asphyxia, sepsis, intraventricular hemorrhage, or other neurologic insult. Before initiating nipple feeding, the nurse observes for signs of stress, such as tachypnea (more than 60 respirations per minute), respiratory distress, or hypothermia, which may increase the risk of aspiration. During the feeding the nurse observes the infant for signs of feeding difficulty (tachypnea, cyanosis, bradycardia, lethargy, uncoordinated suck and swallow). Difficulty in bottle feeding is often associated with a milk bolus that is too large for the infant's oral cavity and can lead to aspiration. Demand feeding protocols, based on the infant's hunger cues, should be considered for a growing premature infant only when there is sufficient caloric intake to promote consistent weight gain.

Breastfeeding.   Mothers who wish to breastfeed their preterm infants are given the opportunity to put the infant to the breast as soon as the infant has demonstrated a coordinated suck and swallow reflex, is showing consistent weight gain, and can control body temperature outside of the incubator, regardless of weight. Preterm infants tolerate breastfeeding with higher transcutaneous oxygen pressures and better maintenance of body temperature than during bottle feeding. Besides breast milk's many benefits for the infant, it allows the mother to contribute actively to the infant's well-being (Figure 27–5 ●). The nurse should encourage mothers to breastfeed if they choose to do so. It is important to be aware of the advantages of breastfeeding, as well as the possible disadvantages of breast milk as the sole source of food for the preterm infant. (For an in-depth discussion of breastfeeding, see Chapter 26 ⊘.)

By initiating skin-to-skin holding of premature infants in the early intensive care phase, mothers can significantly increase milk volume, thereby overcoming lactation problems. Many mothers of preterm infants seem to find the football hold position (see Figure 26–15 ⊘ on page 603) the most convenient breastfeeding position for preterm infants. Feeding may take up to 45 minutes, and babies should be burped as they alternate breasts. The length of feeding time is monitored so that the preterm infant does not expend too many calories.

The nurse should coordinate a flexible feeding schedule so babies can nurse during alert times and be allowed to set their own pace. Feedings should be on demand, but a maximum number of hours between feedings should be set. The mother begins with one feeding at the breast and then gradually increases the number of times during the day that the baby breastfeeds. Even if the infant cannot be put to the breast, mothers can pump their breasts, and the breast milk can be given via gavage. Use of the double-pumping system produces higher levels of prolactin than sequential pumping of the breasts. When breastfeeding is not possible because the infant is too small or too weak to suck at the breast, an option for the mother may be to express her breast milk into a cup. The milk touches the infant's lips and is lapped by the protruding motions of the tongue.

Gavage Feeding.   The gavage feeding method is used with preterm infants (less than 34 weeks' gestation) who lack or have a poorly coordinated suck and swallow reflex or are ill and ventilator dependent. Gavage feeding (see Skill 16–3 in the *Clinical Skills Manual* SKILLS) may be used as an adjunct to nipple feeding if the infant tires easily or as an alternative if an infant is losing weight because of the energy expenditure required for nippling. Gavage feedings are administered by the intermittent bolus or continuous drip method (Figures 27–6 and 27–7 ●). In common practice, bolus feedings are usually initiated, but if intolerance occurs, then the feedings are changed to infuse on a pump over a set amount of time (e.g., over an hour) or continuously (Anderson, Wood, Keller, et al., 2011).

Early initiation of minimal enteral nutrition (MEN) via gavage is now advocated as a supplement to parenteral nutrition. MEN refers to small-volume feedings of formula or human milk (usually less than 24 mL/kg/day) that are designed to "prime" the intestinal tract, thereby stimulating many of its hormonal and enzymatic functions (Cloherty et al., 2012). Benefits of early feeding (as early as 24 to 72 hours of life) include the following: no increased incidence in NEC; fewer days on total parenteral

● **Figure 27–5** This mother is breastfeeding her premature infant.
Source: Carol Harrigan, RN, MSN, NNP-BC

● **Figure 27–6** Measuring gavage tube length.

● **Figure 27–7** Auscultation for placement of gavage tube.

nutrition (TPN), thereby decreasing the incidence of cholestatic jaundice; increased weight gain; increased muscle maturation of the gut function, which can lead to improved feeding tolerance; lower risk of osteopenia; and a possible decrease in the total number of hospital days in the NICU. TPN provides complete nutrition and is used in situations that do not allow the infant to be fed through the GI tract.

SAFETY ALERT!
Orogastric gavage catheter placement is preferable to naso-gastric because most infants are obligatory nose breathers. If nasogastric is used, a #5 French catheter should be used to minimize airway obstruction.

Fluid Requirements
The calculation of fluid requirements must take into account the infant's weight and postnatal age. Recommendations for fluid therapy in the preterm infant of 1500 g are approximately 60 to 80 mL/kg/day for day 1, 80 to 120 mL/kg/day for day 2, and 120 to 160 mL/kg/day by day 3 of life. These amounts may be increased up to 190 mL/kg/day if the infant is very small, receiving pho-totherapy, or under a radiant warmer because of the increased insensible water losses. Fluid losses can be minimized through the use of heat shields and added humidification in the incuba-tor. Daily weights, and sometimes every 6- to 8-hour weights, are the best indicator of fluid status in the less than 1000-g preterm infant. The expected weight loss during the first 5 to 6 days of life in a preterm infant is 15% to 20% of birth weight (Cloherty et al., 2012).

Common Complications of Preterm Newborns and Their Clinical Management
The goals of medical and nursing care are to meet the preterm infant's growth and development needs and to anticipate and manage the complications associated with prematurity. The most common complications associated with prematurity are as follows:

1. Apnea of prematurity. Apnea of prematurity refers to ces-sation of breathing for 20 seconds or longer or for less than 20 seconds when associated with cyanosis, pallor, and bradycardia. Apnea is a common problem in the preterm infant <36 weeks, presenting between day 2 and day 7 of life. The etiology of apnea is multifactorial but is thought to be primarily a result of neuronal immaturity, a factor that contributes to the preterm infant's irregular breathing pat-terns (central apnea). Obstructive apnea can occur when there is cessation of airflow associated with blockage of the upper airway (small airway diameter, increased pharyngeal secretions, altered body alignment and positioning). Gas-troesophageal reflux (GER) is defined as a movement of gastric contents into the lower esophagus caused by poor esophageal sphincter tone, causing laryngospasm, which leads to bradycardia and apnea. Apnea of prematurity is then a diagnosis of exclusion.

2. Patent ductus arteriosus (PDA). The ductus arteriosus fails to close because of decreased pulmonary arteriole musculature and hypoxemia. Symptomatic PDA is often seen around the time when premature infants are recover-ing from RDS. Patent ductus arteriosus often prolongs the course of illness in a preterm newborn and leads to chronic pulmonary dysfunction.

 ### Clinical Tip
A growing premature infant showing clinical signs of worsening re-spiratory status (e.g., increased oxygen needs, increased ventilatory settings), acidosis, and hypotension may be exhibiting signs and symptoms of a patent ductus arteriosus (PDA).

3. Respiratory distress syndrome (RDS). Respiratory distress results from inadequate surfactant production.

4. Intraventricular hemorrhage (IVH). Intraventricular hemor-rhage is the most common type of intracranial hemorrhage in small preterm infants, especially those weighing less than 1500 g or of less than 34 weeks' gestation. Up to 34 weeks' gestation the preterm infant's brain ventricles are lined by the germinal matrix, which is highly susceptible to hypoxic events such as respiratory distress, birth trauma, and birth asphyxia. The germinal matrix is highly vascular, and these blood vessels rupture in the presence of hypoxia (Scher, 2013).

Other common problems of preterm infants such as NEC were briefly discussed in the earlier physiologic sections. (For in-depth discussions of RDS, hyperbilirubinemia, hypoglycemia, anemia of prematurity, and sepsis, see Chapter 28 ✪.)

Long-Term Needs and Outcome

The care of preterm infants and their families does not stop on discharge from the nursery. Within the first year of life, low-birth-weight preterm infants face higher mortality rates than term infants. Causes of death include sudden infant death syndrome (SIDS)—which occurs about five times more frequently in the preterm infant—respiratory infections, and neurologic defects. Morbidity is also much higher among preterm infants, with those weighing less than 1500 g at highest risk for long-term complications.

The most common long-term needs observed in preterm infants include the following:

- *Retinopathy of prematurity (ROP).* Premature newborns are particularly susceptible to characteristic retinal changes, known as ROP, which can result in visual impairment. The disease is now viewed as multifactorial in origin. Increased survival of very-low-birth-weight (VLBW) infants may be the most important factor in the increased incidence of ROP.

- *Bronchopulmonary dysplasia (BPD).* Long-term lung disease is a result of damage to the alveolar epithelium secondary to positive pressure respirator therapy and high oxygen concentration. These infants have long-term dependence on oxygen therapy and an increased incidence of respiratory infection during their first few years of life.

- *Neurologic problems.* The most common neurologic defects include cerebral palsy, hydrocephalus, seizure disorders, lower IQ, and learning disabilities. However, the socioeconomic climate and family support systems are extremely important influences on the child's ultimate school performance in the absence of major neurologic defects. Families can be reminded that risk does not equal injury, injury does not equal damage, and description of damage does not allow a precise prediction about recovery or outcome.

- *Auditory problems.* Preterm infants should have a formal audiologic exam before discharge and at 3 to 6 months (corrected age). Tests currently used to measure hearing functions of the newborn are the evoked otoacoustic emissions (EOAE) or the automated auditory brain response (AABR) test (Figure 27–8 ●). Any infant with repeated abnormal results should be referred to speech/language specialists.

- *Speech problems.* The most frequently observed speech defects involve delayed development of receptive and expressive ability that may persist into the school-age years.

When evaluating the infant's abilities and disabilities, parents must understand that developmental progress must be evaluated based on chronologic age from the expected date of birth,

● **Figure 27–8** Preterm infants should have a formal hearing test prior to discharge.
Source: Carol Harrigan, RN, MSN, NNP-BC

not from the actual date of birth (corrected age). In addition, the parents need the consistent support of healthcare professionals in the long-term management of their infants. Many new and ongoing concerns arise as the high-risk infant grows and develops; the goal is to promote the highest quality of life possible.

NURSING MANAGEMENT *For the Preterm Newborn*

Nursing Assessment and Diagnosis

Assess the physical characteristics and gestational age of the preterm newborn accurately to anticipate the special needs and problems of the baby. Physical characteristics vary greatly depending on gestational age, but the following characteristics are frequently present:

- *Color* is usually pink or ruddy but may show acrocyanosis. (Cyanosis, jaundice, and pallor are abnormal and should be noted.)

- *Skin* is reddened and translucent, blood vessels are readily apparent, there is little subcutaneous fat.

- *Lanugo* is plentiful and widely distributed.

- *Head size* appears large in relation to the body.

- *Skull bones* are pliable; fontanelle is smooth and flat.

- *Ears* have minimal cartilage and are pliable, folded over.

- *Nails* are soft, short.

- *Genitals* are small; testes may not be descended and scrotum nonrugated; clitoris and labia minora are prominent.

- *Resting position* is flaccid, froglike.

- *Cry* is weak, feeble.

- *Reflexes* (sucking, swallowing, gag) are poor.

- *Activity* consists of jerky, generalized movements. (Seizure activity is abnormal.)

Determining gestational age in preterm newborns requires knowledge and experience in administering gestational assessment tools. The tool used should be specific, reliable, and valid.

Nursing diagnoses that may apply to the preterm newborn include the following (NANDA-I © 2012):

- *Gas Exchange, Impaired,* related to immature pulmonary vasculature and inadequate surfactant production

- *Breathing Pattern, Ineffective,* related to immature central nervous system

- *Nutrition, Imbalanced: Less Than Body Requirements,* related to weak suck and swallow reflexes and decreased ability to absorb nutrients

- *Thermoregulation, Ineffective,* related to hypothermia secondary to decreased glycogen and brown fat stores

- *Fluid Volume, Deficient,* related to high insensible water losses and inability of kidneys to concentrate urine

- *Family Processes, Dysfunctional,* related to anger or guilt at having given birth to a premature baby

Planning and Implementation

Maintenance of Respiratory Function

Preterm newborns have an increased danger of respiratory obstruction because their bronchi and trachea are so narrow that mucus can obstruct the airway. Maintain patency through judicious suctioning, but only on an as-needed basis.

Positioning can also affect respiratory function. If the baby is in the supine position, slightly elevate the infant's head to maintain the airway, being careful to avoid hyperextension of the neck because the trachea will collapse. Also, because the newborn has weak neck muscles and cannot control head movement, ensure that this head position is maintained by placing a small roll under the shoulders. Because the prone position splints the chest wall and decreases the amount of respiratory effort used to move the chest wall, it facilitates chest expansion and improves air entry and oxygenation. Weak or absent cough or gag reflexes increase the chance of aspiration in the premature newborn. Ensure that the infant's position facilitates drainage of mucus or regurgitated formula.

Monitor heart and respiratory rates with cardiorespiratory monitors and observe the newborn to identify alterations in cardiopulmonary status. Signs of respiratory distress include the following:

- Cyanosis (serious sign when generalized)

- Tachypnea (sustained respiratory rate greater than 60/minute after first 4 hours of life)

- Retractions

- Expiratory grunting

- Nasal flaring

- Apneic episodes

- Presence of rales or rhonchi on auscultation

- Diminished air entry

If respiratory distress occurs, administer oxygen per physician or nurse practitioner order to relieve hypoxemia. If hypoxemia is not treated immediately, it may result in patent ductus arteriosus or metabolic acidosis. If oxygen is administered to the newborn, monitor the oxygen concentration with devices such as the transcutaneous oxygen monitor ($tcPo_2$) or the pulse oximeter. Periodic arterial blood gas sampling to monitor oxygen concentration in the baby's blood is essential because hyperoxemia may lead to ROP.

Consider respiratory function before initiation of feedings as well as during feeding to prevent aspiration as well as increased energy expenditure and oxygen consumption.

Maintenance of Neutral Thermal Environment

Providing a neutral thermal environment minimizes the oxygen consumption required to maintain a normal core temperature; it also prevents cold stress and facilitates growth by decreasing the calories needed to maintain body temperature. The preterm infant's immature central nervous system, as well as small brown fat stores, provides poor temperature control. A small infant (less than 1200 g) can lose 80 kcal/kg/day through radiation of body heat. Implement all the usual thermoregulation measures discussed in Chapters 26 and 28 🔗.

In addition, to minimize heat loss and temperature instability for preterm and LBW newborns, do the following:

1. Allow skin-to-skin contact between mother and newborn to maintain warmth and faster security (see kangaroo care, described later).

2. Warm and humidify oxygen to minimize evaporative heat loss and decrease oxygen consumption.

3. Place the baby in a double-walled incubator or use a Plexiglas heat shield over small preterm infants in single-walled incubators to avoid radiative heat losses. Some institutions use radiant warmers and plastic wrap over the baby and pipe in humidity ("swamping"). Do not use Plexiglas shields on radiant warmer beds because they block the infrared heat.

4. Avoid placing the baby on cold surfaces such as metal treatment tables and cold x-ray plates (conductive heat loss). Pad cold surfaces with diapers and use radiant warmers during procedures, place the preterm infant on prewarmed mattresses, and warm hands before handling the baby to prevent heat transfer via conduction.

5. Use warmed ambient humidity. Humidity can decrease insensible and transdermal water loss but the optimal level and duration have yet to be determined (Jones, Hayes, Starbuck, et al., 2011). Humidity, however, should only be started once the infant's temperature is within normal limits.

6. Keep the skin dry (evaporative heat loss) and place a cap on the baby's head. The head makes up 25% of the total body size.

7. Keep radiant warmers, incubators, and cribs away from windows and cold external walls (radiative heat loss) and out of drafts (conductive heat loss).

8. Open incubator portholes and doors only when necessary, and use plastic sleeves on portholes to decrease convective heat loss.

9. Use a skin probe to monitor the baby's skin temperature. Correlate ambient temperatures with the skin probe in the

incubator using the servocontrol rather than the manual mode. The temperature should be 36°C to 37°C (96.8°F to 98.6°F). Temperature fluctuations indicate hypothermia or hyperthermia. Be careful not to place skin temperature probes over bony prominences, areas of brown fat, poorly vasoreactive areas such as extremities, or excoriated areas.

10. Warm formula or stored breast milk before feeding.

11. Use reflector patch over the skin temperature probe when using a radiant warmer bed so that the probe does not sense the higher infrared temperature as the baby's skin temperature and therefore decrease the heater output.

Once preterm infants are medically stable, they can be clothed with a double-thickness cap, cotton shirt, and diaper and, if possible, swaddled in a blanket. Familiarize yourself with the individual institution's protocol for weaning preterm infants to a crib.

Maintenance of Fluid and Electrolyte Status

Keep the newborn hydrated by providing adequate intake based on weight, gestational age, chronologic age, and volume of sensible and insensible water losses. Adequate fluid intake should compensate for increased insensible losses and the amount needed for renal excretion of metabolic products. Insensible water losses can be minimized by providing high ambient humidity, humidifying oxygen, using heat shields, covering the skin with plastic wrap, and placing the infant in a double-walled incubator.

Evaluate the hydration status of the baby by assessing and recording signs of dehydration. Identify signs of overhydration by observing the newborn for edema or excessive weight gain and by comparing urine output with fluid intake.

Weigh the preterm infant at least once daily at the same time each day. *Weight change is one of the most sensitive indicators of fluid balance.* Weighing diapers is also important for accurate input and output measurements (1 mL = 1 g). A comparison of intake and output measurements over an 8- or 24-hour period provides important information about renal function and fluid balance. Assessment of patterns and whether they show a net gain or loss over several days is also essential to fluid management. In addition, monitor blood serum levels and pH to evaluate for electrolyte imbalances.

Accurate hourly intake calculations are needed when administering intravenous fluids. Because the preterm infant is unable to excrete excess fluid, it is essential to maintain the correct amount of IV fluid to prevent overload. Accuracy can be ensured by using neonatal or pediatric infusion pumps. Urine-specific gravity and pH are obtained periodically. Hydration is considered adequate when the urine output is 1 to 3 mL/kg/hr.

SAFETY ALERT!

To prevent electrolyte imbalance and dehydration, take care to give the correct intravenous (IV) solutions, as well as the correct volumes and concentrations of formulas.

Provision of Adequate Nutrition and Prevention of Fatigue During Feeding

The feeding method depends on the preterm newborn's feeding abilities and health status. Both nipple and gavage methods are initially supplemented with intravenous therapy until oral intake is sufficient to support growth. Early, small-volume enteral feedings called *minimal enteral nutrition via gavage* have proved to be of benefit to the very-low-birth-weight infant (see *Methods of Feeding* earlier in the chapter). Formula or breast milk (with or without fortifiers to increase caloric content) is incorporated into the feedings slowly. This is done to avoid overtaxing the digestive capacity of the preterm newborn.

Before each feeding, measure abdominal girth and auscultate the abdomen to determine the presence and quality of bowel sounds. Such assessments permit early detection of abdominal distention, visible bowel loops, and decreased peristaltic activity, which may indicate necrotizing enterocolitis (NEC) or paralytic ileus. Check for residual formula in the stomach before feeding when the newborn is fed by gavage. This procedure also can be performed when the nipple-fed newborn presents with abdominal distention. The presence of increasing residual formula is an indication of intolerance to the type or amount of feeding or the increase in amount of feeding. Carefully watch for other signs of feeding intolerance including guaiac-positive stools (occult blood in stools), lactose in the stools (reducing substance in the stools), vomiting, and diarrhea.

Preterm newborns who are ill or who fatigue easily with nipple feedings are usually fed by gavage. The infant is essentially passive with these methods, thus conserving energy and calories. As the baby matures, gavage feedings are replaced with nipple (breast or formula) feedings to assist in strengthening the sucking reflex and in meeting oral and emotional needs. Signs that indicate readiness for oral feedings are a strong gag reflex, presence of nonnutritive sucking, and rooting behavior. Both low-birth-weight and preterm infants nipple-feed more effectively in a quiet state. Establish a gradual nipple-feeding program, such as one nipple feeding per day, then one nipple feeding per shift, and then a nipple feeding every other feeding. Daily weights are monitored because often there is a small weight loss when nipple feedings are started. After feedings, place the baby on the right side (with support to maintain this position) or on the abdomen. These positions facilitate gastric emptying and decrease the chance of aspiration if regurgitation occurs. Gastroesophageal reflux is not uncommon in preterm newborns. Long-term gavage feeding may create nipple aversion that will require developmental occupational therapy interventions.

Involve the parents in feeding their preterm baby (Figure 27–9 ●). This is essential to the development of attachment between parents and infant. In addition, it increases parental knowledge about the care of their infant and helps them cope with the situation.

Prevention of Infection

The nurse bears the responsibility for minimizing the preterm newborn's exposure to pathogenic organisms. The preterm newborn is susceptible to infection because of an immature immune system and thin and permeable skin. Invasive procedures, techniques such as umbilical catheterization and mechanical ventilation, and prolonged hospitalization place the infant at greater risk for infection.

Strict hand washing and use of separate equipment for each infant help minimize the preterm newborn's exposure to

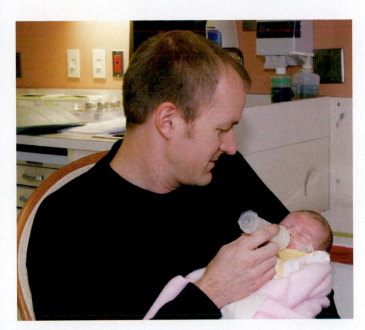

● **Figure 27–9** Father participating in feeding experience with his premature infant.

Source: George Dodson/Lightworks Studio/Pearson Education.

infectious agents. Most nurseries have adopted the Centers for Disease Control and Prevention (CDC) standard precautions of isolating every baby and the Joint Commission requirement that staff members have short-trimmed nails and no artificial nails. Staff members are required to complete a 2- to 3-minute scrub using iodine-containing antibacterial solutions, which inhibit growth of gram-positive cocci and gram-negative rod organisms. Other specific nursing interventions include limiting visitors, requiring visitors to wash their hands, maintaining strict aseptic practices when changing IV tubing and solutions (IV solutions and tubing should be changed every 24 hours or per agency protocols), administering parenteral fluids, and assisting with sterile procedures. Incubators and radiant warmers should be changed weekly. To prevent pressure-area breakdown, change the baby's position regularly, do range-of-motion exercises, and use water-bed pillows or an air mattress. To avoid skin tears, a protective transparent covering can be applied over vulnerable joints; however, this method is used sparingly (Blackburn, 2013). Chemical skin preps and tape may cause skin trauma and should be avoided as much as possible.

If infection (sepsis) occurs in the preterm newborn, you may be the first to identify its subtle clinical signs, such as lethargy and increased episodes of apnea and bradycardia. Inform the clinician of the findings immediately and implement the treatment plan per clinician orders in the presence of infection. (For specific nursing care required for the newborn with an infection, see Chapter 28 🔗.)

Promotion of Parent–Infant Attachment

Preterm newborns can be separated from their parents for prolonged periods after illness or complications that are detected in the first few hours or days following birth. The resultant interruption in parent–newborn bonding necessitates intervention to ensure successful attachment.

Nurses need to take measures to promote positive parental feelings toward the preterm newborn. You can give photographs of the baby to parents to take home. Photos can also be given to the mother if she is in a different hospital or too ill to come to the nursery and visit. Place the infant's first name on the incubator as soon as it is known to help the parents feel that their infant is a unique and special person. Provide a weekly card with the baby's footprint, weight, and length. You also can give parents the telephone number of the nursery or intensive care unit and the names of staff members so that they have access to information about their baby at any time of the day or night. Encourage visits from siblings and grandparents to foster attachment.

Early involvement in the care of and decisions about their baby provides the parents with realistic expectations for their baby. The individual personality characteristics of the infant and the parents influence the bonding and contribute to the interactive process for the family. By observing each infant's patterns of behavior and responses, especially sleep–wake states, you can teach parents optimal times for interacting with their infants. Parents need education to develop caregiving skills and to understand the premature infant's behavioral characteristics. Their daily participation (if possible) is encouraged, as are early and frequent visits.

Skin-to-skin holding (*kangaroo care*) helps parents feel close to their small infant (Figure 27–10 ●). *Skin-to-skin care* is defined as the practice of holding infants skin-to-skin next to their parents. The infant is usually naked, except for a diaper, and placed on his/her parent's bare chest. They are then both covered with a blanket. Benefits of skin-to-skin care as a developmental intervention include the following: improved oxygenation as evidenced by an increase in transcutaneous oxygen levels; enhanced temperature regulation; a decline in episodes of apnea and bradycardia; stabilization of vital signs; improved sleep periods

● **Figure 27–10** Kangaroo (skin-to-skin) care facilitates closeness and attachment between parents and their premature infant.

Source: Carol Harrigan, RN, MSN, NNP-BC

(quiet sleep); positive interaction between parent and infant, which enhances attachment and bonding; parents' improved perception of their caregiving abilities; increased growth parameters; and early discharge (Gardner & Goldson, 2011; Jefferies & Canadian Paediatric Society, Fetus and Newborn Committee, 2012). Limitations to skin-to-skin care may be a result of staff uneasiness or a lack of protocols or guidelines for safely maneuvering, positioning, and holding the infant.

With the parents, plan nursing care around the times when the infant is alert and best able to attend. The more knowledge parents have about the meaning of their infant's responses, behaviors, and cues for interaction, the better prepared they will be to meet their newborn's needs and form a positive attachment with their child. Parental involvement in difficult care decisions is essential and discussed in greater detail in Chapter 28 🔵.

Some parents may progress easily to touching and cuddling their infant; however, others will not. Parents need to know that their feelings are normal and that the progression of acquaintanceship can be slow. Rooming-in can provide another opportunity for the stable preterm infant and family to get acquainted; it offers both privacy and readily available help (Figure 27–11 ●).

Promotion of Developmentally Supportive Care

Prolonged separation and the NICU environment necessitate individualized baby sensory stimulation programs. Determine the appropriate type and amount of visual, tactile, and auditory stimulation.

Some preterm infants are not developmentally able to deal with more than one sensory input at a time. The Assessment of Preterm Infant Behavior (APIB) scale identifies individual preterm newborn behaviors according to five areas of development (Als, Lester, Tronick, et al., 1982). The preterm baby's behavioral reactions to stimulation are observed, and developmental interventions are then based on reducing detrimental environmental stimuli to the lowest possible level and providing appropriate opportunities for development (Blackburn, 2013).

Providing developmentally supportive, as well as family-centered, care has been proven to improve the outcomes of the critically ill newborn. The NICU environment contains many detrimental stimuli that you can help reduce. Noise levels can be lowered by replacing alarms with lights or silencing alarms quickly and keeping conversations away from the baby's bedside. Dimmer switches should be used to shield the baby's eyes from bright lights, and blankets may be placed over the top portion of the incubator. Dimming the lights may encourage infants to open their eyes and be more responsive to their parents. Nursing care should be planned to decrease the number of times the baby is disturbed. Signs (e.g., "Quiet Please") can be placed near the bedside to allow the baby some periods of uninterrupted sleep (Blackburn, 2013). Some other suggested developmentally supportive interventions include the following:

■ Facilitate handling by using containment measures when turning or moving the infant or doing procedures such as suctioning. Use the hands to hold the infant's arms and legs flexed close to the midline of the body. This helps stabilize the infant's motor and physiologic subsystems during stressful activities.

■ Touch the infant gently and avoid sudden postural changes.

■ Promote self-consoling and soothing activities, such as placing blanket rolls or approved manufactured devices next to the infant's sides and against the feet to provide "nesting." Swaddle the infant to maintain extremities in a flexed position while ensuring that the hands can reach the face. This permits the infant to do hand-to-mouth activities (Figure 27–12 ●). Also provide self-consoling objects for the infant to grasp (e.g., a piece of blanket, oxygen tubing, a finger) during caregiving.

■ Simulate the kinesthetic advantages of the intrauterine environment by using sheepskin and approved water beds.

● **Figure 27–11** Family bonding occurs when parents have opportunities to spend time with their infant.
Source: Carol Harrigan, RN, MSN, NNP-BC

● **Figure 27–12** A 2-day-old, 31 weeks' gestational age, IUGR infant is "nested." Hand-to-mouth behavior facilitates self-consoling and soothing activities.
Source: Carol Harrigan, RN, MSN, NNP-BC

Complementary Care Complementary Care in the NICU

As NICUs become more and more "developmentally" friendly, complementary care has become an adjunct to that nurturing environment. This holistic approach in caring for the low-birth-weight infant attempts not only to mimic the intrauterine environment, but also to foster parent–infant bonding by simultaneously caring for the body, spirit, and mind.

- *Aromatherapy* is the use of scent to alter mood or behavior to produce a calming and sedating effect. There is an enhanced bonding process between mothers and newborns associated with the natural body odor emitted from the mother (Gardner & Goldson, 2011). Aromatherapy is utilized in the NICU by placing an article of clothing belonging to the mother next to the infant to produce a soothing and consoling effect on the infant in her absence. Researchers are also investigating other aromatherapies, including peppermint as a respiratory stimulant, chamomile as a method to regulate sleep–wake cycles, Brazilian guava for its analgesic effects, and lavender sitz baths for management of diaper rash.
- *Music therapy* as a noninvasive auditory stimulus has been shown to be advantageous in the premature infant. The music used in NICUs includes primarily lullabies and soft acoustical pieces that are pleasant, soothing, and calming. Such music has been shown to effect newborn physiologic responses, such as improving oxygenation and increasing weight gain. It also has behavioral effects, leading to enhanced parental bonding and increased intervals of nonnutritive sucking periods. Language development is also enhanced if the music is live and sung by the mother or another female, which is preferential to the infant. However, the overall noise level in the NICU needs to be considered before including any extra auditory stimulation, including music therapy (Gardner & Goldson, 2011).
- Infant massage and gentle human touch (GHT) have been practiced for many centuries. The types of stimulation include massage with stroking, gentle touch without stroking, and therapeutic touch or "hands-on" containment. Practitioners report such physiologic benefits as stimulating blood and lymphatic flow, promoting weight gain in premature infants, regulating sleep patterns, and many emotional and behavioral benefits. Massage demonstrates compassion while increasing the parent's empathy and understanding of the baby. It helps parents learn to interpret their baby's behavioral cues such as facial expression, various crying patterns, and other body language. At the same time it helps infants learn about their various body parts and boundaries and feel how they integrate into the whole. Therapeutic Touch reduces motor activity and energy expenditure by the infant and also promotes comfort.

Water bed and pillow use has been reported to improve sleep, decrease motor activity, and lead to more mature motor behavior, fewer state changes, and a decreased heart rate.

- Provide opportunities for nonnutritive sucking with a pacifier. This improves transcutaneous oxygen saturation; decreases body movements; improves sleep, especially after feedings; and increases weight gain.

Teaching the parents to read behavioral cues will help them move at their infant's own pace when providing stimulation. Parents are ideally equipped to meet the baby's need for stimulation. Stroking, rocking, cuddling, quiet singing, and talking to the baby can all be integral parts of the baby's care. Visual stimulation in the form of *en face* interaction with caregivers and mobiles is also important.

Preparation for Home Care

Parents are often anxious when their premature infant is transferred out of the NICU or is discharged home. Parents of preterm babies should receive the same postpartum teaching as any parent taking a new infant home. Prior to discharge, encourage the parents to spend time caring directly for their baby. This familiarizes them with their baby's behavior patterns and helps them establish realistic expectations about the infant. Some hospitals have a special room near the nursery where parents can spend the night with their baby before discharge.

Discharge instruction includes breastfeeding and formula-feeding techniques, formula preparation, and vitamin administration. If the mother wishes to breastfeed, teach her to pump her breasts to keep the milk flowing and provide milk even before discharge. Give information on bathing, diapering, hygiene, and normal elimination patterns and prepare the parents to expect changes in the color of the baby's stool, number of bowel movements, and timing of elimination if the infant is switched from formula to breast milk. This information can prevent unnecessary concern by the parents.

Discuss normal growth and development patterns, reflexes, and activity for preterm infants. In these discussions, emphasize ways to promote bonding behaviors and deal with newborn crying. Care of the preterm infant with complications, feeding problems, prevention of infections, and recognizing signs of a sick baby and the need for continued medical follow-up are other key issues. Also assess if the parents seem unable to cope with an at-risk baby. Family-care conferences with the collaborative care team involved in the care of the preterm infant are often helpful just prior to discharge.

Families with preterm infants usually do not need to be referred to community agencies, such as visiting nurse assistance. However, referral may be necessary if the infant has severe congenital abnormalities, feeding problems, or complications with infections or respiratory problems, or if the parents seem unable to cope with an at-risk baby. Parents of preterm infants can benefit from meeting with others in a similar situation to share common experiences and concerns. Refer parents to support groups sponsored by the hospital or by others in the community and make connections for parents with early education intervention centers.

Preterm and low-birth-weight (LBW) infants are at greater risk of increased morbidity from vaccine-preventable diseases.

Stable preterm infants show consistently high rates of seroconversion following the first dose of hepatitis B vaccine even when the first dose is given as early as 1 month after birth (American Academy of Pediatrics [AAP] Committee on Fetus and Newborn & American College of Obstetricians and Gynecologists [ACOG] Committee on Obstetrics, 2012). The medically stable preterm infant and LBW infant should receive full doses of diphtheria, tetanus, acellular pertussis, *Haemophilus influenzae* type b, poliovirus, and pneumococcal conjugate vaccines at a chronologic age consistent with the schedule recommended for full-term infants. The influenza vaccine should be administered at 6 months of age before the beginning of and during the influenza season. The vaccine for immunoprophylaxis against respiratory syncytial virus (RSV) is given to those high-risk infants prior to discharge from the NICU and monthly thereafter during local RSV season.

Evaluation

Expected outcomes of nursing care include the following:

- The preterm newborn is free of respiratory distress and establishes effective respiratory function.
- The preterm newborn gains weight and shows no signs of fatigue or aspiration during feedings.
- The preterm newborn demonstrates a serial head circumference growth rate of 1 cm (0.4 in.) per week.
- The parents are able to verbalize their anger and guilt feelings about the birth of a preterm baby and show attachment behavior such as frequent visits and growing confidence in their participatory care activities.

CARE OF THE NEWBORN WITH CONGENITAL ANOMALIES

The birth of a baby with a congenital defect places both newborn and family at risk. Many congenital anomalies can be life threatening if not corrected within hours after birth; others are very visible and cause families emotional distress. When one congenital anomaly is found, healthcare providers should look for others, particularly in body systems that develop at the same time during gestation. Table 27–1 identifies common anomalies and their early management and nursing care in the newborn period.

CARE OF THE INFANT OF A SUBSTANCE-ABUSING MOTHER

An **infant of a substance-abusing mother (ISAM)** may be alcohol or drug dependent. After birth, when an infant's connection with the maternal blood supply is severed, the newborn may suffer withdrawal. In addition, the drugs ingested by the mother may be teratogenic, resulting in congenital anomalies or in developmental problems.

Alcohol Dependence

Fetal alcohol syndrome (FAS), a leading cause of mental retardation that is potentially preventable, includes a group of physical, behavioral, and cognitive abnormalities frequently found in infants exposed to alcohol in utero. It is estimated that complete FAS occurs in 0.5 to 2 per 1000 live births annually in the United States (Blackburn, 2013). FAS rates are higher among Native Americans, Alaska natives, African Americans, and women of low socioeconomic status.

A new set of guidelines for diagnosis and referral of infants and children with FAS has been developed. The term *fetal alcohol effects* (FAE) was used to describe children who had some, but not all, of the characteristics of FAS; however, it was vague. Recently the term **fetal alcohol spectrum disorder (FASD)** has been used to include all categories of prenatal alcohol exposure, including FAS. FASD, however, is an umbrella term and not meant to be used as a clinical diagnosis. The new diagnostic categories for FAS take into consideration the various clinical manifestations of FAS, the social and family environment, and, if available, the maternal alcohol history. Five diagnostic categories are used to describe effects of alcohol exposure:

1. FAS with a confirmed history of maternal alcohol intake.
2. FAS with phenotypic features but no confirmed history of maternal alcohol intake.
3. Partial FAS with confirmed history of maternal alcohol intake, some facial abnormalities, and one of the following: CNS abnormalities, growth restriction, or behavioral or cognitive disabilities.
4. *Alcohol-related birth defects (ARBD)* are usually determined only by a positive maternal drinking history. They present with one or more birth defects including malformations and dysplasias of the heart, bone, kidney, vision, or hearing systems and do not exhibit the classic facial dysmorphology of the FAS infant (CDC, 2011).
5. *Alcohol-related neurodevelopmental disorder (ARND)* causes CNS neurodevelopmental abnormalities and complex behavior and cognitive abnormalities. ARBD and ARND can occur together.

Although it is known that ethanol freely crosses the placenta to the fetus, it is still not known whether the alcohol alone or the breakdown products of alcohol cause damage to the fetus. (Chapter 15 ⊘ discusses alcohol abuse in pregnancy.) The effects of other substances often combined with alcohol, such as nicotine, diazepam (Valium), marijuana, and caffeine, as well as poor diet, enhance the likelihood of FAS.

Long-Term Complications for the Infant with FAS

Because of the failure-to-thrive appearance, many FAS infants are often evaluated for deficiencies in organic and inorganic amino acids. These infants have a delay in oral feeding development but have a normal progression of oral motor function. Many FAS infants nurse poorly and have persistent vomiting until 6 to 7 months of age. They have difficulty adjusting to solid foods and show little spontaneous interest in food.

CNS dysfunctions are the most common and serious problem associated with FAS. Hypertonicity and increased placidity are seen in these infants. They also have a decreased ability to block out repetitive stimuli. Children exhibiting FAS can have either severe intellectual disability or normal intelligence. These children

Table 27–1	Congenital Anomalies: Identification and Care in the Newborn Period	

Congenital Anomaly	Nursing Assessments	Nursing Goals and Interventions
CONGENITAL HYDROCEPHALUS (enlarged head)	Enlarged or full fontanelles Split or widened sutures "Setting sun" eyes Head circumference greater than 90% on growth chart	Assess presence of hydrocephalus: Measure and plot occipital-frontal baseline measurements; then measure head circumference once a day. Check fontanelle for bulging and sutures for widening. Assist with head ultrasound and transillumination. Maintain skin integrity: Change position frequently. Clean skin creases after feeding or vomiting. Use sheepskin pillow under head. Postoperatively, position head off operative site. Watch for signs of infection.
CHOANAL ATRESIA (occlusion of posterior nares)	Cyanosis and retractions at rest Noisy respirations Difficulty breathing during feeding Obstruction by thick mucus	Assess patency of nares: Listen for breath sounds while holding baby's mouth closed and alternately compressing each nostril. Assist with passing feeding tube to confirm diagnosis. Maintain respiratory function: Assist with taping airway in mouth to prevent respiratory distress. Position with head elevated to improve air exchange.
CLEFT LIP (unilateral or bilateral visible defect)	May involve external nares, nasal cartilage, nasal septum, and alveolar process Flattening or depression of midfacial contour	Provide nutrition: Feed with special nipple. Burp frequently (increased tendency to swallow air and reflex vomiting). Clean cleft with sterile water (to prevent crusting on cleft before repair). Support parental coping: Assist parents with grief over loss of idealized baby. Encourage verbalization of their feelings about visible defect. Provide role model in interacting with infant: Parents internalize others' responses to their newborn.

Bilateral cleft lip with cleft abnormality involving both hard and soft palates.

Source: Carol Harrigan, RN, MSN, NNP-BC

Congenital Anomaly	Nursing Assessments	Nursing Goals and Interventions
CLEFT PALATE (fissure connecting oral and nasal cavity)	May involve uvula and soft palate May extend forward to nostril involving hard palate and maxillary alveolar ridge Difficulty in sucking Expulsion of formula through nose	Prevent aspiration/infection: Place prone or in side-lying position to facilitate drainage. Suction nasopharyngeal cavity (to prevent aspiration or airway obstruction). During newborn period feed in upright position with head and chest tilted slightly backward (to aid swallowing and discourage aspiration). Provide nutrition: Feed with special nipple that fills cleft and allows sucking. Also decreases chance of aspiration through nasal cavity. Clean mouth with water after feedings. Burp after each ounce (tend to swallow large amounts of air). Thicken formula to provide extra calories. Plot weight gain patterns to assess adequacy of diet. Provide parental support: Refer parents to community agencies and support groups. Encourage verbalization of frustrations because feeding process is long and frustrating. Praise all parental efforts. Encourage parents to seek prompt treatment for upper respiratory infection (URI) and teach them ways to decrease URI.

(continued)

Table 27–1   Congenital Anomalies: Identification and Care in the Newborn Period—continued

Congenital Anomaly	Nursing Assessments	Nursing Goals and Interventions
TRACHEOESOPHAGEAL FISTULA (TYPE 3) (connection between trachea and esophagus)	History of maternal polyhydramnios Excessive oral secretions Constant drooling Abdominal distention beginning soon after birth Periodic choking and cyanotic episodes Immediate regurgitation of feeding Clinical symptoms of aspiration pneumonia (tachypnea, retractions, rhonchi, decreased breath sounds, cyanotic spells) Inability to pass nasogastric tube	Maintain respiratory status and prevent aspiration. Withhold feeding until esophageal patency is determined. Quickly assess patency before putting to breast in birth area. Place on low intermittent suction to control saliva and mucus (to prevent aspiration pneumonia). Place in warmed, humidified incubator (liquefies secretions, facilitating removal). Elevate head of bed 20–40 deg (to prevent reflux of gastric juices). Keep quiet (crying causes air to pass through fistula and to distend intestines, causing respiratory embarrassment). Maintain fluid and electrolyte balance. Give fluids to replace esophageal drainage and maintain hydration. Provide parent education: Explain staged repair—provision of gastrostomy and ligation of fistula, then repair of atresia. Keep parents informed; clarify and reinforce physician's explanations regarding malformation, surgical repair, pre- and postoperative care, and prognosis (knowledge is ego strengthening). Involve parents in care of infant and in planning for future; facilitate touch and eye contact (to dispel feelings of inadequacy, increase self-esteem and self-worth, and promote incorporation of infant into family).

Pharynx
Larynx
Esophageal atresia
Tracheoesophageal fistula
Distal esophagus
Stomach
Palate
Tongue
Trachea

The most frequently seen type of congenital tracheoesophageal fistula and esophageal atresia.

DIAPHRAGMATIC HERNIA (portion of intestines in the thoracic cavity through abnormal opening in diaphragm)	Difficulty initiating respirations Gasping respirations with nasal flaring and chest retraction Barrel chest and scaphoid abdomen Asymmetric chest expansion Breath sounds may be absent, usually on left side Heart sounds displaced to right Spasmodic attacks of cyanosis and difficulty in feeding Bowel sounds may be heard in thoracic cavity.	Nurse should never ventilate with bag and mask O_2 because the stomach will inflate, further compressing the lungs. Maintain respiratory status: Immediately administer oxygen. Initiate gastric decompression. Place in high semi-Fowler's position (to use gravity to keep pressure from abdominal organs off diaphragm). Turn to affected side to allow unaffected lung expansion. Carry out interventions to alleviate respiratory and metabolic acidosis. Assess for increased secretions around suction tube (denotes possible obstruction). Aspirate and irrigate tube with air or sterile water.

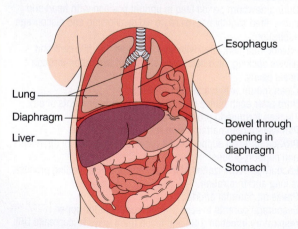

Lung
Diaphragm
Liver
Esophagus
Bowel through opening in diaphragm
Stomach

Diaphragmatic hernia. Note compression of the lung by the intestine on the affected side.

Source: Courtesy Nancy Houck, RNC, BSN, NNP-BC.

Table 27–1	Congenital Anomalies: Identification and Care in the Newborn Period—continued

Congenital Anomaly	Nursing Assessments	Nursing Goals and Interventions
OMPHALOCELE (herniation of abdominal contents into base of umbilical cord)	May have an enclosed transparent sac covering	Maintain hydration and temperature. Provide D$_5$LR and albumin for hypovolemia. Place infant in sterile bag up to and covering defect. Initiate gastric decompression by insertion of nasogastric tube attached to low suction (to prevent distention of lower bowel and impairment of blood flow). Prevent infection and trauma to defect. Position to prevent trauma to defect. Administer broad-spectrum antibiotics.

Newborn with omphalocele.

Source: Carol Harrigan, RN, MSN, NNP-BC

Congenital Anomaly	Nursing Assessments	Nursing Goals and Interventions
GASTROSCHISIS (full-thickness defect in abdominal wall allowing viscera outside the body to the right of an intact umbilical cord)	No sac covering. Intestines exposed to the caustic amniotic fluid. Associated with intestinal atresia, malrotation	Maintain hydration and temperature. Prevent trauma and infection to defect. Provide D$_5$LR normal saline, and/or albumin for hypovolemia. Place infant in sterile bag up to axilla. Initiate gastric decompression by insertion of nasogastric tube attached to low suction. Administer broad-spectrum antibiotics.

Term newborn with gastroschisis. Note the externalized loops of bowel visible through the bag.

Source: Carol Harrigan, RN, MSN, NNP-BC

(continued)

Table 27–1   Congenital Anomalies: Identification and Care in the Newborn Period—continued

Congenital Anomaly	Nursing Assessments	Nursing Goals and Interventions
PRUNE BELLY SYNDROME (congenital absence of one or more layers of abdominal muscles)	Oligohydramnios leading to pulmonary hypoplasia common Deficiency of the abdominal wall musculature causing the abdomen to be shapeless Skin hangs loosely and is wrinkled in appearance Associated with urinary abnormalities (urethral obstruction) In males, cryptorchidism is common; rarely occurs in females	Maintain respiratory status: May need to be immediately intubated and ventilated. Prevent trauma and infection. Administer broad-spectrum antibiotics. Place a urinary catheter and monitor urinary output. Carry out interventions to alleviate respiratory and metabolic acidosis. Keep parents updated and informed about prognosis.

Prune belly syndrome.
Source: Carol Harrigan, RN, MSN, NNP-BC

MYELOMENINGOCELE (saclike cyst containing meninges, spinal cord, and nerve roots in thoracic and/or lumbar area)	Myelomeningocele directly connects to subarachnoid space so hydrocephalus often associated No response or varying response to sensation below level of sac May have constant dribbling of urine Incontinence or retention of stool Anal wink may or may not be present	Prevent trauma and infection. Position on abdomen or on side and restrain (to prevent pressure and trauma to sac). Meticulously clean buttocks and genitals after each voiding and defecation (to prevent contamination of sac and decrease possibility of infection). May put protective covering over sac (to prevent rupture and drying). Observe sac for oozing of fluid. Credé bladder (apply downward pressure on bladder with thumbs, moving urine toward the urethra) as ordered to prevent urinary stasis. Assess amount of sensation and movement below defect. Observe for complications. Obtain occipital-frontal circumference baseline measurements; then measure head circumference once a day (to detect hydrocephalus). Check fontanelle for fullness and bulging.

Newborn with lumbar myelomeningocele.
Source: Carol Harrigan, RN, MSN, NNP-BC

IMPERFORATE ANUS, CONGENITAL DISLOCATED HIP, AND CLUBFOOT	See discussions in the *Anus* and *Extremities* sections in Chapter 25 🔗. Also see Chapters 52 and 57 🔗.	Identify defect and initiate appropriate referral early.

show impulsivity, cognitive impairment, and speech and language abnormalities indicative of CNS involvement. As they progress through the adolescent years, they change from very thin and underweight children to those who are overweight and often obese. Short stature and microcephaly persist.

NURSING MANAGEMENT *For the Newborn with Fetal Alcohol Syndrome (FAS)*

Nursing Assessment and Diagnosis

Newborns with FAS show the following characteristics:

- *Abnormal structural development and CNS dysfunction.* This includes intellectual disability, microcephaly, and hyperactivity.

- *Growth deficiencies.* The growth of infants with FAS is often restricted in regard to weight, length, and head circumference. These infants continue to show a persistent postnatal growth deficiency, with head circumference and linear growth most affected.

- *Distinctive facial abnormalities.* These include short palpebral fissures; epicanthal folds; broad nasal bridge; flattened midfacies; short, upturned, or beaklike nose; micrognathia (abnormally small lower jaw); hypoplastic maxilla; thin upper lip or vermilion border; and smooth philtrum (groove on upper lip) (Cloherty et al., 2012).

- *Associated anomalies.* Abnormalities affecting the heart (primarily septal and valvular defects), eyes (optic nerve hypoplasia), ears (conductive and sensorineural hearing loss), kidneys, and skeleton (especially involving joints, such as congenital dislocated hips) systems are often noted.

An alcohol-exposed newborn in the first week of life may show symptoms that include sleeplessness, excessive arousal states, inconsolable crying, abnormal reflexes, hyperactivity with little ability to maintain alertness and attentiveness to environment, jitteriness, abdominal distention, and exaggerated mouthing behaviors such as hyperactive rooting and increased nonnutritive sucking. Seizures may be common. These symptoms commonly persist throughout the first month of life but may continue longer. Alcohol dependence in the infant is physiologic, not psychologic. Signs and symptoms of withdrawal often appear within 6 to 12 hours and at least within the first 3 days of life. Seizures after the neonatal period are rare.

Nursing diagnoses that may apply to the FAS newborn include the following (NANDA-I © 2012):

- *Nutrition, Imbalanced: Less Than Body Requirements,* related to decreased food intake and hyperirritability

- *Infant Behavior, Disorganized,* related to central nervous system involvement secondary to maternal alcohol use

- *Coping, Ineffective,* related to dysfunctional family dynamics and substance-dependent mother

Planning and Implementation

Hospital-Based Nursing Care

Nursing care of the FAS newborn is aimed at avoiding heat loss, providing adequate nutrition, and reducing environmental stimuli. The FAS baby is most comfortable in a quiet, dimly lit environment. Because of their feeding problems, these infants require extra time and patience during feedings. It is important to provide consistency in the staff working with the baby and parents and to keep personnel and visitors to a minimum at any one time.

Inform the alcohol-dependent mother that breastfeeding is not contraindicated but that excessive alcohol consumption may intoxicate the newborn and inhibit the letdown reflex. Monitor the newborn's vital signs closely and observe for evidence of seizure activity and respiratory distress.

Community-Based Nursing Care

Infants affected by maternal alcohol abuse are also at risk psychologically. Restlessness, sleeplessness, agitation, resistance to cuddling or holding, and frequent crying can be frustrating to parents because their efforts to relieve the distress are unrewarded. Feeding difficulties can also result in frustrations for the caregiver and digestive upsets for the infant. Frustration may cause the parents to punish the baby or result in the unconscious desire to stay away from the infant. Either outcome may create an unstable family environment and result in failure to thrive.

Focus on providing support for the parents and reinforcing positive parenting activity. Before discharge, give parents opportunities to provide baby care so that they can feel confident in their interpretations of their baby's cues and ability to meet the baby's needs. It is essential to refer the family to social services and visiting nurse or public health nurse associations. Follow-up care and teaching can strengthen the parents' skill and coping abilities and help them create a stable, healthy environment for their family. The infant with FAS should be involved in intervention programs that monitor the child's developmental progress, health, and home environment.

Evaluation

Expected outcomes of nursing care include the following:

- The FAS newborn is able to tolerate feedings and gain weight.

- The FAS infant's hyperirritability or seizures are controlled, and the baby has suffered no physical injuries.

- The parents are able to identify the special needs of their newborn and accept outside assistance as needed.

Drug Dependency

Drugs abused by pregnant women can include the following substances, used singularly or in combination: tobacco, cocaine, phencyclidine (PCP), methamphetamines, inhalants, marijuana, heroin, and methadone. The incidence of cocaine (especially "crack") use has stabilized, whereas OxyContin use has risen dramatically. (See *Substances Commonly Abused During Pregnancy* in Chapter 15 🖉 for more discussion of maternal substance abuse.)

Intrauterine drug-exposed infants are predisposed to a number of problems. Because almost all narcotic drugs cross the placenta and enter the fetal circulatory system, the fetus can develop problems in utero or soon after birth. The effects of polydrug use on the newborn must always be taken into consideration.

The greatest risks to the fetus of the drug-abusing mother are as follows:

- *Intrauterine asphyxia.* Asphyxia is often a direct result of fetal withdrawal secondary to maternal withdrawal. Fetal withdrawal is accompanied by hyperactivity, with increased oxygen consumption. Insufficiency of oxygen can lead to fetal asphyxia. Moreover, women addicted to narcotics tend to have a higher incidence of preeclampsia, abruptio placentae, and placenta previa, resulting in placental insufficiency and fetal asphyxia.

- *Intrauterine infection.* Sexually transmitted infection, HIV infection, and hepatitis are often connected with the pregnant addict's lifestyle. Such infections can involve the fetus.

- *Alterations in birth weight.* These alterations may depend on the type of drug the mother uses. Women using predominantly heroin have infants of lower birth weight who are small for gestational age (SGA). Women maintained on methadone have higher-birth-weight infants, some of whom are large for gestational age (LGA).

- *Low Apgar scores.* Low scores may be related to the intrauterine asphyxia or the medication the woman received during labor. The use of a narcotic antagonist (nalorphine or naloxone) to reverse respiratory depression is contraindicated because it may precipitate acute withdrawal in the infant.

Common Complications of the Drug-Exposed Newborn

The newborn of a woman who abused drugs during her pregnancy is predisposed to the following problems:

- *Respiratory distress.* The heroin-addicted newborn frequently suffers respiratory stress, mainly meconium-aspiration pneumonia and transient tachypnea. Meconium aspiration is usually secondary to increased oxygen consumption and activity experienced by the fetus during intrauterine withdrawal. Transient tachypnea may develop secondary to the inhibitory effects of narcotics on the reflex responsible for clearing the lungs. Respiratory

distress syndrome (RDS), however, occurs less often in heroin-addicted newborns, even in those who are premature, because they have tissue-oxygen-unloading capabilities comparable to those of a 6-week-old term infant. In addition, heroin stimulates production of glucocorticoids via the anterior pituitary.

- *Jaundice.* Newborns of methadone-addicted women may develop jaundice because of prematurity. By contrast, infants of mothers addicted to heroin or cocaine have a lower incidence of hyperbilirubinemia because these substances contribute to early maturity of the liver.

- *Congenital anomalies and growth restriction.* Infants of cocaine-addicted mothers exhibit congenital malformations involving bony skull defects, such as microencephaly, and symmetric intrauterine growth restriction (IUGR), cardiac defects, and genitourinary defects. In addition, there is a higher incidence of sudden death syndrome (SIDS). Infants exposed to methamphetamines during gestation may show a higher incidence of cleft lip and palate, cardiac anomalies, microcephaly, and low birth weight (LBW) (Blackburn, 2013). Congenital anomalies, however, are rare.

- *Behavioral abnormalities.* Babies exposed to cocaine have poor state organization. They exhibit decreased interactive behaviors when tested with the Brazelton Neonatal Behavioral Assessment Scale. These infants also have difficulty moving through the various sleep and wake states and have problems attending to and actively engaging in auditory and visual stimuli.

- *Withdrawal.* The most significant postnatal problem of the drug-exposed newborn is opiate withdrawal (usually from heroin or methadone). The onset of the withdrawal manifestations often begins within the first 24 to 48 hours of life. See Table 27–2 for the clinical manifestations of newborn withdrawal.

During the first 2 years of life, many cocaine-exposed infants demonstrate susceptibility to behavior lability and the inability to express strong feelings such as pleasure, anger, or distress, or even a strong reaction to being separated from their parents. As

---

Table 27–2	Clinical Manifestations of Newborn Withdrawal

CENTRAL NERVOUS SYSTEM SIGNS	**GASTROINTESTINAL SIGNS**	**VASOMOTOR SIGNS**
■ Hyperactivity	■ Disorganized, vigorous suck	■ Stuffy nose, yawning, sneezing
■ Hyperirritability (persistent shrill cry)	■ Vomiting	■ Flushing
■ Increased muscle tone	■ Drooling	■ Sweating
■ Exaggerated reflexes	■ Sensitive gag reflex	■ Sudden, circumoral pallor
■ Tremors and myoclonic jerks	■ Hyperphagia	
■ Sneezing, hiccups, yawning	■ Diarrhea	
■ Short, unquiet sleep	■ Poor feeding (less than 15 mL on first day of life; takes longer than 30 min per feeding)	
■ Fever (accompanies the increased neuromuscular activities)		

RESPIRATORY SIGNS	**CUTANEOUS SIGNS**	
■ Tachypnea (greater than 60 breaths per minute when quiet)	■ Excoriated buttocks, knees, elbows	
■ Excessive secretions	■ Facial scratches	
	■ Pressure-point abrasions	

a result, these infants have poor social interaction skills, cannot habitate to external stimuli, become easily overstimulated, and have difficulty sleeping. Cocaine-exposed infants are at higher risk for motor development problems, delays in expressive language skills, and feeding difficulties because of swallowing problems (Blackburn, 2013). Behavioral state control is poorly developed in drug-exposed infants, who tend to rapidly progress from sleep to the awake state of crying without a smooth transition from one state to the next. These infants also have a higher incidence of gastrointestinal and respiratory illnesses related not to drug exposure but to the mother's lack of education regarding proper infant care, feeding, and hygiene. After birth the infant born to a drug-dependent mother may also be subject to neglect, abuse, or both.

Clinical Therapy

For optimal fetal and neonatal outcome, the heroin-addicted woman should receive complete prenatal care as early as possible to reduce maternal morbidity and mortality rates and to promote fetal stability and growth (Weiner & Finnegan, 2011). Methadone maintenance programs have been the standard treatment for mothers who are addicted to heroin to combat the cravings and to prevent withdrawal. For those women dependent on narcotics, it is not recommended that they be withdrawn completely while pregnant because this induces fetal withdrawal with poor newborn outcomes.

Newborn treatment may include management of complications; serologic tests for syphilis, HIV, and hepatitis B; urine drug screen and meconium analysis; and social service referral. Screening of meconium provides a more comprehensive and accurate indication of exposure over a longer gestational period than does screening of neonatal urine (Weiner & Finnegan, 2011). Pharmacologic management for opiate withdrawal may include oral morphine sulfate solution, paregoric, tincture of opium, phenobarbital, and diazepam (Weiner & Finnegan, 2011). Nutritional support is important in light of the increase in energy expenditure that withdrawal may entail.

NURSING MANAGEMENT
For the Substance-Exposed Newborn

Nursing Assessment and Diagnosis

Early identification of the newborn needing clinical or pharmacologic interventions decreases the incidence of neonatal mortality and morbidity. The identification of substance-exposed newborns is determined primarily by clinical indicators in the prenatal period including maternal presentation, history of substance use or abuse, medical history, or toxicology results. During the newborn period, nursing assessment focuses on the following:

- Discovering the mother's last drug intake and dosage level. Women may be reluctant to disclose this information; therefore, a nonjudgmental interview technique is essential (AAP & ACOG, 2012).

- Assessing for congenital malformations and the complications related to intrauterine withdrawal such as SGA, asphyxia, meconium aspiration, and prematurity.

- Identifying the signs and symptoms of newborn withdrawal or neonatal abstinence syndrome (see Table 27–2).

Although many of the signs and symptoms of drug withdrawal are similar to those seen with hypoglycemia and hypocalcemia, glucose and calcium values are reported to be within normal limits.

Neonatal abstinence syndrome (NAS) includes both physiologic and behavioral responses. A number of useful systematic scoring systems are available for assessing the severity of withdrawal, such as the Finnegan scale, which is based on observations and measurement of the responses to neonatal abstinence. It evaluates the infant on potentially life-threatening signs such as vomiting, diarrhea, weight loss, irritability, tremors, and tachypnea (Table 27–3). NAS scoring helps to guide the need for pharmacologic intervention. For example, pharmacologic treatment is recommended for Finnegan scores greater than 8 (Weiner & Finnegan, 2011).

Nursing diagnoses that may apply to drug-dependent newborns include the ones in the nursing care plan as well as the following (NANDA-I © 2012):

- *Breathing Pattern, Ineffective,* related to meconium aspiration syndrome due to fetal stress and hypoxia

- *Skin Integrity, Impaired,* related to constant activity, diarrhea

- *Parenting, Impaired,* related to hyperirritable behavior of the infant and lack of knowledge of infant care

Planning and Implementation
Hospital-Based Nursing Care

Care of the drug-dependent newborn is based on reducing withdrawal symptoms and promoting adequate respiration, temperature, and nutrition. See *Nursing Care Plan: The Newborn of a Substance-Abusing Mother* on pages 658–659 for specific nursing measures. Some general nursing care measures include the following:

- Perform neonatal abstinence scoring per hospital protocol.

- Monitor temperature for hypothermia.

- Monitor pulse and respirations carefully every 15 minutes until stable.

- Provide small, frequent feedings, especially in the presence of vomiting, regurgitation, and diarrhea.

- Position on the right side-lying or in semi-Fowler's to avoid possible aspiration of vomitus or secretions.

- Administer medications as ordered, such as oral morphine, tincture of opium, and paregoric. A sedative, such as phenobarbital, is usually used in combination with an opioid, as the sedative does not control any of the GI symptoms to control irritability associated with NAS (Cloherty et al., 2012).

- Monitor frequency of diarrhea and vomiting, and weigh infant every 8 hours during withdrawal.

- Swaddle infant with hands near mouth to minimize injury and help achieve a more organized behavioral state. Offer a pacifier for nonnutritive, excessive sucking (Figure 27–13 ●). Gentle, vertical rocking can be successful in calming an infant who is out of control.

Table 27–3   Neonatal Abstinence Syndrome (NAS) Score Sheet

NAS Scoring System

System	Signs and Symptoms	Score	AM	PM
Central nervous system disturbances	Excessive high-pitched (or other) cry	2		Daily weight:
	Continuous high-pitched (or other) cry	3		
	Sleeps < 1 hour after feeding	3		
	Sleeps < 2 hours after feeding	2		
	Sleeps < 3 hours after feeding	1		
	Hyperactive Moro reflex	2		
	Markedly hyperactive Moro reflex	3		
	Mild tremors disturbed	1		
	Moderate–severe tremors disturbed	2		
	Mild tremors undisturbed	3		
	Moderate–severe tremors undisturbed	4		
	Increased muscle tone	2		
	Excoriation (specific area)	1		
	Myoclonic jerks	3		
	Generalized convulsions	5		
Metabolic/vasomotor/ respiratory disturbances	Sweating	1		
	Fever < 101°F (37.2–38.2°C [99–100.8°F])	1		
	Fever > 101°F (38.4°C [101.1°F] and higher)	2		
	Frequent yawning (>3 to 4 times/interval)	1		
	Mottling	1		
	Nasal stuffiness	1		
	Sneezing (>3 to 4 times/interval)	1		
	Nasal flaring	2		
	Respiratory rate > 60/min	1		
	Respiratory rate 60/min with retractions	2		
Gastrointestinal disturbances	Excessive sucking	1		
	Poor feeding	2		
	Regurgitation	2		
	Projectile vomiting	3		
	Loose stools	2		
	Watery stools	3		
	Total Score			
	Initials of Scorer			

Source: Permission granted by PMPH-USA, LTD.

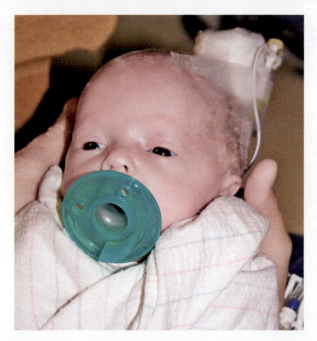

● **Figure 27–13** Nonnutritive sucking on a pacifier has a calming effect on the newborn.

Source: Carol Harrigan, RN, MSN, NNP-BC

- Protect infant's face and extremities from excoriation by using mittens, as well as soft sheets or sheepskin. Apply protective skin emollient to the groin area with each diaper change
- Place the newborn in a quiet, dimly lit area of the nursery

Community-Based Nursing Care

Parents need assistance to prepare for what they can expect for the first few months at home. At the time of discharge, instruct the mother to anticipate mild jitteriness and irritability in the newborn, which may persist from 6 days to 8 weeks, depending on the initial severity of the withdrawal (Blackburn, 2013). Infants with neonatal abstinence syndrome are at significantly higher risk for sudden infant death syndrome (SIDS) when the mother used heroin or cocaine. The infant should sleep supine, and home apnea monitoring should be implemented. Help the mother learn feeding techniques, comforting measures, how to recognize newborn cues, and appropriate parenting responses. Counsel parents regarding available resources, such as support groups, as well as signs and symptoms that indicate the need for further care. Ongoing evaluation is necessary because of the potential for long-term problems. Follow up on missed appointments in order to bring parents back into the healthcare system, thereby improving parent and infant outcomes and promoting a positive, interactive environment after birth.

Evaluation

Expected outcomes of nursing care include the following:

- The newborn tolerates feedings, gains weight, and has a decreased incidence of diarrhea.
- The parents learn innovative ways to comfort their newborn.
- The parents are able to cope with their frustrations and begin to use outside resources as needed.

Infants of Mothers Who Are Tobacco Dependent

Despite increased knowledge about the dangers to the fetus and newborn of smoking mothers, 16% to 25% of these women continue to smoke during pregnancy (Nodine, Arruda, & Hastings-Tolsma, 2011). The common consequence of tobacco use is addiction to nicotine. Most smokers report true enjoyment, associated with a sense of relaxation during stress, especially with the first cigarette of the day.

Risks of Tobacco to the Fetus and Newborn

Preconceptual cigarette smoking has been found to increase infertility. Fortunately, the reduction in fertility is reversible if the woman stops smoking. Smoking during pregnancy has been associated with spontaneous abortion, placenta previa, and abruptio placentae.

The most studied compound found in cigarette smoking that can adversely affect the intrauterine environment is carbon monoxide. Carbon monoxide binds hemoglobin to form carboxyhemoglobin, which reduces the oxygen-carrying capacity of the blood. It also increases the binding of hemoglobin to oxygen, which impairs the release of oxygen to the tissues. Therefore the fetus can experience intrauterine hypoxia and ischemia. Mothers who smoke during pregnancy are more likely to have intrauterine growth restriction (IUGR) infants and preterm infants. These infants typically weigh 150 to 250 g less than infants of nonsmokers (Cloherty et al., 2012). The nicotine in cigarettes acts as a neuroteratogen that interferes with fetal development, specifically the developing nervous system. Additional risks to the fetus and newborn of the mother who smokes include the following (Gleason & Devaskar, 2012):

- *Intrauterine distress* presenting as meconium staining and low Apgar scores
- *Neonatal neurobehavioral abnormalities* such as impaired habituation, orientation, consolability, orientation to sound
- *Hypertonia* or *hypotonia, increase in tremors, increased Moro reflex*
- *Signs of nicotine toxicity* (tachycardia, irritability, poor feeding)
- *Sudden infant death syndrome (SIDS)*

Clinical Therapy

Inquiry into tobacco and smoke exposure should be a routine part of the prenatal history. Preconception and prenatal counseling about the effects of cigarette smoking on pregnancy and the fetus should occur. Mothers should be counseled that eliminating or reducing smoking even late in pregnancy can improve fetal growth. The use of nicotine patches (instead of smoking) reduces the absorption of nicotine and thereby may increase the birth weight of the fetus. See *Tobacco* in Chapter 11 🕮 for further discussion of prenatal smoking cessation and other intervention programs.

Cotinine, a metabolite of nicotine, has been found in fetal body fluids. There is also a positive correlation between the

Intervention	Rationale	Expected Outcome

1. Nursing Diagnosis: *Injury, Risk for,* to the central nervous system (CNS) related to perinatal substance abuse (NANDA-I © 2012)

NIC Priority Intervention:
Newborn monitoring: Measurement and interpretation of physiologic status of the newborn the first 24 hours after birth

NOC Suggested Outcome:
Neurologic status: Extent to which the peripheral and central nervous systems receive, process, and respond to internal and external stimuli

Goal: The newborn will be free of signs and symptoms of CNS injury.

■ Obtain prenatal records and question patient about history of drug addiction. Include duration, type of drug or drugs used, and time and amount of last dose taken prior to birth.	■ Noting the mother's last drug ingestion will provide the medical staff with an approximate time frame to expect the infant to exhibit withdrawal symptoms.	■ Infant will have no signs and symptoms of CNS injury as evidenced by reduced hyperactivity and irritability, normal sleep–wake pattern, no jitteriness, and no seizure activity.
■ Assess newborn for signs and symptoms of withdrawal (e.g., high-pitched shrill cry, sneezing, vomiting, diarrhea, hypertonicity, restlessness, and wakefulness).	■ The average symptoms of withdrawal occur 72 hours after birth; however, symptoms may appear as early as 6–24 hours after birth.	
■ Provide a quiet and calm environment. Swaddle infant tightly and place in a side-lying or prone position.	■ Providing a quiet environment decreases stimuli, therefore reducing CNS symptoms.	
■ Carefully plan tests and treatments to avoid excessive stimuli.	■ Planning care promotes rest and reduces external stimuli.	
■ Use soothing techniques such as rocking, cuddling, soft music, and soft tones when speaking.	■ These activities promote comfort, security, and infant bonding.	
■ Administer appropriate medications as ordered by physician. Monitor efficacy and side effects of these medications, which may include paregoric and phenobarbital.	■ These medications aid patient in alleviating symptoms related to withdrawal.	

2. Nursing Diagnosis: *Airway Clearance, Ineffective,* related to suppression of respiratory system (NANDA-I © 2012)

NIC Priority Intervention:
Respiratory monitoring: Collection and analysis of patient data to ensure airway patency and adequate gas exchange

NOC Suggested Outcome:
Respiratory status: Gas exchange: alveolar exchange of CO_2 or O_2 to maintain arterial blood gas concentrations

Goal: The infant will be free of signs and symptoms of respiratory distress after birth.

■ Obtain maternal prenatal, labor, and birth records.	■ Provides information of fetal stress that may have occurred during the prenatal or intrapartum period. In addition, the birth record will provide information concerning infant's respiratory status at birth; for example, the Apgar score.	■ Infant will maintain adequate respiratory gas exchange as evidenced by respirations of 30–60 breaths/min and arterial blood gases within normal range.
■ Assess infant's respiratory rate and effort, skin color, heart rate, presence or absence of cough reflex, and symptoms of respiratory distress.	■ Maternal narcotic consumption may depress the cough reflex and respiratory center of the infant after birth. Symptoms such as cyanosis, tachycardia, grunting, retractions, and nasal flaring may indicate hypoxia.	
■ Position infant in a side-lying or semi-Fowler's position.	■ Prevents aspiration.	
■ Monitor infant for temperature elevation.	■ Temperature elevation may cause metabolic rate and oxygen needs to increase when associated with CNS stimulation.	
■ **Collaboration:** Obtain arterial blood gases (ABGs) as ordered by physician.	■ Oxygen demands increase with drug withdrawal. Obtaining ABGs will provide medical personnel baseline information about infant's respiratory status, so effective medical interventions can be initiated.	
■ Monitor infant's cardiac status and pulmonary status using ECG and pulse oximetry.	■ Provides medical personnel with cardiac and pulmonary status.	

Nursing Care Plan The Newborn of a Substance-Abusing Mother—continued

Intervention	Rationale	Expected Outcome
3. Nursing Diagnosis: *Nutrition, Imbalanced, Less Than Body Requirements,* related to vomiting and diarrhea, uncoordinated suck and swallow reflex, and hypertonia secondary to withdrawal (NANDA-I © 2012)		

NIC Priority Intervention:
Nutrition therapy: Administration of food and fluids to support metabolic processes of a patient who is malnourished or at high risk for becoming malnourished

Goal: The infant will gain or maintain weight.

NOC Suggested Outcome:
Nutritional status: Extent to which nutrients are available to meet metabolic needs

Intervention	Rationale	Expected Outcome
■ Review gestational age assessment.	■ Oral feeding may be difficult due to CNS hyperactivity and GI hypermobility.	■ Infant will tolerate feedings, maintain weight, or gain weight as evidenced by no regurgitation or aspiration of feedings, and adequate weight gain according to weight graph.
■ Assess infant's sucking and swallowing reflexes.		
■ Monitor regurgitation, vomiting, and diarrhea.	■ GI hypermobility, irritation, and CNS stimulation can increase nutritional needs.	
■ Use bulb syringe before feedings if having problems with nasal stuffiness and congestion.	■ Allows infant to breathe easier by ridding the nasal passages of excessive mucus.	
■ Initiate appropriate feedings per physician's orders (i.e., oral, gavage, or IV feedings).	■ Facilitates nutritional intake because SGA infants require 120–150 kcal/kg/day for adequate nutrition.	
■ Provide small frequent feedings of a high-calorie formula.		
■ Position infant on the side after feedings.	■ Prevents regurgitation and promotes gastric emptying.	
■ Monitor infant's weight and document on graph.	■ Identifies abnormalities in weight gain or loss and allows for early intervention when necessary.	
■ Offer pacifier between feedings for nonnutritive sucking.	■ Nonnutritive sucking allows for sucking practice, management of infant pain, and self-consoling behaviors.	

Intervention	Rationale	Expected Outcome
4. Nursing Diagnosis: *Parenting, Risk for Impaired,* related to lack of knowledge of infant care (NANDA-I © 2012)		

NIC Priority Intervention:
Teaching: Infant care: instruction on nurturing and physical care needed during the first year of life

Goal: The parent will demonstrate ability to independently provide infant care.

NOC Suggested Outcome:
Parenting: Provision of an environment that promotes optimum growth and development of dependent children

Intervention	Rationale	Expected Outcome
■ Assess mother's desire to learn infant care tasks. Evaluate her present physical and emotional stability.	■ Will provide knowledge of mother's ability to care for infant.	■ Parent will demonstrate ability to perform basic infant care tasks as evidenced by exhibiting appropriate attachment behaviors (e.g., talking and holding infant), feeding infant, and bathing infant.
■ Instruct mother on coping strategies (e.g., exercise, listening to music, and discussing concerns openly) to manage stressful situations.	■ Will give mother the tools to handle stress, thereby decreasing the chances of exhibiting abusive behavior.	
■ Assess mother's insight into her own chemical dependency.	■ Assistance in enrollment into a chemical dependency program may be necessary before mother can independently care for infant.	
■ Instruct mother on signs and symptoms of withdrawal and treatment interventions.	■ Assists the mother in understanding infant's behaviors and gives her the tools to intervene without feeling anxious.	
■ Encourage mother and family members to perform basic infant care tasks.	■ Facilitates attachment and increases parenting competence.	

number of cigarettes smoked per day and the concentration of cotinine in maternal urine. Other factors that influence fetal and maternal serum cotinine concentrations are nicotine content of the cigarette and the time elapsed between the last cigarette smoked and the sampling. These findings indicate that cotinine may be used as a marker of maternal–fetal tobacco exposure during pregnancy (Gleason & Devaskar, 2012).

Nursing Management.   Newborns of mothers who are tobacco dependent may be screened with the NICU Network Neurobehavioral Scale (NNNS) to assess their neurologic, behavioral, and stress/abstinence neurobehavioral function.

The potential for long-term respiratory problems such as asthma, as well as cognitive and receptive language delays that may persist into school age, should be evaluated.

CARE OF THE NEWBORN EXPOSED TO HIV/AIDS

In the United States, approximately 6000 pregnant women infected with the HIV virus give birth each year. Preventive strategies have reduced the risk of maternal–child transmission of HIV to approximately 1% to 5% in the United States (Gleason & Devaskar, 2012). Most HIV transmissions during the perinatal and newborn periods can occur across the placenta or through breast milk or contaminated blood. The risk of vertical transmission in mothers not receiving an antiretroviral (ARV) drug regimen such as oral zidovudine (ZDV) during gestation is 15% to 35% depending on whether the mother is in Europe, the United States, or Africa (Gleason & Devaskar, 2012). Pregnant women should be universally tested (with patient notification) for HIV infection as part of the routine battery of prenatal blood tests unless they decline the test (i.e., opt-out approach) as permitted by local and state regulations. Refusal of testing should be documented. (For a discussion of maternal and fetal HIV/AIDS, see Chapter 11 🔗.) Some infants infected by maternal–fetal transmission suffer from severe immunodeficiency, with HIV disease progressing more rapidly during the first year of life.

Early identification of babies with or at risk for HIV/AIDS is essential during the newborn period. HIV-1 diagnostic testing for infants and children younger than 18 months differs from that for older children. Nucleic acid amplification tests (NAATs) are the preferred tests. Results can be made available within 24 hours (Gleason & Devaskar, 2012). The first NAAT tests should be performed on the newborn before 12 hours of age. Umbilical cord blood should not be used for HIV testing because of possible contamination with maternal blood, leading to false-positive results. A repeat should be performed at 1 to 2 months of age and again at 4 to 6 months of age. Most clinicians confirm the absence of HIV-1 infection with a negative HIV-1 antibody assay result at 12 to 18 months of age (Gleason & Devaskar, 2012).

For infants, AZT (zidovudine [ZDV]) is started as soon as possible after birth (by 6 to 12 hours postbirth) and continued for the first 6 weeks of life. Dosage varies depending on gestational age. Nevirapine is also given with the AZT (Glomella, 2013). If the infant is confirmed to be HIV positive, ZDV is changed to a multidrug antiretroviral regimen. Current treatment recommendations for HIV-1-infected children are available at http://aidsinfo.nih.gov.

Nursing Management

Many newborns exposed to HIV/AIDS are premature or small for gestational age (SGA), or both, and show evidence of failure to thrive during neonatal and infant periods. They can show signs and symptoms of disease within days of birth. Signs that may be seen in the early infancy period include enlarged spleen and liver, swollen glands, recurrent respiratory infections, rhinorrhea, interstitial pneumonia (rarely seen in adults), recurrent GI (diarrhea and weight loss) and urinary system infections, persistent or recurrent oral candidiasis infections, and loss of achieved developmental milestones (Glomella, 2013). There is also a high risk of acquiring *Pneumocystis carinii* pneumonia. Opportunistic diseases such as gram-negative sepsis and problems associated with prematurity are the primary causes of mortality in HIV-infected babies.

Nursing care of the newborn exposed to HIV/AIDS includes all the care normally given to any newborn in a nursery. In addition, include care for a newborn suspected of having a bloodborne infection, as with hepatitis B.

SAFETY ALERT!
Standard precautions should be used when caring for the newborn immediately after birth and when obtaining blood samples via vein puncture or heelstick.

The blood of all newborns must be considered potentially infectious because the status of the infant's blood is often not known until after the infant is discharged. Most institutions recommend that their caregivers wear gloves during all diaper changes, especially in the presence of diarrhea, because blood may be in the stool and should be considered part of standard precautions (AAP & ACOG, 2012). There is a window of time before seroconversion occurs when the baby is still considered infectious. See Table 27–4 for some general issues for all caregivers of newborns at risk for HIV/AIDS. In addition, provide for comfort; keep the newborn well nourished and protected from opportunistic infections; administer good skin care to prevent skin rashes; and facilitate growth, development, and attachment. For further discussion of the infant with HIV/AIDS, see *Immunodeficiency Disorders* in Chapter 49 🔗.

CARE OF THE NEWBORN WITH A CONGENITAL HEART DEFECT

Congenital heart defects occur in 3% to 8% of live births (depending on the severity of structural defects). Because accurate diagnosis and surgical treatment are now available, many deaths

---

Clinical Reasoning   Newborn with Possible HIV

Mrs. Jean Corrigan, a 23-year-old G1P1 positive for HIV, has just given birth to a 7 lb, 1 oz baby girl. As she watches you assessing her daughter in the birthing room, she asks why you are wearing gloves and whether her daughter will have to be in isolation. What will your response be?
See www.nursing.pearsonhighered.com for possible responses.

Table 27–4	Issues for Caregivers of Infants at Risk for HIV/AIDS
Resuscitation	For suctioning use a bulb syringe, mucus extractor, or meconium aspirator with wall suction on low setting. Use masks, goggles, and gloves.
Admission care	To remove blood from baby's skin, give warm water–mild soap bath using gloves as soon as possible after admission.
Hand washing	Thorough hand washing is indicated before and after caring for infant. Hands must be washed immediately if contaminated with blood or body fluids. Wash hands after removal of gloves.
Gloves	Gloves are indicated when touching blood or other high-risk fluids. Gloves should also be worn when handling newborns before and during their initial baths, cord care, eye prophylactics, and vitamin K administration.
Mask, goggle, and gown	Not routinely needed unless coming in contact with placenta or the blood and amniotic fluid on the skin of the newborn.
Needles and syringes	Used needles should not be recapped or bent; they should be disposed of in a puncture-resistant plastic container belonging specifically to that baby. After the newborn is discharged the container is discarded.
Specimens	Blood and other specimens should be double bagged and/or sealed in an impervious container and labeled according to agency protocol.
Equipment and linen	Articles contaminated with blood or body fluids should be discarded or bagged according to isolation or agency protocol.
Body fluid spills	Blood and body fluid spills should be cleaned promptly with a solution of 5.25% sodium hypochlorite (household bleach) diluted 1:10 with water. Apply for at least 30 seconds then wipe after the minimum contact time.
Education and support	Provide education and psychologic support for family and staff. Caregivers who avoid contact with a baby at risk or who overdress in unnecessary isolation garb subtly exacerbate an already difficult family situation. Information resources include the National AIDS Hotline (1-800-342-2437) and HIV/AIDS Treatment Enforcement Service website.
Exempted personnel	Immunologically compromised staff (pregnant women may be included in this group) and possibly infectious staff members should not care for these infants.

Source: Adapted from American Academy of Pediatrics Committee on Pediatric AIDS and Committee on Infectious Diseases. (1999). Issues related to human immunodeficiency transmission in schools, child care, medical settings, the home, and community. *Pediatrics, 104*(2), 318–324; Krist, A. H., & Crawford-Faucher, A. (2002). Management of newborns exposed to maternal HIV infection. *American Family Physician, 65*(10), 2049–2056.

can be prevented (Cloherty et al., 2012). Corrective cardiac surgery is being done at earlier ages; for example, more than half the children undergoing surgery are less than 1 year of age, and one fourth are less than 1 month old. It is crucial for the nurse to have comprehensive knowledge of congenital heart disease to detect deviations from normal and initiate interventions.

Overview of Congenital Heart Defects

In the majority of cases of congenital heart malformations, the cause is multifactorial with no specific trigger. Other factors that might influence development of congenital heart malformation can be classified as environmental or genetic. Infections of the pregnant woman, such as rubella, cytomegalovirus, coxsackie B, and influenza, have been implicated. Steroids, alcohol, lithium, and some anticonvulsants have been shown to cause malformations of the heart. Seasonal spraying of pesticides has also been linked to an increase in congenital heart defects. Clinicians are also beginning to see cardiac defects in infants of mothers with phenylketonuria (PKU), an amino acid disorder, who do not follow their diets. Infants with Down syndrome, Turner syndrome, and Holt-Oram syndrome, as well as trisomy 13 and trisomy 18, frequently have heart lesions. Increased incidence and risk of recurrence of specific defects occur in families.

The most common cardiac defects seen in the first 6 days of life are left ventricular outflow obstructions (mitral stenosis, aortic stenosis or atresia), hypoplastic left heart, coarctation of the aorta, patent ductus arteriosus (PDA, the most common defect in premature infants), transposition of the great vessels, tetralogy of Fallot, and large ventricular septal defect or atrial septal defects. Many cardiac defects may not manifest themselves until after discharge from the birthing unit.

Nursing Management

The primary goal of the neonatal nurse is to identify cardiac defects early and initiate referral to the physician. The three most common manifestations of cardiac defect are cyanosis, detectable heart murmur, and congestive heart failure signs (tachycardia, tachypnea, diaphoresis, hepatomegaly, cardiomegaly). See Chapter 48 for a detailed discussion of the clinical manifestations and medical–surgical management of these specific cardiac defects. Initial repair of heart defects in the newborn period is becoming more commonplace. The NICU staff is now involved in both the preoperative and postoperative care of newborns. The benefits for the cardiac infant of being cared for by NICU staff include the staff's knowledge of neonatal anatomy and physiology, experience in supporting the family, and an awareness of the newborn's developmental needs.

After the baby is stabilized, decisions are made about on-going care. The parents need careful and complete explanations and the opportunity to take part in decision making. They also require ongoing emotional support. Families with a baby born with any congenital anomaly also need genetic counseling about future conception. Parents need opportunities to verbalize their concerns about their baby's health maintenance and their understanding of the rationale for follow-up care.

 Clinical Tip

When cyanosis occurs in an otherwise healthy 12- to 24-hour-old newborn displaying no respiratory distress and is not resolved with oxygen, think about cardiac issues, especially a ductal-dependent lesion.

Critical Concept Review

LEARNING OUTCOME 27.1: Explain the factors present at birth that indicate an at-risk newborn.

Factors present at birth that may place an infant at risk include:
1. Maternal low socioeconomic level:
   - Decreased access to health care.
2. Exposure to environmental dangers:
   - Toxic chemicals.
   - Illicit drugs.
3. Preexisting maternal conditions:
   - Heart disease.
   - Diabetes.
   - Hypertension.
   - Renal disease.
4. Maternal age and parity.
5. Pregnancy complications:
   - Abruptio placentae.
   - Placenta previa.
   - Preeclampsia.

LEARNING OUTCOME 27.2: Compare the underlying etiologies of the physiologic complications of small-for-gestational-age (SGA) newborns and preterm appropriate-for-gestational-age (Pr AGA) newborns and the nursing management for each.

Many of the same factors contribute to the common complications of the SGA newborn and the Pr AGA newborn:
1. Maternal factors:
   - Grand multiparity.
   - Multiple-gestation pregnancy.
   - Low socioeconomic status.
   - Poor maternal nutrition.
2. Maternal disease:
   - Heart disease.
   - Hypertension.
   - Preeclampsia.
3. Environmental factors:
   - Maternal use of drugs.
   - Exposure to toxins.
   - High altitude.
4. Placental factors:
   - Small placenta.
   - Placenta previa.
   - Abnormal cord insertions.
5. Fetal factors:
   - Congenital infections.
   - Chromosomal syndromes.

LEARNING OUTCOME 27.3: Explain the impact of maternal diabetes mellitus on the newborn.

The most common complications of maternal diabetes mellitus are:
1. Hypoglycemia.
2. Hypocalcemia.
3. Hyperbilirubinemia.
4. Birth trauma.
5. Polycythemia.
6. Respiratory distress syndrome.
7. Congenital birth defects:
   - Cardiac anomalies.
   - Gastrointestinal anomalies.
   - Sacral agenesis.

LEARNING OUTCOME 27.4: Compare the characteristics and potential complications that influence nursing management of the postterm newborn and the newborn with postmaturity syndrome.

1. Postmaturity:
   - Applies to any newborn born after 42 weeks' gestation.
   - Most are of normal size and health.
   - Large fetus may have difficult time passing through birth passage.
2. Postmaturity syndrome, in which the fetus is exposed to poor placental function, which impairs nutrition and oxygenation and has the following characteristics:
   - Hypoglycemia.
   - Meconium aspiration.
   - Polycythemia.
   - Congenital anomalies.
   - Seizure activity.
   - Cold stress.

LEARNING OUTCOME 27.5: Discuss the physiologic and behavioral characteristics of the preterm newborn that predispose each body system to various complications and that are used in developing a plan of care that includes nutritional management.

1. Respiratory difficulties:
   - Lack of surfactant causes the alveoli to collapse and infant becomes hypoxic.
   - Incomplete development of the muscular coat of the pulmonary blood vessels, which leads to left to right shunting of blood through the ductus arteriosus back into lungs.
2. Cardiac difficulties:
   - Ductus arteriosus remains open due to low oxygen levels and low prostaglandin E levels.
   - Patent ductus remains open, causing more blood to flow to lungs, increased respiratory effort, carbon dioxide retention, and bounding femoral pulses.
3. Temperature control difficulties:
   - Less able to produce heat because of the higher ratio of body surface to body weight.
   - Lack of brown fat.
   - Thin skin, which causes greater insensible water loss.
   - Lack of flexion increases heat loss.
   - Increased chance of aspiration.
   - Decreased ability to convert amino acids.

4. Gastrointestinal difficulties:
   - Poor suck effort.
   - High caloric needs and limited ability to take in nutrition.
   - Increased basal metabolic rate and oxygen needs related to increased effort at sucking.
   - Decreased ability to handle increased osmolarity of formula protein.
   - Difficulty absorbing saturated fats.
   - Difficulty digesting lactose.
   - Diminished blood flow to the intestines resulting in necrotizing enterocolitis.
5. Renal difficulties:
   - Decreased glomerular filtration rate due to decreased renal blood flow.
   - Inability to concentrate urine.
   - Decreased ability of kidney to buffer.
   - Delayed drug excretion time.
   - Spilling of glucose at a lower serum glucose rate.
6. Reactivity and behavioral state difficulties:
   - Delayed or lack of periods of reactivity due to poor condition of newborn.
   - Disorganized sleep–wake cycle.

LEARNING OUTCOME 27.6: Summarize the nursing assessments of and initial interventions for a newborn with selected congenital anomalies.

Nursing assessments and initial interventions focus on:

1. Respiratory:
   - Ability of infant to breathe.
   - Maintain respiratory function.
2. Nutritional:
   - Is infant able to suck and swallow?
   - Does feeding cause respiratory distress?
   - Provide calories by breast, nipple, gastrointestinal tube, or IV.
3. Neurologic:
   - Is infant able to move all extremities?
   - Is there a visible defect present on the spine?

- Is head circumference normal size and does it maintain normal size?
- Keep infant in prone position if necessary.
- Keep defect covered with sterile saline soaks until surgery.
- Keep head of bed elevated if head circumference is larger than normal.
4. Parental involvement:
   - Assess parents' knowledge of infant's anomaly.
   - Keep parents informed about infant's condition.
   - Teach parents appropriate home care of infant.

LEARNING OUTCOME 27.7: Explain the special care needed by an alcohol- or drug-exposed newborn.

Special care of the infant who was exposed to drugs or alcohol focuses on:

1. Assessment of the mother's last drug intake and dosage.
2. Assessment for congenital anomalies and complications.
3. Assessment for signs and symptoms of withdrawal.

LEARNING OUTCOME 27.8: Relate the consequences of maternal HIV/AIDS to the nursing management of infants at risk for HIV/AIDS in the neonatal period and the issues for their caregivers.

Infant of the mother who has HIV/AIDS receives the same care as all newborn infants. The nurse also includes the following aspects of care:

1. Uses standard precautions when drawing blood samples.
2. Uses disposable gloves when changing diapers.
3. Protects infant from opportunistic diseases.
4. Keeps newborn well nourished to prevent failure to thrive.

LEARNING OUTCOME 27.9: Identify the physical examination findings during the early newborn period that would make the nurse suspect a congenital cardiac defect or congestive heart failure.

The three most common manifestations of cardiac defects are:

1. Cyanosis.
2. Detectable heart murmur.
3. Signs of congestive heart failure:
   - Tachycardia.
   - Tachypnea.
   - Diaphoresis.
   - Hepatomegaly.
   - Cardiomegaly.

Clinical Reasoning in Action

As the nurse on duty, you are caring for baby Erin, a 38-week IDM female born by repeat cesarean birth to a 32-year-old G3 now P3 mother. Erin's Apgar scores are 7 and 9 at 1 and 5 minutes. At 2 hours of age, the baby has an elevated respiratory rate of 100 to 110, heart rate of 165 with Grade II/VI intermittent machinery murmur, and mild cyanosis. She is now receiving 30% oxygen and has a respiratory rate of 70 to 80. The baby's clinical course, chest x-ray, and lab results are all consistent with transient tachypnea of the newborn and patent ductus arteriosus. The mother calls you to ask about how her baby is doing. She tells you that her last child was born at 30 weeks and had to be hospitalized for 6 weeks. She says, "I really tried to do it right this time," and asks you if this baby will have the same respiratory problem.

1. What should you tell the mother?
2. What can you do to facilitate mother–infant attachment?
3. Discuss the emotional response of parents to the birth of an ill or at-risk infant.
4. Discuss the four psychologic tasks essential for coping with the stress of an at-risk newborn and providing a basis for the maternal–infant relationship.
5. Baby Erin is being discharged tomorrow. Review the elements of discharge and home care instructions.
6. Design a concept map for one of the diagnoses of an infant of a diabetic mother.

See www.nursing.pearsonhighered.com for possible responses and an interactive template for a concept map.

References

Als, H., Lester, B. M., Tronick, E., & Brazelton, T. B. (1982). Assessment of preterm infant behavior (APIB). In B. M. Fitzgerald Lester & M. W. Yogman (Eds.), *Theory and research in behavioral pediatrics* (Vol. 1). New York, NY: Plenum.

American Academy of Pediatrics (AAP) Committee on Fetus and Newborn & American College of Obstetricians and Gynecologists (ACOG) Committee on Obstetrics. (2012). *Guidelines for perinatal care* (7th ed.). Elk Grove Village, IL: Author.

American Academy of Pediatrics, Committee on Pediatric AIDS and Committee on Infectious Diseases. (1999). Issues related to human immunodeficiency transmission in schools, child care, medical settings, the home, and community. *Pediatrics, 104*(2), 318–324.

Anderson, M. S., Wood, L. L., Keller, J. A., & Hay, W. W. (2011). Enteral nutrition. In S. L. Gardner (Ed.), *Merenstein & Gardner's handbook of neonatal intensive care* (7th ed., pp. 398–433). St. Louis, MO: Mosby.

Blackburn, S. (2013). *Maternal–fetal–neonatal physiology: A clinical perspective* (4th ed.). Philadelphia, PA: Saunders.

Centers for Disease Control and Prevention. (2011). *Fetal alcohol spectrum disorders: Facts about FASDs.* Retrieved from http://www.cdc.gov/ncbddd/fasd/facts.html

Cloherty, J. R., Eichenwald, E. C., Hansen, A. R., & Stark, A. R. (2012). *Manual of neonatal care* (7th ed.). Philadelphia, PA: Lippincott Williams & Wilkins.

Daily, D. K., Carter, A., & Carter, B. S. (2011). Discharge planning and follow-up of the neonatal intensive care unit infant. In S. L. Gardner (Ed.), *Merenstein & Gardner's handbook of neonatal intensive care* (7th ed., pp. 938–961). St. Louis, MO: Mosby.

Gardner, S. L., & Goldson, E. (2011). The neonate and the environment: Impact on development. In S. L. Gardner (Ed.), *Merenstein & Gardner's handbook of neonatal intensive care* (7th ed., pp. 270–331). St. Louis, MO: Mosby.

Gardner, S. L., & Hernandez, J. A. (2011). Initial nursery care. In S. L. Gardner (Ed.), *Merenstein & Gardner's handbook of neonatal intensive care* (7th ed., pp. 78–112). St. Louis, MO: Mosby.

Gleason, C. A., & Devaskar, S. U. (2012). *Avery's diseases of the newborn* (9th ed.). St. Louis, MO: Elsevier/Saunders.

Glomella, T. L. (Ed.). (2013). *Neonatology: Management, procedures, on-call problems, diseases, and drugs* (7th ed.). New York, NY: McGraw-Hill Education.

Jefferies, A. L., & Canadian Paediatric Society, Fetus and Newborn Committee. (2012). Kangaroo care for the preterm infant and family. *Paediatric Child Health, 17*(3), 141–143.

Jones, J. E., Hayes, R. D., Starbuck, A. L., & Porcelli, P. J. (2011). Fluid and electrolyte management. In S. L. Gardner (Ed.), *Merenstein & Gardner's handbook of neonatal intensive care* (7th ed., pp. 333–352). St. Louis, MO: Mosby.

Koops, B. L., Morgan, L. P., & Battaglia, F. C. (1982). Neonatal mortality risk in relationship to birth weight and gestational age. *Journal of Pediatrics, 101*(6), 969.

Krist, A. H., & Crawford-Faucher, A. (2002). Management of newborns exposed to maternal HIV infection. *American Family Physician, 65*(10), 2049–2056.

Liaw, J., Yang, L., Wang, K., Chen, C., Chang, Y., & Ti, Y. (2012). Non-nutritive sucking and facilitated tucking relieve preterm infant pain during heel stick procedures: A prospective randomized controlled

crossover trial. *International Journal of Nursing Studies, 49*(3), 300–309.

Nodine, P. M., Arruda, J., & Hastings-Tolsma, M. (2011). Prenatal environment: Effect on neonatal outcome. In S. L. Gardner (Ed.), *Merenstein & Gardner's handbook of neonatal intensive care* (7th ed., pp. 13–38). St. Louis, MO: Mosby.

Raab, E. L., & Kelly, L. K. (2013). Neonatal resuscitation. In A. H. Decheneny, L. Nathan, N. Laufer, & A. S. Roman (Eds.), *Current diagnosis & treatment: Obstetrics & gynecology* (11th ed., pp. 369–388). New York, NY: McGraw Hill/Lange.

Rozance, P. J., & Rosenberg, A. A. (2012). The neonate. In S. G. Gabbe, J. R Niebyl, J. L. Simpson, M. B. Landon, H. L. Galan, E. R. M. Jauniaux, & D. A. Driscoll (Eds.), *Obstetrics: Normal and problem pregnancies* (6th ed., pp. 481–516). St. Louis, MO: Elsevier.

Ruth, C. A., Roos, N., Hildes-Ripstein, E., & Brownell, M. (2013). The influence of gestational age and socioeconomic status on neonatal outcomes in late preterm and early term gestation: A population based study. BioMed Central *Pregnancy & Childbirth, 12*(1), 62.

Scher, M. S. (2013). Brain disorders of the fetus and neonate. In A. A. Fanaroff & J. M. Fanaroff (Eds.), *Klaus & Fanaroff's care of the high-risk neonate* (6th ed., pp. 476–524). Philadelphia, PA: Elsevier.

Weiner, S. M., & Finnegan, L. P. (2011). Drug withdrawal in the neonate. In S. L. Gardner (Ed.), *Merenstein & Gardner's handbook of neonatal intensive care* (7th ed., pp. 201–222). St. Louis, MO: Mosby.

The Newborn at Risk: Birth-Related Stressors

We watched him breathe every precious breath. He was covered with wires and tubes. The rhythmic tides of his sleeping and feeding spaciously measured his days and nights. We kept watch. He was special to us and we would say over and over, "Daddy and Mommy are here and we love you." —Alan and Claudia, parents of a baby with RDS

Leanne Temme/Getty Images

LEARNING OUTCOMES

28.1 Discuss how to identify infants in need of resuscitation and the appropriate method of resuscitation based on the labor record and observable physiologic indicators.

28.2 Differentiate, based on clinical manifestations, among the various types of respiratory distress (respiratory distress syndrome, transient tachypnea of the newborn, and meconium aspiration syndrome) in the newborn and their related nursing management.

28.3 Discuss selected metabolic abnormalities (including cold stress and hypoglycemia), their effects on the newborn, and the nursing implications.

28.4 Differentiate between physiologic and pathologic jaundice according to timing of onset (in hours), cause, possible sequelae, and specific management.

28.5 Explain how Rh incompatibility or ABO incompatibility can lead to the development of hyperbilirubinemia.

28.6 Identify nursing responsibilities and rationale in caring for the newborn receiving phototherapy.

28.7 Describe the causes and nursing management of infants with anemia.

28.8 Describe the nursing assessments that would lead the nurse to suspect newborn sepsis and the nursing management of the newborn with an infection.

28.9 Relate the consequences of maternally transmitted infections, such as maternal syphilis, gonorrhea, Herpesviridae family (HSV or CMV), and chlamydia, to the nursing management of infants in the neonatal period.

28.10 Describe the interventions to facilitate parental attachment and meet the special initial and long-term needs of parents of at-risk infants.

Marked homeostatic changes occur during the infant's transition from fetal to neonatal life. Because the most rapid anatomic and physiologic changes occur in the cardiopulmonary system, most major problems of the newborn are usually related to this system. These problems include asphyxia, respiratory distress syndrome (RDS), cold stress, jaundice, hemolytic disease, and anemia. Ideally, most problems are anticipated and identified prenatally. Some treatment may be initiated in the prenatal period, whereas other intervention measures are begun at or immediately after birth.

CARE OF THE NEWBORN AT RISK FROM ASPHYXIA

Perinatal asphyxia occurs in 1% to 1.5% of live births, and the incidence increases as the gestational age decreases (Cloherty, Eichenwald, & Stark, 2012). Neonatal asphyxia results in circulatory, respiratory, and biochemical changes. Circulatory patterns that accompany asphyxia indicate an inability of the newborn to make the transition to extrauterine circulation—in effect, a return to fetal circulatory patterns. Failure of lung expansion and establishment of respiration rapidly produces serious biochemical changes, including hypoxemia (decreased oxygen in the blood), metabolic acidosis (increased acidity of blood reflected by low pH), and hypercarbia (excess levels of carbon dioxide in the blood) (Niemeyer & Clarke, 2011).

These biochemical changes produce pulmonary vasoconstriction and high pulmonary vascular resistance, hypoperfusion of the lung, and large right-to-left shunt. However, the most serious biochemical abnormality is a change from aerobic to anaerobic metabolism in the presence of hypoxia. This change results in the buildup of lactate, which combines with hydrogen to form lactic acid, and the development of metabolic acidosis. Lactic acidosis can develop after prolonged tissue hypoxia (oxygen starvation) as active cells rely on anaerobic metabolism.

Simultaneous respiratory acidosis may also occur because of a rapid increase in carbon dioxide (P_{CO_2}) during asphyxia. In response to hypoxia and anaerobic metabolism, the amounts of free fatty acids (FFAs) and glycerol in the blood increase. Glycogen stores are also mobilized to provide a continuous glucose source for the brain. Hepatic and cardiac stores of glycogen may be used up rapidly during an asphyxial incident.

The newborn is supplied with several protective mechanisms against hypoxic insults. These include:

- Relatively immature brain
- Resting metabolic rate lower than that of adults
- Ability to mobilize substances within the body for anaerobic metabolism and to use energy more efficiently
- Intact circulatory system able to redistribute lactate and hydrogen ions in tissues still being perfused

Severe prolonged hypoxia overcomes these protective mechanisms, resulting in brain damage or death of the newborn. The newborn suffering apnea requires immediate resuscitative efforts. The need for resuscitation can be anticipated if specific risk factors are present during the pregnancy or labor and birth period.

Risk Factors Predisposing to Asphyxia

The need for resuscitation may be anticipated if the mother demonstrates the antepartum and intrapartum risk factors described in Table 10–1 on page 198 and Table 18–2 on page 378. Fetal/neonatal risk factors for resuscitation are as follows (Cloherty et al., 2012):

- Nonreassuring fetal heart rate (FHR) pattern/sustained bradycardia
- Anything affecting blood flow through the placenta

- Difficult birth, prolonged labor
- Fetal scalp/capillary blood sample—acidosis pH less than 7.2
- Significant intrapartum bleeding
- Infant of a diabetic mother (IDM)
- Anemia, isoimmunization, fetal–maternal hemorrhage, parvovirus
- Prematurity; small for gestational age (SGA)
- Unexpected congenital anomalies
- Oligohydramnios/polyhydramnios
- Narcotic use during labor

Clinical Therapy

The initial goal of clinical management is to identify the fetus at risk for asphyxia, so that resuscitative efforts can begin at birth.

Fetal biophysical assessment (see Chapter 14 🔗), combined with monitoring of fetal pH, FHR, and fetal oximeter if available during the intrapartum period, may help identify the presence of nonreassuring fetal status. If nonreassuring fetal status is present, appropriate measures can be taken to deliver the fetus immediately, before major damage occurs, and to treat the asphyxiated newborn.

The stress of labor causes an intermittent decrease in exchange of gases in the placental intervillous space, which causes the fall in pH and fetal metabolic acidosis. The acidosis is primarily metabolic. During labor, a fetal pH of 7.25 or higher is considered normal (nonacidemia). A pH value of 7.20 or less is considered an ominous sign of intrauterine asphyxia (acidemia), whereas a pH of less than 7 is considered pathologic acidemia (Cloherty et al., 2012). However, low fetal pH without associated hypoxia can be caused by maternal acidosis secondary to prolonged labor, dehydration, and maternal lactate production.

Assessment of the newborn's need for resuscitation begins at the time of birth. The Apgar score (see Chapter 19 🔗) may be helpful in describing the status of the newborn at birth and his or her subsequent adaptation to the extrauterine environment. If indicated, resuscitation should be started before the 1-minute Apgar score is obtained. The American Academy of Pediatrics (AAP) Committee on Fetus and Newborn and American College of Obstetricians and Gynecologists (ACOG) Committee on Obstetrics (2012) has recommended the use of an assisted Apgar scoring system that documents the assistance the infant is receiving at the time his or her score is assigned.

Resuscitative efforts are required by 5% to 10% of all newborns to begin breathing (Gleason & Devaskar, 2012). The AAP and American Heart Association (AHA) (2011, p. 40) recommend identification of newborns who *do not* require resuscitation by carrying out a rapid assessment of these three characteristics:

1. Is the baby full term?
2. Is the baby breathing or crying?
3. Does the baby have good muscle tone?

If the answers to these questions are "yes," then the baby does not need resuscitation, should not be separated from the mother, and can proceed to routine care. Routine care includes warming the baby (skin-to-skin contact is recommended), clearing the airway by wiping the baby's mouth and nose if necessary, drying the newborn, and providing ongoing evaluation of breathing, activity, and color.

If the answer to *any* of the previous questions is "no," the infant should receive resuscitative assistance (AAP & AHA, 2011).

SAFETY ALERT!
In the birthing room exposure to blood or other body fluids is inevitable. Standard precautions must be practiced by wearing caps, goggles or glasses, gloves, and impervious gowns until the cord is cut and the newborn is dried and wrapped (Cloherty et al., 2012).

Resuscitation Management

After the first few breaths, the nurse places the newborn in a level "sniff" position (head is tilted just far enough back for the infant to look like he or she is sniffing the air with the nose pointed upward) under a radiant heat source and dries the baby quickly with warm blankets to maintain abdominal skin temperature at about 36.5°C to 37°C (97.7°F to 98.6°F). The stable newborn may be placed on the mother's chest or abdomen "skin to skin" as another heat source. If assessment indicates that further assistance and formal resuscitation are necessary, the baby continues in the radiant warmer in a position that facilitates easy access by healthcare providers (Gleason & Devaskar, 2012).

Breathing is established by employing the simplest form of resuscitative measures initially, with progression to more complicated methods as required. For example:

1. Position and clear the airway only as necessary. Simple stimulation is provided by rubbing the newborn's back with a blanket or towel, while simultaneously drying the baby. Suctioning following birth should be reserved for babies who have obvious obstruction to spontaneous breathing or who require positive pressure. Clearing the nasal and oral passages of obstructive fluid, with a bulb syringe or suction catheter attached to low continuous suction, establishes a patent airway. Vigorous suctioning of the posterior pharynx should be avoided because it can produce significant reflex bradycardia and damage the oral mucosa (AAP & ACOG, 2012).

2. Evaluate respirations, heart rate (not color), and oxygenation (per pulse oximetry) (AAP & AHA, 2011). Resuscitation of term newborns may begin with 21% oxygen. Place the oximeter probe on the newborn's right hand or wrist and put on a pulse oximeter. The proper size mask is positioned securely on the face (over nose and mouth, avoiding the eyes), with the infant's head in a "sniffing" or neutral position (Figure 28–1 ●). Hyperextension of the infant's neck obstructs the trachea and must be avoided. An airtight connection is made between the baby's face and the mask (thus allowing the bag to inflate).

● **Figure 28–1** Demonstration of resuscitation of a newborn with bag and mask. Note that the mask covers the nose and mouth, and the head is in a neutral "sniff" position. The resuscitating bag is placed to the side of the baby so that chest movement can be seen.

Source: George Dodson/Lightworks Studio/Pearson Education.

The lungs must be inflated with positive-pressure ventilation (PPV) if there is:

■ Apnea/gasping

■ Heart rate below 100 beats/min, even if breathing

■ Persistent central and low oxygen saturation, despite free-flow oxygen increased to 100%

All positive-pressure devices including adapted self-inflating bags should have a pressure gauge and should be connected to a blender that can deliver an oxygen concentration ranging from 21% to 100%. The lungs are inflated rhythmically by squeezing the bag. The rate of ventilation should be between 40 and 60 breaths per minute. Begin PPV initially at 20 cm H_2O (AAP & AHA, 2011). Pressure should be adequate to move the chest wall. The pressure gauge (manometer) must be in place to avoid overdistention of the newborn's lungs and other problems such as pneumothorax or abdominal distention. When PPV begins, assess for rising heart rate (HR) and improving oxygen saturation (per pulse oximetry). If ventilation is adequate, the chest moves symmetrically with each inspiration, bilateral breath sounds are audible, and the lips and mucous membranes become pink.

If the heart rate is between 60 and 100 beats/min and improving, adjust oxygen, gradually decreasing pressure as HR improves. Distention of the stomach is controlled by inserting a nasogastric tube for decompression.

SAFETY ALERT!

Establishing effective ventilation is the highest priority in neonatal resuscitation. Do not start chest compressions without first establishing effective ventilation (as evidenced by audible bilateral breath sounds and chest movement) (AAP & AHA, 2011).

3. If heart rate is still below 60 beats/min despite 30 seconds of effective positive pressure, increase oxygenation to 100% and begin chest compressions. Air entry and heart rate are checked by auscultation. Heart rate may be quickly checked by palpating the base of the umbilical cord stump and counting the pulsations for 6 seconds and then multiplying by 10.

4. Endotracheal intubation is strongly recommended when chest compressions start in order to coordinate ventilation and chest compressions. However, most newborns, except for very-low-birth-weight (VLBW) (<1500-g) infants, can be resuscitated by bag and mask ventilation. An increasing HR and CO_2 detection are the primary methods for confirming endotracheal tube placement.

Chest compressions are started immediately if there is no detectable heartbeat. The following procedure is used for performing chest compressions:

1. The infant is positioned properly on a firm surface.

2. The resuscitator stands at the foot or head of the infant and places both thumbs over the lower third of the sternum (just below an imaginary line drawn between the nipples), with the fingers wrapped around and supporting the back (Figure 28–2A ●). Alternatively, the resuscitator can use two fingers instead of thumbs (Figure 28–2B ●). The two-thumb method is preferred because it may provide better coronary perfusion pressure; however, it decreases thoracic expansion during ventilation and makes access to the umbilical cord for medication administration more difficult (AAP & AHA, 2011).

3. The sternum is depressed to sufficient depth to generate a palpable pulse or approximately one third of the anterior-posterior diameter of the chest (Niemeyer & Clarke, 2011). Nurses use a 3:1 ratio of heartbeat to assisted ventilation; that is, 90 chest compressions to 30 breaths per minute.

Drugs that should be available in the birthing area include those needed in the treatment of shock, cardiac arrest, and narcosis. Oxygen, because of its effective use in ventilation, is the drug most often used. The most accessible route for administering medications is the umbilical vein (give intravenously [IV]). When the heart rate remains below 60 beats/min despite 45 to 60 seconds of chest compressions and ventilation, then epinephrine, a cardiac stimulant, is indicated (AAP & AHA, 2011). Endotracheal epinephrine administration may be considered while IV access is being established (AAP & AHA, 2011). *Sodium bicarbonate is rarely given in the birthing room.* Sodium bicarbonate is given only to correct metabolic acidosis that results from lactic acid buildup caused by insufficient tissue oxygenation and after effective ventilation is established. Dextrose (2 mL/kg) is given to prevent progression of hypoglycemia. Naloxone hydrochloride (0.1 mg/kg), a narcotic antagonist, is used to reverse known iatrogenic narcotic depression (Young & Mangum, 2012). (See *Drug Guide: Naloxone Hydrochloride [Narcan].*)

If shock develops (low blood pressure, pallor, or poor peripheral perfusion), the baby may be given a volume expander such as normal saline or lactated Ringer's in a dose of 10 mL/kg via umbilical vein route. If there is a known fetal hemorrhage or

A

B

● **Figure 28–2** External cardiac massage. The lower third of the sternum is compressed with two fingertips or thumbs at a rate of 90 beats per minute. *A*, In the thumb method, the fingers support the infant's back and both thumbs compress the sternum. *B*, In the two-fingers method, the tips of two fingers of one hand compress the sternum, and the other hand or a firm surface supports the infant's back.

Source: George Dodson/Lightworks Studio/Pearson Education.

Drug Guide Naloxone Hydrochloride (Narcan)

Overview of Neonatal Action

Naloxone hydrochloride (Narcan) is used to reverse respiratory depression caused by acute narcotic toxicity when the mother received a narcotic within 4 hours of birth. It displaces morphine-like drugs from receptor sites on the neurons, which prevents the narcotics from exerting their depressive effects. It is essentially a pure opioid antagonist. Naloxone reverses narcotic-induced respiratory depression, analgesia, sedation, hypotension, and pupillary constriction.

Route, Dosage, Frequency

Intravenous dose is 0.1 mg/kg of 1 mg/mL solution or 0.25 mL/kg of 0.4 mg/mL concentration at birth, including for premature infants. This drug is usually given through the umbilical vein or endotracheal tube (ET), or can be given intramuscularly (but delays onset of action) if adequate perfusion exists. For IV push, infuse over at least 1 minute. No studies report the efficacy of endotracheal administration (AAP & AHA, 2011).

Reversal of drug depression occurs within 1 to 2 minutes after IV administration and within 15 minutes of IM administration. Duration of narcotic often exceeds that of the naloxone, so watch the infant closely for recurrent respiratory depression. The dose may be repeated in 3 to 5 minutes. If there is no improvement after 2 or 3 doses, discontinue naloxone administration. If the initial reversal occurs, repeat the dose as needed (Young & Mangum, 2012).

Neonatal Contraindications

Naloxone should not be administered to infants of mothers who chronically use narcotics or those on methadone maintenance, because it may precipitate acute withdrawal syndrome (increased heart rate and blood pressure, vomiting, seizures, tremors).

Respiratory depression may result from nonmorphine drugs, such as sedatives, hypnotics, anesthetics, or other nonnarcotic central nervous system (CNS) depressants.

Neonatal Side Effects

Excessive doses may result in irritability, increased crying, and possible prolongation of partial thromboplastin time (PTT). Tachycardia may occur.

Nursing Considerations

■ Monitor respirations—rate and depth—closely for improved respiratory effort.

■ Assess for return of respiratory depression when naloxone effects wear off and effects of longer-acting narcotics.

■ Assess for continued respiratory depression after positive-pressure ventilation has restored normal heart rate and color.

■ Have resuscitative equipment, O$_2$, and ventilatory equipment available.

■ Note that naloxone is incompatible with alkaline solutions such as sodium bicarbonate.

■ Store at room temperature and protect from light.

■ Compatible with heparin.

fetal anemia, whole blood (O Rh-negative cross-matched against the mother's blood) and packed red blood cells (RBCs) given over a 5- to 10-minute period can also be used for volume expansion and treatment of hypovolemic shock.

NURSING MANAGEMENT *For the Newborn Needing Resuscitation*

Nursing Assessment and Diagnosis

Communication between the obstetric (OB) office or clinic and the birthing area nurse facilitates the identification of newborns who may need resuscitation. Check with the OB provider for relevant perinatal and labor history including the answers to these questions:

- What is the gestational age?
- Is the fluid clear?
- How many babies are expected?
- Are there any additional risk factors?

Nursing diagnoses that may apply to the newborn with asphyxia and the newborn's parents include (NANDA-I © 2012):

- *Breathing Pattern, Ineffective,* related to lack of spontaneous respirations at birth secondary to in utero asphyxia
- *Cardiac Output*, *Decreased,* related to impaired oxygenation
- *Coping: Family, Compromised,* related to baby's lack of spontaneous respirations at birth and parents' fear of losing their newborn

Planning and Implementation

Hospital-Based Nursing Care

Following identification of possible high-risk situations, the next step in effective resuscitation is assembling the necessary equipment and ensuring proper functioning.

Check and maintain equipment to ensure its reliability before an emergency arises, and the equipment must be restocked immediately after use and rechecked before every birth. Inspect all equipment—radiant warmer, bag and mask, oxygen, flow meter and blender, pulse oximeter, laryngoscope, and suction machine—for damaged or nonfunctioning parts before a birth or when setting up an admission bed. A systematic check of the emergency cart and equipment is a routine responsibility of each shift. It is desirable to assemble equipment for pH and blood gas determination as well.

During resuscitation, keep the newborn warm. The newborn should be dried quickly with warmed towels or blankets and a hat placed on the newborn's head to prevent evaporative heat loss. Then place the infant under a pre-warmed radiant warmer with servo-control set at 36.5°C (97.7°F). This device provides an overhead radiant heat source. (A thermostatic mechanism that is secured to the infant's abdomen, over a solid organ like the liver, triggers the radiant warmer to turn on or off to maintain a constant temperature.) An open bed is necessary for easy access to the newborn.

Training and knowledge about resuscitation are vital to personnel in the birth setting for both normal and at-risk births. Resuscitation is at least a two-person effort and additional support should be called for as needed. One member must have the skill to perform airway management and ventilation.

Record resuscitative efforts on the newborn's chart so that all members of the healthcare team have access to the information. Postresuscitation care is for newborns who have depressed breathing or activity and/or required supplemental oxygen. They require frequent evaluation to determine if they can be transitioned to routine care or transferred to the neonatal intensive care unit (NICU) as necessary.

Parent Teaching

The new newborn resuscitation guidelines favor family members being present during resuscitation in the birthing room and in the NICU, but be aware that the procedure is particularly distressing for parents (AAP & AHA, 2011). If the need for resuscitation is anticipated, the parents should be assured that a team will be present at the birth to care specifically for their newborn. Advise parents that a support person will be available for them as well if resuscitation is necessary. As soon as the infant's condition has stabilized, a member of the collaborative care team needs to discuss the newborn's condition with the parents. The parents may have many fears about the reasons for resuscitation and the condition of their baby following resuscitation.

Evaluation

Expected outcomes of nursing care include the following:

- The newborn requiring resuscitation is promptly identified, and intervention is started early.
- The newborn's metabolic and physiologic processes are stabilized, and recovery is proceeding without complications.
- The parents can verbalize the reason for resuscitation and what was done to resuscitate their newborn.
- The parents can verbalize their fears about the resuscitation process and potential implications for their baby's future.

CARE OF THE NEWBORN WITH RESPIRATORY DISTRESS

Respiratory distress syndrome (RDS) is an inappropriate respiratory adaptation to extrauterine life. The nurse caring for a baby with respiratory distress needs to understand the normal pulmonary and circulatory physiology (see Chapter 24 ☝), the pathophysiology of the disease process, clinical manifestations, and supportive and corrective therapies. Only with this knowledge can the nurse make appropriate observations about responses to therapy and development of complications. Unlike the verbalizing adult patient, the newborn communicates needs only by behavior or physiologic parameters that must be interpreted by the NICU nurse. The neonatal nurse interprets this behavior as clues about the individual baby's condition. This section discusses respiratory distress syndrome, transient tachypnea of the newborn, and meconium aspiration syndrome.

Respiratory Distress Syndrome

Respiratory distress syndrome (RDS), also referred to as *hyaline membrane disease (HMD)*, is the result of inadequate production of pulmonary surfactant, a substance produced in the lungs that keeps lungs from collapsing on expiration (Cloherty et al., 2012).

RDS affects almost 50% of the premature infants born at less than 30 weeks' gestation (Hallman & Saarela, 2012). The syndrome occurs more frequently in premature Caucasian infants than in infants of African or Hispanic descent and almost twice as often in males as in females.

All the factors precipitating the pathologic changes of RDS have not been determined, but the main factors associated with its development include:

- *Prematurity.* All preterm newborns—whether average for gestational age (AGA), small for gestational age (SGA), or large for gestational age (LGA)—and especially infants of diabetic mothers (IDMs) are at risk for RDS. The incidence of RDS increases with the degree of prematurity, and most deaths occur in newborns weighing less than 1500 g. The maternal and fetal factors resulting in preterm labor and birth, complications of pregnancy, cesarean birth (and its indications), and familial tendency are all associated with RDS.

- *Surfactant deficiency disease.* Normal pulmonary adaptation requires adequate surfactant, a lipoprotein that coats the inner surfaces of the alveoli. Surfactant provides alveolar stability by decreasing the alveoli's surface tension and tendency to collapse. Surfactant is produced by type II alveolar cells starting at about 24 weeks' gestation. In the normal or mature newborn lung, it is continuously synthesized, oxidized during breathing, and replenished. Adequate surfactant levels lead to better lung compliance and permit breathing with less work. RDS is caused by alterations in surfactant quantity, composition, function, or production.

Development of RDS indicates a failure to synthesize surfactant, which is required to maintain alveolar stability (see *Factors Opposing the First Breath* in Chapter 24 🔗). Upon expiration this instability increases atelectasis, which causes hypoxia and acidosis because of the lack of gas exchange. These conditions further inhibit surfactant production and cause pulmonary vasoconstriction. The resulting lung instability causes the biochemical problems of hypoxemia (decreased Po_2), hypercarbia (increased Pco_2), and acidemia (decreased pH), primarily metabolic, which further increase pulmonary vasoconstriction and hypoperfusion; alveolar endothelial and epithelial damage; and subsequent protein-rich interstitial and alveolar edema.

Because of these pathophysiologic conditions, the newborn must expend increasing amounts of energy to reopen the collapsed alveoli with every breath, so that each breath becomes more difficult than the last. The progressive expiratory atelectasis upsets the physiologic homeostasis of the pulmonary and cardiovascular systems and prevents adequate gas exchange. Breathing becomes progressively harder as lung compliance decreases, which makes it more difficult to inflate the lungs and breathe.

The physiologic alterations of RDS produce the following complications:

1. *Hypoxia.* As a result of hypoxia, the pulmonary vasculature constricts, pulmonary vascular resistance increases, and pulmonary blood flow is reduced. Increased pulmonary vascular resistance may precipitate a return to fetal circulation as the ductus opens and blood flow is shunted around the lungs in a right-to-left blood flow. This shunting increases the hypoxia and further decreases pulmonary perfusion. Hypoxia also causes impairment or absence of metabolic response to cold; reversion to anaerobic metabolism, resulting in lactate accumulation (acidosis); and impaired cardiac output, which decreases perfusion to vital organs.

2. *Respiratory acidosis.* Increased Pco_2 and decreased pH are results of alveolar hypoventilation. A persistent rise in Pco_2 is a poor prognostic sign of pulmonary function and adequacy because the increased Pco_2 and decreased pH are results of alveolar hypoventilation.

3. *Metabolic acidosis.* Because of the lack of oxygen at the cellular level, the newborn begins anaerobic metabolism with an increase in lactate levels and a resulting base deficit (loss of bicarbonate). As the lactate levels increase, the pH decreases in an attempt to maintain acid–base homeostasis.

The classic radiologic picture of RDS is diffuse bilateral reticulogranular (ground glass appearance) density, with portions of the air-filled tracheobronchial tree (air bronchogram) outlined by the opaque ("white-out") lungs with widespread atelectasis, potentially obliterating the heart borders (Cloherty et al., 2012). See *Pathophysiology Illustrated: Respiratory Distress Syndrome (RDS)*. The progression of x-ray findings parallels the pattern of resolution, which usually occurs in 7 to 10 days, and the time of surfactant reappearance, unless surfactant replacement therapy has been used (Blackburn, 2013). Echocardiography is a valuable tool in diagnosing vascular shunts that move blood either away from or toward the lungs.

Clinical Therapy

The primary goal of prenatal management is to prevent preterm birth through early assessment of fetal lung maturity, aggressive treatment of preterm labor, and administration of glucocorticoids to enhance fetal lung development (see Chapter 16 🔗). Antenatal steroids reduce the incidence and severity of RDS and improve survivability of the 24 to 34 weeks' gestation and extremely low birth weight newborn (less than 1250 g) (Cloherty et al., 2012).

Postnatal surfactant replacement therapy is available for infants to decrease the severity of RDS in low-birth-weight newborns. This is one of the best studied therapies in newborns. Surfactant replacement therapy is delivered through an endotracheal tube and may be given in either the birthing room or the nursery as indicated by the severity of RDS. Repeat doses are often required. The most frequent reported response to treatment is

---

Teaching Highlights **Understanding Respiratory Distress**

You can help parents understand their baby's respiratory distress by having them think of the air sacs (alveoli) of the lungs as tiny balloons filled with water and no air. When the tiny balloon (alveoli) is emptied (as in expiration), water droplets can remain inside the balloon and the sides of the balloons stick together (increasing the surface tension between the sides of the balloon). This increased surface tension makes the next reinflation very difficult and requires an increased amount of energy.

Pathophysiology Illustrated | Respiratory Distress Syndrome (RDS)

Cycle of events of RDS leading to eventual respiratory failure.
Source: Modified from Gluck, L., & Kulovich, M. V. (1973). Fetal lung development. *Pediatric Clinics of North America, 20,* 375.

RDS chest x-ray. Chest radiograph of respiratory distress syndrome characterized by a reticulogranular pattern with areas of microatelectasis of uniform opacity and air bronchograms.
Source: Carol Harrigan, RN, MSN, NNP-BC

rapidly improved oxygenation and decreased need for ventilatory support, sometimes occurring soon after the dose is administered.

Supportive medical management consists of ventilation therapy, transcutaneous oxygen and carbon dioxide monitoring, blood gas monitoring, pulse oximetry monitoring, correction of acid–base imbalance, environmental temperature regulation, adequate nutrition, and protection from infection (AAP & ACOG, 2012). Ventilation therapy is directed toward preventing hypoventilation and hypoxia. Mild cases of RDS may require only increased humidified oxygen concentrations. Use of continuous positive airway pressure (CPAP) may be required in moderately afflicted infants. Babies with severe RDS require mechanical ventilatory assistance from a respirator (Figure 28–3 ●).

● **Figure 28–3** Mechanical ventilatory assistance. One-day-old, 28 weeks' gestational age, 1450-g baby on respirator and in isolette.
Source: Carol Harrigan, RN, MSN, NNP-BC

 Clinical Tip

In babies with RDS who are on ventilators, increased diuresis or urination (determined by weighing diapers) may be an early clue that the baby's condition is improving. As fluid moves out of the lungs into the bloodstream, alveoli open and kidney perfusion increases; this results in increased voiding. At this point, the nurse must monitor chest expansion closely. If chest expansion is increasing, pulmonary compliance is improving and ventilator settings may have to be decreased, sometimes quite soon after surfactant dosing. A ventilator setting that is too high may "blow the lung," resulting in pneumothorax. If diuresis does not occur, it is a sign that bronchopulmonary dysplasia (BPD), also called *chronic lung disease of prematurity* (CLD), may be developing.

High-frequency ventilation (HFV) can be tried when conventional ventilator therapy has not been successful, and it sometimes can be the primary mode of ventilation to minimize lung injury in very small and/or sick infants (Cloherty et al., 2012).

Nursing Management

The nurse should look for characteristics of RDS such as increasing cyanosis, tachypnea (greater than 60 respirations per minute), grunting respirations, nasal flaring, significant retractions, and apnea. Table 28–1 reviews clinical findings associated with respiratory distress in general. The Silverman-Anderson index is

Table 28–1	Clinical Assessments Associated with Respiratory Distress
Clinical Picture	**Significance**
SKIN COLOR	
Pallor or mottling	These represent poor peripheral circulation caused by systemic hypotension and vasoconstriction and pooling of independent areas (usually in conjunction with severe hypoxia).
Cyanosis (bluish tint)	Depending on hemoglobin concentration, peripheral circulation, intensity and quality of viewing light, and acuity of observer's color vision, this is frankly visible in advanced hypoxia. Central cyanosis is most easily detected by examination of mucous membranes and tongue.
Jaundice (yellow discoloration of skin and mucous membranes caused by presence of unconjugated [indirect] bilirubin)	Metabolic alterations (acidosis, hypercarbia, asphyxia) of respiratory distress predispose a newborn to dissociation of bilirubin from albumin-binding sites and deposition in the skin and central nervous system.
Edema (presents as slick, shiny taut skin)	This is characteristic of preterm infants because their total protein concentration is low, with a decrease in colloidal osmotic pressure and transudation of fluid. Edema of hands and feet is frequently seen within first 24 hours and resolved by fifth day in infants with severe RDS.
RESPIRATORY SYSTEM	
Tachypnea (normal respiratory rate 30 to 60/minute, sustained, elevated respiratory rate 60+/minute)	Increased respiratory rate is the easiest detectable sign of respiratory distress after birth. Because of the premature infant's very compliant chest wall, it is more energy efficient to increase the respiratory rate than the depth of respirations. This compensatory mechanism attempts to increase respiratory dead space to maintain alveolar ventilation and gas exchange in the face of an increase in mechanical resistance. As a decompensatory mechanism it increases workload and energy output by increasing respiratory rate, which causes increased metabolic demand for oxygen and thus increases alveolar ventilation on an already overstressed system. During shallow, rapid respirations, there is an increase in dead space ventilation, thus decreasing alveolar ventilation.

(continued)

Table 28–1 Clinical Assessments Associated with Respiratory Distress—continued

Clinical Picture	Significance
Apnea (episode of nonbreathing for more than 20 seconds; periodic breathing, a common "normal" occurrence in preterm infants, is defined as apnea of 5 to 10 seconds alternating with 10 to 15 seconds of ventilation) that is sometimes quite rapid	This poor prognostic sign indicates cardiorespiratory disease, CNS disease, metabolic alterations, intracranial hemorrhage, sepsis, or immaturity. Physiologic alterations include decreased oxygen saturation, respiratory acidosis, and bradycardia.

CHEST

Chest movement	Inspection of the thoracic cage includes shape, size, and symmetry of movement. Respiratory movements should be symmetrical and diaphragmatic; asymmetry such as seesaw-like movements reflects pathology (pneumothorax, diaphragmatic hernia). Increased anteroposterior diameter indicates air trapping (meconium aspiration syndrome).
Labored respirations indicate severity of retractions (see below), grunting, and nasal flaring, which are signs of labored respirations	Indicates marked increase in the work of breathing.
Retractions (inward pulling of soft parts of the chest cage—suprasternal [above the sternum], substernal, intercostals [between the ribs]—at inspiration)	These reflect the significant increase in negative intrathoracic pressure necessary to inflate stiff, noncompliant lungs. Infants attempt to increase lung compliance by using accessory muscles. Lung expansion markedly decreases. Seesaw respirations are seen when the chest flattens with inspiration and the abdomen bulges. Retractions increase the work of breathing and O_2 need. As a result, assisted ventilation may be necessary because of exhaustion.
Nasal flaring (inspiratory dilation of nostrils)	This compensatory mechanism attempts to lessen the resistance of the narrow nasal passage.
Expiratory grunt (Valsalva maneuver in which the infant exhales against a partially closed glottis, thus producing an audible moan)	This increases intrapulmonary pressure, which decreases or prevents atelectasis, thus improving oxygenation and alveolar ventilation. It allows more time for the passage of oxygen into the circulatory system. Intubation should not be attempted unless the infant's condition is rapidly deteriorating, because it prevents this maneuver and allows the alveoli to collapse.
Rhythmic body movement with labored respirations (chin tug, head bobbing, retractions of anal area)	This is a result of using abdominal and other respiratory accessory muscles during prolonged forced respirations.
Auscultation of chest reveals decreased air exchange, with harsh breath sounds or fine inspiratory rales; rhonchi may be present	Decrease in breath sounds and distant quality may indicate interstitial or intrapleural air or fluid.

CARDIOVASCULAR SYSTEM

Continuous systolic murmur may be audible	Patent ductus arteriosus is a common occurrence with hypoxia, pulmonary vasoconstriction, right-to-left shunting, and congestive heart failure.
Heart rate usually within normal limits (fixed heart rate may occur with a rate of 110 to 120 beats/min)	A fixed heart rate indicates a decrease in vagal control.
Point of maximal impulse usually located at fourth to fifth intercostal space, left sternal border	Displacement may reflect dextrocardia, pneumothorax, or diaphragmatic hernia.

HYPOTHERMIA

	This is inadequate functioning of metabolic processes that require oxygen to produce necessary body heat.

MUSCLE TONE

Flaccid, hypotonic, unresponsive to stimuli Hypertonia and/or seizure activity	These may indicate deterioration in the newborn's condition and possible CNS damage caused by hypoxia, acidemia, or hemorrhage.

a tool that evaluates signs of respiratory distress and may be used in the birthing area.

Based on clinical parameters, the neonatal nurse implements therapeutic approaches to provide the newborn with respiratory distress with a very supportive environment (Figure 28–4 ●) that includes maintaining thermoregulation to decrease respiratory effort and decrease infection secondary to invasive procedures and using standard precautions. (See *Nursing Care Plan: The Newborn with Respiratory Distress Syndrome* on pages 677–679.) Infants with severe respiratory distress are cared for in NICUs by nurses with advanced knowledge and training. Nursing interventions and criteria for instituting mechanical ventilation depend on institutional protocol. Noninvasive oxygen monitoring provides real-time trend information that is particularly useful in infants showing frequent swings in PaO_2 and oxygen saturation. Use of these methods (pulse oximetry, transcutaneous oxygen monitor) can also reduce the frequency of blood gas sampling. Methods of noninvasive oxygen monitoring and nursing interventions are included in Table 28–2. (The nursing care of infants on ventilators or with umbilical artery catheters is not discussed here.) Ventilatory assistance with high-frequency ventilators shows positive results.

Transient Tachypnea of the Newborn

Some newborns, generally term and late preterm infants, may develop progressive respiratory distress that clinically can resemble RDS. Other risk factors include maternal diabetes and asthma, male sex of the fetus, macrosomia (possibly related to maternal diabetes), and cesarean section delivery with or without labor. Delivery with labor has some protective mechanism against transient tachypnea of the newborn (TTN) (Martin & Crowley, 2013). Typically, supplemental oxygen of less than 40% will alleviate the hypoxia (Cloherty et al., 2012). Infants with TTN may have had intrauterine or intrapartum asphyxia due to maternal oversedation or poor uterine perfusion, maternal bleeding, prolapsed cord, or breech presentation. The newborn then fails to clear the airway of lung fluid, mucus, and other debris, or an excess of fluid in the lungs develops due to aspiration of amniotic or tracheal fluid.

Usually the newborn experiences little or no difficulty at the onset of breathing. However, shortly after birth, expiratory grunting, flaring of the nares, and mild cyanosis may be noted in the newborn breathing room air. Air will become trapped and an increase in the anterior-posterior diameter of the chest will be observed (Blackburn, 2013). Tachypnea is usually present by 6 hours of age, with respiratory rates consistently greater than 60 breaths/min and reaching 60 to 120 breaths/min. Mild respiratory and metabolic acidosis may be present at 2 to 6 hours. These clinical signs usually persist for 12 to 24 hours. In mild TTN, the signs can improve within 24 hours but may continue for up to 72 hours when more severe (Cloherty et al., 2012).

Clinical Therapy

Initial x-ray findings may be identical to those showing RDS within the first 3 hours. However, radiographs of infants with TTN usually reveal a generalized overexpansion of the lungs (hyperaeration of alveoli), which is identified principally by flattened contours of the diaphragm. Dense streaks (increased vascularity) radiate from the hilar region and represent engorgement of the lymphatic vessels, which clear alveolar fluid on initiation of air breathing. Within 48 to 72 hours, the chest x-ray examination is normal (Cloherty et al., 2012).

● **Figure 28–4** This baby born at 36 weeks' gestational age had severe RDS. He has ongoing oxygen needs provided by a nasal cannula but still can be held by his proud big brother.

Source: Courtesy of Lisa Smith-Pedersen, RNC, MSN, NNP-BC.

Clinical Reasoning Transient Tachypnea of the Newborn

You are caring for baby girl Linn, who is a 39-week, AGA female born by repeat cesarean birth to a 34-year-old G3, now P3, mother. Baby Linn's Apgar scores were 7 at 1 minute and 9 at 5 minutes. At 2 hours of age, you note an elevated respiratory rate of 70 to 80 and mild cyanosis. The infant is now receiving 30% oxygen and has a respiratory rate of 100 to 120. The baby's clinical course, chest x-ray examination, and lab work are all consistent with transient tachypnea of the newborn. Her mother calls you to ask about her baby. She tells you that her last child was born at 30 weeks' gestation, had respiratory distress syndrome requiring ventilator support, and was hospitalized for 6 weeks. She asks you, "Is this the same respiratory distress?" What will you tell her?

See www.nursing.pearsonhighered.com for possible responses.

Table 28–2	Oxygen Monitors		

Type	Function and Rationale	Nursing Interventions
PULSE OXIMETRY—SPO_2		
Estimates beat-to-beat arterial oxygen saturation.	Calibration is automatic.	Understand and use oxyhemoglobin dissociation curve.
Microprocessor measures saturation by the absorption of red and infrared light as it passes through tissue.	Less dependent on perfusion than TcPO_2 and TcPCO_2; however, functions poorly if peripheral perfusion is decreased due to low cardiac output.	Monitor trends over time and correlate with arterial blood gases. Check disposable sensor at least q8h.
Changes in absorption related to blood pulsation through vessel determine saturation and pulse rate.	Much more rapid response time than TcPO_2— offers real-time readings. Can be located on extremity, digit, or palm of hand, leaving chest free; not affected by skin characteristics. Requires understanding of oxyhemoglobin dissociation curve. Pulse oximeter reading of 88% to 93% reflects a PaO_2 of 50–80 mm Hg (Cloherty et al., 2012). Extreme sensitivity to movement; decreases if average of 7th or 14th beat is selected rather than beat to beat. Poor correlation with extreme hyperoxia.	Use disposable cuffs (reusable cuffs allow too much ambient light to enter, which can result in inaccurate readings).
TRANSCUTANEOUS OXYGEN MONITOR—TcPO_2		
Measures oxygen diffusion across the skin. Clark electrode is heated to 43°C (109.4°F) (preterm) or 44°C (111.2°F) (term) to warm the skin beneath the electrode and promote diffusion of oxygen across the skin surface. PO_2 is measured when oxygen diffuses across the capillary membrane, skin, and electrode membrane (Cloherty et al., 2012).	When transcutaneous monitors are properly calibrated and electrodes are appropriately positioned, they will provide reliable, continuous, noninvasive measurements of PO_2, PCO_2, and oxygen saturation. Readings vary when skin perfusion is decreased. Reliable as trend monitor. Frequent calibration necessary to overcome mechanical drift. Following membrane change, machine must "warm up" 1 hour prior to initial calibration; otherwise, after turning it on, it must equilibrate for 30 minutes prior to calibration. When placed on infant, values will be low until skin is heated; approximately 15 minutes required to stabilize.	Use TcPO_2 to monitor trends of oxygenation with routine nursing care procedures. Clean electrode surface to remove electrolyte deposits; change solution and membrane once a week. Allow machine to stabilize before drawing arterial gases; note reading when gases are drawn and use values to correlate. Ensure airtight seal between skin surface and electrode; place electrodes on clean, dry skin on upper chest, abdomen, or inner aspect of thigh; avoid bony prominences.
	Second-degree burns are rare but can occur if electrodes remain in place too long. Decreased correlations noted with older infants (related to skin thickness), with infants with low cardiac output (decreased skin perfusion), and with hyperoxic infants.	Change skin site and recalibrate at least every 4 hours; inspect skin for burns; if burns occur, use lowest temperature setting and change position of electrode more frequently.
	The adhesive that attaches the electrode may abrade the fragile skin of the preterm infant. May be used for both preductal and postductal monitoring of oxygenation for observations of shunting.	Adhesive disks may be cut to a smaller size, or skin prep may be used under the adhesive circle only; allow membrane to touch skin surface at center.

Nursing Care Plan The Newborn with Respiratory Distress Syndrome

Intervention	Rationale	Expected Outcome

1. Nursing Diagnosis: *Breathing Pattern, Ineffective,* related to immature lung development or inadequate lung surfactant (NANDA-I © 2012)

NIC Priority Intervention:
Respiratory monitoring: Collection and analysis of patient data to ensure airway patency and adequate gas exchange

NOC Suggested Outcome:
Respiratory status: Ventilation: movement of air in and out of the lungs

Goal: The infant will maintain an effective breathing pattern.

- Review maternal birth records noting medications given to mother prior to birth and the infant's condition at birth such as Apgar scores and resuscitative measures.
  - Several drugs suppress respiratory function in the newborn.

- Initiate cardiac and respiratory monitoring and calibrate these monitors every 8 hours.
  - Close monitoring detects periodic apneic spells and allows for medical intervention if necessary.

- Monitor infant's respiratory rate and rhythm, pulse, blood pressure, and activity.
  - Increases in respiratory rate and pulse, alterations in rhythm and blood pressure may indicate respiratory distress.

- Assess skin color; note signs of cyanosis, duskiness, and pallor.
  - Any changes in the normal skin color may indicate a physiologic change is occurring.

- Clear infant's airway by suctioning PRN with bulb syringe.
  - Opens airway by clearing mucus and allows maximum respiratory effort.

- Administer warmed, humidified oxygen by oxygen hood and monitor the oxygen concentrations every 30 minutes or per agency protocol.
  - Prevents mucosal dryness and maintains an even level of oxygen administration.

- Do not allow oxyhood to touch infant's face; maintain a stable oxygen concentration by increasing and decreasing oxygen on 5%–10% increments.
  - Allowing oxyhood to touch infant's face may cause apnea by stimulating the facial nerve.

- **Collaborative:** Obtain arterial blood gases (ABGs) per physician orders.
  - Obtaining arterial blood gases is essential in managing an infant receiving oxygen.

  1. Maintain constant O_2 concentration for 15–30 minutes before sample is obtained.

  2. Avoid stimulating infant 15 minutes prior to obtaining sample.

  3. Avoid suctioning infant prior to obtaining sample.
     - Suctioning may cause a discrepancy in ABG readings and should be avoided.

  4. Obtain sample in heparinized tuberculin syringe and maintain the temperature of the sample.

  5. Assess the patency of the IV line to prevent clot formation, then replace blood used to clear line.

  6. Flush line with 2 mL heparinized solution before restarting flow of IV fluids.

  7. Monitor transcutaneous pulse oximeter continuously or hourly and record. Rotate sensor site every 3–4 hours.

- Assess infant's need for mechanical ventilation: apnea present, hypoxia (Pao_2 50 mm Hg), hypercapnia ($Paco_2$ 60 mm Hg), respiratory acidosis (pH 7.2).
  - Mechanical ventilation improves oxygenation and ventilation, resulting in rise in Pao_2 and decrease in $Paco_2$.

- Administer mechanical ventilation per hospital protocol.
  - CPAP or PEEP can be administered by nasal prongs or by nasopharyngeal or oral intubation.

Expected Outcome:
- Infant will maintain an effective breathing pattern as evidenced by respirations of 30–60 breaths/min, arterial blood gases within normal range, infant free of signs of retractions or nasal flaring, and blood pH of 7.35–7.45.

(continued)

Nursing Care Plan   The Newborn with Respiratory Distress Syndrome—continued

Intervention	Rationale	Expected Outcome

2. Nursing Diagnosis: *Thermoregulation, Ineffective,* related to increased respiratory effort (NANDA-I © 2012)

Intervention	Rationale	Expected Outcome
NIC Priority Intervention: *Temperature regulation:* Attaining or maintaining body temperature within a normal range		**NOC Suggested Outcome:** *Thermoregulation:* Newborn: balance among heat production, heat gain, and heat loss during the neonatal period

Goal: The infant will exhibit no signs of hypothermia.

Intervention	Rationale	Expected Outcome
■ Review maternal prenatal and intrapartum records. Note any medications mother received during these times.	■ Medications such as Demerol and magnesium sulfate used by the mother during the prenatal or intrapartum periods significantly interfere with the infant's ability to retain heat.	■ The infant will not exhibit signs and symptoms of hypothermia as evidenced by temperature maintenance of 97.7°F (36.5°C) to 99.1°F (37.3°C) and no signs and symptoms of respiratory distress.
■ Assess infant's temperature frequently.	■ Hypothermia leads to pulmonary vasoconstriction because of the increase in oxygen consumption.	
■ Observe for signs of increased oxygen consumption and metabolic acidosis.	■ Cold stress leads to increased oxygen needs; thereby, brown fat is used to maintain body temperature. Hypoxia and acidosis further depress surfactant production.	
■ Warm all inspired gases and record temperature of delivered gases.	■ Cold air/oxygen blown in face of newborn is stimulus for consumption of oxygen and glucose and increased metabolic rate.	
■ Use radiant warmers or isolettes with servocontrols, incubators, and open cribs with appropriate clothing.	■ Maintains neutral thermal environment.	
■ Note signs and symptoms of respiratory distress, including tachypnea, apnea, cyanosis, acrocyanosis, bradycardia, lethargy, weak cry, and hypotonia.	■ These signs can predispose the infant to metabolic acidosis.	

3. Nursing Diagnosis: *Nutrition, Imbalanced: Less Than Body Requirements,* related to increased metabolic needs in the infant (NANDA-I © 2012)

Intervention	Rationale	Expected Outcome
NIC Priority Intervention: *Newborn monitoring:* Measurement and interpretation of physiologic status of the newborn the first 24 hours		**NOC Suggested Outcome:** *Nutritional status:* Food and fluid intake: amount of food and fluid taken into the body over a 24-hour period

Goal: The infant will gain weight in a normal curve.

Intervention	Rationale	Expected Outcome
■ Assess suck, swallow, gag, and cough reflexes.	■ Prevents feeding problems and assists in determining the best method of feeding for infant.	■ Infant will maintain steady weight gain as evidenced by no more than 2%/day weight loss, will tolerate oral feedings, and urine output will be 1–3 mL/kg/hour.
■ Assess respiratory status of infant. If problems are noted, notify physician.	■ In the presence of respiratory distress, avoid oral fluids and initiate parenteral nutrition per physician's orders.	
■ Monitor IV rates per infusion pump (starting at 60 mL/kg/day) or as ordered by physician.	■ Allows for close monitoring of fluid intake.	
■ Record hourly intake and output (I&O) and daily weights.	■ IV fluids are administered to replace sensible and insensible water loss, as well as evaporative water loss secondary to infant respiratory distress. Monitoring I&O will prevent circulatory system overload that can lead to pulmonary edema and cardiac problems.	

Nursing Care Plan The Newborn with Respiratory Distress Syndrome—continued

Intervention	Rationale	Expected Outcome
■ Provide total parenteral nutrition (TPN) when indicated.	■ TPN is used as nutritional alternative if bowel sounds are not present and/or infant remains in acute distress.	
■ Advance, based on tolerance, from intravenous to gastrointestinal (GI) feedings. Gavage or nipple feedings are used, and IV is used as supplement (discontinued when oral intake is sufficient).	■ If IV is discontinued before oral intake is established, baby will not receive adequate calories. ■ Formula or breast milk stimulate GI hormones necessary for a functional absorptive GI tract. ■ Avoid complications associated with nutrition by IV route only.	
■ Provide adequate caloric intake: consider amount of intake, type of formula, route of administration, and need for supplementation of intake by other routes.	■ Calories are essential to prevent catabolism of body proteins, and metabolic acidosis due to starvation or inadequate caloric intake.	
■ Assess infusion site for signs and symptoms of infection, including erythema, edema, and drainage with a foul odor.	■ Appropriate intervention can be initiated when signs and symptoms of infection are detected early. Treatment may avoid infection and sepsis in the infant.	

4. Nursing Diagnosis: *Fluid Volume: Imbalanced, Risk for,* related to increased insensible water losses (NANDA-I © 2012)

NIC Priority Intervention: *Fluid monitoring:* Collection and analysis of patient data to regulate fluid balance		NOC Suggested Outcome: *Fluid balance:* Balance of water in the intracellular and extracellular compartments of the body
Goal: The infant will not exhibit signs of dehydration and will display appropriate weight gain.		
■ Observe for weight fluctuations by obtaining daily weights.	■ Fluctuations in weight may indicate water imbalance or inadequate caloric intake.	■ Infant will be free of signs and symptoms of dehydration as evidenced by intake equaling output, urine specific gravity in normal range, and a weight gain of at least 20–30 g/day.
■ Document cumulative balances of intake (IV fluid administration and feedings) and output (urine collection bags, weighing or counting diapers) hourly.	■ Balanced fluid intake and output suggests homeostasis.	
■ Obtain urinalysis, monitor closely specific gravity and nitrites.	■ Specific gravity of 1.013 and nitrites present in the urine are indicative of not enough fluid intake.	
■ Monitor vital signs, including blood pressure, pulse, temperature, and mean arterial pressure (MAP).	■ A MAP of less than 20 mm Hg may indicate hypotension.	
■ Assess patient for signs of dehydration (i.e., poor skin turgor, pale mucous membranes, and sunken anterior fontanelle).	■ Detecting signs and symptoms of dehydration early in the infant is important because early intervention is vital to prevent further damage.	
■ Assess IV site for signs of infection (erythema and edema) and infiltration.	■ If signs and symptoms of infection are noted, intervention is necessary and IV site should be changed.	
■ **Collaborative:** Obtain labs for Hct, serum calcium, serum magnesium, serum potassium, blood urea nitrogen (BUN), creatinine, and uric acid levels.	■ Determines necessity for TPN administration.	
■ Administer fluids, blood products, and electrolytes as ordered by physician.	■ Replaces low nutrient stores and treats anemia if present.	

● **Figure 28–5** Premature infant under oxygen hood. Infant is nested and has a nonnutritive sucking pacifier.
Source: Courtesy of Lisa Smith-Pedersen, RNC, MSN, NNP-BC.

Supplemental oxygen, usually under an oxygen hood, may be required to correct the hypoxemia (Cloherty et al., 2012) (Figure 28–5 ●). Fluid and electrolyte requirements should be met intravenously during the acute phase of the disease. Oral feedings are contraindicated because of rapid respiratory rates and the subsequent risk of aspiration.

When hypoxemia is severe and tachypnea continues, persistent pulmonary hypertension must be considered and treatment measures initiated. If pneumonia or sepsis is suspected initially, antibiotics may be administered prophylactically.

Nursing Management

For nursing actions, see *Nursing Care Plan: The Newborn with Respiratory Distress Syndrome* on pages 677–679.

The Newborn with Meconium Aspiration Syndrome

Because the body's physiologic response to asphyxia is increased intestinal peristalsis, relaxation of the anal sphincter and the presence of meconium in the amniotic fluid indicates that the fetus may be suffering from asphyxia. Head or cord compression may elicit a vagal response in the fetus, thus causing passage of meconium in utero (Gleason & Devaskar, 2012). However, if the fetus is in a breech position, the presence of meconium in the amniotic fluid *does not necessarily* indicate asphyxia.

A significant percentage of all live-born, late preterm or term infants are born through meconium-stained amniotic fluid (MSAF). Of the newborns born through MSAF, an average of 10% develop **meconium aspiration syndrome (MAS)** (Gleason & Devaskar, 2012). This fluid may be aspirated into the tracheobronchial tree in utero or during the first few breaths taken by the newborn. This syndrome primarily affects term, small-for-gestational-age (SGA), and postterm newborns and those who have experienced a long labor (Cloherty et al., 2012).

Presence of meconium in the lungs produces:

- Mechanical obstruction of airways: ball-valve action (air is allowed in but not exhaled), so that alveoli overdistend causing hyperinflation, and air leaks such as pneumothorax are common
- Serious biochemical alterations: (1) extreme metabolic acidosis and respiratory acidosis resulting from cardiopulmonary shunting, hypoperfusion, and hypoventilation, and (2) extreme hypoxia, even in 100% O_2 concentration and with ventilatory assistance
- Chemical pneumonitis leading to the possible development of secondary bacterial pneumonia
- Vasoconstriction of pulmonary vessels; right to left shunting of blood leading to development of persistent pulmonary hypertension of the newborn (PPHN)
- Inactivation of natural surfactant (Cloherty et al., 2012)

Clinical Manifestations of MAS

Clinical manifestations of MAS include:

- Fetal hypoxia in utero a few days or a few minutes before birth, indicated by a sudden increase in fetal activity followed by diminished activity, slowing of fetal heart rate (FHR) or weak and irregular heartbeat, loss of beat-to-beat variability, and meconium staining of amniotic fluid or particulate meconium
- Presence of signs of distress or depression at birth, such as pallor, cyanosis, apnea, slow heartbeat, and low Apgar scores (below 6) at 1 and 5 minutes

After the initial assessment and stabilization, the severity of the ongoing clinical symptoms correlates with the extent of aspiration. Many infants require mechanical ventilation at birth because of immediate signs of distress (generalized cyanosis, tachypnea, and severe retractions). An overdistended, barrel-shaped chest with increased anteroposterior diameter is common. Auscultation reveals diminished air movement, with prominent rales and rhonchi. Abdominal palpation may reveal a displaced liver caused by diaphragmatic depression resulting from the overexpansion of the lungs. Yellowish/pale green staining of the skin, nails, and umbilical cord is usually present, especially if the incident occurred some time before birth.

The MAS chest x-ray film reveals asymmetric, coarse, patchy densities and possible hyperinflation (9 to 11 rib expansion), which may predispose the newborn to air leak syndrome such as pneumothorax or pneumomediastinum (Cloherty et al., 2012).

Clinical Therapy

The combined efforts of the maternity and pediatric team are needed to prevent MAS. If the infant is vigorous even if meconium-stained amniotic fluid is present, no subsequent special resuscitation such as tracheal suctioning is indicated because injury to the vocal cords is possible during attempts to intubate a vigorous newborn.

If the infant has absent or depressed respirations, heart rate less than 100 beats per minute, or poor muscle tone, direct tracheal suctioning by specially trained personnel such as a neonatal nurse practitioner, an experienced NICU nurse trained in those skills, a respiratory therapist, or a nurse anesthetist is recommended. The glottis is visualized and the trachea suctioned to remove meconium or other aspirated material from beneath the glottis with use of a DeLee device attached to low-pressure wall suction to decrease the possibility of human immunodeficiency virus (HIV) transmission.

Further resuscitative efforts are undertaken as indicated, following the same principles of clinical therapy used for asphyxia (discussed earlier in this chapter). Resuscitated newborns should be transferred immediately to the nursery for closer observation. The infant should be maintained in a neutral thermal environment and tactile stimulation should be minimized. An umbilical arterial line may be used for direct monitoring of arterial blood pressures, as well as blood sampling for pH and blood gases. An umbilical venous catheter may be placed for infusion of IV fluids, blood, or medications.

Treatment usually involves delivery of high levels of oxygen and high-pressure ventilation. High pressures may be needed to cause sufficient expiratory expansion of obstructed terminal airways or to stabilize airways that are weakened by inflammation so that the most distal atelectatic alveoli are ventilated. Newborns with respiratory failure who are not responding to conventional ventilator therapy may require treatment with high-frequency ventilation and/or nitric oxide therapy or extracorporeal membrane oxygenation (ECMO). Inhaled nitric oxide has proven successful for newborns with meconium aspiration, pneumonia, and PPHN who are not responding to traditional treatment modalities, and it avoids the need for ECMO.

Naturally occurring surfactant may be inactivated by the presence of meconium and the subsequent inflammatory response that occurs. Providing exogenous surfactant may decrease the incidence of air leaks. Systemic blood pressure and pulmonary blood flow must be maintained.

Prophylactic intravenous antibiotics are frequently given. Continuous infusion of bicarbonate to correct metabolic acidosis may be necessary for several days for severely ill newborns. Mortality in term or postterm infants is very high because the cycle of hypoxemia and acidemia is difficult to break.

NURSING MANAGEMENT *For the Newborn with Meconium Aspiration Syndrome*

Nursing Assessment and Diagnosis

During the intrapartum period observe for signs of fetal hypoxia and meconium staining of amniotic fluid. At birth, assess the newborn for signs of distress. During the ongoing assessment of the newborn, carefully observe for complications such as pulmonary air leaks, PPHN, hypotension and poor cardiac output, inadequate renal function, cerebral and pulmonary edema, sepsis secondary to bacterial pneumonia, and any signs of intestinal necrosis from ischemia.

Nursing diagnoses that may apply to the newborn with MAS and the infants' parents include the following (NANDA-I © 2012):

- *Gas Exchange, Impaired,* related to aspiration of meconium and amniotic fluid during birth
- *Nutrition, Imbalanced: Less Than Body Requirements,* related to respiratory distress and increased energy requirements
- *Coping: Family, Compromised,* related to life-threatening illness in term newborn

Planning and Implementation

Hospital-Based Nursing Care

Initial interventions are aimed at early identification of meconium aspiration. When significant aspiration occurs, therapy is supportive with the primary goals of maintaining appropriate gas exchange and minimizing complications. Nursing interventions after resuscitation should include maintaining adequate oxygenation and ventilation, regulating temperature, performing glucose testing by glucometer to check for hypoglycemia, monitoring calcium levels, observing IV fluid administration, calculating necessary fluids (which may be restricted in the first 48 to 72 hours because of cerebral edema), providing caloric requirements with total parenteral nutrition (TPN), and monitoring IV antibiotic therapy.

Evaluation

Expected outcomes of nursing care include the following:

- The newborn at risk for MAS is promptly identified and early intervention is initiated.
- The newborn is free of respiratory distress and metabolic alterations.
- The parents verbalize their concerns about their baby's health problem and survival and understand the rationale behind the management of their newborn.

CARE OF THE NEWBORN WITH COLD STRESS

Cold stress is excessive heat loss resulting in the use of compensatory mechanisms (such as increased respirations and nonshivering thermogenesis/use of brown fat stores) to maintain core body temperature close to 37.0°C (98.6°F). Heat loss that results in cold stress occurs in the newborn through the mechanisms of evaporation, convection, conduction, and radiation. (See Chapter 24 for types of thermoregulation.) Both preterm and small-for-gestational-age (SGA) newborns are at risk for cold stress because they have decreased adipose tissue, brown fat stores, and glycogen available for metabolism.

As discussed in Chapter 24, the newborn infant's major source of heat production in nonshivering thermogenesis (NST) is brown fat metabolism. The ability of an infant to respond to cold stress by NST is impaired in the presence of several conditions:

- Hypoxemia (PO_2 less than 50 torr)
- Intracranial hemorrhage or any central nervous system (CNS) abnormality
- Hypoglycemia (blood glucose level less than 40 mg/dL)

The metabolic consequences of cold stress can be devastating and potentially fatal to an infant. Oxygen requirements rise; even before noting a change in temperature, glucose use increases, acids are released into the bloodstream, and surfactant production decreases (Blackburn, 2013). These effects are graphically depicted in Figure 28–6 ●.

● **Figure 28–6** Cold stress chain of events. The hypothermic, or cold-stressed, newborn attempts to compensate by conserving heat and increasing heat production. These physiologic compensatory mechanisms initiate a series of metabolic events that results in hypoxemia and altered surfactant production, metabolic acidosis, hypoglycemia, and hyperbilirubinemia.

Nursing Management

The amount of heat an infant loses depends to a large extent on the actions of the nurse or caregiver. During the transfer of a neonatal intensive care unit (NICU) newborn from one bed to another, a transient (although not significant) decrease in temperature may be noted for up to 1 hour. Prevention of heat loss is especially critical in the very-low-birth-weight (VLBW) infant. Use pre-warmed blankets and pre-warm all contact surfaces. Placing the VLBW newborn in a polyethylene wrapping immediately following birth can diminish the postnatal decrease in temperature that normally occurs. Using head coverings made of insulated fabrics, wool, or polyolefin can significantly decrease heat loss after childbirth (Blackburn, 2013). Convective, radiant, and evaporative heat loss can all be reduced. Swaddling and nesting maintain flexion, which reduces exposed surface area and thus convective and radiant losses.

Vasoconstriction is the initial response to cold stress; because it initially decreases skin temperature, monitor and assess skin temperature instead of rectal temperature. A decrease in rectal temperature means that the infant has long-standing cold stress. By monitoring skin temperature, a possible decrease will become apparent before the infant's core temperature is affected.

If the newborn becomes hypothermic, the following nursing interventions should be initiated (Blackburn, 2013):

■ Maintain a neutral thermal environment (NTE); adjust based on the gestational age and postnatal age.

■ Warm the newborn slowly because rapid temperature elevation may cause hypotension and apnea.

■ Increase the air temperature in hourly increments of 0.5°C to 1°C depending on birth weight until the infant's temperature is stable.

■ Monitor skin temperature every 15 to 30 minutes to determine if the newborn's temperature is increasing.

■ Remove plastic wrap, caps, and heat shields while rewarming the infant so that neither cool air nor warm air is trapped.

■ Warm IV fluids before infusion.

■ Initiate efforts to block heat loss by evaporation, radiation, convection, and conduction and maintain the newborn in NTE especially during procedures.

If a decrease in skin temperature is noted, determine whether hypoglycemia is present. Attempts to burn brown fat increase oxygen consumption, lactic acid levels, and metabolic acidosis. Hypoglycemia is a result of the metabolic effects of cold stress and is suggested by glucometer values below 40 to 50 mg/dL, tremors, irritability or lethargy, apnea, or seizure activity. Hypoglycemia may be reversed by adequate glucose intake, as described in the following section.

CARE OF THE NEWBORN WITH HYPOGLYCEMIA

An operational threshold for intervention in newborn **hypoglycemia** is a plasma glucose concentration of less than 40 mg/dL at any time in any newborn. It requires a follow-up glucose measurement to document normal values (Cloherty et al., 2012). Within 1 to 2 hours of life, normal asymptomatic newborns may have a transient glucose level as low as 30 mg/dL that will increase either spontaneously or with feedings (AAP Committee on Fetus and Newborn, 2012). Plasma glucose values of less than 20 to 25 mg/dL should be treated with parenteral glucose $D_{10}W$, regardless of the age or gestation, to raise the plasma glucose level to greater than 45 mg/dL prior to routine feeds. There is no absolute threshold that can be applied to all babies. Glucose concentrations must be looked at in conjunction with clinical manifestations.

Hypoglycemia is the most common metabolic disorder occurring in infants of diabetic mothers (IDMs), small-for-gestational-age

(SGA) infants, the smaller of twins, and male and late preterm infants (Adkin & Committee on Fetus and Newborn, 2011). The pathophysiology of hypoglycemia differs for each classification.

Average-for-gestational-age (AGA) preterm infants have not been in utero a sufficient time to store glycogen and fat. As a result, they have decreased ability to carry out gluconeogenesis. This situation is further aggravated by increased use of glucose by the tissues (especially the brain and heart) during stress and illness (chilling, asphyxia, sepsis, RDS).

IDMs have increased stores of glycogen and fat (see Chapter 27). Circulating insulin and insulin responsiveness are also higher when compared with other newborns. Because the high glucose loads present in utero stop at birth, the newborn experiences rapid and profound hypoglycemia (Blackburn, 2013).

The SGA infant has used up glycogen and fat stores because of intrauterine malnutrition and has a blunted hepatic enzymatic response with which to produce and use glucose. Any newborn stressed at birth from asphyxia or cold also quickly uses up available glucose stores and becomes hypoglycemic. Epidural anesthesia may alter maternal–fetal glucose homeostasis, resulting in hypoglycemia.

Clinical Therapy

The goal of management includes early identification of hypoglycemia through observation and screening of newborns at risk (Gleason & Devaskar, 2012). The newborn may be asymptomatic, or any of the following may occur:

- Lethargy, apathy, and limpness
- Poor feeding, poor sucking, vomiting
- Pallor, cyanosis
- Hypothermia or temperature instability in low-birth-weight (LBW) infants
- Apnea, irregular respirations, respiratory distress
- Tremors, jerkiness, jitteriness, seizure activity
- Weak or high-pitched cry (Cloherty et al., 2012)

In at-risk infants, routine screening should be done frequently during the first 4 hours of life and then at 4-hour intervals until the risk period has passed.

Hypoglycemia may also be defined as a *glucose oxidase reagent strip with reflectance meter* reading below 40 mg/dL, but only when corroborated with laboratory plasma glucose testing (see Skill 10–1: Performing a Capillary Puncture in the *Clinical Skills Manual* SKILLS). Common bedside methods use whole blood, an enzymatic reagent strip, and a reflectance meter or color chart. Bedside glucose reagent strips should not be used by themselves to screen for and diagnose hypoglycemia, because their results depend on the baby's hematocrit (they react to the glucose in the plasma, not the red blood cells) and whole-blood glucose concentrations are 10% to 18% lower than plasma glucose concentrations (Adkin & Committee on Fetus and Newborn, 2011; Cloherty et al., 2012). Newer point-of-care techniques, such as using a glucose analyzer or an optical bedside glucose analyzer, are more reliable for bedside screening but must also be validated with laboratory chemical analysis.

Clinical Tip

Venous blood samples for the laboratory should be placed on ice and analyzed within 30 minutes of drawing to prevent the RBCs from continuing to metabolize glucose and giving a falsely low reading. Also avoid transporting the blood in tubes containing a glycolytic inhibitor such as fluoride.

Early formula feeding or breastfeeding is one of the major approaches for preventing hypoglycemia. If early feeding or IV glucose is started to meet the recommended fluid and caloric needs, the blood glucose concentration is likely to remain above the hypoglycemic level. During the first hours after birth, asymptomatic newborns may also be given oral glucose contained in formula or breast milk (glucose water should not be used because it causes a rapid increase in glucose followed by an abrupt decrease), and then another plasma glucose measurement is obtained within 30 minutes after feeding.

IV minibolus infusions of a dextrose solution of $D_{10}W$ (glucose 10% in water) begun immediately after birth should prevent hypoglycemia. Plasma glucose levels are obtained when the parenteral infusion is started. However, in the very small AGA infant, infusions of 10% dextrose solution may cause hyperglycemia to develop, requiring an alteration in the glucose concentration. An IV glucose solution should be calculated based on the infant's body weight and fluid requirements and correlated with blood glucose tests to determine adequacy of the infusion treatment.

NURSING MANAGEMENT *For the Newborn with Hypoglycemia*

Nursing Assessment and Diagnosis

The objectives of nursing assessment are to identify newborns at risk and to screen symptomatic infants. For newborns diagnosed with hypoglycemia, assessment is ongoing and includes careful monitoring of glucose values. Glucose strips, urine dipstick, and urine volume tests (monitor only if above 1 to 3 mL/kg/hr) may be evaluated frequently for osmotic diuresis and glycosuria.

Nursing diagnoses that may apply to the newborn with hypoglycemia include the following (NANDA-I © 2012):

- *Nutrition, Imbalanced: Less Than Body Requirements,* related to increased glucose use secondary to physiologic stress
- *Breathing Pattern, Ineffective,* related to tachypnea and apnea
- *Pain, Acute,* related to frequent heelsticks secondary to glucose monitoring

Planning and Implementation

Infants in at-risk groups should be monitored within 30 to 60 minutes after birth and before feedings or whenever abnormal clinical manifestations are observed (Cloherty et al., 2012). The IDM should be monitored within 30 minutes of birth. Once an at-risk infant's blood sugar level is stable, glucose testing every

Complementary Care Pain Relief in the NICU

The newborn relies on the nurse's observational, assessment, and interventional skills for anticipation and prevention of pain if possible and then prompt, safe, and effective pain relief. It is vital for the nurse to assist infants to cope with and recover from necessary painful clinical procedures. A variety of nonpharmacologic pain-prevention and relief techniques have been shown to be effective in reducing pain from minor procedures in newborns.

Any unnecessary stimuli (i.e., noise, visual, tactile, and vestibular) of the newborn should be avoided, if possible. Developmental care, which includes limiting environmental stimuli, lateral positioning, the use of supportive bedding, and attention to behavioral cues, assists the newborn to cope with painful procedures (Gardner, Enzman-Himes, & Dickey, 2011).

Containment with swaddling or facilitated tucking (holding the arms and legs in a flexed position) is effective in reducing excessive immature motor responses. Swaddling also may provide comfort through other senses, such as thermal, tactile, and proprioceptive senses. Breastfeeding and skin-to-skin contact with the mother during the painful procedure may help to relieve pain (Gardner et al., 2011).

Nonnutritive sucking (NNS) refers to the provision of a pacifier into the infant's mouth to promote sucking without the provision of breast milk or formula for nutrition. NNS is thought to produce analgesia through stimulation of orotactile and mechanoreceptors when the pacifier is placed into the infant's mouth. Allowing nonnutritive sucking with a pacifier aids in the reduction of procedural pain and stress. Unfortunately, a rebound in distress occurs when the NNS pacifier is removed from the infant's mouth (Gardner et al., 2011).

A wide range of oral sucrose doses has been used for procedural pain relief (heelsticks, venipuncture, IM injections), but no optimal dose has been established. The sweetness of the sucrose, a disaccharide, elevates the pain threshold through endogenous opioid release in the CNS and produces a calming effect. A range of 0.05 to 0.5 mL of 24% sucrose is administered on the anterior part of the tongue via a syringe or nipple approximately 2 minutes before the procedure (Gardner et al., 2011). Some authors have suggested that multiple doses, such as giving a dose 2 minutes before and 1 to 2 minutes after a procedure, are more effective. It is important to be careful with repeated doses of sucrose, because of the concern for hyperglycemia, necrotizing enterocolitis (NEC), and fluid overload. Also, repeated use of sucrose analgesia in preterm infants may affect their neurologic development and behavioral outcomes. Until further research is done, repeated doses of sucrose are not recommended (Gardner et al., 2011). Because oral sucrose reduces but does not eliminate pain, it should be used with other nonpharmacologic measures to enhance effectiveness.

---

2 to 4 hours (or per agency protocol), or before feedings, adequately monitors glucose levels. See Figures 28–7 and 28–8 ●.

The method of feeding greatly influences glucose and energy requirements; thus careful calculation of glucose requirements and attention to glucose monitoring are required during the transition from IV to oral feedings. Titration of IV glucose may be required until the infant is able to take adequate amounts of formula or breast milk to maintain a normal blood sugar level. Enteral feedings are increased to maintain adequate glucose and caloric intake and also normal blood glucose levels.

Evaluation

Expected outcomes of nursing care include the following:

- The newborn at risk for hypoglycemia is identified, and prompt intervention is started.

- The newborn's glucose level is stabilized, and recovery is proceeding without sequelae.

● **Figure 28–7** Potential puncture sites for heelsticks. Avoid gray-shaded areas to prevent injury to arteries and nerves in the foot and the important longitudinally oriented fat pad of the heel, which in later years could impede walking if injured.

Puncture sites

● **Figure 28–8** Heelstick. With a quick, piercing motion, puncture the lateral heel with a microlancet. Be careful not to puncture too deeply.

CARE OF THE NEWBORN WITH JAUNDICE

The most common abnormal physical finding in newborns is jaundice (*icterus neonatorum*). Some degree of jaundice, resulting from elevated unconjugated bilirubinemia, occurs in approximately 85% of healthy term infants and most preterm infants (Cloherty et al., 2012). *Physiologic or neonatal jaundice* is a normal process that occurs during transition from intrauterine to extrauterine life and is caused by the newborn's shortened red blood cell life span (90 days compared with 120 days in the adult), slower uptake by the liver, lack of intestinal bacteria, and/or poorly established hydration from initial breastfeeding. Total bilirubin levels peak around 96 to 120 hours of age, usually after discharge from the hospital.

Jaundice is a yellowish coloration of the skin and sclera of the eyes that develops from deposits of the yellow pigment bilirubin in lipid/fat containing tissues as described in Chapter 24 . Fetal unconjugated (indirect) bilirubin is normally cleared by the placenta in utero, so total bilirubin at birth is usually less than 3 mg/dL unless an abnormal hemolytic process has been present. Postnatally, the infant must conjugate bilirubin (convert a lipid-soluble pigment into a water-soluble pigment) in the liver.

The rate and amount of conjugation of bilirubin depend on the rate of hemolysis, the bilirubin load, the maturity of the liver, and the presence of albumin-binding sites. (See Chapter 24 for discussion of conjugation of bilirubin.) The liver of a normal, healthy term infant is usually mature enough and producing enough glucuronyl transferase that the total serum bilirubin does not reach a pathologic level.

Causes of Hyperbilirubinemia

Serum albumin-binding sites are usually sufficient to conjugate enough bilirubin to meet the normal demands of the newborn. However, certain conditions such as fetal or neonatal asphyxia and neonatal drugs such as indomethacin can decrease the binding affinity of bilirubin to albumin, because acidosis impairs the capacity of albumin to hold bilirubin. Hypothermia and hypoglycemia release free fatty acids that dislocate bilirubin from albumin. Maternal medications such as sulfa drugs and salicylates compete with bilirubin for these sites. Finally, premature infants have less albumin available for binding with bilirubin. Neurotoxicity is possible because unconjugated bilirubin has a high affinity for extravascular tissue, such as fatty tissue (subcutaneous tissue) and cerebral tissue. Other risk factors include predischarge total serum bilirubin (TSB) or transcutaneous bilirubin (TcB) measurement in a high-risk or high-intermediate zone, jaundice in the first 24 hours of age, previous sibling with jaundice, East Asian race, American Indian Greek, and cephalohematoma or significant bruising (Cloherty et al., 2012).

Bilirubin not bound to albumin can cross the blood–brain barrier, damage cells of the CNS, and produce kernicterus or **acute bilirubin encephalopathy (ABE)**. **Kernicterus** (meaning "yellow nucleus") refers to the deposition of indirect or unconjugated bilirubin in the basal ganglia of the brain and to the permanent neurologic sequelae of untreated **hyperbilirubinemia** (elevation of bilirubin level) (Cloherty et al., 2012). The classic acute bilirubin encephalopathy of kernicterus most commonly found with Rh and ABO blood group incompatibility is less common today because of aggressive treatment with phototherapy and exchange transfusions. Kernicterus cases are reappearing as a result of early discharge and the increased incidence of dehydration (as a result of discharge before the mother's milk is established). Unfortunately, current therapy cannot distinguish all infants who are at risk. It is recommended that *all* newborns be screened for bilirubin level prior to leaving the hospital using total serum bilirubin (TSB) or transcutaneous bilirubin (TcB). It is also advised to record information on gestation, birth weight, bilirubin/albumin ratios, and risk factors on the electronic health record (EHR) (Maisels & Watchko, 2012).

Evidence-Based Practice   Use of Transcutaneous Bilirubinometry in Severe Hyperbilirubinemia

Clinical Question
Does the use of transcutaneous bilirubinometry enhance early detection and lower the rates of severe hyperbilirubinemia?

The Evidence
Transcutaneous bilirubinometry (TcB) had been advanced as an early detection tool for hyperbilirubinemia, but its effectiveness in actually preventing severe conditions had not been studied in terms of costs and benefits. TcB is a noninvasive diagnostic tool used to identify babies whose total serum bilirubin should be closely monitored. A group of pediatricians undertook an analysis of outcomes of nearly 15,000 prospectively enrolled healthy infants who were randomized to treatment and control groups. This type of large-sample randomized trial forms the strongest level of evidence for practice. The neonate's chances of advancing to severe hyperbilirubinemia were cut by more than half when TcB was routinely used. Its use was associated with fewer blood draws and lower phototherapy rates, and so procedural costs were reduced.

Readmissions for phototherapy and the subsequent length of treatment were also reduced. In one large cohort study of multiple hospitals, the costs of transcutaneous bilirubin assessment were lower than laboratory measurement, and did not require an invasive procedure (McKenzie & Palmer, 2010). The use of TcB is not limited to acute care facilities; it has the potential to be an effective public health nurse management tool.

Best Practice
Routine use of transcutaneous bilirubinometry reduces the chance that a baby's bilirubinemia will advance to a severe stage. The averted costs associated with its use include the costs of unnecessary blood tests, therapies, and readmissions (Wainer, Parmer, Allegro, et al., 2012).

Clinical Reasoning
What are the triggers that may warrant transcutaneous bilirubinometry? When would its use be most effective in home care and public health settings?

A primary cause of hyperbilirubinemia is **hemolytic disease of the newborn**. All pregnant women who are Rh negative or who have blood type O (possible ABO blood incompatibility) should be asked about outcomes of any previous pregnancies and history of blood transfusion. Prenatal amniocentesis with spectrophotographic examination may be indicated in some cases. Cord blood from newborns is evaluated for bilirubin level, which normally does not exceed 5 mg/dL. Newborns of Rh-negative and O blood type mothers are carefully assessed for appearance of jaundice and levels of serum bilirubin.

Alloimmune hemolytic disease, also known as **erythroblastosis fetalis**, occurs when an Rh-negative mother is pregnant with an Rh-positive fetus and maternal antibodies cross the placenta. Maternal antibodies enter the fetal circulation, then attach to and destroy the fetal RBCs. The fetal system responds by increasing RBC production. Jaundice, anemia, and compensatory erythropoiesis result. A marked increase in immature RBCs (erythroblasts) also occurs, hence the designation erythroblastosis fetalis. Because of the widespread use of Rh immune globulin (RhoGAM), the incidence of erythroblastosis fetalis has dropped dramatically.

Hydrops fetalis, the most severe form of erythroblastosis fetalis, occurs when maternal antibodies attach to the Rh site on the fetal RBCs, making them susceptible to destruction; severe anemia and multiorgan system failure result. Cardiomegaly with severe cardiac decompensation and hepatosplenomegaly occurs. Severe generalized massive edema (anasarca) and generalized fluid effusion into the pleural cavity (hydrothorax), pericardial sac, and peritoneal cavity (ascites) develop. Jaundice is not present until the newborn period because the bilirubin pigments are excreted through the placenta into the maternal circulation. The hydropic hemolytic disease process is also characterized by hyperplasia of the pancreatic islets, which predisposes the infant to neonatal hypoglycemia similar to that of IDMs. These infants have increased bleeding tendencies because of associated thrombocytopenia and hypoxic damage to the capillaries. Hydrops is a frequent cause of intrauterine death among infants with Rh disease.

ABO incompatibility (the mother is blood type O and the baby is blood type A or B) may result in jaundice, although it rarely results in hemolytic disease severe enough to be clinically diagnosed and treated. Hepatosplenomegaly may be found occasionally in newborns with ABO incompatibility, but hydrops fetalis and stillbirth are rare.

The prognosis for a newborn with hyperbilirubinemia depends on the extent of the hemolytic process and the underlying cause. Severe hemolytic disease results in fetal and early neonatal death from the effects of severe anemia—cardiac decompensation, edema, ascites, and hydrothorax. Hyperbilirubinemia that is not aggressively treated may lead to kernicterus. The resultant neurologic damage is responsible for death, cerebral palsy, possible intellectual disability, or hearing loss or, to a lesser degree, perceptual impairment, delayed speech development, hyperactivity, muscle incoordination, or learning difficulties (Maisel & Watchko, 2012).

Clinical Therapy

Laboratory and Diagnostic Assessments

The best treatment for hemolytic disease is prevention by early recognition of prenatal risk factors such as Rh and ABO incompatibility (see Chapter 16 ℰ for discussion of in utero management of this condition), and attention to certain neonatal clinical conditions. Neonatal hyperbilirubinemia can be considered pathologic and requires further investigation if any of the following criteria are met (Maisels & Watchko, 2012):

1. Clinically evident jaundice appears before 24 hours of life or if jaundice seems excessive for the newborn's age in hours.
2. Serum bilirubin concentration rises by more than 0.2 mg/dL per hour.
3. Total serum bilirubin concentration exceeds the 95th percentile on a nomogram.
4. Conjugated bilirubin concentrations are greater than 2 mg/dL or more than 10% to 20% of the total serum bilirubin concentration.
5. Clinical jaundice persists for more than 2 weeks in a term newborn.

Initial diagnostic procedures are aimed at differentiating jaundice resulting from increased bilirubin production, impaired conjugation or excretion, increased intestinal reabsorption, or a combination of these factors.

Transcutaneous bilirubin (TcB) measurements are a noninvasive method of assessing bilirubin levels and may be used for predischarge risk assessment. A TcB can be performed quickly and painlessly, and repeated measures are easily obtained. TcB can quantify the amount of bilirubin pigment in the infant's skin. Nurses need to measure bilirubin levels to confirm the presence, absence, or suspicion of jaundice. However, it is important to remember that total serum bilirubin levels remain the standard of care for confirmation or diagnosis of hyperbilirubinemia (Maisels & Watchko, 2012).

Because of the shorter life span of red blood cells in the newborn, a significant bilirubin load is produced. When bilirubin breaks down, carbon monoxide (CO) is released. This production of carbon monoxide is being investigated as a marker in the study of bilirubin production. Measuring end-tidal CO (ETCO) has been shown to provide results similar to those of laboratory bilirubin; however, devices to measure CO are not widely available.

Essential laboratory evaluations are Coombs' test, serum bilirubin levels (direct and total), hemoglobin, reticulocyte

Developing Cultural Competence
Ethnic Variations and Jaundice

East Asian infants (Japanese, Chinese, and Filipino ethnic groups) have a higher occurrence of hyperbilirubinemia than Caucasian infants. In addition, infants with Asian fathers and Caucasian mothers have a higher incidence of jaundice than if both parents are Caucasian. Other ethnic groups at risk for increased bilirubinemia are Navajo, Eskimo, and Sioux Native American newborns; Greek newborns; Sephardic-Jewish (Asian ancestry) newborns; and some Hispanic newborns.

Clinical Tip

Because of exposure to sunlight, sternal area transcutaneous bilirubin (TcB) measurements may be more accurate than those taken on the forehead. The sternum, in a dressed infant, is less likely to be affected by the influence of ambient light (such as sunlight) on the skin.

percentage, white cell count, and positive smear for cellular morphology.

The Coombs' (direct antiglobulin test [DAT]) test is performed to determine whether jaundice is because of Rh or ABO incompatibility. The indirect Coombs' test measures the amount of Rh-positive antibodies in the mother's blood. Rh-positive red blood cells are added to the maternal blood sample. If the mother's serum contains antibodies, the Rh-positive red blood cells will agglutinate (clump) when rabbit immune antiglobulin is added, which is a positive test result. The direct Coombs' test reveals the presence of antibody-coated (sensitized) Rh-positive red blood cells in the newborn. Rabbit immune antiglobulin is added to the specimen of neonatal blood cells. If the neonatal red blood cells agglutinate, they have been coated with maternal antibodies, a positive result.

If the hemolytic process is caused by Rh sensitization, laboratory findings reveal the following: (1) an Rh-positive newborn with a positive Coombs' test; (2) increased erythropoiesis with many immature circulating red blood cells (nucleated blastocysts); (3) anemia, in most cases; (4) elevated levels (5 mg/dL or more) of bilirubin in cord blood; and (5) a reduction in albumin-binding capacity. Maternal data may include an elevated anti-Rh titer and spectrophotometric evidence of a fetal hemolytic process.

If the hemolytic process is caused by ABO incompatibility, laboratory findings reveal an increase in reticulocytes. The resulting anemia is usually not significant during the newborn period and is rare later on. The direct Coombs' test may be negative or mildly positive, whereas the indirect Coombs' test may be strongly positive. Infants with a positive direct Coombs' test have increased incidence of jaundice, with bilirubin levels in excess of 10 mg/dL. Increased numbers of spherocytes (spherical, plump, mature erythrocytes) are seen on a peripheral blood smear. Increased numbers of spherocytes are not seen on blood smears from infants with Rh disease.

Therapeutic Management

Whatever the cause of hyperbilirubinemia, management of these infants is directed toward alleviating anemia, removing maternal antibodies and sensitized erythrocytes, increasing serum albumin levels, reducing serum bilirubin levels, and minimizing the consequences of hyperbilirubinemia. Early discharge of newborns from birthing centers has significantly influenced the diagnosis and management of neonatal jaundice, increasing the emphasis on outpatient and home care management.

If hemolytic disease is present, it may be treated with phototherapy, exchange transfusion, and drug therapy. When determining the appropriate management of hyperbilirubinemia caused by hemolytic disease, the three relevant variables are the newborn's (1) serum bilirubin level, (2) birth weight, and (3) age in hours. If a newborn has hemolysis with an unconjugated bilirubin level of 14 mg/dL, weighs less than 2500 g (birth weight), and is 24 hours old or less, an exchange transfusion may be the best management. However, if that same newborn is over 24 hours of age, which is past the time during which an increase in bilirubin would occur because of pathologic causes, phototherapy may be the treatment of choice to prevent the possible complication of kernicterus.

Phototherapy

Phototherapy is the exposure of the newborn to high-intensity light. It may be used alone or in conjunction with an exchange transfusion to reduce serum bilirubin levels. Exposure of the newborn to high-intensity light (a bank of fluorescent light bulbs or bulbs in the blue-light spectrum) decreases serum bilirubin levels in the skin by facilitating biliary excretion of unconjugated bilirubin. Phototherapy decreases serum bilirubin levels by changing bilirubin from the non–water-soluble (lipophilic) form to water-soluble by-products that can then be excreted via urine and bile.

Photoisomerization occurs when the natural form of bilirubin is exposed to light at a certain wavelength and the bilirubin is converted to a less toxic form. The new isomer, photobilirubin, is created rapidly but is quite unstable. The photobilirubin is bound to albumin, transported to the liver, and incorporated into bile. If it is not quickly eliminated from the bowel, then it can convert back to its original form and return to the bloodstream. In addition, the photodegradation products formed when light oxidizes bilirubin can be excreted in the urine.

Phototherapy is an intervention that is used to prevent hyperbilirubinemia in order to halt bilirubin levels from climbing dangerously high. The decision to start phototherapy is based on two factors: gestational age and age in hours. Phototherapy does not alter the underlying cause of jaundice, and hemolysis may continue to produce anemia. Many authors have recommended initiating phototherapy "prophylactically" in the first 24 hours of life in high-risk, VLBW, or severely bruised infants. The risk category of newborns requiring follow-up/intervention for their hyperbilirubinemia is evaluated by plotting their serum bilirubin level and age in hours on a nomogram.

Phototherapy can be provided by conventional banks of fluorescent tube phototherapy lights, by a fiberoptic blanket attached to a halogen light source around the trunk of the newborn, by a fiber-optic mattress placed under the baby, or by a combination of these delivery methods. Levels should continue to decline when phototherapy covers a wider surface area. If a drop in bilirubin levels is not reached, then an exchange transfusion should be considered. Most phototherapy units will provide this level of irradiance 45 to 50 cm (18 to 20 in.) below the lamps. The nurse can use a photometer to measure and maintain desired irradiance levels. The nurse keeps track of the number of hours each lamp is used so that each can be replaced before its effectiveness is lost (Bhutani & Committee on Fetus and Newborn, 2011). (See Skill 5–7: Infant Receiving Phototherapy in the *Clinical Skills Manual* SKILLS .)

With the fiber-optic blanket, the light stays on at all times, and the newborn is accessible for care, feeding, and diaper changes; greater surface area is exposed and there are no thermoregulation issues. The eyes are not covered. The babies do not get overheated, and fluid and weight loss are not complications of this system. Furthermore, it makes the infant accessible to the parents and is less alarming to parents than standard phototherapy. Many institutions and pediatricians use fiber-optic blankets for home care. A combination of a fiber-optic light source in the mattress under or around the baby and a standard light source above has also been recommended. This is termed *intensive phototherapy*. Intensive phototherapy should show a drop in total serum bilirubin (TSB) within 4 to 8 hours. Levels should continue to decline when phototherapy covers a wider surface area. If a drop in bilirubin levels is not reached, then an exchange transfusion should be considered. As with the other phototherapy methods, the nurse uses a photometer to measure and maintain desired irradiance levels and keeps track of the number of hours each lamp is used so that each can be replaced before its effectiveness is lost.

Exchange Transfusion

Exchange transfusion is the withdrawal and replacement of the newborn's blood with donor blood. It is used to treat anemia with red blood cells that are susceptible to maternal antibodies, to remove sensitized red blood cells that would soon be lysed, to remove serum bilirubin, to provide bilirubin-free albumin, and to increase the binding sites for bilirubin. Concerns about exchange transfusion are related to the use of blood products and associated potential for HIV infection and hepatitis. If the TSB is at or approaching the exchange level, blood should be sent for immediate typing and cross-matching. Blood for exchange transfusion is modified whole blood (red cells and plasma) cross-matched against the mother and compatible with the infant.

NURSING MANAGEMENT *For the Newborn with Jaundice*

Nursing Assessment and Diagnosis

Assessment is aimed at identifying prenatal and perinatal factors that predispose the newborn to the development of jaundice and at recognizing the jaundice as soon as it is apparent. Significant hyperbilirubinemia in the neonatal population is often due to a multitude of causes, including a genetic basis (Maisels & Watchko, 2012). Clinically, ABO incompatibility presents as jaundice and occasionally as hepatosplenomegaly. Fetal hydrops or erythroblastosis is rare (see Chapter 16 ⬤). Hemolytic disease of the newborn is suspected if one or more of the following are evident:

- The placenta is enlarged.
- The newborn is edematous, with pleural and pericardial effusion plus ascites.
- Pallor or jaundice is noted during the first 24 to 36 hours.
- Hemolytic anemia is diagnosed.
- The spleen and liver are enlarged.

Carefully note changes in behavior and observe for evidence of bleeding. If laboratory tests indicate elevated bilirubin levels, check the newborn for jaundice about every 2 hours and record observations.

To check for jaundice in lighter skinned babies, blanch the skin over a bony prominence (forehead, nose, sternum) by pressing firmly with the thumb. After pressure is released, if jaundice is present, the area appears yellow before normal color returns. Check oral mucosa and the posterior portion of the hard palate and conjunctival sacs for yellow pigmentation in darker skinned babies. Jaundice progresses in a cephalocaudal direction from the face to the trunk and then to the lower extremities. The overall progression of jaundice should be noted. Assessment in daylight gives the best results, because pink walls and surroundings may mask yellowish tints, and yellow light makes differentiation of jaundice difficult. Record and report the time at onset of jaundice. If jaundice appears, careful observation of the increase in depth of color and of the newborn's behavior is mandatory.

In addition to visual inspection, reflectance photometers that measure transcutaneous bilirubin (TcB) should be used to screen and monitor neonatal jaundice. Most hospitals have developed a mandatory screening policy for all newborns before discharge using the TcB monitor, and it is recommended that this screening be done universally (Maisels & Watchko, 2012). If the level comes back elevated, then a follow-up total serum bilirubin (TSB) is performed. Measurements in newborns using the TcB devices are within 2 to 3 mg/dL of the TSB and useful for TSB levels less than 15 mg/dL. When universal screening is performed, there is a reduction in severe hyperbilirubinemia, but there is a significant increase in the use of phototherapy, sometimes at unnecessary levels.

Assess the newborn's behavior for neurologic signs associated with hyperbilirubinemia, which are rare but may include hypotonia, diminished reflexes, lethargy, or seizures.

Nursing diagnoses that may apply to care of a newborn with jaundice include the diagnoses in the nursing care plan and the following (NANDA-I © 2012):

- ***Injury, Risk for,*** related to use of phototherapy
- ***Neurovascular Dysfunction: Peripheral, Risk for,*** related to neurologic damage secondary to kernicterus
- ***Parenting, Risk for Impaired,*** related to deficient knowledge of infant care and prolonged separation of infant and parents secondary to illness

Planning and Implementation
Hospital-Based Nursing Care

Hospital-based care is described in *Nursing Care Plan: The Newborn with Hyperbilirubinemia*. Phototherapy success is measured every 12 hours or with daily serum bilirubin levels (more frequently if there is hemolysis or a higher level before initiation of phototherapy). Turn lights off while blood is drawn to ensure accurate serum bilirubin levels. Because it is not known if phototherapy injures the delicate eye structures, particularly the retina, apply eye patches over the newborn's closed eyes during exposure to banks of phototherapy lights

Nursing Care Plan The Newborn with Hyperbilirubinemia

Intervention	Rationale	Expected Outcome

1. Nursing Diagnosis: *Tissue Integrity, Impaired,* related to predisposing factors associated with hyperbilirubinemia (NANDA-I © 2012)

NIC Priority Intervention: *High-risk newborn care:* Identification and management of a high-risk newborn to promote healthy outcomes for baby		**NOC Suggested Outcome:** *Risk control:* Actions to eliminate or reduce actual, personal, and modifiable health threats

Goal: The infant at risk for jaundice and early signs of jaundice will be identified.

■ Evaluate baby's history for predisposing factors for hyperbilirubinemia.	■ Early identification of risk factors enables the nurse to monitor babies for early signs of hyperbilirubinemia. Acidosis, hypoxia, and hypothermia increase the risk of hyperbilirubinemia at lower bilirubin levels.	■ Infant's jaundice will be identified early.
■ Observe color of amniotic fluid at time of rupture of membranes.	■ Amber-colored amniotic fluid indicates hyperbilirubinemia.	
■ Assess baby for developing jaundice in daylight if possible.	■ Early detection is affected by nursery environment. Artificial lights (with pink tint) may mask beginning of jaundice.	
1. Observe sclera.	1. Most visible sign of hyperbilirubinemia is jaundice noted in skin, sclera, or oral mucosa. Onset is first seen on face and then progresses down trunk.	
2. Observe skin color and assess by blanching.	2. Blanching the skin leaves a yellow color to the skin immediately after pressure is released.	
3. Check oral mucosa, posterior portion of hard palate, and conjunctival sacs for yellow pigmentation in dark-skinned newborns. 4. Report jaundice occurring within 24 hours of birth.	3. Underlying pigment of dark-skinned people may normally appear yellow.	

2. Nursing Diagnosis: *Fluid Volume: Imbalanced, Risk for,* related to phototherapy (NANDA-I © 2012)

NIC Priority Intervention: *Fluid monitoring:* Collection and analysis of patient data to regulate fluid balance		**NOC Suggested Outcome:** *Fluid balance:* Balance of water in the intracellular and extracellular compartments of the body

Goal: The infant will not exhibit signs of dehydration and will display appropriate weight gain.

■ Offer feedings every 2 to 3 hr. Breastfeed on demand with no supplementation unless excessive weight loss or increasing TSB with adequate feeding.	■ Adequate hydration increases peristalsis and excretion of bilirubin.	■ Infant will have good skin turgor, clear amber urine output of 1–3 mL/kg/hr, six to eight wet diapers/day, and will maintain weight.
■ Provide 25% extra fluid intake.	■ Replace fluid losses due to watery stools, if under phototherapy.	

■ Assess for dehydration:
  1. Poor skin turgor
  2. Depressed fontanelles
  3. Sunken eyes
  4. Decreased urine output
  5. Weight loss
  6. Changes in electrolytes
	■ Phototherapy treatment may cause liquid stools and increased insensible water loss, which increases risk of dehydration.	

(*continued*)

Nursing Care Plan   The Newborn with Hyperbilirubinemia—continued

Intervention	Rationale	Expected Outcome

■ Monitor intake and output (I&O).
■ Weigh daily.
■ Report signs of dehydration.
■ Administer IV fluids:
  1. Monitor flow rates.
  2. Assess insertion sites for signs of infection.
	■ Prevents fluid overload. IV fluids may be used if baby is dehydrated or in presence of other complications. IV may be started if exchange transfusion is to be done.	

3. Nursing Diagnosis: *Injury, Risk for,* related to use of banks of phototherapy lights (NANDA-I © 2012)

NIC Priority Intervention:
Newborn monitoring: Measurement and interpretation of physiologic status of the newborn the first 24 hr after birth

NOC Suggested Outcome:
Risk control: Actions to eliminate or reduce actual, personal, and modifiable health threats

Goal: The infant will not have any corneal irritation or drainage, skin breakdown, or major fluctuations in temperature.

■ Cover infant's eyes with eye patches while under banks of phototherapy lights. Cover testes/penis in male infants.	■ Protects retina from damage due to high-intensity light and testes from damage from heat.	■ Infant's eyes will be protected, skin will be intact, and infant will maintain a stable temperature.
■ Make certain that eyelids are closed prior to applying eye patches.	■ Prevents corneal abrasions.	
■ Remove baby from under phototherapy and remove eye patches during feedings.	■ Provides visual stimulation and facilitates attachment behaviors.	
■ Inspect eyes each shift for conjunctivitis, drainage, and corneal abrasions due to irritation from eye patches.	■ Prevents or facilitates prompt treatment of purulent conjunctivitis.	
■ Administer thorough perianal cleansing with each stool or change of perianal protective covering.	■ Frequent stooling increases risk of skin breakdown. Prevents infection.	
■ Provide minimal coverage—only of diaper area.	■ Provides maximal exposure. Shielded areas become more jaundiced, so maximum exposure is essential.	
■ Avoid the use of oily applications on the skin.	■ Prevents superficial burns to skin.	
■ Reposition baby q2h.	■ Provides equal exposure of all skin areas and prevents pressure areas.	
■ Observe for bronzing of skin.	■ Bronzing is related to use of phototherapy with increased direct bilirubin levels or liver damage; may last for 2 to 4 months.	
■ Place Plexiglas shield between baby and light. Monitor baby's skin and core temperature frequently until temperature is stable.	■ Hypothermia and hyperthermia are common complications of phototherapy. Hypothermia results from exposure to lights, subsequent radiation, and convection losses.	
■ Check axillary temperature with readings on servocontrolled unit on incubator. Regulate incubator temperature as needed.	■ Hyperthermia may result from the increased environmental heat. Additional heat from phototherapy lights frequently causes a rise in the baby's and incubator's temperatures. Fluctuations in temperature may occur in response to radiation and convection.	

Nursing Care Plan The Newborn with Hyperbilirubinemia—continued

Intervention	Rationale	Expected Outcome

4. Nursing Diagnosis: *Parenting, Risk for Impaired,* related to deficient knowledge of infant care and prolonged separation of infant and parents secondary to illness (NANDA-I © 2012)

NIC Priority Intervention:
Teaching: Infant care: instruction on nurturing and physical care needed during the first year of life

NOC Suggested Outcome:
Parenting: Provision of an environment that promotes optimum growth and development of dependent children

Goal: The parents will bond with infant and have realistic expectations about their infant. Parents will be comfortable taking their infant home. They will be able to demonstrate normal infant care and assessments of possible complications, and they will know when to return for follow-up.

- Encourage parents to provide tactile stimulation during feeding and diaper changes.
- Encourage cuddling and eye contact during feedings.
- Offer suggestions to comfort restless infant:
  1. Nesting when beneath bili lights
  2. Talking softly and singing quietly to infant
  3. Taped music or tape recording of evening activities from home
  4. Rhythmic patting of buttocks
  5. Firm, nonstroking touch, assisting with control of extremities
  6. Pacifier for nonnutritive sucking

- Encourage family/friend support of mother/parents (e.g., meals, rest, child care for siblings, allow expressions of concerns/feelings).

- Evaluate additional psychosocial needs.

- Discuss rationale for treatment and possible side effects of phototherapy with family (stool changes, increased fluid loss, possible temp instability, slight lethargy, rash, altered sleep–wake patterns). Instruct family on infant's care while undergoing phototherapy:
  1. Safety precautions—bili mask, incubator door closed and latched, covering genitalia per policy if under banks of phototherapy lights.
  2. Skin care, cord care, circumcision care as appropriate.
  3. Lab draws, rationale for intake and output.

- Encourage parent/significant other/sibling involvement in infant care as possible.
- Evaluate family's understanding of information.
- Give explanation of equipment being used and changes in bilirubin levels. Allow parents an opportunity to ask questions; reinforce or clarify information as needed.

- Newborn has normal needs for tactile stimulation.
- Provides opportunity for parents to bond with their newborn.
- Provides comfort and decreases sensory deprivation. Presence of equipment may discourage parents from interacting with newborn.

- Decreases strain on mother/parents by assisting with other responsibilities and allows for additional time with newborn for bonding, care, etc.
- Parents may not understand what is happening or why.

- Physician preference of treatment modalities may vary. Parents may not understand why their newborn is not receiving a treatment that another with the same condition is receiving.

- Parents will demonstrate ability to perform basic infant care tasks as evidenced by exhibiting appropriate attachment behaviors (e.g., talking to and holding infant), feeding infant, and caring for infant under home bili therapy.

- Parents will verbalize understanding of rationale and possible side effects from phototherapy; parents/family members will demonstrate safety precautions when caring for infant; parents will get meals and rest; parents will verbalize support given.

(continued)

Nursing Care Plan   The Newborn with Hyperbilirubinemia—continued

Intervention	Rationale	Expected Outcome
■ As necessary, review role of pumping breasts and offering formula for limited time. ■ Assist mother to pump her breasts to maintain milk supply.	■ The etiology of breast milk jaundice remains uncertain. The serum bilirubin levels begin to fall within 48 hr after discontinuation of breastfeeding. Opinion of physicians varies regarding the need for discontinuing breastfeeding. ■ If breastfeeding is temporarily discontinued, assess mother's knowledge of pumping her breasts and provide information and support as needed.	

(see Figure 28–9 and Skill 5–7 in the *Clinical Skills Manual* SKILLS). Conventional phototherapy is discontinued and the eye patches are removed at least once per shift to assess the eyes for conjunctivitis. Patches are also removed to allow eye contact during feeding (social stimulation) or when parents are visiting (to promote parental attachment).

Some parents may feel guilty about their baby's condition and think they have caused the problem. Under stress, parents may not be able to understand the physician's first explanations. Expect that the parents will need explanations repeated and clarified and that they may need help in voicing their questions and fears. Eye and tactile contact with the newborn are encouraged. Coach parents when they visit with the baby. After the mother's discharge, parents are kept informed of their infant's condition and are encouraged to return to the hospital or telephone at any time so that they can be fully involved in the care of their infant. Parents are advised that after discontinuation of phototherapy, a rebound of 1 to 2 mg/dL can be expected and a follow-up bilirubin test may be done (Cloherty et al., 2012).

Clinical Tip

If the area of jaundice around the eyes begins to disappear, it is probable that the eye patches are allowing light to enter and better eye protection is needed.

While the mother is still hospitalized, phototherapy can also be carried out in the parents' room if the only problem is hyperbilirubinemia and the parents agree to do the following:

■ Keep the baby in the room for 24 hours a day.

■ Take emergency action (e.g., for choking) if necessary.

■ Complete instruction checklists.

■ Sign a consent form per agency protocol.

Instruct the parents but also continue to monitor the infant's temperature, activity, intake and output, and positioning of eye patches (if conventional light banks are used) at regular intervals.

Community-Based Nursing Care

Some studies have shown that the early discharge of newborns and their mothers comes with an increase in hospital readmissions and an elevated risk of pathologic hyperbilirubinemia. Home phototherapy use is recommended only if the bilirubin level is plotted on the nomogram and found to be in the "optional phototherapy" range. Any newborn with a level in the higher range should be hospitalized for continual phototherapy and serum bilirubin levels closely monitored on a regular schedule.

Jaundice and its treatment can be disturbing to parents and may generate feelings of guilt and fear. Reassurance and support are vital, especially for the breastfeeding mother, who may question her ability to adequately nourish her newborn.

It is essential that the impact of cultural beliefs be considered. Some Latina women believe that showing strong maternal emotions during pregnancy and breastfeeding can be detrimental. Some Latina women may blame "bilis" associated with maternal anger for the jaundice. Cultural beliefs lead mothers to interpret illness within their cultural framework, especially when left without clear and understood explanations. The parents' perception of and/or

● **Figure 28–9** Infant receiving phototherapy. The phototherapy light is positioned over the incubator. Bilateral eye patches are always used during photo light therapy to protect the baby's eyes.

Source: Courtesy of Lisa Smith-Pedersen, RNC, MSN, NNP-BC.

misconceptions about jaundice can affect parent–infant interactions. Explain the causes of jaundice and emphasize that it is usually a transient problem and one to which all infants must adapt after birth.

If the baby is to receive phototherapy at home, teach the parents to record the infant's temperature, weight, fluid I&O, stools, and feedings and to use the phototherapy equipment. In addition, if banks of conventional phototherapy lights are being used, parents must agree that the baby will be exposed to the lights for long periods of time; that they will hold the baby for only short periods for feeding, comforting, and cleansing of the perineal area; and that the room temperature will be regulated to minimize heat loss. The best method of home phototherapy depends on the cause of the hyperbilirubinemia and the rate of progression of the jaundice. A combination of phototherapy lights and fiber-optic mattress may be used (Figure 28–10 ●). Ongoing monitoring of bilirubin levels is essential with home phototherapy and can be carried out in the home, in the follow-up clinic, or in the clinician's office.

● **Figure 28–10** Newborn on fiber-optic "bili" mattress and under phototherapy lights. A combination of fiber-optic light source mattress and standard phototherapy light source above may also be used.

Note: The color is distorted because of the reflection of the bili light mattress.

Source: George Dodson/Lightworks Studio/Pearson Education.

Clinical Reasoning Suspected Hyperbilirubinemia

Baby boy Martin is a term male infant born by vaginal delivery with vacuum assist. His mother has blood type O positive, and Baby Martin has blood type A positive. The baby has a normal complete blood count (CBC) with a hematocrit of 60%. While performing a physical examination on Baby Martin on day 2 of life, the nurse notes that he has a large cephalohematoma, an enlarged liver on palpation (hepatomegaly), and is clinically jaundiced. The nurse suspects that Baby Martin has hyperbilirubinemia and discusses her findings with the neonatal nurse practitioner who orders a total bilirubin level be drawn. Results indicate the level is 16 mg/dL. The decision is made to start this infant on phototherapy treatment. What risk factors and clinical findings does this infant have that predispose him to hyperbilirubinemia? How would the nurse explain Baby Martin's hyperbilirubinemia and subsequent treatment and nursing care to his mother?
See www.nursing.pearsonhighered.com for possible responses.

Evaluation

Expected outcomes of nursing care include the following:

- The newborn at risk for development of hyperbilirubinemia is identified, and action is taken to minimize the potential impact of hyperbilirubinemia.

- The baby does not have any corneal irritation or drainage, skin breakdown, or major fluctuations in temperature.

- Parents understand the rationale for, goal of, and expected outcome of therapy.

- Parents verbalize concerns about their baby's condition and identify how they can facilitate their baby's improvement.

CARE OF THE NEWBORN WITH ANEMIA

Neonatal anemia is often difficult to recognize by clinical evaluation alone. The hemoglobin concentration in a full-term newborn is 19.3 ± 2.2 g/dL, which is slightly higher than that in premature newborns (Manco-Johnson, Rodden, & Hays, 2011). The most common causes of neonatal anemia are blood loss (due to lab draws in preterm babies in the neonatal intensive care unit [NICU]), hemolysis/erythrocyte destruction, and impaired red blood cell (RBC) production.

Blood loss (hypovolemia) can also occur in utero from placental bleeding (placenta previa or abruptio placentae). Intrapartum blood loss may be fetomaternal, fetofetal, or the result of umbilical cord bleeding. Birth trauma to abdominal organs (adrenal hemorrhage) or the cranium (subgaleal bleed) may produce significant blood loss, and cerebral bleeding may occur because of hypoxia.

Excessive hemolysis of red blood cells is usually a result of blood group incompatibilities but may be caused by infections. The most common cause of impaired RBC production is a genetically transmitted deficiency in glucose-6-phosphate dehydrogenase (G-6-PD). Anemia and jaundice are the presenting signs.

A condition known as **physiologic anemia of infancy** exists as a result of the normal gradual drop in hemoglobin for the first 8 to 12 weeks of life or corresponds with the decline in fetal hemoglobin (Cloherty et al., 2012). Theoretically, the bone marrow stops production of RBCs in response to higher oxygen levels that result from breathing changes after birth. When the amount of hemoglobin decreases, reaching a nadir of 10 to 11 g/dL in the term infant and a nadir at 6 to 12 weeks and 7 to 9 g/dL in preterm infants at about 5 to 10 weeks of age, the bone marrow begins production of RBCs again, and the anemia disappears (Cloherty et al., 2012). This difference is because of several factors: the preterm infant's rapid growth rate, decreased iron stores, shortened RBC survival time, and an inadequate production of erythropoietin (EPO). Iatrogenic causes occur more often in preterm infants as their condition requires more laboratory assessment.

Clinical Therapy

Hematologic problems can be anticipated based on the pregnancy history and clinical manifestations. The age at which anemia is first noted is also of diagnostic value. Clinically, light-skinned anemic infants are very pale in the absence of other symptoms of shock and usually have abnormally low red blood cell counts. In acute blood loss, symptoms of shock such as pallor, low arterial blood pressure, and a decreasing hematocrit value may be present.

The initial laboratory workup should include hemoglobin and hematocrit measurements, reticulocyte count, examination of peripheral blood smear, direct Coombs' test of infant's blood, and examination of maternal blood smear for fetal erythrocytes (Kleihauer-Betke test). Mild or chronic anemia may be treated adequately with iron supplements alone or with iron-fortified formulas. In severe cases of anemia, transfusions with O-negative or typed and cross-matched irradiated packed red cells are the treatment of choice.

Management of anemia of prematurity includes treating the causative factor (e.g., antibiotics/antivirals used for infection, steroid therapy for disorders of erythrocyte production) and supplemental iron. Blood transfusions (dedicated units of blood) are kept to a minimum.

● **Figure 28–11** Term infant with suspected sepsis.
Source: Courtesy of Valentina Mescolotto.

Nursing Management

Assess the newborn for symptoms of anemia (pallor). If the blood loss is acute, the baby may exhibit signs of shock (a capillary filling time greater than 3 seconds, decreased pulses, tachycardia, low blood pressure). Report promptly any symptoms indicating anemia or shock. Continued observation is necessary to identify physiologic anemia as the preterm newborn grows. Try to prevent iron deficiency by limiting phlebotomy losses and recording blood loss in tenths of a milliliter. The total blood removed is assessed and replaced by transfusion when necessary or by starting iron therapy at 2 weeks of postnatal age. For long-term management, see *Normocytic Anemia* in Chapter 50 🔗.

CARE OF THE NEWBORN WITH INFECTION

Neonatal sepsis is a blood infection that occurs in an infant younger than 90 days old and is caused by organisms that do not cause significant disease in older children. Early-onset sepsis (EOS) is seen in the first week of life. Late-onset sepsis (LOS) occurs between days 8 and 89. The incidence of EOS is 1 to 2 per 1000 live births (0.1% to 0.2%) (Cloherty et al., 2012).

Nosocomial infections are infections acquired while a baby is in the neonatal intensive care unit (NICU). Methicillin-resistant *Staphylococcus aureus* (MRSA) and *Candida* are two of the most common pathogens causing hospital-acquired infections in the NICU population (Venkatesh, Adams, & Weisman, 2011). The general debilitation and underlying illnesses often associated with prematurity necessitate invasive procedures such as umbilical catheterization, intubation, resuscitation, ventilator support, monitoring, parenteral alimentation (especially lipid emulsions), and prior broad-spectrum antibiotic therapy.

However, even full-term infants are susceptible, because their immunologic systems are immature. Their immune systems lack the complex factors involved in effective phagocytosis and the ability to localize infection or to respond with a well-defined, recognizable inflammatory response. In addition, all

newborns lack IgM immunoglobin, which is necessary to protect against bacteria, because it does not cross the placenta (refer to Chapter 24 🔗 for immunologic adaptations in the newborn period). Figure 28–11 ● shows a term infant with suspected sepsis.

Most nosocomial infections in the NICU present as bacteremia/sepsis, urinary tract infections, meningitis, or pneumonia. Maternal antepartum infections such as rubella, toxoplasmosis, cytomegalic inclusion disease, and herpes may cause congenital infections and resulting disorders in the newborn. Intrapartum maternal infections, such as amnionitis, are sources of neonatal infection (see Chapter 16 🔗 for more detailed information). Passage through the birth canal and contact with the vaginal flora (β-hemolytic streptococci, herpes, *Listeria,* gonococci) expose the infant to infection (Table 28–3). With infection anywhere in the fetus or newborn, the adjacent tissues or organs are easily penetrated, and the blood–brain barrier is ineffective. Septicemia is more common in males, except for infections caused by Group B β-hemolytic streptococcus.

Gram-negative organisms (especially *Escherichia coli, Enterobacter, Proteus,* and *Klebsiella*) and the gram-positive organism β-hemolytic streptococcus are the most common causative agents. *Pseudomonas* is a common fomite contaminant of ventilator support and oxygen therapy equipment. Gram-positive bacteria, especially coagulase-negative staphylococci, are common pathogens in nosocomial bacteremias, pneumonias, and urinary tract infections. Other gram-positive bacteria frequently isolated are enterococci and *Staphylococcus aureus* (Cloherty et al., 2012). Protection of the newborn from infections starts prenatally and continues throughout pregnancy and birth.

Clinical Therapy

Cultures should be taken as soon after birth as possible for infants with a history of possible exposure to infection in utero (e.g., premature rupture of membranes [PROM] more than 24 hours before birth, questionable maternal history of infection, maternal fever/chorioamnionitis, or high-risk behavior such as multiple sexual partners or illicit drug use). Cultures are

Table 28–3	Maternally Transmitted Newborn Infections

Infection	Nursing Assessment	Planning and Implementation
GROUP B STREPTOCOCCUS		
1% to 2% colonized with 1 in 10 developing disease. Early onset—usually within hours of birth or within first week. Late onset—1 week to 3 months (Cloherty et al., 2012).	Severe respiratory distress (grunting and cyanosis). May become apneic or demonstrate symptoms of shock. Meconium-stained amniotic fluid seen at birth.	Early assessment of clinical signs necessary. Assist with x-ray examination—shows aspiration pneumonia or respiratory distress syndrome. Immediately obtain blood, gastric aspirate, external ear canal, and nasopharynx cultures. Administer antibiotics, usually aqueous penicillin or ampicillin combined with gentamicin, as soon as cultures are obtained. Early assessment and intervention are essential to survival.
CONGENITAL SYPHILIS		
Spirochetes (*Treponema pallidum*) cross placenta after 16th to 18th week of gestation. The more recent the maternal infection, the higher the likelihood of transmission. Most are asymptomatic at birth but develop symptoms within first 3 months of life.	Check perinatal history for positive maternal serology. Assess infant for: Elevated cord serum IgM and FTA-ABS (fluorescent treponemal antibody absorbed) IgM Rhinitis (sniffles) Fissures on mouth corners and excoriated upper lip Red rash around mouth and anus Copper-colored rash over face, palms, and soles Irritability; generalized edema, particularly over joints; bone lesions; painful extremities, hepatosplenomegaly, jaundice, congenital cataracts, SGA, and failure to thrive.	Initiate standard precautions until infants have been on antibiotics for at least 24 hours. Administer penicillin. Initiate referral to evaluate for blindness, deafness, learning or behavioral problems. Provide emotional support for parents because of their feelings about mode of transmission and potential long-term sequelae.
GONORRHEA		
Approximately 30% to 35% of newborns born vaginally to infected mothers acquire the infection.	Assess infant for: Ophthalmia neonatorum (conjunctivitis) Purulent discharge and corneal ulcerations Neonatal sepsis with temperature instability, poor feeding response, and/or hypotonia, jaundice	Administer prophylaxis ophthalmic antibiotic ointment (see *Drug Guide: Erythromycin Ophthalmic Ointment [Ilotycin Ophthalmic]* on page 588 in Chapter 26 🔗) or tetracycline. If positive maternal test, give single-dose systemic antibiotic therapy. Initiate follow-up referral to evaluate any loss of vision.
HERPES TYPE 2		
Usually transmitted during vaginal birth; a few cases of in utero transmission have been reported.	Check perinatal history for active herpes genital lesions. Small cluster vesicular skin lesions over all the body about 6 to 9 days of life. Disseminated form—pneumonia, DIC, hepatitis with jaundice, hepatosplenomegaly, and neurologic abnormalities. Without skin lesions, assess for fever or subnormal temperature, respiratory congestion, tachypnea, and tachycardia.	Carry out careful handwashing and contact precautions (gown and glove isolation with linen precautions). Obtain skin, eye, and mucocutaneous membrane lesions and cerebrospinal fluid (CSF) cultures to identify herpes virus type 2 antigen-specific antibodies in serum. Cultures positive in 24 to 48 hours after birth. Administer intravenous acyclovir. Make a follow-up referral to evaluate potential sequelae of microcephaly, spasticity, seizures, deafness, or blindness. Encourage parental rooming-in and touching of their newborn. Show parents appropriate handwashing procedures and precautions to be used at home if mother's lesions are active.

(*continued*)

Table 28–3   Maternally Transmitted Newborn Infections—continued

Infection	Nursing Assessment	Planning and Implementation
CYTOMEGALOVIRUS (CMV)		
Most common cause of congenital infection in the United States—approximately 1% of all newborn infants (Cloherty et al., 2012). Transmission occurs in utero, during labor, or may happen postnatally through breast milk.	Congenital CMV disease, including intrauterine growth restriction, jaundice, hepatosplenomegaly, petechiae or purpura (blueberry muffin spots), thrombocytopenia, and pneumonia. CNS manifestations are very common and include lethargy and poor feeding, hypertonia or hypotonia, microcephaly, intracranial calcifications, chorioretinitis, and sensorineural deafness.	Diagnosis of congenital CMV infection is established by isolating virus from urine, saliva, or tissue obtained during the first 3 weeks of life. All infants in whom the diagnosis is suspected should have a viral culture performed; a CT scan of the brain is particularly important to document the extent of CNS involvement; eye exam and hearing test; close long-term follow-up evaluating for developmental effects.
ORAL CANDIDAL INFECTION (THRUSH)		
Acquired during passage through birth canal.	Assess newborn's buccal mucosa, tongue, gums, and inside the cheeks for white plaques (seen 5 to 7 days of age). Check diaper area for bright red, well-demarcated eruptions. Assess for thrush periodically when newborn is on long-term antibiotic therapy.	Differentiate white plaque areas from milk curds by using cotton-tipped applicator (if it is thrush, removal of white areas causes raw, bleeding areas). Maintain cleanliness of hands, linen, clothing, diapers, and feeding apparatus. Instruct breastfeeding mothers on treating their nipples with nystatin. Administer nystatin swabbed on oral lesions 1 hour after feeding or nystatin instilled in baby's oral cavity and on mucosa. Swab skin lesions with topical nystatin.
CHLAMYDIA TRACHOMATIS		
Acquired during passage through birth canal.	Assess for perinatal history of preterm birth. Symptomatic newborns present with conjunctivitis and pneumonia. Chlamydial conjunctivitis presents with inflammation, yellow discharge, and eyelid swelling 5 to 14 days after birth. Chronic follicular conjunctivitis (corneal neovascularization and conjunctival scarring).	Treat chlamydial conjunctivitis or pneumonia with oral erythromycin for 14 days (Cloherty et al., 2012). Monitor for hypertrophic pyloric stenosis. Initiate follow-up referral for eye complications and late development of pneumonia at 4 to 11 weeks postnatally.

Health Promotion Preventing Newborn Infections

The following measures will help to prevent newborn infections.

During the prenatal period:
- Conduct maternal screening for sexually transmitted infections.
- Monitor rubella titers in women who test negative.

During the intrapartum period:
- Sterile technique is essential.
- Visual exam of any lesions should be reported on the labor and birth record to identify a patient with herpes.
- Placenta and amniotic fluid cultures are obtained if amnionitis is suspected.
- Prophylactic antibiotic therapy for asymptomatic women who test positive for Group B streptococcus (GBS) helps prevent early-onset sepsis (Venkatesh et al., 2011).

During the postpartum period:
- Local eye treatment with an antibiotic ophthalmic ointment is given to all newborns to prevent damage from gonococcal infections (occurring 3 days following birth).
- Possibility of chlamydial infection (occurring 7 to 10 days after birth).

obtained before antibiotic therapy is begun (Polin & Committee on Fetus and Newborn, 2012).

1. Anaerobic and aerobic blood cultures are taken from a peripheral site rather than an umbilical vessel, because catheters have yielded false-positive results caused by contamination. The skin is prepared by cleaning with a unit antiseptic solution and allowed to dry; the specimen is obtained with a sterile needle and syringe to lessen the likelihood of contamination. One milliliter of blood is recommended for each culture; do not divide between anaerobic and aerobic bottles.

2. Spinal fluid culture is done following a spinal tap/lumbar puncture if there are concerns about late-onset sepsis (LOS) or CNS symptoms/pathology. The fluid can be analyzed for culture and Gram stain as well as for glucose, protein, and white blood cell (WBC) count (Cloherty et al., 2012).

3. The specimen for urine culture is best obtained by a suprapubic bladder aspiration or sterile catheterization but should not be used in sepsis workup in early-onset sepsis (EOS).

4. Skin cultures are taken of any lesions or drainage from lesions or reddened areas.

5. Tracheal aspirate cultures are taken if they can be obtained immediately after intubation.

Other laboratory investigations include a complete blood count (CBC), C-reactive protein (CRP), chest x-ray examination, serology, and Gram stains of cerebrospinal fluid, urine, skin exudate, and umbilicus. White blood cell (WBC) count with differential may indicate the presence or absence of sepsis. A level of 30,000 to 40,000 mm³ WBCs may be normal in the first 24 hours of life, whereas low WBC (less than 5000 to 7500/mm) may indicate sepsis. A low neutrophil count and a high band (immature white blood cells) count indicate that an infection is present. Stomach aspirate should be sent for culture and smear if a gonococcal infection or amnionitis is suspected. The C-reactive protein, an acute-phase reactant protein, may be helpful in watching for improvement once antibiotic therapy is initiated.

Serum IgM levels are elevated (normal level less than 20 mg/dL) in response to transplacental infections (Blackburn, 2013). If available, counterimmunoelectrophoresis tests for specific bacterial antigens are performed. In the future repetitive sequence-based polymerase chain reactions (rep-PCRs) will be used to identify specific infectious organisms within hours instead of days (Cloherty et al., 2012). Evidence of congenital infections may be seen on skull x-ray films for cerebral calcifications (cytomegalovirus, toxoplasmosis), on bone x-ray films (syphilis, cytomegalovirus), and in serum-specific IgM levels (rubella). Cytomegalovirus infection is best diagnosed by urine culture.

Because neonatal infection causes high mortality, therapy is instituted before results of the septic workup are obtained. A combination of two broad-spectrum antibiotics, such as ampicillin and gentamicin, is given in large doses but only until a culture with sensitivities is obtained.

After the pathogen and its sensitivities have been determined, appropriate specific antibiotic therapy is begun. New kanamycin-resistant enterobacteria and penicillin-resistant staphylococcus necessitate increasing use of gentamicin. Rotating aminoglycosides has been suggested to prevent development of resistance. In treating EOS, use of cephalosporins and, in particular, cefotaxime should be restricted (Polin & Committee of Fetus and Newborn, 2012). Duration of therapy varies from 7 to 14 days (Table 28–4). If cultures are negative and symptoms subside, antibiotics may be discontinued after 2 days/48 hours

Table 28–4	Neonatal Sepsis Antibiotic Therapy			
Drug	**Dose (mg/kg) Total Daily Dose**	**Schedule for Divided Doses**	**Route**	**Comments**
Acyclovir (Zovirax)	20 mg/kg	Every 8 hours	IV	Length of treatment is 14 days for skin/eye/mouth (SEM) or 21 days for CNS and disseminated disease: Herpes.
Ampicillin	50 to 100 mg/kg	Every 12 hours* Every 8 hours† Every 6 hours**	IM or IV	Effective against gram-positive microorganisms, *Haemophilus influenzae*, and most *Escherichia coli* strains. Higher doses indicated for meningitis. Used with aminoglycoside for synergy.
Cefotaxime	50 mg/kg 100 to 150 mg/kg/day	Every 12 hours* Every 6 hours** Every 8 hours†	IM or IV	Active against most major pathogens in infants; is best used against gram-negative meningitis; achieves CSF bactericidal activity; lack of ototoxicity and nephrotoxicity; wide therapeutic index (levels not required); resistant organisms can develop rapidly if used extensively; ineffective against *Pseudomonas, Listeria.*
Gentamicin	2.5 to 3 mg/kg 5 to 7.5 mg/kg/day 4 to 5 mg/kg/dose (first week of life)	Every 12 to 24 hours*‡ Every 8 to 24 hours† Every 24 to 48 hours‡***	IM or IV	Effective against gram-negative rods and staphylococci; may be used instead of kanamycin against penicillin-resistant staphylococci and *E. coli* strains and *Pseudomonas aeruginosa*. May cause ototoxicity and nephrotoxicity. Need to follow serum levels. Must never be given as IV push. Must be given over at least 30 to 60 minutes. In presence of oliguria or anuria, dose must be decreased or discontinued. In infants less than 1000 g or 29 weeks, lower dosage 2.5–3 mg/kg/day. Monitor serum levels before administration of second dose. Peak: 5–12 mcg/mL. Trough: 0.5–1 mcg/mL.
Vancomycin	10 to 20 mg/kg 30 mg/kg/day	Every 12 to 24 hours*‡ Every 8 hours†	IV	Effective for methicillin-resistant strains (*Staphylococcus epidermis*); must be administered by slow intravenous infusion to avoid prolonged cutaneous eruption. In infants less than 1000 g or 29 weeks, lower dosage to 2.5–3 mg/kg/day. Nephrotoxic, especially in combination with aminoglycosides. Slow IV infusion over at least 60 minutes. Peak: 25–40 mcg/mL. Trough: 5–10 mcg/mL.

*Up to 7 days of age. ** >45 weeks postmenstrual age. †Greater than 7 days of age. ‡ Dependent on GA. ***Dependent on postnatal age.

of negative blood cultures. A normal CRP at 48 hours also supports discontinuing antibiotics if blood cultures are negative.

NURSING MANAGEMENT *For the Newborn with Infection*

Nursing Assessment and Diagnosis

Symptoms of infection are most often noticed by the nurse during daily care of the newborn. The infant may deteriorate rapidly in the first 12 to 24 hours after birth if β-hemolytic streptococcal infection is present, with signs and symptoms mimicking RDS. In other cases, the onset of sepsis may be gradual, with more subtle signs and symptoms. The most common signs observed include the following:

- Subtle behavioral changes; the infant "is not doing well" and is often lethargic or irritable (especially after the first 24 hours) and hypotonic; color changes may include pallor, duskiness, cyanosis, or a "shocky" appearance; skin is cool and clammy
- Temperature instability, manifested by either hypothermia (recognized by a decrease in skin temperature) or, rarely in newborns, hyperthermia (elevation of skin temperature), necessitating a corresponding increase or decrease in incubator temperature to maintain a neutral thermal environment
- Feeding intolerance, as evidenced by a decrease in total intake, abdominal distention, vomiting, poor sucking, lack of interest in feeding, and diarrhea
- Jaundice, petechial hemorrhages, hepatosplenomegaly
- Tachycardia initially, followed by spells of apnea or bradycardia

Other signs and symptoms may suggest central nervous system (CNS) disease such as jitteriness, tremors, or seizure activity. A differential diagnosis is necessary because of the similarity of symptoms to other more specific conditions.

Nursing diagnoses that may apply to the infant with sepsis neonatorum and the family include the following (NANDA-I © 2012):

- *Infection, Risk for,* related to newborn's immature immunologic system
- *Fluid Volume, Deficient,* related to feeding intolerance
- *Coping: Family, Compromised,* related to present illness resulting in prolonged hospital stay for the newborn

Planning and Implementation

In the nursery, environmental control and prevention of acquired infection are the responsibilities of the neonatal nurse. An infected newborn can be isolated effectively in an isolette and receive close observation. It is important to promote strict hand washing technique for all who enter the nursery, including nursing colleagues; physicians; laboratory, x-ray, and respiratory therapists; and parents. Visits by unnecessary personnel should be discouraged. Be prepared to assist in the aseptic collection of specimens for laboratory investigations. Scrupulous care of equipment—changing and cleaning of incubators at least every 7 days, removing and sterilizing wet equipment every 24 hours, preventing cross use of linen and equipment, cleaning sinkside equipment such as soap containers periodically, and taking special care with the open radiant warmers (access without prior hand washing is much more likely than with the closed incubator)—will prevent contamination.

Provision of Antibiotic Therapy

Administer antibiotics as ordered by the nurse practitioner or physician. It is your responsibility to be knowledgeable about the following:

- The proper dose to be administered, based on the weight of the newborn and desired peak and trough levels
- The appropriate route of administration, because some antibiotics cannot be given intravenously
- Admixture incompatibilities, because some antibiotics are precipitated by intravenous solutions or by other antibiotics
- Side effects and toxicity

For term infants being treated for infections, neonatal home infusion of antibiotics should be considered as a viable alternative to continued hospitalization. The infusion of antibiotics at home by skilled RNs facilitates parent–infant bonding while meeting the infant's ongoing healthcare needs.

Provision of Supportive Care

In addition to antibiotic therapy, physiologic supportive care is essential in caring for a septic infant. The following care measures should be carried out:

- Observe for resolution of symptoms or development of other symptoms of sepsis.
- Maintain neutral thermal environment with accurate regulation of humidity and oxygen administration.
- Provide respiratory support: administer oxygen, use pulse oximetry, observe and monitor respiratory effort.
- Provide cardiovascular support: observe and monitor pulse and blood pressure; observe for hyperbilirubinemia, anemia, and hemorrhagic symptoms.
- Provide adequate calories, because oral feedings may be discontinued because of increased mucus, abdominal distention, vomiting, and aspiration.
- Provide fluids and electrolytes to maintain homeostasis; monitor weight changes, urine output, and urine specific gravity.
- Observe for the development of hypoglycemia, hyperglycemia, acidosis, hyponatremia, and hypocalcemia.

Restricting parental visits has not been shown to have any effect on the rate of infection and may be harmful for the newborn's psychologic development. With instruction and guidance, both parents should be allowed to handle the baby and participate in daily care. Support of the parents is crucial. They need to be informed of the newborn's prognosis as treatment continues and to be involved in care as much as possible. They also need to understand how infection is transmitted.

Evaluation

Expected outcomes of nursing care include the following:

- The risks for development of sepsis are identified early, and immediate action is taken to minimize the development of the illness.

- Appropriate use of aseptic technique protects the newborn from further exposure to illness.

- The baby's symptoms are relieved, and the infection is treated.

- The parents verbalize concerns about their baby's illness and understand the rationale behind the management of their newborn.

CARE OF THE FAMILY WITH BIRTH OF AN AT-RISK NEWBORN

The birth of a preterm or ill infant or an infant with a congenital anomaly is a serious crisis for a family. Throughout the pregnancy, both parents, together and separately, have felt excitement, experienced thoughts of acceptance, and pictured what their baby would look like. Both parents have wished for a perfect baby and feared an unhealthy one. Each parent and family member must accept and adjust when the fantasized fears become reality.

Parental Responses

Family members have acute grief reactions to the loss of the idealized baby they have envisioned. In a preterm birth, the mother is denied the last few weeks of pregnancy that seem to prepare her psychologically for the stress of birth and the attachment process. Attachment at this time is fragile, and interruption of the process by separation can affect the future mother–child relationship. Parents express grief as shock and disbelief, denial of reality, anger toward self and others, guilt, blame, and concern for the future. Self-esteem and feelings of self-worth are jeopardized.

Feelings of guilt and failure often plague mothers of preterm newborns. Guilt fantasies may lead her to wonder what she might have done to cause the early labor. She might ask herself questions such as "Why did labor start?" "What did I do (or not do)?" "Was it because I had sexual intercourse with my husband (a week, 3 days, a day) ago?" "Was it because I carried three loads of laundry up from the basement?" "Am I being punished for something done in the past—even in childhood?"

The period of waiting between suspicion and confirmation of abnormality or dysfunction is a very anxious one for parents because it is difficult, if not impossible, to begin attachment to the infant if the newborn's future is questionable. During the waiting period, parents need support and acknowledgment that this is an anxious time. They must be kept informed about tests and efforts to gather additional data, as well as efforts to improve their baby's outcome. It is helpful to tell both parents about the problem at the same time, with the baby present. An honest discussion of the problem and anticipatory management at the earliest possible time by health professionals help the parents (1) maintain trust in the physician and nurse, (2) appreciate the reality of the situation by dispelling fantasy and misconception, (3) begin the grieving process, and (4) mobilize internal and external support.

Nurses need to be aware that anger is a universal response by parents to a preterm birth. It is best that the parents direct it outward because holding it in check requires great energy, which is then diverted away from grieving and physical recovery from pregnancy and giving birth. Anger may be directed at the physician and/or nurse, at the food, at nursing care, or at hospital regulations and routines (Discenza, 2012). Parents rarely show anger with the baby; such responses can precipitate guilt feelings. Perceived maternal stress may be lessened and the mother empowered if information is provided regarding preterm behavioral cues. This empowers the mother and allows her to better care for her child. The mother of a preterm baby who has to spend time in a neonatal intensive care unit (NICU) suffers from psychologic distress similar to posttraumatic stress disorder (PTSD). The nurse working with a mother in the NICU setting has the opportunity to encourage maternal competence and confidence, both during and after hospitalization, by teaching interpretation of her infant's behavioral cues, prompting maternal care of the baby while in the NICU, and facilitating expression of her feelings (for more detailed discussion of PTSD see Chapter 31 🔴). The father also may suffer from depression both before and after the birth of the child, adding to the discord in the family unit and compounding the perceived stress experienced by the mother.

A variety of behavioral patterns may occur. For example, one or more members of the family may make a scapegoat of the child. Another may become the youngster's champion to the exclusion of others. One or the other parent may feel pushed aside or denied attention, and thus may withdraw or leave the family unit. Parents or siblings may feel that their own needs (schooling, material goods, freedom of movement) are being set aside when all assets (financial and other) go to support the one child's needs. There may also be an increase in child abuse.

Although reactions and steps of attachment are altered by the birth of at-risk infants, a healthy parent–child relationship can occur. Kaplan and Mason (1974) have identified four psychologic tasks as essential for coping with the stress of an at-risk newborn and for providing a basis for the maternal–infant relationship:

1. Anticipatory grief as a psychologic preparation for possible loss of the child while still hoping for his or her survival

2. Acknowledgment of maternal failure to produce a term or perfect newborn expressed as anticipatory grief and depression and lasting until the chances of survival seem secure

3. Resumption of the process of relating to the infant may be impaired by continuous threat of death or abnormality, and the mother may be slow in her response of hope for the infant's survival

4. Understanding of the special needs and growth patterns of the at-risk newborn, which are temporary and yield to normal patterns

Developmental Consequences

The baby who is born prematurely, is ill, or has a malformation or disorder is at risk for emotional, intellectual, and cognitive developmental delays. The risk is directly proportional to the seriousness of the problem and the length of treatment. Necessary physical separation of family and infant and the tremendous emotional and financial burdens may adversely affect the parent–child relationship. The recent trend to involve the parents with their newborn early, repeatedly, and over protracted periods of time has done much to facilitate positive parent–child relationships.

Parents must have a clear picture of the reality of the handicap and the types of developmental hurdles ahead. Unexpected behaviors and responses from the baby because of his or her defect or disorder can be upsetting and frightening. The demands of care for the child and disputes regarding management of behavior stress family relationships. The entire collaborative care team may need to pool their resources and expertise to help parents of children born with problems or disorders so that both parents and children can thrive.

NURSING MANAGEMENT *For the Family of an At-Risk Newborn*

Nursing Assessment and Diagnosis

A concurrent illness of the mother or other family members or other concurrent stress (lack of health insurance, loss of job, age of parents) may alter the family response to the baby. Feelings of apprehension, guilt, failure, and grief expressed verbally or nonverbally are important aspects of the nursing history. Appropriate nursing observations gathered through continuing contact and development of a therapeutic family relationship let all professionals understand and use the nursing history to provide continuous individual care. Visiting and caregiving patterns indicate the level of parental attachment or lack thereof.

A record of visits, caretaking procedures, affect (in relating to the newborn), and telephone calls indicate the level of parental attachment. Serial observations, rather than just isolated observations that cause concern, must be obtained. Grant (1978) has developed a conceptual framework depicting adaptive and maladaptive responses to parenting of an infant with an actual or potential problem (Table 28–5).

If a pattern of distancing behaviors evolves, the nurse should institute appropriate interventions. Follow-up studies have found that a statistically significant number of preterm, sick, and congenitally defective infants suffer from failure to thrive, battering, or other parenting disorders (Grant, 1978). Early detection and intervention will prevent these aberrations in parenting behaviors from leading to irreparable damage or death.

Nursing diagnoses that may apply to the family of a newborn at risk include the following (NANDA-I © 2012):

- *Grieving, Complicated,* related to loss of idealized newborn
- *Fear* related to emotional involvement with an at-risk newborn
- *Parenting, Impaired,* related to impaired bonding secondary to feelings of inadequacy about caretaking activities

---

Table 28–5	Adaptive and Nonadaptive Parental Responses to an Infant's Health Crisis

Parental tasks at this time include:

- Understanding the infant's medical condition and needs
- Adapting to the NICU environment
- Assuming the main caretaking role
- Taking responsibility for the infant after discharge
- Coping with the death of the infant

ADAPTIVE RESPONSES	NONADAPTIVE RESPONSES
- Frequent visits to infant and calls to the unit	- Failure to visit infant or communicate with unit
- Emotional involvement with infant	- Emotional withdrawal from infant
- Positive interaction with infant during hospitalization	- Lack of interaction with infant during hospitalization
- Eagerness to assume caretaking during infant's hospitalization	- Resistance to providing care of the infant during hospitalization
- Increasing sense of parental competence	- Lack of a sense of parental competence
- Growing attachment to infant	- Failure to achieve attachment to infant
- Realistic interpretation of medical information	- Inability to understand or accept medical information
- Acceptance of infant's condition	- Unhealthy preoccupation with infant's condition
- Understanding of the causes of infant's condition	- Blaming others for infant's condition
- Eagerness to assume total responsibility for infant	- Fear of going home with infant
- Realistic understanding of infant's needs at discharge	- Negative view of infant and his or her needs at discharge
- Open discussion of concerns and needs to staff and family	- Inability to discuss needs and concerns with staff and family
- Fair and realistic expectations of staff	- Distrustful and hostile attitude toward staff

POSITIVE OUTCOME	NEGATIVE OUTCOME
- Healthy parent–child relationship	- Poor parent–child relationship
- Marital and family equilibrium is maintained	- Failure to thrive
	- Vulnerable child syndrome
	- Marital and family equilibrium is compromised

Source: Adapted from Grant, P. (1978). *Family & community health.* Philadelphia, PA: Lippincott Williams & Wilkins.

Planning and Implementation

Hospital-Based Nursing Care

In their sensitive and vulnerable state, parents are acutely perceptive of others' responses and reactions (particularly nonverbal) to the child. Parents can be expected to identify with the responses of others. Nurses may feel uncomfortable, may not know what to say to parents, or may fear confronting their own feelings as well as those of the parents. Each nurse must work out personal reactions with instructors, peers, clergy, parents, or significant others. It is helpful to have a stockpile of therapeutic questions and statements to initiate meaningful dialogue with parents. Opening statements might include the following: "You must be wondering what could have caused this." "Are you thinking that you (or someone else) may have done something?" "How can I help?" and "Are you wondering how you are going to manage?" Avoid statements such as "I understand how you feel," "It could have been worse," "It's God's will," "You have other children," and "You are still young and can have more." This child is important now.

Support of Parents for Initial Viewing of the Newborn

Before parents see their child, prepare them for the visit. It is important to maintain a positive, realistic attitude regarding the infant. All infants exhibit strengths as well as deficiencies; prepare the parents to see both the deviations and the normal aspects of their infant. You may say, "Your baby is small, about the length of my two hands. She weighs 2 lb, 3 oz, but is very active and cries when we disturb her. She is having some difficulty breathing, but is breathing without assistance and is in only 35% oxygen and room air is 21%."

Describe the equipment being used for the at-risk newborn and its purpose before the parents enter the intensive care unit. Many NICUs have booklets for parents to read before entering the units. Through explanations and pictures, the parents are better prepared to deal with the feelings they may experience when they see their infant for the first time (Figure 28–12 ●).

Preparing the parents by having familiar healthcare professionals accompany them to the unit can be reassuring. The primary nurse and physician caring for the newborn need to be with the parents when they first visit their baby. Parental reactions vary, but initially there is usually an element of shock. Providing chairs and time to regain composure assists the parents. Slow, complete, and simple explanations—first about the infant and then about the equipment—allay fear and anxiety.

Concern about the infant's physical appearance is common yet may remain unvoiced. Parents may express concerns such as "He looks so small and red—like a drowned rat." "Why do her genitals look so abnormal?" and "Will that awful-looking mouth [cleft lip and palate] ever be normal?" Anticipate and address such questions. Use of pictures, such as of an infant after cleft lip repair, may be reassuring to doubting parents. Knowledge of the development of a "normal" preterm infant allows you to make reassuring statements such as "The baby's skin may look very red and transparent with lots of visible veins, but it is normal for her maturity. As she grows, subcutaneous fat will be laid down, and these superficial veins will become less visible."

The nursing staff sets the tone of the NICU. Nurses foster the development of a safe, trusting environment by viewing the parents as essential caregivers, not as visitors or nuisances in the unit. It is important to provide parents privacy when needed and

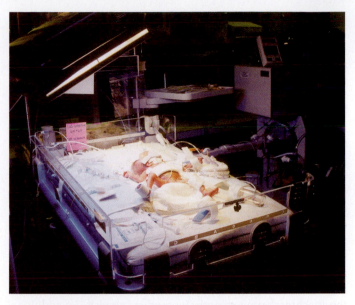

● **Figure 28–12** Preparing parents for first visit to at-risk newborn. This 25 weeks' gestational age infant with respiratory distress syndrome may be frightening for her parents to see for the first time because of the technology that is attached to her.
Source: Courtesy of Lisa Smith-Pedersen, RNC, MSN, NNP-BC.

easy access to staff and facilities. An uncrowded and welcoming atmosphere lets parents know "You are welcome here." However, even in crowded physical surroundings, nurses can convey an attitude of openness and trust. A trusting relationship is essential for collaborative efforts in caring for the infant. Work toward therapeutically using your own responses to relate to the parents on a one-to-one basis. Each individual has different needs, different ways of adapting to crisis, and different means of support. Use techniques that are real and spontaneous to them and avoid words or actions that are foreign to them. Gauge your interventions so that they match the parents' pace and needs.

Implementation of family-centered care, a team approach with healthcare professionals and the family, in which the parents, grandparents, and older siblings are vital members of the team, is important to bonding and the development of the family unit (Chinchilla, 2012). Show concern and support by planning time to spend with the parents, by being psychologically as well as physically present, by encouraging open discussion and grieving, by repetitious explanations (as necessary), by providing privacy as needed, and by encouraging contact with the newborn. Identifying and clarifying feelings and fears decrease distortions in perception, thinking, and feeling. Invest the baby with value in the eyes of the parents by providing meticulous care to the newborn, talk and coo (especially in the face-to-face position) while holding or providing care to the newborn, refer to the child by gender or name, and relate the newborn's activities ("He took a whole ounce of formula," "She took hold of the blanket and just wouldn't let go"). Also note the "normal" characteristics and capabilities of each newborn as well as the newborn's needs. Learn the baby's name and refer to him or her by name. When the baby is physiologically stable and of an appropriate weight, allowing the baby to be dressed in clothes has been determined to aid the mother in perceiving the baby as a "person" or "actual baby".

Facilitation of Attachment If Neonatal Transport Occurs

Transport to a regional referral center some distance from the parents may be necessary. It is essential for the mother to see and touch her infant before the infant is transported. Bring the mother to the nursery or take the infant in a warmed transport incubator to the mother's bedside to allow her to see the infant before transportation to the center. When the infant reaches the referral center, a staff member should call the parents with information about the infant's condition during transport, safe arrival at the center, and present condition.

Support of parents, with explanations from the professional staff, is crucial. Occasionally the mother may be unable to see the infant before transport (e.g., if she is still under general anesthesia or experiencing complications such as shock, hemorrhage, or seizures). In these cases, photograph the infant before transport. The picture should be given to the mother, along with an explanation of the infant's condition, present problems, and a detailed description of the infant's characteristics, to facilitate the attachment process until the mother can visit. An additional photograph is also helpful for the father to share with siblings or extended family. If the mother is hospitalized apart from the infant, the first person to visit the infant should relay information regarding the infant's care and condition to the mother and family. Since the mother has had minimal contact, if any, with her infant, she may mistrust all those who provide information (the father, nurse, physician, or extended family) until she sees the infant for herself. This can put tremendous stress on the relationship between spouses/partners. The parents (and family) should be given information together. This practice helps overcome misunderstandings and misinterpretations and promotes cooperative "working through" of problems.

With the increased attention on improved fetal outcome, prenatal maternal transports, rather than neonatal transports, are occurring more frequently. This practice gives the mother of an at-risk infant the opportunity to visit and care for her infant during the early postpartum period.

Promotion of Touching and Parental Caretaking

Parents visiting a preterm, small-for-gestational-age (SGA), or sick infant may need several visits to become comfortable and confident in their ability to touch the infant without injuring her or him. Barriers such as incubators, incisions, monitor electrodes, and tubes may delay the mother's development of comfort in touching the newborn.

Klaus and Kennell (1982) have demonstrated a significant difference in the amount of eye contact and touching behaviors of mothers of normal newborns and mothers of preterm infants. Whereas mothers of normal newborns progress within minutes to palm contact of the infant's trunk, mothers of preterm infants are slower to progress from fingertip to palm contact and from the extremities to the trunk. The progression to palm contact with the infant's trunk may take several visits to the nursery.

Use support, reassurance, and encouragement to help the mother develop positive feelings about her ability and importance to her infant. Touching facilitates "getting to know" the infant and thus establishes a bond with the infant. Touching and seeing the infant help the mother realize the "normals" and potential of her baby (Figure 28–13 ●).

● **Figure 28–13** Beginnings of attachment. Mother of this 26-week-gestational-age 600-g baby begins attachment through fingertip touch.
Source: Courtesy of Lisa Smith-Pedersen, RNC, MSN, NNP-BC.

The nurse can also encourage parents to meet their newborn's need for stimulation. Stroking, rocking, cuddling, singing, and talking should be an integral part of the parents' caretaking responsibilities. Bonding can be facilitated by encouraging parents to visit and become involved in their baby's care (Figure 28–14 ●). When visiting is impossible, the parents should feel free to phone when they wish to receive information about their baby. A nurse's warm, receptive attitude provides support. Facilitate parenting by personalizing a baby to the parents, by referring to the infant by name, or relating personal behavioral characteristics. Remarks such as "Jenny loves her pacifier" help make the infant seem individual and unique.

The variety of equipment needed for life support is hardly conducive to anxiety-free caretaking by the parents. However,

● **Figure 28–14** Facilitating bonding. This mother of a 31-week-gestational-age infant with respiratory distress syndrome is spending time with her newborn and meeting the baby's need for cuddling.
Source: Courtesy of Lisa Smith-Pedersen, RNC, MSN, NNP-BC.

even the sickest infant may be cared for, if only in a small way, by the parents. Demonstration and explanation, followed by support of the parents in initial caretaking behaviors, positively reinforce parents' sense of success. Changing their infant's diaper, providing skin or oral care, or helping the nurse turn the infant may at first provoke anxiety, but the parents will become more comfortable and confident in caretaking and feel satisfied by the baby's reactions and their ability "to do something." Complimenting the parents' competence in caretaking also increases their self-esteem, which has received recent "blows" of guilt and failure. *Never give the parents a task that they might not be able to accomplish.* Cues that the parents are ready to become involved with the child's care include their reference to the baby by name and their questioning as to the amount of feeding taken, sleeping patterns, appearance today, and the like.

Often parents of high-risk infants have ambivalent feelings toward the nurse. These feelings may take the form of criticism of the care of the infant, manipulation of staff, or personal guilt. You should accept this behavior, but continue to remind the parents that it is okay and natural to feel disappointment, a sense of failure, helplessness, or anger about the birth. The overprotectiveness and overoptimism are defense mechanisms. To deny the negative feelings only entrenches them further, delays their resolution, and delays realistic planning. Instead of fostering (by silence), you need to intervene appropriately to enhance parent–infant attachment. Learn to deal with ambivalent feelings that contribute to a competitive atmosphere. For example, avoid making unfavorable comparisons between the baby's responses to parental and nursing caretaking. Verbalizations that improve parental self-esteem are essential and easily shared. You can point out that, in addition to physiologic use, breast milk is important because of the emotional investment of the mother. Pumping, storing, labeling, and delivering quantities of breast milk is a time-consuming "labor of love" for mothers. Positive remarks about breast milk reinforce the maternal behavior of caretaking and providing for her infant: "Breast milk is something that only you can give your baby," "You really have brought a lot of milk today," "Look how rich this breast milk is," or "Even small amounts of milk are important, and look how rich it is."

If the infant begins to gain weight while being fed breast milk, it is important to point this correlation out to the mother. Advise parents that initial weight loss with beginning nipple feedings is common because of the increased energy expended when the infant begins active rather than passive nutritional intake.

During a quiet time it may help to encourage the parents to talk about their hopes and fears and to facilitate their involvement in parent groups. Encourage parents to provide care for their infant even if the baby is very sick and likely to die. Detachment is easier after attachment, because the parents are comforted by the knowledge that they did all they could for their child while he or she was alive.

Facilitation of Family Adjustment During Crisis

During crisis, it is difficult to maintain interpersonal relationships. Yet in a newborn intensive care area, the parents are expected to relate to many different care providers. It is important that parents have as few professionals as possible relaying information to them. A primary nurse should coordinate care and provide continuity for parents. Care providers are individuals and thus will use different terms, inflections, and attitudes. These subtle differences are monumental to parents and may confuse, confound, and produce anxiety. The transfer of the baby from the NICU to a step-down unit or transport back to the home hospital provokes parental anxiety because they must now deal with new healthcare professionals. The nurse not only functions as a liaison between the parents and the various professionals interacting with the infant and parents but also offers clarification, explanation, interpretation of information, and support to the parents.

Encourage parents to deal with the crisis with help from their support system. The support system attempts to meet the emotional needs and to provide support for the family members in crisis and stress situations. Biologic kinship is not the only valid criterion for a support system; an emotional kinship is the most important factor. In our mobile society of isolated nuclear families, the support system may be a next-door neighbor, a best friend, or perhaps a schoolmate. Search out the significant others in the lives of the parents and help them understand the problems so that they can be a constant parental support.

The impact of the crisis on the family is individual and varied. To institute appropriate interventions, view the birth of any infant (normal newborn, preterm infant, infant with congenital anomaly) as defined by the family.

It is important to encourage open intrafamily communication. Discourage the family from keeping secrets from one another, especially between spouses/partners, because secrets undermine the trust of relationships. Well-meaning rationales such as "I want to protect her," "I don't want him to worry about it," and so on can be destructive to open communication and to the basic element of a relationship—trust.

The needs of siblings should not be overlooked. Siblings have been looking forward to the new baby, and they, too, suffer a degree of loss. Young children may react with hostility and older ones with shame at the birth of an infant with an anomaly. Both reactions may make siblings feel guilty. Parents, who may be preoccupied with working through their own feelings, often cannot give the other children the attention and support they need. Sometimes another child becomes the focus of family tension. Anxiety thus directed can take the form of finding fault or of overconcern. This is a form of denial; the parents cannot face the real worry—the infant at risk. After observing and assessing the situation, ensure that another family member or friend steps in to support the siblings of the affected baby.

Parents from minority cultures must deal with language barriers and cultural differences that can make feelings of isolation and uncertainty more acute. Healthcare providers have the professional responsibility to be aware of the cultural needs of all patients and to ensure those needs are met. Feelings of isolation and uncertainty influence not only the parent's emotional responses to the ill newborn, but also the utilization of services and their interaction with health professionals. Hospital cultural interpreter programs can assist families with interactions with staff, as well as provide translation during family meetings, collaborative care family conferences, and parent support groups.

Families with children in the NICU may become friends and support one another. To encourage the development of these friendships and to provide support, many units have established parent groups. The core of the groups consists of parents whose infants were once in the intensive care unit. Most groups make contact with families within a day or two of the infant's admission to the unit, through either phone calls or visits to the hospital. Early one-on-one parent contacts are more effective than discussion groups in helping families work through their feelings. This personalized method gives the grieving parents an opportunity to express personal feelings about the pregnancy, labor, and birth and their "different from expected" infant with others who have experienced the same feelings and with whom they can identify.

Community-Based Nursing Care

Predischarge planning begins once the infant's condition becomes stable and it seems likely the newborn will survive. These medically fragile infants remain vulnerable for several years (Holditch-Davis, Miles, Burchinal, et al., 2011). Discharge preparation and care conferences should involve a collaborative care team approach. The NICU nursing staff is the fulcrum for aiding in the transition of high-risk infants from the intensive care unit to the home. Effective open communication with the families during the entire discharge planning phase of care empowers the families to assume the role of primary caregiver for their children.

Adequate predischarge teaching helps parents transform any feelings of inadequacy they may have into feelings of self-assurance and attachment. From the beginning the parents should be taught about their infant's special needs and growth patterns. This teaching and involvement are best facilitated by a nurse who is familiar with the infant and his or her family over a period of time and who has developed a comfortable and supportive relationship with them.

Cobedding of twins is often used in the NICU to provide comfort, decrease stress to the twins, and provide a form of developmentally supportive care. Cobedding is also a strategy to maximize the synchronization of sleep–wake cycles (Gardner & Goldson, 2011). Parents of multiples may desire cobedding at home to allow for clustering of care and to facilitate the parents' ability to spend time with both of their children (Figure 28–15 ●). If twins or other multiples experienced cobedding in the NICU, discuss the advantages and disadvantages of continuing the practice at home. Currently, there is no evidence to establish cobedding of multiples outside the NICU as a safe or unsafe sleep practice (Gardner & Goldson, 2011).

SAFETY ALERT!

The high incidence of prematurity and low birth weight (LBW) in multiple-birth infants and the corresponding risks for sudden infant death syndrome (SIDS) should be considered. As with all families at discharge, parents of multiples should be taught SIDS risk-reduction practices, which include supine positioning, babies sleeping in parents' room, firm bedding surface, no loose coverings/items, and no barriers between infants.

Provide home care instructions in an optimal environment for parental learning. Learning should take place over time,

● **Figure 28–15** Cobedding of twins facilitates delivery of care and parent interaction with healthcare members. These twins were born at 33 weeks' gestation and required oxygen and gavage feeding while in the NICU.
Source: Courtesy of Lisa Smith-Pedersen, RNC, MSN, NNP-BC.

to avoid bombarding the parents with instructions in the day or hour before discharge. Parents often enjoy performing minimal caretaking tasks, with gradual expansion of their role. Many NICUs provide facilities for parents to room in with their infants for a few days before discharge. This allows parents a degree of independence in the care of their infant with the security of nursing help nearby. This practice is particularly helpful for anxious parents, parents who have not had the opportunity to spend extended time with their infant, or parents who will be giving complex physical care at home, such as gastrostomy feeding and medication administration (Lopez, Anderson, & Feutchinger, 2012; Schlittenhart, Smart, Miller, et al., 2012). According to Lopez et al. (2012), parents of NICU graduates do not feel adequately prepared for the transition from the NICU to home with their babies. Teaching that occurs with daily interaction of the NICU staff is not always perceived by the family as adequate, and the stress levels of the family while in the NICU can be a barrier to a learning environment.

Families interact with staff while gradually transitioning to sole caretakers of their medically complex high-risk infant. When discharging a medically fragile infant to home, schedule a predischarge home visit by a public health nurse or home health agency. This discharge visit evaluates the home for any possible issues that may complicate the parents' ability to care for their at-risk infant, especially if there are multiple monitoring equipment needs (AAP Committee on Fetus and Newborn, 2010). The basic elements of discharge and home care instruction are as follows:

1. Teach the parents routine well-baby care, such as bathing, taking a temperature, preparing formula, and breastfeeding.

2. Help parents learn to do special procedures as needed by the newborn, such as gavage or gastrostomy feedings, tracheostomy or enterostomy care, medication administration, CPR, and operation of the apnea monitor. Before discharge, the parents should be as comfortable as possible

with these tasks and should demonstrate independence. Written tools and instructions are useful for parents to refer to once they are home with the infant, but they should not replace actual participation in the infant's care.

3. Make sure that all applicable screening (metabolic, vision, hearing) tests, immunizations, and respiratory syncytial virus (RSV) prophylaxis are done before discharge and that all records are given to the primary care provider and parents.

4. Refer parents to community health and support organizations. The Visiting Nurse Association, public health nurses, or social services can assist the parents in the stressful transition from hospital to home by providing the necessary home teaching and support. Some NICUs have their own parent support groups to help bridge the gap between hospital and home care. Parents can also find support from a variety of community organizations, such as mothers-of-twins groups, March of Dimes Birth Defects Foundation, services for children with disabilities, and teen mother and child programs. Each community has numerous agencies capable of assisting the family in adapting emotionally, physically, and financially to the chronically ill infant. The nurse should be familiar with community resources and help the parents identify which agencies may benefit them.

5. Help parents recognize the growth and development needs of their infant. A development program begun in the hospital can be continued at home, or parents may be referred to an infant development program in the community.

6. Arrange medical follow-up care before discharge. The infant will need to be followed up by a family pediatrician, a well-baby clinic, or a specialty clinic. The first appointment should be made before the infant is discharged from the hospital.

7. Evaluate the need for special equipment for infant care (such as a respirator, oxygen, apnea monitor, feeding pump) in the home. Any equipment or supplies should be placed in the home before the infant's discharge.

8. Ensure that a medical home for continuing medical care for the infant has been identified and a plan for transfer of information and care has been completed as needed.

9. Arrange for neonatal hospice for parents of the medically fragile infant as needed.

Further evaluation after the infant has gone home is useful in determining whether the crisis has been resolved satisfactorily. The parents are usually given the intensive care nursery's telephone number to call for support and advice. The staff can follow up with each family with visits or telephone calls at intervals for several weeks to assess and evaluate the infant's (and parents') progress (Figure 28–16 ●).

Evaluation

Expected outcomes of nursing care include the following:

■ The parents are able to verbalize their feelings of grief and loss.

● **Figure 28–16** Discharge day. These 33 weeks' gestational age twins are being held by staff in the NICU on the happy day of discharge. This is what is so rewarding about working in the NICU: healthy babies going home to their families.

Source: Courtesy of Lisa Smith-Pedersen, RNC, MSN, NNP-BC.

■ The parents verbalize their concerns about their baby's health problems, care needs, and potential outcome.

■ The parents are able to participate in their infant's care and show attachment behaviors.

Considerations for the Nurse Who Works with At-Risk Newborns

The birth of a baby with a problem is a traumatic event with the potential for either disruption and growth, or both, of the involved family. NICU staff nurses may never see the long-term results of the specialized sensitive care they give to parents and their newborns. Their only immediate evidence of effective care may be the beginning resolution of parental grief; or discharge of a recovered, thriving infant to the care of happy parents; and the beginning of reintegration of family life.

Nurses cannot provide support unless they themselves are supported. Working in an emotional environment of "lots of living and lots of dying" takes its toll on staff. NICUs are among the most stressful areas in health care for patients, families, and nurses. Nurses bear most of the stress and largely determine the atmosphere of the NICU. The nurse's ability to cope with stress is the key to creating an emotionally healthy environment and a positive working atmosphere. The emotional needs and feelings of the staff must be recognized and dealt with so that the staff can support the parents. An environment of openness to feelings and support in dealing with their human needs and emotions is essential for the staff.

As caregivers, nurses may be unaware of their need to grieve for their own losses in the NICU. Nurses must also go through the grief work that parents experience. Techniques such as group meetings, individual support, and primary care nursing may assist in maintaining staff mental health. Reunions in some nurseries are beneficial for the families and healthcare professionals so they are able to see the children after discharge.

Critical Concept Review

LEARNING OUTCOME 28.1: Discuss how to identify infants in need of resuscitation and the appropriate method of resuscitation based on the labor record and observable physiologic indicators.

1. Infants at risk for resuscitation include those with:
   - Nonreassuring fetal heart pattern, meconium-stained amniotic fluid and/or acidosis detected by fetal scalp sample.
   - Cardiac disease diagnosed prenatally.
   - Other congenital abnormality diagnosed prenatally.
   - Premature birth.
   - Infant of multiple pregnancy.
   - Prolonged or difficult delivery.
2. Infants needing resuscitation:
   - Weak cry at birth.
   - Poor respiratory effort at birth.
   - Retractions at birth.

3. Resuscitation methods:
   - Stimulation by rubbing the newborn's back. (Done initially to all infants.)
   - Use of positive pressure to inflate the lungs. (Used if respirations are inadequate or have not been initiated.)
   - Endotracheal intubation. (Used immediately for severely premature infants, infants with known congenital anomalies, and infants who do not respond to stimulation or bag and mask.)
   - Medications: Naloxone (Narcan) may be used to reverse effects of narcotics given to mother prior to birth.

LEARNING OUTCOME 28.2: Differentiate, based on clinical manifestations, among the various types of respiratory distress (respiratory distress syndrome, transient tachypnea of the newborn, and meconium aspiration syndrome) in the newborn and their related nursing management.

1. Respiratory distress syndrome:
   - Lack of sufficient surfactant causes labored respirations and increased work at breathing.
   - Seen most frequently in premature newborns.
   - Nursing care involves administration of surfactant, close assessment, and supportive care if mechanical ventilation is needed.
2. Transient tachypnea of the newborn (TTNB):
   - Usually results from excess fluid in the lungs.
   - Infant breathes normally at birth, but develops symptoms of respiratory distress by 4–6 hours of age.
   - Nursing care involves initiating oxygen therapy and restricting oral feedings until respiratory status improves.

3. Meconium aspiration syndrome:
   - Signs and symptoms of respiratory distress beginning at birth.
   - May depend on the amount of meconium that is aspirated and the activity level of the newborn.
   - Initial nursing care involves:
     - If infant is vigorous even in presence of meconium—no subsequent special resuscitation.
     - If infant has absent or depressed respirations, HR less than 100 beats per minute, or poor muscle tone—direct tracheal suctioning by specially trained personnel.
   - After initial suctioning and/or resuscitation efforts, nursing care involves ongoing assessment for signs and symptoms of respiratory distress and supportive care of the infant requiring mechanical ventilation or ECMO.

LEARNING OUTCOME 28.3: Discuss selected metabolic abnormalities (including cold stress and hypoglycemia), their effects on the newborn, and the nursing implications.

1. Cold stress sets up the chain of physiologic events of hypoglycemia, pulmonary vasoconstriction, hyperbilirubinemia, respiratory distress, and metabolic acidosis.
2. Nursing interventions include:
   - Keep infant warm during any transport.

   - Observe for any signs of hypoglycemia.
   - Have infant go to breast or feed early in neonatal period.
   - Assess blood glucose frequently.

LEARNING OUTCOME 28.4: Differentiate between physiologic and pathologic jaundice according to timing of onset (in hours), cause, possible sequelae, and specific management.

1. Physiologic jaundice:
   - Occurs in 50% of all newborns.
   - Appears after 24 hours of age.
   - Not visible after 10 days of age.
   - May require phototherapy.

2. Pathologic jaundice:
   - Usually caused by ABO or Rh incompatibility.
   - Jaundice may be present within 24 hours of birth.
   - Treatment begins with phototherapy, but may progress to exchange transfusions.
3. Untreated hyperbilirubinemia (due to either type of jaundice) may result in neurotoxicity.

LEARNING OUTCOME 28.5: Explain how Rh incompatibility or ABO incompatibility can lead to the development of hyperbilirubinemia.

1. Rh incompatibility:
   - Maternal antibodies enter the fetal circulation, then attach to and destroy fetal red blood cells.
   - Fetal system produces more RBCs.
   - Hyperbilirubinemia, anemia, and jaundice result.

2. ABO incompatibility:
   - Mother is type O and infant is type A or B.
   - Less severe than Rh incompatibility.

LEARNING OUTCOME 28.6: Identify nursing responsibilities and rationale in caring for the newborn receiving phototherapy.

Nursing responsibilities for the newborn receiving phototherapy include:

1. Expose maximum amount of skin surface for optimal therapeutic results.
2. Apply eye patches while banks of phototherapy lights are in progress.
3. Assess eyes for signs/symptoms of conjunctivitis per agency protocol.
4. Frequently monitor temperature.
5. Offer infant water and formula frequently to assist in excretion of bilirubin.
6. Keep parents informed of need for phototherapy and encourage parents to hold and care for infant while undergoing phototherapy.

LEARNING OUTCOME 28.7: Describe the causes and nursing management of infants with anemia.

1. Anemia in newborns results from prenatal blood loss, birth trauma, infection, or blood group incompatibility:
   - Nursing assessments for signs and symptoms of anemia.
   - Record all amounts of blood taken during laboratory testing.

LEARNING OUTCOME 28.8: Describe the nursing assessments that would lead the nurse to suspect newborn sepsis and the nursing management of the newborn with an infection.

The most common signs of newborn sepsis include:

1. Lethargy or irritability.
2. Pallor or duskiness.
3. Hypothermia.
4. Feeding intolerance.
5. Hyperbilirubinemia.
6. Tachycardia, bradycardia, or apneic spells.

The nursing care includes:

- Obtain cultures before antibiotic therapy starts.
- Carry out laboratory sepsis workup.
- Administer antibiotics as prescribed.
- Provide supportive care to include NTE, respiratory and cardiovascular support, nutrition, monitor fluid and electrolyte homeostasis, and observe for complications.

LEARNING OUTCOME 28.9: Relate the consequences of maternally transmitted infections, such as maternal syphilis, gonorrhea, Herpesviridae family (HSV or CMV), and chlamydia, to the nursing management of infants in the neonatal period.

1. All infants receive eye prophylaxis with ophthalmic antibiotic due to possibility of transmission of gonorrhea or chlamydia during the birth process.
2. Maternal syphilis requires that the infant be isolated from other newborns and receive antibiotics at birth.
3. Maternal herpes virus infection requires administration of IV antiviral medications in the immediate newborn period as well as multiple cultures (skin, spinal fluid) for presence of herpesvirus.

LEARNING OUTCOME 28.10: Describe the interventions to facilitate parental attachment and meet the special initial and long-term needs of parents of at-risk infants.

1. Assess the parent's level of understanding of the infant's problem. Initially, the parents need to understand the infant's problem, including expected treatments.
2. Prepare and facilitate the parents' viewing of the infant.
3. Promote touching and facilitate parental participation in care of the infant.
4. Ensure parents understand routine well-baby care, normal growth and development of infants and have referral for normal infant screening procedures.
5. Have medical follow-up arranged.
6. Facilitate parental adjustment to the infant's special needs.
7. Parents have referral for any special equipment required at home and understand how to perform any special procedures needed to care for the infant.

Clinical Reasoning in Action

Rebecca Prince, age 21, G2 now P2, gives birth to a 5-pound baby at 38 weeks' gestation by primary cesarean birth for fetal distress. The infant's Apgars are 7 and 9 at 1 and 5 minutes. The infant is suctioned and given free-flow oxygen at birth, then is admitted to the newborn nursery for transitional care and does well. You are the nurse caring for Baby Prince at 36 hours old. You review the newborn's record and note that the baby's blood type is A+ and his mother is O+. Rebecca wants to breastfeed. You are performing a shift assessment on Baby Prince when you observe that the infant has a unilateral cephalohematoma and is lethargic. You blanch the skin over the sternum and observe a yellow discoloration of the skin. Lab tests reveal a serum bilirubin level of 12 mg/dL, hematocrit 55%, a mildly positive direct Coombs' test, and a positive indirect Coombs' test.

Baby Prince is diagnosed with hyperbilirubinemia secondary to ABO incompatibility and cephalohematoma. You provide phototherapy by fiber-optic blanket around the trunk of the infant and take the baby to his mother's room.

1. How would you explain the purpose of phototherapy to the mother?
2. Describe the care the mother can give to the newborn.
3. Discuss the advantage of fiber-optic blanket phototherapy for the newborn.
4. Newborns up to 1 month of age are susceptible to organisms that do not cause significant disease in older children. Explore the circumstances that cause susceptibility to infection.
5. Describe how to distinguish between oral thrush and milk curds.
6. Develop a concept map for the care of an infant with a cephalhematoma.

See www.nursing.pearsonhighered.com for possible responses and an interactive template for a concept map.

References

Adkin, D. H., & Committee on Fetus and Newborn. (2011). Postnatal glucose homeostasis in late-preterm and term infants. *Pediatrics, 127*, 575–579. doi:10.1542/peds. 2010-3851

American Academy of Pediatrics (AAP) & American Heart Association (AHA). (2011). *Textbook of neonatal resuscitation* (6th ed.). Elk Grove Village, IL: Author.

American Academy of Pediatrics (AAP) Committee on Fetus and Newborn. (2010). Policy statement: Hospital stay for healthy term newborns. *Pediatrics, 125*(2), 405–409. doi:10.1542/peds.2009-3119

American Academy of Pediatrics (AAP) Committee on Fetus and Newborn & American College of Obstetricians and Gynecologists (ACOG) Committee on Obstetrics. (2012). *Guidelines for perinatal care* (7th ed.). Evanston, IL: Author.

Bhutani, V. K., & Committee on Fetus and Newborn. (2011). Phototherapy to prevent severe neonatal hyperbilirubinemia in the newborn infant 35 or more weeks of gestation. *Pediatrics, 128,* e1046–1052. doi:10.1542/peds.2011-1494.

Blackburn, S. T. (2013). *Maternal, fetal, & neonatal physiology: A clinical perspective* (4th ed.). St. Louis, MO: Saunders.

Chinchilla, M. K. (2012). Patient family-centered care: A bedside RN's perspective. *Neonatal Network, 31*(5), 341–344.

Cloherty, J. P., Eichenwald, E. C., & Stark, A. R. (2012). *Manual of neonatal care* (7th ed.). Philadelphia, PA: Lippincott Williams & Wilkins.

Discenza, D. (2012). Helping babies therapeutically post-NICU. *Neonatal Network,* 31(5), 339–340.

Gardner, S. L., Enzman-Hines, M., & Dickey, L. A. (2011). Pain and pain relief. In S. L. Gardner, B. S. Carter, M. Enzman-Hines, & J. A. Hernandez (Eds.), *Merenstein & Gardner's handbook of neonatal intensive care* (7th ed., pp. 223–269). St. Louis, MO: Mosby/Elsevier.

Gardner, S. L., & Goldson, E. (2011). The neonate and the environment: Impact on development. In S. L. Gardner,

B. S. Carter, M. Enzman-Hines, & J. A. Hernandez (Eds.), *Merenstein & Gardner's handbook of neonatal intensive care* (7th ed., pp. 270–332). St. Louis. MO: Mosby/Elsevier.

Gleason, C. A., & Devaskar, S. U. (2012). *Avery's diseases of the newborn* (9th ed.). St. Louis, MO: Elsevier/Saunders.

Grant, P. (1978). Psychological needs of families of high-risk infants. *Family and Community Health, 11*(3), 93–97.

Hallman, M., & Saarela, T. (2012). Respiratory distress syndrome: Predisposing factors, pathophysiology and diagnosis. In G. Buonocore, R. Bracci, & M. Weindling (Eds.), *Neonatalogy: A practical approach to neonatal management* (pp. 441–454). Milan, Italy: Springer-Verlag.

Holditch-Davis, D., Miles, M. S., Burchinal, M. R., & Goldman, B. D. (2011). Medical role attainment with medically fragile infants: Part 2. Relationship to the quality of parenting. *Research in Nursing Health, 34*(1), 35–48. doi:10.1002/nur.20418

Kaplan, D. M., & Mason, E. A. (1974). Maternal reactions to premature birth viewed as an acute emotional disorder. In H. J. Parad (Ed.), *Crisis intervention* (pp. 118–128). New York, NY: Family Services Association of America.

Klaus, M. H., & Kennell, J. H. (1982). *Maternal–infant bonding* (2nd ed.). St. Louis, MO: Mosby.

Lopez, G. L., Anderson, K. H., & Feutchinger, J. (2012). Transition of premature infants from hospital to home life. *Neonatal Network, 31*(4), 207–214.

Maisels, M. J., & Watchko, J. F. (2012). Treatment of hyperbilirubinemia. In G. Buonocore, R. Bracci, & M. Weindling (Eds.), *Neonatalogy: A practical approach to neonatal management* (pp. 629–640). Milan, Italy: Springer-Verlag.

Manco-Johnson, M., Rodden, D. J., & Hays, T. (2011). Newborn hematology. In S. L. Gardner, B. S. Carter, M. Enzman-Hines, & J. A. Hernandez (Eds.), *Merenstein & Gardner's handbook of neonatal intensive care* (7th ed., pp. 503–530). St. Louis, MO: Mosby/Elsevier.

Martin, R. J., & Crowley, M. A. (2013). Respiratory problems. In A.A. Fanaroff & J. M. Fanaroff (Eds.), *Klaus & Fanaroff's care of the high-risk neonate* (6th ed., pp. 244–269). St. Louis, MO: Saunders/Elsevier.

McKenzie, J., & Palmer, B. (2010). Cost comparison of heel stick procedures and transcutaneous sample methods for bilirubin evaluation. *Neonatal Intensive Care, 23*(5), 39–42.

Niemeyer, S., & Clarke, S. B. (2011). Delivery room care. In S. L. Gardner, B. S. Carter, M. Enzman-Hines, & J. A. Hernandez (Eds.), *Merenstein & Gardner's handbook of neonatal intensive care* (7th ed., pp. 52–77). St. Louis, MO: Mosby/Elsevier.

Polin, R. A., & Committee on Fetus and Newborn. (2012). Management of neonates with suspected or proven early-onset bacterial sepsis. *Pediatrics, 129,* 1006–1015. doi:10.1542/peds.2012-0541

Schlittenhart, J. M., Smart, D., Miller, K., & Severtson, B. (2012). Preparing parents for NICU discharge: An evidence-based teaching tool. *Nursing for Women's Health. 15*(6), 484–496.

Solnit, A., & Stark, M. (1961). Mourning and the birth of a defective child. *Psychoanalytic Study of the Child, 16,* 505.

Venkatesh, M. P., Adams, K. M., & Weisman, L. E. (2011). Infection in the newborn. In S. L. Gardner, B. S. Carter, M. Enzman-Hines, & J. A. Hernandez (Eds.), *Merenstein & Gardner's handbook of neonatal intensive care* (7th ed., pp. 553–786). St. Louis. MO: Mosby/Elsevier.

Wainer, S., Parmar, S., Allegro, D., Rabi, Y., & Lyon, M. (2012). Impact of a transcutaneous bilirubinometry program on resource utilization and severe hyperbilirubinemia. *Pediatrics, 129*(1), 77–86.

Young, T. E., & Mangum, O. B. (2012). *Neofax®: A manual of drugs used in neonatal care* (25th ed.). Raleigh, NC: Acorn.

Postpartum Adaptation and Nursing Assessment

I acutely felt the fatigue and sense of loss of the relationship with my baby that I had during pregnancy. But then the wonderful part happened with the reuniting with my new daughter. Holding her, having her latch on to my breast to get nourishment, and her looking into my eyes to say "Hello, Mom."
—Susan, 34

Kevin Peterson/Getty Images

LEARNING OUTCOMES

29.1   Describe the basic physiologic changes that occur in the postpartum period as a woman's body returns to its prepregnant state.

29.2   Describe the psychologic adjustments that normally occur during the postpartum period.

29.3   Describe the physiologic and psychologic components of a systematic postpartum assessment.

29.4   Describe the common concerns of the mother that are considered in a postpartum assessment.

29.5   Examine the physical and developmental tasks that the mother must accomplish during the postpartum period.

29.6   Identify the factors that influence the development of a positive parent–infant attachment in the nursing assessment of early attachment.

During the **puerperium**, or postpartum period, the woman readjusts, physically and psychologically, from pregnancy and birth. The period begins immediately after birth and continues for approximately 6 weeks, or until the body has returned to a near prepregnant state.

This chapter describes the physiologic and psychologic changes that occur postpartum and the basic aspects of a thorough postpartum assessment.

POSTPARTUM PHYSICAL ADAPTATIONS

Comprehensive nursing assessment is based on a sound understanding of the normal anatomic and physiologic processes of the puerperium. These processes involve the reproductive organs and other major body systems.

Reproductive System

Involution of the Uterus

The term **involution** is used to describe the rapid reduction in size and the return of the uterus to a nonpregnant state. Following separation of the placenta, the decidua of the uterus is irregular, jagged, and varied in thickness. The spongy layer of the decidua is cast off as lochia, and the basal layer of the decidua remains in the uterus to become differentiated into two layers. This occurs within the first 48 to 72 hours after birth. The outermost layer becomes necrotic and is sloughed off in the lochia. The layer closest to the myometrium contains the fundi of the uterine endometrial glands, and these glands lay the foundation for the new endometrium. Except at the placenta site, this process is completed in approximately 3 weeks. The placental site can take up to 6 weeks to be completely healed (Pessel & Tsai, 2013). Bleeding from the larger uterine vessels of the placental site is controlled by compression of the retracted uterine muscle fibers. The clotted blood is gradually absorbed by the body. Some of these vessels are eventually obliterated and replaced by new vessels with smaller lumens.

The placental site heals by a process of exfoliation and growth of endometrial tissue. This occurs with upward endometrial growth in the decidua basalis under the placental site, with simultaneous growth of endometrial tissue from the margins of the site. The infarcted superficial tissue then becomes necrotic and is sloughed off (Blackburn, 2013). *Exfoliation* is a very important aspect of involution; if healing of the placental site leaves a fibrous scar, the area available for future implantation is limited, as is the number of possible pregnancies.

With the dramatic decrease in the levels of circulating estrogen and progesterone following placental separation, the uterine cells atrophy, and the hyperplasia of pregnancy begins to reverse. Proteolytic enzymes are released, and macrophages migrate to the uterus to promote autolysis (self-digestion). Protein material in the uterine wall is broken down and absorbed. Factors that enhance involution include an uncomplicated labor and birth, complete expulsion of the placenta or membranes, breastfeeding, manual removal of the placenta during a cesarean birth, and early ambulation. Factors that slow uterine involution and the rationale for each factor are listed in Table 29–1.

Changes in Fundal Position

The **fundus** (top portion of the uterus) is situated in the midline midway between the symphysis pubis and the umbilicus (Figure 29–1 ●). Immediately following the birth of the placenta, the uterus contracts to the size of a large grapefruit. The walls of the contracted uterus are in proximity, and the uterine blood vessels are firmly compressed by the myometrium. Within 6 to 12 hours after birth, the fundus of the uterus rises to the level of the umbilicus because of blood and clots that remain within the uterus and changes in support of the uterus by the ligaments. A fundus that is above the umbilicus and boggy (feels soft and spongy rather than firm and

Table 29-1	Factors That Retard Uterine Involution
Factor	**Rationale**
Prolonged labor	Muscles relax because of prolonged time of contraction during labor.
Anesthesia	Muscle relaxation results in a "boggy uterus."
Difficult birth	The uterus is manipulated excessively causing muscle fatigue.
Grand multiparity	Repeated distention of uterus during pregnancy and labor leads to muscle stretching, diminished tone, and muscle relaxation.
Full bladder	As the uterus is pushed up and usually to the right, pressure on it interferes with effective uterine contraction.
Incomplete expulsion of placenta or membranes	The presence of even small amounts of tissue interferes with the ability of the uterus to remain firmly contracted.
Infection	Inflammation interferes with the uterine muscle's ability to contract effectively.
Overdistention of uterus	Overstretching of uterine muscles with conditions such as multiple gestation, hydramnios, or a very large baby may set the stage for slower uterine involution.

● **Figure 29–1** Involution of the uterus. *A,* Immediately after delivery of the placenta, the top of the fundus is in the midline and approximately halfway between the symphysis pubis and the umbilicus. About 6 to 12 hours after birth, the fundus is at the level of the umbilicus. *B,* The height of the fundus then decreases about one finger breadth (approximately 1 cm) each day.

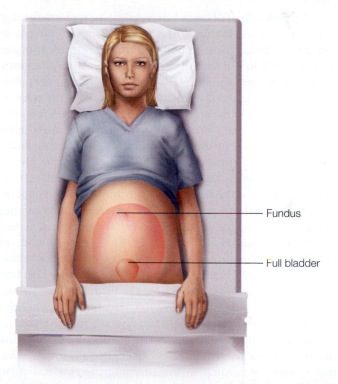

● **Figure 29–2** Displacement and deviation of the uterus. The uterus becomes displaced and deviated to the right when the bladder is full.

well contracted) is associated with excessive uterine bleeding. As blood collects and forms clots within the uterus, the fundus rises; firm contractions of the uterus are interrupted, causing a **boggy uterus (uterine atony)**.

When the fundus is higher than expected on palpation and is not in the midline (usually deviated to the right), distention of

the bladder should be suspected; the bladder should be emptied immediately and the uterus remeasured (Figure 29–2 ●). If the woman is unable to void, in-and-out catheterization of the bladder may be required. In the immediate postpartum period, many women may not be aware of a full bladder. Because the uterine ligaments are still stretched, a full bladder can move the uterus. By the end of the puerperium these ligaments have regained their nonpregnant length and tension.

After birth the top of the fundus remains at the level of the umbilicus for about half a day. On the first postpartum day, the top of the fundus is located about 1 cm below the umbilicus. The top of the fundus descends approximately one finger breadth (width of index, second, or third finger), or 1 cm, per day until it descends into the pelvis on about the 10th day.

If the mother is breastfeeding, the release of endogenous oxytocin from the posterior pituitary in response to suckling hastens involution of the uterus. Barring complications, such as infection or retained placental fragments, the uterus approaches its prepregnant size and location by 5 to 6 weeks. In women who had an oversized uterus during the pregnancy (because of hydramnios, birth of a large-for-gestational-age [LGA] infant, or multiple gestation), the time frame for an immediate uterine involution process is lengthened. If intrauterine infection is present, in addition to foul-smelling lochia or vaginal discharge, the uterine fundus descends much more slowly. When infection is suspected, other clinical signs such as fever and tachycardia in addition to delay in involution must be assessed. Any slowing of descent is called **subinvolution** (for further discussion of subinvolution, see Chapter 31 🔗).

Lochia

The uterus rids itself of the debris remaining after birth through a discharge called **lochia**, which is classified according to its appearance and contents. **Lochia rubra** is dark red. It occurs for the first 2 to 3 days and contains epithelial cells, erythrocytes, leukocytes, shreds of decidua, and occasionally fetal meconium, lanugo, and vernix. Clotting is often the result of pooling of blood in the upper portion of the vagina. A few small clots (no larger than a nickel) are common, particularly in the first few days after birth. However, lochia should not contain large (plum-size) clots; if it does the cause should be investigated without delay. **Lochia serosa** is a pinkish color. It follows from about day 3 until day 10. Lochia serosa is composed of serous exudate (hence, the name), shreds of degenerating decidua, erythrocytes, leukocytes, cervical mucus, and numerous microorganisms (Blackburn, 2013). The red blood cell (RBC) component decreases gradually, and a creamy or yellowish discharge persists for an additional week or two. This final discharge, termed **lochia alba** from the Latin word for "white," is composed primarily of leukocytes, decidual cells, epithelial cells, fat, cervical mucus, cholesterol crystals, and bacteria.

Recent studies examining lochia patterns have found that the lochia rubra phase lasts longer than generally assumed and that it varies according to breastfeeding practice and parity (Blackburn, 2013). Variation in the duration of lochia discharge is not uncommon; however, the trend should be toward a lighter amount of flow and a lighter color of discharge. When the lochia flow stops, the cervix is considered closed, and chances of infection ascending from the vagina to the uterus decrease.

Like menstrual discharge, lochia flow has a musty, stale odor that is not offensive. Microorganisms are always present in the vaginal lochia, and by the second day following birth the uterus is contaminated with the vaginal bacteria. It is thought that an infection does not develop because the organisms involved are relatively nonvirulent. Any foul smell to the lochia or used peripad suggests infection and the need for prompt additional assessment, such as white blood cell (WBC) count and differential and assessment for uterine tenderness and fever.

The total average volume of lochia is about 225 mL, and the daily volume gradually decreases (Blackburn, 2013). Discharge is greater in the morning because of pooling in the vagina and uterus while the mother lies sleeping. The amount of lochia may also be increased by exertion or breastfeeding. Multiparous women usually have more lochia than first-time mothers. Women who undergo a cesarean birth typically have less lochia than women who give birth vaginally (Blackburn, 2013).

Evaluation of lochia is necessary not only to determine the presence of hemorrhage but also to assess uterine involution. The type, amount, and consistency of lochia determines the stage of healing of the placental site, and a progressive change from bright red at birth to dark red to pink to white or clear discharge should be observed. Persistent discharge of lochia rubra or a return to lochia rubra indicates subinvolution or late postpartum hemorrhage (see Chapter 31 🔗).

The nurse should exercise caution when evaluating bleeding immediately after birth. The continuous seepage of blood is consistent with cervical or vaginal lacerations and may be effectively diagnosed when the bleeding is evaluated in conjunction with the consistency of the uterus. Lacerations should be suspected if the uterus is firm and of expected size and if no clots are expressed.

Cervical Changes

Following birth the cervix is flabby, formless, and may appear bruised. The lateral aspects of the external os are frequently lacerated during the birth process (Cunningham et al., 2010). The external os is markedly irregular and closes slowly. It admits two fingers for a few days following birth, but by the end of the first week it admits only a fingertip.

The shape of the external os is permanently changed by the first childbearing. The characteristic dimple-like os of the nullipara changes to the transverse slit (fish-mouth) os of the multipara (Pessel & Tsai, 2013). After significant cervical laceration or several lacerations, the cervix may appear lopsided. Because of the slight change in the size of the cervix, a diaphragm or cervical cap will need to be refitted if the woman is using one of these methods of contraception.

Vaginal Changes

Following birth the vagina appears edematous and may be bruised. Small superficial lacerations may be evident, and the rugae are obliterated. The apparent bruising is caused by pelvic congestion and trauma and will quickly disappear. The hymen, torn and jagged, heals irregularly, leaving small tags called *carunculae myrtiformes*.

Clinical Reasoning   **Variation in Fundus Status**

You have completed your assessment of Patty Clark, a 24-year-old, G2P2 woman who is 24 hours past childbirth. The fundus is just above the umbilicus and slightly to the right. Lochia rubra is present, and a pad is soaked every 2 hours. What would you do?

See www.nursing.pearsonhighered.com for possible responses.

The size of the vagina decreases and rugae return within 3 to 4 weeks (Blackburn, 2013; Whitmer, 2011). This facilitates the gradual return to smaller, although not nulliparous, dimensions. By 6 weeks the nonbreastfeeding woman's vagina usually appears normal. The lactating woman is in a hypoestrogenic state because of ovarian suppression, and her vaginal mucosa may be pale and without rugae; the effects of the lowered estrogen level may lead to dyspareunia (painful intercourse), which may be reduced by the addition of a water-soluble personal lubricant. Tone and contractility of the vaginal orifice may be improved by perineal tightening exercises such as Kegel exercises (see Chapter 11 🔗), which may begin soon after birth. The labia majora and labia minora are more flaccid in the woman who has borne a child than in the nullipara woman.

Perineal Changes

During the early postpartum period, the soft tissue in and around the perineum may appear edematous, with some bruising. If an episiotomy or a laceration is present, the edges should be drawn together. Occasionally, ecchymosis occurs, and this may delay healing. Initial healing of the episiotomy or laceration occurs in 2 to 3 weeks after the birth, although complete healing may take up to 4 to 6 months (Blackburn, 2013). Perineal discomfort may be present during this time.

Recurrence of Ovulation and Menstruation

The return of ovulation and menstruation varies for each postpartum woman. Menstruation generally returns as soon as 7 weeks in 70% and by 12 weeks in all nonlactating mothers or as late as 3 years in 70% of breastfeeding mothers (Pessel & Tsai, 2013). The return of ovulation is directly associated with a rise in the serum progesterone level. In nonlactating mothers the average time to first ovulation can occur within 70 to 75 days, with a mean time of 6 months in lactating women (Pessel & Tsai, 2013).

The return of ovulation and menstruation in breastfeeding mothers is usually prolonged and is associated with the length of time the woman breastfeeds and whether formula supplements are used. If a mother breastfeeds for less than 1 month, the return of menstruation and ovulation is similar to that of the nonbreastfeeding mother. In women who exclusively breastfeed, menstruation is usually delayed for at least 3 months. Suckling by the infant typically results in alterations in the gonadotropin releasing hormone (GnRH) production, which is thought to be the cause of amenorrhea (Blackburn, 2013). Although exclusive breastfeeding helps to reduce the risk of pregnancy for the first 6 months after birth, it should be relied on only temporarily and if it meets the observed criteria for the lactational amenorrhea method (LAM). Furthermore, because ovulation precedes menstruation and women often supplement breastfeeding with bottles and pacifiers, breastfeeding is not considered a reliable means of contraception.

Abdomen

The uterine ligaments (notably the round and broad ligaments) are stretched and require the length of the puerperium to recover. Although the stretched abdominal wall appears loose and flabby, it responds to exercise within 2 to 3 months. **Diastasis recti abdominis**, a separation of the abdominal muscle, may occur with pregnancy, especially in women with poor abdominal muscle tone (Figure 29–3 ●). If diastasis occurs, part of the

Normal location of rectus muscles of the abdomen

Diastasis recti: separation of the rectus muscles

● **Figure 29–3** Diastasis recti abdominis, which involves a separation of the abdominal musculature, commonly occurs after pregnancy.

abdominal wall has no muscular support but is formed only by skin, subcutaneous fat, fascia, and peritoneum. This may be especially pronounced in women who have undergone a cesarean section, because the rectus abdominis muscles are manually separated to access the uterine muscle. Improvement depends on the physical condition of the mother, the total number of pregnancies, pregnancy spacing, and the type and amount of physical exercise. This may result in a pendulous abdomen and increased maternal backache. Fortunately, diastasis responds well to exercise, and abdominal muscle tone can improve significantly.

The striae (stretch marks), which occur as a result of stretching and rupture of the elastic fibers of the skin, take on different colors based on the mother's skin color. The striae of Caucasian mothers are red to purple at the time of birth and gradually fade to silver or white. The striae of mothers with darker skin, in contrast, are darker than the surrounding skin and remain darker. These marks gradually fade after a time but remain visible.

Lactation

During pregnancy, breast development in preparation for lactation results from the influence of both estrogen and progesterone. After birth, the interplay of maternal hormones leads to milk production. (For further details, see *Breastfeeding* in Chapter 26 .)

Gastrointestinal System

Hunger following birth is common, and the mother may enjoy eating a light meal. Frequently, she is quite thirsty and will drink large amounts of fluid. Drinking fluids helps replace fluids lost during labor, in the urine, and through perspiration.

The bowels tend to be sluggish following birth because of the lingering effects of progesterone, decreased abdominal muscle tone, and bowel evacuation associated with the labor and birth process. Women who have had an episiotomy, lacerations, or hemorrhoids may tend to delay elimination for fear of increasing their pain or because they believe their stitches will be torn if they bear down. In refusing or delaying the bowel movement, the woman may cause increased constipation and more pain when bowel elimination finally occurs.

The woman with a cesarean birth may receive clear liquids shortly after surgery; once bowel sounds are present, her diet is quickly advanced to solid food. In addition, the woman may experience some initial discomfort from flatulence, which is relieved by early ambulation and use of antiflatulent medications. Chamomile tea and peppermint tea may also be helpful in reducing discomfort from flatulence. It may take a few days for the bowel to regain its tone, especially if general anesthesia was used. The woman who has had a cesarean or a difficult birth may benefit from stool softeners.

Urinary Tract

The postpartum woman has an increased bladder capacity, swelling and bruising of the tissue around the urethra, decreased sensitivity to fluid pressure, and a decreased sensation of bladder filling. Consequently, she is at risk for overdistention, incomplete bladder emptying, and a buildup of residual urine. Women who have had an anesthetic block have inhibited neural functioning of the bladder and are more susceptible to bladder distention, difficulty voiding, and bladder infections. In addition, immediate postpartum use of oxytocin to facilitate uterine contractions following expulsion of the placenta has an antidiuretic effect. Following cessation of the oxytocin, the woman will experience rapid bladder filling.

Urinary output increases during the early postpartum period (first 12 to 24 hours) because of *puerperal diuresis*. The kidneys must eliminate an estimated 2000 to 3000 mL of extracellular fluid with the normal pregnancy, which causes rapid filling of the bladder. Thus adequate bladder elimination is an immediate concern. Women with preeclampsia, chronic hypertension, and diabetes experience greater fluid retention than other women, and postpartum diuresis is increased accordingly.

If urine stasis exists, chances for urinary tract infection increase because of bacteriuria and the presence of dilated ureters and renal pelves, which persist for about 6 weeks after birth. A full bladder may also increase the tendency of the uterus to relax by displacing the uterus and interfering with its contractility, leading to hemorrhage. In the absence of infection, the dilated ureters and renal pelves return to prepregnant size by the end of the sixth week.

Vital Signs

During the postpartum period, with the exception of the first 24 hours, the woman should be afebrile. A maternal temperature of up to 38°C (100.4°F) may occur after childbirth as a result of the exertion and dehydration of labor. An increase in temperature to between 37.8°C and 39°C (100°F to 102.2°F) may also occur during the first 24 hours after the mother's milk comes in (Cunningham et al., 2010). However, in women not meeting these criteria, infection must be considered in the presence of an increased temperature (see discussion in Chapter 31).

Immediately following childbirth, many women experience a transient rise in both systolic and diastolic blood pressure, which spontaneously returns to the prepregnancy baseline during the next few days. A decrease may indicate physiologic readjustment to decreased intrapelvic pressure, or it may be related to uterine hemorrhage. Orthostatic hypotension, as indicated by feelings of faintness or dizziness immediately after standing up, can develop in the first 48 hours as a result of abdominal engorgement that may occur after birth. A low or decreasing blood pressure may reflect hypovolemia secondary to hemorrhage, but it is a late sign. Blood pressure elevations may result from excessive use of oxytocin or vasopressor medications. Because preeclampsia can persist into or occur first in the postpartum period, routine evaluation of blood pressure is needed. If a woman complains of headache, hypertension must be ruled out before analgesics are administered.

Clinical Tip

During the first few hours after birth, the woman may have some orthostatic hypotension; it will cause her to have a lower blood pressure reading in a sitting position. For the most accurate reading, be sure to measure the woman in the same position each time, preferably lying on her back with her arm at her side.

Puerperal bradycardia with rates of 50 to 70 beats per minute (beats/min) commonly occurs during the first 6 to 10 days of the postpartum period. It may be related to decreased cardiac effort, the decreased blood volume following placental separation and contraction of the uterus, and increased stroke volume. A pulse rate greater than 100 beats/min may be indicative of hypovolemia, infection, fear, or pain and requires further assessment.

Blood Values

Blood values should return to the prepregnant state by the end of the postpartum period. Pregnancy-associated activation of coagulation factors may continue for variable amounts of time after birth. This condition, in conjunction with trauma, immobility, or sepsis, predisposes the woman to the development of thromboembolism. The incidence of thromboembolism is reduced by early mobilization.

Nonpathologic leukocytosis often occurs during labor and in the immediate postpartum period, with white blood cell (WBC) counts of 25,000 to 30,000/mm^3. WBC values typically return to normal levels by the end of the first postpartum week. Leukocytosis combined with the normal increase in erythrocyte sedimentation rate may obscure the diagnosis of acute infection at this time (Whitmer, 2011).

Hemoglobin and hematocrit levels may be difficult to interpret in the first 2 days after birth because of the changing blood volume. This loss in blood in the first 24 hours accounts for half of the red blood cell (RBC) volume gained during the course of the pregnancy. Blood loss averages 200 to 500 mL with a vaginal birth and nearly 1000 mL with a cesarean birth (Pessel & Tsai, 2013). Lochia constitutes less than 25% of this blood loss. As extracellular fluid is excreted, hemoconcentration occurs, with a concomitant rise in hematocrit. A drop in values indicates an abnormal blood loss. The following is a convenient rule to remember: A two to three percentage point drop in hematocrit equals a blood loss of 500 mL (Whitmer, 2011). After 3 to 4 days, mobilization of interstitial fluid leads to a slight increase in plasma volume. This hemodilution leads to a decrease in hemoglobin, hematocrit, and plasma protein by the end of the first postpartum week. Decreases in plasma volume reach nonpregnant levels by 4 to 6 weeks postpartum (Blackburn, 2013).

Platelet levels typically fall as a result of placental separation. They then begin to increase by the third to fourth postpartum day, gradually returning to normal by the sixth postpartum week. Fibrinolytic activity typically returns to normal during the hours following birth. The hemostatic system as a whole reaches its normal prepregnant status by 3 to 4 weeks postpartum; however, the diameter of deep veins can take up to 6 weeks to return to prepregnant levels (Blackburn, 2013). This is why there is a prolonged risk of thromboembolism in the first 6 weeks following birth.

Cardiovascular Changes

The cardiovascular system undergoes dramatic changes during the birth that can result in cardiovascular instability because of an increase in the cardiac output. The cardiac output typically stabilizes and returns to prepregnancy levels within an hour following birth (Whitmer, 2011). Maternal hypervolemia acts to protect the mother from excessive blood loss. Cardiac output declines by 30% in the first 2 weeks and reaches normal levels by 6 to 12 weeks (Blackburn, 2013). Diuresis in the first 2 to 5 days assists to decrease the extracellular fluid and results in a weight loss of 3 kg. Failure of diuresis to occur in the immediate postpartum period can lead to pulmonary edema and subsequent cardiac problems.

Neurologic and Immunologic Changes

Neurologic problems and disorders can predispose women to higher rates of morbidity and mortality during pregnancy and in the postpartum period. Headaches are the most common neurologic symptoms encountered by postpartum women. Headaches may result from fluid shifts in the first week after birth, leakage of cerebrospinal fluid into the extradural space during spinal anesthesia, gestational hypertension, or stress (Carhuapoma, Tomlinson, & Levine, 2011). Migraine headaches, although less frequent during pregnancy, tend to resume in the postpartum period. In women with epilepsy, 1% to 2% are likely to have a seizure in the first 24 hours after birth rather than during the pregnancy (Carhuapoma et al., 2011). Women with epilepsy are more likely to be diagnosed with depression, and need referrals to therapists or support groups. Women with multiple sclerosis are more likely to have symptoms during the postpartum period than during pregnancy (Carhuapoma et al., 2011). Myasthenia gravis is an autoimmune disease that affects the neuromuscular junctions. The exacerbation of symptoms during pregnancy is variable; however, the first month of pregnancy and the first month of the postpartum period are the most critical (Kalayjian, Goodwin, & Lee, 2013).

Weight Loss

An initial weight loss of about 10 to 12 lb occurs as a result of the birth of the infant, placenta, and amniotic fluid. Diuresis accounts for the loss of an additional 5 lb during the early puerperium. By the sixth to eighth week after birth, many women have returned to approximately their prepregnant weight if they gained the average 25 to 30 lb. For others, a return to prepregnant weight may take longer. Women often express concern about the slow pace of their postpartum weight loss. Multiparas tend to be more positive than primiparas, probably because the multipara's previous experience has prepared her for the fact that the body does not immediately return to a prepregnant state.

Postpartum Chill

Frequently the mother experiences intense tremors that resemble shivering from a chill immediately after birth. Several theories have been offered to explain this shivering: It is the result of the sudden release of pressure on the pelvic nerves after birth, a response to a fetus-to-mother transfusion that occurred during placental separation, a reaction to maternal adrenaline production during labor and birth, or a reaction to epidural anesthesia. If not followed by fever, this chill is of no clinical concern, but it is uncomfortable for the woman. The nurse can increase the woman's comfort by covering her with a warmed blanket and reassuring her that the shivering is a common, self-limiting situation. If she allows herself to go with the shaking, the shivering will last only a short time. Some women may also find a warm beverage helpful. Later in the puerperium, chill and fever indicate infection and require further evaluation.

Postpartum Diaphoresis

The elimination of excess fluid and waste products via the skin during the puerperium produces increased perspiration. Diaphoretic (sweating) episodes frequently occur at night, and the woman may awaken drenched with perspiration. This perspiration is not significant clinically, but the mother should be protected from chilling.

Afterpains

Afterpains are more common in multiparas than in primiparas and are caused by intermittent uterine contractions. Although the uterus of the primipara usually remains consistently contracted, the lost tone of the multiparous uterus results in alternate contraction and relaxation. This phenomenon also occurs if the uterus has been markedly distended, as with a multiple-gestation pregnancy or hydramnios, or if clots or placental fragments were retained. These afterpains may cause the mother severe discomfort for 2 to 3 days after birth. The administration of oxytocic agents (intravenous infusion with Pitocin or oral administration of Methergine) stimulates uterine contraction and increases the discomfort of the afterpains. Because endogenous oxytocin is released when the infant suckles, breastfeeding also increases the frequency and severity of the afterpains.

A warm water bottle placed against the low abdomen may reduce the discomfort of afterpains. In addition, the breastfeeding mother may find it helpful to take a mild analgesic agent approximately 1 hour before feeding her infant. The nurse can assure the nursing mother that the prescribed analgesics are not harmful to the newborn and help improve the quality of the breastfeeding experience. An analgesic is also helpful at bedtime if the afterpains interfere with the mother's rest.

POSTPARTUM PSYCHOLOGIC ADAPTATIONS

The postpartum period is a time of readjustment and adaptation for the entire childbearing family, but especially for the mother. The woman experiences a variety of responses as she adjusts to a new family member, postpartum discomforts, changes in her body image, and the reality that she is no longer pregnant.

Taking-In and Taking-Hold

Initially after birth during the *taking-in* period, the woman tends to be passive and somewhat dependent. She follows suggestions, hesitates to make decisions, and is still rather preoccupied with her needs (Rubin, 1984). She may have a great need to talk about her perceptions of her labor and birth. This helps her work through the process, sort out the reality from her fantasized experience, and clarify anything that she did not understand. Food and sleep are major needs.

By the second or third day after birth, the new mother is often ready to resume control of her body, her mothering, and her life in general. Rubin (1984) labeled this the *taking-hold* period. If she is breastfeeding, she may worry about her technique or the quality of her milk. If her baby spits up after a feeding, she may view it as a personal failure. She may also feel demoralized by the fact that the nurse or an older family member handles her baby proficiently while she feels unsure and tentative. She requires assurance that she is doing well as a mother. Today's mothers seem to be more independent and adjust more rapidly, exhibiting behaviors of "taking-in" and "taking-hold" in shorter time periods.

Becoming a Mother (BAM)

Maternal role attainment (MRA) is the process by which a woman learns mothering behaviors and becomes comfortable with her identity as a mother. As the mother grows to know her child and forms a relationship, the mother's maternal identity gradually and systematically evolves and she "binds in" to the infant (Rubin, 1984). In most cases, maternal role attainment occurs within 3 to 10 months after birth.

In 2004, Mercer proposed replacing the term *maternal role attainment* with the term **becoming a mother (BAM)**. She stated that BAM "more accurately encompasses the dynamic transformation and evolution of a woman's persona than does MRA, and the term MRA should be discontinued" (Mercer, 2004, p. 226). BAM more accurately reflects the transition process of becoming a mother that changes throughout the maternal–child relationship. Postpartum nurses need to be aware of the long-term adjustments and stresses that the childbearing family faces as its members adjust to new and different roles. Nursing interventions that foster the process of becoming a mother include the following categories: instructions for infant caregiving, building awareness of and responsiveness to infant interactive capabilities, promoting maternal–infant attachment, maternal social role preparation, and interactive therapeutic nurse–patient relationships. Maternal/social role preparation and interactive therapeutic nurse–patient relationships have a greater impact on the progress of becoming a mother than formal teaching.

Postpartum Blues

The **postpartum blues** consist of a transient period of depression that occurs during the first few days of the puerperium. It may be manifested by mood swings, anger, weepiness, anorexia, difficulty sleeping, and a feeling of being letdown. This mood change frequently occurs while the woman is still hospitalized, but it may occur at home as well. Changing hormone levels are certainly a factor; psychologic adjustments, an unsupportive environment, and insecurity also have been identified as potential causes. In addition, fatigue, discomfort, and overstimulation may play a role. The postpartum blues usually resolve naturally within 10 to 14 days, but if they persist or symptoms worsen, the woman may need evaluation for postpartum depression (see Chapter 31 ✏). Ideally a depression assessment should be completed each trimester to update a pregnant woman's risk status for postpartum depression (Beck, 2008; Davey, Tough, Adair, et al., 2011).

Importance of Social Support

After the birth of a baby, a woman and her partner may find that family relationships become increasingly important. The attention that their infant receives from family members is a source of satisfaction to the new parents. In many cases, the ties to the woman's family become especially good. A new father may report that his relationship with his in-laws becomes far more positive and supportive. However, the increased family interaction can be a source of stress, especially for the new mother, who tends to have more contact with the families.

The new parents may also have increasing contact with other parents of small children while contact with coworkers declines.

Of great concern are women and their partners who have no families or friends with whom to form social networks. Isolation at a time when women feel an increased need for support can result in tremendous stress and is often a contributing factor in situations of postpartum depression, child neglect, or abuse. New mother support groups are helpful for women who lack a social support system.

DEVELOPMENT OF FAMILY ATTACHMENT

Some parents may lack any experience with babies and may feel overwhelmed by the infant. Bonding is a series of steps in which the mother, father, and infant develop relationships.

Maternal–Infant Attachment Behavior

A mother's first interaction with her infant is influenced by many factors, including her involvement with her family of origin, her relationships, the stability of her home environment, the communication patterns she developed, and the degree of nurturing she received as a child. These factors have shaped the person she has become. The following personal characteristics are also important.

- *Level of trust.* What level of trust has this mother developed in response to her life experiences? What is her philosophy of childrearing? Will she be able to treat her infant as a unique individual with changing needs that should be met as much as possible?

- *Level of self-esteem.* How much does she value herself as a woman and as a mother? Does she feel generally able to cope with the adjustments of life?

Developing Cultural Competence
Middle Eastern Initial Postpartum Experience

In many countries in the Middle East that follow a patriarchal system, the new mother and her infant stay with the husband's family following the birth of the infant. Frequent visits from the woman's family are discouraged and may even be viewed as burdensome by the husband's family. Typically, only women visit the new mother during the postpartum period. For the birth of the first baby, the wife's parents are expected to purchase all of the baby's supplies and clothing.

- *Capacity for enjoying herself.* Is the mother able to find pleasure in everyday activities and human relationships?

- *Adequacy of knowledge about childbearing and childrearing.* What beliefs about the course of pregnancy, the capabilities of newborns, previous experiences with infants/children, and the nature of her emotions may influence her behavior at first contact with her infant and later?

- *Prevailing mood or usual feeling tone.* Is the woman predominantly content, angry, depressed, or anxious? Is she sensitive to her own feelings and those of others? Will she be able to accept her own needs and to obtain support in meeting them?

- *Reactions to the present pregnancy.* Was the pregnancy planned? Did it go smoothly? Were there ongoing life events that enhanced her pregnancy or depleted her reserves of energy? How have other life roles changed because of her pregnancy and motherhood?

By the time of birth each mother has developed an emotional orientation of some kind to the baby based on these factors.

Initial Maternal Attachment Behavior

After labor and birth, a new mother will demonstrate a fairly regular pattern of maternal behaviors as she continues to familiarize herself with her newborn. In a progression of touching activities, the mother proceeds from fingertip exploration of the newborn's extremities toward palmar contact with larger body areas and finally to enfolding the infant with the whole hand and arm. The time taken to accomplish these steps varies from minutes to days. The mother increases the proportion of time spent in the *en face* position (Figure 29–4 ●). She arranges herself or the newborn so that she has direct face-to-face and eye-to-eye contact. There is an intense interest in having the infant's eyes open. When the infant's eyes are open, the mother characteristically greets the newborn and talks in high-pitched tones to him or her.

In most instances the mother relies heavily on her senses of sight, touch, and hearing in getting to know what her baby is really like. She tends also to respond verbally to any sounds

● **Figure 29–4** The mother has direct face-to-face and eye-to-eye contact in the *en face* position.
Source: Courtesy of Joanna Allen.

emitted by the newborn, such as cries, coughs, sneezes, and grunts. The sense of smell may be involved as well.

While interacting with her newborn, the mother may be experiencing shock, disbelief, or denial. She may state, "I can't believe she's finally here" or "I feel like he is a stranger." On the other hand, feelings of connectedness between the newborn and the rest of the family can be expressed in positive or negative terms: "She's got your cute nose, Daddy" or "Oh, no! He looks just like Matthew, and he was an impossible baby." A mother's facial expressions or the frequency and content of her questions may demonstrate concerns about the infant's general condition or normality, especially if her pregnancy was complicated or if a previous baby was not healthy.

During the first few days after her child's birth, the new mother applies herself to the task of getting to know her baby. This is termed the *acquaintance phase*. If the infant gives clear behavioral cues about needs, the infant's responses to mothering will be predictable, which will make the mother feel effective and competent. Other behaviors that make an infant more attractive to caretakers are smiling, grasping a finger, nursing eagerly, and being easy to console.

During this time the newborn is also becoming acquainted. Within a few days after birth, infants show signs of recognizing recurrent situations and responding to changes in routine. To the extent that their mother is their world, it can be said that they are actively acquainting themselves with her.

During the *phase of mutual regulation,* mother and infant seek to determine the degree of control each partner in their relationship will exert. In this phase of adjustment, a balance is sought between the needs of the mother and the needs of the infant. The most important consideration is that each should obtain a good measure of enjoyment from the interaction. During this phase, negative maternal feelings are likely to surface or intensify. Because "everyone knows that mothers love their babies," these negative feelings often go unexpressed and are allowed to build up. If they are expressed, the response of friends, relatives, or healthcare personnel is often to deny the feelings to the mother: "You don't mean that." Some negative feelings are normal in the first few days after birth, and the nurse should be supportive when the mother vocalizes these feelings.

When mutual regulation arrives at the point where both mother and infant primarily enjoy each other's company, reciprocity has been achieved. **Reciprocity** is an interactional cycle that occurs simultaneously between mother and infant.

Clinical Tip

Newborns are sometimes taken from their parents immediately after birth and placed in a special care or intensive care nursery. This separation can interfere with the normal attachment process. If this occurs, parents should be brought to the nursery as soon as possible to interact with their infants, and should be allowed to hold and care for their infant as much as possible. If the infant is in an incubator and cannot be held, encourage the parents to stroke the infant's hand, foot, or cheek. Provide reassurance that this will not hurt the infant and is in fact beneficial.

It involves mutual cuing behaviors, expectancy, rhythmicity, and synchrony. The mother develops a new relationship with an individual who has a unique character and evokes a response entirely different from the fantasy response of pregnancy. When reciprocity is synchronous, the interaction between mother and infant is mutually gratifying and is sought and initiated by both partners (Feldman, 2010; Reyna & Pickler, 2009).

Father–Infant Interactions

In Western cultures, commitment to family-centered maternity care has fostered interest in understanding the feelings and experiences of the new father. Evidence suggests that the father has a strong attraction to his newborn and that the feelings he experiences are similar to the mother's feelings of attachment (Figure 29–5 ●). The characteristic sense of absorption, preoccupation, and interest in the infant demonstrated by fathers during early contact is termed **engrossment**. Differences in involvement still exist among fathers in Western culture and may be influenced by factors other than culture (e.g., previous experience with paternal role or exposure to male/father role models).

Siblings and Others

Infants are capable of maintaining a number of strong attachments without loss of quality. These attachments may include siblings, grandparents, aunts, and uncles. The social setting and personality of the individual seem to be significant factors in the development of multiple attachments. Birth centers are especially geared toward the inclusion of the family in the birth

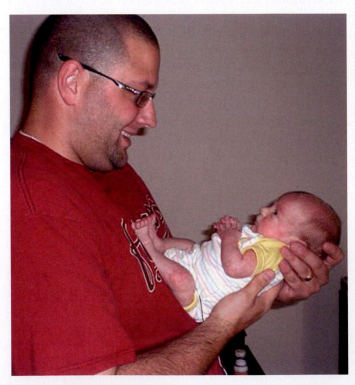

● **Figure 29–5** The father experiences strong feelings of attraction during engrossment.
Source: Courtesy of Christopher Allen.

Developing Cultural Competence
Muslim Paternal Attachment

In some cultures, there may be little involvement of the father in new-born care. In the Muslim culture, for example, emphasis on childrearing and infant care activities is on the mother and extended female family members. Nurses need to be aware of cultural differences when evaluating a father's interaction with his newborn.

process. In the hospital setting, the advent of open visiting hours and rooming-in permits siblings and others to participate in the attachment process.

Cultural Influences in the Postpartum Period

Whereas Western culture places primary emphasis on the events of birth, many other cultures place greater emphasis on the postpartum period. For women not of the dominant American culture, the new mother's culture and personal values influence her beliefs about her postpartum care. Her expectations about food, fluids, rest, hygiene, medications, relief measures, support, and counsel—as well as other aspects of her life—will be influenced by the beliefs and values of her family and cultural group. Sometimes, a new mother's wishes will differ from the expectations of the certified nurse-midwife (CNM), physician, or nurse. (See Chapter 2 for an in-depth discussion of cultural factors ⊘.) Nurses belong to their particular ethnoculture and also share in the culture of health care. Thus their nursing care practices may tend to support the general beliefs of their own groups. Nurses need to be aware of these tendencies and allow the mother to exercise her choices when possible and support those choices, with the help of cultural awareness and a sound knowledge base.

The woman of European heritage may expect to eat a full meal and have large amounts of iced fluids after the birth, in the belief that the food restores energy and the fluids help replace fluid lost during the labor. She may want to ambulate shortly after the birth, shower, wash her hair, and put on a fresh gown. She may expect a short stay in the hospital and may or may not be interested in educational classes. Women of the Islamic faith may have specific modesty requirements; the woman must be completely covered, with only her feet and hands exposed, and no man, other than the husband or a family member, may be alone with her.

Some cultures emphasize certain postpartum routines or rituals for mother and baby that are designed to restore the hot–cold balance of the body. Some women of Hispanic, African, and Asian cultures may avoid cold after birth. This prohibition includes cold air, wind, and all water (even if heated). On the other hand, some women of traditional Mexican descent may avoid eating "hot" foods such as pork just after the birth of a baby (considered a "hot" experience). It is important to note that each individual or cultural group may define hot and cold conditions and foods differently. The nurse should ask each woman what she can eat and what foods she thinks would be helpful for healing. The nurse may encourage family members to bring preferred foods and drinks for the mother. For more detailed discussion of the hot–cold balance concept, see *Cultural Influences Affecting the Family* in Chapter 2 ⊘.

In many cultures, the extended family plays an essential role during the puerperium. The grandmother is often the primary helper to the mother and newborn. She brings wisdom and experience, allowing the new mother time to rest and giving her ready access to someone who can help with problems and concerns as they arise. African American mothers often model their mothering skills after their older female relatives. In addition, these same older female relatives frequently provide child care as needed (Lauderdale, 2012).

It is important to ensure access of all family members to the mother and newborn. Visiting hours may be waived to allow family members or authority figures access to the mother and newborn. These practices show respect and foster a blending of old and new behaviors to meet the goals of all concerned (Lauderdale, 2012).

Developing Cultural Competence
Caring for the Orthodox Jewish Couple

The orthodox Jewish couple's beliefs and practices are strictly adhered to in their dress, communication, dietary practices, and activities of daily living in the postpartum time. The nurse should assist the woman in maintaining her modesty in her dress and keeping her hair covered at all times. For the first 7 days after delivery, the woman will be given special treatment and will be cared for by family members. Jewish patients may request a kosher diet. Some traditional Jewish couples avoid physical contact while the woman is experiencing any vaginal discharge; unfortunately, the man following this custom may be viewed as unsupportive by the staff during the postpartum period. Resting after childbirth is considered crucial for the first 6 weeks. The woman will breastfeed her newborn. The baby will not be named nor will the newborn male be circumcised until a later date after discharge from the hospital. The Sabbath is sacred and begins at sundown on Friday evening and ends after dark on Saturday. During this time neither the man nor the woman will use electricity, travel, or write. They will not tear or cut anything. So if the woman is in the hospital during the Sabbath, the nurse should be sensitive to the fact that any forms that may need to be signed will have to be signed before or after the Sabbath. The woman will need the nurse to adjust an electric bed, turn off/on lights, tear pieces of toilet paper for her to use, etc. The woman will not leave the hospital and travel home until after the Sabbath (Lauderdale, 2012).

POSTPARTUM NURSING ASSESSMENT

Comprehensive care is based on a thorough assessment that identifies individual needs or potential problems.

Risk Factors

Ongoing assessment and patient education during the puerperium is designed to meet the needs of the childbearing family and to detect and treat possible complications. Table 29–2 identifies factors that may place the new mother at risk during the postpartum period. The nurse uses this knowledge during the assessment and is particularly alert for possible complications associated with identified risk factors.

Table 29–2	Postpartum High-Risk Factors
Factor	**Maternal Implication**
Preeclampsia	↑ Blood pressure ↑ CNS irritability ↑ Need for bed rest → ↑ risk thrombophlebitis
Diabetes	Need for insulin regulation Episodes of hypoglycemia or hyperglycemia ↓ Healing
Cardiac disease	↑ Maternal exhaustion
Cesarean birth	↑ Healing needs ↑ Pain from incision ↑ Risk of infection ↑ Length of hospitalization Exacerbation of carpal tunnel syndrome
Overdistention of uterus (multiple gestation, hydramnios)	↑ Risk of hemorrhage ↑ Risk of thrombophlebitis (C/S risk) ↑ Risk of anemia ↑ Risk of breastfeeding problems (C/S risk) ↑ Stretching of abdominal muscles ↑ Incidence and severity of afterpains
Abruptio placentae, placenta previa	Hemorrhage → anemia ↓ Uterine contractility after birth → ↑ infection risk
Precipitous labor (less than 3 hours)	↑ Risk of lacerations to birth canal → hemorrhage
Prolonged labor (greater than 24 hours)	Exhaustion ↑ Risk of hemorrhage Nutritional and fluid depletion ↑ Bladder atony and/or trauma ↑ Pain and bruising from prolonged time in stirrups
Difficult birth	Exhaustion ↑ Risk of perineal lacerations ↑ Risk of hematomas ↑ Risk of hemorrhage → anemia
Extended period of time in stirrups at birth	↑ Risk of thrombophlebitis
Retained placenta	↑ Risk of hemorrhage ↑ Risk of infection

Physical Assessment

The nurse should remember several principles when preparing for and completing the assessment of the postpartum woman:

- Select a time that will provide the most accurate data. Palpating the fundus when the woman has a full bladder, for example, may give false information about the progress of involution. Ask the woman to void before assessment.

- Consider the patient's need for possible premedication before any painful assessment such as fundal massage.

- Explain the purpose of regular assessment.

- Ensure that the woman is relaxed before starting; perform the procedures as gently as possible to avoid unnecessary discomfort.

- Document and report the results as clearly as possible.

- Take appropriate precautions to prevent exposure to body fluids.

While performing the physical assessment, the nurse should also be teaching the woman. For example, when assessing the breasts of a lactating woman, the nurse can discuss breast care, breast milk production, the letdown reflex, and breast self-examination. A new mother may be very receptive to instruction on postpartum abdominal tightening exercises when the nurse assesses the woman's fundal height and diastasis. The assessment provides an excellent time to provide information about the body's postpartum physical and anatomic changes as well as danger signs to report. See *Health Promotion: Common Postpartum Concerns*. Because the time new mothers spend in the postpartum unit is limited, nurses need to use every available opportunity for patient education about self-care. To assist nurses in recognizing these opportunities, examples of patient teaching during the assessment are provided throughout the following discussion.

Vital Signs

Many nurses begin by assessing vital signs because the findings are more accurate when they are obtained with the woman at rest. In addition, establishing whether the vital signs are within the expected normal range will assist the nurse in determining if other assessments are needed. For instance, if the temperature is elevated, the nurse considers the time since birth and gathers information to determine whether the woman is dehydrated or whether an infection is developing.

Temperature elevations (less than 38°C [100.4°F]) caused by normal processes should last for only 24 hours. The nurse evaluates any elevation of temperature in light of associated signs and symptoms and carefully reviews the woman's history to identify other factors, such as premature rupture of membranes (PROM) or prolonged labor, that might increase the incidence of infection in the genital tract.

Alterations in vital signs may indicate complications, so the nurse assesses them at regular intervals. After an immediate, transient rise after birth, the blood pressure should remain stable. The pulse often shows a characteristic slowness that is no cause for alarm. Pulse rates return to prepregnant norms very quickly unless complications arise.

SAFETY ALERT!
During the first few hours after birth, the woman may have some orthostatic hypotension. This will cause her to have a lower blood pressure reading in a sitting position. For the most accurate reading, measure the woman's blood pressure with her in the same position each time, preferably lying on her back with her arm at her side. Because of the propensity for hypotension, the nurse should assist the mother the first few times she attempts to ambulate after childbirth.

Health Promotion   Common Postpartum Concerns

Several postpartum occurrences cause special concern for mothers. The nurse will frequently be asked about the following events.

Source of Concern	Explanation
Gush of blood that sometimes occurs when she first arises	Results from normal pooling of blood in the vagina when the woman lies down to rest or sleep. Gravity causes blood to flow out when she stands.
Passing clots	Blood pools at the top of the vagina and forms clots that are passed upon rising or sitting on the toilet.
Night sweats	Normal physiologic occurrence that results as the body attempts to eliminate excess fluids that were present during pregnancy. May be aggravated by a plastic mattress pad.
Afterpains	More common in multiparas. Caused by contraction and relaxation of uterus. Increased by oxytocin, breastfeeding. Relieved with mild analgesics and time.
"Large stomach" after birth and failure to lose all weight gained during pregnancy	The baby, amniotic fluid, and placenta account for only a portion of the weight gained during pregnancy. The remainder takes approximately 6 weeks to lose. Abdomen also appears large because of decreased muscle tone. Postpartum exercises will help.

The nurse informs the woman of her vital signs and provides information about the normal changes in blood pressure and pulse. This may present an opportunity to determine whether the mother knows how to assess her own and her infant's temperature, how to read a thermometer, and how to select a thermometer from the wide variety now available.

Auscultation of Lungs

The breath sounds should be clear. Women who have been treated for preterm labor or preeclampsia are at higher risk for pulmonary edema. (See *Care of the Woman with a Hypertensive Disorder* in Chapter 16 for further discussion.)

Breasts

Before examining the breasts, the nurse dons gloves and then assesses the fit and support provided by the woman's bra and, if appropriate, offers information about how to select a supportive bra. A properly fitting bra supports the breasts and helps maintain breast shape by limiting stretching of supporting ligaments and connective tissue. If the mother is breastfeeding, the straps of the bra should be cloth, not elastic (because cloth has less stretch and provides more support), and easily adjustable. The back should be wide and have at least three rows of hooks to adjust for fit. Traditional nursing bras have a fixed inner cup and a separate half cup that can be unhooked for breastfeeding while the cup continues to support the breast. Purchasing a nursing bra one size larger than the prepregnant size will usually result in a good fit because the breasts increase in size with milk production.

Clinical Tip

An easy way to remember the components specific to the postpartum examination is to remember the term BUBBLEHE: B–breast, U–uterus, B–bladder, B–bowel, L–lochia, E–episiotomy/laceration/edema, H–Homans'/hemorrhoids, E–emotional.

The nurse can then ask the woman to remove her bra so the breasts can be examined. The nurse notes the size and shape of the breasts and any abnormalities, reddened or hot areas, or engorgement. The breasts are also lightly palpated for softness, slight firmness associated with filling, firmness associated with engorgement, warmth, and tenderness. The nipples are assessed for fissures, cracks, soreness, and inversion. The nurse teaches the woman the characteristics of the breast and explains how to recognize problems such as fissures and cracks in the nipples.

The nonbreastfeeding mother is assessed for evidence of breast discomfort, and relief measures are instituted if necessary. (See discussion of lactation suppression in the nonbreastfeeding mother in Chapter 30.) Breast assessment findings for a nonbreastfeeding woman may be recorded as follows: "Breasts soft, filling, no evidence of nipple tenderness or cracking, nipples everted."

Abdomen and Fundus

Before examination of the abdomen, the woman should void. This practice ensures that a full bladder is not displacing the uterus or causing any uterine atony; if atony is present, other causes (such as uterine relaxation associated with a regional block, overstretched uterus, or distended bladder) must be investigated.

The nurse determines the relationship of the fundus to the umbilicus and also assesses the firmness of the fundus. The top of the fundus is measured in finger breadths above, below, or at the umbilicus (Figure 29–6 ●). See Skill 4–1: Assessing the Status of the Uterine Fundus After Vaginal or Cesarean Birth in the *Clinical Skills Manual* SKILLS . The nurse notes whether the fundus is in the midline or displaced to either side of the abdomen. If not midline, the uterus position should be located. The most common cause of displacement is a full bladder; this finding requires further assessment. If the fundus is in midline but higher than expected, it is usually associated with clots within the uterus. The nurse should then record the results of the assessment.

In the woman who has had a cesarean birth, the abdominal incision is extremely tender. The nurse should palpate the

● **Figure 29–6** Measurement of descent of fundus for the woman with a vaginal birth. The fundus is located two finger breadths below the umbilicus.

Scant amount
Blood only on tissue when wiped or less that 1-inch stain on peripad.

Light amount
Less that 4-inch stain on peripad.

Moderate amount
Less that 6-inch stain on peripad.

Heavy amount
Saturated peripad within 1 hour.

● **Figure 29–7** Suggested guideline for assessing lochia volume.

fundus with extreme care and inspect the abdominal incision for signs of healing, such as approximation (edges of incision appear "glued" together), bleeding, and any signs of infection, including drainage, foul odor, or redness. The nurse should document whether internal sutures, Steri-Strips, or staples are intact. The nurse can also review characteristics of normal healing, incision care, and discuss signs of infection.

Lochia

The nurse then evaluates the lochia, including character, amount, odor, and the presence of clots. Nurses must don disposable gloves just before assessing the abdomen and fundus, or when they are ready to assess the perineum and lochia. During the first 1 to 3 days, the lochia should be rubra. A few small clots are normal and occur as a result of blood pooling in the vagina. However, the passage of numerous or large clots is abnormal, and the cause should be investigated immediately. After 2 to 3 days, the lochia flow becomes serosa.

Lochia should never exceed a moderate amount, such as that needed to partially saturate perineal pads daily, with an average of six. However, because this number is influenced by an individual woman's pad-changing practices, as well as the absorbency of the pad, the nurse needs to question her about the length of time the current pad has been in use, whether the amount is normal compared with her typical menstrual period, and whether any clots were passed before this examination, such as during voiding. If heavy bleeding is reported but not seen, the nurse asks

the woman to put on a clean perineal pad and then reassesses the woman's pad in 1 hour (Figure 29–7 ●). See Skill 4–2: Evaluating Lochia in the *Clinical Skills Manual* `SKILLS`.

SAFETY ALERT!
If blood loss exceeds the guidelines given in this chapter, weigh the perineal pads and the chux pads to estimate the blood loss more accurately. Typically, 1 g = 1 mL blood. Because blood can pool below the woman on the chux pad make sure you elevate the buttocks as part of your assessment.

Clots and heavy bleeding may be caused by uterine relaxation (atony), retained placental fragments, or rarely, an unknown cervical laceration, seen as heavy bleeding but with firm fundus, that may require further assessment (Table 29–3). Because of the evacuation of the uterine cavity during cesarean birth, women with such surgery usually have less lochia after the first 24 hours than mothers who give birth vaginally. If the woman is at increased risk for bleeding, or is actually experiencing heavy flow of lochia rubra, her blood pressure, pulse, and uterus need to be assessed frequently, and the physician/CNM may prescribe oxytocin (Pitocin) or methylergonovine maleate (Methergine). (See *Drug Guide: Methylergonovine Maleate [Methergine]* on page 735 in Chapter 30 ●.)

The odor of the lochia is inoffensive and never foul. If a foul odor is present, so is an infection. When using narrative nursing notes, chart the amount of lochia first, followed by character. For example:

■ Lochia: moderate rubra
■ Lochia: small rubra/serosa

Patient teaching that the nurse may address during assessment of the lochia may center on normal changes, effect of position changes, or what can be expected in the amount and color of the flow. Hygienic measures, such as wiping the perineum from front to back and washing her hands after toileting and changing pads, may be reviewed if appropriate. The nurse should approach

 Clinical Tip

Assessing the status of the uterine fundus may cause discomfort for the mother. In addition to explaining the importance of assessing the fundal position and how to determine firmness to the mother, you can show her how to perform frequent light massage of the fundus herself to promote uterine involution. Involving her in her own care encourages her participation. In addition, having her massage her own uterus may lessen bleeding and reduce the need for more thorough massage.

Table 29–3	Changes in Lochia That Cause Concern	
Change	**Possible Problem**	**Nursing Action**
Presence of clots	Inadequate uterine contractions that allow bleeding from vessels at the placental site	Assess location and firmness of fundus. Assess voiding pattern. Record and report findings.
Persistent lochia rubra	Inadequate uterine contractions; retained placental fragments; infection; undetected cervical laceration	Assess location and firmness of fundus. Assess activity pattern. Assess for signs of infection. Record and report findings.

the timing of teaching hygienic practices delicately, along with the content to be included. By establishing positive goals for the teaching—promoting comfort, enhancing tissue healing, and preventing infection—the nurse can avoid value-laden statements regarding personal beliefs about the need for cleanliness or control of body odor. The nurse should review with the mother the need to notify a healthcare professional if there is regression in the lochia flow pattern (e.g., color or amount).

Perineum

The perineum is inspected with the woman lying in a Sims' position. The nurse lifts the buttock to expose the perineum and anus.

If an episiotomy was done or a laceration required suturing, the nurse assesses the wound. To evaluate the state of healing, the nurse inspects the wound for **r**edness, **e**dema, **e**cchymosis, **d**ischarge/drainage, and **a**pproximation (REEDA scale). After 24 hours some edema may still be present, but the skin edges should be well approximated so that gentle pressure does not separate them. Gentle palpation should elicit minimal tenderness, and there should be no hardened areas suggesting infection. Ecchymosis interferes with normal healing, as does infection. Foul odors associated with drainage indicate infection. Hematomas sometimes occur, although these are considered abnormal.

The nurse next assesses whether hemorrhoids are present around the anus. If present, they are assessed for size, number, and pain or tenderness. (See Figure 29–8 ● and Skill 4–3: Postpartum Perineal Assessment in the *Clinical Skills Manual* SKILLS .)

During the assessment, the nurse talks with the woman to determine the effectiveness of comfort measures that have been used. The nurse provides teaching about the episiotomy

● **Figure 29–8** Intact perineum with hemorrhoids.

or perineal laceration. Some women do not thoroughly understand what and where an episiotomy is, and they may believe that the stitches must be removed as with other types of surgery. Frequently, when women fear that the stitches must be removed manually, they are afraid to ask about them. While explaining the findings of the assessment, the nurse provides information about the episiotomy, its location, and the signs that are being assessed. In addition, the nurse can add that the sutures are special and will dissolve slowly over the next few weeks as the tissues heal. By the time the sutures are dissolved, the tissues are strong and the incision edges will not separate. This is also an opportunity to teach comfort measures that may be used and reinforce the need to consult with the healthcare provider before using over-the-counter (OTC) medications/supplements if breastfeeding (see *Relief of Perineal Discomfort* in Chapter 30 ✪).

Clinical Tip

In evaluating the perineum, use the REEDA scale as a quick reminder of what to assess. Specifically:

R = redness

E = edema or swelling

E = ecchymosis or bruising

D = discharge/drainage

A = approximation (how well the edges of an incision—the episiotomy—or a repaired laceration seem to be holding together)

Complementary Care Lysine Following Episiotomy

Lysine, an essential amino acid, has been identified as a supplement that decreases the incidence of pain following an episiotomy. The recommended adult dosage is 12 mg/kg of body weight per day. It is also present in dietary sources, including meat, cheese, fish, eggs, soybeans, and nuts.

An example of documenting a perineal assessment might read: "Midline episiotomy; no edema, tenderness, or ecchymosis present. Skin edges well approximated"; or, if a perineal laceration repair, "Skin edges intact, no edema, tenderness, or ecchymosis, pain meds helpful. Woman reports sitz bath and Tucks pads or pain relief measures are controlling discomfort."

Lower Extremities

Postpartum women are at increased risk for *thrombophlebitis,* thrombus formation, and inflammation involving the leg vein (see Chapter 31 🔗 for a discussion of thrombophlebitis). To assess for thrombophlebitis, the nurse should have the woman stretch her legs out with the knees slightly flexed and the legs relaxed. The nurse then grasps the woman's foot and sharply dorsiflexes it. The second leg is assessed in the same way. No discomfort or pain should be present. If pain is elicited, the nurse notifies the physician/CNM that the woman has a positive Homans' sign (Figure 29–9 ●). The pain is caused by inflammation of the vessel. The nurse also evaluates the legs for edema by comparing both legs, because usually only one leg is involved. Any areas of redness, tenderness, and increased skin temperature are also noted.

● **Figure 29–9** Homans' sign: With the woman's knee flexed, the nurse dorsiflexes the foot. Pain in the foot or leg is a positive Homans' sign.
Source: © Image Source/Getty Images.

Some facilities have discontinued performing a Homans' sign in the nursing assessment, stating it is not diagnostic and could lead to emboli if a clot is dislodged during assessment. Supporters advocate its use as a screening tool, and there are no published reports of an emboli occurring as a result of performing a Homans' sign. In the event of a positive Homans' sign, diagnosis is made by compression or duplex ultrasonography. Low-dose heparin therapy is used in postpartum women who do develop a deep venous thrombosis (Cunningham et al., 2010).

Early ambulation is an important aspect in the prevention of thrombophlebitis. Most women are able to be up shortly after birth or once they have fully recovered from the effects of regional anesthetic agents, if one has been used. The mother's legs should be assessed for return of sensation following regional anesthesia. The cesarean birth patient requires range-of-motion exercises until she is ambulating more freely.

Patient teaching associated with assessment of the lower extremities focuses on the signs and symptoms of thrombophlebitis. In addition, the nurse may review self-care measures to promote circulation and measures to prevent thrombophlebitis, such as leg exercises that may be performed in bed, dorsiflexion on an hourly basis while on bed rest, ambulation, and avoiding pressure behind the knees and crossing the legs.

Usually, the nurse records the results of the assessment on a flowsheet or a summary nursing note. If tenderness and warmth have been noted, they might be recorded as follows: "Tenderness, warmth, slight edema, and slight redness noted on posterior aspect of left calf—positive Homans'. Woman advised to avoid pressure to this area; lower leg elevated and moist heat applied per agency protocol. Call placed to Dr. Garcia to report findings."

Elimination

During the hours after birth, the nurse carefully monitors a new mother's bladder status. A boggy uterus, a displaced uterus, or a palpable bladder are signs of bladder distention and require nursing intervention.

The postpartum woman can quickly show signs of bladder distention, possibly as soon as 1 to 2 hours after childbirth. This distention results because of normal postpartum diuresis. The nurse should assess the bladder for distention until the woman demonstrates complete emptying of the bladder with each voiding. The nurse may employ techniques to facilitate voiding, such as helping the woman out of bed to void or pouring warm water on the vulva, running water in the sink, and encouraging the woman to relax and take deep breaths. The physician will order catheterization when the bladder is distended and the woman cannot void, when she is voiding small amounts (less than 100 mL) frequently, or when no voiding has occurred in 8 hours. Although many physicians/CNMs write orders stating that the woman can be catheterized in 8 hours if she has not voided, the nurse needs to assess the bladder and any voiding pattern frequently before the end of the 8-hour period. Some women require catheterization sooner. The mother who has had a cesarean birth may have an indwelling catheter inserted prophylactically. The same assessments should be made in evaluating bladder emptying once the catheter has been removed.

The nurse elicits information from the woman about the adequacy of her fluid intake, whether she feels she is emptying her bladder completely when she voids, and any signs of urinary tract infection (UTI) she may be experiencing.

In the same way, the nurse obtains information about the new mother's intestinal elimination and any concerns she may have about it. Many mothers fear that the first bowel movement will be painful and possibly even damaging if an episiotomy has been done. Often, women have defecated during labor or childbirth; therefore, bowel movements normally return within 2 to 3 days after a vaginal childbirth. Stool softeners may be ordered to increase bulk and moisture in the fecal material and to allow more comfortable and complete evacuation. Constipation should be avoided to prevent pressure on sutures and increased discomfort. To enhance bowel elimination and help the woman reestablish her normal bowel pattern, the nurse can encourage ambulation, increased fluid intake (up to 2000 mL/day or more), and additional fresh fruits and roughage in her diet.

During the assessment, the nurse may provide information about postpartum diuresis and explain why the woman may be emptying her bladder so frequently. Information about the need for additional fluid intake, with suggestions of specific amounts, may be helpful. The woman should drink at least eight 8-oz glasses of water or juice daily in addition to other fluids. Breastfeeding mothers will have a higher requirement. The nurse discusses signs of urinary retention and overflow voiding and may review symptoms of UTI if it seems an appropriate moment for teaching. The nurse can also review methods of assisting bowel elimination and provide opportunities for the woman to ask questions.

Rest and Sleep Status

Physical fatigue often affects other adjustments and functions of the new mother. The mother requires energy to make the psychologic adjustments to a new infant and to a new role. Fatigue is often a highly significant factor in a new mother's apparent disinterest in her newborn. Frequently, the woman is so tired from a long labor and birth that everything seems to be an effort. To avoid inadvertently classifying a very tired mother as one with a potential attachment problem, the nurse should do a psychologic assessment on more than one occasion. After a nap the new mother is often far more receptive to her baby and her surroundings. During the postpartum assessment, the nurse evaluates the amount of rest a new mother is getting. If the woman reports difficulty sleeping at night, the nurse should try to determine the cause. If it is simply the strange environment, a warm drink and back rub may prove helpful. Appropriate nursing measures are indicated if the woman is bothered by normal postpartum discomforts such as afterpains, diaphoresis, or episiotomy or hemorrhoidal pain. The impact of rooming-in on the mother's ability to rest should be assessed. See Chapter 30 🔴 for more detailed discussion of comfort/pain relief measures.

The nurse should encourage a daily rest period and schedule hospital activities to allow time for napping. The nurse can also provide information about the fatigue a new mother experiences, strategies to promote rest/sleep at home, and the impact it can have on a woman's emotions and sense of control.

Nutritional Status

As a part of the nutritional assessment, the nurse can provide teaching about the nutritional needs of the woman during the postpartum period. See the postpartum nutrition discussion in Chapter 12 🔴. Visiting the mother during mealtime provides an opportunity for unobtrusive nutritional assessment and counseling.

During pregnancy the daily recommended dietary allowances call for increased amounts of calories, protein, and most vitamins and minerals. After birth, the nonbreastfeeding mother should be advised about the need to reduce her caloric intake by about 300 kcal daily and to return to prepregnancy levels for other nutrients. The breastfeeding mother should increase her daily caloric intake by about 200 kcal over the pregnancy requirements, or a total of 500 kcal over the prepregnant requirement. New mothers are advised that it is common practice to prescribe iron supplements for 3 months after birth. The hemoglobin and hematocrit values are then checked at the postpartum visit to detect any anemia.

Basic discussion often proves helpful, followed by referral as needed. In all cases, literature on nutrition should be provided, so that the woman will have a source of information after discharge. The nurse should inform the dietitian of any mother who is a vegetarian, has food allergies or lactose intolerance, or whose cultural or religious beliefs require specific foods. Appropriate meals can then be prepared for her. Many women, especially those who gained more than the recommended number of pounds during their pregnancy, are interested in losing weight after birth. The dietitian can design weight-reduction diets to meet nutritional needs and food preferences. The nurse may also refer women with unusual eating habits or numerous questions about good nutrition to the dietitian.

As part of a nutritional assessment, the nurse can provide teaching about the nutritional needs of the woman during the postpartum period.

Psychologic Assessment

During the first several postpartum weeks, the woman must accomplish certain physical, psychologic, and developmental tasks:

- Restoring physical condition
- Developing competence in caring for and meeting the needs of her infant

- Establishing a relationship with her new child
- Adapting to altered lifestyles and family structure resulting from the addition of a new member

Adequate assessment of the mother's psychologic adjustment is an integral part of postpartum evaluation. Some new mothers have little or no experience with newborns and may feel totally overwhelmed. They may show these feelings by asking questions and reading all available material or by becoming passive and quiet because they simply cannot deal with their feelings of inadequacy. Unless a nurse questions the woman about her plans and previous experience in a supportive, nonjudgmental way, the nurse might conclude that the woman is disinterested, withdrawn, or depressed. Clues indicating adjustment difficulties include excessive continued fatigue, marked depression, excessive preoccupation with physical status or discomfort, evidence of low self-esteem, lack of support systems, marital problems, inability to care for or nurture the newborn, and current family crises (illness or unemployment). These characteristics frequently indicate a potential for maladaptive parenting, which may lead to child abuse or neglect (physical, emotional, intellectual) and cannot be ignored. Referrals to public health nurses or other available community resources may provide greatly needed assistance and alleviate potentially dangerous situations.

Assessment of Early Attachment

The beginnings of parent–newborn attachment may be observed in the first few hours after birth. Continued assessments may occur during the postpartum stay and during home visits after discharge. A nurse in any of the postpartum settings should note progress toward attachment. See Table 29–4 for behaviors related to attachment.

The assessment should include both parents when possible; however, in this section, these behaviors focus primarily on the mother's attachment process. As discussed previously, research shows that fathers experience similar attachment feelings to those experienced by mothers. The following questions can be addressed in the course of nurse–patient interaction:

- Is the mother attracted to her newborn? To what extent does she seek face-to-face contact and eye contact? Has she progressed from fingertip touch, to palmar contact, to enfolding the infant close to her own body? Is attraction increasing or decreasing? If the mother does not exhibit increasing attraction, why not? Do the reasons lie primarily within her, with the baby, or with the environment?
- Is the mother inclined to nurture her infant? Is she progressing in her interactions with her infant?
- Does the mother act consistently? If not, is the source of unpredictability within her or her infant?
- Is her mothering consistently carried out? Does she seek information and evaluate it objectively? Does she develop solutions based on adequate knowledge of valid data? Does she evaluate the effectiveness of her maternal care and adjust appropriately?

Table 29–4	Parent Attachment Behaviors	
Assessment Area	**Attachment**	**Behavior Requiring Assessment and Information**
Caretaking	Talks with baby. Demonstrates and seeks eye-to-eye contact. Touches and holds baby. Changes diapers when needed. Baby is clean. Clothing is appropriate for room temperature. Feeds baby as needed and baby is gaining weight. Positions baby comfortably and checks on baby.	Does not refer to baby. Completes activities without addressing the baby or looking at the baby. Lacks interaction with baby. Does not recognize need for or demonstrate concern for baby's comfort or needs. Feeding occurs intermittently. Baby does not gain weight. Waits for baby to cry and then hesitates to respond.
Perception of the baby	Has knowledge of expected child development. Understands that the baby is dependent and cannot meet parents' needs. Accepts gender of child and characteristics.	Has unrealistic expectations of the baby's abilities and behaviors. Expects love and interaction from the baby. Believes that the baby will fulfill parents' needs. Is strongly distressed over gender of baby or feels that some aspect of the baby is unacceptable.
Support	Has friends who are available for support. Seems to be comfortable with being a parent. Has realistic beliefs of parenting role.	Is alone or isolated. Is on edge, tense, anxious, and hesitant with the baby. Demonstrates difficulty incorporating parenting with own wants and needs.

Note: These are a few of the behaviors that may be associated with attachment. It is vitally important for the nurse to observe the parents on more than one occasion and to take into consideration individual characteristics, values, beliefs, and customs.

■ Is she sensitive to the newborn's needs as they arise? How quickly does she interpret her infant's behavior and react to cues? Does she seem happy and satisfied with the infant's responses to her efforts? Is she pleased with feeding behaviors? How much of this ability and willingness to respond is related to the baby's nature and how much to her own?

■ Does she seem pleased with her baby's appearance and gender? Does she experience pleasure when interacting with her infant? What interferes with the enjoyment? Does she speak to the baby frequently and affectionately? Does she call him or her by name? Does she point out family traits or characteristics she sees in the newborn?

■ Are there any cultural factors that might modify the mother's response? For instance, is it customary for the grandmother to assume most of the childcare responsibilities while the mother recovers from childbirth?

When the nurse has addressed these questions and assembled the facts, the nurse's intuition and knowledge should combine to answer three more questions: Is there a problem in attachment? What is the problem? What is its source? The nurse can then devise a creative approach to the problem as it presents itself in the context of a unique, developing mother–infant relationship. See *Assessment Guide: Postpartum—First 24 Hours After Birth.*

DISCHARGE ASSESSMENT AND FOLLOW-UP

The final discharge assessment should include a physical examination and appropriate discharge teaching that includes both maternal and newborn care guidelines. The optimal time for a home visit or follow-up phone call is 3 to 4 days after birth; this provides opportunities for further assessment of mothers and their infants and teaching. (See *Assessment Guide: Postpartum—First Home Visit and Anticipated Progress at 6 Weeks* on pages 757–759 in Chapter 30 .)

Assessment Guide　Postpartum—First 24 Hours After Birth

Physical Assessment/Normal Findings	Alterations and Possible Causes*	Nursing Responses to Data†
Vital Signs		
Blood pressure (BP): Should remain consistent with baseline BP during pregnancy.	High BP (preeclampsia, essential hypertension, renal disease, anxiety). Drop in BP (may be normal; uterine hemorrhage).	Evaluate history of preexisting disorders and check for other signs of preeclampsia (edema, proteinuria). Assess for other signs of hemorrhage (↑ pulse, cool clammy skin).
Pulse: 60 to 100 beats/minute. May be bradycardia of 50 to 70 beats/minute.	Tachycardia (difficult labor and birth, hemorrhage).	Evaluate for other signs of hemorrhage (↓ BP, cool clammy skin).
Respirations: 12 to 20/minute.	Marked tachypnea (respiratory disease).	Assess for other signs of respiratory disease.
Temperature: 36.6°C to 38°C (98°F to 100.4°F).	After first 24 hours temperature of 38°C (100.4°F) or above suggests infection.	Assess for other signs of infection; notify physician/CNM.
Breasts		
General appearance: Smooth, even pigmentation; changes of pregnancy still apparent; one may appear larger.	Reddened area (mastitis).	Assess further for signs of infection.
Palpation: Depending on postpartum day, may be soft, filling, full, or engorged.	Palpable mass (caked breast, mastitis). Engorgement (venous stasis). Tenderness, heat, edema (engorgement, caked breast, mastitis).	Assess for other signs of infection: If blocked duct, consider heat, massage, position change for breastfeeding. Assess for further signs. Report mastitis to physician/certified nurse-midwife.
Nipples: Supple, pigmented, intact; become erect when stimulated.	Fissures, cracks, soreness (problems with breastfeeding), not erectile with stimulation (inverted nipples).	Reassess technique; recommend appropriate interventions.
Lungs		
Sounds: clear to bases bilaterally.	Diminished (fluid overload, asthma, pulmonary embolus, pulmonary edema).	Assess for other signs of respiratory distress.

(continued)

Assessment Guide Postpartum—First 24 Hours After Birth—continued

Physical Assessment/Normal Findings	Alterations and Possible Causes*	Nursing Responses to Data†
Abdomen		
Musculature: Abdomen may be soft, have a "doughy" texture; rectus muscle intact.	Separation in musculature (diastasis recti abdominis).	Evaluate size of diastasis; teach appropriate exercises for decreasing the separation.
Fundus: Firm, midline; following expected process of involution.	Boggy (full bladder, uterine bleeding).	Massage until firm; assess bladder and have woman void if needed; attempt to express clots when firm. If bogginess remains or recurs, report to physician/certified nurse-midwife.
May be tender when palpated. Cesarean section incision dressing; dry and intact.	Constant tenderness (infection). Moderate to large amount of blood or serosanguineous drainage on dressing.	Assess for evidence of endometritis. Assess for hemorrhage. Reinforce dressing and notify healthcare provider.
Lochia		
Scant to moderate amount, earthy odor; no clots.	Large amount, clots (hemorrhage). Foul-smelling lochia (infection).	Assess for firmness, express additional clots; begin peripad count. Assess for other signs of infection; report to physician/certified nurse-midwife.
Normal progression: First 1 to 3 days: rubra.	Failure to progress normally or return to rubra from serosa (subinvolution).	Report to physician/certified nurse-midwife.
Following rubra: Days 3 to 10: serosa (alba seldom seen in hospital).		
Perineum		
Slight edema and bruising in intact perineum.	Marked fullness, bruising, pain (vulvar hematoma).	Assess size; apply ice glove or ice pack; report to physician/certified nurse-midwife.
Episiotomy: No redness, edema, ecchymosis, or discharge; edges well approximated.	Redness, edema, ecchymosis, discharge, or gaping stitches (infection).	Encourage sitz baths; review perineal care, appropriate wiping techniques.
Hemorrhoids: None present; if present, should be small and nontender.	Full, tender, inflamed hemorrhoids.	Encourage sitz baths, side-lying position; Tucks pads, anesthetic ointments, manual replacement of hemorrhoids, stool softeners, increased fluid intake.
Costovertebral Angle (CVA) Tenderness		
None.	Present (kidney infection).	Assess for other symptoms of urinary tract infection (UTI); obtain clean-catch urine specimen; report to physician/certified nurse-midwife.
Lower Extremities		
No pain with palpation; negative Homans' sign.	Positive findings (thrombophlebitis).	Report to physician/certified nurse-midwife.
Elimination		
Urinary output: Voiding in sufficient quantities at least every 4 to 6 hours; bladder not palpable.	Inability to void (urinary retention). Symptoms of urgency, frequency, dysuria (UTI).	Employ nursing interventions to promote voiding; if not successful, obtain order for catheterization. Report symptoms of UTI to physician/certified nurse-midwife.
Bowel elimination: Should have normal bowel movement by second or third day after birth.	Inability to pass feces (constipation caused by fear of pain from episiotomy, hemorrhoids, perineal trauma).	Encourage fluids, ambulation, roughage in diet; sitz baths to promote healing of perineum; obtain order for stool softener.

Assessment Guide Postpartum—First 24 Hours After Birth—continued

Cultural Assessment‡	Variations to Consider	Nursing Responses to Data†
Determine customs and practices regarding postpartum care. Ask the mother whether she would like fluids, and ask what temperature she prefers. Ask the mother what foods or fluids she would like.	Individual preference may include room-temperature or warmed fluids rather than iced drinks. Special foods or fluids to hasten healing after childbirth.	Provide for specific request if possible. If woman is unable to provide specific information, the nurse may draw from general information regarding cultural variation. Mexican women may want food and fluids that restore hot–cold balance to the body. Women of European background may ask for iced fluids.
Ask the mother whether she would prefer to be alone during breastfeeding.	Some women may be hesitant to have someone with them when their breast is exposed.	Provide privacy as desired by mother.

Psychologic Adaptation

During first 24 hours: Passive; preoccupied with own needs; may talk about her labor and birth experience; may be talkative, elated, or very quiet.	Very quiet and passive; sleeps frequently (fatigue from long labor; feelings of disappointment about some aspect of the experience; may be following cultural expectation).	Provide opportunities for adequate rest; provide nutritious meals and snacks that are consistent with what the woman desires to eat and drink; provide opportunities to discuss birth experience in nonjudgmental atmosphere if the woman desires to do so.
Usually by 12 hours: Beginning to assume responsibility; some women eager to learn; easily feels overwhelmed.	Excessive weepiness, mood swings, pronounced irritability (postpartum blues; feelings of inadequacy; culturally proscribed behavior).	Explain postpartum blues; provide supportive atmosphere; determine support available for mother; consider referral for evidence of profound depression.

Attachment

En face position; holds baby close; cuddles and soothes; calls by name; identifies characteristics of family members in infant; may be awkward in providing care.	Continued expressions of disappointment in gender, appearance of infant; refusal to care for infant; derogatory comments; lack of bonding behaviors (difficulty in attachment, following expectations of cultural/ethnic group).	Provide reinforcement and support for infant caretaking behaviors; maintain nonjudgmental approach and gather more information if caretaking behaviors are not evident.
Initially may express disappointment over gender or appearance of infant but within 1 to 2 days demonstrates attachment behaviors.		

Patient Education

Has basic understanding of self-care activities and infant care needs; can identify signs of complications that should be reported.	Unable to demonstrate basic self-care and infant care activities (knowledge deficit; postpartum blues; following prescribed cultural behavior and will be cared for by grandmother or other family member).	Identify dominant learning style. Determine whether woman understands English and provide interpreter if needed; provide reinforcement of information through conversation and through written material (remember that some women and their families may not be able to understand written materials because of language difficulties or inability to read); provide information regarding infant care skills that are culturally consistent; give woman opportunity to express her feelings; consider social service home referral for women who have no family or other support, are unable to take in information about self-care and infant care, and demonstrate no caretaking activities.

*Possible causes of alterations are identified in parentheses.

†This column provides guidelines for further assessment and initial nursing actions.

‡ These are only a few suggestions. It is not our intent to imply this is a comprehensive cultural assessment.

Critical Concept Review

LEARNING OUTCOME 29.1: Describe the basic physiologic changes that occur in the postpartum period as a woman's body returns to its prepregnant state.

1. Uterus is at the level of umbilicus within a few hours after childbirth. Decreases by about one finger breadth per day.
2. Placental site heals by a process of exfoliation, so no scar formation occurs.
3. Lochia flow progresses from rubra to serosa to alba.
4. Ovarian function and menstruation return in approximately 6–12 weeks in the nonlactating mother.
5. Breasts begin milk production.
6. Intestines are sluggish for a few days, leading to constipation, but return to prepregnant state within a week.

7. Postpartum diuresis occurs, bladder tone is decreased, and bladder takes approximately 6 weeks to return to prepregnant state.
   - A higher-than-usual boggy uterus, which deviates to the side, usually indicates a full bladder.
8. Bradycardia is normal for the first 6–10 days.
9. Hemostatic system reaches prepregnant state in 3–4 weeks. WBC count is often elevated. Activation of clotting factors predisposes to thrombus formation.

LEARNING OUTCOME 29.2: Describe the psychologic adjustments that normally occur during the postpartum period.

1. Psychologic adjustment includes:
   - Taking-in.
   - Taking-hold.
   - Maternal role attainment.
   - Possibility of postpartum blues.

LEARNING OUTCOME 29.3: Describe the physiologic and psychologic components of a systematic postpartum assessment.

1. Systematic postpartum assessment includes:
   - Vital signs.
   - Breast examination.
   - Assessment of fundus, incision, episiotomy, and perineum.
   - Assessment of lochia in terms of type, quantity, and characteristics.
   - Assessment of bladder and bowels.
   - Assessment of lower extremities.
   - Psychologic assessment.
     - Expected phase of adjustment to parenthood.
     - Expected level of attachment to infant.
   - Patient education concerning self-care.

LEARNING OUTCOME 29.4: Describe the common concerns of the mother that are considered in a postpartum assessment.

1. The nurse will often be asked about these common postpartum concerns:
   - A gush of blood that sometimes occurs when the woman first arises.
   - Passing clots.
   - Night sweats.
   - Afterpains.
   - "Large stomach" after birth and failure to lose all the weight gained during pregnancy.

2. Review the *Health Promotion* feature on page 721 for an explanation of these common postpartum concerns.

LEARNING OUTCOME 29.5: Examine the physical and developmental tasks that the mother must accomplish during the postpartum period.

1. The woman's physical condition returns to a nonpregnant state.
2. The woman gains competence and confidence in herself as a parent by:
   - Developing competence in caring for and meeting the needs of her infant.
   - Establishing a relationship with her new child.
   - Adapting to altered lifestyles and family structure resulting from the addition of a new member.

LEARNING OUTCOME 29.6: Identify the factors that influence the development of a positive parent–infant attachment in the nursing assessment of early attachment.

1. Parent–infant attachment is influenced by:
   - Involvement with woman's own family.
   - Stability of relationships and home environment.
   - Mother's ability to trust.
   - Mother's level of self-esteem.
   - Mother's ability to enjoy herself.
   - Mother's knowledge of expectations of childbearing and childrearing.
   - Positive reaction to present pregnancy.

Clinical Judgment in Action

Janet Burns, a 25-year-old G3P3, is 2 hours past a low forceps vaginal birth with a right medial lateral episiotomy of a live 8-pound baby boy. You obtain vital signs of BP 118/70, T 98.8°F, P 76, R 14. You observe the fundus is +1 finger breadth above the umbilicus and slightly to the right. Her episiotomy is slightly ecchymotic and well approximated without edema or discharge. Ice has been applied to the episiotomy for the last 20 minutes. Lochia rubra is present and a pad was saturated in 90 minutes. Janet has an intravenous of Ringer's lactate with 10 units of Pitocin infusing at 100 mL/hr in her lower left arm and is complaining of moderate abdominal cramping. Janet's baby is sleeping peacefully in the bassinet next to her bed. She tells you that she is very tired and requests some pain medication so she can sleep for a while.

1. What nursing assessment is of immediate concern?
2. Discuss care of her episiotomy and perineum.
3. What other self-care measures could you advise?
4. Discuss postpartum occurrences that may cause special concern for the mother.
5. Janet expressed concern about her episiotomy healing. What information can you offer?
6. Develop a concept map for episiotomy care.

See www.nursing.pearsonhighered.com for possible responses and an interactive template for a concept map.

References

Beck, C. T. (2008). *Postpartum mood and anxiety disorders: Case studies, research, and nursing care* (2nd ed.). Washington, DC: Association of Women's Health, Obstetric and Neonatal Nurses.

Blackburn, S. T. (2013). *Maternal, fetal, & neonatal physiology: A clinical perspective* (4th ed.). St. Louis, MO: Saunders.

Carhuapoma, J. R., Tomlinson, M. W., & Levine, S. R. (2011). Neurologic complications. In D. James, P. J. Steer, C. P. Weiner, B. Gonik, C. C. Crowther, & S. C. Robson, *High risk pregnancy: Management options* (4th ed., pp. 861–891). St. Louis, MO: Elsevier/Saunders.

Cunningham, F. G., Leveno, K. J., Bloom, S. L., Hauth, J. C., Rouse, D. J., & Spong, C. Y. (2010). *Williams obstetrics* (23rd ed.). New York, NY: McGraw-Hill.

Davey, H. L., Tough, S. C., Adair, C. E., & Benzies, K. M. (2011). Risk factors for sub-clinical and major postpartum depression among a community cohort of Canadian women. *Maternal Child Health Journal, 15,* 866–875. doi:10.1007/s10995-008-0314-8

Feldman, R. (2010). The relational basis of adolescent adjustment: Trajectories of mother–child interactive behaviors from infancy to adolescence shape adolescents' adaptation. *Attachment & Human Development 12,* (1–2), 173–192.

Kalayjian, L., Goodwin, T. M., & Lee, R. H. (2013). Nervous system & autoimmune disorders in pregnancy. In A. H. DeCherney, L. Nathan, N. Laufer, & A. S. Roman (Eds.), *Current diagnosis & treatment: Obstetrics & gynecology* (11th ed., pp. 533–542). New York, NY: McGraw-Hill.

Lauderdale, J. (2012). Transcultural perspectives in childbearing. In M. M. Andrews & J. S. Boyle (Eds.), *Transcultural concepts in nursing care* (6th ed., pp. 91–122). Philadelphia, PA: Wolters Kluwer/Lippincott Williams & Wilkins.

Mercer, R. T. (2004). Becoming a mother versus maternal role attainment. *Journal of Nursing Scholarship, 36*(3), 226–232.

Pessel, C., & Tsai, M. C. (2013). The normal puerperium. In A. H. DeCherney, L. Nathan, N. Laufer, & A. S. Roman (Eds.), *Current diagnosis & treatment: Obstetrics & gynecology* (11th ed., pp. 190–213). New York, NY: McGraw-Hill.

Reyna, B. A., & Pickler, R. H. (2009). Mother–infant synchrony. *Journal of Obstetric, Gynecologic, and Neonatal Nursing, 38*(4), 470–477. doi:10.1111/j.1552-6909.2009.01044.x

Rubin, R. (1984). *Maternal identity and the maternal experience.* New York, NY: Springer.

Whitmer, T. (2011). Physical and psychologic changes. In S. Mattson & J. E. Smith (Eds.), *Core curriculum for maternal–newborn nursing* (4th ed., pp. 301–314). St. Louis, MO: Saunders/Elsevier.

CHAPTER 30

The Postpartum Family: Early Care Needs and Home Care

More than anything else that happened after my baby was born, I was surprised by the fatigue I felt. In the first few weeks, I spent every minute that my baby slept cleaning, doing laundry, and the like. Then, during my checkup, the nurse-midwife told me that I had to rest when my baby slept. What a difference that made. Suddenly I was less overwhelmed and more able to enjoy being a mother. —Mai Ling, 26

© pressmaster/Fotolia.com

LEARNING OUTCOMES

30.1 Formulate nursing diagnoses and nursing care based on the findings of the normal postpartum assessment and teaching needs.

30.2 Describe appropriate nursing interventions to promote postpartum maternal comfort, rest, and well-being.

30.3 Explain factors that affect postpartum family wellness in the provision of nursing care and patient teaching.

30.4 Compare the postpartum nursing needs of the woman who experienced a cesarean birth with the needs of a woman who gave birth vaginally.

30.5 Examine the nursing needs of the childbearing adolescent during the postpartum period.

30.6 Describe possible approaches to sensitive, holistic nursing care for the woman who relinquishes her newborn.

30.7 Explain the specific postpartum needs for women with obesity, developmental disabilities, or history of sexual abuse.

30.8 Identify postpartum teaching needs that should be modified to provide sensitive care to meet the needs of lesbian mothers.

30.9 Identify teaching topics related to postpartum discharge.

30.10 Identify the main purposes and components of home visits during the postpartum period.

30.11 Summarize actions a nurse should take to ensure personal safety as well as fostering a caring relationship during a home visit.

30.12 Describe maternal and family assessment and anticipated progress after birth.

30.13 Delineate interventions to address the common concerns of breastfeeding mothers following discharge.

30.14 Describe the assessment and care of the newborn during postpartum home care.

733

Chapter 29 ⊘ provided a thorough discussion of postpartum adaptation and nursing assessment. This chapter describes how the nurse can use the remaining steps of the nursing management process effectively to plan and provide care. Specific nursing responses to the mother's physical needs and the family's psychosocial needs are described at length.

NURSING CARE DURING THE EARLY POSTPARTUM PERIOD

For most postpartum women, physical recovery goes smoothly and is considered a healthy process. Because of this perception, caregivers too often assume that the woman and her family have no real needs and that no care plan is needed. Nothing could be further from the truth. Every member of the family has needs, although the needs may not be obvious, especially if they are psychologic or educational.

Nursing Diagnosis

The postpartum family's needs, which should be identified during assessment, are the basis for developing nursing diagnoses. Many nurses have suggested that nursing diagnoses are difficult to make in a wellness setting because of their emphasis on "problems." Nurses involved in the effort to formulate standardized diagnoses recognize this difficulty and continue working to develop nursing diagnoses that are more congruent with wellness settings.

Many agencies that use nursing diagnoses prefer to use only the NANDA diagnoses. Consequently, physiologic alterations form the basis of many postpartum diagnoses. Examples of such diagnoses include (NANDA-I © 2012):

- *Breastfeeding, Ineffective,* related to postpartum pain from a cesarean birth or maternal fatigue
- *Constipation* related to fear of tearing stitches or pain
- *Pain, Acute,* related to perineal trauma secondary to episiotomy or birth

Diagnoses related to family coping or instructional needs are also used frequently. Examples of these diagnoses include (NANDA-I © 2012):

- *Knowledge, Readiness for Enhanced,* about infant care related to an expressed desire to improve parenting skills
- *Anxiety* related to self and infant care secondary to lack of knowledge of appropriate care practices
- *Coping: Family, Readiness for Enhanced,* related to successful adjustment to new baby
- *Self-Health Management, Readiness for Enhanced,* related to desire to obtain optimal health in the postpartum period

Nursing Plan and Implementation

An important component of postpartum nursing care is patient teaching, which must be individualized to the learning capability and readiness of the parent(s). As part of the teaching role, the nurse discusses desired outcomes and goals with the mother and family members as soon as possible following the birth. Interventions can then be designed to achieve optimal health promotion. Strategies for promoting effective learning are discussed shortly, and specific teaching content is provided throughout the rest of this chapter. Home care visits and phone contacts help ensure that new parents have the necessary skills and resources to care for their infant.

PROMOTION OF MATERNAL COMFORT AND WELL-BEING

The nurse can promote and restore maternal physical well-being by monitoring uterine status, vital signs, cardiovascular status, elimination patterns, nutritional needs, sleep and rest, and learning needs. Some women also require medication to relieve pain, treat anemia, provide immunity to rubella, and prevent development of antibodies in a nonsensitized Rh-negative woman. Most postpartum women need nursing interventions to promote their comfort and relieve stress. During the postpartum period, ongoing assessments are warranted to assess the physiologic changes that have occurred and ensure that adequate return to a nonpregnant state is occurring. After birth, the examination of the uterine status, lochia, and episiotomy is performed every 15 minutes for 1 hour, then every 30 minutes × 2, then every hour × 2, then every 4 hours × 2, and then every 8 hours until the woman is discharged home.

Postpartum Examination

A complete assessment for the postpartum woman should include assessing the breasts, uterus, bowels, bladder, lochia, episiotomy, hemorrhoids, and emotional status. The mnemonic BUBBLE-HE provides the nurse with a means to memorize these components of a postpartum assessment. Table 30–1 provides the normal and abnormal findings that can be identified in the postpartum period and interventions for routine care.

Occasionally medications are needed to promote uterine contractions. These include oxytocin, discussed in Chapter 23 🔗, and methylergonovine maleate (Methergine) (see the accompanying *Drug Guide*). The nurse also monitors the amount, consistency, color, and odor of the lochia on an ongoing basis. Continued assessment is warranted during the first 24 hours because early postpartum hemorrhage typically occurs in the 24 hours after birth and is most commonly related to uterine atony (the top portion of the uterus is soft and spongy rather than firm and well contracted) (Lowe, 2012). Table 30–2 describes the position of the uterine fundus following birth. See Chapter 31 🔗 for treatment of uterine atony.

Relief of Perineal Discomfort

Before selecting a method to help relieve perineal discomfort, the nurse needs to assess the perineum to determine the degree of edema and other problems. It is also important to ask the woman if she believes any special measures will be particularly effective and to offer her choices when possible. The nurse uses disposable gloves while applying all relief measures and washes hands before and after using the gloves. At all times it is

---

 ## Drug Guide Methylergonovine Maleate (Methergine)

Overview of Action

Methylergonovine maleate (Methergine) is an ergot alkaloid that stimulates smooth muscle tissue. Because the smooth muscle of the uterus is especially sensitive to this drug, it is used postpartum to stimulate the uterus to contract in order to decrease blood loss by clamping off uterine blood vessels and to promote the involution process. In addition, the drug has a vasoconstrictive effect on all blood vessels, especially the larger arteries. This may result in hypertension, particularly in a woman whose blood pressure is already elevated.

Route, Dosage, Frequency

Methergine has a rapid onset of action and may be given orally or intramuscularly.

> Usual IM dose: 0.2 mg following expulsion of the placenta. The dose may be repeated every 2 to 4 hours if necessary.
> Usual oral dose: 0.2 mg every 4 hours (six doses).

Maternal Contraindications

Pregnancy, hepatic or renal disease, cardiac disease, hypertension, or preeclampsia contraindicate this drug's use. Methylergonovine maleate must be used with caution during lactation (Wilson, Shannon, & Shields, 2013).

Maternal Side Effects

Hypertension, nausea, vomiting, headache, bradycardia, dizziness, tinnitus, abdominal cramps, palpitations, dyspnea, chest pain, and allergic reactions may be noted.

Effects on Fetus/Newborn

Because Methergine has a long duration (3 hours [Wilson et al., 2013]) and action and can thus produce tetanic contractions, it *should never be used during pregnancy or in labor*, when it may result in a sustained uterine contraction that may cause amniotic fluid embolism (increased pressure in uterus may allow entry of amniotic fluid under the edge of the placenta and thus entry into the maternal venous system), uterine rupture, cervical and perineal lacerations (resulting from tetanic contractions and rapid birth of the baby), and hypoxia and intracranial hemorrhage in the baby (because of tetanic contractions, which severely decrease the maternal–placental–fetal blood flow, or uterine rupture, which causes cessation of blood flow to the unborn baby) (Wilson et al., 2013).

Nursing Considerations

- Monitor fundal height and consistency and the amount and character of the lochia.
- Assess the blood pressure before and routinely throughout drug administration.
- Observe for adverse effects or symptoms of ergot toxicity (ergotism) such as nausea and vomiting, headache, muscle pain, cold or numb fingers and toes, chest pain, and general weakness (Wilson et al., 2013).
- Provide patient and family teaching regarding importance of not smoking during Methergine administration (nicotine from cigarettes leads to constricted vessels and may lead to hypertension) and signs of toxicity.

Table 30–1 BUBBLE-HE Mnemonic for Postpartum Examination

Area to Be Assessed	Normal Findings	Abnormal Findings	Interventions for Routine Care
Breasts	Soft or filling No cracking or bleeding from nipples Nipples erect with stimulation Colostrum present	Nipples flat or inverted Unable to obtain erect nipples with feeding or use of breast pump Reddened, tender area warm to touch (possible mastitis or engorgement) Cracked, bleeding nipples (possible trauma from breastfeeding, fissure, infection)	Advise use of a supportive bra. Suggest that breast shells be worn for flat or inverted nipples. Obtain an order for a lactation consult as needed. Note that cracking and bleeding are most commonly related to improper positioning with feeding. Contact healthcare provider immediately if symptoms of infection are present.
Uterus	Fundus firm, midline, position dependent on time since birth but should at or below umbilicus (see Table 30–2)	Uterus boggy, soft, shifted to the right or not midline, position above umbilicus (possible full bladder, subinvolution) Excessive tenderness with palpation (possible endometritis)	Teach woman to monitor her uterus for firmness. Advise frequent voiding to reduce incidence of bleeding. Suggest use of ibuprofen for any afterbirth pains. Inform woman that breastfeeding aids with involution process. For heavier than expected bleeding, try uterine massage.
Bowels	Abdomen soft, nondistended Normal bowel sounds in all quadrants Passing flatus Bowel movements occur without difficulty	Abdomen distended with discomfort noted No flatus Constipation, reduced bowel sounds	Encourage ambulation, fluids, diet high in fiber, stool softeners. Enema may be needed. Note that women with third- or fourth-degree lacerations need stool softeners.
Bladder	Nondistended, nonpalpable on exam Adequate voiding Urine clear yellow (may contain lochia)	Distended Unable to void or inadequate voiding pattern that does not fully empty bladder	Encourage frequent voiding. Measure first three voids after birth to ensure adequate bladder emptying.
Lochia	Lochia rubra immediately after birth until 3 days Lochia serosa from 3 days to 10 days Lochia alba after that Scant to moderate amount with earthy odor	Heavy amount Clotting Foul smelling Persistent lochia rubra that does not change to serosa	Teach that perineal hygiene includes frequent voiding and cleaning self from front to back. Instruct on consistent use of a peri-bottle while lochia present. Provide sitz bath if ordered.
Episiotomy	Episiotomy or perineum with mild edema Laceration or episiotomy should be intact and well approximated	Excessive edema Bruising Hematoma Discharge Sutures not well approximated or loose	Apply ice to perineum for 20 minutes on then 20 minutes off for first 24 hours. Give local perineal medication preparations. Provide sitz baths after first 24 hours. Review perineal hygiene measures.
Hemorrhoids	Rectum intact Hemorrhoids may be present but are small and nontender	Full Tender Inflamed	Teach patient about helpful topical agents: witch hazel pads, anesthetic ointments or creams. Try manual replacement of hemorrhoids. Increase fluids and fiber. Encourage sitz baths and side-lying position.
Emotional status	Adequate maternal–newborn attachment is observed Verbalization on proper care of infant Some anxiety is normal	Lack of interest in newborn Lack of expected maternal–infant attachment behaviors Excessive worrying Depression	Provide education on infant care practice, postpartum needs. Explore support system availability. Refer to support groups and new mother groups. Encourage frequent rest periods. Review baby blues and signs of postpartum depression.

Table 30–2	Position of the Uterine Fundus Following Birth
Time	**Position of Fundus**
Immediately after birth	Top of fundus is in the midline about midway between the symphysis pubis and umbilicus.
Six to twelve hours after birth	Top of fundus is in the midline and at the level of the umbilicus.
One day after birth	Top of fundus is in the midline and one finger breadth below the umbilicus.
Second day after birth and thereafter	Top of fundus remains in the midline and descends about one finger breadth per day.

essential for the nurse to remember hygienic practices, such as moving from the front of the perineum (area of the symphysis pubis) to the back (area around the anus). Avoiding contamination between the anal area and the urethral/vaginal area is vital to the prevention of infection. It is important to remember that in some cultures or religions, such as Orthodox Judaism, women are prohibited from touching or changing their own perineal pads and will require the nurse or a family member to do so.

Perineal Care

Perineal care after each elimination cleanses the perineum, prevents infection, and helps promote comfort. The woman should be instructed to wash her hands before and after changing peripads or performing pericare. The nurse demonstrates how to cleanse the perineum and assists the woman as necessary. Many agencies provide "peri-bottles" that the woman can use to squirt warm tap water over her perineum following elimination. To cleanse her perineum, the woman should use moist antiseptic towelettes or toilet paper in a blotting (patting) motion and should be taught to start at the front and proceed toward the back to prevent contamination from the anal area.

Many women have never used perineal pads and will need teaching and assistance in using them during the postpartum period. To prevent contamination, the perineal pad should be applied from front to back (place the front portion against the

perineum first) and changed when saturation occurs or after each perineal cleansing. The woman is advised to hold the pad on the sides to prevent contamination. The pad needs to be placed snugly against the perineum but should not produce pressure. If the pad is worn too loosely, it may rub back and forth, irritating perineal tissues and causing contamination between the anal and vaginal areas. The pad should be changed after urination and defecation. Women should be advised to cleanse the perineal area with soap and water at least one time per day in addition to using the peri-bottle after each void or pad change (Peterson, 2011). Advise the woman that the pad should be changed at least 4 times per day to prevent contamination from bacteria (Peterson, 2011). Women should be advised that perineal pain is common and will decrease gradually each day. Most women note complete resolution within 8 weeks of birth (Peterson, 2011). (For information regarding the care of the perineum following an episiotomy, see *Teaching Highlights: Episiotomy Care.*)

Ice Pack

If an episiotomy is done at the time of birth, an ice pack is generally applied to the perineum to reduce edema and provide numbing of the tissues, which promotes comfort. In some agencies, chemical ice bags are used. These are usually activated by folding both ends toward the middle. The nurse can create inexpensive ice bags by filling a disposable glove with ice chips or crushed ice and then taping the top of the glove closed. To protect the perineum from burns caused by contact with such an ice pack, the glove needs to be rinsed under running water to remove any powder and then wrapped in an absorbent towel or washcloth before placing it against the perineum. To attain the maximum effect of this cold treatment, a pattern of applying the ice pack for approximately 20 minutes and then removing it for about 10 minutes should be followed during the first 2 hours to reduce edema. Usually ice packs are needed for the first 24 hours to reduce pain (Peterson, 2011). The nurse

---

Complementary Care **Lavender Oil for Perineal Pain**

For centuries, lavender oil has been infused into warm water for relief of perineal pain associated with childbirth. Lavender is grown in Africa, Russia, the Arabic peninsula, and the Mediterranean region. The fragrance of lavender is said to promote a calming effect. The antianxiety qualities, combined with its soothing properties when diffused in water, make it a popular alternative therapy modality for postpartum women. Lavender may also have some antibacterial effects that may prevent infection in postpartum women.

Teaching Highlights **Episiotomy Care**

- Describe the process of wound healing.
- Discuss the risks of contamination of the episiotomy by bacteria from the anal area.
- Describe techniques that are used to keep the episiotomy clean and promote healing:
  - Sitz bath
  - Use of peri-bottle following each voiding or defecation
  - Pad change following each elimination and at regular intervals
  - Ice pack or ice-filled glove to perineum immediately following childbirth
  - Judicious use of analgesics or topical anesthetics
  - Tightening buttocks before sitting
- Identify signs of episiotomy infection (redness, edema, drainage, incomplete approximation of the edges).
- Advise the woman to contact her caregiver if signs of infection develop.

provides information about the purpose of the ice pack, as well as anticipated effects, benefits, and possible problems, and explains how to prepare an ice pack for home use if edema is present and early discharge is planned.

Sitz Bath

The warmth of the water in a sitz bath provides comfort, decreases pain, and promotes circulation to the tissues, which promotes healing and reduces the incidence of infection (Figure 30–1 ●). In some facilities, the use of the sitz bath has declined and is reserved only for women who have third- and fourth-degree lacerations (see Chapter 31 🖉 for further discussion of lacerations of the genital tract), whereas in other facilities, it is offered to all women who have edema or a laceration following birth. Sitz baths may be ordered three times a day (TID) and as needed (PRN). The nurse prepares the sitz bath by cleaning the equipment and adding water at 38.9°C to 40.6°C (102°F to 105°F). The woman is encouraged to remain in the sitz bath for about 20 minutes. It is important for the woman to have a clean, unused towel to pat dry her perineum after the sitz bath and to have a clean perineal pad to apply. Care needs to be taken during the first sitz bath because the moist heat may cause the woman to faint. The nurse places a call bell well within reach and asks the woman to use it if she feels dizzy or light-headed or develops difficulty hearing. The nurse also checks on the woman at frequent intervals.

● **Figure 30–1** A sitz bath promotes healing and provides relief from perineal discomfort during the initial weeks following birth.

Cool sitz baths have been used because they are effective in reducing perineal edema and reducing the response of nerve endings that cause perineal discomfort (Peterson, 2011). In administering a cool sitz bath, have the woman start with the water at room temperature and add ice according to the woman's comfort. Some women may prefer a warm sitz bath and achieve greater comfort levels from warmed water so personal preference should be valued.

The nurse provides information about the purpose and use of the sitz bath; anticipated effects, benefits, and possible problems; and safety measures to prevent overheating, scalds, chills, or injury from fainting or slipping while getting into or out of the tub. Home use of sitz baths may be recommended for the woman with an extensive episiotomy. The woman may use a portable sitz bath or her bathtub. It is important for the nurse to emphasize that in using a bathtub, the woman should draw only 4 to 6 in. of water, assess the temperature, and use the water only for the sitz and not for bathing. If the woman takes a sitz bath, she should release the water, have a helper clean the tub, and draw new water before bathing to prevent infection.

Topical Agents

Topical anesthetics such as Dermoplast aerosol spray and Americaine spray may be used to relieve perineal discomfort. The woman is advised to apply the anesthetic after a sitz bath or perineal care. Witch hazel compresses may be used to relieve perineal discomfort and edema. Nupercainal ointment or Tucks or witch hazel pads may be ordered for relief of both hemorrhoidal and perineal pain. The nurse should emphasize the need for the woman to wash her hands before and after using the topical treatments.

The nurse provides information about the anesthetic spray or topical agent. The woman needs to understand the purpose, use, anticipated effects and benefits, and possible problems associated with the product. The nurse can combine a demonstration of application with teaching. A return demonstration is a useful method of evaluating the woman's understanding.

Relief of Hemorrhoidal Discomfort

Some mothers experience hemorrhoidal pain after giving birth. (See Figure 29–8 🖉 on page 723.) Relief measures include the use of sitz baths, topical anesthetic ointments, rectal suppositories, or witch hazel pads applied directly to the anal area. The woman may be taught to digitally replace external hemorrhoids in her rectum. Handwashing to prevent contamination to the vagina is essential. She may also find it helpful to maintain a side-lying position when

> ### Teaching Highlights Self-Evaluation of the Perineum
>
> After the mother completes the sitz bath, teach her to inspect the perineal area for burns (that could be related to using water that is too hot), edema, and approximation by using a handheld mirror. If the mother routinely inspects the area, she will be aware of changes that may indicate an infection, such as redness, poor approximation, drainage, or odor.

possible and to avoid prolonged sitting. The mother is encouraged to maintain an adequate fluid intake, and stool softeners are administered to ensure greater comfort with bowel movements. Mothers should be advised to avoid straining with bowel movements because this can increase the severity and discomfort associated with hemorrhoids. The hemorrhoids usually disappear a few weeks after birth if the woman did not have them before her pregnancy.

Relief of Afterpains

Afterpains are the result of intermittent uterine contractions. A primipara may not experience afterpains because her uterus is able to maintain a contracted state. However, multiparous women and those who have had a multiple-gestation pregnancy or hydramnios frequently experience discomfort from afterpains

as the uterus contracts intermittently. Breastfeeding women are also more likely to experience afterpains than formula-feeding women because of the release of oxytocin when the infant suckles.

The nurse can suggest that the woman lie prone, with a small pillow under her lower abdomen, and explain that the discomfort may feel intensified for about 5 minutes but then diminishes greatly if not completely. The prone position applies pressure to the uterus and therefore stimulates contractions. When the uterus maintains a constant contraction, the afterpains cease. Additional nursing interventions include a sitz bath (for warmth), positioning, ambulation, or administration of an analgesic agent. For breastfeeding mothers, an analgesic administered 30 minutes to an hour before nursing helps promote comfort and enhances maternal–infant interaction (Table 30–3).

Table 30–3	**Essential Information for Common Postpartum Drugs**

TYLENOL NO. 3 (300 MG ACETAMINOPHEN AND 30 MG CODEINE)

Drug Class: Narcotic analgesic. *Dose/Route:* Usual adult dose: 1 to 2 tablets PO every 4 hours PRN. *Indication:* For relief of mild to moderate pain. *Adverse Effects:* Respiratory depression, apnea, light-headedness, dizziness, nausea, sweating, dry mouth, constipation, facial flushing, suppression of cough reflex, ureteral spasm, urinary retention, pruritus, hepatotoxicity (overdose). *Nursing Implications:* Determine whether woman is sensitive to acetaminophen or codeine; has history of impaired hepatic or renal function. Monitor bowel sounds, respirations, urine output. Administer with food or after meals if GI upset occurs; encourage woman to drink one full glass (240 mL) with the tablet to reduce the risk of the tablet lodging in the esophagus. Encourage increased fluids, raw fruits and vegetables, and use of a stool softener as needed should constipation occur.	*Patient Teaching:* Inform patient about name of drug, expected action, possible side effects, that it is secreted in breast milk, and can cause constipation for the mother. (*Note:* Some physicians/CNMs may avoid ordering this medication for breastfeeding mothers.) Review safety measures (assess for dizziness, use side rails, call for assistance when getting out of bed and ambulating, report to nurse any signs of adverse effects) and ask if she has any questions. *Nursing Diagnoses (NANDA-I © 2012) Related to Drug Therapy:* *Self-Health Management, Readiness for Enhanced,* related to information regarding drug therapy *Injury, Risk for,* related to dizziness secondary to effect of drug *Constipation* related to slowed gastrointestinal activity secondary to effects of medications

PERCOCET (325 MG ACETAMINOPHEN AND 5 MG OXYCODONE)

Drug Class: Narcotic analgesic. *Dose/Route:* 1 to 2 tablets PO every 4 hours PRN. *Indication:* For moderate to moderately severe pain. Can be used in aspirin-sensitive women. *Adverse Effects:* *Acetaminophen:* Hepatotoxicity, headache, rash, hypoglycemia. *Oxycodone:* Respiratory depression, apnea, circulatory depression, euphoria, facial flushing, constipation, suppression of cough reflex, ureteral spasm, urinary retention. *Nursing Implications:* Determine whether woman is sensitive to acetaminophen or codeine; has bronchial asthma, respiratory depression, convulsive disorder. Observe woman carefully for respiratory depression if given with barbiturates or sedative/hypnotics. Consider that post–cesarean birth woman may have depressed cough reflex, so teaching and encouragement to deep breathe and cough are needed. Monitor bowel sounds, urine and bowel elimination.	*Patient Teaching:* Teaching should include name of drug, expected effect, possible adverse effects, that drug is secreted in the breast milk, encouragement to report any signs of adverse effects immediately. *Nursing Diagnoses (NANDA-I © 2012) Related to Drug Therapy:* *Breathing Pattern, Ineffective,* related to respiratory depression *Constipation* related to slowed gastrointestinal activity secondary to the effects of medications

(continued)

Table 30–3   Essential Information for Common Postpartum Drugs—continued

RUBELLA VIRUS VACCINE, LIVE (MERUVAX 2)

Dose/Route:
Single-dose vial, inject subcutaneously in outer aspect of the upper arm.

Indication:
Stimulate active immunity against rubella virus. Rubella titer of less than 1:10 or antibody negative on ELISA test.

Adverse Effects:
Burning or stinging at the injection site; about 2 to 4 weeks later may have rash, malaise, sore throat, or headache.

Nursing Implications:
Obtain informed consent. Determine whether woman has sensitivity to neomycin (vaccine contains neomycin); is immunosuppressed, or has received blood transfusions (not to be administered within 3 months of blood transfusion, plasma transfusion, or serum immune globulin). To be given at discharge.

Patient Teaching:
Name of drug, expected effect, possible adverse effects, possible comfort measures to use if adverse effects occur; rubella titer will be assessed in about 3 months. Instruct woman to AVOID PREGNANCY FOR 3 MONTHS following vaccination. Provide information regarding contraceptives and their use.

Nursing Diagnoses (NANDA-I © 2012) Related to Drug Therapy:
Knowledge, Deficient, regarding drug therapy
Self-Health Management, Readiness for Enhanced, related to information about postpartum contraception regarding an expressed desire to avoid pregnancy following rubella vaccination
Pain related to rash and malaise

RHOGAM (RH IMMUNE GLOBULIN SPECIFIC FOR D ANTIGEN)

Dose/Route:
Postpartum: One vial IM within 72 hours of birth. *Antepartum:* One vial microdose RhoGAM IM at 28 weeks in Rh-negative women; after amniocentesis, spontaneous or therapeutic abortion, or ectopic pregnancy.

Indication:
Prevention of sensitization to the Rh factor in Rh-negative women and to prevent hemolytic disease in the newborn in subsequent pregnancies (see Chapter 15 🔴). Mother must be Rh negative, not previously sensitized to Rh factor. Infant must be Rh positive, direct antiglobulin negative.

Adverse Effects:
Soreness at injection site.

Nursing Implications:
Confirm criteria for administration are present. Ensure correct vial is used for the patient (each vial is cross-matched to the specific woman and must be carefully checked).
Inject entire contents of vial.

Patient Teaching:
Name of drug, expected action, possible side effects; report soreness at injection site to nurse; woman should carry information regarding Rh status and dates of RhoGAM injections with her at all times; explain use of RhoGAM with subsequent pregnancies.

Nursing Diagnoses (NANDA-I © 2012) Related to Drug Therapy:
Self-Health Management, Readiness for Enhanced, related to information about future need for Rh immune globulin regarding an expressed desire to understand the long-term implications of her Rh-negative status
Pain related to soreness at injection site

AMBIEN (ZOLPIDEM TARTRATE)

Drug Class:
Hypnotic, sedative.

Dose/Route:
5 to 10 mg PO at bedtime.

Indication:
Promote sleep.

Adverse Effects:
Dizziness, daytime drowsiness, diarrhea, drugged feelings, amnesia.

Nursing Implications:
Determine if woman has compromised respiratory function. Monitor respirations, blood pressure, pulse. Modify environment to increase relaxation and promote sleep. Monitor for drug interaction if woman is taking other CNS depressants.

Patient Teaching:
Name of drug, expected effect, possible adverse effects, safety measures (side rails, use call bell, ask for assistance when out of bed); medication is secreted in breast milk.

Nursing Diagnoses Related to Drug Therapy (NANDA-I © 2012):
Injury, Risk for, related to possible ataxia or vertigo
Confusion, Risk for Acute, related to drug-induced drowsiness
Health-Seeking Behavior related to information regarding drug therapy

---

The nurse provides information about the cause of afterpains and methods to decrease discomfort. She or he explains any medications that are ordered, including their expected effect, benefits, and possible side effects, and any special considerations such as the possibility of dizziness or sleepiness with particular medications.

Relief of Discomfort from Immobility and Muscle Strain

Discomfort may be caused by immobility. The woman who has been in stirrups or has pulled back on her legs for an extended period of time may experience muscular aches from such extreme positioning. It is not unusual for women to experience joint pains and muscular pain in both arms and legs, depending on the effort they exerted during the second stage of labor.

Early ambulation is encouraged to help reduce the incidence of complications such as constipation and thrombophlebitis. It also helps promote a feeling of general well-being. The nurse provides information about ambulation and the importance of monitoring any signs of dizziness or weakness. Assist the woman the first few times she gets up during the postpartum period. Fatigue, effects of medications, loss of blood, and lack of food intake may cause feelings of dizziness or faintness when the woman stands up. Because this may be a problem during the woman's first shower, the nurse should remain in the room, check the woman frequently, and have a chair close by in case she becomes faint. During this first shower the nurse instructs the woman in the use of the emergency call button in the bathroom; she is advised that, if she becomes faint during a future shower, she should sit down and press the call button for assistance immediately.

Relief of Discomfort from Postpartum Diaphoresis

Postpartum diaphoresis (excessive perspiration) may cause discomfort for new mothers. The nurse can offer a fresh, dry gown and change bed linens to enhance the mother's comfort. Some women may feel refreshed by a shower. For women experiencing hot flashes as a result of changing hormones, a cool shower may be preferable over a warm or hot shower. It is necessary to consider cultural practices and realize that some Hispanic and Asian women prefer to delay showering. Nurses can offer these women a warm or cool washcloth to increase comfort. The nurse provides information about the normal physiologic changes that cause diaphoresis and methods to increase comfort.

Because diaphoresis may also increase thirst, the nurse can offer fluids as the woman desires. Again, the nurse needs to ask the woman about her preferred beverage. Women of western European background may prefer iced drinks, whereas Asian women may prefer hot tea or water at room temperature. It is important to ascertain the woman's wishes rather than operate from one's own values or cultural beliefs.

Suppression of Lactation in the Non-Breastfeeding Mother

For the woman who chooses not to breastfeed, lactation may be suppressed by mechanical inhibition. Although signs of engorgement do not usually appear until the second or third postpartum day, engorgement is best prevented by beginning mechanical methods of lactation suppression as soon as possible after birth. Ideally, this involves having the woman begin wearing a supportive, well-fitting bra within 6 hours after birth. A tight-fitting sports bra may be preferred by some women. The bra is worn continuously until lactation is suppressed (usually about 5 to 7 days) and is removed only for showers. The bra provides support and eases the discomfort that can occur with tension on the breasts because of fullness. Ice packs should be applied over the axillary area of each breast for 20 minutes four times daily.

This practice should begin soon after birth. In addition, ice is useful in relieving discomfort if engorgement occurs.

The mother is advised to avoid any stimulation of her breasts by her baby, herself, breast pumps, or her sexual partner until the sensation of fullness has passed (usually about 5 to 7 days). Such stimulation increases milk production and delays the suppression process. Heat is avoided for the same reason; therefore, the mother is encouraged to let shower water flow over her back rather than her breasts.

Some mothers may inquire about suppression medications used in the past for non-nursing mothers. Women should be informed that, because of concerns related to side effects, these medications are no longer used. Mechanical, rather than pharmacologic, methods are now employed.

Relief of Emotional Stress

The birth of a child, with the changes in role and the increased responsibilities it produces, is a time of emotional stress for the new mother. During the early postpartum period, the mother may be emotionally labile, and mood swings and tearfulness are common. Initially the mother may repeatedly discuss her experiences of labor and birth. This allows the mother to integrate her experiences. If she believes that she did not cope well with labor, she may have feelings of inadequacy and may benefit from reassurance that she did well. Some women feel that they did not have any perception of time during the labor and birth and want to know how long it really lasted, or they may not remember the entire experience. In this case, it is helpful for the nurse to talk with the woman and provide the information that she is missing and desires.

During this time the new mother must also adjust to the loss of her fantasized child and accept the child she has borne. This task may be more difficult if the child is not of the desired sex or if he or she has birth defects (see Chapter 27). Women who deliver prematurely may experience guilt or have feelings of inadequacy. Immediately after the birth (the taking-in period) the mother is focused on bodily concerns and may not be fully ready to learn about personal and infant care. Following the initial dependent period, the mother becomes very concerned about her ability to be a successful parent (the taking-hold period). During this time the mother requires reassurance that she is effective. She also tends to be receptive to teaching and demonstration designed to assist her in mothering successfully. The depression, weepiness, and "let-down feeling" that characterize the postpartum blues are often a surprise for the new mother. She requires reassurance that these feelings are normal, an explanation of why they occur, and a supportive environment that permits her to cry without feeling guilty.

PROMOTION OF MATERNAL REST AND ACTIVITY

Following childbirth some women feel exhausted and in need of rest. Other women may be euphoric and full of psychic energy, ready to relive and recount the experience of birth repeatedly. The nurse can provide a period for airing of feelings and then encourage a period of rest. Nurses also promote rest by organizing their activities to avoid frequent interruptions for the woman.

Relief of Fatigue

Physical fatigue often affects other adjustments and functions of the new mother. For example, fatigue can reduce milk flow, thereby increasing problems with establishing breastfeeding. Energy is also needed to make the psychologic adjustments to a new infant and to assume new roles. It is helpful for the new mother to know that fatigue may persist for several weeks or even months. Persistent fatigue is especially common when mothers attempt to perform activities while the baby is napping, instead of resting themselves. The nurse teaches women that this practice can lead to chronic fatigue and should be avoided. Mothers who have other children may feel overwhelmed with trying to meet the needs of their other child(ren) (Hunter, Rychnovsky, & Yount, 2009). Severe ongoing fatigue can also be a symptom of a thyroid disorder and should be evaluated by a clinician. Although most new mothers feel tired, if they have perceived the pregnancy and birth as a natural process, they tend to view themselves as healthy and well. Fatigue can also be a symptom of postpartum depression and should be discussed with the healthcare provider if symptoms continue or are accompanied by other signs of depression.

Specific groups of mothers are at a higher risk for postpartum fatigue. These include mothers of multiples, mothers with hospitalized infants who must make multiple trips to the hospital to visit their babies, mothers of infants with birth defects or special needs, mothers who lack social support, and mothers who return to work before the advised 6-week time period. A mother who has been on extended bed rest during the pregnancy may also be more at risk for fatigue. Because many families are now geographically separated and may be unable to come and spend time with the mother and new baby, fatigue may also be more common in these women when the mother is left to care for herself and baby in the early postpartum period.

Developing Cultural Competence
Postpartum Recuperation

Most mothers view the postpartum period as a time for recuperation. In many non-Western cultures, the 40 days following a birth are a time of recovery when female relatives or friends assist the new mother in her daily activities (Wong, 2008). In Northern Africa, for example, the 40-day period after birth is considered a time of transition for the mother. The mother and infant are not separated during this time. This practice is known to prevent postpartum psychosis and facilitate bonding (Wong, 2008). This is also the custom in India, where it is believed that the mother and new baby need protection from evil spirits as well as from exposure to illness, because they are both considered vulnerable during this time period (Lynn-McDonough, 2010).

In Mexico, this period is briefer, lasting only 20 days. During the first 7 days, nonhousehold members are not permitted to visit or enter the home. The mother gradually increases activity after the first week. The end of the postpartum period is marked by a *sobada*, a massage performed by the midwife on the 20th day after birth (Lynn-McDonough, 2010).

Resumption of Activity

Ambulation and activity may gradually increase after birth. The new mother should avoid heavy lifting, excessive stair climbing, and strenuous activity. One or two daily naps are essential and are most easily achieved if the mother sleeps when her baby does. Women with older children often find it difficult to get adequate rest because they want to spend time with their older children when the infant is napping. The woman should be cautioned that fatigue and exhaustion can become a vicious cycle and should be avoided. Assistance in the household can help prevent this and can enable the mother to spend special time with older children while others take over household tasks.

By the second week at home, the woman may resume light housekeeping. Although it is customary to delay returning to work for 6 weeks, most women are physically able to resume practically all activities by 4 to 5 weeks. In some cases, if bleeding returns, it is often a sign that the mother is overdoing her activities and should decrease some activity. Delaying the return to work until after the final postpartum examination minimizes the possibility of problems.

Postpartum Exercises

The woman should be encouraged to begin simple exercises while in the birthing unit and to continue them at home. Kegel exercises should be reviewed and begun while the woman is still in the hospital (see Chapter 11 and Figure 11–8 on page 232). She is advised that increased lochia or pain means she should reevaluate her activity and make necessary alterations. Most agencies provide a booklet describing suggested postpartum exercises. (Exercise routines vary for women undergoing cesarean birth or tubal ligation after childbirth.)

Exercise during the postpartum period has several health benefits for new mothers. Exercise can help maintain insulin and high-density lipoprotein (HDL) cholesterol levels, as well as improve aerobic fitness. The postpartum woman is more likely to have positive views of her well-being, more self-esteem, and less fatigue if she continues to do stretching and her own pattern of exercise after she is home. The addition of pelvic floor exercises can also decrease such problems as urinary leakage or incontinence. Exercise also helps facilitate postpartum weight loss, reduces stress, and provides the mother with needed time alone.

Sexual Activity and Contraception

Typically, postpartum couples resume sexual intercourse once the episiotomy is healed and the lochial flow has stopped (Leeman & Rogers, 2012). Because this usually occurs by the end of the third week, before the 6-week check, it is important that the woman and her partner have information about what to expect. The nurse may inform the couple that, because the vaginal vault is "dry" (lacking estrogen), some form of water-soluble lubrication such as K-Y jelly or Astroglide may be necessary during intercourse. The female-superior and side-lying coital positions may be preferable because they allow the woman to control the depth of penile penetration. Couples should be counseled that intercourse may be uncomfortable for the woman for some time and that patience is imperative.

Breastfeeding couples should be forewarned that during orgasm milk may spurt from the nipples because of the release of oxytocin. Some couples find this spurt pleasurable or amusing, but others choose to have the woman wear a bra during sexual activity. Nursing the baby before lovemaking reduces the chance of milk release (Leeman & Rogers, 2012).

Other factors may inhibit satisfactory sexual experiences: the baby's crying may "spoil the mood," the woman's changed body may seem unattractive to her or her partner, maternal sleep deprivation may reduce the woman's desire, and the woman's physiologic response to sexual stimulation may be altered because of hormonal changes. By 3 months postpartum, many couples have returned to prepregnant levels of sexual interest and activity; however, this is highly variable. It is not abnormal for women, especially when breastfeeding, to experience decreased libido for several months (Leeman & Rogers, 2012). Decreased libido can be associated with hormonal changes, fatigue, stress, and lack of time because of family and work demands.

With anticipatory guidance during the prenatal and postpartum periods, the couple can be forewarned of potential temporary problems. Anticipatory guidance is enhanced if the couple can discuss their feelings and reactions as they are experienced. (See *Teaching Highlights: Resumption of Sexual Activity After Childbirth*.)

Information on contraception is often provided as part of discharge teaching if it is permissible within the healthcare agency. The nurse can also be an important resource for the woman and her partner during postpartum follow-up. Couples typically choose to use contraception to control the number of children they will have or to determine the spacing of future children. However, some religious-based hospital facilities prohibit nurses and other healthcare providers from discussing contraception. If the nurse is discussing birth control, it is important to emphasize that in choosing a specific method, consistency of use is essential. The nurse needs to identify the advantages, disadvantages, risks, and contraindications of the various methods to help the couple, or the single mother, make an informed choice about the most practical and compatible method. (For a more detailed discussion of contraceptive methods, see Chapter 5 🔗.) Breastfeeding women are commonly concerned that a contraceptive method will interfere with their ability to breastfeed. Breastfeeding women should be given available options and choose the method that best fits their lifestyle, financial situation, and personal preference.

Pharmacologic Interventions

Pharmacologic preparations, including pain medications, vaccinations (rubella and Tdap), and Rh immune globulin, are frequently administered in the postpartum period (see Table 30–3).

PROMOTION OF EFFECTIVE PARENT LEARNING

Meeting the educational needs of the new mother and her family is a primary challenge facing the postpartum nurse. Each woman's educational needs vary based on her age, background, educational level, experience, and expectations. However, because the mother spends only a brief period of time in the postpartum area, identifying and addressing individual instructional needs can be difficult. Effective education provides the childbearing family with sufficient knowledge to meet many of their own health needs and to seek assistance if necessary.

The nurse first assesses the learning needs of the new mother through observation, sensitivity to nonverbal cues, and tactfully phrased questions. For example, "What plans have you made for handling things when you get home?" may elicit a response of several words and may provide the opportunity for some information sharing and guidance. Some agencies also use checklists of common concerns for new mothers. The woman can check the concerns that are of interest to her.

Teaching during the postpartum period is a continuous process in which the nurse takes opportunities throughout interactions with the new parents to identify learning opportunities and offer teaching interventions. The nurse can also plan and implement teaching in a logical, nonthreatening way based on knowledge and respect of the family's cultural values and beliefs.

Teaching Highlights   Resumption of Sexual Activity After Childbirth

- Delay intercourse until no lochia is present because lochia indicates that healing is not yet complete.
- Tenderness of the vagina and perineum may cause discomfort. The partner may test the woman's level of comfort by slipping a lubricated finger inside her vagina. The female-superior and side-lying positions may be preferable because they let the woman control the depth of penetration of the penis.
- Vaginal dryness may occur because the vagina is "hormone poor." Discomfort as a result of dryness can be avoided by using a water-soluble lubricant.
- Based on the amount of breast engorgement and tenderness present, the partner may need to avoid breast stimulation during foreplay or use a very gentle approach.
- Escape of milk during sexual activity can be minimized by breastfeeding immediately beforehand.
- Fatigue and the new baby's schedule may have a negative impact on the woman's feelings of desire. Napping when the baby sleeps helps decrease fatigue. However, fatigue may be a reality couples need to accept during the early postpartum months.
- Contraception is important even during the early postpartum period. The woman's body needs adequate time to heal and recover from the stress of pregnancy and childbirth. Couples opposed to contraception may choose abstinence at this time.

Health Promotion   Postpartum Tdap Vaccination

It is recommended by the Advisory Committee on Immunization Practices (2008) that postpartum women should receive Tdap (reduced diphtheria toxoid, and acellular pertussis) vaccine if they have not received it earlier.

Unless the nurse believes a culturally related activity would be harmful, it can be supported and encouraged.

Nurses need to consider the mother's physical and psychosocial needs when conducting postpartum teaching. Initially, women may be exhausted from the birth experience and their concentration may be impaired. Later, the new mother may be preoccupied with visitors and phone calls. Information should be delivered a little at a time and repeated to make sure that the parents understand what the nurse has discussed with them. Repetition is a valuable tool in the postpartum environment. In addition, many women are discharged during the first 48 hours after birth, making postpartum education difficult (Fink, 2011). When performing teaching sessions, the father's schedule must also be considered. If the father returns to work during the immediate postpartum period, he may be more likely to attend teaching sessions scheduled in the late afternoon or early evening (Figure 30–2 ●). In some cultures, such as the Hispanic culture, female relatives often assist the new mother and baby. It is important to include any care providers in the teaching session.

Postpartum units use a variety of instructional methods, including handouts, formal classes, videotapes, and individual interaction. Printed materials are helpful for new mothers to consult if questions arise at home. Some facilities offer a hotline service that new mothers can call with questions or concerns. As the cultural diversity in the United States continues to grow, the need for culturally sensitive information is imperative. Along with culturally diverse material, teaching aids should be presented in the woman's native language when possible. Written materials should be available and translators or language lines should be utilized. Many patients are now accustomed to using the Internet and may prefer to use online support groups and access educational materials found online. As technology expands, the nurse must remain current with the changing technology and the resources it creates. Evaluation of learning may also take several forms: return demonstrations, question-and-answer sessions, and even formal evaluation tools. Follow-up phone calls after discharge provide additional evaluative information and continue the helping process for the family.

Teaching content should include information on role changes and psychologic adjustments as well as skills. Risk factors and signs of postpartum depression should be reviewed with all women. Information is also essential for women with specialized educational needs such as the mother who has had a cesarean birth, the parents of twins, the parents of an infant with congenital anomalies, parents with other young children, and parents with a child that will require long-term hospitalization. Because more and more women with disabilities are now having children, they may require additional support and education. Anticipatory guidance can help prepare parents for the many changes they will experience with a new family member.

PROMOTION OF FAMILY WELLNESS

A positive maternity experience is likely to have a positive effect on the entire family. The family that receives appropriate information and has adequate time to interact with its newest member in a supportive environment will feel more comfortable and secure at home.

Today most facilities support *family-centered care* that is focused on keeping the mother and baby together as much as the mother desires. This type of care is called **mother–baby care**, or **couplet care**, and provides increased opportunities for parent–child interactions because the newborn shares the mother's room and they are cared for together. Mother–baby care provides the mother with time to bond with her baby and to learn to care for her or him in a supportive environment. It is especially conducive to a hunger-demand feeding schedule for both breastfeeding and formula-feeding babies. This arrangement also allows the father, siblings, grandparents, and others to participate in the care of the new baby. Women who give birth in a facility that offers mother–baby care are often more satisfied with their postpartum experience than women who are cared for under different care models. The World Health Organization (WHO) (2009) advocates for a "rooming-in" model of care where the mother and infant remain together as much as possible.

Mother–baby unit policies must be flexible enough to permit the mother to return the baby to the nursery if she finds it necessary because of fatigue or physical discomfort. Some mother–baby units also return the newborns to a central nursery at night so the mothers can get more rest.

Reactions of Siblings

Mother–baby care provides excellent opportunities for family bonds to grow when the mother, father/partner, newborn, and

● **Figure 30–2** Postpartum teaching. The nurse provides educational information to both parents.

> ### Clinical Tip
>
> Because siblings may feel left out with the addition of a new family member, provide positive feedback to promote attachment. For example, pointing out to the older child that "Carlos is looking at you" or asking, "Do you think he knows you're his big sister?" can help make siblings feel accepted and valued. Also identify ways in which siblings can help the new mother, for example, by bringing her a cup of water or singing the baby a favorite lullaby.

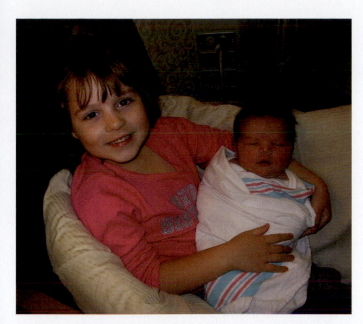

● **Figure 30–3** Siblings and the newborn. The sister of this newborn becomes acquainted with the new family member during a nursing assessment.

Source: Courtesy of Wilson Garcia.

siblings begin functioning as a family unit immediately after the birth. When mother–baby care is not available, liberal sibling visitation policies can help meet the family's needs. A visit to the mother–baby unit reassures children that their mother is well and still loves them. It also provides an opportunity for the children to become familiar with the new baby. For the mother, the pangs of separation are lessened as she interacts with her children and introduces them to the newest family member (Figure 30–3 ●). Even infants who require intensive care nursery admissions should be allowed to have sibling visits whenever possible. Although preventing preemies and other infants who require intensive care services from infection is a valid concern, policies that involve taking the sibling's temperature before each visit and documenting the sibling's health status can provide a safeguard that still promotes family bonding. Some of these infants may be hospitalized for weeks or months. Sibling visitation allows the early incorporation of the infant into the family unit for siblings.

Teach parents that, although they may have prepared their children for the presence of a new brother or sister, the actual arrival of the infant in the home requires some adjustments. Although it may be more chaotic for the parents, allowing the children to come to the hospital to pick up mom and the new baby can signify their importance in the family process. If small children are waiting at home, it is helpful if the father carries the baby inside. This practice keeps the mother's arms free to hug and touch her older children. Many mothers bring a doll home with them for an older child. Caring for the doll alongside the mother or father helps the child to identify with the parents. This identification helps decrease anger and the need to regress to gain attention.

Parents may also provide supervised times when older children can hold the new baby and perhaps even help with a

feeding or diapering. Many parents may have concerns about the children "hurting" the new baby, but with proper supervision, the siblings are more likely to develop an attachment to their new sibling. The other children feel a sense of accomplishment and learn tenderness and caring. The nurse also suggests that parents spend one-to-one quality time with each of their older children each day. This may require some careful planning, but it confirms the parents' continuing love for the other children and promotes siblings' acceptance of the newborn.

Promotion of Parent–Infant Attachment During the Postpartum Period

Nursing interventions to enhance the quality of parent–infant attachment should be designed to promote feelings of well-being, comfort, and satisfaction. Although many new mothers lack experience and feel overwhelmed with their infants, certain groups of women are at higher risk for alterations in parent–infant attachment. These include women who are unemployed, single, living in poverty, or have a previous history of mental health issues, parents with developmental disabilities, parents with substance abuse issues, low-birth-weight infants, and first-born infants (Michigan Department of Community Health, 2012). Other factors such as an infant's temperament and genetic factors may also impact parent–infant bonding (Geravi, 2009). These mothers warrant additional assessment and support from the nurse to ensure proper bonding is taking place.

Following are some suggestions for ways the nurse can promote parent–infant attachment during the postpartum stay:

- Determine the parenting style and goals of the infant's mother and father/partner and adapt them when possible in planning nursing care for the family. This includes giving the parents choices about their initial time with their new infant.
- Provide time and as much privacy as possible for the new family to become acquainted. Allow siblings to visit throughout the postpartum stay if requested by the parents.
- Arrange the healthcare setting so that the individual nurse–patient relationship can be developed. A primary nurse can develop rapport and assess the mother's strengths and needs.
- Use anticipatory guidance to prepare the parents for expected problems of adjustment. Model appropriate behaviors based on the infant's cues and behaviors.
- Include parents in any nursing intervention, planning, and evaluation. Give choices when possible.
- Initiate and support measures to alleviate fatigue in the parents.
- Help parents identify, understand, and accept both positive and negative feelings related to the overall parenting experience.
- Support and assist parents in determining the personality and unique needs of their infant.

The beginnings of parent–newborn attachment may be observed in the first few hours after birth (see Chapter 26 ⊘ for a discussion of early attachment behaviors). Continued assessments may occur during the postpartum stay (Chapter 29 🔗 discusses the development of family attachment) and during home visits after discharge. As the nurse assesses attachment, it is important to remember that cultural values, beliefs, and practices will direct the childcare activities and self-care practices. (See Table 29–4 🔗 on page 726 for behaviors related to attachment and behaviors that may be cause for concern.)

NURSING CARE FOLLOWING CESAREAN BIRTH

After a cesarean birth the new mother has postpartum needs similar to those of women who have given birth vaginally. Because she has undergone major abdominal surgery, however, the woman's nursing care needs are also similar to those of other surgical patients.

Promotion of Maternal Physical Well-Being After Cesarean Birth

The chances of pulmonary infection are increased because of immobility after the use of narcotics and sedatives and because of the altered immune response in postoperative patients. Therefore, the woman is encouraged to cough and deep breathe every 2 to 4 hours while awake until she is ambulating frequently. Leg exercises are also encouraged every 2 hours until the woman is ambulating. These exercises increase circulation, help prevent thrombophlebitis, and also aid intestinal motility by tightening abdominal muscles.

Early ambulation, eating a low roughage diet shortly after birth, and breastfeeding or infant feeding soon after birth all enhance the recovery of the mother and decrease complications in the postoperative period. Even though a cesarean birth is an operative procedure, most women giving birth are relatively healthy and therefore are less likely to experience postoperative complications when compared with other surgical patients.

Health Promotion   Reducing Cesarean Births
Healthy People 2020 objectives (U.S. Department of Health and Human Services [USDHHS], 2013) include reducing the number of cesarean births in low-risk women. Nurses can explain to women that even though a cesarean birth was performed for this birth, a trial of labor after cesarean (TOLAC) may be a viable option in the future.

The nurse monitors and manages the woman's pain experience during the postpartum period. Sources of pain include incisional pain, gas pain, referred shoulder pain, periodic uterine contractions (afterbirth pains), discomfort related to breastfeeding, and pain from voiding, defecation, or constipation.

Nursing interventions are oriented toward preventing or alleviating pain or helping the woman cope with pain. The nurse should undertake the following measures:

- Administer analgesics as needed, especially during the first 24 to 72 hours after childbirth. Use of analgesics relieves the woman's pain and enables her to be more mobile and active. Some facilities administer ibuprofen on a continuous basis in the early postpartum period to decrease swelling, reduce pain, and decrease the need for, or frequency of, narcotic agents.

- Promote comfort through proper positioning, frequent position changes, massage, back rubs, oral care, and the reduction of noxious stimuli such as noise and unpleasant odors.

- Encourage visits by significant others, including the newborn and older children. These visits distract the woman from the painful sensations and help reduce her fear and anxiety.

- Encourage the use of breathing, relaxation, guided imagery, and distraction (e.g., stimulation of cutaneous tissue) techniques taught in childbirth preparation class.

Epidural analgesia administered just after the cesarean birth is an effective method of pain relief for most women in the first 24 hours following birth (see *Drug Guide: Postpartum Epidural Morphine*).

The physician may order **patient-controlled analgesia (PCA)**. With this approach the woman is given a bolus of analgesia, usually morphine or fentanyl, at the beginning of therapy. Using a special intravenous (IV) pump system, the woman presses a button to self-administer small doses of the medication as needed. For safety, the pump is preset with a time lockout so that the woman cannot deliver another dose until a specified period of time has elapsed. The use of a PCA helps women feel a greater sense of control and less dependence on nursing staff. The frequent, smaller doses help the woman experience rapid pain relief without grogginess and avoid the discomfort associated with injections.

Another technique of pain control that is sometimes used is the **continuous epidural infusion (CEI)** technique, in which the epidural catheter is left in place following the cesarean birth and medication is continually administered via an electric pump. The device also has a button that the woman can depress if additional pain relief is needed. Fentanyl is the most commonly used drug because it tends to provide good pain relief (Palmer, D'Angelo, & Paech, 2011). Nursing assessments are hourly for women with a CEI in place and include vital signs, level of pain, amount of drug received, and amount of self-administration. The tubing is inspected to ensure connections are maintained because movement by the woman in bed could disrupt the line. The epidural site should also be assessed to ensure the catheter has not been displaced.

Another technique used for pain control for post–cesarean birth is the use of a continuous peripheral nerve block that delivers a local anesthetic through a tiny catheter that is positioned directly into the wound site. An external balloon allows medication to be delivered at a steady rate for up to 5 days after the birth and creates a numbing effect at the incision site. After a specified time period, the catheter is displaced by gently pulling it from the site. Additional surgical intervention is not required to remove the device. The use of one of these devices can reduce the amount of systemic analgesia that is needed in the postpartum period (Palmer et al., 2011). Most recently, ultrasound guidance

Drug Guide Postpartum Epidural Morphine

Overview of Obstetric Action

Epidural morphine is used to provide relief of pain associated with cesarean birth, extensive episiotomies (mediolaterals), or third- and fourth-degree lacerations. Epidural morphine pain relief results directly from its effect on the opiate receptors in the spinal cord (it depresses pain impulse transmission). Morphine binds opiate receptors, thereby altering both the perception of and emotional response to pain. Women experience little or no discomfort or pain during recovery and for up to 24 hours afterward. There is no motor or sympathetic block or associated hypotension. Onset of analgesia is slower, but duration is longer.

Route, Dosage, Frequency

Morphine (5 to 7.5 mg) is injected through a catheter into the epidural space, providing pain relief for about 24 hours (Wilson et al., 2013).

Maternal Contraindications

Allergy to morphine, narcotic addiction, chronic debilitating respiratory disease, infection at the injection site, or administration of parenteral corticosteroids in past 14 days (Wilson et al., 2013).

Maternal Side Effects

Late-onset respiratory depression (rare but may occur 8 to 12 hours after administration), nausea and vomiting (occurring between 4 and 7 hours after injection), itching (begins within 3 hours and lasts up to 10 hours), urinary retention, and rarely somnolence. Side effects can be managed with naloxone.

Neonatal Effects

No adverse effects because medication is injected after the birth of the baby.

Nursing Considerations

- Obtain history: sensitivity (allergy) to morphine, presence of any contraindications (Wilson et al., 2013).
- Assess orientation, reflexes, skin color, texture, breath sounds, presence of lesions or infection over area of lumbar spine, voiding pattern, urinary output within normal limits (Wilson et al., 2013).
- Monitor and evaluate analgesic effect. Ask patient about comfort level and notify anesthesiologist of inadequate pain relief.
- Check catheter for obvious knots, breaks, and leakage at insertion site and catheter hub.
- Assess for pruritus (scratching and rubbing, especially around face and neck).
- Administer comfort measures for narcotic-induced pruritus, such as lotion, back rubs, cool/warm packs, or diversional activities. If the itching can be tolerated, naloxone should be avoided, especially because it counteracts the pain relief.
- If allergic reaction (urticaria, edema, or respiratory difficulties) occurs, administer naloxone or diphenhydramine per physician order.
- Provide comfort measures for nausea/vomiting, such as frequent oral hygiene or gradual increase of activity; administer naloxone, trimethobenzamide (Tigan), or metoclopramide HCl per physician order.
- Assess postural blood pressure and heart rate before ambulation.
- Assist patient with her first ambulation and then as needed.
- Assess respiratory function every hour for 24 hours, then every 2 to 8 hours as needed. Also assess level of consciousness and mucous membrane color. May need to monitor patient via apnea monitor for 24 hours.
- Monitor urinary output and assess bladder for distention. Assist patient to void.

---

has been utilized to produce better pain relief results (Mariano & Ilfeld, 2011). Although these devices are not widely used, they can be an option for a woman who has undergone a cesarean birth.

Although the use of general anesthesia continues to decline, women who receive general anesthesia warrant additional assessments in the immediate postpartum period. Vital signs should be monitored continually until the woman has regained consciousness. Cardiopulmonary equipment should be in close range with cardiac monitoring available as needed. The pulse oximeter should be used to determine the woman's oxygen status.

If a general anesthetic was used, abdominal distention may produce marked discomfort for the woman during the first few postpartum days. Measures to prevent or minimize abdominal distention include leg exercises, abdominal tightening, ambulation, avoiding carbonated or very hot or cold beverages, and avoiding the use of straws. Women can be started on a regular low-residue diet as tolerated. In one study that examined resumption of solid foods after emergency cesarean births, only 6% of the women experienced nausea, vomiting, or bloating and patient satisfaction scores were significantly higher (92%) than a comparison group (42%) who were only given clear liquids after birth (Zoumenou et al., 2011). Medical intervention for gas pain includes using rectal suppositories and enemas to stimulate

passage of flatus and stool and encouraging the woman to lie on her left side. Lying on the left side allows the gas to pass from the descending colon to the sigmoid colon so that it can be expelled more readily.

Many physicians also order a nonsteroidal anti-inflammatory drug (NSAID) in addition to the previously mentioned agents once the woman is tolerating oral fluids well. NSAIDs assist with decreasing inflammation and do not have the negative side effects associated with many narcotics, such as sedation and constipation. NSAIDs are often given in combination with narcotic agents in the immediate postpartum period and often result in a decreased intake of narcotic agents.

Sometimes women who have had a cesarean birth have other discomforts that can be relieved with pharmacologic interventions. The nurse assesses the woman for other symptoms, such as nausea, itching (which is typically related to the morphine used in the epidural), and headache. If the woman is experiencing nausea, an antiemetic can be administered. Itching can also be relieved with pharmacologic interventions. NSAIDs are effective in managing headaches and other body aches.

The nurse can minimize discomfort and promote satisfaction as the mother assumes the activities of her new role. Instruction and assistance in assuming comfortable positions when holding or breastfeeding the infant will do much to increase the mother's sense of competence and comfort. The woman should be taught to splint her incision when she ambulates to decrease pulling on the incision and the discomfort created by contraction of the abdominal muscles.

Other measures are aimed at other needs that are unique to the woman who has had an operative birth. These include (Fowles, Cheng, & Mills, 2012):

- Assessing the consistency of the abdomen. Women with a firm, distended abdomen may be having difficulty passing flatus or stool.
- Assessment of the intravenous (IV) site, flow rate, and patency of the IV tubing.
- Monitoring the condition of surgical dressings or the incision site using the REEDA scale (redness, edema, ecchymosis, discharge, and approximation of the suture line) along with skin temperature at and around the incision line.

The cesarean birth mother usually does extremely well postoperatively. Most women are ambulating by the day after the surgery. Usually by the second postpartum day the woman can shower, which seems to provide a mental as well as physical lift. Most women are discharged by the third day after birth.

Promotion of Parent–Infant Interaction After Cesarean Birth

Many factors associated with cesarean birth may hinder successful and frequent parent–infant interaction. These factors include the physical condition of the mother and newborn and maternal reactions to stress, anesthesia, and medications. The father or significant other may be concerned about the mother and preoccupied with her condition, resulting in less interaction with the newborn. The mother and her infant may be separated after birth because of birthing unit routines, prematurity, or neonatal complications or a birth defect. A healthy infant born by uncomplicated cesarean is no more fragile than one born vaginally.

In some cases, signs of depression, anger, or withdrawal may indicate a grief response to the loss of the fantasized birth experience. Fathers as well as mothers may experience feelings of "missing out," guilt, or even jealousy toward another couple who had a vaginal birth. The cesarean birth couple may need the opportunity to tell their story repeatedly to work through these feelings. The nurse can provide factual information about their situation and support the couple's effective coping behaviors.

Clinical Reasoning Repeat Cesarean

You walk into her room and find Dana Sullivan, a 29-year-old G2P2, crying 48 hours after a repeat cesarean birth. She states "I'm not ready to go home. With my first baby they made me go home after two days. Can they make me go home so early again?"

What therapeutic nursing questions would you ask Dana to assess her reluctance to go home?

See www.nursing.pearsonhighered.com for possible responses.

The nurse should acknowledge their feelings while emphasizing the importance of a healthy birth outcome. Enhanced communication during the labor, birth, and in the immediate period after birth, along with specific teaching related to issues regarding a cesarean birth, is associated with less maternal distress and improved satisfaction with the birth experience (Nilsson, Lundgren, Karlström, et al., 2012). It is also important to remember that some women may feel more comfortable with a cesarean birth and may have requested a primary or repeat cesarean birth (Tschudin et al., 2009).

During the initial taking-in phase, the new parents are processing their new role and may be nurturing themselves and each other. This is normal and expected. By the second or third day, the cesarean birth mother moves into the "taking-hold" period and is usually receptive to learning how to care for herself and her infant. During this period, the focus shifts from the mother and father/partner to the baby. Vulnerability can occur during this period and the parents may feel overwhelmed. The need for nursing intervention to guide the new parents is essential. Special emphasis should be given to home management. The nurse can encourage the mother to let others assume responsibility for housekeeping and cooking. Fatigue not only prolongs recovery but also interferes with breastfeeding and mother–infant interaction, increases the risk of prolonged postpartum blues, and leads to feelings of being overwhelmed.

The presence of the father or significant other during the birth process positively influences the woman's perception of the birth event. The partner's presence reduces the woman's fears, enhances her sense of control, and enables the couple to share feelings and respond to each other with touch and eye contact. Later, they have the opportunity to relive the experience and fill in any gaps or missing pieces. The presence of the father or significant other is especially valuable if the mother has had general anesthesia. The partner can take pictures, hold the baby, and foster the discovery process by directing the mother's attention to the details of the newborn. Sometimes, during the taking-hold phase, the father/partner can feel neglected or excluded. This will soon pass as the letting-go stage begins. During this transition, the family incorporates the baby into the family unit and other family members, such as grandparents and siblings, get to know the baby and be included in the new family routine.

The infant born by cesarean is typically removed from the operating room before the mother is able to hold the newborn. Separation of the family unit is not medically necessary unless the infant needs to be stabilized or there is a complication occurring in the operating room. The practice is typically historical in nature. Agencies that embrace family-centered care can advocate to keep the mother–baby couple together as much as possible. The nurse can play a crucial role in facilitating interaction by encouraging the father or support person to stand beside the warmer and interact with the infant. Often, the infant can be given to the father or support person to hold. The father or support person can hold the infant close to the mother and place the infant against the mother's cheek so direct eye contact can occur. The nurse can also arrange for the infant to stay with the parents in the recovery area in the immediate postoperative period. This gives the family time to interact when the infant is in an alert state.

Often new parents perceive the parenting role as an extension of the childbearing role. Inability to fulfill expected childbearing behavior (vaginal birth) may lead to parental feelings of role failure and frustration. If the parents' attitude is more positive than negative, successful resolution of subsequent stressful events is more likely. The nurse can help families alter their negative definitions of cesarean birth and bolster and encourage positive perceptions.

NURSING CARE OF THE POSTPARTUM ADOLESCENT

The adolescent mother may have special postpartum needs, depending on her level of maturity and her support system. The nurse needs to assess maternal–infant interaction, roles of support people, plans for discharge, knowledge of childrearing, and plans for follow-up care. It is imperative that a community health service contact the adolescent shortly after discharge.

Contraception counseling is an important part of teaching. *Healthy People 2020* objectives (USDHHS, 2013) include using contraception as a means of pregnancy planning. The incidence of repeat pregnancies during adolescence is high. The younger the adolescent, the more likely she is to become pregnant again. Nurses should be aware of the state laws that govern their jurisdiction in order to determine if providing contraception without parental consent is allowed. In states where adolescents can obtain birth control without parental consent, it is often more comfortable for the adolescent to address these issues without others present. (Chapter 13 discusses adolescent pregnancy in depth.) Adolescents may encounter obstacles when attempting to obtain contraceptives. These may include embarrassment about discussing the topic; concerns about confidentiality, such as not wanting their parents to know or having to give permission; and lack of knowledge regarding available methods (Coles, Makino, & Stanwood, 2011). Nurses can play a key role in overcoming these obstacles by providing teaching and referrals that address these barriers.

The nurse has many opportunities for teaching the adolescent about her newborn in the postpartum unit. Because the nurse is a role model, the manner in which she handles the newborn greatly influences the young mother. If he is present, the father should be included in as much of the teaching as possible. If the grandparents are going to take an active role in caring for the infant, they should also be included in teaching *if* desired by the new mother.

As with older parents, a newborn examination done at the bedside gives adolescents information about their baby's health and shows possible positions for handling the baby. The nurse can also use this time to provide information about newborn and infant behavior. Parents who have some idea of what to expect from their infant are less frustrated with the newborn's behavior.

The adolescent mother appreciates positive feedback about her newborn and her developing maternal responses. Praise and encouragement will increase her confidence and self-esteem. Young mothers with low self-esteem, family conflict, and few social supports are more likely to encounter postpartum depression (Clare & Yeh, 2012). Careful assessment of these factors should be made during the postpartum period so appropriate referrals can be provided before discharge.

Group classes for adolescent mothers should include information about infant care skills, such as taking the baby's temperature, clearing the nose and mouth, monitoring growth and development, feeding the infant, providing well-baby care, and identifying danger signals in the ill newborn. These classes can also address unique needs of teen mothers, such as peer relationships, added responsibilities, and goal setting.

Ideally, teenage mothers should visit adolescent clinics for assessment of themselves and their newborn for several years after birth. In this way, the adolescent's enrollment in classes on parenting, need for vocational guidance, and school attendance can be supported and followed closely. School systems' classes for young mothers are an excellent way of helping adolescents finish school and learn how to parent at the same time. Some public high schools have on-site childcare centers to

---

Evidence-Based Practice · Encouraging Adolescent Mothers to Continue Breastfeeding

Clinical Question
How can adolescent mothers be encouraged to continue breastfeeding at home?

The Evidence
Adolescent mothers have one of the lowest rates of continued breastfeeding; more than half of adolescents are not breastfeeding their baby at all 6 weeks after giving birth. A systematic review and a retrospective cohort review were conducted to determine strategies most likely to be successful in encouraging persistence in breastfeeding among adolescent mothers. These reviews included 18 research studies and a cohort study with more than 500 subjects. These multiple-study reviews and large-sample cohort studies provide the strongest evidence for practice. Support for adolescent breastfeeding must be multivariate to be effective. Strategies applied through peer support, such as group counseling, education, and peer-to-peer sponsors, were the most

effective in changing behavior (Glass, Tucker, Stewart, et al., 2010). Support for self-esteem, informational materials, and emotional support were also important determinants of persistence. Home care visits were effective in providing informational support and access to resources for these teens (Grassley, 2010).

Best Practice
Providing multiple sources and kinds of support will help adolescents persist in breastfeeding their baby, which is an ideal source of nutrition for the first 6 months. Developing peer systems of support may be the most powerful method for enhancing the desirability of breastfeeding and success.

Clinical Reasoning
What are the elements of a support system for teens who want to breastfeed? How can the nurse help adolescents access and use these supports in a timely way?

assist with childcare needs and to provide an opportunity for adolescents to learn important child development principles and childcare tasks.

NURSING CARE OF THE WOMAN WHO RELINQUISHES HER INFANT

Women who choose to give their infants up for adoption typically are single, white, never-married adolescents. It is much less common in black and Hispanic cultures to consider adoption. Less than 1% of all births in the United States result in an adoption (Center for American Progress, 2010). The majority of young women who relinquish their children have higher education and income levels, higher future educational or career goals, and mothers and fathers who favor adoption. Still others may feel that they are not emotionally ready for the responsibilities of parenthood, or their partner may strongly disapprove of the pregnancy. These and many other reasons may prompt the woman to relinquish her baby.

Some mothers are forced to relinquish their infants because of lifestyle choices such as illicit drug use, past history of abusing children, and incarceration. The number of infants placed for adoption because of these circumstances is unknown. Many of these infants may be placed with relatives or in the foster care system. Several factors must be met, including clear evidence that the parent is unfit and that severing the parental rights is in the best interest of the child (Center for American Progress, 2010).

Starting in 1997, Infant Safe Haven Acts were enacted to protect newborns from death caused by abandonment; to provide a means for a mother to place her baby up for adoption anonymously; and to ensure that relinquished babies are left with safe providers who can care for them and provide medical services. The relinquishing mother is protected from prosecution for neglect or abandonment under the law (Child Welfare Information Gateway, 2012).

Surrogacy is also becoming more common in the United States, resulting in relinquishment agreements that may not show up in the adoption statistics. Even though the mother has entered a legal agreement to give up the child she is carrying, she still faces grief issues. The mother who chooses to let her child be adopted usually experiences intense ambivalence. Several factors contribute to this ambivalence. First, there are social pressures against giving up one's child. Additionally, the woman has usually made considerable adjustments in her lifestyle to carry and give birth to this child, and may be unaware of the growing bond between her and her child. Her attachment feelings may peak upon seeing her baby. At the same time, she may not have told friends and relatives about the pregnancy and so may lack a support system to help her work through her feelings and support her decision making. After childbirth, the mother needs to complete a grieving process to work through her loss and its accompanying grief, loneliness, guilt, and other feelings. Mothers who relinquish their infants often experience disenfranchised grief, that is, grief that is unrecognized or not socially accepted. Nurses may unintentionally exacerbate this grief by not acknowledging the women's need to grieve (Aloi, 2009). When the relinquishing mother is admitted to the birthing unit, the nurse should be informed about the mother's decision to relinquish the baby. The nurse needs to respect any special requests for the birth and encourage the woman to express her emotions. After the birth the mother should have access to the baby; she will decide whether she wants to see the newborn. Seeing the newborn often aids the grieving process and provides an opportunity for the birth mother to say goodbye. When the mother sees her baby, she may feel strong attachment and love. The nurse needs to assure the woman that these feelings do not mean that her decision to relinquish the child is wrong; relinquishment is often a painful act of love (Aloi, 2009).

Postpartum nursing care also includes arranging ongoing care for the relinquishing mother. Some mothers may request an early discharge or a transfer to another medical unit. When possible, the nurse supports these requests.

POSTPARTUM CARE FOR SPECIAL POPULATIONS

Nursing Care of the Postpartum Patient with Obesity

As obesity increases in the United States, the postpartum nurse will care for a growing number of patients who are obese or morbidly obese. The patient with obesity has needs similar to those of other postpartum patients, but she needs special attention to prevent injury, respiratory complications, thromboembolic disease, and infection, for which she is at high risk.

The nurse should carefully assess the woman for airway obstruction and hypoxia, particularly if she received opioids. Ambulation should be encouraged as soon as possible to prevent pneumonia. The use of sequential compression devices (SCDs) and early ambulation is essential to the prevention of deep vein thrombosis, especially if the patient had a cesarean birth. If mechanical vacuum devices are used to facilitate drainage from her incision following a cesarean birth, the patient should be educated about them. The mother should demonstrate how to visualize, clean, and completely dry her incision prior to discharge. The use of a mirror may be helpful. She needs to recognize and promptly report signs of infection or dehiscence of her surgical incision or episiotomy repair.

SAFETY ALERT!
The nurse needs to utilize adequate personnel and appropriate assistive devices to maintain safety for both the patient who is obese and staff members during position changes, transport, and ambulation. Additionally, the new mother may need extra supervision and assistance when breastfeeding her baby to ensure newborn safety.

Nursing Care of the Lesbian Mother

Although the literature regarding gay and lesbian families is growing, much of it is focused on options for conception, challenges experienced by gay parents, and legal issues. Little has been published about the labor, delivery, and postpartum experiences of lesbian mothers. Spidsberg and Sørlie (2012) examined lesbian couples and found that lesbian couples have a unique and different bond compared to heterosexual couples. In general, most lesbian partners often feel more at ease in the delivery room than many fathers. The nonpregnant partner often assumes a co-mothering role in the family unit. The main needs of lesbian couples identified in Spidsberg and Sørlie's qualitative study were to have an open relationship with healthcare providers who were accepting of their differences and to be able to build a rapport between the nurse and the couple. Nurses need to examine their own feelings about how they perceive alternative families and be mindful of their nonverbal expressions when interacting with these families (Spidsberg & Sørlie, 2012).

The nurse should maintain an attitude that is respectful, caring, and open to sexual diversity when working with all patients. Providing quality patient-centered care for any postpartum woman involves acknowledging, welcoming, and involving her intimate partner in care and decision making. The nurse should be aware that standardized postpartum instructions, particularly those related to intercourse and contraception, might need to be individualized and amended.

Nursing Care of the Postpartum Mother with a Developmental Disability

The postpartum time period is one of great growth in the maternal mothering role. New mothers are faced with various challenges and different learning opportunities. Women with developmental or intellectual disabilities are at particular risk during this time period. Material should be presented to them in an easy-to-understand format. Peer mentors are often helpful role models for these women. Teaching should be conducted at a level that is achievable for the individual woman. A needs assessment should be performed to determine what needs the mother and new family may have. Community and private resources should be available to make the transition to the postpartum period as flawless as possible.

Nursing Care of the Mother with a History of Sexual Abuse

Women who have been sexually abused tend to have more anxiety and stress related to hospital procedures, interactions with unfamiliar staff, and being touched in general. The postpartum woman who has a history of sexual abuse may have difficulty establishing trust and may feel uncomfortable when private demonstrations are being performed. The nurse should treat the woman with respect by providing draping whenever possible. Speaking to the woman in private protects her fragile emotions from being observed by others. Support groups may offer the mother with a history of sexual abuse a safe haven to share her experiences and the impact they have on her mothering.

PREPARATION FOR DISCHARGE

In preparation for discharge, the nurse evaluates the mother and newborn's progress toward identified outcomes and provides discharge teaching.

Discharge Criteria

Ideally, preparation for discharge begins the moment a woman is admitted to the birthing unit. Before discharge, the nurse assesses the mother's physical and psychologic condition, the newborn's adjustment to extrauterine life, the family's overall adjustment, and the need for outside resources. Nursing efforts should be directed toward assessing the parents' knowledge, expectations, and beliefs and then providing anticipatory guidance and teaching accordingly. Because teaching is one of the primary responsibilities of the postpartum nurse, many agencies have elaborate teaching programs and videos. The nurse should spend time with the parents to determine if they have any last-minute questions. A sample postpartum discharge teaching checklist is found on this text's website. In general, the following criteria should be assessed and met before discharge:

- Normal vital signs
- Appropriate involution of the uterus
- Appropriate amount of lochia without evidence of infection
- Knowledge of signs of infection
- Episiotomy or laceration well approximated with a decrease in edema or bruising
- Ability to perform pericare and apply medications to perineal or anal area if ordered
- Ability to void and pass flatus (some facilities' criteria may include having a bowel movement before discharge)
- Ability to take fluids and foods without difficulty
- Ability to care for self and newborn
- Has received rubella vaccine or RhoGAM if indicated (see Table 30–3)

Additional outcomes for the cesarean birth mother include the following:

- States in own words the reason for the cesarean birth
- Maintains desired pain control
- Maintains moderate mobility level

Ensuring that the woman has met the criteria before discharge decreases the incidence of complications or readmission in the postpartum period.

Discharge Teaching

In general, discharge teaching includes at least the following information and maternal activities:

1. Review of literature and videos the woman has received or viewed that explains recommended postpartum exercises, the need for adequate rest, the need to avoid overexertion initially, and the recommendation to abstain from sexual intercourse until lochia has ceased. (If the family desires information about birth control methods, the nurse can provide such information at this time.)

2. Information geared to the specific nutritional needs of breastfeeding or formula-feeding mothers. (If the mother

has been receiving vitamins and/or iron supplements, the nurse encourages her to continue until the first postpartum examination.) Demonstrates proper breastfeeding techniques and breast care or describes formula preparation, formula-feeding techniques, and nonlactating breast care.

3. How to provide basic care for the infant; when to anticipate that the cord will fall off; when the infant can have a tub bath; when the infant will need her or his first immunizations; and so on. (Parents should also be comfortable feeding and handling the baby, and should practice basic principles of safety, including the need to use a car seat when the infant is in a car.) See more detailed discussion later in the home care section.

4. Procedure for obtaining copies of her infant's birth certificate.

5. When to schedule the first appointment for her postpartum examination and for her newborn's first well-baby examination.

6. Signs of possible complications (see Table 30–4) and encouragement for the woman to contact her caregiver if she develops any of them. Signs and symptoms that indicate possible problems in the infant and who the parents should contact about them.

7. Information on local agencies and/or support groups, such as La Leche League, Mothers of Twins, adolescent groups, or new mother support groups, that might be of particular assistance to the family. Displays appropriate interaction with baby. Identifies the symptoms of postpartum depression and available resources.

8. Phone number of the mother–baby unit or information hotline and encouragement to call if she has any questions or concerns. Plans for home care visits so that the parents know when to expect the visit and what it entails.

The nurse can also use this final opportunity to reassure the couple of their ability to be successful parents. The nurse can stress the infant's need to feel loved and secure and urge parents to talk to each other and work together to solve any problems that arise.

Considerations for Follow-Up Care

In 1998, the Newborns' and Mothers' Health Protection Act went into effect. This federal law ensures that all insurance companies cover a 48-hour stay for vaginal deliveries and a 96-hour stay for women who have undergone a cesarean birth (U.S. Department of Labor, 2009). In consideration of the risks associated with voluntary early discharge, more than half of all U.S. states have passed legislation mandating a home visit if the family was discharged before 48 hours.

Early discharges have implications for the mother, including the risk of postpartum hemorrhage and difficulties with breastfeeding. In addition, opportunities for the mother to become comfortable with her new baby may be compromised. The risk of postpartum depression commonly occurs in the first month following the birth. Women who receive some type of follow-up assessment from a nurse experience less depression than those who do not receive postpartum follow-up (Surkan, Gottlieb, McCormick, et al., 2012). In addition, extended family members who live at a distance and have agreed to assist the new family in the first few weeks after birth may not have arrived yet. Furthermore, in the first 24 hours after childbirth, the mother may be too tired or may not be ready emotionally to participate in learning activities. In all cases of early discharge, a home visit by an experienced postpartum nurse can be invaluable.

These early discharges present a challenge to nurses because the time available for nursing assessments and patient teaching is greatly reduced. In addition, many conditions in the newborn, such as jaundice, ductal-dependent cardiac lesions, and gastrointestinal obstructions, may take longer than 2 days to develop, and identification of these problems depends on a skilled, experienced professional (American Academy of Pediatrics [AAP] Committee on Fetus and Newborn, 2010). Other experts contend that breastfeeding may not be well established before 48 hours and discharge before this time can lead to increased rates of dehydration and poor breastfeeding outcomes (AAP Committee on Fetus and Newborn, 2010).

The need for follow-up postpartum care is essential. Most women who had a vaginal birth are seen at 6 weeks while women undergoing a cesarean birth are evaluated at the 2-week visit. *Healthy People 2020* objectives (USDHHS, 2013) include increasing the number of women who receive medical care at a 6-week-postpartum visit.

Table 30–4	When to Contact the Primary Care Provider

After discharge, a woman should contact her physician/CNM if any of the following develop:

- Sudden, persistent, or spiking fever
- Change in the character of the lochia—foul smell, return to bright-red bleeding, excessive amount, passage of large clots
- Pain at the site of a laceration, episiotomy, or abdominal incision
- Evidence of wound infection including redness, swelling, severe or worsening pain, or foul-smelling discharge
- Evidence of mastitis, such as breast tenderness, reddened areas, malaise
- Evidence of thrombophlebitis, such as calf pain, tenderness, redness
- Evidence of urinary tract infection, such as urgency, frequency, burning on urination
- Continued severe or incapacitating postpartum depression
- Inability to care for self or baby for any physical or psychologic reason

---

Health Promotion *Healthy People 2020*
Birth Weight Goals

Healthy People 2020 goals (USDHHS, 2013) include reducing the incidence of low weight, very low weight, and premature infants, including later preterm births.

Special emphasis has also been placed on the needs of the **late preterm infant**, born between 34 and 37 weeks (Association of Women's Health, Obstetric and Neonatal Nurses [AWHONN], 2010). Late preterm infants are at a greater risk for increases in mortality and morbidity because they are physically not mature and are more prone to have physiologic and metabolic complications (AWHONN, 2010). Readmissions for infection and jaundice are more common in later preterm infants than in term infants (AWHONN, 2010). The American Academy of Pediatrics (AAP) has identified specific risk factors in late preterm infants that increase the likelihood of readmission and neonatal mortality. These include being first born, breastfeeding at the time of discharge, having a mother who has had labor and childbirth complications, having public insurance as your source of payment, and being an Asian/Pacific Islander (Barfield & Lee, 2012). Special attention by the home health nurse is warranted for these infants to ensure a proper home transition and to identify possible early complications (AWHONN, 2010).

Following discharge, various services are available in most communities to meet the needs of the postpartum family. The goal is to help ensure that all family members have the opportunity to meet healthcare needs, regardless of their resources. Some types of follow-up care include telephone follow-up and home visits.

Telephone Follow-Up

Telephone follow-up is offered to families before discharge, and a mutually agreed-on time is set for the call. Typically the call is made within 3 days after discharge or earlier if desired, lasts about 20 minutes, and is goal directed. To perform effective telephone assessment, the nurse must be able to listen skillfully, ask open-ended questions, and project an attitude of caring. If the assessment reveals any signs of a postpartum complication, the nurse refers the woman to her healthcare provider for further evaluation. The plan of care developed and implemented during a telephone conversation is limited to supportive counseling, teaching, and referral.

It is also fairly common for a home care nurse to make a telephone follow-up call to a family a few days after a home visit to provide additional information, address questions or areas of confusion, and make referrals if indicated. The mother may have multiple questions and is generally at a high level of learning readiness. Some women may prefer a telephone-based follow-up because it requires less preparation and time than a home visit.

In addition to these scheduled follow-up telephone calls, nurses in birthing, newborn, and postpartum units, as well as clinic nurses, often receive phone calls from postpartum families seeking advice or care. These calls must be triaged immediately. Calls with urgent or life-threatening implications should be referred appropriately, either by initiating an immediate call to the practitioner or, in rare circumstances, calling 9-1-1.

Finally, many communities have established 24-hour help lines for new parents to call when they have questions or need support. In areas where help lines are not available, parents may be directed to call the birthing center. In either case, the nurse provides the number so that it is readily accessible for the family.

Home Visit

If the mother, family, and physician/CNM have chosen discharge earlier than 48 hours after vaginal birth, in some states, the mother may request a total of three home visits. The home setting provides an opportunity for the nurse and family to interact in a more relaxed environment in which the family has control. In some instances, the challenges of assessing and enhancing self-care and infant care may be unique in the home, and the nurse will have many opportunities to exercise critical thinking to develop creative options with the family. The nurse should explain that, unlike community health visits, only one or two home visits are typically planned and spaced out over the next week, and long-term follow-up by the postpartum nurse is not anticipated. Occasionally the nurse may schedule additional home visits based on the findings of the first home visit and the follow-up phone call.

Evaluation

Anticipated outcomes of comprehensive postpartum nursing care of the family include the following:

- The mother is reasonably comfortable and has learned pain relief measures.
- The mother is rested and understands how to add more activity over the next few days and weeks.
- The mother's physiologic and psychologic well-being have been supported.
- The mother verbalizes her understanding of self-care measures.
- The new parents demonstrate how to care for their baby.
- The new parents have had opportunities to form attachment with their baby.
- Follow-up care contacts have been initiated as needed.

CONSIDERATIONS FOR THE HOME VISIT

Before the home visit, the nurse (who is experienced in postpartum maternal and newborn care) prepares by identifying the purpose of the home visit and gathering needed materials and equipment. A personal contact while the woman is still in the birth setting or a previsit telephone call is used to arrange the appointment with the woman and her family. During the previsit contact, it is important for the nurse to clearly identify the purpose and goals of the visit and to begin establishing rapport.

Purpose and Timing of the Home Visit

Postpartum home care is focused more on assessment, teaching, facilitating learning, and counseling than on physical care. First, it provides an opportunity to assess the status of the mother and infant for signs of any complications. The established guidelines for discharge of the mother and baby mean the nurse can expect certain levels of health and wellness. However, because the status of the mother and newborn can change, the nurse should stay alert for deviations from the norm and identify conditions that may warrant further medical evaluation or rehospitalization. The nurse can also complete follow-up blood work if needed.

In addition, the nurse assesses adaptation of the family to the new baby and adjustment of any siblings. The nurse also assesses the parents' skill in bathing, dressing, handling, and comforting their newborn, and the appropriateness and safety of the home environment.

Another purpose of the home visit is to ascertain current informational needs and to offer requested information in a more relaxed setting. Postpartum home care provides opportunities for enhancing self- and infant-care techniques initially presented in the birth setting. Many times, questions and concerns arise at home that were not identified in the hospital.

In addition, the nurse answers questions about breast-feeding, provides support and encouragement, and addresses the need for referrals to clinics, classes, or postpartum support groups.

Maintaining Safety

In the past, nurses were perceived as a mainstay of communities and could move in most settings without fear or concern for safety. Today, some communities are not safe for visiting nurses. It is important for the nurse to follow basic safety rules when conducting a home visit, including the following:

- Know the specific address and ask for directions during the previsit contact. If the area is not familiar, trace out the route on a map or use an Internet program to provide directions before leaving for the visit and take a map along. Even with a global positioning system (GPS), some newer areas may not be included or found within the system, so always have a backup plan in place.

- Carry a fully charged cellular phone and a working flashlight, especially for night visits.

- Notify an instructor or supervisor when leaving for a visit and check in as soon as the visit is completed.

Many agencies that provide home care services have established violence prevention programs to help ensure safety. Nurses in the community need to be aware of their environment and alert to environmental cues, whether overt or subtle. In addition, the following recommendations are important (McPhaul, Lipscomb, & Johnson, 2010):

- Invest time in personal safety by driving around a neighborhood before making an initial visit to identify potential cues to violence. Avoid walking through a crowd or staying in an elevator with others if it makes you uneasy.

- In high-risk areas, visit the family during daylight hours. Inform the family when you plan to arrive and advise them to call a supervisor if you do not arrive within 15 minutes of the arranged time. Provide them with a contact name and phone number.

- Do not park in deserted or unlit areas. Make sure your car is in good working order and has gas. Keep doors locked and windows closed.

- Before leaving for the visit, lock personal belongings in the trunk of the car, out of sight. Do not carry a purse, medications, or other items.

- In accordance with agency policy, wear scrubs, a lab coat, or other uniform that identifies you as a nurse. Wear a name tag and carry identification. Avoid wearing expensive jewelry or pins of a religious or political nature that might be seen as offensive.

- Be aware of personal body language and how it might be interpreted. (For example, avoid crossing arms or shoving hands in pockets, which may suggest hostility; remain calm and convey a sense of respect at all times.)

- Pay attention to the body language of anyone present during the visit, not just the patient.

- Be alert for signs that a person is becoming enraged (reddened neck and/or face, clenched fists, pacing). If any family member is violent, or if drug or alcohol abuse is occurring, leave the home and report the incident to your supervisor.

- Leave the home immediately if a gun or knife is visible. Do not confront the patient or family member.

- If a situation arises that feels unsafe, or a "gut feeling" tells you something is not right, terminate the visit immediately.

If the visit is in an area that seems unsafe, it may be wise for two nurses to go together. Nurses should avoid entering areas where violence is in progress. In such cases, they should return to the car and contact the police or dial 9-1-1. Most people are more comfortable in familiar neighborhoods and have some hesitation when entering homes in other residential areas. First home visits may feel uncomfortable because they are unfamiliar, but with experience comfort increases (Figure 30–4 ●).

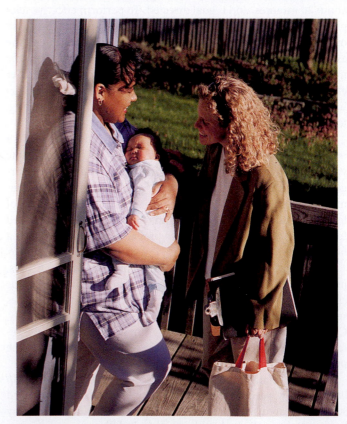

● **Figure 30–4** Nurse arriving for a home visit.

Source: George Dodson/Pearson Education.

Fostering a Caring Relationship with the Family

Although the nurse in the birthing center strives to enhance family autonomy and control, the atmosphere of the institutional environment may cause the new mother and family to feel disempowered. It is important for the professional nurse to recognize that the parameters of the home visit are different. In the home, the family members have control of their environment and the nurse is an invited visitor. The nurse can rely on the same characteristics of a caring relationship that have been integral to hospital-based practice—regard for patients, genuineness, empathy, and establishment of trust and rapport—when providing care in the home setting (Table 30–5). Evidence of these characteristics forms the foundation for a caring relationship.

When the door is answered, the nurse should introduce herself or himself and confirm that the location is correct. If a place to sit is not indicated, the nurse may inquire, "Where is the best place to sit so that we can talk for a while?" In some families, offering refreshments may be an important aspect of welcoming a visitor. In this case, it is beneficial to the relationship for the nurse to accept the refreshment graciously. Many cultures have strong ties to certain foods and beverages during the postpartum period. Accepting the food or beverage conveys acceptance of cultural norms. It is helpful for the nurse to be familiar with various cultural norms and traditions (Spector, 2012).

The maternal psychologic assessment focuses on attachment, adjustment to the parental role, sibling adjustment, the mother's perception of her new role and coping, and educational needs.

In ideal situations a family approach involving the presence of the father and any siblings provides an opportunity to observe family interactions and opportunities for all family members to ask questions and express concerns. In addition, any questionable family interaction pattern such as one suggestive of abuse or neglect may be evident and further referral could be considered if needed.

HOME CARE: THE MOTHER AND FAMILY

During the first home visit, the nurse completes a physical assessment of the mother and a psychosocial assessment of the family. Teaching for self-care is commonly required for new mothers, especially breastfeeding mothers with nipple soreness, engorgement, and other concerns. Family teaching related to resumption of sexual activity and contraception may also be required.

Assessment of the Mother and Family

Before performing the physical assessment, the nurse should ensure the mother's privacy. The physical assessment focuses on maternal physical adaptation, which is assessed by focusing

---

Developing Cultural Competence
Role of Extended Family

In some cultures, extended family members such as grandmothers and aunts play a major role in the care of the postpartum woman and her family. Sometimes, these family members take full responsibility for running the household throughout the postpartum period. In other families, they concentrate entirely on the mother's or newborn's care. When culturally appropriate, include these extended family members in postpartum education sessions.

Table 30–5	Fostering a Caring Relationship
Demonstrated Goal	**Approaches to Achieve Goal**
Regard	Introduce yourself to the family. Call the family members by their surnames until you have been invited to use the given or a less formal name.
	Ask to be introduced to other members of the family who are present. Allow the mother or spokesperson to assume this role. Remember, in some cultures, it may be a male figure or a mother figure who assumes the primary role. Use active listening. Maintain objectiveness.
	Ask permission before sitting.
Genuineness	Mean what you say. Make sure that your verbal and nonverbal messages are congruent.
	Be nonjudgmental. Do not make assumptions about individuals or settings.
	Always strive to demonstrate caring behaviors.
	Be prepared for the visit, honestly answer questions and provide information, and be truthful. If you do not know the answer to a question, tell the patient you will find the information and report back.
Empathy	Listen to the mother and family "where they are" without judgment. Be attentive to what the birthing experience is for them so that you will understand from their perspective.
	Remember that empathy denotes understanding, not sympathy.
Trust and rapport	Do what you say you will do.
	Be prepared for the visit and be on time.
	Follow-up on any areas that are needed.

on vital signs, breasts, abdominal musculature, elimination patterns, reproductive tract, and laboratory values. The nurse also talks with the mother about her diet, fatigue level, ability to rest and sleep, pain management, and signs of postpartum complications. In addition, for breastfeeding mothers, the nurse assesses the woman's feeding technique and presents information about possible problems that may occur. (See *Assessment Guide: Postpartum—First Home Visit and Anticipated Progress at 6 Weeks* on pages 757–759.) Generally the new mother has a final postpartum examination with her caregiver about 6 weeks after childbirth. However, if the nurse's assessment indicates a need, the nurse refers the woman to her healthcare provider for care before the 6-week check and for appropriate follow-up.

Many new mothers are concerned about weight loss. Women who have gained excess weight during the pregnancy are at risk for obesity in later life. Counseling the mother about proper diet and exercise is an effective strategy to lose weight in the postpartum period. Nursing women should be counseled that extreme weight loss strategies are not advised, but that healthy food choices and exercise can aid in weight reduction. There are also weight loss programs designed specifically for nursing mothers that can offer counseling, group support, and monitoring in the postpartum period.

Breastfeeding Concerns Following Discharge

Because mothers are discharged from the birthing unit before breastfeeding is well established, they are frequently alone when they encounter changes in the breastfeeding process. Many women stop nursing if the situations they encounter seem problematic. For this reason, the nurse providing a home visit is in a unique position to positively impact the duration and success of breastfeeding (Kronborg, Vaeth, & Kristensen, 2012). Table 30–6 on page 760 summarizes self-care measures the nurse can suggest to a woman with a breastfeeding problem.

Regardless of feeding method (newborn feeding is discussed in detail in Chapter 26 🔗), it is important for the nurse to assess the newborn's fluid and nutritional intake. As part of the physical assessment, the newborn's nude weight is determined. If the weight loss since birth is 10% or more, the nurse assesses the baby for signs of dehydration such as loose skin with decreased skin turgor, dry mucous membranes, sunken anterior fontanelle, and decreased frequency and amount of voiding and stooling. Risk factors for suboptimal breastfeeding include maternal obesity, primiparity, young maternal age, use of formula supplementation, use of pacifiers, cesarean birth, second stage of labor greater than 1 hour, low birth weight, breastfeeding difficulty, and flat or inverted nipples (Chapman & Pérez-Escamilla, 2012).

Nipple Soreness

Some discomfort often occurs initially with breastfeeding; it peaks between days 3 and 6 and then recedes. Breastfeeding difficulty and nipple soreness are often causes for women to discontinue breastfeeding. The nurse should counsel the mother not to switch to formula feeding or delay feedings because these measures cause engorgement and more soreness (Riordan & Wambach, 2010). Discomfort that lasts throughout the feeding or past the first week demands attention.

The baby's position at the breast is a critical factor in nipple soreness. The mother's hand should be off the areola, and the baby should be facing the mother's chest, with ear, shoulder, and hip aligned (see Figure 26–15 🔗 on page 603). Because the area of greatest stress to the nipple is in line with the newborn's chin and nose, nipple soreness may be decreased by encouraging the mother to rotate positions when feeding the infant. Changing positions alters the focus of greatest stress and promotes more complete breast emptying.

Nipple soreness may also develop if the infant has faulty sucking habits. Nipples may have injured tips that are bruised, scabbed, or blistered from the nipple entering the baby's mouth at an upward angle and rubbing against the roof of the mouth or from poor latch-on (Riordan & Wambach, 2010). Soreness may also result from continuous negative pressure if the infant falls asleep with the breast in his or her mouth.

Chewed nipples, which result from improper positioning, are cracked or tender at or near the base. In these cases, the baby's jaws close only on the nipple instead of on the areola, or the baby's mouth is not opened wide enough or has slipped down to the nipple from the areola as a result of engorgement. Soreness on the underside of the nipple is caused by the infant nursing with her or his bottom lip tucked in rather than out, causing a friction burn. In such cases, even vigorous sucking produces little milk because the milk sinuses under the areola are not compressed. This situation results in a frustrated infant and marked soreness for the mother. The problem is overcome by manipulating the baby's bottom lip with a fingertip before beginning the feeding, positioning the infant with as much areola as possible in his or her mouth, and rotating the baby's positions at the breast.

Nipple soreness is especially pronounced during the first few minutes of a feeding. If the mother is not expecting this discomfort, she may become discouraged and quickly stop. The let-down reflex may take a few minutes to activate, and it may not occur if the mother stops nursing too quickly. The infant is unsatisfied, and the possibility of breast engorgement increases.

Nipple soreness can also result from the vigorous feeding of an overeager infant. Thus the mother may find it helpful to nurse more frequently. Again, promoting let-down just before feeding may help. Other self-care measures include applying ice to the nipples and areola for a few minutes before feeding to promote nipple erectness and numb the tissue initially. To promote dryness, the mother may leave her bra flaps down for a few minutes after feeding (Figure 30–5 ●) or expose her nipples to sunlight or ultraviolet light for 30 seconds at first, gradually increasing to 3 minutes. Drying the nipples with a hair dryer on a low heat setting also facilitates drying and promotes healing (Riordan & Wambach, 2010). The use of petroleum-based products such as Vaseline, A & D, cocoa butter, and baby oil to lubricate the nipples is discouraged because the petroleum interferes

Assessment Guide   Postpartum—First Home Visit and Anticipated Progress at 6 Weeks

Physical Assessment/Normal Findings	Alterations and Possible Causes*	Nursing Responses to Data†
Vital Signs		
Blood pressure: return to normal prepregnant level	Elevated blood pressure (anxiety, essential hypertension, renal disease), preeclampsia (can occur postpartum)	Review history, evaluate normal baseline; refer to physician/CNM if necessary.
Pulse: 60–100 beats/min (or prepregnant normal rate)	Increased pulse rate, tachycardia, chest pain (excitement, anxiety, cardiac disorders)	Count pulse for full minute, note irregularities; marked tachycardia or beat irregularities require additional assessment and possible physician/CNM referral.
Respirations: 12–20/min	Marked tachypnea or abnormal patterns (respiratory disorders)	Evaluate for respiratory disease; refer to physician/CNM if necessary.
Temperature: 36.6–37.6°C (98–99.6°F).	Increased temperature (infection)	Assess for signs and symptoms of infection or disease state.
Weight		
2 days: possible weight loss of 12–20+ lb	Minimal weight loss (fluid retention, preeclampsia)	Evaluate for fluid retention, edema, deep tendon reflexes, and blood pressure elevation.
6 weeks: returning to normal prepregnant weight	Retained weight (excessive caloric intake)	Determine amount of daily exercise. Provide dietary teaching. Refer to dietitian if necessary for additional dietary counseling.
	Extreme weight loss (excessive dieting, inadequate caloric intake)	Discuss appropriate diets, refer to dietitian for additional counseling if necessary.
Breasts		
Nonbreastfeeding: 2 days: may have mild to moderate tenderness; small amount of milk may be expressed 6 weeks: soft, with no tenderness; return to prepregnant size	Some engorgement (incomplete suppression of lactation) Redness; marked tenderness (mastitis) Palpable mass (tumor)	Engorgement may be seen in nonbreastfeeding mothers. Advise patient to wear a supportive, well-fitted bra; avoid very warm showers; avoid pumping or any stimulation of breasts; use ice packs for comfort; evaluate for signs and symptoms of mastitis (rare in nonbreastfeeding mothers). Parcooked cabbage leaves can be placed against the breast to relieve engorgement.
Breastfeeding: full, with prominent nipples; lactation established	Cracked, fissured nipples (feeding problems) Redness, marked tenderness, or even abscess formation (mastitis) Palpable mass (full milk duct, tumor)	Counsel about nipple care. Observe infant feeding. Evaluate patient condition, evidence of fever, redness, or tender area, refer to physician/CNM for initiation of antibiotic therapy, if indicated. Opinion varies as to value of breast examination for breastfeeding mothers; some feel a breastfeeding mother should examine her breasts monthly, after feeding, when breasts are empty; if palpable mass is felt, refer to physician for further evaluation. For breast inflammation instruct the mother to: 1. Keep breast empty by frequent feeding. 2. Rest when possible. 3. Take prescribed pain relief medication. 4. Force fluids. 5. Take antibiotics if ordered. If symptoms are accompanied by fever, flulike symptoms, or redness, instruct woman to call her physician/CNM and take an analgesic.

*Possible causes of alterations are identified in parentheses.

†This column provides guidelines for further assessment and initial nursing intervention.

(*continued*)

Physical Assessment/Normal Findings	Alterations and Possible Causes*	Nursing Responses to Data†
Abdominal Musculature		
2 days: improved firmness, although "bread dough" consistency is not unusual, especially in multipara; striae pink and obvious	Marked relaxation of muscles	Evaluate exercise level; provide information on appropriate exercise program.
Cesarean incision healing	Use the REEDA scoring system: redness, ecchymosis, edema, discharge from incision site, and approximation. Assess for tenderness and pain.	Evaluate for infection; refer to physician/CNM if necessary.
6 weeks: muscle tone continues to improve; striae may be beginning to fade, may not achieve a silvery appearance for several more weeks; linea nigra fading		
Elimination Pattern		
Urinary tract: return to prepregnant urinary elimination routine	Urinary incontinence, especially when lifting, coughing, laughing, and so on (urethral trauma, cystocele)	Assess for cystocele; instruct in appropriate muscle tightening exercises; refer to physician/CNM.
	Pain or burning when voiding, urgency and/or frequency, pus, blood, or white blood cells (WBC.) in urine, pathogenic organisms in culture (urinary tract infection)	Evaluate for urinary tract infection; obtain clean-catch urine; refer to physician/CNM for treatment if indicated.
Routine urinalysis within normal limits (proteinuria disappeared)	Sugar or ketone in urine—may be some lactose present in urine of breastfeeding mothers (diabetes)	Evaluate diet; assess for signs and symptoms of diabetes; refer to physician/CNM.
Bowel habits: 2 days: May be some discomfort with defecation, especially if patient had severe hemorrhoids or third- or fourth-degree extension	Severe constipation or pain when defecating (trauma or hemorrhoids)	Discuss dietary patterns; encourage fluids and high-fiber diet, adequate roughage. Counsel on the effects of medications. Continue use of stool softener if necessary to prevent pain associated with straining; continue sitz baths, periods of rest for severe hemorrhoids; assess healing of episiotomy and/or lacerations; severe constipation may require administration of laxatives, stool softeners, and an enema if not contraindicated (check with physician/CNM).
6 weeks: return to normal prepregnancy bowel elimination	Marked constipation (inadequate fluid/fiber intake)	See previous discussed interventions.
	Fecal incontinence or constipation (rectocele)	Assess for evidence of rectocele; instruct in muscle tightening exercises; refer to physician/CNM.
Reproductive Tract		
Lochia: 2 days: lochia rubra or lochia serosa, scant amounts, fleshy odor	Excessive amounts and/or large clots (nonfirm uterus), foul odor (infection), passing tissue (possible retained placenta)	Assess for evidence of infection and/or failure of the uterus to decrease in size; refer to physician/CNM. See above.
6 weeks: no lochia, or return to normal menstruation pattern	See above	
Fundus and perineum: 2 days: Fundus is at least two finger breadths below the umbilicus; uterine muscles still somewhat lax; introitus of vagina lacks tone—gapes when intra-abdominal pressure is increased by coughing or straining	Uterus not decreasing in size appropriately (infection)	Assess fundus for firmness and/or signs of infection; refer to physician/CNM if indicated.
Episiotomy and/or lacerations healing; no signs of infection; may have some bruising and tenderness	Evidence of redness, severe pain, poor tissue approximation in episiotomy and/or laceration (wound infection)	Utilize cool or warm sitz baths, topical medications.
6 weeks: uterus almost returned to prepregnant size with almost completely restored muscle tone	Continued flow of lochia, failure to decrease appropriately in size (subinvolution)	Assess for evidence of subinvolution and/or infection; refer to physician for further evaluation and treatment if necessary.

*Possible causes of alterations are identified in parentheses.

†This column provides guidelines for further assessment and initial nursing intervention.

Assessment Guide Postpartum—First Home Visit and Anticipated Progress at 6 Weeks—continued

Physical Assessment/Normal Findings	Alterations and Possible Causes*	Nursing Responses to Data†
Hemoglobin and Hematocrit Levels 6 weeks: hemoglobin (Hb) 12 g/dL; hematocrit (Hct) 37% ± 5%	Hb less than 12 g/dL; Hct 32% (anemia)	Assess nutritional status, assess for signs or symptoms of anemia, begin (or continue) supplemental iron; for marked anemia (Hb less than or equal to 9 g/dL) additional assessment and/or physician/CNM referral may be necessary.
Attachment Bonding process demonstrated by soothing, cuddling, and talking to infant; appropriate feeding techniques; eye-to-eye contact; calling infant by name.	Failure to bond demonstrated by lack of behaviors associated with bonding process, calling infant by nickname that promotes ridicule, inadequate infant weight gain, infant is dirty, hygienic measures are not being maintained, severe diaper rash, failure to obtain adequate supplies to provide infant care (malattachment).	Provide counseling; talk with the woman about her feelings regarding the infant; provide support for the caretaking activities that are being performed; refer to public health nurse for continued home visits; refer if abuse or neglect is suspected.
Parent interacts with infant and provides soothing, caretaking activities.	Parent is unable to respond to infant needs (inability to recognize needs, inadequate education and support, fear, family stress).	Provide support for caretaking activities observed; provide information regarding caretaking activities, such as responding to infant cry; methods of wrapping infant; methods of soothing the infant such as swaddling, rocking, increasing stimuli by singing to the infant or decreasing stimuli by putting infant to rest in quiet room; methods of holding the infant; differences in the cry. Identify support system such as friends, neighbors; provide information regarding community resources and support groups.
Parents express feelings of comfort and success with the parent role.	Evidence is seen of stress and anxiety (difficulty moving into or dealing with the parent role).	Provide support and encouragement; provide information regarding progression into parent role and assist parents in talking through their feelings; refer to community resources and support groups.
Woman is in the informal or personal stage of maternal role attainment.	Woman is still greatly influenced by others, has not developed an image or style of her own (woman remains in the anticipatory stage).	Provide role modeling for the woman in working through problem solving with the infant, provide encouragement as she thinks through decisions and develops her sense of problem solving; encourage her to make decisions regarding infant care.
Adjustment to Parental Role Parents are coping with new roles in terms of division of labor, financial status, communication, readjustment of sexual relations, and adjusting to new daily tasks.	Inability to adjust to new roles (immaturity, inadequate education and preparation, ineffective communication patterns, inadequate support, current family crisis).	Provide counseling, refer to parent groups.
Education Mother understands self-care measures.	Knowledge of self-care is inadequate (inadequate education).	Provide education and counseling.
Parents are knowledgeable regarding infant care.	Knowledge of infant care is inadequate (inadequate education).	
Siblings are adjusting to new baby. Parents have a method of contraception.	Sibling rivalry is excessive. Birth control method has not been chosen.	

*Possible causes of alterations are identified in parentheses.

†This column provides guidelines for further assessment and initial nursing intervention.

Table 30–6	Common Breastfeeding Problems and Remedies	
Problem	**Possible Cause**	**Remedies**
NIPPLES NOT GRASPABLE	Flat or inverted nipples	■ Use Hoffman technique to break adhesions. ■ Wear breast shells to encourage nipples to protrude. ■ Grasp nipples and roll gently between the fingers to increase protractility. ■ Form the nipple before breastfeeding by hand shaping, ice, or wearing nipple shells a half-hour before feeding. ■ Use a breast pump to draw nipples out so that the mother can then put the baby to the breast.
	Engorged breasts	■ Treat engorgement by feeding the baby more frequently. ■ A hand or electric pump or manual emptying of the breast can be done if the baby in unable to grasp the nipple.
	Large breasts	■ Support breast with opposite hand, or use rolled towel under breast to bring nipple to the level of baby's mouth. ■ Avoid having the nipple pointing downward because this makes latch-on more difficult. ■ Use C-hold to make nipple accessible to baby.
ENGORGEMENT	Missed or infrequent feedings	■ Breastfeed frequently (every 1½ hours). ■ Massage and hand express or pump to empty breasts completely when feedings are missed or when a full feeling develops in breasts and baby is not available or willing to feed. ■ Avoid excessive stimulation or pumping between feedings because this will increase milk production. ■ Place warm compresses on breast just before feeding to soften breast. ■ Use cold applications between feedings to slow milk production (frozen bagged vegetables, ice packs, and par-cooked cabbage leaves) (Arora, Vatsa, & Dadhwal, 2008).
	Breasts not emptied at feedings	■ Massage breasts and use warm cloths before feedings. ■ Breastfeed long enough to empty breasts (10 to 15 minutes on each side at each feeding). ■ If baby will not feed long enough to empty breasts, hand express or pump after feeding.
	Inadequate let-down	■ Use relaxation techniques, massage, and warm compresses before breastfeeding. ■ Relax in warm shower with water running from back over shoulders and breasts, hand expressing to relieve fullness. ■ Use hand or electric pump before placing baby on breast to encourage let-down. ■ Listen to soothing music; use visualization or breathing techniques. ■ If caused by anxiety, try to eliminate the source of tension.
	Baby sleepy or not eager to feed	■ Use rousing techniques (e.g., hold baby upright, unwrap blanket, change diaper). ■ Pre-express milk onto nipple or baby's lips to entice baby. ■ Avoid use of bottles of water or formula; these will decrease baby's willingness to suckle.
INADEQUATE LET-DOWN	Let-down not well established	■ Give the baby ample time at the breast (at least 15 minutes per side) to allow for let-down and complete emptying. ■ Breastfeed in a quiet spot away from distractions. ■ Massage breasts and apply warm compresses before breastfeeding. ■ Drink juice, water, or tea (no caffeine) before and during breastfeeding. ■ Condition let-down by setting up a routine for beginning feedings. ■ Use relaxation, visualization, and breathing techniques. ■ Stimulate the nipple manually before breastfeeding. ■ Concentrate thought on the baby and milk flow; turn on a faucet so that the sound of running water helps stimulate let-down. ■ Take a warm shower before feedings. ■ Use breast pump to stimulate the let-down. ■ Avoid waiting to put baby to breast until the baby is famished because this may increase maternal anxiety. ■ Assess for maternal pain, cold temperature, or anxiety before feeding.
	Mother overtired or overextended	■ Nap or rest when the baby rests. ■ Limit distractions, limit visitors, focus on personal needs. ■ Lie down to breastfeed. ■ Simplify daily chores; set priorities.

Table 30–6 Common Breastfeeding Problems and Remedies—continued

Problem	Possible Cause	Remedies
	Mother tense, pressured	■ Identify the causes of tensions and eliminate or minimize them. ■ Decrease fatigue. ■ Have others assist with other household duties or tasks. ■ Use relaxation, visualization, and breathing exercises to promote relaxation and comfort.
	Mother caught in cycle of little milk, worry, less milk	■ Try all of the actions listed above. ■ Counsel mother that most women do produce enough milk. ■ Have infant weighed to ensure adequate weight gain, which is a reflection of milk supply. ■ Encourage frequent, uninterrupted feedings. ■ Consult a lactation consultant as needed.
CRACKED NIPPLES	All causes of sore nipples carried to extreme	■ Refer to all actions for sore nipples. ■ Ensure infant is properly positioned. ■ Feed infant more frequently. ■ Avoid soaps, perfumes, or other cleaning products that can dry out nipples and predispose them to cracking. ■ Express milk post-feeding and rub into nipple allowing it to air dry. ■ Use emollients or lanolin as directed by physician/CNM/lactation consultant. ■ Consult doctor about using ibuprofen (Motrin), acetaminophen (Tylenol), or other painkiller. ■ Improve nutritional status, increasing protein, vitamin C, zinc.
	Local infection (baby with staph or other organism may have infected mother's nipples)	■ Refer to physician.
PLUGGED DUCTS	Poor positioning	■ Try a variety of positions for complete emptying. ■ Alternate positions so that different areas of the nipple have different compression pressure. ■ Avoid incomplete emptying of breast. ■ Breastfeed at least 10 minutes per side after let-down. ■ Alternate breastfeeding positions. ■ If baby does not empty breasts, pump or express milk after feedings.
	External pressure on breast	■ Use larger-size bra, insert bra extender, or go braless. ■ Wear a sports bra instead of a traditional bra. ■ Use nursing bra instead of pulling up conventional bra to breastfeed to avoid pressure on ducts. ■ Avoid bunching up sweater or nightgown under arm during breastfeeding.
SORE NIPPLES	Poor positioning	■ Alternate breastfeeding positions throughout the day. ■ Bring the baby close to feed so the baby does not pull on the breast. ■ Place the nipple and some of the areola in the baby's mouth. ■ Check to ensure the baby is put on and off the breast properly. ■ Check to ensure the nipple is back far enough in the baby's mouth. ■ Hold the baby closely during feeding so the nipple is not constantly being pulled. ■ Ensure that shoulder, hip, and knees are all properly aligned and facing the mother.
	Baby chewing or nuzzling onto nipple	■ Form the nipple for the baby. ■ Set up a pattern of getting the baby onto the breast using the rooting reflex.
	Baby sucking on end of nipple	■ Ensure the nipple is way back in the baby's mouth by getting the baby properly onto the breast. ■ Check for an inverted nipple. ■ Check for engorgement. ■ If baby is initially placed incorrectly on the end of the nipple, break the suction using a fish hook motion with your index finger and reposition baby on nipple properly. ■ Do not allow baby to nurse on end of nipple, reposition immediately.

(continued)

Table 30–6	Common Breastfeeding Problems and Remedies—continued	
Problem	Possible Cause	Remedies
	Baby chewing his or her way off the nipple (nipple being pulled out of baby's mouth at end of feeding)	■ Remove the baby from the breast by placing a finger between the baby's gums to ensure suction is broken. ■ End feeding when the baby's suckling slows, before he or she has a chance to chew on the nipple.
	Baby overly eager to nurse	■ Breastfeed more often. ■ Pre-express milk to hasten let-down, avoiding vigorous suckling.
	Dry colostrum or milk causing nipple to stick to bra or breast pads	■ Moisten bra or pads before taking off so as not to remove keratin. ■ Ensure that nipples are dry before replacing bra or clothing against nipples.
	Nipples not allowed to dry	■ Remove plastic liners from milk pads. ■ Air dry breast completely after nursing. ■ Change nursing pads frequently. ■ Switch to cotton nursing pads.
	Nipple skin not resistant to stress	■ Improve diet, especially adding fresh fruits and vegetables and vitamin supplements. ■ Eliminate or decrease use of sugary foods, alcohol, caffeine, cigarettes. ■ Check use of cleansing or drying agents.
	Natural oils removed or keratin layers broken down by drying agents (soap, alcohol, shampoo, deodorant)	■ Eliminate irritants. ■ Wash breasts with water only.

● **Figure 30–5** Mothers with sore nipples can leave bra flaps down after feedings to promote air drying and prevent chapping.

with skin respiration and may prolong soreness. Because of the risk of allergic reactions, Massé cream (risk of peanut allergy) is discouraged. In addition, products that are washed off before breastfeeding are avoided because of the irritation that washing produces. During bathing, mothers should be advised to only rinse their nipples with water and to avoid soap because this can dry the nipple out and lead to soreness.

Current research as to the effectiveness of nipple lubricants is inconclusive. Thus many lactation experts recommend that the mother's own milk be applied to the nipples and allowed to air dry. Breast milk is high in fat, fights infection, and will not irritate the nipples. Moreover, it is readily available at no cost to the mother. For some women with very dry or severely sore nipples, hypoallergenic medical-grade anhydrous lanolin cream or peppermint gel may help prevent or aid in healing cracked nipples. This product poses a low risk of allergy because the alcohols that contribute to the allergic response have been removed.

If the woman finds that her bra or clothing rubs against her nipples and adds to her discomfort, she may insert shells into her bra. Medela Shells relieve friction and promote air circulation. If a woman uses breast pads inside her bra to keep milk from leaking onto her clothes, she should change the pads frequently so the nipples remain dry. Some women may be sensitive to the plastic liner within the disposable pad, so the plastic can be removed or they can be encouraged to try cotton pads.

Complementary Care Remedies for Nipple Soreness

Older remedies for nipple soreness are receiving renewed acceptance. For instance, tea bags may be moistened in warm water and applied to the nipples. The tannic acid seems to help toughen the nipples, and the warmth is soothing and promotes healing. Tannic acid also has anti-inflammatory properties that can help relieve discomfort. Other therapies have included warm compresses and heat applications (Strong, 2011).

Clinical Tip

If the mother continually has soreness because of a delay in let-down, encourage her to massage the breast in a circular pattern and apply warm compresses just before each breastfeeding session. These activities encourage let-down, increasing the chance that it will occur at the same time that the infant is placed on the breast.

If nipple soreness persists, the woman should be advised to consult a certified lactation consultant to determine the etiology of the soreness. Nipple dermatitis, which causes swollen, reddened, burning nipples, is most commonly caused by thrush or by allergic response to breast cream preparations. If the nipple soreness has a sudden onset and is accompanied by burning or itching, shooting pains through the breast, and a deep pink coloration of the nipple, it may be caused by a thrush infection transmitted from the infant to the mother. White patches or streaks in the infant's mouth indicate a need for treatment of the mouth and nipple infection. The infection can be treated with a variety of antifungal preparations and does not preclude breastfeeding. It is important for both the mother and the infant to receive treatment to prevent cross-transfer of the fungus.

Cracked Nipples

When a breastfeeding mother complains of soreness, the nurse carefully examines the nipples for fissures or cracks and observes the mother during breastfeeding to see whether the infant is correctly positioned at the breast. If the positioning is correct and cracks exist, interventions are necessary. All the interventions described for sore nipples may be used. It may also help the mother to begin nursing on the breast that is less sore. This approach allows the let-down reflex to occur in the affected breast and permits the infant to do more vigorous sucking on the less tender breast, which decreases trauma to the cracked nipple. For the mother's comfort, analgesics may be taken approximately 1 hour before nursing.

Breast Engorgement

A distinction exists between breast fullness and engorgement. All lactating women experience a transitional fullness at first, initially caused by venous congestion and later caused by accumulating milk. However, this fullness generally lasts only 24 hours, the breasts remain soft enough for the newborn to suckle, and there is no pain. Engorged breasts are hard, painful, and warm and appear taut and shiny. The consistency is like gravel.

The infant should suckle for an average of 15 minutes per feeding and should feed at least 8 to 12 times in 24 hours (Riordan & Wambach, 2010). If the baby is unable to nurse more frequently, the mother may express some milk manually or with a pump, taking care to avoid traumatizing the breast tissue. As just noted, warm compresses before nursing stimulate let-down and soften the breast so that the infant can grasp the areola more easily. Cool compresses after nursing can help slow refilling of the breasts and provide comfort to the mother. Ice packs may also be used as a comfort measure. The mother should wear a well-fitted nursing bra 24 hours a day to support the breasts and prevent discomfort from tension.

Plugged Ducts

Some mothers experience plugging of one or more ducts, especially in conjunction with or following engorgement. When breast milk pools within a duct and then dries, it forms a white, hardened plug that is typically visible at the outlet of the duct at the nipple surface. Because milk accumulates behind a plugged duct, women also experience an area of fullness, tenderness, and/or lumpiness in the associated region of the breast.

Self-care measures include the use of heat and massage. The nurse can encourage the mother to massage her breasts from her chest wall forward to the nipple while standing in a warm shower or following the application of moist heat to the breast. Warm compresses can be used and changed as temperature requires. The mother should then nurse her infant starting on the unaffected breast if the plugged breast is tender. Some lactation consultants advocate starting on the affected side because the more vigorous sucking may help dislodge the plug. A breast pump may also be effective in unplugging the duct.

Prevention of plugged ducts involves frequent nursing and the use of a variety of positions to ensure complete emptying. Some mothers discover that pressure from a shoulder strap on a purse, their infant sling, or a car seat belt causes recurring plugged ducts in the compressed area. Repositioning the device may help prevent plugged ducts in these women. Prevention and prompt correction of plugged ducts is important because a plugged duct could lead to mastitis (inflammation of the breast) (mastitis is discussed in detail in Chapter 31 🔗).

Clinical Reasoning Difficulties with Breastfeeding

Ann Nyembe calls you from home in tears on her third postpartum day. She states breastfeeding was going well in the hospital but now her breasts are swollen, hard, and very painful, and her baby is refusing to suckle. Ann expresses some disappointment that "the breastfeeding didn't work" because she truly believes that breastfeeding is best for babies, and she enjoyed her breastfeeding experience in the hospital, especially breastfeeding the baby immediately after birth. But she also states she has been crying all day and can no longer tolerate her painful breasts. In addition, she says the baby "seems happier" with the bottle. What actions can the nurse recommend to Ann to increase the likelihood she will continue breastfeeding and to decrease her discomfort? ***See www.nursing.pearsonhighered.com for possible responses.***

Effects of Alcohol and Medications

Mothers may ask the home care nurse about the use of alcohol and medications when breastfeeding. According to the American College of Obstetricians and Gynecologists (ACOG) (2011), alcohol consumption among breastfeeding women should be limited to occasional use after breastfeeding is well established. Breastfeeding mothers should not consume alcohol for at least 3 to 4 hours before nursing (ACOG, 2011). Alcohol levels in breast milk parallel those found in the maternal plasma, peaking 30 to 60 minutes after consumption. Mothers who do occasionally drink while lactating should be advised to consume the alcohol after breastfeeding rather than shortly before a feeding in order to minimize the amount the infant receives. Alcohol consumption is associated with a reduction of milk consumption by the infant. Ongoing use is associated with alterations in infant growth, sleep pattern disturbances, and altered psychomotor behaviors (ACOG, 2011). Mothers with alcoholism who consume large quantities of alcohol daily should be advised not to breastfeed.

It has long been recognized that medications taken by the breastfeeding mother may penetrate breast milk to some degree. But we now have a better understanding of the kinetics of drug entry into breast milk, as well as factors influencing its bioavailability to the nursing infant. This is important, because use of medication has been identified as a barrier to breastfeeding and a major reason women cite for discontinuing it (Hale, 2010). Note that (1) most drugs pass into breast milk, (2) almost all medications appear in only small amounts in human milk (usually less than 1% of the maternal dosage), and (3) very few drugs are contraindicated for breastfeeding women (AAP Committee on Drugs, 2001; Briggs, Freeman, & Yaffe, 2012; Hale, 2010). The properties of a drug influence its passage into breast milk, as does the amount of the drug taken, the frequency and route of administration, and the timing of the dose in relationship to infant feeding. The drug's effects are influenced by the infant's age, the feeding frequency, the volume of milk taken, and the degree of absorption through the gastrointestinal tract. If the medication is not compatible with breastfeeding but is needed for only a short time, the mother can use a breast pump to maintain lactation and discard the milk.

SAFETY ALERT!
The mother should be advised to inform her healthcare provider and her infant's healthcare provider that she is breastfeeding when a drug is prescribed for her.

Breastfeeding and the Working Mother

The best preparation for maintaining lactation after returning to work is frequent, unlimited breastfeeding. Even when well planned, the first day back to work may be fraught with emotional and physical distress. Anticipatory guidance from the nurse may facilitate the transition from maternity leave to work. The earlier the breastfeeding mother returns to work, the more often she will need to pump her breasts to express the breast milk. Because milk production follows the principle of supply and demand, if breasts are not pumped, the milk supply will decrease. *Healthy People 2020* objectives (USDHHS, 2013) include increasing the number of employers that have worksite lactation support programs.

An electric breast pump and double collection system are considered the optimal means of milk expression. However, this is not the only method; mechanical means may not suit some women. Sometimes a mother has a flexible schedule and can return home or have the baby brought to her to nurse at lunch time. If this is not possible, the infant may be fed expressed milk via bottle or spoon. (For proper storage of breast milk, see *Bottle-Feeding Breast Milk* in Chapter 26 .) The mother should wait until lactation is well established before introducing the bottle. Most babies adjust to the bottle within 7 to 10 days.

To maintain a milk supply, the working mother must pay special attention to her fluid intake. She can ensure adequate intake by drinking extra fluid at each break and when possible during the day. It is also helpful to nurse more on weekends, nurse during the night, eat a nutritionally sound diet, and continue manual expression or pumping when not nursing.

Night nursing presents a dilemma: It may help a working mother maintain her milk supply, but it may also contribute to fatigue. Some women choose to have the infant sleep nearby so that breastfeeding is more easily accomplished; other women find it difficult to sleep soundly when the infant is close by. For the mother who works long hours or has a rigid work schedule, the best alternative may be to limit breastfeeding to morning and evening feedings, with supplemental feedings at other times. This choice allows her to maintain a close relationship with the infant and provides some of the unique benefits of breast milk.

Maternal Concerns About Breastfeeding

Table 30–7 summarizes concerns new mothers may have about breastfeeding and ways the nurse can respond.

Clinical Tip

Infants with special needs sometimes benefit from a longer duration of breastfeeding. Infants who are prone to allergies, gastrointestinal reflux, or impaired motility of the gastrointestinal tract may receive benefits from continued breastfeeding that their mothers may be unaware of. These women should be counseled to discuss weaning with their pediatricians or infant specialists before weaning because the benefits of breastfeeding may influence their choice of timing regarding weaning (see Chapter 33 for a discussion of weaning).

HOME CARE: THE NEWBORN

In the home, a newborn physical examination is performed as described in Chapter 25. The nurse also assesses and reinforces knowledge related to infant care as detailed in the following paragraphs.

Handling and Positioning

The nurse demonstrates methods of positioning and handling the newborn as needed. As the family members provide care, the nurse can instill confidence by giving them positive feedback. If a family member encounters problems, the nurse can suggest alternatives and serve as a role model.

When holding the newborn, one of the following positions can be used (Figure 30–6 ●). The *cradle hold* is frequently used

Table 30–7	Maternal Concerns About Breastfeeding
Concern	**Response**
Pain	Breastfeeding with proper technique should not hurt. Instruct the mother on proper technique and if she still has difficulty encourage her to seek assistance from a lactation specialist.
Leaking milk	Instruct the mother on how to apply gentle pressure directly over her nipple for a minute or so to gradually stop the leaking. The use of nursing pads (with instructions to change wet pads frequently), wearing printed tops that camouflage small leaks, and reassurance that the problem lessens with time may help alleviate this problem.
Embarrassment	An unfriendly social environment may make it difficult to breastfeed in public. Classes and support groups can teach the mother how to breastfeed discreetly while in public, such as draping a blanket or shawl over her chest to provide more coverage.
Father feels left out	Inform the parents that it is advisable for the father to wait to bottle-feed the baby with expressed breast milk until after breastfeeding is established. In the meantime, encourage the father to be supportive of the breastfeeding mother, to have a lot of skin-to-skin contact with his infant, and to share the responsibilities of all other aspects of infant care (bathing, dressing, diapering, burping, rocking, etc.).
Limited hormonal birth control options	Using birth control pills containing progesterone and estrogen can cause a decrease in milk volume and may affect the quality of breast milk. It is preferred that the mother who wants to use a hormonal birth control method consider using the progestin-only mini pill (i.e., Nicronor, Nor-QD, Aygestin, or Norlutate); receive Depo-Provera, a progestin-only injection administered every 90 days; or have a progestin-only implant. Although progestin-only hormonal birth control is compatible with lactation, it should not be started at the time of discharge. It is recommended that the mother wait 6 weeks before taking the hormonal medication to ensure a good milk supply. Mothers can be reassured that barrier methods of birth control and natural family planning do not interfere with lactation at all and are good options to consider as well.
Vaginal dryness	Give reassurance that this is only a temporary side effect of a low level of estrogen while lactating. A water-based lubricant such as K-Y jelly or Astroglide can be used during intercourse until the mother weans and estrogen levels increase again.

A   B   C

● **Figure 30–6** Various positions for holding an infant. *A,* Cradle hold. *B,* Upright position. *C,* Football hold.

during feeding. It provides a sense of warmth and closeness, permits eye contact, frees one of the adult's hands, and provides security because the cradling protects the newborn's body. Extra security is provided by gripping the baby's thigh with the hand while the arm supports the newborn's body. This grip is important to use when the infant is being carried. The *upright position* provides security and a sense of closeness and is ideal for burping the infant. One hand should support the neck and shoulders, while the other hand holds the buttocks or is placed between the newborn's legs. The newborn may also be held upright in a cloth sling carrier that gently holds the baby against the parent's chest and frees the hands for other tasks. The *football hold* frees one of the caregiver's hands and permits eye contact. This hold is ideal for shampooing, carrying, or breastfeeding. It frees the caregiver to talk on the telephone, answer the door, or do the myriad tasks that await attention at this busy time.

The infant's position should be changed periodically throughout the early months of life, because skull bones are soft, and permanently flattened areas may develop if the newborn consistently lies in one position. The awake newborn is frequently positioned on her or his side with the dependent arm forward to provide support and to prevent rolling. The side-lying position aids drainage of mucus and allows air to circulate around the cord. It is also comfortable for the newly circumcised male. After feeding, the newborn may be placed on the right side to aid digestion and to prevent aspiration of regurgitated feedings; this position also makes it easier to expel air bubbles from the stomach.

Although the side-lying position is appropriate when the infant is awake and under observation, infants should always sleep on their backs (Figure 30–7 ●). The American Academy of Pediatrics has recommended sleeping in nonprone positions since 1992 to reduce the risk of sudden infant death syndrome (SIDS). *Healthy People 2020* goals (USDHHS, 2013) are aimed at

● **Figure 30–7** Infants should be placed on their backs when sleeping.

> ### Health Promotion SIDS Prevention
>
> Newborns should be placed in the supine position during sleep to reduce the risk of SIDS (AAP, 2011).

increasing the number of infants who are placed on their backs for sleep. Since the initiation of the "Back to Sleep" campaign, there has been an increase in malformation of the skull caused by a decrease in tummy time. The syndrome is also known as *deformational plagiocephaly,* or positional plagiocephaly. These infants commonly have a flat spot on their skull, usually on the back or side, that is caused by continued placement in the same position. Infants who are not placed on their stomachs while awake at least three times daily are at risk for this skull malformation. Often these malformations will resolve on their own by 1 year of age, but sometimes infants need to wear a specially fitted helmet to correct the malformation (Flannery, Looman, & Kemper, 2012).

Prone positioning while awake, also known as **tummy time**, is important for all babies because it assists them with learning developmentally appropriate skills; builds muscle strength for their shoulders, neck, and back; and prevents deformational plagiocephaly (Flannery et al., 2012). Infants should be placed on their tummies only when they are under direct supervision of a parent or adult.

Bathing

An actual bath demonstration is the best way for the nurse to provide information about bathing to parents. Because excess bathing and the use of soap remove natural skin oils and dry out the newborn's sensitive skin, bathing should be done every other day or twice a week. Sponge baths are recommended for the first 2 weeks or until the umbilical cord completely falls off and the umbilicus has healed. Some agencies use a tub bath for the bath demonstration. See Skill 5–6, Initial Newborn Bath, in the *Clinical Skills Manual* SKILLS.

At home, bath supplies can be kept in a plastic bag or some type of container to eliminate the necessity of hunting for them each time. For the baby's tub, the family may want to use a plastic dishpan, a clean kitchen or bathroom sink, or a large bowl. If using a sink, care should be taken to keep the infant away from faucets via which accidental burns could occur. Expensive baby tubs are not necessary, but some prefer to purchase them.

Before starting, if no one else is at home, the parent may want to take the phone off the hook and put a sign on the door to prevent being disturbed. Having someone home during the first few baths will be helpful, because that person can get forgotten items, attend to interruptions, and provide moral support. The room should be warm and free of drafts.

Sponge Baths

After the supplies are gathered, the tub (or any of the containers mentioned) is filled with water that is warm to the touch. Even though the newborn will not be placed in the tub, the bath giver carefully tests the water temperature with an elbow or forearm. Families may also choose to purchase a thermometer to help them determine when the bath water is at approximately 37.8°C (100°F) and safe to use. An unperfumed, mild soap such as Castile or Neutrogena should be used and kept on a soap dish or paper towel, not added to the water. Before the bath, the newborn should be wrapped in a blanket, with a T-shirt and diaper on, to keep her or him warm and secure.

To start the bath, the adult wraps a washcloth once around the index finger and wets it with water. *Soap is not used on the face.* Each eye is gently wiped from inner to outer corner. This direction prevents the potential for clogging the tear duct at the inner corner, where the eye naturally drains. A different portion of the washcloth is used for each eye to prevent cross contamination. Cotton balls can also be used for this purpose, a new one for each eye. Some swelling and drainage may be present the first few days after birth because of eye prophylaxis.

The bath giver washes the ears next by wrapping the washcloth once around an index finger and gently cleaning the external ear and behind the ear. Cotton swabs are never used in the ear canal because it is possible to put the swab too far into the ear and damage the ear drum. In addition, the swab may push any discharge farther down into the ear canal. The caregiver then wipes the remainder of the baby's face. Many babies start to cry at this point. The face should be washed every day and the mouth and chin wiped off after each feeding.

The neck is washed carefully but thoroughly with the washcloth. Soap may now be used. Formula or breast milk and lint collect in the skin folds of the neck, so it may be helpful to sit the newborn up, supporting the neck and shoulders with one hand while washing the neck with the other hand.

Next the bath giver unwraps the blanket, removes the T-shirt, and wets the chest, back, and arms with the washcloth. The bath giver may then lather the hands with soap and wash the baby's chest, back, and arms. The umbilical cord should be kept clean and dry. Wetting the cord is avoided, if possible, because it delays drying. The proximity of the umbilical vessels makes the cord a possible entry area for infection. See Chapter 26 ❷ for care of the umbilical cord and signs and symptoms of problems. Soap is rinsed off with the wet washcloth, and the upper part of the body is dried with a towel or blanket. The newborn's upper body is then wrapped with a clean, dry blanket to prevent a chill.

The bath giver then unwraps the newborn's legs, wets them with the washcloth, and lathers, rinses, and dries them well. If the newborn has dry skin, a small amount of unscented lotion or ointment (petroleum jelly or A & D ointment) may be used. Ointments are thought to be better than lotions for dry, cracked feet and hands. Baby oil is not recommended, because it clogs skin pores. Powders are not currently recommended. Families should be warned that baby powder can cause serious respiratory problems if inhaled. If parents want to use powder, they should be advised to use one that is talc free. The powder should be shaken into the hand and then placed on the newborn rather than shaken directly onto the baby.

The genital area is cleansed with soap and water daily and with water after each wet or dirty diaper. Females are washed from the front of the genital area toward the anus to prevent fecal contamination of the urethra and thus the bladder. Newborn females often have a thick, white mucous discharge or a slight bloody discharge from the vaginal area. This discharge is normal for the first 1 to 2 weeks after birth and should be wiped off with a damp cloth during diaper changes. The labia should be wiped, but the inner labial folds should not be aggressively cleaned.

Parents of uncircumcised males should cleanse the penis daily. Even minimal retraction of the foreskin is not advised (see in-depth discussion of care of uncircumcised male babies in Chapter 26 ❷). Males who have been circumcised also need daily gentle cleansing. Squeeze warm water over the baby's penis, letting the warm water run over the circumcision site. The area is rinsed off with warm water and lightly patted dry. A small amount of petroleum jelly, A & D ointment, or bactericidal ointment may be put on the circumcised area until the healing is complete, but excessive amounts may block the meatus and should be avoided. It is important to avoid using ointments if a Plastibell is in place because use of ointments may cause the Plastibell ring to slip off the penis too early. The Plastibell usually falls off within 5 to 8 days.

It is important to cleanse the diaper area with each diaper change to prevent diaper rash. Although this cleansing is done on a routine basis, a diaper rash may occasionally occur. Baby powder or cornstarch is not recommended for diaper rash. Baby powder may cake with urine and irritate the perineal area; cornstarch may promote fungal infection. Ointments that provide a barrier, such as zinc oxide, A & D ointment, and petroleum jelly, are effective for diaper rash. If the ointment does not help the rash, families using single-use (disposable) diapers should try another brand. If they use cloth diapers, a different detergent or fabric softener, more thorough rinsing, and hanging them in the sun to dry may alleviate the problem. If the rash persists, parents should discuss the problem with their nurse practitioner or physician, because it may be caused by a fungal infection.

The last step in bathing is washing the hair (a step some suggest doing first). The newborn is swaddled in a dry blanket, leaving only the head exposed, and held in the football hold with the head tilted slightly downward to prevent water from running into the eyes. Water should be brought to the head by a cupped hand. The infant should never be placed under running water because extreme changes in temperature can lead to burns. The hair is moistened and lathered with a small amount of mild shampoo. A very soft brush may be used to massage the shampoo over the entire head, including the fontanelles. The hair is then rinsed and toweled dry. Oils or lotions are not used on the newborn's head unless there is evidence of cradle cap. Moistening the scaly area with lotion or mineral oil half an hour or more before shampooing softens the crusts or scales and makes it easier to remove them with a soft brush during the shampoo.

Tub Baths

The baby may be put in a small tub after the cord has fallen off and, for males, when the circumcision site is healed (approximately 2 weeks) (Figure 30–8 ●). Newborns usually enjoy a tub bath more than a sponge bath, although some cry during either type. Only 3 or 4 inches of water is needed in the tub. To prevent slipping, a washcloth is placed in the bottom of the tub or sink. Some parents choose to bring the newborn into the tub with them.

● **Figure 30–8** When bathing the newborn, the caregiver must support the head. Wet babies are very slippery.

The baby's face is washed in the same manner as for a sponge bath. The parent then places the newborn in the tub using the cradle hold and grasping the distal thigh. The neck is supported by the parent's elbow in the cradle position. An alternative hold is to support the newborn's head and neck with the forearm while grasping the distal shoulder and arm.

Because wet newborns are slippery, some parents pull a cotton sock (with holes cut out for the fingers) over the supporting arm to provide a "nonskid" surface. The newborn's body may be washed with a soapy washcloth or hand. To wash the back, the bath giver places his or her noncradling hand on the newborn's chest with the thumb under the newborn's arm closest to the adult. Gently tipping the newborn forward onto the supporting hand frees the cradling arm to wash the back. After the bath, the

newborn is lifted out of the tub in the cradle position, dried well, and wrapped in a dry blanket. The hair is then washed in the same way as for a sponge bath.

Nail Care

The nails of the newborn are seldom cut in the birthing center. During the first days of life, the nails may adhere to the skin of the fingers, and cutting is contraindicated. Within a week the nails separate from the skin and frequently break off. If the nails are long or if the newborn is scratching his or her face, the nails may be trimmed. Trimming is most easily done while the infant is asleep. Nails should be cut straight across using adult cuticle scissors or blunt-ended infant cuticle scissors. Infant nails may also be filed.

Dressing the Newborn

Newborns need to wear a T-shirt, diaper (diaper cover or plastic pants if using cloth diapers), and a sleeper. On a fairly cool day, they should be wrapped in a light blanket while being fed. Newborns should be covered with a blanket in air-conditioned buildings. The blanket should be unwrapped or removed when inside a warm building. At home, the amount of clothing the newborn wears is determined by the temperature. Families who maintain their home at 15.5°C to 18.3°C (60°F to 65°F) should dress the infant more warmly than those who maintain a temperature of 21.1°C to 23.9°C (70°F to 75°F).

Newborns should wear head coverings outdoors to protect their sensitive ears from drafts. A blanket can be wrapped around the baby, leaving one corner free to place over the head while outdoors or in crowds for added protection. The nurse must advise families about the ease with which a newborn's skin can burn when exposed to the sun. To prevent sunburn, the newborn should remain shaded, wear a light layer of clothing, and avoid being directly exposed to sun during peak hours between 10 a.m. and 4 p.m.

Diaper shapes vary and are subject to personal preference (Figure 30–9 ●). Prefolded and disposable diapers are usually

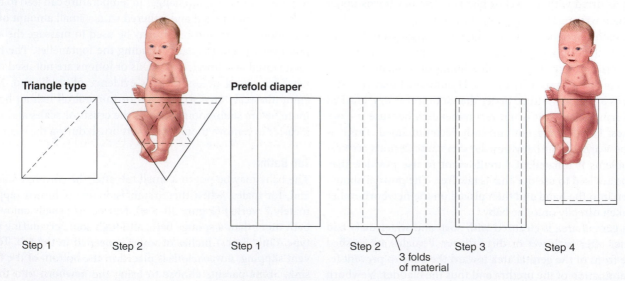

Triangle type   Step 1   Step 2   Prefold diaper   Step 1   Step 2   3 folds of material   Step 3   Step 4

● **Figure 30–9** Two basic cloth diaper shapes. Dotted lines indicate folds.

rectangular. Cloth diapers may also be triangular or kite folded. Extra material is placed in front for males and toward the back for females to increase absorbency. Cloth diapers, some of which now use Velcro and highly absorbent materials, have been used more frequently in recent years because of the environmental concerns related to disposable diapers.

Baby clothing should be laundered separately with a mild soap or detergent. Diapers may be presoaked before washing. All clothing should be rinsed twice to remove soap and residue and to decrease the possibility of rash. Some newborns may not tolerate clothing treated with fabric softeners added to the washer or dryer.

Temperature Assessment

As the nurse prepares to teach parents about taking their baby's temperature, it is important to provide opportunities for discussion and demonstration. Families often need a review of how to take the baby's temperature and when to call their primary healthcare provider.

The nurse discusses the different types of thermometers available for home use. It is important that parents understand the differences and how to select the appropriate one. Tympanic membrane (ear) thermometers use infrared temperature scanning techniques to determine the infant's temperature. Infrared forehead thermometers are also available, but these devices may be less accurate than internal monitoring techniques (Fadzil, Choon, & Arumugam, 2010). Other parents elect to use a digital thermometer. The nurse reviews the correct procedure for using the chosen thermometer.

Parents need to take the newborn's temperature only when signs of illness are present. They should call their pediatrician or pediatric nurse practitioner immediately if the temperature exceeds 38.4°C (101°F) rectally or 38°C (100.4°F) axillary. In premature infants, a low temperature may be a sign of infection; therefore, if the temperature is below 36.1°C (97°F) rectally or 36.6°C (97.8°F) axillary, the pediatrician should be notified.

Parents should discuss management of flu, colds, teething, constipation, diarrhea, gas discomfort, and other common ailments with their clinician before they occur. When analgesic or antipyretic medication is needed, clinicians frequently recommend acetaminophen or ibuprofen drops. Parents should not give any form of aspirin for an illness unless specifically directed to do so by their healthcare provider; use of aspirin in viral illnesses has been linked to Reye's syndrome in children.

 Clinical Tip

Healthcare facilities no longer use glass thermometers because of the risks associated with resulting mercury spillage should one break. Parents should be advised not to use mercury thermometers and should be encouraged to discard them at a hazardous materials site specific to mercury thermometers. Before teaching families about temperature taking, you might find it helpful to visit a local pharmacy and review the types of thermometers available, the costs of the most commonly used methods, and the instructions provided. This will enable you to answer questions accurately when you work with parents or caregivers.

Stools and Urine

The appearance and frequency of a newborn's stools can cause concern for parents. The nurse prepares them by discussing and showing pictures of meconium stools and transitional stools and by describing the difference between breast milk and formula stools. Although each baby develops his or her own stooling patterns, parents can expect the following (see Figure 26–23 on page 607):

- Breastfed newborns may have 6 to 10 small, semiliquid, yellow stools per day by the third or fourth day, when milk production is established, unless the mother is having problems with her milk supply. Once breastfeeding is well established, usually by 1 month, the newborn may have only one stool every few days because of the increased digestibility of breast milk. However, they may still have several daily. Constipation is unlikely to occur in newborns receiving only breast milk. Infrequent stooling in the first few weeks may indicate inadequate milk intake.

- Formula-fed babies may have only one or two stools a day; they are more formed and yellow or yellow-brown.

The parents may also be shown pictures of a constipated stool (small, pelletlike) and diarrhea (loose, green, or perhaps blood tinged). Families should understand that a green color is common in transitional stools, so that transitional stools are not confused with diarrhea during the first week of a newborn's life. Constipation may indicate that the newborn needs additional fluid intake. Parents may try offering additional water in an attempt to reverse the constipation. Parents should be counseled that each baby develops his or her own stooling pattern, and some babies may not pass a stool daily. As long as the infant appears comfortable and is not in distress, this can be normal for that infant and is not a cause for concern.

Babies normally void five to eight times per day. Fewer than six to eight wet diapers a day may indicate that the newborn needs more fluids. Frequency of voiding is easy to assess with cloth diapers. Parents who use superabsorbent single-use disposable diapers may have difficulty determining voiding patterns because the surface of the diaper feels dry. The liquid pools inside the filling of the diaper.

Sleep and Activity

The newborn demonstrates several different sleep–wake states after the initial periods of reactivity described in Chapter 24 . Six newborn sleep–wake states have been identified (see Table 30–8). It is not uncommon for a newborn to sleep almost continuously for the first 2 to 3 days following birth, awakening

 Clinical Tip

If parents using disposable diapers are unable to determine if the diaper is wet, advise them to tear off the top layer of the diaper and examine the cotton batting beneath the absorbent layer. It is easier for parents to see urine saturation and a change of color on this portion of the diaper in order to determine if the infant has voided.

| Table 30–8 | Infant Sleep and Awake States* | | |

Infant States	Physical Characteristics	Body Activity	Eye Movements
SLEEP STATES			
Quiet sleep (also known as deep sleep)	Anabolic, restorative sleep, increased cell mitosis and replication, lowered oxygen consumption, release of growth hormone.	Typically still, may occasionally startle or twitch.	None.
Active sleep (also known as light sleep or rapid eye movement [REM] state)	Processing and recording information. Often linked to learning. Is the highest proportion of sleep and precedes awakening.	Some body movements.	REM, closed eyelids may flutter.
AWAKE STATES			
Drowsy (also known as semi-dozing)	May return to sleep or awaken further.	Smooth movements with variable activity level. May experience mild startles intermittently.	Eyes may open and close. May appear heavy lidded, or eyes may appear like slits.
Quiet alert	Attentive to environment, focus attention on stimuli.	Minimal.	Eyes bright and wide.
Active alert	Infant's eyes are open, not as bright as in quiet alert. More body activity than in a quiet alert state.	Smooth movements may be interspersed with mild startles from time to time.	Eyes open with a gazed, dull appearance.
Crying	Communication tool, response to unpleasant stimuli from environment or internal stimuli. Characterized by intense crying for more than 15 seconds.	Increased motor activity, skin color changes to darkened appearance, red, or ruddy.	Eyes may be tightly closed or open.

Source: March of Dimes. (2003). *Understanding the behavior of term infants.* White Plains, NY: Author.

Note: *A state is a group of characteristic behaviors and physiologic changes that occur together in a regular pattern.

Facial Movements	Breathing Pattern	Responses	Caregiver Implications
None or may have occasional sucking movements.	Slow and regular.	Only intense or disturbing stimuli will arouse infant, threshold to stimuli is high.	Difficult to arouse for feedings. Teach parents to time feedings when infant is in a more responsive state. Infant may arouse slightly if an attempt is made to awaken but typically returns to the quiet sleep state.
May smile or make fussing or crying noises.	Irregular.	More responsive to internal stimuli (hunger) and external stimuli (such as being picked up by caregiver). When stimulated may arouse, return to quiet sleep, or remain in active sleep.	Inexperienced care providers may attempt to feed when infant makes normal crying sounds.
May have no facial movements and appear still, or may have some facial movements.	Irregular.	Usually reacts to stimuli but may be slowed. May change to other states such as quiet alert, active alert, or crying.	To stimulate infant, provide verbal, sight, or oral stimulation. If left alone, infant may return to a sleep state.
Attentive appearance.	Regular.	Most attentive, focus attention on stimuli.	In the first hours after birth, may experience intense alertness before going into a long sleeping period. This state increases in intensity as the infant becomes older. Providing stimuli will help maintain a quiet alert or active alert state. Infant provides pleasure and positive feedback to care providers. Good time to feed infant.
May be still with or without facial movements.	Irregular.	Reacts to stimuli with delayed responses to stimuli, or may change to quiet alert or crying state.	Infant may be fussy and become sensitive to stimuli, may become more and more active and start crying. If fatigue or caregiver interventions disturb this state, infant may return to a drowsy or sleep state.
Grimaces.	More irregular than in other states.	Very responsive to internal or external unpleasant stimuli.	Indicates that the infant's limits have been reached. May be able to console himself or herself and return to an alert or sleep state, or may need intervention from caregiver.

only for feedings every few hours. Indeed, it is not uncommon to have difficulty feeding the infant during the first 24 to 48 hours because of this deep sleep. Some newborns bypass this stage and require only 12 to 16 hours of sleep. The parents need to know that this pattern is normal.

Infants typically do not sleep through the night until they are at least 3 months of age or weigh 12 to 13 lb (5443 to 5897 g). Some infants sleep through the night as early as 8 weeks, whereas others do not sleep through the night until 6 months of age or beyond. It is estimated that two thirds of infants sleep through the night by the age of 6 months. Although newborns typically sleep up to 16 hours per day, they do so in short time intervals. Some parents may be tempted to try home remedies, such as giving infants cereal in their bottles or other additives that are said to assist their children in sleeping through the night. Parents should be counseled that these remedies are not recommended.

Crying

For the newborn, crying is the only means of expressing needs vocally. Families learn to distinguish different tones and qualities of the newborn's cry. The amount of crying is highly individual. Some cry as little as 15 to 30 minutes in 24 hours, and others cry as long as 2 hours every 24 hours. When crying continues after causes such as discomfort and hunger are eliminated, the newborn may be comforted by swaddling or by rocking and other reassuring activities. There is some indication that newborns who are held more tend to be calmer and cry less when not being held. Some parents are afraid that holding may "spoil" the newborn and need reassurance that this is not the case. Picking babies up when they cry teaches them that adults are responsive to them. This helps build a sense of trust in humankind. Excessive crying should be noted and assessed, taking other factors into consideration. After the first 2 or 3 days, newborns settle into individual patterns.

Coping with prolonged crying may be a challenge for new parents, who may respond by withdrawing their affection from the newborn, providing routine care and feeding, but not becoming emotionally attached. Other parents may respond by neglecting, abandoning, or even hitting or shaking their newborn. Parents need to understand the serious, even life-threatening consequences of such behavior. For example, a neglected or abandoned newborn can quickly become dehydrated, and hitting can cause internal hemorrhage, bruising, and fractures. Shaking can cause brain hemorrhage, spinal cord injury, retinal hemorrhage or detachment, long-term developmental problems, mental retardation, or even death. This collection of symptoms that are caused by vigorously shaking an infant is known as **shaken baby injuries** or *shaken baby syndrome* and is a form of abusive head trauma (AHT) and inflicted traumatic brain injury (ITBI). Shaken baby syndrome is also sometimes referred to as *intentional injuries*. (For more information on child abuse, see Chapters 43 and 55 .)

To increase parents' coping abilities, suggest that they initially respond to the baby's crying by checking for hunger, a wet or soiled diaper, excessive cold or heat, restrictive or chafing clothing or blankets, or other comfort concerns. If these are not present, suggest holding or rocking the infant as previously discussed. Other calming measures include burping the infant (which provides repetitive tactile stimulation and disperses air bubbles), placing the infant in a mechanized infant swing, or taking the infant for a ride in a stroller or car. Some infants are soothed by white noise such as the sound of a dryer or the static on an untuned radio, whereas others are soothed when bound "papoose style" on the mother's or father's chest, swaddled, bathed, or massaged.

Crying can also be associated with gastrointestinal upset in infants. The parents should discuss concerns with the physician or nurse practitioner to ensure the crying is not associated with a physical cause, such as acid reflux, ear infections, or other physical conditions. In addition, it is not uncommon for infants to cry after feedings because of pain from a buildup of air bubbles in the stomach and an inability to pass flatus. Some practitioners recommend simethicone after each feeding to decrease the incidence of flatus pain. Placing the infant in a prone position across the lap while burping the infant can also aid in passing flatus.

Safety Considerations

Newborns should not have pillows, blankets, bumper pads, or stuffed animals in the crib while they sleep; these items could cause suffocation. Mattresses should fit snugly in a crib to prevent entrapment and suffocation, and the crib should be inspected regularly to determine whether it is in safe working order. Crib slats should be no more than 2⅜ in. apart. Parents can be encouraged to attend infant cardiopulmonary resuscitation (CPR) classes, especially if there is a family history of SIDS or the infant requires special care.

Many families, especially breastfeeding families, practice **co-sleeping**, in which the infant sleeps with the mother or both parents during the night. The American Academy of Pediatrics does not recommend co-sleeping because it is considered a risk factor for SIDS. Some families and cultures, however, may still participate in this practice and thus warrant appropriate teaching measures.

Co-sleeping families should be counseled to follow these safety guidelines:

- Place the infant on a firm mattress, never on comforters, pillows, or a waterbed.

- Never sleep with your infant if you have been using drugs or have become intoxicated.

- Ensure that the infant is protected from rolling off the bed or becoming entrapped in bed rails or a space between the frame and the mattress.

Clinical Tip

Advise parents that if they become frustrated with a crying baby, they should put the baby in the crib or in a safe location and allow themselves time to calm down. Sometimes going outside the door, counting to 10, doing deep breathing, or calling a friend can help. Remind parents that crying never hurts a baby, but shaking can seriously injure the baby. Reassure parents that all new parents have times when they feel frustrated and do not know what to do. This is a normal part of parenting a newborn.

■ As with crib sleeping, remove all decorative pillows, stuffed animals, toys, or blankets that could impair the baby's breathing. Do not cover the baby with blankets, sheets, or down comforters.

■ Make sure the baby is sleeping on his or her back.

■ Ensure plenty of ventilation to the infant.

■ Avoid overdressing the infant because the parent's body heat will reduce the need for excess clothing.

■ Never smoke in bed with the infant. Family members should smoke outdoors and not in the household with the infant.

■ If additional children are sleeping in the bed, make sure they are not sleeping directly next to the infant.

Smoking poses multiple risks to the newborn and any older children living in the household. Infants living in a household with a smoker have a higher rate of hospital admissions during the first year of life. They are more prone to ear infections, asthma, allergies, and other respiratory problems (see Chapter 47 ⊘). The AAP (2011) recommends that the safest place for the infant to sleep is in the parents' room with the infant in a crib in proximity to the parents for the first 6 months of life. The use of pacifiers has also been associated with a reduction in SIDS deaths (AAP, 2011).

Smoking also creates a fire hazard within the household. Smoking is the primary cause of household fires in the United States. The incidence of such fires increases dramatically when other intoxicating agents are ingested, such as alcohol or drugs. Parents should be counseled to smoke outdoors; use large, heavy ashtrays to avoid tipping; ensure that all cigarette butts are properly extinguished; and never smoke in bed. *Healthy People 2020* goals (USDHHS, 2013) aim to reduce the number of women who start smoking again after giving birth.

POSTPARTUM CLASSES AND SUPPORT GROUPS

Services for families range from educational, such as classes on nutrition, exercise, infant care, and parenting, to specific healthcare programs, such as well-baby checks, immunization clinics, family-planning services, new mother support groups, and more.

Postpartum classes are becoming more common as caregivers recognize the continuing needs of the childbearing family. In many instances, classes are prepared to meet the specific needs of a variety of families so that, for example, single mothers and adolescent mothers can attend class with peers. A series of structured classes may focus on topics such as parenting, postpartum exercise, or nutrition, or there may be loosely structured group sessions that address mothers' concerns as they arise. Such classes offer chances for the new mother to socialize, share her concerns, and receive encouragement. Because baby-sitting arrangements may be difficult or expensive, it is desirable to provide child care for newborns and siblings; in some instances infants may remain with mothers during the class.

Many communities offer support groups through birthing centers, hospitals, or other facilities. La Leche League, an excellent support group for breastfeeding mothers, typically meets monthly and is open to all pregnant and breastfeeding mothers of infants and toddlers. The Women, Infants, and Children (WIC) Supplemental Nutrition Program may have a lactation consultant on staff or may have a contract with a lactation consultant in private practice in the community. Some military facilities provide lactation services to their service members and dependents. It is very helpful to have a handout listing available services.

Women who have children with special needs may need additional support. Referring them to peer counselors or support groups is an effective way to help them find both support and information.

Many parents today look to the Internet for information on parenting and newborn care. Nurses have an opportunity to assist parents in evaluating the reliability of the information they find. Criteria that suggest that Internet information is reliable and of high quality include affiliation with a university medical or nursing school or a government agency; inclusion of authors' credentials, education, board certification, and affiliations; referencing of information; currency of information; similarity of information when compared with other sources; and easy accessibility.

Critical Concept Review

LEARNING OUTCOME 30.1: Formulate nursing diagnoses and nursing care based on the findings of the normal postpartum assessment and teaching needs.

1. Nursing diagnoses focus on the normal and expected postpartum course.

2. Nursing diagnoses allow the nurse to identify expected outcomes and select nursing interventions that will help the family meet the expected outcomes and achieve optimal health promotion.

3. The nurse should discuss desired outcomes and goals with the mother and family members.

LEARNING OUTCOME 30.2: Describe appropriate nursing interventions to promote maternal comfort, rest, and well-being.

1. The nurse can promote and restore maternal physical well-being by monitoring uterine status, vital signs, cardiovascular status, elimination patterns, nutritional needs, sleep and rest, and support and educational needs.
2. The nurse should:
   - Encourage the new mother to rest when the infant rests.
   - Counsel the new mother to resume activities gradually.
   - Recommend exercise to provide health benefits to the new mother.
3. In addition, the postpartum woman may need medications to promote comfort, treat anemia, provide immunity to rubella, and prevent development of antigens (in the nonsensitized Rh-negative woman).

LEARNING OUTCOME 30.3: Explain factors that affect postpartum family wellness in the provision of nursing care and patient teaching.

1. Possible reactions of siblings.
2. Resumption of sexual activity:
   - Discuss possible temporary problems such as sleep deprivation, vaginal dryness, and lack of time together.
3. Contraception.
4. Parent–infant attachment:
   - Help parents realize there will be both positive and negative feelings about parenthood.
   - New parents need to understand that the infant is unique with a distinctive personality.

LEARNING OUTCOME 30.4: Compare the postpartum nursing needs of the woman who experienced a cesarean birth with the needs of a woman who gave birth vaginally.

1. A woman who has experienced a cesarean birth has all the needs of the woman who had a vaginal birth:
   - Assessment of the fundus.
   - Assessment of breasts.
   - Perineal evaluation (may have varicose veins or hemorrhoids from pregnancy).
   - Assessment of lochia flow.
   - Assessment of bowel and bladder.
2. After a cesarean birth the woman needs assessment of the abdomen:
   - Incision.
   - Turn, cough, and deep breathe.
   - Bowel sounds.
3. After a cesarean birth the mother will have a greater need for pain medication. She will also have increased fatigue because of the surgical intervention. The mother may need encouragement to interact with the infant.

LEARNING OUTCOME 30.5: Examine the nursing needs of the childbearing adolescent during the postpartum period.

1. The nurse should evaluate the adolescent mother in terms of her level of maturity, available support systems, cultural back ground, and existing knowledge, and then plan care accordingly.

LEARNING OUTCOME 30.6: Describe possible approaches to sensitive, holistic nursing care for the woman who relinquishes her newborn.

1. The mother who decides to relinquish her baby needs emotional support. She should be able to decide whether to see and hold her baby, and any special requests regarding the birth should be honored.

LEARNING OUTCOME 30.7: Explain the specific postpartum needs for women with obesity, developmental disabilities, or history of sexual abuse.

1. Women with obesity need special attention to prevent injury, respiratory complications, thromboembolic disease, and infection.
2. Women with developmental disabilities should be presented with educational materials that are in an easy-to-understand format. Teaching should be conducted at a level that is achievable for the individual.
3. Women with a history of sexual abuse tend to have more anxiety and stress related to hospital procedures, interactions with unfamiliar staff, and being touched in general. Treat the woman with respect by providing draping and speaking to her in private. Support groups may be helpful.

LEARNING OUTCOME 30.8: Identify postpartum teaching needs that should be modified to provide sensitive care to meet the needs of lesbian mothers.

1. Maintain an attitude that is respectful, caring, and open to sexual diversity; acknowledge, welcome, and involve her intimate partner in care and decision making.
2. Standardized postpartum instructions, particularly those related to intercourse and contraception, might need to be individualized and amended.

LEARNING OUTCOME 30.9: Identify teaching topics related to postpartum discharge.

1. Prior to discharge the couple should be given any information necessary for the woman to provide appropriate self-care.
2. Parents should have a beginning skill in caring for their newborn and should be familiar with warning signs of possible complications for mother or baby.
3. Printed information is valuable in helping couples deal with questions that may arise at home.
4. Available types of follow-up care and community resources (telephone calls, home visits, baby care/postpartum classes, new mother support groups).

LEARNING OUTCOME 30.10: Identify the main purposes and components of home visits during the postpartum period.

The main purposes of the home visit:
1. Assess the status of the mother and infant.
2. Assess adaptation and adjustment of the family to the new baby.
3. Determine current informational needs.
4. Provide teaching as needed.
5. Use as an opportunity to answer additional questions related to infant care and feeding, and to provide emotional support to the mother and family.

The components of the postpartum home visit include:

1. Establish contact with the mother prior to the visit.
2. Identify the purpose and goals of the visit.
3. Establish rapport with the mother.
4. Maintain safety during the visit.
5. Assess the status of the mother, newborn, and family.
6. Reinforce teaching concerning maternal and newborn care.

LEARNING OUTCOME 30.11: Summarize actions a nurse should take to ensure personal safety as well as fostering a caring relationship during a home visit.

Nurses need to act proactively to maintain their safety when making home visits by exercising reasonable caution and remaining alert to environmental cues.

Fostering a caring relationship in the home involves:

1. Evidence of genuineness and empathy.
2. Establishment of trust and rapport.
3. Positive regard for the mother and family.

LEARNING OUTCOME 30.12: Describe maternal and family assessment and anticipated progress after birth.

1. Expected maternal assessments:
   - Vital signs. (Should be at prepregnancy level.)
   - Weight. (Expect weight to be near prepregnancy level at 6 weeks postpartum.)
   - Condition of the breasts.
   - Condition of the abdomen, including a healing cesarean incision, if applicable.
   - Elimination pattern. (Should return to normal by 4 to 6 weeks postpartum.)
   - Lochia. (Should progress from lochia rubra to lochia serosa to lochia alba. If not breastfeeding, menstrual pattern should return at 6 weeks postpartum.)
   - Fundus. (Fundus should decrease in size one finger breadth per day after the birth of the baby. Uterus should return to normal size by 6 weeks postpartum.)
   - Perineum. (Episiotomy and lacerations should show signs of healing.)

2. Family assessment:
   - Bonding. (Appropriate demonstration of bonding should be apparent.)
   - Level of comfort. (Parents should display appropriate levels of comfort with the infant.)
   - Siblings are adjusting to new baby.
   - Parental role adjustment. (Parents should be working on division of labor, changes in financial status, communication changes, readjustment of sexual relations, and adjustment to new daily tasks.)
   - Contraception. (Parents understand need to choose and use a method of contraception.)

LEARNING OUTCOME 30.13: Delineate interventions to address the common concerns of breastfeeding mothers following discharge.

1. Common concerns of the breastfeeding mother include:
   - Nipple soreness.
   - Cracked nipples.
   - Engorgement.
   - Plugged ducts.

2. Breastfeeding mothers are encouraged to:
   - Nurse frequently.
   - Change the infant's position regularly.
   - Allow nipples to air dry after breastfeeding.

LEARNING OUTCOME 30.14: Describe the assessment and care of the newborn during postpartum home care.

1. Assess the infant's weight, length, heart rate, head circumference, and any signs of jaundice.
2. Watch the mother feed the baby and discuss any concerns she has about feeding.
3. Reinforce teaching in the following areas:
   - Positioning and handling.
   - Bathing.
   - Dressing.
   - Temperature assessment.
   - Stool and urine.
   - Sleep and activity.
   - Crying.
   - Safety considerations.
   - Newborn screening and necessary immunizations.

Clinical Reasoning in Action

Wendy Calahan, a 31-year-old G3P2, gave birth to an 8.5-pound baby boy by primary cesarean birth for failure to progress. The baby's Apgar scores were 9 and 9 at 1 and 5 minutes. The baby was admitted to the newborn nursery for transitional observation. Wendy was transferred to the postpartum unit, where you assume her care. You introduce yourself and orient her to the room, call bell, and safety measures. You perform an initial assessment, with all findings within normal limits. Wendy tells you she is very tired and would like to rest while her baby is in the nursery. Her husband and family have left the hospital after spending time with her in the recovery room but will return later. She admits she is disappointed that she could not give birth vaginally even though she pushed for 2 hours. She says, "This baby was just too big."

1. How would you discuss with Wendy the need for frequent assessments after birth?
2. Explain "maternity blues" or "baby blues."
3. Explore activities to minimize maternity blues.
4. Discuss concerns of a woman experiencing her second pregnancy.
5. Discuss behaviors that inhibit paternal attachment.
6. Develop a concept map for the mother with a medical diagnosis of postpartum depression, cesarean birth, or secondary macrosomia.

See www.nursing.pearsonhighered.com for possible responses and an interactive template for a concept map.

References

Advisory Committee on Immunization Practices (ACIP) Centers for Disease Control and Prevention. (2008). Prevention of pertussis, tetanus, and diphtheria among pregnant and postpartum women and their infants. Recommendations of the Advisory Committee on Immunization Practices (ACIP). *MMWR Recomm Rep* 2008 May 30; 57(RR-4), 1–51.

Aloi, J. A. (2009). Nursing the disenfranchised: Women who have relinquished an infant for adoption. *Journal of Psychiatric and Mental Health Nursing, 16,* 27–31.

American Academy of Pediatrics (AAP). (2011, October). *Policy statement: SIDS and other sleep-related infant deaths: Expansion of recommendations for a safe infant sleeping environment.* doi:10.1542/peds.2011-2284

American Academy of Pediatrics (AAP) Committee on Drugs. (2001). Transfer of drugs and other chemicals into human milk. *Pediatrics, 108*(3), 776–789. Retrieved from http://www.aap.org/healthtopics/breastfeeding.cfm

American Academy of Pediatrics (AAP) Committee on Fetus and Newborn. (2010). Hospital stay for healthy term newborns. *Pediatrics, 125*(2), 405–409. doi:10.1542/peds.2009-3119

American College of Obstetricians & Gynecologists (ACOG). (2011). At-risk drinking and alcohol dependence—Obstetric and gynecologic implications (ACOG Committee Opinion No. 496). Washington, DC: Author.

Arora, S., Vatsa, M., & Dadhwal, V. (2008). A comparison of cabbage leaves vs. hot and cold compresses in the treatment of breast engorgement. *Indian Journal of Community Medicine, 33*(3),160–162.

Association of Women's Health, Obstetric and Neonatal Nurses (AWHONN). (2010). *Assessment and care of the late preterm infant. Evidence-based clinical practice guideline.* Washington, DC: Author.

Barfield, W. D., & Lee, K. G. (2012). *Late preterm infants.* Retrieved from http://www.uptodate.com/contents/late-preterm-infants

Briggs, G. G., Freeman, R. K., & Yaffe, S. J. (2012). *Drugs in pregnancy and lactation: A reference guide to fetal and neonatal risk* (9th ed.). Baltimore, MD: Lippincott Williams & Wilkins.

Center for American Progress. (2010). *The adoption option.* Retrieved from http://www.americanprogress.org/issues/women/report/2010/10/18/8460/the-adoption-option

Chapman, D. J., & Pérez-Escamilla, R. (2012). Breastfeeding among minority women: Moving from risk factors to interventions. *Advances in Nutrition, 3*(1), 95–104.

Child Welfare Information Gateway. (2012). *Infant safe haven laws: Summary of state laws.* Retrieved from http://www.childwelfare.gov/systemwide/laws_policies/statutes/safehaven.cfm

Clare, C. A., & Yeh, J. (2012). Postpartum depression in special populations: A review. *Obstetrical & Gynecological Survey, 67*(5), 313–323.

Coles, M. S., Makino, K. K., & Stanwood, N. L. (2011). Contraceptive experiences among adolescents who experience unintended birth. *Contraception, 84*(6), 578–584.

Fadzil, F. M., Choon, D., & Arumugam, K. (2010). A comparative study on the accuracy of noninvasive thermometers. *Australian Family Physician, 39*(4), 237–239.

Fink, A. M. (2011). Early hospital discharge in maternal and newborn care. *Journal of Obstetric, Gynecologic, & Neonatal Nursing, 40*(2), 149–156. doi:10.1111/j.1552-6909.2011.01225.x

Flannery, A. B., Looman, W. S., & Kemper, K. (2012). Evidence-based care of the child with deformational plagiocephaly, Part II: Management. *Pediatric Health Care, 26*(5), 320–331.

Fowles, E. R., Cheng, H. R., & Mills, S. (2012). Postpartum health promotion interventions: A systematic review. *Nursing Research, 61*(4), 269–282. doi:10.1097/NNR.0b013e3182556d29

Geravi, J. (2009). Environmental and genetic influences on early attachment. *Child and Adolescent Psychiatry and Mental Health, 3,* 25. doi:10.1186/1753-2000-3-25

Glass, T., Tucker, K., Stewart, R., Baker, T., & Kauffman, R. (2010). Infant feeding and contraceptive practices among adolescents with a high teen pregnancy rate: A 3-year retrospective study. *Journal of Women's Health, 19*(9), 1659–1661.

Grassley, J. (2010). Adolescent mothers' breastfeeding social support needs. *Journal of Obstetric, Gynecologic & Neonatal Nursing, 39*(6), 713–722.

Hale, T. W. (2010). *Medications and mothers' milk* (14th ed.). Amarillo, TX: Pharmasoft.

Hunter, L., Rychnovsky, J., & Yount, S. (2009). A selective review of maternal sleep characteristics in the postpartum period. *Journal of Obstetric, Gynecologic, and Neonatal Nursing,* 38(1), 60–68.

Kronborg, H., Vaeth, M., & Kristensen, I. (2012). The effect of early postpartum home visits by health visitors: A natural experiment. *Public Health Nurse, 29*(4), 289–301.

Leeman, L. M., & Rogers, R. G. (2012). Sex after childbirth: Postpartum sexual function. *Obstetrics & Gynecology, 119*(3), 647–655. doi:10.1097/AOG.0b013e3182479611

Lowe, N. K. (2012). The persistent problem of postpartum hemorrhage. *Journal of Obstetric, Gynecologic, & Neonatal Nursing, 41*(4), 459–460. doi:10.1111/j.1552-6909.2012.01397.x

Lynn-McDonough, V. (2010). *A month of rest: Global practices of postpartum recuperation.* Retrieved from http://www.mypostpartumwellness.com/a-month-of-res

March of Dimes. (2003). *Understanding the behavior of term infants.* White Plains, NY: Author.

Mariano, E. R., & Ilfeld, B. M. (2011). Ultrasound-guided continuous peripheral nerve blocks. *Atlas of Ultrasound-Guided Procedures in Interventional Pain Management, 4,* 259–272. doi:10.1007/978-1-4419-1681-5_19

McPhaul, K., Lipscomb, J., & Johnson, J. (2010). Assessing risk for violence on home health visits. *Home Healthcare Nurse, 28*(5), 278–289.

Michigan Department of Community Health. (2012). *Infant mental health.* Retrieved from http://

www.michigan.gov/mdch/0,4612,7-132-2941_4868_7145-14659--,00.html

Nilsson, C., Lundgren, I., Karlström, A., & Hildingsson, I. (2012). Self reported fear of childbirth and its association with women's birth experience and mode of delivery: A longitudinal population-based study. *Women and Birth: Journal of the Australian College of Midwives, 25*(3), 114–121.

Palmer, C. M., D'Angelo, R., & Paech, M. J. (2011). *Obstetric anesthesia.* Oxford, UK: Oxford University Press.

Peterson, M. R. (2011). Review of interventions to relieve postpartum pain from perineal trauma. *American Journal of Maternal–Child Nursing, 36*(4), 241–245. doi:10.1097/NMC.0b013e3182182579

Riordan, J., & Wambach, K. (2010). *Breastfeeding and human lactation* (4th ed.). Boston, MA: Jones & Bartlett.

Spector, R. E. (2012). *Cultural diversity in health and illness* (8th ed.). Upper Saddle River, NJ: Prentice Hall Health.

Spidsberg, B. D., & Sørlie, V. (2012). An expression of love—Midwives' experiences in the encounter with lesbian women and their partners. *Journal of Advanced Nursing, 68*(4), 796–805. doi:10.1111/j.1365-2648.2011.05780.x

Strong, G. D. (2011). Provider management and support for breastfeeding pain. *Journal of Obstetric, Gynecologic, and Neonatal Nursing, 40*(6), 753–764.

Surkan, P. J., Gottlieb, B. R., McCormick, M. C., Hunt, A., & Peterson, K. E. (2012). Impact of a health promotion intervention on maternal depressive symptoms at 15 months postpartum. *Maternal and Child Health Journal, 16*(1),139–148.

Tschudin, S., Alder, J., Hendriksen, S., Bitzer, J., Popp, K. A., Zanetti, R., . . . Geissbühler, V. (2009). Previous birth experience and birth anxiety: Predictors of caesarean section on demand. *Journal of Psychosomatic Obstetrics and Gynaecology, 30*(3), 175–180. doi:10.1080/01674820902789233

U.S. Department of Health and Human Services (USDHHS). (2013). *Healthy People 2020: Topics and objectives.* Retrieved from http://www.healthypeople.gov/2020/topicsobjectives2020/default.aspx

U.S. Department of Labor. (2009). *Fact sheet: Newborn & mother's health protection act.* Retrieved from http://www.dol.gov/ebsa/newsroom/fsnmhafs.html

Wilson, B. A., Shannon, M. T., & Shields, K. M. (2013). *Nurse's drug guide 2013.* Upper Saddle River, NJ: Pearson Education.

Wong, W. Y. (2008). *Postpartum care in eastern cultures.* Retrieved from http://suite101.com/article/postpartum-care-in-eastern-cultures-a73434

World Health Organization (WHO). (2009). *Baby-friendly hospital initiative: Revised, updated and expanded for integrated care.* Retrieved from http://apps.who.int/iris/browse?type=mesh&authority=Rooming-in+Care

Zoumenou, E., Denakpo, J. L., Assouto, P., Tchaou, B., Lokossou, T., & Chobli, M. (2011). Early resumption of food intake after cesarean section in black African women: Liquid versus solid food. *Medecine Tropicale,71*(2), 165–168.

The Postpartum Family at Risk

We are surviving. Maybe just. I was told that babies ate at six-ten-two-six-ten-two, but no one said that he would eat at five-seven-nine-eleven or so it seems. I am either getting ready to feed him or just finished feeding and changing him. But I love him without bounds. I feel a need to protect him from ever being hurt or wounded. During that first week, when I was tired and recovering from the emergency cesarean, I was afraid that I would not be able to shelter and help this young son grow up. —Kate, 34

Ryan McVay/Getty Images

LEARNING OUTCOMES

31.1 Identify the causes, contributing factors, signs and symptoms, clinical therapy, and nursing interventions for early and late postpartum hemorrhage.

31.2 Explain the causes, contributing factors, signs and symptoms, clinical therapy, and nursing interventions for reproductive tract infection.

31.3 Develop a nursing care plan that reflects knowledge of etiology, pathophysiology, clinical therapy, and nursing and preventive management for the woman experiencing urinary tract infection, mastitis, or a postpartum psychiatric disorder.

31.4 Identify the causes, contributing factors, signs and symptoms, clinical therapy, and nursing interventions for postpartum thromboembolic disease.

31.5 Evaluate the woman's knowledge of healthcare promotion measures and signs of postpartum complications to be reported to the primary care provider.

The postpartum period is typically viewed as a smooth, uneventful transition time—and often it is, even with the challenges of new parenthood and the integration of a new person into the family. However, it is important for the nurse to be aware of physical or emotional complications that may develop postpartum. The nurse should teach the family the signs of postpartum complications, findings to report to the physician/certified nurse-midwife (CNM), and preventive measures, if available.

Written instructions to supplement any discussion will be of great value in the early weeks at home with a newborn when life can be chaotic and instructions may be forgotten. The family should be given telephone numbers for postpartum follow-up services and other resources that can respond to questions. By communicating an attitude of willingness to answer questions and listen to concerns, the nurse enhances the parents' comfort in making calls later for what they might otherwise perceive as issues "too trivial to bother someone about."

When a telephone follow-up or an examination during the home visit provides evidence of a developing complication, the nurse shares these findings or impressions with the woman, and they mutually plan an appropriate next step. In the case of telephone follow-up, the nurse usually counsels the woman about when to notify her physician/CNM and is prepared to schedule an appointment immediately if risk assessment indicates. The nurse who identifies a complication at the home visit will need to communicate the clinical findings to the physician/CNM and document them, as well as any interventions, for the permanent record. (See Chapter 30 🔗 for a more detailed discussion of home care for the postpartum family.)

Complications, by their very nature, suggest the need for immediate collaborative management and are inherently stressful. Postpartum complications sometimes necessitate readmission of the postpartum patient to the hospital, thereby disrupting the family and adding concerns not only about the mother's health but about how infant care will be managed. The most common complications of the postpartum period are hemorrhage, infection, thromboembolic disease, and postpartum psychiatric disorders. This chapter will focus on these issues.

CARE OF THE WOMAN WITH POSTPARTUM HEMORRHAGE

Hemorrhage in the postpartum period is described as either early (immediate or primary) or late (delayed or secondary). **Early (primary) postpartum hemorrhage** occurs in the first 24 hours after childbirth. **Late (secondary) postpartum hemorrhage** occurs from 24 hours to 6 weeks after birth. Postpartum hemorrhage continues to be a cause of significant maternal mortality and morbidity and accounts for approximately one sixth of all maternal deaths attributed to pregnancy-related hemorrhage in the United States (Brown & Smrtka, 2011; Poggi, 2013).

The traditional definition of postpartum hemorrhage has been a blood loss of greater than 500 mL following childbirth. That definition is currently being questioned, however, because careful quantification indicates that the average blood loss in a vaginal birth is actually greater than 500 mL, the average blood loss after a cesarean childbirth exceeds 1000 mL, and the average blood loss is more than 1500 mL during repeat cesarean birth (Harvey & Dildy, 2013). Clinical estimates of blood loss tend to underestimate actual loss by up to 50%. Clinical estimation of blood loss at childbirth is difficult because blood mixes with amniotic fluid and is obscured as it oozes onto sterile drapes or is sponged away. As the amount of blood loss increases, as in the case of hemorrhage, estimates are likely to be even less accurate than with normal childbirth. Moreover, postpartum hemorrhage may occur intra-abdominally, into the broad ligament, or into hematomas arising from genital tract trauma, wherein the blood loss is concealed. Given the increased blood volume of pregnancy, the clinical signs of hemorrhage—such as increasing pulse, decreased blood pressure, and decreasing urinary output—do not appear until as much as 1000 to 2000 mL has been lost, shortly before the woman becomes hemodynamically unstable (Gilbert, 2011).

SAFETY ALERT!
To meet the standard of care in cases of postpartum hemorrhage, rapid response systems are needed in every obstetric setting that enable nurses to respond quickly to implement certain actions independently based on evidence-based protocols, similar to a call for coding someone experiencing a cardiac arrest.

Early (Primary) Postpartum Hemorrhage

At term, blood volume and cardiac output have increased so that 20% of cardiac output, or 600 mL per minute, perfuses the pregnant uterus, supporting the developing fetus. When the placenta separates from the uterine wall, the many uterine vessels that have carried blood to and from the placenta are severed abruptly. The normal mechanism for hemostasis after delivery of the placenta is contraction of the interlacing uterine muscles to occlude the open sinuses that previously brought blood into the placenta. Absence of prompt and sustained uterine contractions (uterine atony) can result in significant blood loss. Other causes of postpartum hemorrhage include laceration of the genital tract; episiotomy; retained placental fragments; vulvar, vaginal, or subperitoneal hematomas; uterine inversion; uterine rupture; problems of placental implantation; and coagulation disorders.

Uterine Atony

Uterine atony (relaxation of the uterus) is a common cause of early postpartum hemorrhage. As many as 50% of cases of hemorrhage are due to atony. Although uterine atony can occur after any childbirth, its contributing factors include the following (Poggi, 2013):

- Overdistention of the uterus caused by multiple gestation, hydramnios, or a large infant (macrosomia)
- Dysfunctional or prolonged labor, which indicates that the uterus is contracting abnormally
- Oxytocin augmentation or induction of labor
- Grand multiparity, because stretched uterine musculature contracts less vigorously
- Use of anesthesia (especially halothane) or other drugs, such as magnesium sulfate, calcium channel blockers such as nifedipine, or tocolytics, any of which cause the uterus to relax
- Prolonged third stage of labor—more than 30 minutes
- Preeclampsia
- Asian or Hispanic heritage
- Operative birth (includes vacuum extraction or forceps-assisted births)
- Retained placental fragments
- Placenta previa

Hemorrhage from uterine atony may be slow and steady rather than sudden and massive. The blood may escape the vagina or collect in the uterus, where it is evident as large clots. The uterine cavity may distend with up to 1000 mL or more of blood,

although the perineal pad and linen protectors remain suspiciously dry. A treacherous feature of postpartum hemorrhage is that maternal vital signs may not change until significant blood loss has occurred because of the increased blood volume associated with pregnancy.

SAFETY ALERT!
It is critical to remember that a woman with no identifiable risk factors may hemorrhage after childbirth as well.

The woman and her partner may wish to have some private time engaging with the newborn when he or she is appropriately warm and ready for an early visit. But postpartum women must be assessed at frequent intervals, especially in the initial hours after delivery of the placenta when most deaths from hemorrhage occur.

Ideally, postpartum hemorrhage is prevented. Review of maternal records for risk factors will help nurses to plan assessment timelines to maximize early identification and management of excessive bleeding. Any woman at risk should be typed and cross-matched for blood and have intravenous (IV) lines in place with needles suitable for blood transfusion (18-gauge minimum). After expulsion of the placenta, the fundus is palpated to ensure that it is firmly contracted. If it is boggy (not firm), fundal massage is performed until the uterus contracts. Fundal massage is painful for the woman who has not received regional anesthesia; consequently, the nurse will need to explain why this procedure is necessary and give verbal support as massage is initiated.

Clinical Therapy.   If bleeding is excessive, the clinician will likely order IV oxytocin at a rapid infusion rate and may elect to do a bimanual massage (Figure 31–1*A* ●). Table 31–1 summarizes critical nursing information about the use of uterine stimulants. The need for IV fluid replacement and blood transfusion is determined on the basis of hemoglobin and hematocrit results as well as coagulation studies.

Conservative management includes uterine stimulants to contract the atonic musculature. Oxytocin, ergotamine, and prostaglandin are most often used. Misoprostol, best known to the obstetric community for its use in labor induction, is being used to prevent and treat uterine atony after failed attempts to control bleeding with oxytocics. Sublingual misoprostol (800 mcg) has been found to be as effective as oxytocin (40 units/L) (Poggi, 2013). When conservative measures do not successfully control bleeding, surgical intervention is required. In order of increasing invasiveness, surgical procedures include uterine balloon tamponade, selective radiographic-guided pelvic arterial embolization, uterine suturing techniques, ligation of the uterine or hypogastric arteries, and, as a last resort, hysterectomy, which clearly ends childbearing (Harvey & Dildy, 2013).

Lacerations of the Genital Tract

Early postpartum hemorrhage is associated with lacerations of the perineum, vagina, or cervix. Several factors predispose women to higher risk of reproductive tract lacerations:

- Nulliparity
- Epidural anesthesia
- Precipitous childbirth (less than 3 hours)

A

B

● **Figure 31–1** Manual compression of uterus and removal of placenta. *A,* Manual compression of the uterus and massage with the abdominal hand usually will effectively control hemorrhage from uterine atony. *B,* Manual removal of placenta. The fingers are alternately abducted, adducted, and advanced until the placenta is completely detached. Both procedures are performed only by the medical clinician.

- Forceps- or vacuum-assisted birth
- Macrosomia
- Use of oxytocin

Genital tract lacerations should be suspected when vaginal bleeding persists in the presence of a firmly contracted uterus. The nurse who suspects a laceration should notify the clinician so that the laceration can be immediately sutured to control the hemorrhage and restore the integrity of the reproductive tract. The woman may be moved to a delivery or surgical area for access to special lighting to facilitate treatment.

Table 31–1   Uterine Stimulants Used to Prevent and Manage Uterine Atony

Drug	Dosing Information	Contraindications	Expected Effects	Side Effects
Oxytocin (Pitocin, Syntocinon)	IV use: 10 to 40 units in 500 to 1000 mL crystalloid fluid at 50 milliunits/min administration rate. Onset: immediate. Duration: 1 hr. *IV bolus administration not recommended.* IM use: 10 units. Onset: 3 to 5 min. Duration: 2 to 3 hr.	None for use in postpartum hemorrhage. Avoid undiluted rapid IV infusion, which causes hypotension.	Rhythmic uterine contractions that help to prevent or reverse postpartum hemorrhage caused by uterine atony.	Uterine hyperstimulation, mild transient hypertension, water intoxication rare in postpartum use.
Methylergonovine maleate (Methergine)	IM use: 0.2 mg q2–4hr. Onset: 2 to 5 min. Duration: 3 hr (for 5 dose maximum). PO use: 0.2 mg q4hr (for 6 doses). Onset: 7 to 15 min. Duration: 3 hr (for 1 week). IV administration not recommended.	Women with labile or high blood pressure, known sensitivity to drug, or cardiac disease. Use with caution during lactation.	Sustained uterine contractions that help to prevent or reverse postpartum hemorrhage caused by uterine atony; management of postpartum subinvolution.	Hypertension, dizziness, headache, flushing/hot flashes, tinnitus, nausea and vomiting, palpitations, chest pain. Overdose or hypersensitivity is recognized by seizures; tingling and numbness of fingers and toes.
Ergonovine maleate (Ergotrate Maleate)	IM use: 0.2 mg q2–4hr. Onset: 7 min. Duration: 3 hr (5 dose maximum). PO use: 0.2 mg q6–12hr. Onset: 15 min. Duration: 3 hr (for 2–7 days). *IV administration not recommended.*	Women with labile or high blood pressure or known sensitivity to drug.	Sustained uterine contractions that help to prevent or reverse postpartum hemorrhage caused by uterine atony; management of postpartum subinvolution.	Hypertension, dizziness, headache, nausea and vomiting, chest pain. Hypersensitivity is noted by systemic vasoconstrictive effects: seizure, chest pain, general weakness, and tingling and numbness of fingers and toes that leads rarely to gangrene.
Prostaglandin (PGF₂, carboprost tromethamine [Hemabate], Prostin/15M)	IM use: 0.25 mg 15–90 min, repeated up to maximum 8 doses. Physician may elect to administer by direct intramyometrial injection.	Women with active cardiovascular, renal, liver disease, or asthma or with known hypersensitivity to drug.	Control of refractory cases of postpartum hemorrhage caused by uterine atony; generally used after failed attempts at control of hemorrhage with oxytocic agents.	Nausea, vomiting, diarrhea, headache, flushing, bradycardia, bronchospasm, wheezing, cough, chills, fever.
Misoprostol (Cytotec)	800–1000 mcg rectally.	History of allergies to prostaglandins.	Used to prevent and treat uterine atony after failed attempts to control bleeding with oxytocics.	Diarrhea, abdominal pain, headache.
Dinoprostone (Prostin E2)	Suppository (vaginally or rectally) 20 mcg every 2 hr. Store frozen—must be thawed to room temperature.	Avoid if woman is hypotensive, or has asthma or acute inflammatory disease.	Stimulate uterine contractions.	Fever is common and occurs within 15–45 min of insertion; bleeding, abdominal cramps, N/V.

IMPLICATIONS FOR NURSING MANAGEMENT OF THE POSTPARTUM WOMAN RECEIVING UTERINE STIMULANTS

- Assess fundus for evidence of contraction and amount of uterine bleeding at least q10–15 min × 1–2 hr after administration, then q30–60min until stable. *More frequent assessments are determined by the woman's condition or by orders of the physician/CNM.*
- Assess blood loss by hematocrit and hemoglobin levels.
- Monitor pulse and blood pressure q15min for at least 1 hr after administration, then q30–60min until stable.
  - Apply pulse oximeter and administer oxygen according to agency protocol.
  - Weigh peripads or chux dressing.
- Note expected duration of action of drug being administered, and take care to recheck fundus at that time.
- When the drug is ineffective, the fundus remains atonic (boggy or uncontracted), and bleeding continues. Massage the fundus. If massage fails to cause sustained contraction, notify the physician/CNM immediately.
- Monitor woman for signs of known side effects of the drug; report to physician/CNM if side effects occur.
  - Continuous EKG monitoring may be indicated for hypotension, continuous bleeding, tachycardia, or shock.
  - Elevate the legs to a 20- to 30-degree angle to increase venous return.
- Remind the woman and her support person that uterine cramping is an expected result of these drugs and that medication is available for discomfort. Administer analgesic medications as needed for pain relief. Provide nonpharmacologic comfort measures. If analgesic medication ordered is insufficient for pain relief, notify the physician/CNM. Provide information to patient and family regarding importance of not smoking during Methergine administration (nicotine from cigarettes leads to constricted vessels and may lead to hypertension) and signs of toxicity.

WHEN PROSTAGLANDIN IS USED

- Check temperature q1–2hr and/or after chill. Administer antipyretic medication as ordered for prostaglandin-induced fever.
- Auscultate breath sounds frequently for signs of adverse respiratory effects.
- Assess for nausea, vomiting, and diarrhea. Administer antiemetic and antidiarrheal medications as ordered. (In some settings, women are premedicated with these drugs.)

Episiotomy is an often underappreciated source of postpartum blood loss because of slow, steady bleeding, especially if it was done early in the birth process. The risk for bleeding is increased with mediolateral episiotomies. To fully assess the episiotomy site, the nurse must position the woman on her side. (See discussion of episiotomy in Chapter 23 🔗.)

Retained Placental Fragments

Retained placental fragments may be a cause of early postpartum hemorrhage and are also the most common cause of late hemorrhage. Retention of fragments is usually attributable to partial separation of the placenta during massage of the fundus before spontaneous placental separation. Therefore, this practice should be avoided.

SAFETY ALERT!

Postpartum nurses are wise to appreciate that most deaths from postpartum hemorrhage are not caused by catastrophic bleeding episodes but by ineffective management of slow, steady blood loss.

Following birth, the placenta should always be inspected for intactness and for evidence of missing fragments or cotyledons on the maternal side and for vessels that transverse to the edge of the placenta outward along the membranes of the fetal side, which may indicate succenturiate placenta and a retained lobe. Uterine exploration may be required to remove missing fragments (Figure 31–1B ●). This cause should be immediately suspected if bleeding persists and no lacerations are noted. Sonography may be used to diagnose retained placental fragments. Curettage, formerly standard treatment, is now thought by some to traumatize the implantation site, thereby increasing bleeding and the potential for uterine adhesions. However, it may be necessitated by the degree of hemorrhage (Poggi, 2013).

Vulvar, Vaginal, and Pelvic Hematomas

Hematomas occur as a result of injury to a blood vessel from birth trauma, often without noticeable trauma to the superficial tissue, or from inadequate hemostasis at the site of repair of an incision or laceration. The soft tissue in the area offers no resistance, and hematomas containing 250 to 500 mL of blood may develop rapidly. Signs and symptoms vary somewhat with the type of hematoma. Hematomas may be vulvar (involving branches of the pudendal artery), vaginal (especially in the area of the ischial spines), vulvovaginal, or subperitoneal. The latter are rare; however, they are the most dangerous because of the large amount of blood loss that can occur without clinical symptoms until the woman becomes hemodynamically unstable. Subperitoneal hematomas involve the uterine artery branches or vessels in the broad ligaments and require laparotomy for surgical correction.

Risk factors for hematomas include preeclampsia, use of pudendal anesthesia, first full-term birth, precipitous labor, prolonged second stage of labor, macrosomia, forceps- or vacuum-assisted births, and history of vulvar varicosities. Hematomas less than 3 cm in size and nonexpanding are managed expectantly with ice packs and analgesia. Small hematomas usually resolve over several days. For larger hematomas and those that

expand, surgical management is usually required; the hematoma is evacuated, the bleeding vessel ligated, and the wound closed, with or without vaginal packing. A temporary indwelling urinary catheter may be necessary because voiding may be impossible with packing in place.

The hematoma site is an ideal medium for the growth of flora normally present in the genital tract. Consequently, broad-spectrum antibiotics are usually ordered to prevent infection or abscess.

Uterine Inversion

Uterine inversion—a prolapse of the fundus to or through the cervix so that the uterus is, in effect, turned inside out after birth—is a rare but life-threatening cause of postpartum hemorrhage. Although not always preventable, uterine inversion is often associated with factors such as fundal implantation or abnormal adherence of the placenta, protracted labor, weakness of the uterine musculature, uterine relaxation secondary to anesthesia or drugs such as magnesium sulfate, and excess traction on the umbilical cord or vigorous manual removal of the placenta. Most cases of uterine inversion are managed by immediate repositioning of the uterus within the pelvis by the physician.

Late (Secondary) Postpartum Hemorrhage

Although early postpartum hemorrhage usually occurs within hours after birth, delayed hemorrhage generally occurs within 1 to 2 weeks after childbirth, most frequently as a result of **subinvolution** (failure to return to normal size) of the placental site or retention of placental fragments. Blood loss at this time may be excessive but rarely poses the same risk as that from immediate postpartum hemorrhage. Late postpartum hemorrhage is much less common but can be extremely stressful for the woman and her family who are at home by this time.

The site of placental implantation is always the last area of the uterus to regenerate after childbirth. In the case of subinvolution, adjacent endometrium and the decidua basalis fail to regenerate to cover the placental site. Deficiency of immunologic factors has been implicated as a cause. Faulty implantation in the less vascular lower uterine segment, retention of placental tissue, or infection may contribute to subinvolution. With subinvolution, the postpartum fundal height is greater than expected. In addition, lochia flow often fails to progress from rubra to serosa to alba normally. Lochia rubra that persists longer than 2 weeks postpartum is highly suggestive of subinvolution. Some women report scant brown lochia or irregular heavy bleeding. Leukorrhea, backache, and foul-smelling lochia may occur if infection is a cause. There may be a history of heavy early postpartum bleeding or difficulty with expulsion of the placenta. When portions of the placenta have been retained in the uterus, bleeding continues because normal uterine contractions that constrict the bleeding site are prohibited. Presence of placental tissue within the uterus can be confirmed by pelvic ultrasound.

Subinvolution is most commonly diagnosed during the routine postpartum examination at 4 to 6 weeks. The woman may relate a history of irregular or excessive bleeding or describe the symptoms listed previously. An enlarged, softer-than-normal uterus palpated bimanually is an objective indication of subinvolution. Treatment includes oral administration of methylergonovine maleate (Methergine) 0.2 mg every 4 hours for 24 to 48 hours (see Table 31–1). When uterine infection is present, antibiotics are also administered. The woman is reevaluated in 2 weeks.

NURSING MANAGEMENT *For the Woman at Risk for Postpartum Hemorrhage*

Nursing Assessment and Diagnosis

Careful and ongoing assessment of the woman during labor and birth and evaluation of her prenatal history will help identify factors that put her at risk for postpartum hemorrhage. Following birth, assess periodically for evidence of vaginal bleeding. Regularly and frequently assess fundal height and uterine tone or contractility; such assessments will alert you to the possible development or recurrence of hemorrhage. Monitor the bladder for evidence of increasing distention. Immediate intervention can sometimes help to prevent excessive bleeding that occurs when a full bladder displaces the uterus and interferes with contractility. This assessment can be done visually, by pad counts, or by weighing the perineal pads. In cases of excessive bleeding, be alert for signs of impending hypovolemic shock and the development of coagulation problems, such as disseminated intravascular coagulation (DIC) (see Chapter 16 for a discussion of DIC).

For all complaints of perineal pain, examine the perineal area for signs of hematomas: ecchymosis, edema, tenseness of tissue overlying the hematoma, a fluctuant mass bulging at the introitus, and extreme tenderness to palpation. Estimating the size on first assessment of the perineum will enable you to better identify increases in size and the potential blood loss. Notify the physician/CNM if a hematoma is suspected. Decrease the risk of vulvar or vaginal hematoma by applying an ice pack to the woman's perineum during the first hour after birth and intermittently thereafter for the next 8 to 12 hours. If a small hematoma develops despite preventive measures, a sitz bath after the first 12 hours will aid fluid absorption once bleeding has stopped and will promote comfort, as will the judicious use of analgesic agents. Close monitoring of the woman who has had excessive bleeding is important during sitz baths to ensure safety.

Nursing diagnoses that may apply to a woman experiencing postpartum hemorrhage include the following (NANDA-I © 2012):

- *Fluid Volume, Deficient,* related to blood loss secondary to uterine atony, lacerations, or retained placental fragments
- *Bleeding, Risk for,* related to lack of information about signs of delayed postpartum hemorrhage

Planning and Implementation

Hospital-Based Nursing Care

Upon detection of a soft, boggy uterus, massage it until firm. If the uterus is not contracting well and appears larger than anticipated, you may express clots during fundal massage. Once clots have been expressed, the uterus tends to contract more effectively. Overly aggressive massage should be avoided so as not to injure the vessels in the broad ligaments or cause reactive relaxation of the musculature.

If the woman seems to have a slow, steady, free flow of blood, do pad counts and if possible begin to weigh the perineal pads (1 mL = 1 g) (Harvey & Dildy, 2013). Monitor the woman's vital signs every 15 minutes, or more frequently if indicated. If the fundus is displaced upward or to one side because of a full bladder, encourage the woman to empty her bladder—or catheterize her if she is unable to void—to allow for efficient uterine contractions.

When there are risk factors for postpartum hemorrhage, or frequent fundal massage has been necessary to sustain uterine contractions, maintain any vascular access (IV) started during labor and anticipate the need for a second IV in case additional fluids, medications, or blood is necessary. Sometimes physicians/CNMs write orders that specify "discontinue IV after present bottle." It is nonetheless still important to assess the consistency of the fundus and the presence of normal versus excessive lochia before discontinuing the infusion. If the assessments are not reassuring, continue the intravenous (IV) infusion and notify the physician/CNM.

Review postpartum hemoglobin and hematocrit values when available, compare them to the admission baseline, and notify the physician/CNM if the hematocrit has decreased by 10 percentage points or more. In cases where there is risk of postpartum hemorrhage (e.g., women with prenatal anemia or labor and delivery complications) and blood has been cross-matched earlier, check that blood is available in the blood bank. Assess the woman for signs of anemia, such as fatigue, pallor, headache, thirst, and orthostatic changes in pulse or blood pressure, and review the results of all hematocrit determinations. All medical interventions, intravenous infusions, blood transfusions, oxygen therapy, and medications such as uterine stimulants should be monitored as necessary and evaluated for effectiveness. Also monitor urinary output to determine adequacy of fluid replacement and renal perfusion and report amounts less than 30 mL/hr to the physician/CNM (Gilbert, 2011).

SAFETY ALERT!

Good hand washing using standard precautions throughout the hospitalization and emphasizing proper hand washing for home care is important to minimize risk of postpartum infection.

Help the woman plan activities so that adequate rest is possible. The woman who is experiencing anemia and fatigue

Clinical Tip

Bogginess indicates that the uterus is not contracting well, which results in increased uterine bleeding. This blood may remain in the uterus and form clots or may result in increased flow. In assessing the amount of blood loss, first massage the uterus until it is firm and then express clots. Do not be misled by the fact that a woman has a firm uterus. Significant bleeding can occur from causes other than uterine atony. To accurately determine the amount of blood loss, it is not sufficient to assess only the peripads. You should also ask the woman to turn on her side so you can assess underneath her for pooling of blood.

related to hemorrhage may need assistance with self-care and progressive ambulation for several days. When she is able to be out of bed to shower, use of a shower chair permits independence while providing a measure of safety in case the woman experiences weakness or dizziness.

SAFETY ALERT!
The emergency call light should be easily accessible whenever nurses have left the bedside, even temporarily.

The mother may find it difficult to care for her baby because of the fatigue associated with blood loss. Try to find ways to promote maternal–infant attachment while accommodating the mother's health needs. The mother may require additional assistance in caring for her infant. If she has intravenous lines in place, even carrying the newborn may be awkward. For the mother who feels compelled to do as much as possible, you may also need to give the mother "permission" to return her infant to the nursery so she can have adequate periods of uninterrupted rest.

If the father of the child or the woman's partner is involved in the birth experience, including that person in the plan of care is a productive strategy. This person can support the mother's recovery by helping to meet her physical needs while encouraging her to rest. The mother is likely to feel less concern over her limited opportunities for the newborn's care if she can witness the father/partner interacting with and caring for the newborn. The extent to which the father/partner becomes involved with the care of the mother and baby must be carefully balanced with the need to be rested for the extra responsibilities the support person will assume when the mother and newborn child are discharged from the hospital.

Community-Based Nursing Care
For postpartum women, the usual discharge instructions include advice such as "You take care of your baby, and let someone else

Health Promotion Preventing Postpartum Bleeding

The woman and her family or other support persons should receive clear, preferably written, explanations of the normal postpartum course, including changes in the lochia and fundus and signs of abnormal bleeding. Instructions for the prevention of bleeding should include fundal massage, ways to assess the fundal height and consistency, and inspection of any episiotomy and lacerations, if present. The woman should receive instruction in perineal care (see discussion on perineal care in Chapter 30 🔗). The mother and her family are advised to contact her caregiver if any of the signs of postpartum hemorrhage occur (Table 31–2). If iron supplementation is ordered, instructions for proper dosage should be provided along with patient teaching to enhance absorption and avoid constipation and nausea.

Table 31–2	Signs of Postpartum Hemorrhage
Excessive or bright-red bleeding (saturation of more than one pad per hour)	
A boggy fundus that does not respond to massage	
Abnormal clots	
High temperature	
Any unusual pelvic discomfort or backache	
Persistent bleeding in the presence of a firmly contracted uterus	
Rise in the level of the fundus of the uterus	
Increased pulse or decreased BP	
Hematoma formation or bulging/shiny skin in the perineal area	
Decreased level of consciousness	

Clinical Reasoning Postpartum Hemorrhage

Betsy Lambert is a primigravida who had a spontaneous vaginal delivery at 0941 today. An overview of her history reveals the following: 23 years old, married, G1P0 on admission to Labor Unit. Pregnancy normal. Rh positive. No drug allergies. Labs on admission to L&D normal with exception of hemoglobin 11 grams and hematocrit 32%. Labor: 13 hours. Estimated blood loss: 450 mL. Delivered female (7 lb 7 oz) spontaneously after epidural anesthesia. APGAR 9/10. Newborn exam was within normal limits and routine newborn orders were implemented. Day shift reports firm fundus; voided 210 mL around 1100; vital signs stable. Baby visited and breastfed briefly with help from lactation nurse. Ate lunch and had Tylenol #3 at 1300 for perineal pain. Has been sleeping for long intervals.

You find Mrs. Lambert still dozing but awaken her for exam and note the following: BP 112/60, HR 116, R 20, T 100. Breasts—soft, nontender, wearing support bra. Uterus—fundus firm and 2 cm below umbilicus slightly left of midline. Bladder—possibly slightly distended but she feels no urge to void. Lochia—the two perineal pads and blue absorbent underpads are covered with bright red blood. Perineum—covered

with blood, as are thighs. Some of the blood has dried on the skin. Slight edema noted—midline episiotomy intact. Ice pack in place but ice melted. Homans' sign—negative. Emotional status—reports her husband went home to rest and will be back at dinnertime. Talks with excitement about first attempt to nurse baby. Asks for something cold to drink. The patient cannot remember when she was last checked for bleeding. You don gloves and wash her perineum gently and her thighs and change all her pads so you can better assess her degree of bleeding. An IV is in place with 10 units of Pitocin (100 mL is left in the IV bag).

You return, as promised, in 15 minutes to reevaluate her lochia and find that her perineal pads are again covered in blood. Based on your assessments and Mrs. Lambert's lab findings, what actions will you take first? If one of your anticipated actions is to inform the physician/CNM, what specific information will you report and what management should you anticipate initially? What follow-up care will you anticipate performing during the remainder of your shift?
See www.nursing.pearsonhighered.com for possible responses.

care for you, the family, and the household." Because of her fatigue and weakened condition, the woman who experiences postpartum hemorrhage may be unable even to care for her newborn unassisted. The caregivers at home need clear, concise explanations of her condition and needs for recovery. For example, they should understand the woman's need to rest and to be given extra time to rest after any necessary activity.

To ensure her safety, advise the woman to rise slowly to minimize the likelihood of orthostatic hypotension. Until she regains strength, she should be seated when holding the newborn.

The person who assumes responsibility for grocery shopping and meal preparation needs advice about the importance of including foods high in iron in the daily menus. Having the woman indicate her preferences from a list of such foods will promote cooperation with the diet. Also explain the rationale for continuing medications containing iron and remind the woman that vitamin C–containing fluids maximize absorption of iron, and tea or milk products prevent absorption (Gilbert, 2011).

The woman should continue to count perineal pads for several days so that she can recognize any recurring problems with excessive blood loss. The debilitated condition and anemia associated with hemorrhage increase the woman's risk of puerperal infection. She and her caregivers should use good hand washing technique and minimize exposure to infection in the home. Give the woman's caregiver a list of the signs of infection and ensure that she or he understands the importance of alerting the physician/CNM immediately if signs occur.

In addition to meeting the woman's physical needs, you will need to assess the couple's coping strategies and resources for dealing with the impending crisis. Providing realistic information, offering to call those in their support network, and exploring effective coping strategies can be of immeasurable value as the couple tries to maintain a sense of balance in this difficult situation. A sense of emergency often accompanies late postpartum hemorrhage. Because it commonly occurs 1 to 2 weeks after birth, the couple is generally at home, involved in the day-to-day activities demanded by their new roles, when the unexpected, excessive bleeding begins. Quick decisions about childcare arrangements must often be made so that the mother can return to the hospital. Both mother and father are likely to be alarmed by the excessive bleeding and concerned about her prognosis. There may be additional worries about separation from the newborn, especially when the mother is breastfeeding. The father may find himself torn between the needs of the mother and those of the newborn. Ideally, arrangements can be made to minimize separation of the family members.

Complementary Care Adjunct Therapy for Controlling Postpartum Bleeding

The Western herb shepherd's purse can be used in tea or tincture form to help control postpartum bleeding. Yarrow is often used with shepherd's purse as a homeostatic agent. Cinnamon and cayenne have also been used. Always report bleeding to a healthcare provider.

Evaluation

Expected outcomes of nursing care include the following:

- Signs of postpartum hemorrhage are detected quickly and managed effectively.
- Maternal–infant attachment is maintained successfully.
- The woman is able to identify abnormal changes that might occur following discharge and understands the importance of notifying her caregiver if they develop.

CARE OF THE WOMAN WITH A REPRODUCTIVE TRACT INFECTION OR WOUND INFECTION

Puerperal infection is an infection of the reproductive tract associated with childbirth that occurs any time up to 6 weeks postpartum. The most common postpartum infection is endometritis (metritis), which is infection limited to the uterine lining. Indeed, the cause of postpartum fever is presumed to be metritis until proven otherwise. However, infection can be spread by way of the lymphatic and circulatory systems to become a progressive disease resulting in parametrial cellulitis and peritonitis. The woman's prognosis is directly related to the stage of the disease at the time of diagnosis, the causative organism, and the state of her health and immune system.

The standard definition of **puerperal morbidity**, established by the Joint Committee on Maternal Welfare, is *a temperature of 38°C (100.4°F) or higher, with the temperature occurring on any 2 of the first 10 postpartum days, exclusive of the first 24 hours, and when taken by mouth by standard technique at least four times a day.* During today's short obstetric hospital stays, the temperature is measured every 6 hours in most settings, consistent with the definition for puerperal morbidity. However, serious infections can occur in the first 24 hours or may cause only persistent low-grade temperatures. Therefore, careful assessment of all postpartum women with elevated temperatures is essential.

The vagina and cervix of approximately 70% of all healthy pregnant women contain pathogenic bacteria that, alone or in combination, are sufficiently virulent to cause excessive infection. Although the uterus is considered a sterile cavity before rupture of the fetal membranes, bacterial contamination of amniotic fluid with membranes still intact at term is more common than previously believed and may contribute to premature labor. Following rupture of membranes and during labor, contamination of the uterine cavity by vaginal or cervical bacteria can easily occur. Other factors must also be present for infection to occur such as the change to an alkaline pH of the vagina postpartum that favors growth of aerobes. Uterine infections are relatively uncommon following uncomplicated vaginal births, but they continue to be a major source of morbidity for women who give birth by cesarean.

Routine antibiotic prophylaxis for cesarean childbirth in conjunction with aseptic technique, fewer traumatic operative births, a better understanding of labor dystocia, improved surgical intervention, and a population that is generally at less risk from malnutrition and chronic debilitative disease has contributed to a reduction in overall postpartum morbidity and mortality.

Postpartum Uterine Infection

Postpartum uterine infection is known variously as *metritis* and *endometritis*. Postpartum infection involves the decidual lining of the uterus, the myometrium, and parametrial tissue. Risk factors for postpartum uterine infection include the following:

- Cesarean deliveries prior to onset of labor—the single most significant risk (5% to 15% increased incidence) (Ambrose & Repke, 2011)
- Prolonged premature rupture of the amniotic membranes (PPROM)
- Prolonged labor preceding cesarean birth
- Multiple vaginal examinations during labor
- Compromised health status (low socioeconomic status, poor nutritional intake, anemia, obesity, smoking, and use of illicit drugs or alcohol)
- Use of fetal scalp electrode or intrauterine pressure catheter for internal monitoring during labor
- Obstetric trauma—episiotomy and lacerations of perineum, vagina, or cervix
- Chorioamnionitis
- Diabetes
- Preexisting bacterial vaginosis or *Chlamydia trachomatis* infection
- Instrument-assisted childbirth—vacuum or forceps
- Manual removal of the placenta
- Lapses in aseptic technique by surgical staff or prolonged duration of surgery

Endometritis (Metritis)

Endometritis (metritis), an inflammation of the endometrium portion of the uterine lining, may occur postpartum in 1% to 3% of women who give birth vaginally and ranges from 5% to 15% of those who give birth by cesarean (Ambrose & Repke, 2011).

Postpartum infection from vaginal delivery primarily affects the placental implantation site, decidua, and adjacent myometrium. Bacteria that colonize the cervix and vagina gain access to the amniotic fluid during labor and postpartum begin to invade devitalized tissue (the lower uterine segment, lacerations, and incisions). The same pathogenesis, polymicrobial proliferation and tissue invasion, is associated with cesarean delivery, but surgical trauma; additional devitalization of tissue, blood and serum accumulation; and foreign bodies (sutures, staples) provide additional favorable anaerobic bacterial conditions. For highly indigent populations, the risk remains high (Poggi, 2013). Both aerobic and anaerobic organisms cause endometritis, which is often polymicrobial. See Table 31–3 for a list of common causative organisms.

Clinical findings of metritis in the initial 24 to 36 hours postpartum tend to be related to Group B streptococcus (GBS).

Table 31–3	Common Causative Organisms in Metritis

Aerobes	Anaerobes
■ Group A, B, D streptococcus	■ *Peptostreptococcus*
■ *Enterococcus*	■ *Clostridium* species
■ *Staphylococcus* species	■ *Bacteroides* species
■ *Escherichia coli*	■ *Chlamydia* trachomatis
■ *Klebsiella pneumoniae*	■ Genital mycoplasma
■ *Proteus mirabilis*	
■ *Gardnerella vaginalis*	
■ *Neisseria gonorrhoeae*	

Source: Data from Duff, W. P., Sweet, R. L., & Edwards, R. K. (2009). Maternal and fetal infectious disorders. In R. K. Creasy & R. Resnik (Eds.), *Maternal–fetal medicine: Principles and practice* (6th ed., pp. 739–796). Philadelphia, PA: Saunders; Poggi, S. B. H. (2013). Postpartum hemorrhage & the abnormal puerperium. In A. H. DeCherney, L. Nathan, N. Laufer, & A. S. Roman (Eds.), *Current diagnosis & treatment: Obstetrics & gynecology* (11th ed., pp. 349–368). New York, NY: McGraw-Hill.

Late-onset postpartum metritis is most commonly associated with genital mycoplasmas and *Chlamydia trachomatis*. These microbes have a longer replication time and latency period than other bacteria and are not consistently eradicated by antibiotics used for early postpartum infections.

In mild cases of metritis, the woman generally has vaginal discharge that is bloody, foul smelling, and either scant or profuse. In more severe cases, she also has uterine tenderness; sawtooth temperature spikes, usually between 38.3°C (101°F) and 40°C (104°F) on two separate assessments at least 6 hours apart; tachycardia that parallels the temperature increase; and chills. Purulent and foul-smelling lochia is cited as a classic sign of endometritis (Ambrose & Repke, 2011).

Pelvic Cellulitis (Parametritis)

Pelvic cellulitis (parametritis) is infection involving the connective tissue of the broad ligament or, in more severe forms, the connective tissue of all the pelvic structures. The infection generally ascends upward in the pelvis by way of the lymphatics in the uterine wall, but may also occur if pathogenic organisms invade a cervical laceration that extends upward into the connective tissue of the broad ligament—a direct pathway into the pelvis. Infection involving the peritoneal cavity is **peritonitis**. A pelvic abscess is most commonly found as a palpable mass in the uterine ligaments, the cul-de-sac of Douglas, and the subdiaphragmatic space. Parametritis may be a secondary result of pelvic vein thrombophlebitis. This condition occurs when the clot, usually in the right ovarian vein, becomes infected and the wall of the vein breaks down from necrosis, spilling the infection into the connective tissues of the pelvis.

A woman suffering from parametritis may demonstrate a variety of symptoms, including marked high temperature (38.9°C to 40°C [102°F to 104°F]), chills, malaise, lethargy, abdominal pain, subinvolution of the uterus, tachycardia, and local and referred rebound tenderness (Poggi, 2013). If peritonitis develops, the woman becomes acutely ill, with severe pain, marked anxiety, high fever, rapid and shallow respirations, pronounced tachycardia, excessive thirst, abdominal distention, nausea, and vomiting.

Perineal Wound Infections

Given the degree of bacterial contamination that occurs with normal vaginal birth, it is surprising that more women do not have infections of the episiotomy or repaired lacerations of the perineum, vagina, or vulva. Good aseptic technique is the likely rationale. When perineal wound infection occurs, it is recognized by the classic signs: redness, warmth, edema, purulent drainage, and, later, gaping of the wound that had previously been well approximated. Local pain may be severe.

Cesarean Wound Infections

After cesarean delivery, wound infection is most often associated with concurrent endometritis. The wound is typically red, indurated, tender at the margins, and draining purulent exudate. Some women have cellulitis without actual purulent drainage. Clinical exam is usually sufficient for diagnosis but culture of the exudate should be routinely done since methicillin-resistant *Staphylococcus aureus* (MRSA) infections are possible (Thurman, 2010).

Clinical Therapy

The infection site and causative organism are diagnosed by careful history and complete physical examination, blood tests, aerobic and anaerobic endometrial cultures (although cultures may be of limited value because multiple organisms are usually present), and urinalysis to rule out urinary tract infection (UTI).

Localized wound infection is treated with broad-spectrum antibiotics, sitz baths, and analgesics as necessary for pain relief. Wounds with evidence of pus or serosanguineous effusion or an infected stitch site are opened and drained completely. Once the incision and drainage (I&D) of the wound is complete, it may be packed with saline-dampened gauze, repacked 2 to 3 times daily, and covered with clean gauze using aseptic technique. This allows removal of necrotic debris when packing is removed. When the infection is resolved and there is evidence of healthy granulation tissue, secondary closure is considered. Antibiotics with coverage against *Staphylococcus aureus* should be given. Nafcillin, 2 grams IV every 6 hours is a common choice. For allergy to β-lactam antibiotics, an appropriate alternative is vancomycin 1 gram IV every 12 hours. Antibiotics are typically continued until the wound base is clean and any signs of cellulitis have resolved.

The incidence of metritis has been reduced by prophylactic administration of antibiotics to women undergoing cesarean childbirth. Metritis, once diagnosed, is treated by the administration of parenteral broad-spectrum antibiotics. Common standard treatment regimens consist of clindamycin for gram-positive and anaerobic coverage in combination with an aminoglycoside, typically gentamicin once a day, and for gram-negative coverage ampicillin and sulbactam every 6 hours (Poggi, 2013). The route and dosage are determined by the severity of the infection. Careful monitoring is also necessary to prevent the development of a more serious infection. Parametritis and peritonitis are treated with aggressive IV therapy. Broad-spectrum antibiotics

effective against the most common causative organisms are chosen initially until the results of culture and sensitivity reports are available. If multiple organisms are present, the approach to antibiotic therapy is continued unless no improvement is observed; then the antibiotic is changed. With appropriate antibiotic coverage, improvement should occur within a few days. Antibiotics are generally continued until the woman is afebrile for 24 to 48 hours. Follow-up with oral antibiotics is not necessary (Poggi, 2013). Approximately 90% of women with postpartum infection respond quickly to antibiotic therapy and experience complete recovery and no long-term sequelae (Ambrose & Repke, 2011).

NURSING MANAGEMENT *For the Postpartum Woman with Puerperal Infection*

Nursing Assessment and Diagnosis

Inspect the woman's perineum every 8 to 12 hours for signs of early infection. The REEDA scale helps in remembering to consider *r*edness, *e*dema, *e*cchymosis, *d*ischarge, and *a*pproximation. Immediately report any degree of induration (hardening) to the clinician.

Note and report the presence of fever, malaise, abdominal pain, foul-smelling lochia, larger than expected uterus, tachycardia, and other signs of infection so that treatment can begin. The white blood cell (WBC) count, a usual objective measure of infection, cannot be used reliably because of the normal increase in WBCs during the postpartum period; a WBC count of 14,000 to 16,000 mm^3 is not an unusual finding. An increase in WBC level of more than 30% in a 6-hour period, however, is indicative of infection.

Nursing diagnoses that may apply to the woman with a puerperal infection include the following (NANDA-I © 2012):

- *Injury, Risk for,* related to the spread of infection
- *Pain* related to the presence of infection
- *Parenting, Risk for Impaired,* related to delayed parent–infant attachment secondary to malaise and other symptoms of infection

Planning and Implementation
Hospital-Based Nursing Care

Careful attention to standard precautions and aseptic techniques during labor, birth, and postpartum is essential. As the nurse caring for a woman during the postpartum period, you are responsible for teaching her self-care measures that are helpful in preventing infection. If the woman has a draining wound or purulent lochia, it is especially important that those in contact with soiled items and linens practice good hand hygiene. Provide clear, concise instructions about wound care and how to discard soiled dressings appropriately to safeguard the woman and her caregivers.

If the woman is seriously ill, ongoing assessment of urine-specific gravity, as well as intake and output, is necessary. It is also necessary to carefully administer antibiotics as ordered and regulate the intravenous fluid rate. Ongoing assessment of the woman's condition is vital to detect subtle changes in her health status. Address the woman's comfort needs related to hygiene, positioning, oral hygiene, and pain relief.

Promoting maternal–infant attachment can be difficult with the acutely ill woman. You can provide pictures of the infant and keep the mother informed of the infant's well-being. Mementos, such as a footprint, a note written by the father "from the baby," or a videotape of the baby can be comforting to the mother during their separation. If she feels up to it, the new mother will also benefit from brief visits with her newborn. The woman who wishes to breastfeed when her condition allows can maintain lactation by pumping her breasts regularly. Understanding that the opportunity to breastfeed is simply delayed, not eliminated, by the infectious process may improve the woman's morale. The partner of a seriously ill woman will be concerned about her condition and torn about spending time with her and with their newborn. Because maternal–infant bonding may be compromised, allow for privacy with limited interruptions to facilitate father–newborn bonding. See *Nursing Care Plan: The Woman with a Puerperal Perineal Wound Infection* for specific nursing care measures.

 ## Nursing Care Plan The Woman with a Puerperal Perineal Wound Infection

Intervention	Rationale	Expected Outcome

1. Nursing Diagnosis: *Infection, Risk for,* spread of related to traumatized tissues (NANDA-I © 2012)

NIC Priority Intervention: *Infection control:* Minimizing the acquisition and transmission of infectious agents		**NOC Suggested Outcome:** *Risk control:* Actions to eliminate or reduce actual, personal, and modifiable health threats

Goal: The patient will be free of complications associated with infection.

▪ Encourage patient, staff, and family members to adhere to a strict hand-washing policy.	▪ Hand washing kills bacteria and prevents cross-contamination.	▪ Patient will remain free of complications associated with infection as evidenced by practicing behaviors that prevent the spread of infection and promote timely wound healing.
▪ Review the patient's prenatal, intrapartum, and postpartum records for underlying problems that could contribute to poor wound healing or increase risk for spread of infection.	▪ Identifying underlying problems gives the caregiver an opportunity to initiate preventive measures that will promote healthy wound healing and stop the spread of infection.	
▪ Monitor blood pressure, pulse, respiration, and temperature.	▪ Obtain baseline data; signs and symptoms of septic shock produce a ↓ in blood pressure and an ↑ in respirations.	
▪ Instruct patient on proper perineal care, including wiping perineum front to back after voiding, perineal washes after voiding and defecating, and changing peripads frequently.	▪ Proper perineal care techniques enhance good hygiene and assist in removing urine and fecal contaminants from perineum. Changing peripads frequently decreases skin contact with a moist medium that favors bacteria growth.	
▪ Encourage patient to consume 2000 mL of fluid a day.	▪ Maintains hydration and increases circulating volume.	
▪ Encourage use of the sitz bath, surgigator, or the perineal light 2 to 4 times a day for at least 10–15 minutes.	▪ Moist or dry heat to the perineum increases blood flow and promotes healing.	
▪ Encourage early ambulation.	▪ Enhances circulation and drainage of lochia.	
▪ Assess and report signs and symptoms of infection in perineum, including erythema, edema, discharge, approximation of wound edges (REEDA), and pain.	▪ Identifying signs and symptoms of infection early allows for prompt treatment and healing.	
▪ Collaborative: Obtain lab work as ordered by physician, including culture and sensitivity, CBC with differential, and WBC count.	▪ Identifies abnormal lab values for early intervention. In addition, identifies infection and its causative organism for appropriate antibiotic treatment.	

Nursing Care Plan   The Woman with a Puerperal Perineal Wound Infection—continued

Intervention	Rationale	Expected Outcome
■ Administer antibiotic therapy as ordered by the physician.	■ Fights present infection and helps prevent the spread of further infection.	
■ Promote wound drainage by assisting physician in opening wound if necessary. If wound is greater than 2–3 cm, pack with iodoform gauze.	■ Iodoform gauze is used to maintain patency of wound opening. This promotes drainage and prevents abscesses from developing.	
■ Report signs and symptoms of severe infections: foul-smelling lochia, uterine subinvolution, uterine tenderness, severe lower abdominal pain, elevated temperature, elevated WBC count, general malaise, chills, lethargy, tachycardia, nausea and vomiting, and abdominal rigidity.	■ Reporting signs and symptoms of severe infections early allows for initiation of appropriate therapy by physician and prevents further spread of the invading pathogen.	

2. Nursing Diagnosis: *Pain* related to the infection process (NANDA-I © 2012)

NIC Priority Intervention:
Pain management: Alleviation of pain or a reduction in pain to a level of comfort that is acceptable to the patient

NOC Suggested Outcome:
Pain level: Amount of reported or demonstrated pain

Goal: The patient will be free of pain.

■ Assess pain location and intensity, have patient describe on a scale from 1 (mild) to 10 (severe). Assess nonverbal signs of pain, including facial grimacing and agitation.	■ Assesses the need for pain management and evaluates interventions already implemented.	■ Patient will be free of pain as evidenced by verbalization of pain relief and the exhibition of a relaxed demeanor.
■ Encourage patient to discuss anxiety and fears.	■ Reduces anxiety and fear and may decrease the patient's perception of pain.	
■ Encourage frequent rest periods and decrease disturbing environmental stimuli.	■ Uses frequent rest periods to conserve patient's energy. Increasing environmental stimuli may increase patient's pain perception.	
■ Encourage use of exercises and diversional activities, including radio/television, reading, guided imagery, deep breathing techniques, massage, visualization, and meditation.	■ Promotes relaxation and refocuses patient's attention away from the intensity of pain.	
■ Collaborative: Administer analgesics as ordered by the physician.	■ Relieves pain and reduces anxiety.	

3. Nursing Diagnosis: *Attachment, Risk for Impaired (Parent–Infant),* related to pain secondary to maternal infection (NANDA-I © 2012)

NIC Priority Intervention:
Attachment promotion: Facilitation of the development of the parent–infant relationship

NOC Suggested Outcome:
Parent–infant attachment: Behaviors that demonstrate an enduring affectionate bond between a parent and infant

Goal: Mother will have no problems bonding with infant and assuming responsibility for the care of the infant.

■ Provide quality time for mother and infant contact.	■ Aids in the bonding process.	■ Mother will bond with infant as evidenced by exhibiting appropriate attachment behaviors when interacting with infant, providing care to self and infant, and verbalization of understanding of the parenting role.

(continued)

Nursing Care Plan   The Woman with a Puerperal Perineal Wound Infection—continued

Intervention	Rationale	Expected Outcome
■ Encourage partner or family members to give patient videos and pictures of the infant if the mother's condition requires separation from the infant.	■ Promotes bonding and gives the mother reassurance that the infant is being cared for.	
■ Encourage partner and family members to become involved with the care of the infant and verbalize interaction to the mother.	■ Allows mother to feel as though she is involved in the care of the infant.	
■ Encourage mother to feed (breast or bottle) infant if her condition is stable. If mother is unable to breastfeed, encourage and assist her in pumping her breasts to maintain milk production.	■ Gives mother a positive outlook through hands-on participation in the infant's care.	
■ Assess maternal support systems.	■ As mother is recovering, she will need assistance in household organization and personal care.	
■ Collaborative: Offer referrals to home health services, doula services, and support groups.	■ Ensures patient's well-being, and identifies problems that may require intervention.	

Community-Based Nursing Care

The woman with a puerperal infection needs assistance when she is discharged from the hospital. If the family cannot provide this home assistance, a referral to home care services is needed. Home care services should be contacted as soon as puerperal infection is diagnosed so that a nurse can meet with the woman for a family and home assessment and development of a home care plan.

The family needs instruction in the care of a newborn, including feeding, bathing, cord care, immunizations, and significant observations that should be reported (see Chapter 30 🔗). A well-baby appointment should be scheduled. The woman who wishes to breastfeed when her condition allows can maintain lactation by pumping her breasts regularly. Breastfeeding mothers receiving antibiotics should be instructed to inspect the infant's mouth for signs of thrush and to report the finding to their physician.

The mother should be instructed regarding activity, rest, medications, diet, and signs and symptoms of complications. She should also be scheduled for a return medical visit. She needs to know the importance of taking the entire course of prescribed antibiotics even though she may begin to feel better before the bottle is empty. She also needs to be informed about the importance of pelvic rest; that is, she should not use tampons or douches nor have intercourse until she has been examined by the physician/CNM and told it is safe to resume those activities.

Evaluation

Expected outcomes of nursing care include the following:

■ The infection is quickly identified and treated successfully, without further complications.

■ The woman understands the infection and the purpose of therapy; she cooperates with ongoing antibiotic therapy after discharge.

■ Maternal–infant attachment is maintained.

CARE OF THE WOMAN WITH A URINARY TRACT INFECTION

The postpartum woman is at increased risk of developing a urinary tract infection (UTI) caused by the normal postpartum diuresis, increased bladder capacity, decreased bladder sensitivity from stretching or trauma, and possible inhibited neural control of the bladder following the use of general or regional anesthesia and contamination from catheterization. The number of catheterizations performed during labor has increased. It is essential that the mother empty the bladder completely with each voiding.

Overdistention of the Bladder

Overdistention occurs postpartum when the woman is unable to empty her bladder, usually because of trauma or the effects of anesthesia. Women who have not sufficiently recovered from the effects of anesthesia cannot void spontaneously, and catheterization is necessary. After the effects of regional anesthesia have worn off, if the woman cannot void, postpartum urinary retention is highly indicative of UTI. Other risk factors for urinary retention after childbirth include nulliparity, instrumental childbirth, and prolonged labor (Pessel & Tsai, 2013).

Clinical Therapy

Overdistention in the early postpartum period is often managed by draining the bladder with a straight catheter as a one-time measure. If the overdistention recurs or is diagnosed later in the postpartum period, an indwelling catheter is generally ordered for 24 hours. An alternative urinary retention protocol involves bladder ultrasound scans with intervention based on the amount of urine volume.

NURSING MANAGEMENT *For the Postpartum Woman with a Urinary Tract Infection*

Nursing Assessment and Diagnosis

The overdistended bladder appears as a large mass, reaching sometimes to the umbilicus and displacing the uterine fundus upward. Increased vaginal bleeding occurs, the fundus is boggy, and the woman may complain of cramping as the uterus attempts to contract. Some women also experience backache and restlessness.

Nursing diagnoses that may apply when a woman has difficulties with overdistention of the bladder include the following (NANDA-I © 2012):

- *Infection, Risk for,* related to urinary stasis secondary to overdistention
- *Urinary Retention* related to decreased bladder sensitivity and normal postpartum diuresis

Planning and Implementation

Diligent monitoring of the bladder during the recovery period and preventive health measures greatly reduce the chances for overdistention of the bladder. Encourage the mother to void spontaneously and help her use the toilet, if possible, or the bedpan, if she has received conductive anesthesia. This will help prevent overdistention in most cases. Help the woman to a normal position for voiding (i.e., sitting with the legs and feet lower than the trunk) and provide privacy to encourage voiding. The woman should receive medication for whatever pain she may be having before she attempts to void, because pain may cause a reflex spasm of the urethra. Applying perineal ice packs after childbirth helps minimize edema, which may interfere with voiding. Pouring warm water over the perineum or having the woman void in the sitz bath may also be effective. Some women note that hearing running water nearby, blowing bubbles through a straw into a glass of water, or voiding onto a bedpan into which a few drops of tincture of peppermint have been added helps stimulate voiding.

If catheterization becomes necessary, careful, meticulous aseptic technique is employed during catheter insertion. The vagina and vulva are traumatized to some degree by vaginal birth, and edema is common. This edema may obscure the urinary meatus; therefore, be extremely careful when cleansing the vulva and inserting the catheter. It is imperative to discard a catheter that has inadvertently been introduced into the vagina and thus contaminated. Catheterization is an uncomfortable procedure because of the postpartum trauma and edema of the tissue, so be careful and gentle not only when inserting the catheter but also when handling and cleaning the perineal area.

If the amount of urine drained from the bladder reaches 900 to 1000 mL, the catheter is clamped and taped firmly to the woman's leg. Take the woman's vital signs before and after the procedure and note the woman's responses. After an hour, the catheter may be unclamped and placed on gravity drainage. This technique protects the bladder and prevents rapid intra-abdominal decompression. When the indwelling catheter is removed, a urine specimen is often sent to the laboratory. The tip of the catheter is also removed and may be sent for culture.

Evaluation

Expected outcomes of nursing care include the following:

- The woman voids adequately to meet the demands of the increased fluid shifts during the postpartum period.
- The woman does not develop infection caused by stasis of urine.
- The woman actively incorporates self-care measures to decrease bladder overdistention.

Cystitis (Lower Urinary Tract Infection)

Retention of residual urine, bacteria introduced at the time of catheterization, and a bladder traumatized by birth combine to provide an excellent environment for the development of cystitis. *Escherichia coli* has been demonstrated to be the causative agent in most cases of postpartum cystitis and pyelonephritis (in both lower and upper UTI). *Klebsiella pneumoniae* and *Proteus* species are significant pathogens, especially in women with histories of recurrent UTIs (Poggi, 2013). Generally, the infection ascends the urinary tract from the urethra to the bladder and then to the kidneys because vesicoureteral reflux (backward flow of urine) forces contaminated urine into the renal pelvis.

Clinical Therapy

When cystitis is suspected, a clean-catch midstream urine sample is obtained for microscopic examination, culture, and sensitivity tests. The specimen may require collection by the nurse with the woman on a bedpan because few postpartum women can collect a true midstream, clean-catch specimen without contaminating the specimen with lochia. A catheterized specimen is avoided when possible because of the increased risk of infection. When the bacterial concentration is greater than 100,000 colonies of the same organism per milliliter of fresh urine, infection is generally present. Counts between 10,000 and 100,000 suggest infection, particularly if clinical symptoms are noted.

In the clinical setting, antibiotic therapy is often initiated before culture and sensitivity reports are available. Frequently used antibiotics include a preparation of trimethoprim-sulfamethoxazole double strength (Bactrim DS, Septra DS), one

Clinical Tip

Postpartum urinary retention is often defined as "the absence of spontaneous urination within 6 hours of a vaginal delivery or within 6 hours after removal of an indwelling catheter post–cesarean delivery." The astute nurse will watch the woman's bladder—not the clock!—for signs of retention. Because urinary retention promotes uterine atony and a subsequent increase in bleeding and also contributes to the possibility of UTI, timely intervention is crucial.

of the short-acting sulfonamides, nitrofurantoin (Macrobid), and, in the case of sulfa allergy, ampicillin or amoxicillin–clavulanic acid (Augmentin). The antibiotic is changed later if indicated by the results of the sensitivity report. Antispasmodics or urinary analgesic agents, such as Pyridium, may be given to relieve discomfort.

NURSING MANAGEMENT *For the Postpartum Woman with Cystitis*

Nursing Assessment and Diagnosis

Symptoms of cystitis often appear 2 to 3 days after childbirth and may include frequency, urgency, dysuria, and nocturia. Gross hematuria may be noted but high fever and systemic symptoms are not expected.

When a UTI progresses to pyelonephritis, systemic symptoms usually occur, and the woman becomes acutely ill. Symptoms include chills, high fever, flank pain (unilateral or bilateral), nausea, and vomiting, in addition to the signs of lower UTI. Costovertebral angle tenderness on palpation may be noted on exam but is not required for diagnosis. Clean-catch urine specimens show large numbers of white blood cells and are positive for infection (Vidaeff & Ramin, 2011).

Nursing diagnoses that may apply if a woman develops postpartum cystitis include the following (NANDA-I © 2012):

- *Pain, Acute,* with voiding related to dysuria secondary to infection
- *Self-Health Management, Ineffective,* related to need for information about self-care measures to prevent UTI

Planning and Implementation

Screening for asymptomatic bacteriuria in pregnancy should be routine. Encourage frequent emptying of the bladder during labor and postpartum to prevent overdistention and trauma to the bladder. Catheterization technique and nursing actions to prevent overdistention (previously discussed) also apply. The woman with pyelonephritis must understand the importance of follow-up care after discharge to prevent recurrence or further complications.

Health Promotion   Avoiding Postpartum UTIs

Advise the postpartum woman to continue good perineal hygiene after discharge. Also advise the woman to maintain a good fluid intake (at least eight to ten 8-oz glasses daily), especially of water, and to empty her bladder whenever she feels the urge to void, but at least every 2 to 4 hours while awake. Once sexual intercourse is resumed, the new mother should void before (to prevent bladder trauma) and following intercourse (to wash contaminants from the vicinity of the urinary meatus). Wearing underwear with a cotton crotch to facilitate air circulation also reduces the risk of UTI. Acidification of the urine is thought to aid in preventing and managing UTI. Therefore advise the woman to avoid carbonated beverages, coffee, citrus fruits, tomatoes, and chocolate, which increase the alkalinity of urine, and to drink low-sugar juices such as cranberry, plum, apricot, and prune and take vitamin C, which increase the acidity of urine.

Evaluation

Expected outcomes of nursing care include the following:

- The woman identifies the signs of UTI and her condition is treated successfully.
- The woman incorporates self-care measures to prevent the recurrence of UTI as part of her personal hygiene routine.
- The woman cooperates with any long-term therapy or follow-up.
- Maternal–infant attachment is maintained and the woman is able to care for her newborn effectively.

CARE OF THE WOMAN WITH MASTITIS

Mastitis is an infection of the breast connective tissue that occurs primarily in lactating women. The usual causative organisms are *Staphylococcus aureus, Haemophilus parainfluenzae, H. influenzae, Escherichia coli,* and *Streptococcus* species (Poggi, 2013). Infectious mastitis is a very serious infection, with fever, chills, headache, flulike muscle aches and malaise, and a warm, reddened, painful area of the breast, often wedge shaped because of the connective tissue septal divisions of the breast (Newton, 2012) (Figure 31–2 ●).

The infection usually begins when bacteria invade the breast tissue after it has been traumatized in some way (see the factors commonly associated with mastitis in Table 31–4). Milk

● **Figure 31–2** Mastitis. Erythema and swelling are present in the upper outer quadrant of the breast. Axillary lymph nodes are often enlarged and tender. The segmental anatomy of the breast accounts for the demarcated, often V-shaped wedge of inflammation.

Table 31–4	Factors Associated with Development of Mastitis

MILK STASIS

Failure to change infant position to allow emptying all lobes

Failure to alternate breasts at feedings

Poor suck

Poor let-down

ACTIONS THAT PROMOTE ACCESS/MULTIPLICATION OF BACTERIA

Poor hand-washing technique

Improper breast hygiene

Failure to air dry breasts after breastfeeding

Use of plastic-lined breast pads that trap moisture against nipple

BREAST/NIPPLE TRAUMA

Incorrect positioning for breastfeeding

Poor latch-on

Failure to rotate position on nipple

Incorrect or aggressive pumping technique

Cracked nipples

OBSTRUCTION OF DUCTS

Restrictive clothing

Constricting bra

Underwire bra

CHANGE IN NUMBER OF FEEDINGS/FAILURE TO EMPTY BREASTS

Attempted weaning

Missed feeding

Prolonged sleeping, including sleeping through night

Favoring side of nipple soreness

LOWERED MATERNAL DEFENSES

Fatigue

Stress

serves as a favorable medium for the invasive bacteria; thus, milk stasis is another risk factor. The most common sources of pathogenic organisms are the infant's nose and throat, although other sources include the hands of the mother or birthing unit personnel and the woman's circulating blood. Infants of women with mastitis generally remain well unless the causative organism is *Candida albicans*.

When *Candida albicans* is the causative organism of mastitis, entering the breast through a small fissure or abrasion on the nipple, the baby will often have thrush, a candidal infection of the mouth. There may be a history of a recent course of antibiotics in the woman. Signs include late-onset nipple pain and burning pain of the nipple/areola, followed by stabbing pain of the breast during and between feedings, often radiating to the chest wall (Newton, 2012). Eventually, the skin of the affected breast becomes pink, shiny, flaking, and pruritic. Women may notice a yeasty odor to their milk. Unless the mother and her newborn are treated for *Candida*, recolonization will occur when breastfeeding is resumed.

Clinical Therapy

Clinical diagnosis is usually based on history and physical examination; a culture and sensitivity testing of breast milk obtained by a midstream-type collection process may be done. The nipple is washed first; then the first 3 mL of breast milk are manually expressed and discarded, after which the actual specimen is collected. A leukocyte count of 1 million/mL and a bacterial count of greater than 10,000/mL are diagnostic (Newton, 2012).

Treatment of mastitis involves bed rest for at least 24 hours; increased fluid intake (at least 2 to 2.5 L/day); a supportive bra; frequent breastfeeding; local application of warm, moist-heat compresses; and analgesics that are compatible with breastfeeding (Riordan & Wambach, 2010). Nonsteroidal anti-inflammatory agents are recommended to treat both fever and inflammation. Also, a course of 7 to 10 days of antibiotics is appropriate, usually with a penicillinase-resistant penicillin, such as dicloxacillin 250 mg every 6 hours or a cephalosporin 500 mg every 6 hours (Newton, 2012).

Candidal infections can be especially stubborn. Initial treatment generally involves antifungal creams or ointments once or twice daily. Oral Diflucan for the mother is excreted in breast milk but is not considered toxic to the infant and can be used if other agents fail. Women should be instructed to cleanse their nipples with warm water and allow to air dry before application of the antifungal medication. For women who prefer to avoid medication, an alternative treatment is cleansing of the nipples with a solution of 1 tablespoon of vinegar in 1 cup of water or 1 teaspoon of baking soda in 1 cup of water, followed by air drying.

Complementary Care Probiotics

Probiotics are a category of dietary supplements consisting of beneficial microorganisms (*pro* means "for" and *biotic* means "life" versus *antibiotic*, which literally means "against life"). Probiotics compete with disease-causing microorganisms in the gastrointestinal tract. When antibiotics are taken, they kill many of the beneficial bacteria that exist naturally in the digestive tract. Supplementing with probiotics after a course of antibiotics is frequently prescribed by nutritionists and complementary practitioners. Commonly used probiotics include *Lactobacillus acidophilus* and *Bifidobacterium bifidum*; other species of *Lactobacillus* and *Bifidobacterium* have been shown to be effective in such conditions as diarrhea and vaginal infections. *Bifidobacterium* also competes against *Candida albicans*. Probiotics can be taken in the form of powder, capsules, and suppositories, or in fermented milk products such as yogurt or *kefir*.

Other complementary therapies used for mastitis include belladonna, acupuncture, oxytocin nasal spray to improve milk ejection, a traditional Chinese herb known as extracts of *Fructus gleditsiae*, and application of cabbage leaves over the affected area to relieve engorgement.

Ten percent of cases will progress to abscess formation if mastitis remains untreated, treatment fails, or the infant is abruptly weaned (Newton, 2012). Abscess is more common when there is a lag of 24 hours or more between onset of symptoms and when the woman seeks care. Abscesses are associated with exquisite tenderness of the breast and an indurated area with possible fluctuation. Breast abscess may require incision and drainage (I&D) and intravenous (IV) antibiotics; analgesics and antipyretics are commonly ordered. Community-acquired methicillin-resistant *Staphylococcus aureus* (MRSA) is likely to cause abscess formation (Poggi, 2013).

Improved outcome, decreased duration of symptoms, and decreased incidence of breast abscess result if the breasts continue to be emptied by either nursing or pumping. Thus continued breastfeeding is recommended in the presence of mastitis. The woman should be contacted within 24 hours of initiation of treatment to ensure that symptoms are subsiding.

NURSING MANAGEMENT *For the Postpartum Woman with Mastitis*

Nursing Assessment and Diagnosis

Each day assess the mother's breast consistency, skin color, surface temperature, nipple condition, and presence of pain to detect early signs of problems that may predispose her to mastitis. Observe the mother breastfeeding her baby to ensure proper technique (see Chapter 26 🔗).

If an infection develops, assess for contributing factors such as cracked nipples, poor hygiene, engorgement, supplemental feedings, change in routine or infant feeding pattern, abrupt weaning, and lack of proper breast support so that these factors can be corrected as part of the treatment plan.

Nursing diagnoses that may apply to the woman with mastitis include the following (NANDA-I © 2012):

- *Trauma, Risk for,* related to lack of information about appropriate breastfeeding practices
- *Breastfeeding, Ineffective,* related to pain secondary to development of mastitis

Planning and Implementation

Preventing mastitis is far simpler than treating it. Ideally mothers are instructed in proper breastfeeding technique prenatally. Assist the mother to breastfeed soon after childbirth and review correct technique. Comanagement of breastfeeding between the nurse and a certified lactation specialist is often possible. Encourage new mothers, even those not breastfeeding, to wear a good supportive bra at all times to prevent milk stasis, especially in the lower lobes.

Meticulous hand washing by the breastfeeding mother and all personnel is the primary measure in preventing epidemic nursery infections and subsequent maternal mastitis. Prompt attention to mothers who have blocked milk ducts eliminates stagnant milk as a growth medium for bacteria. If the mother finds that one area of her breast feels distended, she can rotate the position of her infant for nursing, manually express milk remaining in the breast after feeding (usually necessary only if the infant is not sucking well), or massage the caked area toward the nipple as the infant nurses. Mothers who develop mastitis can apply warm, moist compresses to the affected area before and during breastfeeding. Encourage the mother to breastfeed frequently, starting with the unaffected breast until let-down occurs in the affected breast, then switching to the affected breast until it is emptied completely. Early identification of and intervention for sore nipples are also essential, as is prompt assessment of the breastfeeding mother's breast when thrush is discovered in her newborn's mouth. For a detailed discussion of breastfeeding problems, see *Breastfeeding Concerns Following Discharge* in Chapter 30 🔗.

Discharge Planning and Home Care Teaching

Make sure the woman is aware of the importance of regular, complete emptying of the breasts to prevent engorgement and stasis. She should also understand the role of let-down in successful breastfeeding, correct positioning of the infant on the nipple, proper latch-on, and the principle of supply and demand. If the mother is taking antibiotics, she needs to understand the importance of completing the full course of antibiotics, even if the infection seems to clear quickly. Infants tolerate the small amount of antibiotics in breast milk without difficulty. Breastfeeding mothers who are returning to work outside the home need information on how to do so successfully. Because mastitis tends to develop after discharge, it is important to include information about signs and symptoms in the discharge teaching and printed materials (Table 31–5). All flulike symptoms should be considered a sign of mastitis until proven otherwise. If symptoms develop, the woman should contact her caregiver immediately because prompt treatment helps to prevent abscess formation.

Community-Based Nursing Care

Because symptoms seldom occur before the second to fourth week postpartum, birthing unit nurses often are not fully aware of how uncomfortable and acutely ill the woman can be. The home care nurse who suspects mastitis on the basis of assessment findings refers the woman to her physician/CNM, and may be asked to obtain a sample of breast milk to be cultured for the causative organism.

If the mother feels too ill to breastfeed or develops an abscess that prevents nursing, help the mother obtain a breast pump to help her maintain lactation and provide opportunities for demonstration and return demonstration of pumping. Assist the mother in dealing with her feelings about temporarily being unable to breastfeed. Referral to a lactation consultant or the La Leche League can be invaluable to the woman's physical and emotional adjustment to mastitis.

Evaluation

Expected outcomes of nursing care include the following:

- The woman is aware of the signs and symptoms of mastitis.
- The woman reports the mastitis signs and symptoms early and is treated successfully.
- The woman resumes breastfeeding if she chooses.
- The woman understands self-care measures she can employ to prevent the recurrence of the mastitis.

Table 31–5	Symptoms of Engorgement, Plugged Duct, and Mastitis				
Onset	**Location**	**Heat/Swelling**	**Temperature**	**Pain**	**General Symptoms**
ENGORGEMENT					
Gradual; postpartum	Entire breast	Breast is hot and swollen	<38.4°C (101.1°F)	Entire breast	None
PLUGGED DUCT					
Gradual; after feedings	One side of breast	Little or no heat; there may be swelling	<38.4°C (101.1°F)	Mild pain on affected side	None
MASTITIS					
Sudden; usually after about 10 days	Generally one side of breast	Swelling on affected side; skin is red and hot	>38.4°C (101.1°F)	Intense pain on affected side	Similar to flu

Source: Data from Lawrence, R. A., & Lawrence, R. M. (2005). *Breastfeeding: A guide for the medical profession* (6th ed.). Philadelphia, PA: Elsevier Mosby.

CARE OF THE WOMAN WITH POSTPARTUM THROMBOEMBOLIC DISEASE

Thromboembolic disease may occur during the antepartum, but it is generally considered a postpartum complication. *Venous thrombosis* refers to blood clot (thrombus formation) at an area of impeded blood flow in a superficial or deep vein, usually in the legs. When the thrombus is formed in response to inflammation in the vein wall, it is termed **thrombophlebitis**. Pulmonary embolism, a rare, life-threatening condition, occurs when thrombi formed in the deep leg veins are carried to the pulmonary artery, obstructing pulmonary blood flow to one or both lungs.

Three major causes of thromboembolic disease, often referred to as *Virchow's triad*, are hypercoagulability of blood, venous stasis, and injury to the epithelium of the blood vessel. Changes in the woman's coagulation system in pregnancy contribute to hypercoagulability and compression of the common iliac vein by the gravid uterus, which leads to venous stasis (Witcher & Hamner, 2013). These factors increase the risk of thromboembolic disease in pregnant and postpartum women approximately 2 to 6 times. Venous thrombophlebitis complicates the general childbearing period for 0.5 to 3 per 1000 women (Witcher & Hamner, 2013). In contrast, deep vein thrombosis (DVT), which is more serious, occurs most commonly in postpartum women between postpartum days 10 and 20.

Factors contributing directly to the development of thromboembolic disease postpartum include (1) increased amounts of certain blood-clotting factors; (2) postpartum thrombocytosis (increased quantity of circulating platelets and their increased adhesiveness); (3) release of thromboplastin substances from the tissue of the decidua, placenta, and fetal membranes; and (4) increased amounts of fibrinolysis inhibitors. Because all women are at risk for thromboembolic disease during the childbearing period, attention should be given to conditions that increase risk of thromboembolic disease (Table 31–6).

Table 31–6	Factors Associated with Increased Risk of Thromboembolic Disease

- Major pelvic or abdominal surgery at time of cesarean birth
- Previous thromboembolic disease or strong personal or family history
- Obesity (BMI > 30)
- Thrombophilia, acquired or inherited (protein C and protein S deficiency)
- Age greater than 35 years
- Operative delivery or instrumentation
- Gross varicose veins
- Prolonged immobility
- Multiparity
- Active infection or inflammatory process

Superficial Leg Vein Disease

Superficial thrombophlebitis is far more common postpartum than during pregnancy. Often the clot involves one of the saphenous veins. This disorder is more common in women with preexisting varices (enlarged veins), although it is not limited to these women. They may also occur as a sequelae to IV catheterization. Symptoms usually become apparent about postpartum day 3 or 4 and include tenderness in a portion of the vein, some local heat and redness, normal temperature or low-grade fever, and occasionally slight elevation of the pulse. A tender palpable cord may be noted along a portion of the veins. Treatment involves application of local heat, elevation of the affected limb, bed rest, analgesics, and the use of elastic support hose. Anticoagulants are usually not necessary unless complications develop. Pulmonary embolism is extremely rare.

Deep Vein Thrombosis

Deep vein thrombosis (DVT) is more frequently seen in women with a history of thrombosis. Obstetric complications, such as hydramnios, preeclampsia, and operative birth, are also associated with an increased incidence. After a clinical diagnosis of DVT, a woman's risk in a subsequent pregnancy increases.

Clinical manifestations may include edema of the ankle and leg and an initial low-grade fever often followed by high temperature and chills. Other findings include tenderness or pain, a palpable cord, changes in limb color, and difference in limb circumference of more than 2 cm (0.8 in.). Depending on the vein involved, the woman may complain of pain in the popliteal and lateral tibial areas (popliteal vein), pain in the entire lower leg and foot (anterior and posterior tibial veins), inguinal tenderness (femoral vein), or pain in the lower abdomen (iliofemoral vein). The Homans' sign (Figure 29–9 🔗 on page 724) may or may not be positive. A positive Homans' sign is a specific finding but has low sensitivity for helping diagnose DVT (Pettker & Lockwood, 2012). Most DVTs occur in the left leg. Because of reflex arterial spasm, sometimes the limb is pale and cool to the touch and peripheral pulses may be diminished or difficult to palpate.

Clinical Therapy

Treatment involves the immediate intravenous (IV) administration of either standard unfractionated heparin or low-molecular-weight heparin (LMWH) using an infusion pump to permit continuous, accurate infusion to stabilize the clot. An example of a possible regimen is a subcutaneous injection of enoxaparin 1 mg/kg twice daily (Witcher & Hamner, 2013). Heparin therapy is continued until the international normalized ratio (INR) with oral warfarin is achieved at 2.0 to 3.0 for 2 consecutive days. Advantages of LMWH include its safe profile and the fact that dosing is not reliant on monitoring the *activated partial thromboplastin time* (aPTT) at a laboratory. In some cases thrombolytics (streptokinase or urokinase) or an embolectomy may be used. Maintenance with warfarin sodium (Coumadin) is started at 1 to 5 days. An initial dose of 10 to 15 mg/daily PO is titrated based on the prothrombin time (PT) with the INR target rate cited above. Analgesics are given as necessary to relieve discomfort. If fever is present, the woman may also be given an antibiotic. In most cases thrombectomy (surgical removal of the clot) is not necessary.

Once the symptoms have subsided (usually in several days), the woman may begin walking while wearing elastic support stockings. The woman will continue on warfarin sodium (Coumadin) for 4 to 6 weeks postpartum or up to 3 months (Witcher & Hamner, 2013). While taking warfarin sodium, prothrombin times are assessed periodically to maintain correct

dosage levels. Periodic assessment for signs of bleeding is essential, including those for hematuria and fecal occult blood. In those who cannot be given anticoagulants, a vena cava filtering device may be considered. To prevent recurrence in subsequent pregnancies, prophylactic treatment will be considered.

NURSING MANAGEMENT *For the Postpartum Woman with Thromboembolic Disease*

Nursing Assessment and Diagnosis

Carefully assess the woman's history for factors predisposing her to development of thrombosis or thrombophlebitis. In addition, as part of regular postpartum assessment, be alert to any complaints of pain in the legs, inguinal area, or lower abdomen because such pain may indicate deep vein thrombosis (DVT). Also assess the woman's legs for evidence of edema, temperature change, or pain with palpation.

Nursing diagnoses that may apply to a postpartum woman with a thrombotic disease include the following (NANDA-I © 2012):

- ■ *Tissue Perfusion: Peripheral, Ineffective,* related to obstructed venous return
- ■ *Pain, Acute,* related to tissue hypoxia and edema secondary to vascular obstruction
- ■ *Knowledge, Deficient,* related to self-care after discharge on anticoagulant therapy

Planning and Implementation

Hospital-Based Nursing Care

Women are at risk for thromboembolic disease during the childbearing period especially during labor and the postpartum period. Attention should be given to nursing measures that might prevent or deal with this complication (Table 31–7).

Once DVT is diagnosed, maintain the heparin therapy, provide appropriate comfort measures, and monitor the woman closely for signs of pulmonary embolism. Assess for evidence of bleeding related to heparin and keep the antagonist for heparin, protamine sulfate, readily available. Remind the woman to mention her history of thrombosis or thrombophlebitis to her physician/CNM during subsequent pregnancies so that preventive measures can be instituted early.

Patients on warfarin need to be educated about foods high in vitamin K (a nutrient that lessens warfarin's effectiveness) and the need to strive for consistent daily intake so that accurate dosage of the drug can be achieved. When the dietary intake of these foods, such as cauliflower, soybean and canola oil, mayonnaise, broccoli, green and black tea, peppers, spinach, and collard greens, decreases significantly, there is a risk of bleeding. Favorite foods that are high in vitamin K can be consumed in moderation, while nonfavorites are avoided daily. Cranberry juice increases the effects of the drug and, if desired, should be consumed in moderation and with consistency. Many multivitamins contain vitamin K; patients on warfarin may take them but should do so consistently. Vitamin C doses up to 500 mg/day and vitamin E doses up to 400 International Units/day are considered safe; higher doses can affect coagulation.

> ### Clinical Reasoning Postpartum Leg Pain
>
> Wanda Sugiyama, G1P1, had a cesarean birth after a prolonged labor and failure to progress. As she is walking in the hallway with her husband, you notice that Wanda is limping slightly, and you comment on that observation. Wanda responds that she is having pain in her right lower leg. She says, "Maybe I pulled a muscle during labor." What would you do?
>
> *See www.nursing.pearsonhighered.com for possible responses.*

Table 31–7	Measures to Decrease Risk of Thromboembolic Disease in Childbearing Women	
Antepartum Measures	**Intrapartum Measures**	**Postpartum Measures**
■ Advise woman to avoid sedentary lifestyle and to exercise as possible (walking is ideal). ■ Advise to quit smoking. ■ Teach to avoid prolonged standing or sitting in one position or sitting with legs crossed. ■ Encourage elevation of legs when sitting. ■ Teach to avoid tight knee-high hose or other constrictive garments. ■ Encourage to take frequent breaks during long car trips to walk around and while working if she sits most of the day, thereby preventing prolonged venous stasis.	■ Encourage ambulation unless contraindicated in early labor; later, encourage leg exercises. ■ Do not gatch bed or use pillows under knees. ■ Pad stirrups prevent pressure on popliteal vessels. ■ Ensure correct positioning in stirrups to minimize pressure on the popliteal area. ■ Limit time in stirrups as possible because trauma is a factor. ■ After cesarean birth, initiate leg/foot exercises as soon as possible (in recovery) to promote venous return. ■ Use antiembolism stockings for women at risk for DVT.	■ Encourage early ambulation. ■ For patients on bed rest, advise or assist with turning and leg exercises every 2 hours (woman may be encouraged to rotate ankles and to "write baby's name in the air with her toes"). ■ Encourage fluids to avoid dehydration. ■ Advise no smoking. ■ Use antiembolism stockings with those at risk, including after cesarean birth. ■ Advise against prolonged sitting and crossing of legs. ■ Encourage elevation of legs while sitting.

Women who are discharged on warfarin must understand the purpose of the medication and be alert for signs of bleeding such as bleeding gums, epistaxis, petechiae or ecchymosis, and evidence of blood in the urine or stool. Certain medications such as aspirin and other nonsteroidal anti-inflammatory drugs increase anticoagulant activity and should be avoided. When taking warfarin the woman should check for possible medication interaction before taking *any* other medication. She should also have vitamin K available in case bleeding occurs. Women should be cautious about using sharp objects such as knives or razor blades to avoid injury. Risky behaviors that could contribute to falls should be avoided. Wearing protective gloves during gardening or heavy housework and always wearing shoes can keep hands and feet safe from injury.

Because careful monitoring is important, the woman should clearly understand the need to keep scheduled appointments for prothrombin time (PT) assessment to guide dosing. Point-of-care testing is now available to decrease the inconvenience of going to the laboratory. Home self-testing involves a single capillary fingerstick (CoaguChek, ProTime, Avocet) to test thromboplastin-mediated clotting expressed as PT or INR. The risk of bleeding increases significantly when the INR is greater than 3 (Pettker & Lockwood, 2012). Bleeding should be reported if it fails to stop within 10 minutes. (See *Nursing Care Plan: The Woman with Thromboembolic Disease* for specific nursing care measures.)

Community-Based Nursing Care

Because the mother with postpartum thromboembolic disease will depend on others for much of her initial home care, it is helpful for the father of the newborn to be involved in preparations for discharge. Provide ample time to answer questions and clarify instructions, verbally and in writing. It is especially important to assess the couple's plans to ensure complete bed rest for the mother. They might explore ways for her to maintain bed rest and still spend quality time with her newborn and any other children. For example, young children can sit on the bed for storytelling or play quiet games, and the newborn's crib can be placed next to the mother's bed.

The father/partner may be assuming multiple roles in these circumstances—household manager, parent, worker, and caregiver. Fatigue is inevitable. There may also be financial concerns as a result of prolonged health care or his extended time away from work to care for the family. Many concerns will not surface until the couple actually returns home and fully comprehends the reality of their situation. For that reason, it is valuable to provide them with an accessible resource person and to plan telephone or home visit follow-up care.

Signs of postpartum thrombophlebitis may not occur until after discharge from the birthing unit. Consequently all couples must be taught to recognize its signs and symptoms and appreciate the importance of reporting them immediately and not massaging the affected leg. If signs and symptoms occur after discharge, a short readmission may be required. In that case every effort is made to allow mother, father, and newborn to remain together.

After DVT, some women continue to have leg pain, edema, and dermatitis of the affected extremity for prolonged periods caused by a residual venous abnormality. This situation can significantly affect quality of life. Continuing use of compression stockings for a minimum of 1 year after diagnosis will help to prevent this complication of DVT.

Evaluation

Expected outcomes of nursing care include the following:

■ The woman seeks treatment for her thrombophlebitis early and is managed successfully, without further complications.

■ At discharge the woman is able to explain the purpose, dosage regimen, and necessary precautions associated with any prescribed medications such as anticoagulants.

■ The woman can discuss the self-care measures and ongoing therapies (such as need for rest and the use of elastic stockings) that are indicated.

■ The woman has bonded successfully with her newborn and is able to care for her baby effectively.

Nursing Care Plan The Woman with Thromboembolic Disease

Intervention	Rationale	Expected Outcome

1. Nursing Diagnosis: *Tissue Perfusion: Peripheral, Ineffective,* related to interruption of venous blood flow secondary to complications of labor and birth (NANDA-I © 2012)

NIC Priority Intervention:
Embolus care: peripheral: Limitation of complications for a patient experiencing, or at risk for, occlusion of peripheral circulation

Goal: The patient's presenting signs and symptoms will be relieved.

NOC Suggested Outcome:
Tissue perfusion: peripheral: Extent to which blood flows through the small vessels of the extremities and maintains tissue function

- Assess, record, and report signs of thrombophlebitis.

  - Early detection of developing thrombophlebitis permits prompt treatment. As the thrombus increases in size, signs of obstruction also increase.

  - Patient will have increased venous return from lower leg as evidenced by decreased edema in lower leg, negative Homans' sign, and no pain or tenderness in lower leg.

- Assess leg for edema, peripheral pulse, temperature, color, and tenderness every 8 hours.

  - Assessment provides baseline data that may be used to monitor success of treatment. Edema/swelling, diminished or absent peripheral pulse, pallor, cool skin temperature, and tenderness are symptoms of deep vein thrombosis (DVT) and indicate dysfunction of peripheral circulation in the lower extremities. Measure circumference of lower leg to monitor for swelling. Peripheral pulses in both legs should be palpated for pulse rate and pulse strength to allow for comparison. Lower extremities that are cool to the touch may be due to reflex arterial spasm.

- Assess Homans' sign every 8 hours.

  - Normally there is no pain or discomfort associated with this procedure. Pain is caused by inflammation of the vessel. If pain is elicited, the nurse documents the response as a positive Homans' sign and reports findings to the physician.

- Maintain bed rest during the acute phase.

  - Bed rest is ordered to decrease possibility that portion of clot will dislodge and result in pulmonary embolism.

- Provide warm, moist soaks as ordered.

  - Warmth promotes blood flow to affected area.

- Maintain limb in elevated position.

  - Elevation of affected limb promotes venous return and helps decrease edema.

- Initiate progressive ambulation following the acute phase and provide properly fitting elastic stockings prior to ambulation.

  - Elastic stockings or "Teds" help prevent pooling of venous blood in lower extremities.
  - Patient may begin to ambulate within a few days when symptoms subside.

- **Collaborative:** Administer intravenous heparin as ordered, by continuous intravenous drip, heparin lock, or subcutaneously, including:
  1. Monitor IV or heparin lock site for signs of infiltration.

  - Heparin does not dissolve blood clot but is administered to prevent further clotting and improve tissue perfusion. It is safe for breastfeeding mothers because heparin is not excreted in mother's milk.

Nursing Care Plan   **The Woman with Thromboembolic Disease—continued**

Intervention	Rationale	Expected Outcome

2. Obtain international normalized ratio (INR) and partial thromboplastin time (PTT) per physician order and review prior to administering heparin.
3. Observe for signs of anticoagulant overdose with resultant bleeding, including:
   a. Hematuria
   b. Epistaxis
   c. Ecchymosis
   d. Bleeding gums		

4. Provide protamine sulfate, per physician order, to combat bleeding problems related to heparin overdose.	■ Protamine sulfate is a heparin antagonist, given intravenously, which is almost immediately effective in counteracting bleeding complications caused by heparin overdose.	
5. Monitor and report any signs of pulmonary embolism.	■ Pulmonary embolism is a major complication of DVT/thrombophlebitis.	
6. Initiate or support any emergency treatment.	■ Signs and symptoms may occur suddenly and require immediate emergency treatment; prognosis is related to size and location of embolism.	
7. Obtain prothrombin time (PT) and review prior to beginning warfarin. Repeat periodically per physician order.	■ PT is the test most commonly used to monitor the blood of patients receiving warfarin.	

2. Nursing Diagnosis: *Pain* related to tissue hypoxia and edema secondary to vascular obstruction (NANDA-I © 2012)

NIC Priority Intervention: *Pain management:* Alleviation of pain or a reduction in pain to a level of comfort that is acceptable to the patient		**NOC Suggested Outcome:** *Pain: disruptive effects:* Observed or reported disruptive effects of pain on emotions and behavior
Goal: The patient will obtain relief of pain.		
■ Administer analgesics per physician order. Notify physician if pain is not relieved.	■ Analgesics act to relieve pain and enable the woman to rest. Aspirin or ibuprofen products are contraindicated because they inhibit platelet adhesiveness. Acetaminophen may be ordered by the physician.	■ Patient will have reduction in pain as evidenced by a pain level < 5 at all times.
■ Provide supportive nursing comfort measures such as back rubs, quiet time for sleep, and diversional activities.	■ Once pain decreases, patient is more likely to ambulate, which will help increase venous return and decrease edema.	

3. Nursing Diagnosis: *Parenting, Risk for Impaired,* related to decreased maternal–infant interaction secondary to bed rest and IVs (NANDA-I © 2012)

NIC Priority Intervention: *Attachment promotion:* Facilitation of the development of the parent–infant relationship		**NOC Suggested Outcome:** *Parent–infant attachment:* Behavior that demonstrates an enduring affectionate bond between a parent and infant

Goal: The patient will demonstrate evidence of positive physical and social interaction with newborn.

(continued)

Nursing Care Plan   The Woman with Thromboembolic Disease—continued

Intervention	Rationale	Expected Outcome
■ Maintain mother–infant attachment when mother is on bed rest: 1. Provide frequent contacts for mother and infant; use modified rooming-in if possible by having the crib placed close to the mother's bed and nurse checks often to help mother lift or move infant. 2. Encourage mother to continue feeding infant.	■ Maternal–infant attachment is enhanced by frequent contact and opportunities to interact.	■ Patient will develop attachment bonds as evidenced by physical interactions (good eye contact, touching the baby, holding baby close, attempting to comfort baby, kissing baby) and social interactions (calling baby by name, making positive comments about baby, asking questions about baby, asking questions about baby care, and talking to baby).

4. Nursing Diagnosis: *Knowledge, Deficient,* related to lack of information about DVT/thrombophlebitis, its treatment, preventive measures, and the medication warfarin (NANDA-I © 2012)

NIC Priority Intervention:
Health education: Development and provision of instruction and learning experiences to facilitate voluntary adaptation of behavior conducive to health in individuals, families, groups, or communities

NOC Suggested Outcome:
Knowledge: health promotion: Extent of understanding conveyed about the promotion and protection of health

Goal: The patient will understand her condition, its treatment, and long-term implications.

■ Discuss ways of avoiding circulatory stasis such as avoiding prolonged standing, sitting, and crossing legs.	■ Such discussion is essential to help the woman understand the condition, her medication, and its implications. She must have a clear understanding to be able to provide effective self-care. ■ Prolonged sitting, standing, and crossing legs should be avoided because these activities decrease venous return.	■ Patient will gain health promotion knowledge as evidenced by: 1. Woman verbalizes understanding of ways to avoid circulatory stasis, need to wear supportive stockings, medication's dosage and side effects, and the importance of a balanced diet, which includes vitamin K foods. 2. Woman verbalizes understanding of signs and symptoms of bleeding that need to be reported to healthcare provider.
■ Review need to wear support stockings and to plan for rest periods with legs elevated. ■ In the presence of DVT, discuss the following: 1. The use of warfarin, its side effects, possible interactions with other medications, and the need to have dosage assessed through periodic checks of the prothrombin time. 2. Signs of bleeding, which may be associated with warfarin sodium and need to be reported immediately, include the following: hematuria, epistaxis, ecchymosis, bleeding gums, and rectal bleeding. 3. Monitor menstrual flow: bleeding may be heavier.	■ Patient placed on warfarin (Coumadin) therapy for 2–6 months at home.	

Nursing Care Plan	The Woman with Thromboembolic Disease—continued

Intervention	Rationale	Expected Outcome
4. Review need for woman to eat a consistent amount of leafy green vegetables (lettuce, cabbage, brussels sprouts, broccoli) every day.	■ These foods are high in vitamin K and will affect balance between dose of warfarin and prothrombin time.	
5. Instruct the woman to report any bleeding that continues more than 10 minutes.		
6. Instruct the woman to do the following: ■ Routinely inspect the body for bruising. ■ Carry medical alert card indicating she is on anticoagulant therapy. ■ Use electric razor to avoid scratching skin. ■ Use soft-bristle toothbrush. ■ Avoid binge alcohol intake or keep at minimum. ■ Avoid taking certain herbs such as ginger, garlic, and ginkgo and any other drugs that can prolong PT without checking with the physician. ■ Note that stools may change color to pink, red, or black as a result of anticoagulant use. ■ Advise all health providers, including dentists, that she is taking anticoagulants.		

CARE OF THE WOMAN WITH A POSTPARTUM PSYCHIATRIC DISORDER

Types of Postpartum Psychiatric Disorders

The classification of postpartum psychiatric disorders is a subject of some controversy. The *Diagnostic and Statistical Manual of Mental Disorders* (DSM-V-TR) (American Psychiatric Association [APA], 2013) contains a peripartum onset specifier to the mood disorder diagnostic category of psychiatric disorders. It is proposed that postpartum psychiatric disorders be considered one diagnosable syndrome with three subclasses: (1) adjustment reaction with depressed mood, (2) postpartum mood episodes with psychotic features, and (3) peripartum major mood episodes (also known as postpartum depression). The incidence, etiology, symptoms, treatment, and prognosis vary with each subclass.

Adjustment Reaction with Depressed Mood

Adjustment reaction with depressed mood is also known as **postpartum blues** or as *maternal blues* or *baby blues*. It occurs in as many as 50% to 70% of mothers and is characterized by mild depression interspersed with happier feelings (Pessel & Tsai, 2013). Postpartum blues typically occur within a few days

after the baby's birth, are self-limiting, and can last up to 6 weeks (Katz, 2012). The depression is more severe in primiparas than in multiparas and seems related to the rapid alteration of estrogen, progesterone, and prolactin levels after birth. New mothers experiencing postpartum blues commonly report feeling overwhelmed, unable to cope, fatigued, anxious, irritable, and oversensitive. A key feature is episodic tearfulness, often without an identifiable reason. Often, when the woman is asked why she is crying, she will respond that she does not know. Cunningham et al. (2010) identify several factors that contribute to the postpartum blues:

■ Emotional letdown that follows labor and childbirth

■ Physical discomfort typical in the early postpartum

■ Fatigue

■ Anxiety about caring for the newborn after discharge

■ Severe PMS (premenstrual syndrome)

■ Depression during pregnancy or previous depression unrelated to pregnancy

Validating the existence of this phenomenon, labeling it as a real but normal adjustment reaction, and providing reassurance can offer a measure of relief. Assistance with self-care and infant care, rest, good nutrition, information, and family support aid recovery. Helping the new mother anticipate a transient emotional letdown after discharge is important guidance from the nurse, as is talking with her about her view of "the perfect mother." Trying to achieve that image can contribute to fatigue and exacerbate the letdown feeling. The partner should be encouraged to watch for and report signs that the new mother is not returning to a more normal mood but slipping into a deeper depression or that happier times are no longer interspersed with the blues.

Postpartum Mood Episodes with Psychotic Features

Postpartum mood episodes with psychotic features, which have an incidence of 0.5 to 1 per 1000 births, usually becomes evident within the first 4 weeks after childbirth (APA, 2013). Although relatively rare, new-onset postpartum psychosis gains considerable national attention in the media when there is an incident of infanticide associated with it. Symptoms include agitation, hyperactivity, insomnia, mood lability, confusion, irrationality, difficulty remembering or concentrating, poor judgment, delusions, and hallucinations that tend to be related to the infant (Wisner et al., 2012). The woman with psychosis may experience delusions or hallucinations that support her perceptions that the infant should not be allowed to live. Illogical thinking or evidence of bonding difficulties may serve as cues to infanticide and suicide risk; however, this assessment is often challenging because of the lucidity seen in some patients with psychosis. With appropriate treatment, improvement should be seen in 2 to 3 months.

Peripartum Major Mood Episodes

The rate of **peripartum major mood episodes**, also known as **postpartum depression (PPD)**, is about 8% to 15% of postpartum women and is higher for women with history of previous mood disorder (APA, 2013; Katz, 2012).

Risk factors for postpartum depression include the following:

- Primiparity
- Ambivalence about maintaining the pregnancy
- History of postpartum depression or bipolar illness
- Lack of social support

- Lack of a stable and supportive relationship with parents or partner
- Lack of a supportive relationship with her parents, especially her father, as a child
- The woman's dissatisfaction with herself, including body image problems and eating disorders

Although it may occur at any time during the first postpartum year, the periods of greatest risk occur around the fourth week, just before the initiation of menses, and upon weaning. Women with postpartum depression are at risk for suicide, most prominently as they enter or exit the deeply depressed state. In a deep depression, the woman is unlikely to be able to plan and carry out suicide. For that reason, signs of improvement in depression should be celebrated with some caution. Whereas the woman with postpartum mood episodes with psychotic features may attempt suicide because of illogical thought processes, the woman with major depression attempts suicide because her suffering is so great that dying seems a more favorable option than continuing to live in such pain. She may also attempt suicide to save her newborn from some perceived or real threat—including the possibility that she herself might harm the baby. The risk of suicide is greater in those who have attempted suicide previously, have a specific plan, and can access the means or weapon identified within the plan. The more specific the plan, the greater the probability of an attempt.

Post-Traumatic Stress Disorder

Many women envision their own labor and delivery unfolding in a particular way and may experience angst if their labor reality fails to match their expectations. Labor and birth situations that go awry, including those associated with complications, may cause **post-traumatic stress disorder (PTSD)** (also called *post-traumatic stress syndrome*), which the DSM-V-TR (APA, 2013) describes as "exposure to actual or threatened death, serious injury, or sexual violence in one (or more) of the following ways: 1. directly experiencing the traumatic event(s); 2. witnessing, in person, the event(s) as it occurred to others; 3. learning that the traumatic event occurred to a close family member or close friend; 4. experiencing

---

 Evidence-Based Practice Identifying and Managing Postpartum Depression

Clinical Question
How can public health systems be most effective in identifying and managing postpartum depression?

The Evidence
Public health nurses are in an ideal position to identify postpartum depression and propose effective interventions. A study was conducted of 228 women who were provided community-based supportive counseling by public health nurses who were specially trained to identify signs of depression and provide supportive counseling. A second, redesigned study of more than 2200 women investigated a community-based postpartum program intended to help mothers manage their emotional responses in the postpartum period. These large-sample randomized trials provide some of the strongest evidence for practice. The redesigned community-based care was useful in reducing the effects of postpartum

depression. Supportive counseling based on a nondirective method provided the most effective treatments in the public health setting (Glavin, Smith, Sorum, et al., 2010). Van Dinter and Graves (2012) found, more specifically, that psychosocial support includes offering mental health counseling services in community settings.

Best Practice
Training public health nurses to identify early signs of depression and to intervene using supportive counseling may be effective in reducing the incidence of this postpartum disorder. Providing this service as part of a community-based effort is most successful in helping new mothers manage the postpartum period.

Clinical Reasoning
What is supportive nondirective counseling? What are the early signs of postpartum depression that might be part of a public health campaign?

repeated or extreme exposure to adverse details of the traumatic events" (p. 271). These extreme traumatic situations are typically ones outside the realm of usual human experience—situations that would be distressing for anyone.

At particular risk for PTSD are women who are especially anxious or fearful about childbirth or who have low coping capacity and/or prior psychiatric histories (Beck, Gable, Sakala, et al., 2011). For the woman, the facts of the labor and birth have become distorted, perhaps because of pain or change in consciousness related to medications she received. Perhaps she underwent an emergency cesarean delivery or her baby had a serious physical anomaly. Perhaps her labor coach could not make the trip to the hospital in time for the birth or she experienced a postpartum hemorrhage. Her perceptions of what occurred and the actions of those involved are frequently far different from the reality, perhaps even seeming delusional.

Clinical features of PTSD include feeling numb, seeming dazed and unaware of her environment, intrusive thoughts and flashbacks to the threatening event, difficulty thinking, difficulty sleeping, irritability, and avoidance of others and reminders of the traumatic event. Tachycardia, hyperventilation, and nausea may occur. These signs and symptoms may not be evident until after the woman has left the birth setting. Distress associated with the original traumatic event can recur at anniversaries, and some women are hesitant to consider future pregnancies because of this birth trauma (Beck, 2008).

Based on her qualitative research and the work of others related to traumatic birth experiences, Beck (2008, p. 8) suggests the following implications for nursing care:

1. Intervene, whenever possible, to prevent traumatic birth experiences.
2. Provide technically competent, concerned care for the woman and family.
3. Assess for anxiety and fears on admission to labor and provide information to dispel myths.
4. Debrief the woman and family after a stressful traumatic childbirth experience.
5. Visit the woman during her hospitalization to assess for evidence of signs of early trauma.

Women should be asked to tell their birth story, to compare and contrast the actual experience with their birth plan or prior visions of the special day, and to tell what went well for them and what part, if any, of the experience was unexpected, troublesome, disappointing, or distressing.

Clinical Therapy

Women with a history of postpartum psychosis or depression or other risk factors should be referred to a mental health professional for counseling and biweekly visits between the second and sixth week postpartum for evaluation. Medication, individual or group psychotherapy, and practical assistance with child care and other demands of daily life are common treatment measures for both disorders; however, the specific therapies used may vary.

It is important for the nurse to realize that many of the drugs used in treating postpartum psychiatric conditions are contraindicated in breastfeeding women. All currently prescribed antidepressant agents are excreted into breast milk. Zoloft, Lustral, Paxil, Seroxat, and Deroxat are considered first-line agents. Because of its prolonged half-life, fluoxetine (Prozac) is not recommended for nursing mothers. Physicians will wish to educate their breastfeeding postpartum patients who need antidepressants about the different alternatives and help them to balance the risks and benefits with the safety profiles. The final decision about continuing to breastfeed and to take antidepressants is the informed woman's choice. When making the decision, she and her partner need to be helped to consider how she will respond without pharmacologic therapy and how unmedicated depression will affect the maternal–infant relationship and the infant's well-being and development. An invaluable online resource for prescribers with current information on drug safety and toxic effects during pregnancy and lactation is the LacMed Database.

Treatment of postpartum psychosis is directed at the specific type of psychotic symptoms displayed and may include lithium, antipsychotics, or electroconvulsive therapy in combination with psychotherapy, removal of the infant, and social support.

Support groups are successful adjuncts to the previously discussed treatments. Within a support group of postpartum women and their partners, a couple may feel consolation that they are not alone in their experience. Moreover, the group provides a forum for exchanging information about postpartum depression, learning stress reduction measures, and experiencing renewed self-esteem and support. The most effective support groups provide for safe child care to facilitate attendance. If a support group is not available locally, the woman and her family may be encouraged to contact Depression after Delivery (DAD), now a national Web-based support network that provides education and volunteers, or Postpartum Support International. The Mills Depression and Anxiety Symptom-Feeling Checklist is also available online.

NURSING MANAGEMENT *For the Postpartum Woman with a Psychiatric Disorder*

Nursing Assessment and Diagnosis

Assessment for factors predisposing a patient to postpartum depression or psychosis should begin prenatally. Questions designed to detect problems can be included as part of the routine prenatal history interview or questionnaire. Women with a personal or family history of psychiatric disease, particularly postpartum depression or psychosis, need prenatal instructions on the signs and symptoms of depression and may need additional emotional support. Ideally a depression assessment should be completed each trimester to update a pregnant woman's risk status.

If not done previously, assess the woman for predisposing factors during labor and the postpartum stay. Several depression scales are available for assessing postpartum depression. The routine use of a screening tool in a matter-of-fact approach significantly increases the diagnosis. The Edinburgh Postnatal Depression Scale (EPDS) is the most widely used screening tool for postpartum depression in large populations of women. The tool has been validated, computerized, and used in telephone screening. Mothers who score above 12 on the EPDS are likely to be suffering from postpartum depression. Another tool is Beck's (2002) revised Postpartum Depression Predictors Inventory (PDPI–Revised). This tool is also a practical and simple screening checklist to use during routine care with all postpartum women to identify those who might be experiencing postpartum depression so that early management might be initiated (Table 31–8).

Table 31–8	Postpartum Depression Predictors Inventory (PDPI)—Revised and Guide Questions for Its Use

During Pregnancy

MARITAL STATUS	Check One	
1. Single	❏	
2. Married/cohabitating	❏	
3. Separated	❏	
4. Divorced	❏	
5. Widowed	❏	
6. Partnered	❏	

SOCIOECONOMIC STATUS		
Low	❏	
Middle	❏	
High	❏	

SELF-ESTEEM	Yes	No
Do you feel good about yourself as a person?	❏	❏
Do you feel worthwhile?	❏	❏
Do you feel you have a number of good qualities as a person?	❏	❏

PRENATAL DEPRESSION		
1. Have you felt depressed during your pregnancy?	❏	❏
If yes, when and how long have you been feeling this way?		
If yes, how mild or severe would you consider your depression?		

PRENATAL ANXIETY		
Have you been feeling anxious during your pregnancy?	❏	❏
If yes, how long have you been feeling this way?		

UNPLANNED/UNWANTED PREGNANCY		
Was the pregnancy planned?	❏	❏
Is the pregnancy unwanted?	❏	❏

HISTORY OF PREVIOUS DEPRESSION		
1. Before this pregnancy, have you ever been depressed?	❏	❏
If yes, when did you experience this depression?		
If yes, have you been under a physician's care for this past depression?	❏	❏
If yes, did the physician prescribe any medication for your depression?	❏	❏

SOCIAL SUPPORT		
1. Do you feel you receive adequate emotional support from your partner?	❏	❏
2. Do you feel you receive adequate instrumental support from your partner (e.g., help with household chores or babysitting)?	❏	❏
3. Do you feel you can rely on your partner when you need help?	❏	❏
4. Do you feel you can confide in your partner? (Repeat same questions for family and again for friends.)	❏	❏

Table 31–8	Postpartum Depression Predictors Inventory (PDPI)—Revised and Guide Questions for Its Use—continued		

During Pregnancy

MARITAL SATISFACTION

1. Are you satisfied with your marriage (or living arrangement)?	❏	❏
2. Are you currently experiencing any marital problems?	❏	❏
3. Are things going well between you and your partner?	❏	❏

LIFE STRESS

1. Are you currently experiencing any stressful events in your life such as:

Financial problems?	❏	❏
Marital problems?	❏	❏
Death in the family?	❏	❏
Serious illness in the family?	❏	❏
Moving?	❏	❏
Unemployment?	❏	❏
Job change?	❏	❏

After Delivery, Add the Following Items

CHILDCARE STRESS

	Yes	No
1. Is your infant experiencing any health problems?	❏	❏
2. Are you having problems with your baby feeding?	❏	❏
3. Are you having problems with your baby sleeping?	❏	❏

INFANT TEMPERAMENT

1. Would you consider your baby irritable or fussy?	❏	❏
2. Does your baby cry a lot?	❏	❏
3. Is your baby difficult to console or soothe?	❏	❏

MATERNITY BLUES

1. Did you experience a brief period of tearfulness and mood swings during the first week after delivery?	❏	❏

COMMENTS:

Source: Beck, C. T. (2002). Revision of the Postpartum Predictors Inventory. *Journal of Obstetric, Gynecologic, and Neonatal Nursing, 31*(4), 394–402 (Table 2 on PDPI, pp. 399–400). Washington, DC: AWHONN. © 2002 by the Association of Women's Health, Obstetric and Neonatal Nurses. All rights reserved.

No matter what approach is used to assess for postpartum depression, enabling the woman's voice to be heard about her feelings of maternal role transition and how she is adjusting in this vulnerable time is of inestimable value (Beck, 2008). Listening to her story provides a critical emie (insider's) view of her circumstances as opposed to an etic (outsider's) view.

In providing daily care, observe the woman for objective signs of depression—anxiety, irritability, poor concentration, forgetfulness, sleep difficulties, appetite change, fatigue, and tearfulness—and listen for statements indicating feelings of failure and self-accusation. Severity and duration of symptoms should be noted. Report as soon as possible for further evaluation any behaviors and/or verbalizations that are bizarre or seem to indicate a potential for violence against herself or others, including the infant.

Be aware that many normal physiologic changes of the puerperium are similar to symptoms of depression (lack of sexual interest, appetite change, fatigue). It is essential that observations be as specific and as objective as possible and that they are carefully documented.

Beck (2008) found that anxiety was a prominent feature of illness for some women and suggested that women be assessed for their level of anxiety, particularly regarding infant care. Because of the strong association between interrupted sleep and postpartum depression and the finding that severe fatigue was an excellent predictor of postpartum depression, assessing fatigue level at 2 weeks postpartum by telephone may be helpful in predicting depression risk early. Restorative sleep improves one's ability to cope and make decisions, thereby producing a sense of better self-control.

A central challenge for nursing is identifying women at risk of suicide. Family members of the depressed woman should also be alert to signals that she may be intent on self-harm; advise them that threats should always be taken seriously. Tell family members to be especially vigilant for suicide when the woman seems to be feeling better.

Possible nursing diagnoses that may apply to a woman with a postpartum psychiatric disorder include the following (NANDA-I © 2012):

- *Coping, Ineffective,* related to postpartum depression
- *Parenting, Risk for Impaired,* related to postpartum mental illness
- *Violence, Self-Directed,* possible suicide and/or violence directed at newborn, and other children related to depression

Planning and Implementation

Nurses working in antepartum settings or teaching childbirth classes play indispensable roles in helping prospective parents appreciate the lifestyle changes and role demands associated with parenthood. Offer realistic information and anticipatory guidance and debunk myths about the perfect mother or perfect newborn to help prevent postpartum depression. Social support teaching guides are available for nurses to help postpartum women explore their needs for postpartum support.

Alert the mother, spouse/partner, and other family members to the possibility of postpartum blues in the early days after birth and reassure them of the short-term nature of the condition. Describe the symptoms of postpartum depression and encourage the mother to call her healthcare provider if symptoms become severe, if they fail to subside quickly, or if at any time she feels she is unable to function. Encouraging the mother to plan how she will manage at home and providing concrete suggestions on how to cope will aid in her adjustment to motherhood. Table 31–9 provides suggestions that serve as primary prevention measures for postpartum depression.

Information, emotional support, and assistance in providing or obtaining care for the infant may be needed. Assist family members by identifying community resources, making referrals to public health nursing services and social services, and providing a list of telephone numbers as well as emergency services that they may need. Postpartum follow-up is especially important, as well as visits from a psychiatric home health nurse.

Table 31–9	Primary Prevention Strategies for Postpartum Depression
1. Celebrate childbirth but appreciate that it is a life-changing transition that can be stressful—at times it can seem overwhelming. Share your feelings with each other and/or others.	
2. Consider keeping a journal in which you write down feelings. Not only is it emotionally cathartic, it provides a great memory book.	
3. Appreciate that you do not have to know everything to be a good parent—it is okay to seek advice during this transition.	
4. Connect with others who are parents—use them as a support and information network.	
5. Set a daily schedule and follow it even if you do not feel like it. Structuring activity helps counteract the inertia that comes with feeling sad or unsettled.	
6. Prioritize daily tasks. Decide what must be done and what can wait. Try to get one major thing done every day. Remember, you do not always have to look like a magazine fashion model.	
7. Remember that you do not have to entertain or care for everyone who drops by. Doing something for someone else, however, often tends to make you feel better.	
8. If someone volunteers to help you with tasks or baby care, take him or her up on it. While your volunteer is in action, do something pleasurable or get some rest.	
9. Maintain outside interests. Plan some time every day—even if it's just 15 minutes—to do something exclusively for "you" that is pleasurable.	
10. Eat a healthful diet. Limit alcohol. Quit smoking. Get some exercise. (All of these can positively affect the immune system.)	
11. Get as much sleep as possible. Rest whenever you can, such as when the baby is napping. If you have other young children, bring them onto your bed to read or play quietly while you lie down.	
12. Limit major changes (moves, job changes, etc.) the first year insofar as possible.	
13. Spend time with others.	
14. If things get overwhelming, and you feel yourself slipping into depression, reach out to someone for help.	
15. Attend a local postpartum support group if one is available. Consider also an international program such as Postpartum Support International.	

A diagnosis of postpartum depression or other psychiatric disorder poses major problems for the family, especially the father/partner. The symptoms of these disorders are difficult to witness and may be harder to understand than physical problems such as hemorrhage and infection. The father/partner may feel hurt by the new mother's hostility, worry that she is becoming insane, or be baffled by her mood swings and lack of concern about herself, the newborn, or household responsibilities. Certainly, he has cause for concern about how the newborn and any other children are being affected. Very real practical matters—running the household; managing the children, including the totally dependent newborn; and caring for the mother—may be added to his usual routines and work responsibilities. It is not surprising that, even in the most supportive families, relationships may suffer in response to these circumstances. It is often the father/partner or another close family member who in desperation makes contact with the healthcare agency. This is especially difficult when the mother is reluctant to admit she is suffering emotional difficulty or is too ill to recognize her own needs.

The integration of the newborn into the family and care of the newborn and other children can be further compromised by concurrent postpartum depression in fathers/partner. With both parents having depressive symptoms, the infant and other children are further at risk.

Evaluation

Expected outcomes of nursing care include the following:

- The woman's signs of depression are identified and she receives therapy quickly.
- The newborn is cared for effectively by the father or another support person until the mother is able to provide care.
- The mother and newborn will remain safe.
- The newborn is integrated into the family.

Critical Concept Review

LEARNING OUTCOME 31.1: Identify the causes, contributing factors, signs and symptoms, clinical therapy, and nursing interventions for early and late postpartum hemorrhage.

1. Thorough nursing history for any contributing factors:
   - Overdistention of uterus due to a large baby, multiple gestation, or multiparity.
   - Rapid or prolonged labor.
   - Oxytocin induction of labor.
   - C-section.
2. Nursing assessments of body systems include:
   - Frequent fundal checks and massage of fundus if bogginess is detected.
   - Frequent perineal pad checks.
   - Assessment for normal changes in lochia.
3. Signs and symptoms:
   - Postpartum hemorrhage: excessive vaginal bleeding.

4. The main causes of postpartum hemorrhage and the appropriate nursing interventions include:
   - Uterine atony: perform fundal massage and check for clots.
   - Laceration of vagina and cervix (suspect if mother is bleeding heavily in presence of firmly contracted fundus): contact physician to suture the laceration.
   - Retained placental fragments (suspect if patient is bleeding, fundus is firm and no lacerations are present): thoroughly inspect placenta.
   - Subinvolution (usually occurs 1–2 weeks after birth): provide mother with discharge instructions, including information about possible complications.
5. To prevent complications the nurse will:
   - Assess fundus for signs of bogginess.
   - Assess perineal pads for excessive bleeding.

LEARNING OUTCOME 31.2: Explain the causes, contributing factors, signs and symptoms, clinical therapy, and nursing interventions for reproductive tract infection.

1. Thorough nursing history for causes and contributing factors for reproductive tract infection:
   - C-section.
   - Prolonged labor preceding C-section.
   - Prolonged premature rupture of the amniotic membranes.
   - Oxytocin induction of labor.
   - Chorioamnionitis.
   - Obstetric trauma: episiotomy laceration of perineum, vagina, or cervix.
   - Multiple vaginal exams.

2. Nursing assessments of body systems include:
   - Temperature elevation.
   - Assessment for abnormal changes in lochia.
   - Inspection of the perineum, all incisions.

3. Signs and symptoms:
   - Temperature of 38°C (100.4°F) or higher, with temperature occurring on any 2 of the first 10 postpartum days; exclusive of the first 24 hr.
   - Foul, bloody discharge from vagina or incision.
   - Uterine tenderness
   - Chills, malaise, lethargy, subinvolution of the uterus
   - Lack of wound healing (REEDA).

4. To prevent postpartum reproductive tract infections, the nurse will:
   - Assess incisions for signs of infection.
   - Implement standard precautions; aseptic technique during labor, birth, and postpartum period.
   - Use good hand-washing techniques to prevent transmission of infective material.
   - Provide clear instructions about wound care.
   - Administer antibiotics.
   - Address comfort needs related to hygiene, positioning, oral hygiene, and pain.
   - Review *Nursing Care Plan: The Woman with a Puerperal Perineal Wound Infection* beginning on page 788.

LEARNING OUTCOME 31.3: Develop a nursing care plan that reflects knowledge of etiology, pathophysiology, clinical therapy, and nursing and preventive management for the woman experiencing urinary tract infection, mastitis, or a postpartum psychiatric disorder.

1. Thorough nursing history for any predisposing factors for these postpartum complications:
   - Mastitis.
   - Depression.
   - Urinary catheterization.
2. Nursing assessments of body systems include:
   - Prevention of overdistention of the bladder.
   - Frequent vital sign assessments.
   - Inspection of the breasts and nipples each shift.
   - Assessment for signs of postpartum "blues" or depression.
3. Signs and symptoms:
   - Infection: burning during urination, redness and pain in the breast about fourth postpartum week.
   - Postpartum depression: feelings of overwhelming sadness and lack of desire to care for infant.

4. To prevent these postpartum complications, the nurse will:
   - Assess bladder for signs of distention and encourage woman to void frequently.
   - Assess breasts for cracking, plugged ducts, and signs of mastitis. Teach mother proper latching-on techniques and breast care.
   - Assess woman for signs of depression.
   - Assess the newborn's integration into the family.

LEARNING OUTCOME 31.4: Identify the causes, contributing factors, signs and symptoms, clinical therapy, and nursing interventions for postpartum thromboembolic disease.

1. Thorough nursing history for causes and contributing factors that increase the risk of thromboembolic disease:
   - Previous thromboembolic disease or strong personal or family history.
   - Thrombophilia, acquired or inherited (protein C and protein S deficiency).
   - Operative delivery or instrumentation.
   - Age over 35 years.
   - Obesity (BMI > 30).
   - Gross varicose veins.
2. Nursing assessments of all body systems include:
   - Frequent vital signs and peripheral pulses assessments.
   - Check CMS.
   - Assessment for Homans' sign each shift.

3. Signs and symptoms:
   - Thrombophlebitis: pain and swelling in the lower extremities.
   - Localized heat and redness.
4. To prevent thromboembolic disease, the nurse will:
   - Assess lower extremities for signs of thrombophlebitis, encourage early ambulation, and assess for pulmonary embolus.
   - Review *Nursing Care Plan: The Woman with Thromboembolic Disease* beginning on page 798.

LEARNING OUTCOME 31.5: Evaluate the woman's knowledge of healthcare promotion measures and signs of postpartum complications to be reported to the primary care provider.

1. Teaching for self care includes:
   - Knowledge of progress of involution.
   - Care of the breasts.
   - Prevention of infection.
   - Expected emotional changes.
   - Need for extra rest.
   - Nutritional needs.
   - Knowledge of dosage regimens and side effects of prescribed medication.

   - Signs and symptoms of complications:
     - Increased vaginal bleeding.
     - Fever.
     - Foul-smelling vaginal discharge.
     - Pain and/or redness in an incision.
     - Pain, redness, or swelling in the breasts and/or legs.
     - Overwhelming feelings of sadness or inability to care for infant.
2. Assess the newborn's integration into the family.

Clinical Reasoning in Action

Betty Jones, a 32-year-old G4P2012, is admitted to the postpartum unit after the precipitous birth of a preterm (35 weeks' gestation) 4-pound baby girl followed by a postpartum tubal ligation. Betty's vital signs and postpartum assessment are within normal limits. She has an abdominal dressing that is dry and intact and she is able to void. Her IV with 10 units of Pitocin is infusing well in her lower left arm. She admits to 3 on a pain scale of 10. Betty admits to active use of crack cocaine throughout her pregnancy, and smoked it most recently 5 hours before she gave birth. She is HIV positive with a CD4 count of 726 cells/mm^3 and was treated with zidovudine during the pregnancy, labor, and birth. She also has a history of genital herpes and was treated for chlamydia during the pregnancy. Her infant has been admitted to the special care nursery because of her preterm status. Betty anticipates her baby will be taken into foster care when discharged from the nursery. Wishing to establish as much of a relationship with her infant as possible before that happens, she asks if she can breastfeed the baby while she is in the hospital.

1. What is your response to Betty's request to breastfeed her infant?
2. Over the course of the first postpartum day, Betty appears lethargic and spends most of her time sleeping. After her evening visitors leave, you observe that she is highly energetic and excitable. Would urine testing be useful to help determine if Betty has used cocaine this evening?
3. Develop a concept map for infants born of mothers who are HIV positive.
4. Betty wishes for an early discharge from the hospital. What physical criteria must be met before leaving the hospital?
5. Discuss when she should contact her physician/CNM after her discharge for follow-up.

See www.nursing.pearsonhighered.com for possible responses and an interactive template for a concept map.

References

Ambrose, A., & Repke, J. T. (2011). Puerperal problems. In D. James, P. J. Steer, C. P. Weiner, B. Gonik, C. C. Crowther, & S. C. Robson (Eds.), *High risk pregnancy: Management options* (4th ed., pp. 1313–1329). St. Louis, MO: Elsevier/Saunders.

American Psychiatric Association (APA). (2013). *Diagnostic and statistical manual of mental disorders* (5th ed., text rev.). Washington, DC: Author.

Beck, C. T. (2002). Revision of the Postpartum Depression Predictors Inventory. *Journal of Obstetric, Gynecologic, and Neonatal Nursing, 31*(4), 394–402.

Beck, C. T. (2008). *Postpartum mood and anxiety disorders: Case studies, research, and nursing care* (Practice Bulletin) (2nd ed.). Washington, DC: Association of Women's Health, Obstetric and Neonatal Nurses.

Beck, C. T., Gable, R. K., Sakala, C., & Declercq, E. R. (2011). Posttraumatic stress disorder in new mothers: Results from a two-stage U.S. national survey. *Birth, 38*(3), 216–227.

Brown, H. L., & Smrtka, M. (2011). Postpartum hemorrhage: Emergency management and treatment. *The Female Patient, 36*, 16–22.

Cunningham, F. G., Leveno, K. J., Bloom, S. L., Hauth, J. C., Rouse, D. J., & Spong, C. Y. (2010). *Williams obstetrics* (23rd ed.). New York, NY: McGraw-Hill.

Duff, W. P., Sweet, R. L., & Edwards, R. K. (2009). Maternal and fetal infectious disorders. In R. K. Creasy & R. Resnik (Eds.), *Maternal–fetal medicine: Principles and practice* (6th ed., pp. 739–796). Philadelphia, PA: Saunders.

Gilbert, E. S. (2011). *Manual of high risk pregnancy and delivery* (5th ed.). St. Louis, MO: Elsevier/Mosby.

Glavin, K., Smith, L., Sorum, R., & Ellefsen, B. (2010). Redesigned community postpartum care to prevent and treat postpartum depression in women—A one-year follow-up study. *Journal of Clinical Nursing, 19*(21/22), 3051–3062.

Harvey, C. J., & Dildy, G. A. (2013). Obstetric hemorrhage. In N. H. Troiano, C. J. Harvey, & B. F. Chez (Eds.), *AWHONN's high-risk & critical care obstetrics* (3rd ed., pp. 246–273). Philadelphia, PA: Lippincott.

Katz, V. L. (2012). Postpartum care. In S. G. Gabbe, J. R. Niebyl, J. L. Simpson, M. B. Landon, H. L. Galan, E. R. M. Jauniaux, & D. A. Driscoll (Eds.). *Obstetrics: Normal and problem pregnancies* (6th ed., pp. 517–532). St. Louis, MO: Elsevier.

Lawrence, R. A., & Lawrence, R. M. (2005). Breastfeeding: *A guide for the medical profession* (6th ed.). Philadelphia, PA: Elsevier Mosby.

Newton, E. R. (2012). Lactation and breastfeeding. In S. G. Gabbe, J. R Niebyl, J. L. Simpson, M. B. Landon, H. L. Galan, E. R. M. Jauniaux, & D. A. Driscoll (Eds.). *Obstetrics: Normal and problem pregnancies* (6th ed., pp. 533–564). St. Louis, MO: Elsevier.

Pessel, C., & Tsai, M. C. (2013). The normal puerperium. In A. H. DeCherney, L. Nathan, N. Laufer, & A. S. Roman (Eds.), *Current diagnosis & treatment: Obstetrics & gynecology* (11th ed., pp.190–213). New York, NY: McGraw-Hill.

Pettker, C. M., & Lockwood, C. J. (2012). Thromboembolic disorders. In S. G. Gabbe, J. R Niebyl, J. L. Simpson, M. B. Landon, H. L. Galan, E. R. M. Jauniaux, & D. A. Driscoll (Eds.). *Obstetrics: Normal and problem pregnancies* (6th ed., pp. 980–993). St. Louis, MO: Elsevier.

Poggi, S. B. H. (2013). Postpartum hemorrhage & the abnormal puerperium. In A. H. DeCherney, L. Nathan, N. Laufer, & A. S. Roman (Eds.), *Current diagnosis & treatment: Obstetrics & gynecology* (11th ed., pp. 349–368). New York, NY: McGraw-Hill.

Riordan, J., & Wambach, K. (2010). *Breastfeeding and human lactation* (4th ed.). Sudbury, MA: Jones & Bartlett.

Thurman, A. R. (2010). Post-cesarean delivery infectious morbidity: Focus on preoperative antibiotics and methicillin-resistant Staphylococcus aureus. *American Journal of Infection Control, 38*, 612–616.

Van Dinter, M. C., & Graves, L. (2012). Managing adverse birth outcomes: Helping patients and families cope. *American Family Physician, 85*(9), 900–904.

Vidaeff, A. C., & Ramin, S. M. (2011). Renal disorders. In D. James, P. J. Steer, C. P. Weiner, B. Gonik, C. C. Crowther, & S. C. Robson (Eds.), *High risk pregnancy: Management options* (4th ed., pp. 893–915). St. Louis, MO: Elsevier/Saunders.

Wisner, K. L., Sit, D. K. Y., Altemus, M., Bogen, D. L., Famy, C. S., Pearlstein, T. B., . . . Perel, J. M. (2012). Mental health and behavioral disorders in pregnancy. In S. G. Gabbe, J. R Niebyl, J. L. Simpson, M. B. Landon, H. L. Galan, E. R. M. Jauniaux, & D. A. Driscoll (Eds.), *Obstetrics: Normal and problem pregnancies* (6th ed., pp. 1156–1188). St. Louis, MO: Elsevier/Saunders.

Witcher, P. M., & Hamner, L. (2013). Venous thromboembolism in pregnancy. In N. H. Troiano, C. J. Harvey, & B. F. Chez (Eds.), *AWHONN's high-risk & critical care obstetrics* (3rd ed., pp. 285–301). Philadelphia, PA: Lippincott.

CHAPTER
32

Growth and Development

We want to help our adopted daughter Irena grow into a healthy and special child. She had challenges in her short life in Romania that we can only imagine. We worry about how we can help her grow and develop. —Mother of Irena, 2

LEARNING OUTCOMES

32.1 Describe the major theories of development as formulated by Freud, Erikson, Piaget, Kohlberg, social learning theorists, and behaviorists.

32.2 Recognize risks to developmental progression and factors that protect against those risks.

32.3 Plan nursing interventions for children that are appropriate for each child's developmental state, based on theoretical frameworks.

32.4 Explain contemporary developmental approaches such as temperament theory, ecologic theory, and the resilience framework.

32.5 Identify major developmental milestones for infants, toddlers, preschoolers, school-age children, and adolescents.

32.6 Synthesize information from several theoretical approaches to plan assessments of the child's physical growth and developmental milestones.

32.7 Describe the role of play in the growth and development of children.

32.8 Use data collected during developmental assessments to implement activities that promote development of children and adolescents.

Children develop as they interact with their surroundings. They learn skills at different ages, but the order in which they learn them is universal. Development is affected by factors such as nutrition and cultural practices, as well as the social situation in the country or neighborhood. While each child will develop in a unique manner influenced by genetic makeup, life experiences, and the interactions among these factors, certain principles of development assist parents and the nurse in fostering positive adaptations for the child.

This chapter covers general principles of growth and development and explores several theories related to childhood development, as well as their nursing applications. Each age group, from infancy through adolescence, is described in detail. Developmental milestones, physical and cognitive characteristics, play patterns, and communication strategies are presented, as are conditions that interfere with usual developmental progression. The information provided helps guide developmentally appropriate care for children in each age group and in a variety of situations. These concepts can be applied when caring for all children, including those in special situations.

PRINCIPLES OF GROWTH AND DEVELOPMENT

It is essential to understand the concepts of growth and development when learning to care for children. A skilled pediatric nurse integrates knowledge of physical growth and psychosocial development into each child healthcare encounter. **Growth** refers to an increase in physical size. Growth represents quantitative changes such as height, weight, blood pressure, and number of words in the child's vocabulary. **Development** refers to a qualitative increase in capability or function. Developmental skills, such as the ability to sit without support or to throw a ball overhand, unfold in a complex manner influenced by the relationship between the child's innate capabilities and the stimuli and support provided in the environment. The quantitative and qualitative changes in body organ functioning, ability to communicate, and performance of motor skills develop over time and are key components in the process of planning pediatric health care.

Each child displays a unique maturational pattern during the process of development. Although the exact age at which skills emerge differs, the sequence or order of skill performance is uniform among children. Skill development proceeds according to two processes: from the head downward; and from the center of the body outward.

- **Cephalocaudal development** (Figure 32–1 ●) proceeds from the head downward through the body and toward the feet. For example, at birth an infant's head is much larger proportionately than the trunk or extremities. Similarly, infants learn to hold up their heads before sitting and to sit before standing. Skills such as walking that involve the legs and feet develop last in infancy.

- **Proximodistal development** (see Figure 32–1) proceeds from the center of the body outward toward the extremities. For example, infants are first able to control the trunk, then the arms; only later are fine motor movements of the fingers possible. As the child grows, both physical and cognitive skills differentiate from general to more specific skills. Pediatric nurses use these concepts of predictable and sequential developmental direction to analyze the infant's and child's present state and to partner with parents to plan ways to encourage and support the next emerging developmental abilities.

During the childhood years, extraordinary changes occur in all aspects of development. Physical size, motor skills, cognitive ability, language, sensory ability, and psychosocial patterns all undergo major transformations. Nurses study normal patterns of development to identify children who demonstrate unexpected developmental findings. These assessments can guide the nurse in planning interventions for the child and family, such as referring the child for a diagnostic evaluation or

Cephalocaudal growth occurs from the head down.

Proximodistal growth occurs from the center of the body out.

● **Figure 32–1** Cephalocaudal and proximodistal development. In normal cephalocaudal growth, the child gains control of the head and neck before the trunk and limbs. In normal proximodistal growth, the child controls arm movements before hand movements. For example, the child reaches for objects before being able to grasp them. Children gain control of their hands before their fingers; that is, they can hold things with the entire hand before they can pick something up with just their fingers.

rehabilitation, or teaching the parents how to provide adequate stimulation for the child. Nurses use **anticipatory guidance** to predict upcoming developmental tasks or needs of a child and to perform appropriate teaching related to them. When development is proceeding normally, the nurse uses his or her knowledge of these normal patterns to provide approaches based on the child's cognitive and language ability, to offer appropriate toys and activities during illness, and to respond therapeutically

during interactions with the child. For situations with special challenges, such as in adoptions, additional interventions may be needed (see *Growth and Development*).

MAJOR THEORIES OF DEVELOPMENT

Child development is a complex process. Many theorists have attempted to organize their observations of behavior into a description of principles or a set of stages. Each theory focuses on a particular facet of development. Most developmental theorists separate children into age groups by common characteristics (Table 32–1).

Freud's Theory of Psychosexual Development
Theoretical Framework
Sigmund Freud (1856–1939) was a physician in Vienna, Austria. His work with adults experiencing a variety of neurologic disorders led him to develop an approach called psychoanalysis, which explored the driving forces of the unconscious mind. These psychoanalytic techniques led Freud to believe that early childhood experiences form the unconscious motivation for actions in later life. He believed that sexual energy is centered in specific parts of the body at certain ages. Unresolved conflict and unmet needs at a certain stage lead to a fixation of development at that stage (Craig & Dunn, 2010).

Freud viewed the personality as a structure with three parts: The *id* is the basic sexual energy that is present at birth and drives the individual to seek pleasure; the *ego* is the realistic part of the person, which develops during infancy and searches for acceptable methods of meeting impulses; and the *superego* is the moral/ethical system, which develops in childhood and contains a set of values and a conscience (Craig & Dunn, 2010). The ego diverts impulses and protects itself from excess anxiety by use of **defense mechanisms**, including regression to earlier stages

Growth and Development

About 15% of annual adoptions in the United States, or over 22,000, are international adoptions. China, South Korea, Russia, and Ethiopia are frequent countries of origin for orphans being adopted in the United States (Smit, 2010; U.S. Department of Health and Human Services, 2011). While all adoptions can be stressful for the new parents and child, international adoptions pose a unique set of circumstances that influence the child's development.

Parents need to protect themselves and others from infectious diseases when traveling to bring home a child from another country. They should consult their local health district and healthcare providers for a list of recommended immunizations for the country they are visiting. They should also obtain a list of medications and supplies to carry for themselves and the child, such as antidiarrheal medicine, decongestants, analgesics, bandages, and hand sanitizer (Children's Hospital of Philadelphia, 2012).

Parents require counseling to learn about cultural practices, language, and other differences they may encounter. Once they bring the child home, they will need support as the child grows to integrate the

child's history and culture into their family. The moment when the child meets an adoptive parent may be seen as joyous by the parent but can be traumatic for the young child, who is separated from familiar adults. Parents need preparation for establishing trust with the child (Children's Hospital of Philadelphia, 2012; Smit, 2010). Several agencies offer information to prepare new parents for their adoption experience (see www.nursing.pearsonhighered.com).

The adopted child should be examined once home for length, weight, and head circumference. If growth is delayed, continued monitoring and dietary interventions may be needed. The psychosocially based problem of eating disorder of infancy and childhood (also called failure to thrive) should also be considered. (See Chapter 33 ⊘ for a thorough discussion of this condition.) Parasitic infection and chronic diseases are possible causes of continuing growth abnormalities. Perform developmental screening to provide a baseline for future developmental observations. Frequent physical and psychosocial assessments will be needed, and teaching is provided for parents to enhance development.

Table 32–1	Developmental Age Groups	
Developmental Stage	**Age Group**	**Characteristics**
Infancy	Birth to 12 months	Includes infants or babies up to 1 year of age, all of whom require a high level of care in daily activities.
Toddlerhood	1 to 3 years	Characterized by increased motor ability and independent behavior.
Preschool	3 to 6 years	The preschooler refines gross and fine motor ability and language skills and often participates in a preschool learning program.
School age	6 to 12 years	Begins with entry into a school system and is characterized by growing intellectual skills, physical ability, and independence.
Adolescence	12 to 18 years	Begins with entry into the teen years. Mature cognitive thought, formation of identity, and influence of peers are important characteristics of adolescence.

Clinical Reasoning   International Adoption Counseling

Michael and Alyssa had tried for several years to have a biologic child. After an unsuccessful in vitro fertilization, they decided to try to adopt a child. They explored opportunities with adoption agencies and learned that international adoption would be possible for them. They adopted 2-year-old Irena from Romania several months ago. Irena appears small for her age, but she seems to be thriving in her new environment. She is learning to say a few English words and is responding appropriately to care and interactions.

Despite thorough investigation of Michael and Alyssa by the adoption agency, they received only scant information about Irena's history. They were told that she was left at an orphanage by her birth mother when she was about 7 months old; the birth mother stated that the pregnancy and birth were normal. According to reports, the birth mother had decided to relinquish the child because she had two older children to care for and her husband had left home nearly a year before and had not been heard from since.

How can you work with Michael and Alyssa to ensure special attention to Irena's growth and healthcare needs, such as physical growth, language, and social skills? Consider both assessment and planned interventions.

What will Irena's cultural needs be as she grows older? How can Michael and Alyssa prepare to tell her about her adoption and background someday?

See www.nursing.personhighered.com for possible responses.

and repression or forgetting of painful experiences such as child abuse (Table 32–2).

Stages

Oral (Birth to 1 Year).   The infant derives pleasure largely from the mouth, with sucking and eating as primary desires.

Anal (1 to 3 Years).   The young child's pleasure is centered in the anal area, with control over body secretions as a prime force in behavior.

Table 32–2	Common Defense Mechanisms Used by Children	
Defense Mechanism	**Definition**	**Example**
Regression	Return to an earlier behavior	A previously toilet trained child becomes incontinent when a new infant is born into the family.
Repression	Involuntary forgetting of uncomfortable situations	An abused child cannot consciously recall episodes of abuse.
Rationalization	An attempt to make unacceptable feelings acceptable	A child explains hitting another because "he took my toy."
Fantasy	A creation of the mind to help deal with unacceptable fear	A hospitalized child who is weak pretends to be Superman.

Phallic (3 to 6 Years).   Sexual energy becomes centered in the genitalia as the child works out relationships with parents of the same and opposite sexes.

Latency (6 to 12 Years).   Sexual energy is at rest in the passage between earlier stages and adolescence.

Genital (12 Years to Adulthood).   Mature sexuality is achieved as physical growth is completed and relationships with others occur.

Nursing Application

Freud emphasized the importance of meeting the needs of each stage in order to move successfully into future developmental stages. The crisis of illness can interfere with normal developmental processes and add challenges for the nurse striving to meet an ill child's needs. For example, the importance of sucking in infancy guides the nurse to provide a pacifier for the infant who cannot have oral fluids. The preschool child's concern about sexuality guides the nurse to provide privacy and clear explanations during any procedures involving the genital area. It may be necessary to teach parents that masturbation by the young child is normal and to help parents deal with it through distraction or refocusing. The adolescent's focus on relationships suggests that the nurse should include questions about significant friends during history taking. Table 32–3 summarizes techniques the nurse can use to apply these theoretical concepts to the care of children.

Age Group	Theorist/Developmental Stage	Characteristics of Stage	Nursing Applications
Infant (birth to 1 year)	Freud: Oral stage.	The baby obtains pleasure and comfort through the mouth.	When a baby is not able to take foods or fluids, offer a pacifier if not contraindicated. After painful procedures, offer a baby a bottle or pacifier or have the mother breastfeed.
	Erikson: Trust versus mistrust stage.	The baby establishes a sense of trust when basic needs are met.	Hold the hospitalized baby often. Offer comfort after painful procedures. Meet the baby's needs for food and hygiene. Encourage parents to room in. Manage pain effectively with use of pain medications and other measures.
	Piaget: Sensorimotor stage.	The baby learns from movement and sensory input.	Use crib mobiles, manipulative toys, wall murals, and bright colors to provide interesting stimuli and comfort. Use toys to distract the baby during procedures and assessments.
Toddler (1–3 years)	Freud: Anal stage.	The child derives gratification from control over body excretions.	Ask about toilet training and the child's rituals and words for elimination during admission history. Continue child's normal patterns of elimination in the hospital. Do not begin toilet training during illness or hospitalization. Accept regression in toileting during illness or hospitalization. Have potty chairs available in hospital and childcare centers.
	Erikson: Autonomy versus shame and doubt stage.	The child is increasingly independent in many spheres of life.	Allow self-feeding opportunities. Encourage child to remove and put on own clothes, brush teeth, or assist with hygiene. (A) If immobilization for a procedure is necessary, proceed quickly, providing explanations and comfort.
	Piaget: Sensorimotor stage (end); preoperational stage (beginning).	The child shows increasing curiosity and explorative behavior. Language skills improve.	Ensure safe surroundings to allow opportunities to manipulate objects. Name objects and give simple explanations.
Preschooler (3–6 years)	Freud: Phallic stage.	The child initially identifies with the parent of the opposite sex but by the end of this stage identifies with the same-sex parent.	Be alert for children who appear more comfortable with male or female nurses, and attempt to accommodate them. Encourage parental involvement in care. Plan for playtime and offer a variety of materials from which to choose.
	Erikson: Initiative versus guilt stage.	The child likes to initiate play activities.	Offer medical equipment for play to lessen anxiety about strange objects. (B) Assess children's concerns as expressed through their drawings. Accept the child's choices and expressions of feelings.

A

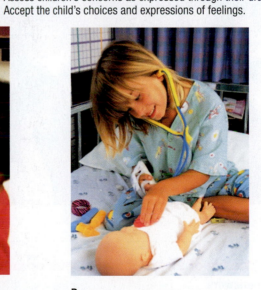

B

(continued)

Table 32–3	Nursing Applications of Theories of Freud, Erikson, and Piaget—continued		
Age Group	**Theorist/Developmental Stage**	**Characteristics of Stage**	**Nursing Applications**
	Piaget: Preoperational stage.	The child is increasingly verbal but has some limitations in thought processes. Causality is often confused, so the child may feel responsible for causing an illness.	Offer explanations about all procedures and treatments. Clearly explain that the child is not responsible for causing an illness in self or family member.
School age (6–12 years)	Freud: Latency stage.	The child places importance on privacy and understanding the body.	Provide gowns, covers, and underwear. Knock on door before entering. Explain treatments and procedures.
	Erikson: Industry versus inferiority stage.	The child gains a sense of self-worth from involvement in activities.	Encourage the child to continue schoolwork while hospitalized. Encourage the child to bring favorite pastimes to the hospital. (*C*) Help the child adjust to limitations on favorite activities.
	Piaget: Concrete operational stage.	The child is capable of mature thought when allowed to manipulate and see objects.	Give clear instructions about details of treatment. Show the child equipment that will be used in treatment.
Adolescent (12–18 years)	Freud: Genital stage.	The adolescent's focus is on genital function and relationships.	Ensure access to gynecologic care for adolescent females and testicular examinations for adolescent males. Provide information on sexuality. Ensure privacy during health care. Have brochures and videos available for teaching about sexuality.
	Erikson: Identity versus role confusion stage.	The adolescent's search for self-identity leads to independence from parents and reliance on peers.	Provide a separate recreation room for teens who are hospitalized. (*D*) Take health history and perform examinations without parents present. Introduce adolescent to other teens with same health problem.
	Piaget: Formal operational stage.	The adolescent is capable of mature, abstract thought.	Give clear and complete information about health care and treatments. Offer both written and verbal instructions. Continue to provide education about the disease to the adolescent with a chronic illness, as mature thought now leads to greater understanding.

C

D

Erikson's Theory of Psychosocial Development

Theoretical Framework

Erik Erikson (1902–1994) studied Freud's theory of psychoanalysis under Freud's daughter, Anna. He later established his own developmental theory, which describes psychosocial stages during eight periods of human life. Five of Erikson's eight stages apply to children and are described below. For each stage, Erikson identified a crisis, that is, a particular challenge that exists for healthy personality development to occur (Erikson, 1963, 1968). The word "crisis" in this context refers to normal maturational social needs rather than to a single critical event. Each developmental crisis has two possible outcomes. When needs are met, the consequence is healthy and the individual moves on to future stages with particular strengths. When needs are not met, an unhealthy outcome occurs that will influence future social relationships.

Stages

Trust Versus Mistrust (Birth to 1 Year).   The task of the first year of life is to establish trust in the people providing care. Trust is fostered by provision of food, clean clothing, touch, and comfort. If basic needs are not met, the infant will eventually learn to mistrust others.

Autonomy Versus Shame and Doubt (1 to 3 Years).   The toddler's sense of autonomy or independence is shown by controlling body excretions, saying no when asked to do something, and directing motor activity and play. Children who are consistently criticized for expressions of autonomy or for lack of control—for example, during toilet training—will develop a sense of shame about themselves and doubt in their abilities.

Initiative Versus Guilt (3 to 6 Years).   The young child initiates new activities and considers new ideas. This interest in exploring the world creates a child who is involved and busy. Constant criticism, on the other hand, leads to feelings of guilt and a lack of purpose.

Industry Versus Inferiority (6 to 12 Years).   The middle years of childhood are characterized by development of new interests and by involvement in activities. The child takes pride in accomplishments in sports, school, home, and community. If the child cannot accomplish what is expected, however, the result will be a sense of inferiority.

Identity Versus Role Confusion (12 to 18 Years).   In adolescence, as the body matures and thought processes become more complex, a new sense of identity or self is established. The self, family, peer group, and community are all examined and redefined. The adolescent who is unable to establish a meaningful definition of self will experience confusion in one or more roles of life.

Nursing Application

Erikson's theory is directly applicable to the nursing care of children. Health promotion and health maintenance visits in the community provide opportunities for helping caregivers meet children's needs. Parents benefit from learning what the child's developmental tasks are at each stage and from discussing ideas about how to encourage healthy psychosocial development. Such discussions also may highlight parental concerns and provide a forum for reassurance about normal developmental characteristics, such as a child who does not follow through on each activity as a preschooler or tries different hairstyles each month as an adolescent.

The child's usual support from family, peers, and others is interrupted by hospitalization. The challenge of hospitalization also adds a situational crisis to the normal developmental crisis a child is experiencing. Although the nurse may meet many of the hospitalized child's needs, continued parental involvement is necessary both during and after hospitalization to ensure progression through expected developmental stages (see Table 32–3).

Piaget's Theory of Cognitive Development

Theoretical Framework

Jean Piaget (1896–1980) was a Swiss scientist who wrote detailed observations of the behavior of his own and other children. Based on these observations, Piaget formulated a theory of cognitive (or intellectual) development. He believed that the child's view of the world is influenced largely by age and maturational ability. Given nurturing experiences, the child's ability to think matures naturally (Ginsberg & Opper, 1988; Piaget, 1972). The child incorporates new experiences via **assimilation** and changes to deal with these experiences by the process of **accommodation**. An example of assimilation occurs when the infant uses reflexes to suck on objects that touch the lips. With more experience the infant accommodates to learn that not all objects are pleasant to suck and cognitive structures change to integrate and learn from the experiences.

Stages

Sensorimotor (Birth to 2 Years).   Infants learn about the world by input obtained through the senses and by their motor activity. Six substages are characteristic of this stage.

Use of reflexes (birth to 1 month).   The infant begins life with a set of reflexes such as sucking, rooting, and grasping. By using these reflexes, the infant receives stimulation via touch, sound, smell, and vision. The reflexes thus pave the way for the first learning to occur.

Primary circular reactions (1 to 4 months).   Once the infant responds reflexively, the pleasure gained from that response causes repetition of the behavior. For example, if a toy grasped reflexively makes noise and is interesting to look at, the infant will grasp it again.

Secondary circular reactions (4 to 8 months).   Awareness of the environment grows as the infant begins to connect cause and effect. The sounds of bottle preparation will lead to excited behavior. If an object is partially hidden, the infant will attempt to uncover and retrieve it.

Coordination of secondary schemes (8 to 12 months).   Intentional behavior is observed as the infant uses learned behavior to obtain objects, create sounds, or engage in other pleasurable activity. **Object permanence** (the knowledge that something continues to exist even when out of sight) begins when the infant remembers where a hidden object is likely to be found; it is no longer "out of sight, out of mind." The concept of object permanence is not fully developed, however. The infant knows the parent well, objects to new people, and seems very worried when the parent leaves. Other caretakers may be rejected because the infant does not understand that the parent will return. This phase of "stranger anxiety" is quite common and heralds the infant's growing recognition of and desire to be cared for by the parent.

Tertiary circular reactions (12 to 18 months).   Curiosity, experimentation, and exploration dominate as the toddler tries out actions to learn results. The child turns objects in every direction, places them in the mouth, uses them for banging, and inserts them in containers as he or she explores their qualities and uses.

Mental combinations (18 to 24 months). Language provides a new tool for the toddler to use in understanding the world. Language enables the child to think about events and objects before or after they occur. Object permanence is now fully developed as the child actively searches for objects in various locations and out of view. The child who has had successful separations from the parents followed by return, such as hours spent in another's home or childcare center, begins to understand that the missing parent will return.

Preoperational (2 to 7 Years).
The young child thinks by using words as symbols, but logic is not well developed.

Preconceptual substage. During the preconceptual substage (2 to 4 years), vocabulary and comprehension increase greatly but the child is egocentric (that is, unable to see things from the perspective of another).

Intuitive substage. In the intuitive substage (4 to 7 years), the child relies on transductive reasoning (drawing conclusions from one general fact to another). For example, when a child disobeys a parent and then falls and breaks an arm that day, the child may ascribe the broken arm to bad behavior. Cause-and-effect relationships are often unrealistic or a result of magical thinking (the belief that events occur because of thoughts or wishes).

Additional characteristics noted in the thought of preschoolers include centration, or the ability to consider only one aspect of a situation at a time, and animism, or giving life to inanimate objects because they move, make noise, or have certain other qualities.

Concrete Operational (7 to 11 Years).
Transductive reasoning has given way to a more accurate understanding of cause and effect. The child can reason quite well if concrete objects are used in teaching or experimentation. The concept of conservation (that matter does not change when its form is altered) is learned at this age.

Formal Operational (11 Years to Adulthood).
Fully mature intellectual thought has now been attained. The adolescent can think abstractly about objects or concepts and consider different alternatives or outcomes.

Nursing Application
Piaget's theory is essential to pediatric nursing. The nurse must understand a child's thought processes in order to design stimulating activities and meaningful, appropriate teaching plans. What activities could be planned for a hospitalized child based on his or her expected cognitive level? How can cognitive development be encouraged in a school-age child receiving home health services? Understanding a child's concept of time suggests how far in advance to prepare that child for procedures. Similarly, decisions about offering manipulative toys, reading stories, drawing pictures, or giving the child reading material to explain healthcare measures depend on the child's cognitive stage of development (see Table 32–3).

Kohlberg's Theory of Moral Development
Theoretical Framework
Lawrence Kohlberg (1927–1987) was a German theorist who used Piaget's cognitive theory as a basis for his theory of moral development. He presented stories involving moral dilemmas to children and adults and asked them to solve the dilemmas. Kohlberg then analyzed the motives they expressed when making decisions about the best course to take. Based on the explanations given, Kohlberg established three levels of moral reasoning. Although he provided age guidelines, he stated that they are approximate and that many people never reach the highest (postconventional) stage of development (Santrock, 2011).

Stages
Preconventional (4 to 7 Years).
Decisions are based on the desire to please others and to avoid punishment.

Conventional (7 to 12 Years).
Conscience, or an internal set of standards, becomes important. Rules are important and must be followed to please other people and "be good."

Postconventional (12 Years and Older).
The individual has internalized ethical standards on which to base decisions. Social responsibility is recognized. The value in each of two differing moral approaches can be considered and a decision made.

Nursing Application
Decision making is required in many areas of health care. Children can be assisted to make decisions about health care and to consider alternatives when available. Keep in mind that young children may agree to participate in research simply because they want to comply with adults and appear cooperative. Guidelines for child participation in research are available (see Chapter 1).

Parents can be provided with information so that they can assist their children in moral judgments. Encourage talking with a child or adolescent about how a particular decision was made. Parents can then add information and help the child learn to integrate more factors into decision making. Talking about the process is important in helping children progress to higher moral development stages. Focusing on the feelings of others, using positive discipline techniques, and clearly identifying positive and negative behaviors are important.

Social Learning Theory
Theoretical Framework
Originally from Canada, psychologist Albert Bandura (1925–) has conducted research at Stanford University for many years. He believes that children learn attitudes, beliefs, customs, and values through their social contacts with adults and other children. Children imitate (or model) the behavior they see; if the behavior is positively reinforced, they tend to repeat it. The external environment and the child's internal processes are key elements in social learning theory (Bandura, 1986, 1997a).

Bandura believes that an important determinant of behavior is self-efficacy, or the expectation that someone can produce a desired outcome. For example, if adolescents believe they can avoid use of drugs or alcohol, they are more likely to do so. A child who has confidence in his or her ability to exercise regularly or

Evidence-Based Practice Concept of Self-Efficacy

Clinical Question

How can nurses use the concept of self-efficacy when planning interventions for children and families?

The Evidence

Parental self-efficacy is the belief that parents can manage a range of tasks and situations in caring for their children. Parents with higher self-efficacy scores were significantly more likely to manage conduct problems of their adolescents successfully, and their adolescents displayed fewer behavioral problems than adolescents of parents with lower parental self-efficacy. This study was carried out with Mexican American families, demonstrating the cross-cultural applicability of the concept of self-efficacy (Dumka, Gonzalez, Wheeler, et al., 2010).

Mothers who have a greater degree of self-efficacy about ability to breastfeed are significantly more likely to begin and to continue breastfeeding. A Breastfeeding Self-Efficacy Scale has been developed to identify risk and protective factors that influence the self-efficacy of new mothers. A network of support for breastfeeding is important, and evaluating breastfeeding self-efficacy can identify women at risk for early discontinuation of breastfeeding (McCarter-Spaulding & Dennis, 2010).

An intervention with over 1000 students in grades 5 and 6 was effective in increasing self-efficacy regarding television viewing time and decreasing television viewing time (Salmon, Jorna, Hume, et al., 2011).

Best Practice

In addition to providing information about health behaviors, nurses need to integrate methods to increase self-efficacy in teaching projects with families. Assessments should be designed to identify self-efficacy of parents and children around health topics of interest. When planning interventions to encourage health behaviors in children and adolescents, assess the youth's beliefs that the new behaviors are important and that they can be adopted. Include interventions that demonstrate that others have adopted the health behaviors and plan approaches to enhance the child's belief in ability to change.

Clinical Reasoning

Plan a teaching project about the importance of physical activity and healthy eating for presentation to a group of 12-year-olds. What approaches will enhance the self-efficacy of the children? How would interventions to enhance self-efficacy differ for young elementary-school children from those in middle or high school? What theoretical approaches discussed earlier in this chapter help you to understand the cognitive abilities of children at various ages and suggest ways to influence their self-efficacy?

---

lose weight has a greater chance of success with these behavior changes. Parents who have confidence in their ability to care adequately for their infants are more likely to do so (Bandura, 1997b). See *Evidence-Based Practice: Concept of Self-Efficacy* for further examples of application of the concept of self-efficacy.

Nursing Application

The importance of modeling behavior can readily be applied in health care. Children are more likely to cooperate if they see adults or other children performing a task willingly. A frightened child may watch another child perform vision screening or have blood drawn and then decide to allow the procedure to take place. Contact with positive role models is useful when teaching children and adolescents self-care for chronic diseases such as diabetes. Give positive reinforcement for desired performance.

Nurses can use the concept of self-efficacy to increase the chance of success with lifestyle behavior changes. For example, encouraging youth who are trying to quit smoking, providing them with role models, and pointing out parental successes with their children all demonstrate methods of fostering self-efficacy.

Behaviorism

Theoretical Framework

John Watson (1878–1958) was an American scientist who applied the research of animal behaviorists like Pavlov and Skinner to children. Pavlov and, later, Skinner worked with animals, presenting a stimulus such as food and pairing it with another stimulus such as a ringing bell. Eventually the animal being fed began to salivate when the bell rang. As Skinner and then Watson began to apply these concepts to children, they showed that

behaviors can be elicited by positive reinforcement, such as a food treat, or extinguished by negative reinforcement, such as scolding or withdrawal of attention. Watson believed that he could make a child into anyone he desired—from a professional to a thief or beggar—simply by reinforcing behavior in certain ways (Santrock, 2011).

Nursing Application

Behaviorism has been criticized for being simplistic and for its denial of people's inherent capacity to respond willfully to events in the environment. This theory does, however, have some use in health care. When particular behaviors are desired, health-care providers can establish positive reinforcement to encourage these behaviors. Using behavioral techniques, nurses may influence the behavior of children by giving a sticker to a child after a physical examination or blood draw. Parents often use reinforcement in toilet training and other skills learned in childhood.

Ecologic Theory

Theoretical Framework

There is controversy among theorists concerning the relative importance of heredity versus environment—or nature versus nurture—in human development. **Nature** refers to the genetic or hereditary capability of an individual. **Nurture** refers to the effects of the environment on a person's performance (Figure 32–2 ●). Piaget believed in the importance of internal cognitive structures that unfold at their appointed times, given any environment that provides basic opportunities. He emphasized the strength of nature. The behaviorist John Watson, on the other hand, believed that behaviors are primarily shaped by environmental responses;

● **Figure 32–2** An example of nurturing. Children exposed to pleasant stimulation and who are supported by an adult will develop and refine their skills faster. Group activities such as these provide an opportunity for both motor skill and psychosocial development. Can you identify which skills are being developed?

he thus stressed the predominance of nurture. Contemporary developmental theories increasingly recognize the interaction of nature and nurture in determining the child's development.

Urie Bronfenbrenner (1917–2005), a professor at Cornell University, formulated the ecologic theory of development to explain the unique relationship of the child with all of life's experiences or systems (Bronfenbrenner, 1986, 2005; Bronfenbrenner, McClelland, Ceci, et al., 1996). **Ecologic theory** emphasizes the presence of mutual interactions between the child and these various settings or systems. Neither nature nor nurture is considered of more importance. Bronfenbrenner believed each child brings a unique set of genes—as well as specific attributes such as age, gender, health, and other characteristics—to his or her interactions with the environment. The child then interacts in many settings at different levels or systems (Figure 32–3 ●).

Levels/Systems

Microsystem.   This level is defined as the daily, consistent, close relationships such as home, child care, school, friends, and neighbors. For the child with a chronic illness requiring regular care, the healthcare providers may even be part of the microsystem. In the ecologic model, the child influences each of the settings in the microsystem, in addition to being influenced by them, with reciprocal interactions.

Mesosystem.   This level includes relationships of microsystems with one another. For example, two microsystems for most children are the home and the school. The relationships between these microsystems are shown by parents' involvement in their children's school. This involvement, in turn, influences the effects of the home and school settings on the children.

Exosystem.   This level is composed of those settings that influence the child even though the child is not in close daily contact with the system. Examples include the parents' jobs and the governing board of the local school district. Although the child may not go to the parents' workplaces, he or she can be influenced by policies related to health care, sick leave, inflexible work hours, overtime, or travel, or even by the mood of the boss (through its impact on the parent). Likewise, when a local school board votes to ban certain books or to finance a field trip, the child is influenced by these decisions; the child, in turn, can help establish an atmosphere that will guide future school board decisions.

Macrosystem.   This level includes the beliefs, values, and behaviors expressed in the child's environment. Culture is a powerful influence in the macrosystem, as is the political system. For instance, a democratic system creates different beliefs, values, and even eating practices than an anarchic system.

Chronosystem.   This final level brings the perspective of time to the previous settings. The time period during which the child grows up influences views of health and illness. For example, the experiences of children with influenza in the 19th versus the 20th century were quite different. The age of the parent, child, and other family members also influences views of health.

Nursing Application

Nurses use ecologic theory when they assess the child's settings to identify influences on development. Table 32–4 provides an assessment tool based on this theory. Interventions are planned to enhance the strengths of the child's settings and to improve on areas that are not supportive.

Table 32–4   Assessment of Ecologic Systems in Childhood—Bronfenbrenner

Microsystems	Mesosystems	Exosystems	Macrosystems	Chronosystems
Parents	Parents' involvement in child care or school	Community centers	Cultural group membership	Child's and parents' ages
Significant others in close contact	Parents' involvement in community	Local political influences	Beliefs and values of group	Period in historic time
Childcare arrangements		Parents' work	Political structure	
School	Parents' relationships with significant others (e.g., grandparents, care providers)	Parents' friends and activities		
Neighborhood contacts		Social services		
Clubs		Health care		
Friends, peers	Influences of religious community (e.g., church, synagogue, mosque) or parents and school	Libraries		
Religious community (e.g., churches, synagogues, mosques)				

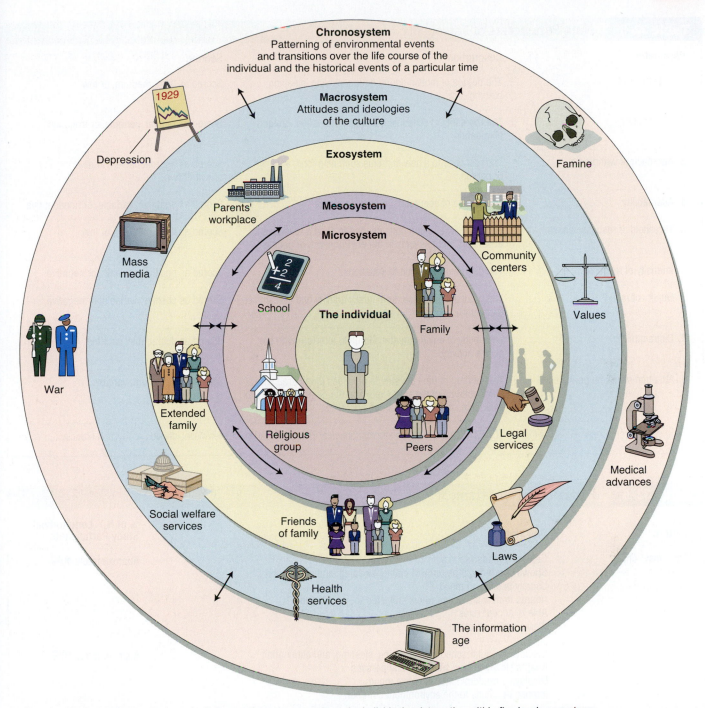

● **Figure 32–3** Bronfenbrenner's ecologic theory of development views the individual as interacting within five levels or systems.

Source: Data from Santrock, J. W. (2007). *Life span development.* Madison, WI: Brown & Benchmark. Based on Bronfenbrenner's (1979, 1986) works in Contexts of child rearing: Problems and prospects. *American Psychologist, 34,* 844–850; Ecology of the family as a context for human development: Research perspectives. *Developmental Psychology, 22,* 723–742.

Temperament Theory

Theoretical Framework

In contrast to behaviorists such as Watson or maturational theorists such as Piaget, Stella Chess and Alexander Thomas recognize the innate qualities of personality that each individual brings to the events of daily life. They, like Bronfenbrenner, believe the child is an individual who both influences and is influenced by the environment. However, Chess and Thomas focus on one specific aspect of development—the wide spectrum of behaviors possible in children—identifying nine parameters of response to daily events (Table 32–5). Their theory is based on a research study entitled the New York Longitudinal Study, which began with infants in 1956 and has continued into the adulthood of these participating individuals. By careful observations of responses to life events, Chess and Thomas identified characteristics of personality that provide the basis for the study on temperament. Infants generally display clusters of responses, which are classified into three major personality types (Table 32–6). Although most children do not demonstrate all behaviors described for a particular type, they usually show a grouping indicative of one personality type (Chess & Thomas, 1995, 1996, 1999).

Table 32–5	Nine Parameters of Personality	
Parameter	**Description**	**Scoring**
1. Activity level	The degree of motion during eating, playing, sleeping, bathing.	Scored as high, medium, or low.
2. Rhythmicity	The regularity of schedule maintained for sleep, hunger, elimination.	Scored as regular, variable, or irregular.
3. Approach or withdrawal	The response to a new stimulus such as a food, activity, or person.	Scored as approachable, variable, or withdrawn.
4. Adaptability	The degree of adaptation to new situations.	Scored as adaptive, variable, or nonadaptive.
5. Threshold of responsiveness	The intensity of stimulation needed to elicit a response to sensory input, objects in the environment, or people.	Scored as high, medium, or low.
6. Intensity of reaction	The degree of response to situations.	Scored as positive, variable, or negative.
7. Quality of mood	The predominant mood during daily activity and in response to stimuli.	Scored as positive, variable, or negative.
8. Distractibility	The ability of environmental stimuli to interfere with the child's activity.	Scored as distractible, variable, or nondistractible.
9. Attention span and persistence	The amount of time devoted to activities (compared with other children of the same age) and the degree of ability to stick with an activity in spite of obstacles.	Scored as persistent, variable, or nonpersistent.

Source: Data from Chess, S., & Thomas, A. (1996). *Temperament: Theory and practice.* Philadelphia, PA: Brunner/Mazel, division of Taylor & Francis.

Table 32–6	Patterns of Temperament	
Pattern	**Description**	**% of N.Y. Longitudinal Study Participants**
The "easy" child	Generally moderate in activity Shows regularity in patterns of eating, sleeping, and elimination Usually positive in mood Adapts to new situations when subjected to new stimuli Able to accept rules Works well with others	Approximately 40%
The "difficult" child	Displays irregular schedules for eating, sleeping, and elimination Adapts slowly to new situations and persons Displays a predominantly negative mood Intense reactions to the environment common	Approximately 10%
The "slow-to-warm-up"	Initial withdrawal, followed by gradual, quiet, slow interaction with the environment Adapts slowly to new situations Mild reactions to environment	Approximately 15%
Mixed	Some of each personality type's characteristics apparent	Approximately 35%

Source: Chess, S., & Thomas, A. (1995). *Temperament in clinical practice.* New York, NY: Guilford Press.

Recent research demonstrates that personality characteristics displayed during infancy are often consistent with those seen later in life. Predicting future characteristics is not possible, however, because of the complex and dynamic interaction of personality traits and environmental reactions.

Many other researchers have expanded the work of Chess and Thomas, developing assessment tools for temperament types. The concept of "goodness of fit" is an outgrowth of this theory. Goodness of fit refers to whether parents' expectations of their child's behavior are consistent with the child's temperament type. There is a "good fit" when the properties of the environment are in accord with the child's capabilities, characteristics, and style of behavior (Burney & Leerkes, 2010). For example, an infant who is very active and reacts strongly to verbal stimuli may be unable to sleep well when placed in a room with older siblings. A child who is slow to warm up may not perform well in the first few months at a new school, much to the parents' disappointment. When parents understand a child's temperament characteristics, they are better able to shape the environment to meet the child's needs.

Nursing Application

The concept of personality type or temperament is a useful one for nurses. Nurses can assess the temperament of young children and alter the environment to meet their needs. This may involve moving a hospitalized child to a single room to ensure adequate rest if the child is easily stimulated, or allowing a shy child time to become accustomed to new surroundings and equipment before beginning procedures or treatments.

Parents are often relieved to learn about temperament characteristics. They learn to appreciate their children's qualities and to adapt the environment to meet the children's needs. A burden of guilt can also be lifted from parents who feel that they are responsible for their child's actions. Parents may be taught ways to enhance goodness of fit between the child's personality and the environment (Chess & Thomas, 1999) (Table 32–7).

Resiliency Theory

Theoretical Framework

Why do some children coming from similar backgrounds have such different behavioral outcomes? The resiliency theory examines the individual's characteristics as well as the interaction of these characteristics with the environment. **Resilience** is the ability to function with healthy responses, even when faced with significant stress and adversity (Henderson, Bernard, & Sharp-Light, 2007). In this model the individual or family members experience a crisis that provides a source of stress, and the family interprets or deals with the crisis based on resources available. Families and individuals have **protective factors**, which are characteristics that provide strength and assistance in dealing with crises, and **risk factors**, which are characteristics that promote or contribute to their challenges (Daly, Shin, Thakral, et al., 2009). Risk and protective factors can be identified in children, in their families, and in their communities. (See Chapter 43 🔗 for further description of the interplay of social and environmental factors with individual characteristics.) A crisis for a young child might be a transfer to a new childcare provider. Protective factors could involve past positive experiences with new people, an "easy" temperament, and the new childcare provider's awareness of adaptation needs of young children to new experiences. Risk factors for a similar child might be repeated moves to new care providers, limited close relationships with adults, and a "slow-to-warm-up" temperament.

Once confronted by a stress or crisis, the child and family first experience the **adjustment phase**, characterized by disorganization and unsuccessful attempts at meeting the crisis. In the **adaptation phase**, the child and family meet the challenge and use resources to deal with the crisis. Adaptation may lead to increasing resilience as well when the child and family learn about new resources and inner strengths and develop the ability to deal more effectively with future crises. Components and examples are described in Table 32–8.

Nursing Application

Nurses gather information about the individual characteristics, prior life experiences, and environmental factors that

Table 32–7	Ways to Improve Goodness of Fit Between Parents and Child
Child's Behavior	**Parents' Adaptations**
Extremely active	Plan periods of active play several times a day. Have restful periods before bedtime to foster sleep.
Shy	Allow time to adapt at own pace to new people and situations.
Easily stimulated	Have quiet room for sleeping for an infant. Have quiet room for homework for a school-age child.
Short attention span	Provide projects that can be completed in a short period. Gradually encourage longer periods at activities.

Table 32–8	Components of Resiliency Model	
Component	**Example**	
Internal risk/protective factors	Health	
	Developmental level	
	Genetic traits	
	Temperament	
	Coping ability	
External risk/protective factors	Family members	
	Quality of relationships	
	Knowledge level	
	Environmental characteristics	
	Community services	
Interventions	Enhance knowledge	
	Minimize risk factors	
	Enhance protective factors	
	Enhance supportive resources	
	Strengthen family and community resources	

Source: Data from Daly, B. P., Shin, R. Q., Thakral, C., Selders, M., & Vera, E. (2009). School engagement among urban adolescents of color: Does perception of social support and neighborhood safety really matter? *Journal of Youth and Adolescence, 38*(1), 63–74.

Table 32–9	Assessment Questions to Determine Resilience Capability
Category	**Questions**
To determine risk factors, ask:	■ Describe the event that occurred and what it has been like for your family. ■ What other stressors do you have in your family right now? ■ Are there financial worries? ■ Are there things you think and worry about late at night? ■ Describe your job, your friends. ■ What is a typical day like? ■ Describe your neighborhood. ■ Do you have friends, people to call in emergencies?
To determine protective factors, ask:	■ What gives you strength? ■ How do you deal with this stress? ■ What do you think you do well in your family? ■ Who do you call when you need help? ■ Do you have a computer? Internet access? ■ Are you religious? Spiritual? ■ Do you exercise regularly? ■ How do you spend free time?

● **Figure 32–4** A child with fetal alcohol syndrome.

Source: © 2012—Custom Medical Stock Photo, All Rights Reserved.

act as protective and risk factors for children. Table 32–9 lists questions that can be helpful as the nurse gathers information from a child or family members. Nurses then use concepts of resiliency theory in planning interventions for children and families. Nursing strategies can target risk factors, such as encouraging gun safety in families with firearms, and by teaching about use of gun trigger locks and locked gun cabinets. In addition, protective factors can be emphasized, such as encouraging holding and verbalization to parents of infants to provide an environment that allows for trust establishment and speech development.

INFLUENCES ON DEVELOPMENT

Both nature and nurture are important in determining individual patterns of development. The interaction of these two forces can explain differences in time frames for acquisition of developmental skills, personality variations between identical twins, and other unique characteristics of individuals. Genetic and environmental factors interact and contribute to individual differences in rates and outcomes of child development.

Genetic inheritance plays an important part in the child's potential and the unfolding of developmental milestones. See Chapters 4 and 7 ✪ for a description of chromosomes and genes. Every chromosome carries many genes that determine physical characteristics, intellectual potential, personality type, and other traits. Children are born with the potential for certain features; however, their interaction with the environment influences how and to what extent particular traits are manifested.

Some Asian cultures calculate age from the time of conception. This practice acknowledges the profound influence of the prenatal period. The mother's nutrition and general state of health play a part in pregnancy outcome. Poor nutrition can lead to small infants and infants with compromised neurologic performance, slow development, or impaired immune status with resultant high disease rates. Low maternal stores of iron can result in anemia in the infant (American Academy of Pediatrics, 2009). Maternal smoking is associated with low-birth-weight infants. Ingestion of alcoholic beverages, including beer and wine, during pregnancy may lead to fetal alcohol syndrome (Figure 32–4 ●). Illicit drug use by the mother may result in neonatal addiction, convulsions, hyperirritability, poor social responsiveness, and other neurologic disturbances.

Even prescription or over-the-counter drugs may adversely affect the fetus. This was brought to general attention with the drug thalidomide, commonly used in Europe to treat nausea during the 1950s. This drug resulted in the birth of infants with limb abnormalities to women who used the drug during pregnancy. Differences in physiology related to gastric emptying, renal clearance, drug distribution, and other factors contribute to variations in pharmacokinetics during pregnancy. Drugs can cause teratogenesis (abnormal development of the fetus) or mutagenesis (permanent changes in the fetus's genetic material). See Chapter 11 ✪ for a description of the FDA's established risk categories for drugs in pregnancy.

Some maternal illnesses are harmful to the developing fetus. An example is rubella (German measles), which is rarely a serious disease for adults but can cause deafness, vision defects, heart defects, and intellectual disability in the fetus if it is acquired by a pregnant woman. A fetus can also acquire diseases such as acquired immunodeficiency syndrome (AIDS)/human immunodeficiency virus (HIV) infection or hepatitis B from the mother.

Radiation, chemicals, and other environmental hazards may adversely affect a fetus when the mother is exposed to these influences during her pregnancy. The best outcomes for infants occur when mothers eat well; exercise regularly; seek early prenatal care; refrain from use of drugs, alcohol, tobacco, and excessive caffeine; and follow general principles of good health.

As we have seen, both nature and nurture are important in determining individual patterns of development. These two forces interact in unique ways in each individual, explaining differences in time frames for acquisition of developmental skills among children, personality variations between identical twins, and other unique characteristics of individuals. An environmental factor that is extremely important in the development of children is the profile of family characteristics. The family is an important component in the lives of all children and plays an essential role in fostering the development of youth. A significant concept in families is that of parenting. How children are parented interacts with their individual characteristics to influence risk and protective factors, personality characteristics, and developmental outcomes. The families into which children are born influence them profoundly. Children are supported in different ways and acquire different worldviews depending on such factors as whether one or both parents work, how many siblings are present, and whether an extended family is close by. Note should be made of variations in family structure such as single parent, homosexual parents, extended family, and stepparents. How might a nontraditional "family" setting, such as an adoptive home with many children, influence a child's development?

Another factor that influences child development is that of culture. The traditional customs of the many cultural groups represented in North American society influence the development of the children in these groups. Foods commonly eaten vary among people with different cultural backgrounds and influence the incidence of health problems such as cardiovascular disease in these groups. The Native American practice of carrying infants on boards often delays walking when measured against the norm for walking on some developmental tests. Children who are carried by straddling the mother's hips or back for extended periods have a low incidence of developmental dysplasia of the hip since this keeps their hips in an abducted position. It is important for nurses to take cultural practices into account when performing developmental screening; some tests may not be culturally sensitive and can inaccurately label a child as delayed when the pattern of development is simply different in the group, perhaps due to childrearing practices in the family.

In addition, certain ethnic or racial groups are more prone to develop certain diseases due to genetic variations. Examples include Hispanics, who have a high incidence of diabetes; African Americans, who more commonly have sickle cell disease; and Northern European Americans, who have a higher incidence of phenylketonuria.

All cultural groups have rules regarding patterns of social interaction. Schedules of language acquisition are determined by the number of languages spoken and the amount of speech in the home. The particular social roles assumed by men and women in the culture affect school activities and ultimately career choices. Attitudes toward touching and other methods of encouraging developmental skills vary among cultures. Chapter 38 🔗 includes further description of other factors that influence child development such as school and child care, community services, and additional community and family factors.

INFANT (BIRTH TO 1 YEAR)

Imagine the experience of tripling body weight in 1 year, or becoming proficient in understanding fundamental words in a new language and even speaking a few. These and many more accomplishments take place in the first year of life. Starting the year as a mainly reflexive creature, the infant can walk and communicate by the year's end. Never again in life is development so rapid and profound.

Physical Growth and Development

The first year of life is one of rapid change for the infant. The birth weight usually doubles by about 5 months and triples by the end of the first year (Figure 32–5 ●). Height increases by about a foot during this year. Teeth begin to erupt at about 6 months, and by the end of the first year the infant has six to eight deciduous teeth (see Chapter 35 🔗). Physical growth is closely associated with type and quality of feeding. (See Chapter 33 🔗 for a discussion of nutrition in infancy.)

Body organs and systems, although not fully mature at 1 year, function differently than they did at birth. Kidney and liver

3 mo. fetus   Newborn   2 yr   5 yr   13 yr   Adult

● **Figure 32–5** Body proportions at various ages.

maturation helps the 1-year-old excrete drugs or other toxic substances more readily than in the first weeks of life. The changing body proportions mirror changes in developing internal organs. Maturation of the nervous system is demonstrated by increased control over body movements with growing differentiation from general to specific skills, thus enabling the infant to sit, stand, and walk. Sensory function also increases as the infant begins to discriminate visual images, sounds, and tastes (Table 32–10).

Table 32–10	Physical Growth and Development Milestones During Infancy			
Age	**Physical Growth**	**Fine Motor Ability**	**Gross Motor Ability**	**Sensory Ability**
Birth to 1 month	Gains 140–200 g (5–7 oz)/ week Grows 1.5 cm (1/2 in.) in first month Head circumference increases 1.5 cm (1/2 in.)/month	Holds hand in fist (A) Draws arms and legs to body when crying	Inborn reflexes such as startle and rooting are predominant activity May lift head briefly if prone (B) Alerts to high-pitched voices Comforts with touch (C)	Prefers to look at faces and black-and-white geometric designs Follows objects in line of vision (D)

A Holds hand in fist

B May lift head

C Comforts with touch

D Follows objects

| 2–4 months | Gains 140–200 g (5–7 oz)/ week
Grows 1.5 cm (1/2 in.)/month
Head circumference increases 1.5 cm (1/2 in.)/month
Posterior fontanelle closes
Ingests 120 mL/kg/24 hr (2 oz/lb/24 hr) | Holds rattle when placed in hand (E)
Looks at and plays with own fingers
Brings hands to midline | Moro reflex fading in strength
Can turn from side to back and then return (F)
Decrease in head lag when pulled to sitting position; sits with head held in midline with some bobbing
When prone, holds head and supports weight on forearms (G) | Follows objects 180 degrees
Turns head to look for voices and sounds |

E Holds rattle

F Can turn from side to back

G Holds head up and supports weight with arms

Table 32–10	Physical Growth and Development Milestones During Infancy—continued			
Age	**Physical Growth**	**Fine Motor Ability**	**Gross Motor Ability**	**Sensory Ability**
4–6 months	Gains 140–200 g (5–7 oz)/ week Doubles birth weight at 5–6 months Grows 1.5 cm (1/2 in.)/month Head circumference increases 1.5 cm (1/2 in.)/month Teeth may begin erupting by 6 months Ingests 100 mL/kg/24 hr (1 1/2 oz/lb/24 hr)	Grasps rattles and other objects at will; drops them to pick up another offered object (*H*) Mouths objects Holds feet and pulls to mouth Holds bottle Grasps with whole hand (palmar grasp) Manipulates objects (*I*)	Head held steady when sitting No head lag when pulled to sitting Turns from abdomen to back by 4 months and then back to abdomen by 6 months When held standing supports much of own weight (*J*)	Examines complex visual images Watches the course of a falling object

H Grasps objects at will

I Manipulates objects

J Supports most of weight when held standing

6–8 months	Gains 85–140 g (3–5 oz)/week Grows 1 cm (3/8 in.)/month Growth rate slower than first 6 months	Bangs objects held in hands Transfers objects from one hand to the other Beginning pincer grasp at times	Most inborn reflexes extinguished Sits alone steadily without support by 8 months (*K*) Likes to bounce on legs when held in standing position	Responds readily to sounds Recognizes own name and responds by looking and smiling Enjoys small and complex objects at play

K Sits alone without support

(continued)

Table 32–10   Physical Growth and Development Milestones During Infancy—continued

Age	Physical Growth	Fine Motor Ability	Gross Motor Ability	Sensory Ability
8–10 months	Gains 85–140 g (3–5 oz)/week Grows 1 cm (3/8 in.)/month	Picks up small objects (*L*) Uses pincer grasp well (*M*)	Crawls or pulls whole body along floor by arms (*N*) Creeps by using hands and knees to keep trunk off floor Pulls self to standing and sitting by 10 months Recovers balance when sitting	Understands words such as "no" and "cracker" May say one word in addition to "mama" and "dada"

L Picks up small objects

M Uses pincer grasp well

N Crawls or pulls body by arms

Age	Physical Growth	Fine Motor Ability	Gross Motor Ability	Sensory Ability
10–12 months	Gains 85–140 g (3–5 oz)/week Grows 1 cm (3/8 in.)/month Head circumference equals chest circumference Triples birth weight by 1 year	May hold crayon or pencil and make mark on paper Places objects into containers through holes (*O*)	Stands alone (*P*) Walks holding onto furniture Sits down from standing (*Q*)	Plays peek-a-boo and patty cake

O Places objects in container through holes

P Stands alone

Q Sits down from standing

Cognitive Development

The brain continues to increase in complexity during the first year. Most of the growth involves maturation of cells, with only a small increase in number of cells. This growth of the brain is accompanied by development of its functions. One only has to compare the behavior of an infant shortly after birth with that of a 1-year-old to understand the incredible maturation of brain function. The newborn's eyes widen in response to sound; the 1-year-old turns to the sound and recognizes its significance. The 2-month-old cries and coos; the 1-year-old says a few words and understands many more. The 6-week-old grasps a rattle for the first time; the 1-year-old reaches for toys and feeds himself or herself.

The infant's behaviors provide clues about thought processes. Piaget's work outlines the infant's actions in a set of rapidly progressing changes in the first year of life. The infant receives stimulation through sight, sound, and feeling, which the maturing brain interprets. This input from the environment interacts with internal cognitive abilities to enhance cognitive functioning.

Psychosocial Development

Play

An 8-month-old infant is sitting on the floor, grasping blocks and banging them on the floor. Infants spend much of their time engaging in **solitary play**, or playing by themselves. When a parent walks by, the infant laughs and waves hands and feet wildly. Physical capabilities enable the infant to move toward and reach out for objects of interest. Cognitive ability is reflected in manipulation of blocks to create different sounds. Social interaction enhances play. The presence of a parent or other person increases interest in surroundings and teaches the infant different ways to play.

The play of infants begins in a reflexive manner. When an infant moves extremities or grasps objects, the foundations of play are established. The feel and sound of these activities give pleasure to the infant, who gradually performs them purposefully. For example, when a parent places a rattle in the hand of a 6-week-old infant, the infant grasps it reflexively. As the hands move randomly, the rattle makes an enjoyable sound. The infant learns to move the rattle to create the sound and then finally to grasp the rattle at will to play with it.

The next phase of infant play focuses on manipulative behavior. The infant examines toys closely, looking at them, touching them, and placing them in the mouth. The infant learns a great deal about texture, qualities of objects, and all aspects of the surroundings. At the same time, interaction with others becomes an important part of play. The social nature of play is obvious as the infant plays with other children and adults.

Toward the end of the first year, the infant's ability to move in space enlarges the sphere of play (Table 32–11). Once the infant is crawling or walking, he or she can get to new places, find new toys, discover forgotten objects, or seek out other people for interaction. Play is a reflection of every aspect of development, as well as a method for enhancing learning and maturation.

Personality and Temperament

Why does one infant frequently awaken at night crying while another sleeps for 8 to 10 hours undisturbed? Why does one infant smile much of the time and react positively to interactions while another is withdrawn with unfamiliar people and frequently frowns and cries? Such differences in responses to the environment are believed to be inborn characteristics of temperament. Infants are born with a tendency to react in certain ways to noise and to interact differently with people. They may display varying degrees of regularity in activities of eating and sleeping, and manifest a capacity for concentrating on tasks for different amounts of time.

Nursing assessment identifies personality characteristics of the infant that the nurse can share with the parents. With this information the parents can appreciate more fully the uniqueness of their infant and design experiences to meet the infant's needs. Parents can learn to modify the environment to promote adaptation. For example, an infant who does not adapt easily to new situations may cry, withdraw, or develop another way of coping when adjusting to new people or places. Parents might be advised to use one or two babysitters rather than engaging new sitters frequently. If the infant is easily distracted when eating, parents can feed the infant in a quiet setting to encourage a focus on eating. Although the infant's temperament is unchanged, the ability to fit with the environment is enhanced. See Chapter 35 🔗 for further application of this information to health promotion of the infant.

Communication

Even at a few weeks of age, infants communicate and engage in two-way interaction. Comfort is expressed by soft sounds, cuddling, and eye contact. The infant displays discomfort by thrashing the extremities, arching the back, and crying vigorously. From these rudimentary skills, communication ability continues to develop until the infant speaks several words at the end of the first year of life (Table 32–11).

Nurses assess communication to identify possible abnormalities or developmental delays. Language ability may be assessed with the Denver II Developmental Test and other specialized language screening tools (see Chapters 35 and 36 🔗). Normal infants understand (receptive speech) more words than they can speak (expressive speech). Abnormalities may be caused by a hearing deficit, developmental delay, or lack of verbal stimulation from caretakers. Further assessment may be required to pinpoint the cause of the abnormality.

Nursing interventions focus on providing a stimulating environment. Encourage parents to speak to infants and teach words. Hospital nurses should include the infant's known words when providing care.

Complementary Care Infant Massage

Infant massage is a technique for communicating with and soothing infants. This technique has been used in many cultures throughout history, but it is not traditional within most families in the United States. It has many benefits for both infants and parents and can be taught to families who are interested. Some of the benefits for infants include improved sleep, soothability, decreased stress hormones, and positive parent–child interaction. Premature infants are particularly benefited by this intervention, with positive weight gain and decreased heart rate variability observed. Massage periods of 10 to 15 minutes daily can be encouraged and facilitated. Such episodes will enhance bonding and attachment between parents and infant.

Source: Field, T., Diego, M., & Hernandez-Reif, M. (2010). Preterm infant massage therapy research: A review. *Infant Behavior and Development, 33,* 115–124; McGrath, J. M. (2009). Touch and massage in the newborn period. *Journal of Perinatal & Neonatal Nursing, 23,* 304–306; Smith, S. L., Lux, R., Haley, S., Slater, H., Beechy, J., & Moyer-Mileur, L. J. (2012). The effect of massage on heart rate variability in preterm infants. *Journal of Perinatology.* doi:10.1038/jp.2012.47.

Table 32–11	Psychosocial Development During Infancy	
Age	Play and Toys	Communication
Birth–3 months	Prefers visual stimuli of mobiles, black-and-white patterns, mirrors Auditory stimuli are music boxes, tape players, soft voices Responds to rocking and cuddling Moves legs and arms while adult sings and talks Likes varying stimuli—different rooms, sounds, visual images	Coos Babbles Cries
3–6 months	Prefers noise-making objects that are easily grasped like rattles Enjoys stuffed animals and soft toys with contrasting colors	Vocalizes during play and with familiar people Laughs
6–9 months	Likes teething toys Increasingly desires social interaction with adults and other children Soft toys that can be manipulated and mouthed are favorites	Cries less Squeals and makes pleasure sounds Babbles multisyllabically (mamamamama) Increases vowel and consonant sounds Links syllables together Uses speechlike rhythm when vocalizing with others
9–12 months	Enjoys large blocks, toys that pop apart and go back together, nesting cups and other objects Laughs at surprise toys like jack-in-the-box Plays interactive games like peek-a-boo Uses push-and-pull toys	Understands "no" and other simple commands Says "dada" and "mama" to identify parents Learns one or two other words Receptive speech surpasses expressive speech

Growth and Development

Strategies for communicating with infants include the following:

- Hold for feedings.
- Hold, rock, and talk to infant often.
- Talk and sing frequently during care.
- Tell names of objects.
- Use high-pitched voice with newborns.
- When the infant is upset, swaddle and hold securely.

TODDLER (1 TO 3 YEARS)

Toddlerhood is sometimes called the first adolescence. An infant only months before, the child from 1 to 3 years is now displaying independence and negativism. Pride in newfound accomplishments emerges.

Physical Growth and Development

The rate of growth slows during the second year of life. Parents may become concerned because the child has a limited food intake. They may need reassurance that this is normal. (See Chapter 33 for further discussion of nutrition in toddlerhood.) By age 2 years, the birth weight has usually quadrupled and the child is about one half of the adult height. Body proportions begin to change, with the legs longer and the head smaller in proportion to body size than during infancy (see Figure 32–5). The toddler has a pot-bellied appearance and stands with feet apart to provide a wide base of support. By approximately 33 months, eruption of deciduous teeth is complete, with 20 teeth present.

Gross motor activity develops rapidly (Table 32–12), as the toddler progresses from walking to running, kicking, and riding a Big Wheel tricycle (Figure 32–6 ●). As physical maturation occurs, the toddler develops the ability to control elimination patterns (see *Growth and Development* and *Developing Cultural Competence: Childrearing Practices*).

Table 32-12   Physical Growth and Development Milestones During Toddlerhood

Age	Physical Growth	Fine Motor Ability	Gross Motor Ability	Sensory Ability
1–2 years	Gains 227 g (8 oz) or more per month Grows 9–12 cm (3.5–5 in.) during this year Anterior fontanelle closes	By end of second year, builds a tower of four blocks (A) Scribbles on paper (B) Can undress self (C) Throws a ball	Runs Shows growing ability to walk and finally walks with ease Walks up and down stairs a few months after learning to walk with ease (E) Likes push-and-pull toys (F)	Visual acuity 20/50
2–3 years	Gains 1.4–2.3 kg (3–5 lb)/year Grows 5–6.5 cm (2–2.5 in.)/year	Draws a circle and other rudimentary forms Learns to pour Learning to dress self (D)	Jumps Kicks ball Throws ball overhand	

Fernando Cortes/Shutterstock

A Builds tower of four blocks

B Scribbles on paper

C Can undress self

D Learning to dress self

E Walks up and down stairs

F Likes push-and-pull toys

Cognitive Development

During the toddler years, the child moves from the sensorimotor to the preoperational stage of development. The early use of language awakens in the 1-year-old the ability to think about objects or people when they are absent. Object permanence is well developed.

At about 2 years of age, the increasing use of words as symbols enables the toddler to use preoperational thought. Rudimentary problem solving, creative thought, and an understanding of cause-and-effect relationships are now possible.

Psychosocial Development

Play

Many changes in play patterns occur between infancy and toddlerhood. Developing motor skills enable toddlers to bang pegs into a pounding board with a hammer, for example. The social nature of toddler play is also readily seen. Toddlers find the company of other children pleasurable, even though socially interactive play may not occur. Two toddlers tend to play with similar objects side by side, occasionally trading toys and words. This is called **parallel play**. This playtime with other children helps

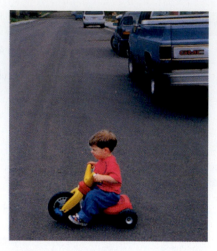

● **Figure 32–6** Gross-motor activity. This toddler has learned to ride a Big Wheel, which he is doing right into the street. Toddlers must be closely watched to prevent injury.

Developing Cultural Competence
Childrearing Practices

In traditional Native American families, children are allowed to unfold and develop naturally at their own pace. Children thus wean and toilet train themselves with little interference or pressure from parents. In other groups, toilet training is accomplished at an early age. The nurse should be sensitive to the childrearing practices of the family and support them in these culturally accepted practices, rather than imposing a more structured approach to toilet training.

toddlers develop social skills. Toddlers engage in play activities they have seen at home, such as pounding with a hammer and talking on the phone. This imitative behavior teaches them new actions and skills.

Physical skills are manifested in play as toddlers push and pull objects, climb in and out and up and down, run, ride a Big Wheel, turn the pages of books, and scribble with a pen. Both gross motor and fine motor abilities are enhanced during this age period.

Cognitive understanding enables the toddler to manipulate objects and learn about their qualities. Stacking blocks and placing rings on a building tower teach spatial relationships and other lessons that provide a foundation for future learning. Various kinds of play objects should be provided for the toddler to meet play needs. These play needs can easily be met whether the child is hospitalized or at home (Table 32–13).

Personality and Temperament

The toddler retains most of the temperamental characteristics identified during infancy but may demonstrate some changes. The normal developmental progression of toddlerhood also plays a part in responses. For example, the infant who previously responded positively to stimuli, such as a new babysitter, may appear more negative in toddlerhood. The increasing independence characteristic of this age is shown by the toddler's use of the word "no." The parent and child constantly adapt their responses to each other and learn anew how to communicate with each other.

Communication

Because of the phenomenal growth of language skills during the toddler period, adults should communicate frequently with

Growth and Development

Strategies for toilet training include the following:

■ When are children ready to learn toileting?
■ Are parents responsible for the differences in ages at which toilet training is accomplished?
■ Does toilet training provide clues to a child's intellectual ability?

We know that children are not ready for toilet training until several developmental capabilities exist: to stand and walk well, to pull pants up and down, to recognize the need to eliminate and then to be able to wait until in the bathroom. Once this readiness is apparent, the child can be given a small potty chair and the procedure explained.

Children often prefer their own chairs on the floor to using a large toilet. The child should be placed on the chair at regular intervals for a few moments and can be given a reward or praise for successes. If the child seems not to understand or does not wish to cooperate, it is best to wait a few weeks and then try again. Just as all of development is subject to individual timetables, toilet training occurs with considerable variability from one child to another. Identify for parents the developmental characteristics of their child and encourage them to appreciate without anxiety the unfolding of skills. These timetables are not predictive of future development.

The child who is ill or hospitalized or has other stress often regresses in toilet-training activities. It is best to quietly reinstitute

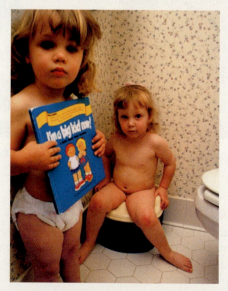

attempts at training after the trauma. Potty chairs should be available on pediatric units and toileting habits identified during initial assessment so that regular routines can be followed and the child's usual words for elimination can be used.

Table 32–13	Psychosocial Development During Toddlerhood	
Age	Play and Toys	Communication
1–3 years	Refines fine motor skills by use of cloth books, large pencil and paper, wooden puzzles	Increasingly enjoys talking
	Facilitates imitative behavior by playing kitchen, grocery shopping, toy telephone	Exponential growth of vocabulary, especially when spoken and read to
	Learns gross motor activities by riding Big Wheel tricycle, playing with soft ball and bat, molding water and sand, tossing ball or bean bag	Needs to release stress by pounding board, frequent gross motor activities, and occasional temper tantrums
	Cognitive skills develop with exposure to educational television shows, music, stories, and books	Likes contact with other children and learns interpersonal skills

children in this age group. Toddlers imitate words and speech intonations, as well as the social interactions they observe.

At the beginning of toddlerhood, the child may use four to six words in addition to "mama" and "dada." Receptive speech (the ability to understand words) far outpaces expressive speech. By the end of toddlerhood, however, the 3-year-old has a vocabulary of almost 1000 words and uses short sentences.

Communication occurs in many ways, some of which are nonverbal. Toddler communication includes pointing, pulling an adult over to a room or object, and speaking in expressive jargon. **Expressive jargon** is using unintelligible words with normal speech intonations as if truly communicating in words. Another communication method occurs when the toddler cries, pounds feet, displays a temper tantrum, or uses other means to illustrate dismay. These powerful communication methods can upset parents, who often need suggestions for handling them. It is best to verbalize the feelings shown by the toddler, for example, by saying, "You must be very upset that you cannot have that candy. When you stop crying you can come out of your room," and then ignore further negative behavior. The toddler's search for autonomy and independence creates a need for such behavior. Sometimes an upset toddler responds well to holding, rocking, and stroking.

Parents and nurses can promote a toddler's communication by speaking frequently, naming objects, explaining procedures in simple terms, expressing feelings that the toddler seems to be

Growth and Development

Strategies for communicating with toddlers include the following:

- Give short, clear instructions.
- Do not give choices if none exist. For example, do not ask "Do you want to take your medicine now?" but rather say "What juice do you want after you take your medicine—apple or orange?"
- Offer a choice of two alternatives when possible.
- Approach positively and slowly, allowing time for the toddler to adjust.
- Tell toddler what you are doing, and say the names of objects.

Table 32–14	Communicating with a Toddler

Procedures such as drawing blood can be frightening for a toddler. Effective communication minimizes the trauma caused by such procedures:

- Avoid telling toddlers about the procedure too far in advance. They do not have an understanding of time and can become quite anxious.
- Use simple terminology. "We need to get a little blood from your arm. It will help us to find out if you are getting better." If the parent is willing, say, "Your mom will hold your arm still so we can do it quickly."
- Allow the toddler to cry. Acknowledge that it must be frightening and that you understand.
- Perform the procedure in a treatment room so that the toddler's bed and room are a safe haven.
- Be sure the toddler is restrained, with the joints above and below the procedure immobilized.
- Use a Band-Aid to cover up the site. This can reassure the toddler that the body is still intact.
- Allow the toddler to choose a reward such as a sticker after the procedure.
- Praise the toddler for cooperation and acknowledge that you know this was difficult.
- Comfort the toddler by rocking, offering a favorite drink, playing music, and holding. If parents are present, they can offer the comfort needed.

displaying, and encouraging speech. The toddler from a bilingual home is at an optimal age to learn two languages. If the parents do not speak English, the toddler will benefit from a daycare experience in which the providers do, so that he or she can learn both languages.

The nurse who understands the communication skills of toddlers is able to assess expressive and receptive language and communicate effectively, thereby promoting positive healthcare experiences for these children (Table 32–14).

PRESCHOOL CHILD (3 TO 6 YEARS)

The preschool years are a time of new initiative and independence. Most children are in a childcare center or school for part of the day and learn a great deal from this social contact.

Table 32–15   Physical Growth and Development Milestones During the Preschool Years

Physical Growth

Gains 1.5–2.5 kg (3–5 lb)/year   Grows 4–6 cm (1 1/2–2 1/2 in.)/year

Fine Motor Ability

Uses scissors (A)
Draws circle, square, cross (B)
Draws at least a six-part person
Enjoys art projects such as pasting, stringing beads, using clay
Learns to tie shoes at end of preschool years (C)
Buttons clothes (D)
Brushes teeth (E)
Uses spoon, fork, knife

A Uses scissors

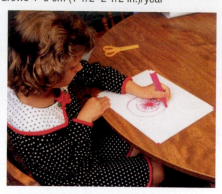

B Draws circle, square, cross

C Ties shoes

D Buttons clothes

E Brushes teeth

Gross Motor Ability	Sensory Ability	Fine Motor Ability
Throws a ball overhand Climbs well (F) Rides bicycle (G)	Visual acuity continues to improve Can focus on and learn letters and numbers (H)	Eats three meals with snacks Uses spoon, fork, and knife

F Climbs well

G Rides bicycle or bicycle with training wheels

H Learns letters and numbers

Language skills are well developed, and the child is able to understand and speak clearly. Endless projects characterize the world of busy preschoolers. They may work with play dough to form animals, then cut out and paste paper, then draw and color.

Physical Growth and Development

Preschoolers grow slowly and steadily, with most growth taking place in the long bones of the arms and legs. The short, chubby toddler gradually gives way to a slender, long-legged preschooler (Table 32–15).

Physical skills continue to develop (Figure 32–7 ●). The preschooler runs with ease, holds a bat, and throws balls of various types. Writing ability increases, and the preschooler enjoys drawing and learning to write a few letters.

The preschool period is a good time to encourage good dental habits. Children can begin to brush their own teeth with parental supervision and help to reach all tooth surfaces. Parents should floss children's teeth, give fluoride as prescribed if the water supply is not fluoridated, and schedule the first dental visit so the child can become accustomed to the routine of periodic dental care.

Cognitive Development

The preschooler exhibits characteristics of preoperational thought. Symbols or words are used to represent objects and people, enabling the young child to think about them. This is a milestone in intellectual development; however, the preschooler still has some limitations in thought (Table 32–16).

Psychosocial Development

Play

The preschooler has begun playing in a new way. Toddlers simply play side by side with friends, each engaging in his or her own activities, but preschoolers interact with others during play. One child cuts out colored paper, for example, while her friend glues it on paper in a design. This new type of interaction is called **associative play** (Figure 32–8 ●). The child life therapist in hospital settings recognizes the therapeutic value of play in planning activities for children that enable them to work through feelings about procedures and separation, as well as facilitating the normal developmental need for interaction with other children.

● **Figure 32–7** Development of physical skills in preschoolers. Preschoolers continue to develop advanced skills such as kicking a ball without falling down.

● **Figure 32–8** These preschoolers are participating in associative play, which means they can interact. One child is cutting out shapes, and the other is gluing them in place.

Table 32–16	Characteristics of Preoperational Thought	
Characteristic	**Definition**	**Example**
Egocentrism	Ability to see things only from one's own point of view	The child who cannot understand why parents may need to leave the hospital for work when the child wishes them to be present
Transductive reasoning	Connecting two events in a cause-and-effect relationship simply because they occur together in time	A child who, awakening after surgery and feeling pain, notices the intravenous infusion and believes that it is causing the pain
Centration	Focusing on only one particular aspect of a situation	The child who is concerned about breathing through an anesthesia mask and will not listen to any other aspects of preoperative teaching
Animism	Giving lifelike qualities to nonliving things	The child who views a monitoring machine as alive because it beeps

In addition to this social dimension of play, other aspects of play also differ. The preschooler enjoys large motor activities such as swinging, riding a tricycle, and throwing a ball. Increasing manual dexterity is demonstrated in greater complexity of drawings and manipulation of blocks and modeling. These changes necessitate planning of playtime to include appropriate activities. Preschool programs and child life departments in hospitals help meet this important need.

Materials provided for play can be simple but should guide activities in which the child engages. Since fine motor activities are popular, paper, pens, scissors, glue, and a variety of other such objects should be available. The child can use them to create important images such as pictures of people, hospital beds, or friends. A collection of dolls, furniture, and clothing can be manipulated to represent parents and children, nurses and physicians, teachers, or other significant people. Because fantasy life is so powerful at this age, the preschooler readily uses props to engage in **dramatic play**, that is, the living out of the drama of human life (Figure 32–9 ●).

The nurse can use playtime to assess the preschool child's developmental level, knowledge about health care, and emotions related to healthcare experiences. Observations about objects chosen for play, content of dramatic play, and pictures drawn can provide important assessment data. The nurse can also use play periods to teach the child about healthcare procedures and offer an outlet for expression of emotions (Table 32–17).

Personality and Temperament

Characteristics of personality observed in infancy tend to persist over time. The preschooler may need assistance as these characteristics are expressed in the new situations of preschool or nursery school. An excessively active child, for example, will need gentle, consistent handling to adjust to the structure of a classroom. Encourage parents to visit preschool programs to choose the one that would best foster growth in their child. Some preschoolers enjoy the structured learning of a program that focuses on cognitive skills, whereas others are happier and more open to learning in a small group that provides much time for free play. Nurses can help parents to identify their child's personality or temperament characteristics and to find the best environment for growth.

Communication

Language skills blossom during the preschool years. The vocabulary grows to over 2000 words, and children speak in complete sentences of several words and use all parts of speech. They practice these newfound language skills by endlessly talking and asking questions.

● **Figure 32–9** Jasmine is participating in dramatic play with a nurse while her mother looks on. In dramatic play the child uses props to play out the drama of human life. It can be an excellent way for a nurse to assess the developmental level of children while talking to them. Notice that the child and the nurse are on the floor at the same level and the atmosphere is informal. Why is it important to be at the same level as the child?

Table 32–17	Psychosocial Development During the Preschool Years	
Age	**Play and Toys**	**Communication**
3–6 years	Associative play is facilitated by simple games, puzzles, nursery rhymes, songs Dramatic play is fostered by dolls and doll clothes, play houses and hospitals, dress-up clothes, puppets	All parts of speech are developed and used, occasionally incorrectly Communicates with a widening array of people
	Stress is relieved by pens, paper, glue, scissors Cognitive growth is fostered by educational television shows, music, stories, and books	Play with other children is a favorite activity Health professionals can: ■ Verbalize and explain procedures to children ■ Use drawings and stories to explain care ■ Use accurate names for body functions ■ Allow the child to talk, ask questions, and make choices

Growth and Development

Strategies for communicating with preschoolers include the following:

- Allow time for child to integrate explanations.
- Verbalize frequently to the child.
- Use drawings and stories to explain care.
- Use accurate names for body functions.
- Allow choices.

A

B

The sophisticated speech of preschoolers mirrors the development occurring in their minds and helps them to learn about the world around them. However, this speech can be quite deceptive. Although preschoolers use many words, their grasp of meaning is usually literal and may not match that of adults. These literal interpretations have important implications for healthcare providers. For example, the preschooler who is told she will be "put to sleep" for surgery may think of a pet recently euthanized; the child who is told that a dye will be injected for a diagnostic test may think he is going to die; mention of "a little stick" in the arm can cause images of tree branches rather than of a simple immunization.

The child may also have difficulty focusing on the content of a conversation. The preschooler is egocentric and may be unable to move from individual thoughts to those the nurse is proposing in a teaching situation.

Concrete visual aids such as pictures of a child undergoing the same procedure or a book to read together enhance teaching by meeting the child's developmental needs. Handling medical equipment such as intravenous bags and stethoscopes increases interest and helps the child to focus. Teaching may have to be done in several short sessions rather than one long session.

SCHOOL-AGE CHILD (6 TO 12 YEARS)

Errol, 10 years old, arrives home from school shortly after 3 P.M. each day. He immediately calls his friends and goes to visit one of them. They are building models of cars and collecting baseball cards. Endless hours are spent on these projects and on discussions of events at school that day (Figure 32–10 ●).

Nine-year-old Karen practices soccer two afternoons a week and plays in games each weekend. She also is learning to play the flute and spends her free time at home practicing. Although practice time is not her favorite part of music, Karen enjoys the performances and wants to play well in front of her friends and teacher. Her parents now allow her to ride her bike unaccompanied to the store or to a friend's house.

These two school-age children demonstrate common characteristics of their age group. They are in a stage of industry in which it is important to the child to perform useful work. Meaningful activities take on great importance and are usually carried out in the company of peers. A sense of achievement in these activities is important to develop self-esteem and to prevent a sense of inferiority or poor self-worth.

● **Figure 32–10** *A,* School-age children may take part in activities that require practice. This is a consideration when children are hospitalized and unable to practice or perform. Why? *B,* School-age children enjoy spending time with others the same age on projects and discussing the activities of the day. This is an important consideration when they are in an acute care setting. When you are in the clinical setting, look for examples of this type of interaction taking place.

Physical Growth and Development

School age is the last period in which girls and boys are close in size and body proportions. As the long bones continue to grow, leg length increases (see Figure 32–5). Fat gives way to muscle, and the child appears leaner. Jaw proportions change as the first deciduous tooth is lost at 6 years and permanent teeth begin to erupt. Body organs and the immune system mature, resulting in fewer illnesses among school-age children. Medications are less likely to cause serious side effects, since they can be metabolized more easily. The urinary system can adjust to changes in fluid status. Physical skills are also refined as children begin to play sports, and fine motor skills are well developed through school activities (Table 32–18 and Figure 32–11 ●).

Table 32–18	Physical Growth and Development Milestones During the School-Age Years			

Physical Growth	Fine Motor Ability	Gross Motor Ability	Sensory Ability
Gains 1.4–2.2 kg (3–5 lb)/year	Enjoys craft projects	Rides two-wheeler (A)	Can read
Grows 4–6 cm (1 1/2–2 1/2 in.)/year	Plays card and board games	Jumps rope (B) Roller skates or ice skates	Able to concentrate for longer periods on activities by filtering out surrounding sounds (C)

A Rides two-wheeler   B Jumps rope   C Concentrates on activities for longer periods

Although it is commonly believed that the start of adolescence (age 12 years) heralds a growth spurt, the rapid increases in size commonly occur during school age. Girls may begin a growth spurt by 9 or 10 years and boys a year or so later. Nutritional needs increase dramatically with this spurt.

The loss of the first deciduous teeth and the eruption of permanent teeth usually occur at about age 6 years, or at the beginning of the school-age period. Of the 30 permanent teeth, 22 to 26 erupt by age 12 years and the remaining molars follow during the teenage years. The school-age child should be closely monitored to ensure that brushing and flossing are adequate, that fluoride is taken if the water supply is not fluoridated, that dental care is obtained to provide for examination of teeth and alignment, and that loose teeth are identified before surgery or other events that may lead to loss of a tooth.

Cognitive Development

The child enters the stage of concrete operational thought at about 7 years. This stage enables school-age children to consider alternative solutions and solve problems. However, school-age

● **Figure 32–11** School-age children's physical development. *Left*, Front teeth are lost around age 6 years. The family may have rituals associated with the loss of teeth that could affect the child's behavior if he loses a tooth while in the hospital. *Right*, School-age girls and boys enjoy participating in sports. They begin to lose fat while developing their muscles, so they appear leaner than at earlier ages.

children continue to rely on concrete experiences and materials to form their thought content.

During the school-age years, the child learns the concept of **conservation** (that matter is not changed when its form is altered). At earlier ages a child believes that when water is poured from a short, wide glass into a tall, thin glass, there is more water in the taller glass. The school-age child recognizes that although it may look like the taller glass holds more water, the quantity is the same. The concept of conservation is helpful when the nurse explains medical treatments. The school-age child understands that an incision will heal, that a cast will be removed, and that an arm will look the same as before once the intravenous infusion is removed.

Psychosocial Development

Play

When the preschool teacher tries to organize a game of baseball, both the teacher and the children become frustrated. Not only are the children physically unable to hold a bat and hit a ball, but they seem to have no understanding of the rules of the game and do not want to wait for their turn at bat. By 6 years of age, however, children have acquired the physical ability to hold the bat properly and may occasionally hit the ball. School-age children also understand that everyone has a role—the pitcher, the catcher, the batter, the outfielders. They cooperate with one another to form a team, are eager to learn the rules of the game, and want to ensure that these rules are followed exactly (Table 32–19).

The characteristics of play exhibited by the school-age child are cooperation with others and the ability to play a part in order to contribute to a unified whole. This type of play is called **cooperative play**. The concrete nature of cognitive thought leads to a reliance on rules to provide structure and security. Children have an increasing desire to spend much of playtime with friends, which demonstrates the social component of play. Play is an extremely important method of learning and living for the school-age child. Active physical play has decreased in recent years as television viewing and playing of computer games have

● **Figure 32–12** The nurse can help the hospitalized school-age child and family accept and adjust to new circumstances. Encouraging the child in a wheelchair to participate in group activities can help build confidence in physical skills. Good self-esteem, goal attainment, personal satisfaction, and general health are the continued benefits.

increased, leading to poor nutritional status and a high rate of overweight among children. See Chapter 33 🔗 for further discussion of nutrition and physical activity in children.

When a child is hospitalized, the separation from playmates can lead to feelings of sadness and purposelessness. School-age children often feel better when placed in multibed units with other children. Games can be devised even when children are wheelchair bound (Figure 32–12 ●). Normal, rewarding parts of play should be integrated into care. Friends should be encouraged to visit or call a hospitalized child. Discharge planning for the child who has had a cast or brace applied should address the activities the child can engage in and those the child must avoid. Reinforce the importance of playing games with friends.

Table 32–19	Psychosocial Development During the School-Age Years	
Age	**Activities**	**Communication**
6–12 years	Gross motor development is fostered by ball sports, skating, dance lessons, water and snow skiing/boarding, biking A sense of industry is fostered by playing a musical instrument, gathering collections, starting hobbies, playing board and video games Cognitive growth is facilitated by reading, crafts, word puzzles, schoolwork	Mature use of language Ability to converse and discuss topics for increasing lengths of time Spends many hours at school and with friends in sports or other activities Health professionals can: ■ Assess child's knowledge before teaching ■ Allow the child to select rewards following procedures ■ Teach techniques such as counting or visualization to manage difficult situations ■ Include both parent and child in healthcare decisions

Personality and Temperament

The enduring aspects of temperament continue to be manifested during the school years. The child classified as "difficult" at an earlier age may now have trouble in the classroom. Advise parents to provide a quiet setting for homework and to reward the child for concentration. For example, after homework is completed, the child can watch a television show. Creative efforts and alternative methods of learning should be valued. Encourage parents to see their children as individuals who may not all learn in the same way. The "slow-to-warm-up" child may need encouragement to try new activities and to share experiences with others, while the "easy" child will readily adapt to new schools, people, and experiences.

Communication

During the school-age years, the child should learn how to correct any lingering pronunciation or grammatical errors. Vocabulary increases, and the child is taught about parts of speech in school. School-age children enjoy writing and can be encouraged to keep a journal of their experiences while in the hospital as a method of dealing with anxiety. It is uncommon for school-age children to understand words as literally as preschoolers.

Sexuality

While children become aware of sexual differences between genders during preschool years, they deal much more consciously with sexuality as school-age children. As children mature physically, they need information about their body changes so that they can develop a healthy self-image and an understanding of the relationships between their bodies and sexuality. Children become interested in sexual issues and are often exposed to erroneous information on television shows, in magazines, or from friends and siblings. Schools and families need to find opportunities to teach school-age children factual information about sex and to foster healthy concepts of self and others. It is advisable to ask occasional questions about sexual issues to learn how much the child knows and to provide correct information when answers demonstrate confusion. Both friends and the media are common sources of erroneous ideas. Appropriate and inappropriate touch should be discussed, with lists of trusted people who can be approached (teachers, clergy, school counselors, family members, neighbors) to discuss any episodes with which the child feels uncomfortable. Even these trusted people can be implicated in inappropriate episodes, so encourage the child to go to more than one person, an important approach if the child is uncomfortable about a relationship with any individual.

ADOLESCENT (12 TO 18 YEARS)

Adolescence is a time of passage signaling the end of childhood and the beginning of adulthood. Although adolescents differ in behaviors and accomplishments, they are in a period of identity formation. If a healthy identity and sense of self-worth are not developed in this period, role confusion and purposeless struggling will ensue. The adolescents encountered in nursing practice represent various degrees of identity formation, and each will offer unique challenges.

 Growth and Development

Strategies for communicating with school-age children include the following:

■ Provide concrete examples of pictures or materials to accompany verbal descriptions.
■ Assess knowledge before planning teaching.
■ Allow child to select rewards following procedures.
■ Teach techniques such as counting or visualization to manage difficult situations.
■ Include child in discussions and history with parent.
■ Be honest in explanations and all communications.

Physical Growth and Development

The physical changes ending in **puberty**, or sexual maturity, begin near the end of the school-age period. The prepubescent period is marked by a growth spurt at an average age of 10 years for girls and 13 years for boys. The increase in height and weight is generally remarkable and is completed in 2 to 3 years (Table 32–20). The growth spurt in girls is accompanied by an increase in breast size and growth of pubic hair. Menstruation occurs last and signals achievement of puberty. In boys the growth spurt is accompanied by growth in size of the penis and testes and by growth of pubic hair. Deepening of the voice and growth of facial hair occur later, at the time of puberty. See Chapter 34 for a description of the pubertal stages.

During adolescence children grow stronger and more muscular and establish characteristic male and female patterns of fat distribution. The apocrine and eccrine glands mature, leading to increased sweating and a distinct odor to perspiration. All body organs are now fully mature, enabling the adolescent to take adult doses of medications.

The adolescent must adapt to a rapidly changing body for several years. Height, weight, and body proportions increase. Such changes occur with great variability so an adolescent may be at different points of maturation than peers. These physical changes, hormonal variations, and differences in timing offer challenges to identity formation. The adolescent must incorporate the new body, its functions, and retain a healthy sense of self in relationship to peers. The formation of self-identity is a psychologic process but is necessarily closely connected with the bodily changes occurring.

Cognitive Development

Adolescence marks the beginning of Piaget's last stage of cognitive development, the stage of formal operational thought. The adolescent no longer depends on concrete experiences as the basis of thought but develops the ability to reason abstractly. Such concepts as justice, truth, beauty, and power can be understood. The adolescent revels in this newfound ability and spends a great deal of time thinking, reading, and talking about abstract concepts.

The ability to think and act independently leads many adolescents to rebel against parental authority and experiment with risky behaviors. Through these actions, adolescents seek to establish their own identity and values.

Table 32–20 — Physical Growth and Development Milestones During Adolescence

Physical Growth	Fine Motor Ability	Gross Motor Ability	Sensory Ability
Variation in age of growth spurt During growth spurt, girls gain 7–25 kg (15–55 lb) and grow 2.5–20 cm (2–8 in.); boys gain approximately 7–29.5 kg (15–65 lb) and grow 11–30 cm (4 1/2–12 in.)	Skills are well developed (*A*)	New sports activities attempted and muscle development continues (*B*) Some lack of coordination common during growth spurt	Fully developed

A Skills are well developed

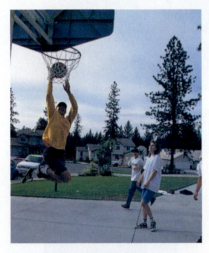

B New sports activities attempted

Psychosocial Development

Activities

Maturity leads to new activities. Adolescents may drive, ride buses, or bike independently. They are less dependent on parents for transportation and spend more time with friends. Activities include participation in sports and extracurricular school activities, as well as "hanging out" and attending movies or concerts with friends (Table 32–21). The peer group becomes the focus of activities (Figure 32–13 ●), regardless of the teen's interests. Peers are important in establishing identity and providing meaning. Although same-sex interactions dominate, boy–girl relationships are more common than at earlier stages. Adolescents thus participate in and learn from social interactions fundamental to adult relationships.

Table 32–21 — Psychosocial Development During Adolescence

Age	Activities	Communication
12–18 years 	Sports—ball games, gymnastics, water and snow skiing/boarding, swimming, school sports School activities—drama, yearbook, class office, club participation Quiet activities—reading, schoolwork, television, computer, video games, music	Increasing communication and time with peer group—movies, dances, driving, eating out, attending sports events Applying abstract thought and analysis in conversations at home and school

● **Figure 32–13** Peer group activities in adolescence. Social interaction between children of same and opposite sex is as important inside the acute care setting as it is outside. *A*, Teenagers enjoy playing together. *B*, Emotional relationships form during adolescence.

Personality and Temperament

Characteristics of temperament manifested during childhood usually remain stable in the teenage years. For instance, the adolescent who was a calm, scheduled infant and child often demonstrates initiative to regulate study times and other routines. Similarly the adolescent who was an easily stimulated infant may now have a messy room, a harried schedule with assignments always completed late, and an interest in many activities. It is also common for an adolescent who was an easy child to become more difficult because of the psychologic changes of adolescence and the need to assert independence.

As during the child's earlier ages, the nurse's role may be to inform parents of different personality types and to help them support the teen's uniqueness while providing necessary structure and feedback. Nurses can help parents understand their teen's personality type and work with the adolescent to meet expectations set by teachers and others in authority.

Communication

The adolescent uses and understands all parts of speech. Colloquialisms and slang are commonly used with the peer group. The adolescent often studies a foreign language in school, having the ability to understand and analyze grammar and sentence structure.

The adolescent increasingly leaves the home base and establishes close ties with peers. These relationships become the basis for identity formation. There is generally a period of stress or crisis before a strong identity can emerge. The adolescent may try out new roles by learning a new sport or other skills, experimenting with drugs or alcohol, wearing different styles of clothing, or trying other activities. It is important to provide positive role models and a variety of experiences to help the adolescent make wise choices.

The adolescent also has a need to leave the past, to be different, and to change from former patterns to establish his or her own identity. Rules that are repeated constantly and dogmatically will probably be broken in the adolescent's quest for self-identity. This poses difficulties when the adolescent has a health problem, such as diabetes, or a heart problem that requires ongoing care. Introducing the adolescent to other teens who manage the same problem appropriately is usually more successful than telling the adolescent what to do.

Ensure privacy during the taking of health histories or interventions with teens. Even if a parent is present for part of a history or examination, the adolescent should be given the opportunity to relay information or ask questions alone with the healthcare provider. Give the adolescent a choice of whether to have a parent present during an examination or while care is provided. Most information shared by an adolescent is confidential. Some states mandate disclosure of certain information to parents, such as an adolescent's desire for an abortion. In these cases the adolescent should be informed of what will be disclosed to the parent.

Setting up teen rooms (recreation rooms for use only by adolescents) or separate adolescent units in hospitals can provide necessary peer support during hospitalization. Most adolescents are not pleased when placed on a unit or in a room with young children. Choices should be allowed whenever possible. These might include preference for evening or morning bathing, the type of clothes to wear while hospitalized, timing of treatments, and who should be allowed to visit and for how long. Use of negotiations and agreements with adolescents may increase compliance. Firmness, gentleness, choices, and respect must all be balanced during care of adolescent patients.

Sexuality

With maturation of the body and increased secretion of hormones, the adolescent achieves sexual maturity. This complex process involves a growing interest in sexuality and romantic or sexual relationships, an interplay of the forces of society and family, and identity formation. The early adolescent progresses from dances and other social events with members of the opposite sex; the late adolescent is mature sexually and may have regular sexual encounters. About one half of all high-school students in the United States have had intercourse, but only 63% of these youths used a condom at their last sexual encounter, putting this age group at high risk of acquiring sexually transmitted infections (Eaton, Kann, Kinchen, et al., 2010).

Growth and Development

Strategies for communicating with adolescents include the following:

- Provide written as well as verbal explanations.
- Direct history and explanations to teen alone; then include parent.
- Allow for safe exploration of topics by suggesting that teen is similar to other teens. ("Many teens with diabetes have questions about how to eat foods they and their friends like and still stay within their diet needs. How about you?")
- Arrange meetings for discussions with other teens.

Teenagers need information about their bodies and emerging sexuality. To make informed decisions about their behavior, teenagers should understand the interests and forces they experience. Including sex education in school classes and healthcare encounters is important. Information on how to prevent sexually transmitted infections (STIs) is given, with most school districts now providing some teaching on AIDS. Far more common risks to teens, however, are diseases such as gonorrhea and herpes. Health histories should include questions on sexual activity, STIs, and birth control use and understanding. Most hospitals routinely perform pregnancy screening on adolescent girls before elective procedures.

Adolescents benefit from clear information about sexuality, an opportunity to develop relationships with adolescents in various settings, an open atmosphere at home and school where problems and issues can be discussed, and previous experience in problem solving and self-decision making. Sexual issues should be among topics that adolescents can discuss openly in a variety of settings. Alternatives and support for their decisions should be available.

Some adolescents identify with a sexual minority group such as lesbian, gay, bisexual, or transgender. They are at particular risk of being stigmatized and harassed by other youth or adults. They are more likely to suffer a variety of problems, such as isolation, rejection by family and friends, violence, and suicide, and to take sexual risks (Dowshen & Garofalo, 2009). Nurses are instrumental in helping these youth by providing information for them and their parents, integrating sexual minority content into school sexual curricula, and providing referrals for health care and social care when needed. See Chapter 43 for further information about the health issues related to homosexuality and other sexual minority practices.

Critical Concept Review

LEARNING OUTCOME 32.1: Describe the major theories of development as formulated by Freud, Erikson, Piaget, Kohlberg, social learning theorists, and behaviorists.

1. Freud:
   - Early childhood experiences form the unconscious motivation for action in later life.
2. Erikson:
   - There are eight periods that determine an individual's future social relationships.
3. Piaget:
   - Child's view of the world is influenced largely by age, experience, and maturational ability.
4. Kohlberg:
   - Moral decision making proceeds in a developmental fashion.
5. Social learning theorists:
   - Children learn attitudes, beliefs, and customs through social contact with adults and other children.
6. Behaviorists:
   - Behavior can be elicited by positive reinforcement and extinguished by negative reinforcement.

LEARNING OUTCOME 32.2: Recognize risks to developmental progression and factors that protect against those risks.

1. Risk factors:
   - Financial problems.
   - Stresses and worries.
   - Family and job instability.
   - Neighborhood and home hazards.
   - Lack of resources.
2. Protective factors:
   - Coping mechanisms.
   - Access to community, Internet, and other resources.
   - Family and friend support.
   - Religion, spirituality, and life meaning.
   - Positive health behaviors.

LEARNING OUTCOME 32.3: Plan nursing interventions for children that are appropriate for each child's developmental state, based on theoretical frameworks.

1. Infant:
   - Encourage parents to hold and stay with infant.
   - Provide opportunities for sucking.
   - Provide infant with toys that give comfort or stimulate interest.
2. Toddler:
   - Maintain toilet-training procedures.
   - Encourage appropriate independent behavior.
   - Give short explanations.
   - Provide rewards for appropriate behaviors.

3. Preschooler:
   - Encourage parents to be involved in care of child.
   - Provide safe versions of medical equipment for playtime.
   - Give clear explanations about procedures and illnesses.
4. School-age child:
   - Provide for privacy and modesty.
   - Explain treatments and procedures clearly.
   - Encourage continuation of schoolwork.

5. Adolescent:
   - Provide privacy.
   - Interview and examine adolescent without parents present, if possible.
   - Encourage adolescent participation in treatment and decision making.
   - Encourage visitation of peers.

LEARNING OUTCOME 32.4: Explain contemporary developmental approaches such as temperament theory, ecologic theory, and the resilience framework.

1. Ecologic theory:
   - Emphasizes the presence of mutual interactions between the child (who is unique) and various settings.
2. Temperament theory:
   - All children can be categorized into three patterns of temperament, which can be used to assist in adaptation of the child's environment and for a better understanding of the child.

3. Resiliency theory:
   - All individuals experience crises that lead to adaptation and development of inner strengths and the ability to handle future crises.

LEARNING OUTCOME 32.5: Identify major developmental milestones for infants, toddlers, preschoolers, school-age children, and adolescents.

1. Infant:
   - Rolls over.
   - Sits up.
   - Stands.
   - Able to say one to two words.
   - Uses pincer grasp well.
2. Toddler:
   - Walks up and down stairs.
   - Undresses self.
   - Scribbles on paper.
   - Kicks a ball.
   - Has a vocabulary of 1000 words and uses short sentences.
3. Preschooler:
   - Uses scissors.

   - Rides bicycle with training wheels.
   - Throws a ball.
   - Writes a few letters.
   - All parts of speech well developed.
4. School-age child:
   - Possesses reading ability.
   - Rides a two-wheeled bike.
   - Jumps rope.
   - Plays organized sports.
   - Mature use of language.
5. Adolescent:
   - Fine motor skills well developed.
   - Gross motor skills improve due to growth spurts.
   - Able to apply abstract thought and analysis.

LEARNING OUTCOME 32.6: Synthesize information from several theoretical approaches to plan assessments of the child's physical growth and developmental milestones.

The nurse plans assessments of the child's:
1. Physical growth and development and prenatal influences.
2. Cognitive development.
3. Psychosocial development.
4. Personality and temperament.
5. Communication.
6. Sexuality.

LEARNING OUTCOME 32.7: Describe the role of play in the growth and development of children.

1. Infant:
   - Engages primarily in solitary play, although social interaction enhances play.
   - Learns and matures through feel and sound of activities and objects.
   - As the infant begins to crawl and walk, the sphere of play enlarges and the effect of play on growth and development increases.
2. Toddler:
   - Increased motor skills enable the toddler to engage in new ways of playing.
   - Play becomes more social, and often includes parallel play with other toddlers.
   - Engages in imitative behavior, which teaches them new actions and skills.
   - Increased cognitive abilities enable the toddler to manipulate objects and learn about their qualities.

3. Preschooler:
   - Interacts with others in associative play.
   - Enjoys large motor activities.
   - Increased manual dexterity is demonstrated in greater complexity of play activities.
   - Fantasy play enhances growth and development.
4. School-age child:
   - Increased physical abilities allow greater range and complexity of activities.
   - Engages in cooperative play, which increases social and cognitive skills.
5. Adolescent:
   - Increased maturity leads to new activities and ways to play.
   - The peer group—as the focus of activities—plays an important role in establishing the adolescent's identity.
   - Participate in and learn from social interactions fundamental to adult relationships.

LEARNING OUTCOME 32.8: Use data collected during developmental assessments to implement activities that promote development of children and adolescents.

1. Discuss proper nutrition and feeding techniques.
2. Conduct health teachings and screenings that are appropriate for child's age.
3. Encourage family to discover child's personality characteristics and temperament.
4. Instruct parents in expected language skills and refer to appropriate providers for assistance.
5. Give parents information regarding appropriate and normal sexual behavior in young children.
6. Instruct school-age children concerning the expected body changes of puberty.
7. Give adolescent information concerning birth control and sexually transmitted infections.

Clinical Reasoning in Action

You encounter a 12-month-old child, Julia, while working in the developmental clinic. Her mother tells you that their family practice physician had concerns that Julia might have a developmental delay. She was a full-term baby and there were no complications throughout her mother's pregnancy or delivery. Julia's mother tells you that she has a generally shy and slow-to-warm-up temperament. She makes little eye contact with you and prefers to sit on her mother's lap and cling to her arms if a stranger gets close. She is able to pick up small objects, babble, crawl, and use her pincer grasp. She is not able to walk, hold a crayon, or speak any words. Julia clearly has a developmental delay.

1. What are some examples of toys you can suggest to Julia's parents based on her developmental level (not based on her age)?
2. What are some examples of hazards you can advise Julia's parents about avoiding based on her developmental level?
3. What is a suggestion you can give the parents about dealing with a child like Julia who has a shy or slow-to-warm-up temperament?

See www.nursing.pearsonhighered.com for possible responses.

References

American Academy of Pediatrics. (2009). *Pediatric nutrition handbook* (6th ed.). Elk Grove Village, IL: Author.

Bandura, A. (1986). *Social foundations of thought and actions: A social cognitive theory*. Englewood Cliffs, NJ: Prentice Hall.

Bandura, A. (1997a). *Self efficacy in changing societies*. New York, NY: Cambridge University Press.

Bandura, A. (1997b). *Self efficacy: The exercise of control*. New York, NY: Freeman.

Bronfenbrenner, U. (1986). Ecology of the family as a context for human development: Research perspectives. *Developmental Psychology, 22*, 723–742.

Bronfenbrenner, U. (Ed.). (2005). *Making human beings human: Bioecological perspectives on human development*. Thousand Oaks, CA: Sage.

Bronfenbrenner, U., McClelland, P. D., Ceci, S. J., Moen, P., & Wethington, E. (1996). *The state of Americans*. New York, NY: Free Press.

Burney, R. V., & Leerkes, E. M. (2010). Links between mothers' and fathers' perceptions of infant temperament and coparenting. *Infant Behavior and Development, 33*(2), 125–135.

Chess, S., & Thomas, A. (1995). *Temperament in clinical practice*. New York, NY: Guilford Press.

Chess, S., & Thomas, A. (1996). *Temperament: Theory and practice*. Philadelphia, PA: Brunner/Mazel.

Chess, S., & Thomas, A. (1999). *Goodness of fit: Clinical applications from infancy through adult life*. Philadelphia, PA: Brunner/Mazel.

Children's Hospital of Philadelphia. (2012). *International adoption health program*. Retrieved from http://www.chop.edu/service/adoption/health-considerations

Craig, G. J., & Dunn, W. L. (2010). *Understanding human development* (2nd ed.). Upper Saddle River, NJ: Pearson Prentice Hall.

Daly, B. P., Shin, R. Q., Thakral, C., Selders, M., & Vera, E. (2009). School engagement among urban adolescents of color: Does perception of social support and neighborhood safety really matter? *Journal of Youth and Adolescence, 38*(1), 63–74.

Dowshen, N., & Garofalo, R. (2009). Optimizing primary care for LGBTQ youth. *Contemporary Pediatrics, 26*(10), 58–66.

Dumka, L. E., Gonzales, N. A., Wheeler, L. A., & Millsay, R. E. (2010). Parenting self-efficacy and parenting practices over time in Mexican American families. *Journal of Family Psychology, 24*(5), 522–531.

Eaton, D. K., Kann, L., Kinchen, S., Shanklin, S., Ross, J., Hawkins, J., & Wechsler, H. (2010). Youth Risk Behavior Surveillance—United States, 2009. *Morbidity and Mortality Weekly Report, 59*(SS-5), 1–146.

Erikson, E. (1963). *Childhood and society*. New York, NY: Norton.

Erikson, E. (1968). *Identity: Youth and crisis*. New York, NY: Norton.

Field, T., Diego, M., & Hernandez-Reif, M. (2010). Preterm infant massage therapy research: A review. *Infant Behavior and Development, 33*, 115–124.

Ginsberg, H., & Opper, S. (1988). *Piaget's theory of intellectual development* (3rd ed.). Paramus, NJ: Prentice Hall.

Henderson, N., Benard, B., & Sharp-Light, M. (2007). *Resiliency in action*. Ojai, CA: Resiliency in Action.

McCarter-Spaulding, D. E., & Dennis, C. L. (2010). Psychometric testing of the Breastfeeding Self-Efficacy Scale-Short Form in a sample of black women in the United States. *Research in Nursing and Health, 33*(2), 111–119.

McGrath, J. M. (2009). Touch and massage in the newborn period. *Journal of Perinatal & Neonatal Nursing, 23*, 304–306.

Piaget, J. (1972). *The child's conception of the world*. Totowa, NJ: Littlefield, Adams.

Salmon, J., Jorna, M., Hume, C., Arundell, L., Dhahine, J., Tienstra, J., & Crawford, C. (2011). A translational research intervention to reduce screen behaviours and promote physical activity among children: Switch-2-Activity. *Health Promotion International, 26*, 311–321.

Santrock, J. (2011). *Life-span development* (11th ed.). Boston, MA: McGraw-Hill.

Smit, E. M. (2010). International adoption families: A unique health care journey. *Pediatric Nursing, 36*, 253–258.

Smith, S. L., Lux, R., Haley, S., Slater, H., Beechy, J., & Moyer-Mileur, L. J. (2012). The effect of massage on heart rate variability in preterm infants. *Journal of Perinatology*. doi:10.1038/jp.2012.47

U.S. Department of Health and Human Services. (2011). *Immigrant orphans adopted by U.S. citizens by gender, age, and region and country of birth: Fiscal year 2010*. Retrieved from http://www.childwelfare.gov/systemside/statistics/adoption.cfm#inter

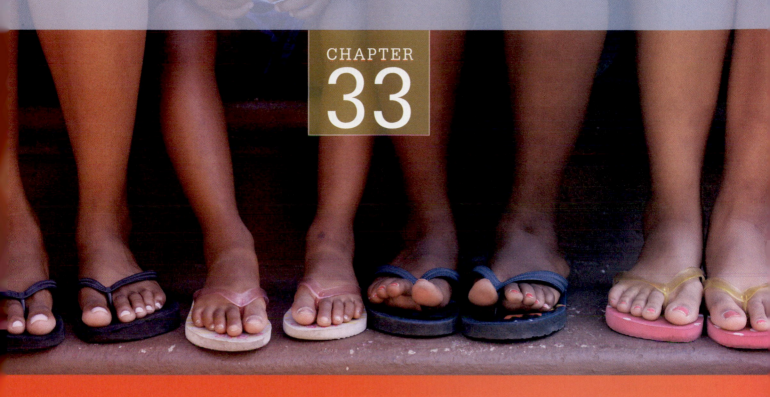

Infant, Child, and Adolescent Nutrition

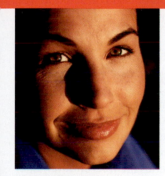

It is exciting to see Joey progressing into the school setting. Being with children his age will really help him develop in many ways. We're just worried because he needs to get only foods he can chew and swallow so he does not choke. He also needs his tube feedings during school to be sure he gets enough energy to do well. —Mother of Joey, 11 years old

Ryan McVay/Getty Images

LEARNING OUTCOMES

33.1 Discuss major nutritional concepts pertaining to the growth and development of children.

33.2 Describe and plan nursing interventions to meet nutritional needs for all age groups from infancy through adolescence.

33.3 Integrate methods of nutritional assessment into nursing care of infants, children, and adolescents.

33.4 Identify and explain common nutritional problems of children.

33.5 Develop nursing interventions for children with nutritional disorders.

Adequate nutrition is an essential component of growth and development. The child's nutritional status begins before birth and is related to the mother's nutritional state. All children must be assessed for nutritional status, followed by teaching or other interventions to enhance health. Nurses are instrumental in giving parents information about normal nutritional needs of infants, children, and adolescents. Common techniques to assess nutrition, such as measuring growth and monitoring hematocrit, provide needed information about whether intake of nutrients is adequate.

All children and their parents can benefit from information about nutritional needs, but some children have additional concerns that must be considered. The nurse recognizes the special requirements of children with conditions such as feeding disorder, food allergies, cystic fibrosis, cerebral palsy, or diabetes. Nutrition monitoring is provided throughout childhood so that dietary counseling can be integrated with other teaching to promote development. How can the nurse bridge the various settings in which children's nutritional needs are met? These might include the home, childcare settings, schools, and hospitals. How can the nurse help the family prepare for meeting the nutritional needs of a child who has special needs during car or plane travel?

Some children have unique nutritional needs due to their social environments. Parents may not be knowledgeable about child nutritional requirements. Perhaps the family is vegetarian and needs extra help to ensure intake of essential nutrients. If finances are limited, the family may need resources such as food stamps, food banks, or budget planning. The nurse considers the high rate of childhood obesity and common nutritional deficits when applying concepts of health promotion with families. Whatever the nurse's setting, knowledge of nutrition must be integrated within nursing care.

GENERAL NUTRITION CONCEPTS

Nutrition refers to taking in food and assimilating it metabolically for use by the body. It is an essential component of life and therefore an important body of knowledge to consider in discussions of child growth and development. The body requires a wide array of nutrients. **Macronutrients**, or the major building blocks of the body, are carbohydrates, protein, and fat. Vitamins and minerals are **micronutrients**, or substances needed in small quantities for healthy body functioning. The need for nutrients is dependent on activity level, state of health, and presence of disease or other stress- and age-related requirements.

The **Dietary Reference Intakes (DRIs)** are a set of values established by the Food and Nutrition Board of the Institute of Medicine (IOM) and the National Academy of Science that can be used to assess and plan intake for individuals of different ages (Institute of Medicine, 2011). They commonly include Estimated Average Requirement, or EAR (intake needed to meet requirements of 50% of the population); Recommended Dietary Allowance, or RDA (intake needed to meet requirements of 97% to 98% of the population); Adequate Intake, or AI (used when data to support EAR are not available); and Upper Intake, or UI (maximum level unlikely to pose health risk). Although the DRI approach is used in the United States, other countries have developed their own approaches to dietary standards. For example, Canada uses Adequate Intake and Reference Nutrient Intake, while the United Kingdom uses Recommended Daily Nutrient Intakes. The aims of these standards are to provide a method to evaluate individual and population diets and to plan nutrition programs and education. DRIs are generally specific to males and females in several age categories. See Appendix G ✪ for a list of DRIs for children and adolescents.

Although the DRIs provide useful information when evaluating diets, their use can be time consuming. What "quick check" can provide feedback about the daily diets of children? The nurse should be familiar with the U.S. MyPlate food guide

● **Figure 33–1** The U.S. MyPlate food guide is used to provide teaching about amounts of foods recommended for daily intake.

Source: From U.S. Department of Agriculture and U.S. Department of Health and Human Services. (2011). Retrieved from http://www.choosemyplate.gov

and hang posters that illustrate its healthy choices in schools, clinics, and hospitals. It is a fast way to examine children's intakes for one day and evaluate whether they meet most requirements. Instead of calculating amounts of nutrients ingested, the MyPlate program focuses on categories of foods, which readily reflects the actual intake. The numbers of servings from various categories stay constant throughout childhood, while the serving sizes increase as the child gets older. See Figure 33–1 ● for MyPlate, and consult the U.S. Department of Agriculture (USDA) website for ethnic/cultural food guides for vegetarians and those from various ethnic groups, such as Hispanic and Native American.

NUTRITIONAL NEEDS

Nutritional needs evolve during all of infancy and childhood. They support growth and development and influence the progression of the child along the developmental path. Nutritional intake helps to maintain the health of the child and fosters a state of maximal potential or health promotion. Specific needs during each developmental stage are discussed in this section. A detailed description of breast and bottle feeding for the newborn can be found in Chapter 26 🔗, while additional pertinent information about infant nutrition is discussed below.

Infancy

Fluid and Macronutrients

Fluid requirements during the neonatal period are high (140 to 160 mL/kg/day) because of the newborn's decreased ability to concentrate urine and increased overall metabolic rate. Although the infant's total body water content is high (75% to 80%) compared with an adult (60%), the infant has an increased surface area–to–mass ratio and decreased renal absorptive capacity that makes the infant more susceptible to dehydration from insufficient fluid intake or increased fluid loss caused by diarrhea, vomiting, or another source of fluid loss. Parents and caretakers should be aware of the signs of dehydration. See Chapter 45 🔗 for further information about fluid needs in infancy.

The basal metabolic rate (BMR) refers to the energy needed for thermoregulation, cardiorespiratory function, cellular activity,

and growth. A newborn requires 100 to 115 kcal/kg/day at 1 month. In breast milk, the primary carbohydrate is lactose. In addition to providing energy, lactose also functions to enhance the absorption of calcium, magnesium, and zinc (Lawrence & Lawrence, 2011). Human milk also contains trace amounts of other carbohydrates such as glucosamines and nitrogen-containing oligosaccharides. Glucosamines are one of the building blocks for connective tissues and help to strengthen ligaments and tendons. Oligosaccharides promote the growth of *Lactobacillus bifidus,* which promotes an intestinal acidic environment that is hostile to bacteria, making it difficult for them to thrive (Riordan & Wambach, 2010).

Infants receive approximately 50% of their calories from fat. Fats also help the body absorb the fat-soluble vitamins A, D, E, and K. Fats are a precursor of prostaglandins and other hormones. Fatty acids are a key component to brain development. Their derivatives, docosahexaenoic acid (DHA) and arachidonic acid (ARA), are long-chain polyunsaturated fatty acids (LCPUFAs) needed for myelination of the spinal cord and other nerves, and for development of visual acuity and cognitive and behavioral functions (Cloherty, Eichenwald, & Stark, 2012).

Approximately 98% of human milk fat is in the form of triglycerides, and a small amount is from cholesterol. Cholesterol levels in breast milk may also stimulate the production of enzymes that lead to more efficient metabolism of cholesterol, thereby reducing its harmful long-term effects on the cardiovascular system.

Fat content is the most variable component in breast milk, ranging from 30 to 50 g/L. It is influenced by maternal parity, duration of pregnancy, the stage of lactation, diurnal regulation, and changes in fat content even during a single feeding. Multiparous mothers produce milk with a lower content of fatty acids than primiparous women. Mothers of preterm infants have a greater concentration of LCPUFAs in their milk compared with mothers of term infants. By receiving this preterm breast milk, preterm infants receive the increased concentrations of DHA and ARA intended for their growth (Lawrence & Lawrence, 2011).

Phospholipids and cholesterol levels are higher in colostrum compared with mature milk, although overall fat content is higher in mature breast milk compared with colostrum. Fat content is generally higher in the evening and lower in the early morning. Within a single feeding session, an infant initially receives the low-fat foremilk before receiving the higher calorie, high-fat hindmilk. Finally, the fat content of breast milk is also affected by maternal diet and maternal fat stores. Mothers on low-fat diets have increased production of medium-chain fatty acids (C6–C10), and mothers with high levels of body fat produce breast milk with a higher fat content (Lawrence & Lawrence, 2011).

The fats in milk-based formulas are modified in an attempt to parallel the fat profile of breast milk by removing the butterfat from cow's milk and adding vegetable oils. The different blends of fats all provide a fatty acid profile that is similar to breast milk in terms of amount of saturated, monounsaturated, and polyunsaturated fats present. Since 2002, infant formulas have been supplemented with DHA and ARA. However, breast milk also contains 167 other fatty acids of uncertain function that are absent from formula (Cloherty et al., 2012).

Weblink · USDA

Proteins are the building blocks for muscle and organ structure. They are key to the body's metabolic processes including energy metabolism, cell signaling, growth, and immune function. Milk proteins are often grouped into casein and whey proteins. Whey protein is the predominant dietary protein in human milk. During digestion this type of protein creates soft curds that are easily and quickly broken down. Because of this, breastfeeding babies digest their meals in 90 minutes and need to feed often, receiving about 8 to 12 feedings per day. Casein is the major phosphoprotein found in milk. Cow's milk contains a high amount of casein (a low ratio of whey to casein—approximately 20:80) compared with mature human milk (60:40 whey:casein). Because of its tendency to form curds, milk with high amounts of casein is less easily digested. Cow's milk–based formulas are usually modified to get closer to the whey:casein ratio of human milk.

Micronutrients

The fat-soluble vitamins (vitamins A, D, E, and K) are found in both cow's milk–based formula and breast milk. After absorption via the lymphatic system, vitamins enter the blood and are transported to the various tissues. Excessive amounts of fat-soluble vitamins may result in toxicity, and there is general agreement that no routine fat-soluble vitamin supplementation is needed with the exception of vitamin D. See *Teaching Highlights: Supplements for Breastfed Babies* for recommendations regarding vitamin D and other nutrients.

The vitamin B complex and vitamin C are water-soluble vitamins that pass readily from serum to breast milk. However, mothers who follow a strict vegetarian or macrobiotic diet may have insufficient vitamin B_{12} in their milk. In that case the exclusively breastfed infant should receive vitamin B_{12} supplementation. Formula is fortified with adequate amounts of the water-soluble vitamins to meet the DRIs. Unlike fat-soluble vitamins, any excess water-soluble vitamins ingested are simply excreted and the threat of toxicity is low (Lawrence & Lawrence, 2011).

Both human milk and infant formulas contain several major and trace minerals to satisfy the needs of the growing infant. The mineral content of breast milk does not appear to be influenced by maternal diet.

Dental Health

Early childhood caries, the presence of one or more decayed, lost, or filled tooth surfaces in a primary tooth from birth to 6 years of age, can occur when a young child is allowed to breastfeed or drink from a bottle for long periods, especially when sleeping (American Academy of Pediatrics [AAP] Committee on Nutrition, 2009) (Figure 33–2 ●). The milk, juice, or other fluid pools around the upper anterior teeth, salivary flow decreases, and acid buffering is decreased, resulting in tooth decay. Nurses should teach parents to avoid putting the child to bed with a bottle and encourage pacifier use or a bottle of water instead. The child should not walk around with a bottle during the day. Mothers who breastfeed should also be cautioned to limit feeding to specific times rather than letting the infant breastfeed every few minutes (sometimes done when infant and mother co-sleep) so that milk will not pool in the mouth during sleep. When sleepy the infant does not swallow well and the milk is in constant contact with the teeth where milk sugars can decay erupting teeth.

Parents can be taught beginning dental care for the infant, which includes wiping the teeth off daily once they erupt with a piece of moist gauze or a small infant toothbrush. Some pediatric dentists like to see the child for a first dental visit at about 1 year of age, while others wait until the child is older. The nurse should encourage the parents to select and establish contact with a dental provider when the child is nearing the end of infancy.

Weaning

Weaning is the term used when infants stop breast or bottle feeding and obtain most liquids by cup. At about 8 to 9 months, a cup should be offered to the infant with assistance provided so that learning about drinking from a cup can begin. By about 1 year of age, infants are usually able to drink most liquids from a cup with a lid, so bottles can be slowly withdrawn and replaced by cups.

Teaching Highlights   Supplements for Breastfed Babies

1. Each baby receives a vitamin K injection after birth to promote adequate blood clotting. After that, no further vitamin K is needed since the child manufactures this vitamin in the gut once he or she begins eating.
2. Vitamin D is recommended at a minimum of 400 International Units/day for all infants (AAP Section on Breastfeeding, 2012).
3. Iron is not needed unless the infant is not eating food with iron by 4 to 6 months. The baby may need an iron source earlier if the mother was anemic during pregnancy or while breastfeeding.
4. Fluoride 0.25 mg is given after 6 months of age if water is not fluoridated to a level of 0.3 part per million (ppm), or if the baby is not drinking any water.

● Figure 33–2 Early childhood caries. This child has had major tooth decay related to sleeping as an infant and toddler while sucking bottles of juice and milk.
Source: Everst/Alamy

The decision to wean the baby from the breast may be made for a variety of reasons, including family or cultural pressures, changes in the home situation, pressure from the woman's partner, or a personal opinion about when weaning should occur. Some infants wean themselves spontaneously, despite the wishes of the mother. For the woman who is comfortable with breastfeeding and well informed about the process, the appropriate time to wean her infant will become evident if she is sensitive to the child's cues (Centers for Disease Control and Prevention [CDC], 2011a). The infant who is weaned before 12 months should be given iron-fortified infant formula rather than cow's milk.

If weaning is timed to respond to the child's cues, and if the mother is comfortable with the timing, it can be accomplished with less difficulty than if the process begins before mother and child are ready emotionally. Nevertheless, weaning is a time of emotional separation for mother and baby; it may be difficult for them to give up the closeness of their nursing sessions. The nurse who understands this possibility can help the mother see that her infant is growing up and plan other comforting, consoling, and play activities to replace breastfeeding. A gradual approach is the easiest and most comforting way to wean the child from breastfeeding.

During weaning, the mother should substitute one cup feeding or bottle feeding for one breastfeeding session over a few days to a week so that her breasts gradually produce less milk.

Eliminating the breastfeedings associated with meals first facilitates the mother's ability to wean the infant, because satiation with food lessens the desire for milk. Over a period of several weeks she can substitute more cup feedings or bottle feedings for breastfeedings. The slow method of weaning prevents breast engorgement, allows infants to alter their eating methods at their own rates, and provides time for psychologic adjustment.

Introduction of Complementary Foods

When should other foods be added to the infant's diet? Although some parents add other foods when the infant is only days or weeks old and such practices are often culturally derived, it is best to take cues from the infant's developmental milestones. The American Academy of Pediatrics recommends introducing complementary foods at about 6 months (AAP Committee on Nutrition, 2009). At this age the extrusion reflex (or tongue thrust) decreases and the infant can sit well with support. The infant is also developing the ability to appreciate texture and swallow nonliquid foods and can indicate desire for food or turn away when full. At 6 to 12 months, complementary foods are offered in addition to the intake of breast milk or formula, rather than replacing that essential nutrient (Hagan, Shaw, & Duncan, 2008) (see Table 33–1).

The first complementary food added to the infant's diet is often rice cereal. The advantages of introducing cereal first is that it provides iron at an age when the infant's prenatal iron

Table 33–1	Introduction of Solid Foods in Infancy
Recommendation	**Rationale**
Introduce rice cereal at about 6 months.	Rice cereal is easy to digest, has low allergenic potential, and contains iron.
Introduce fruits or vegetables at 6–8 months. Some healthcare providers recommend vegetable introduction before fruits.	Fruits and vegetables provide needed vitamins. Vegetables are not as sweet as fruits; introducing them first may enhance acceptability to the infant.
Introduce meats at 8–10 months.	Meats are harder to digest, have high protein load, and should not be fed until close to 1 year of age.
Use single-food prepared baby foods rather than combination meals.	Combination meals usually contain more sugar, salt, and fillers.
Introduce one new food at a time, waiting at least 3–4 days to introduce another. Delay feeding eggs, strawberries, wheat, corn, fish, and nut products until close to 2–3 years of age.	If a food allergy or intolerance develops, it will be easy to identify. The foods listed are those most commonly associated with food allergies.
Avoid carrots, beets, and spinach before 6 months of age. Have well water evaluated for nitrates (the recommended level is less than 10 mg/L).	Nitrates in these foods and in water near agricultural runoff can be converted to nitrite by young infants, causing methemoglobinemia.
Infants can be fed mashed portions of table foods such as carrots, rice, and potatoes.	This is a less expensive alternative to jars of commercially prepared baby food; it allows parents of various cultural groups to feed ethnic foods to infants.
Avoid adding sugar, salt, and spices when preparing baby foods at home.	Infants need not become accustomed to these flavors; they may get too much sodium from salt or develop gastric distress from some spices.
Avoid honey until at least 1 year of age.	Infants cannot detoxify *Clostridium botulinum* spores sometimes present in honey and can develop botulism.

● **Figure 33–3** Introducing finger foods. The baby who has developed the ability to grasp with thumb and forefinger should receive some foods that can be held in the hand.

Table 33–2	Infant Nutritional Patterns
Age	**Pattern**
Birth–1 month	■ Eats every 2–3 hours, breast or bottle ■ 2–3 ounces (60–90 mL) per feeding
2–4 months	■ Has coordinated suck–swallow ■ Eats every 3–4 hours ■ 3–4 ounces (90–120 mL) per feeding
4–6 months	■ Begins baby food, usually rice cereal, 2–3 T, twice daily ■ Consumes breast milk or formula 4 or more times daily ■ 4–5 ounces (100–150 mL) per feeding
6–8 months	■ Eats baby food such as rice cereal, fruits, and vegetables, 2–5 T, three times daily ■ Consumes breast milk or formula 4 times daily ■ 6–8 ounces (160–225 mL) per feeding
8–10 months	■ Enjoys soft finger foods three times daily ■ Consumes breast milk or formula 4 times daily ■ 6 ounces (160 mL) per feeding ■ Uses cup with lid
10–12 months	■ Eats most soft table foods with family three times daily ■ Uses cup with or without lid ■ Attempts to feed self with spoon though spills often ■ Consumes breast milk or formula 4 times daily ■ 6–8 ounces (160–225 mL) per feeding

stores begin to decrease, it seldom causes allergy, and it is easy to digest. A tablespoon or two is fed to the infant once or twice daily just before formula or breastfeeding. The infant may appear to spit out food at first because of normal back-and-forth tongue movement. Parents should not interpret this early feeding behavior as indicating dislike for the food. With a little practice the infant becomes adept at spoon feeding.

Once the infant eats 1/4 cup of cereal twice daily, usually at 6 to 8 months of age, vegetables or fruits can be introduced, at a rate of one new food every several days (Table 33–1). By 8 to 10 months of age, most fruits and vegetables have been introduced and strained meats or other protein (e.g., tofu, cheese, mashed cooked beans) can be added to the infant's diet. Finger foods are introduced during the second half of the first year as the infant's palmar and then finger grasp develops and as teeth begin to erupt (Figure 33–3 ●). Infants enjoy toast, O-shaped cereal, finely sliced meats, cheese and tofu, and small pieces of cooked, softened vegetables. Certain foods are associated with choking and should be avoided.

SAFETY ALERT!

Advise parents to use caution when providing finger foods to the infant. Hard foods and some soft and malleable ones slip easily into the throat and may cause choking. Avoid hot dogs, hard vegetables, candy, and chunks of peanut butter. Infants and other young children should always be supervised while eating. Be sure parents are familiar with techniques for airway obstruction removal and have emergency numbers clearly listed on their phones.

Certain foods are more commonly associated with development of food allergies, and avoiding them in infancy may decrease allergy incidence. Recommendations for infants at risk

due to family history of allergy are to delay feeding of cow milk until 1 year, eggs until 2 years, and peanuts, nuts, fish, and shellfish until 3 years (AAP Committee on Nutrition, 2009). As food and juice intake increase, formula- or breastfeedings decrease in amount and frequency (Table 33–2).

If breastfeeding is not chosen, or if supplemental feedings are provided, only iron-fortified infant formula should be used during the first year of life. Cow's milk (including evaporated milk) can lead to bleeding and anemia (see content on iron and anemia on page 864 in this chapter), can interfere with absorption of some nutrients, and has a high solute load, which immature kidneys can have difficulty excreting. Iron-fortified formula should always be used when the infant under 12 months drinks formula. When breastfed babies are not eating foods with iron by 6 months, supplemental iron may need to be added. Careful dietary assessment and discussion of intake by the nurse at health visits helps the practitioner decide if supplemental iron is needed.

Parents who want to make baby foods at home can be encouraged and instructed to do so. Some commercially prepared foods have unnecessary additives such as salt, sugar, and food starch, and they may be costly for some families. Parents can easily blend fruits and vegetables the family is eating without adding salt, sugar, or seasoning. Prepared foods should be used promptly and stored in the refrigerator between feedings. Foods can also be placed into ice cube trays and frozen; a cube or two can be defrosted at mealtime. Nurses should caution parents not to use honey in foods for infants as it can lead to infant botulism since infants cannot detoxify the *Clostridium botulinum* spores sometimes present in honey. If foods or fluids are microwaved, they should be shaken, stirred, and checked for temperature so that hot areas in the food do not burn the infant.

Toddlerhood

Why do parents of toddlers frequently become concerned about the small amount of food their children eat? Why do toddlers seem to survive and even thrive with minimal food intake? The toddler often displays the phenomenon of **physiologic anorexia**, caused when the extremely high metabolic demands of infancy slow to keep pace with the more moderate growth rate of toddlerhood. Although it can appear that the toddler eats nothing at times, intake over days or a week is generally sufficient and balanced enough to meet the body's demands for nutrients and energy.

Parents often need knowledge about the types of foods that constitute a healthy diet. Some easy-to-prepare foods are high in salt and other additives and can lead to exceeding the recommendation of *Healthy People 2020* for sodium intake (U.S. Department of Health and Human Services [USDHHS], 2011). The nurse can offer alternatives to hot dogs, microwave meals, or fast foods by providing information about easy preparation of sliced meats, cheese, tofu, fruits, and vegetables. Healthy snacks for young children include yogurt, cheese, milk, slices of bread with peanut butter, thinly sliced fruits, and soft vegetables.

Parents should be advised to offer a variety of nutritious foods several times daily (three meals and two snacks) and let the toddler make choices from the foods offered. They should offer foods only at mealtimes and have the child sit in a high chair or on a special seat at the table to eat (Figure 33–4 ●). Small portions are most appealing to the toddler. A general guideline

for food quantity at a meal is one tablespoon of each food per year of age.

The toddler should drink 16 to 24 oz (1/2 to 3/4 L) of milk daily. Parents should be cautioned against giving the toddler more than a quart (1 L) of milk daily, since this interferes with the desire to eat other foods, leading to dietary deficiencies. Recall that the child should not be put to bed with a bottle or allowed to carry a bottle of milk or juice around during the day, due to the risk of early childhood caries (see earlier discussion). In addition, parents should be advised to use only 100% fruit juice and to limit consumption of this juice to 4 to 6 ounces daily for children ages 1 to 6 years to decrease the opportunity for becoming overweight, developing dental caries, or experiencing abdominal discomfort (AAP, 2011). Unpasteurized juice should never be used since it may contain pathogens particularly harmful to young children. Drinking water and eating whole fruits, which provide fiber, are healthier alternatives. Avoid more than one meal weekly from a fast-food restaurant due to the generally high-fat, high-sugar, and low-fiber content of such meals.

Learning how to eat with others is an important task of toddlerhood. The toddler displays characteristic autonomy or independence during mealtime. Advise parents to provide opportunities for self-feeding of food with fingers and utensils and to allow some simple choices, such as type of liquid or cup to use. Young children should eat at a table with others, not be allowed to run and play while eating, and eat at specified meal and snack times. Toddlers should be taught to brush teeth after each meal, and care providers should offer assistance and supervision. A dental visit should occur during toddlerhood.

Because social skills are developing, the hospitalized toddler may eat better if allowed to have meals with parents or other hospitalized children. See Chapter 40 🔗 for further suggestions about management of nutrition in hospitalized children.

Preschool

The diet of the preschooler is similar to that of the toddler, but mealtime is now a more social event. Preschoolers like the company of others while they eat, and they enjoy helping with food preparation and table setting (Figure 33–5 ●). Involving them in these tasks can provide a forum for teaching about nutritious foods and principles of preparation, such as the need for refrigeration, safety around stoves, and cleanliness. Visits to fast-food restaurants should be limited to about once weekly, and parents can use the opportunity to assist the child in making wise choices of nutritionally adequate foods in that setting.

● **Figure 33–4** Fostering healthy eating habits. Toddlers should sit at a table or in a high chair to eat, to minimize the chance of choking and to foster positive eating patterns.

 Growth and Development

Toddlers generally eat three meals and two to three snacks daily. Toddlers can drink 2% milk or "follow-up" formula starting at 2 years of age. Cups are recommended, and bottle use should be discontinued. Drinks should be consumed at mealtimes and for snacks while sitting at a table; carrying cups during the day while playing or at other activities is not recommended. The child is learning to use utensils but may prefer fingers and still needs small serving sizes.

● **Figure 33–5** Preschoolers learn food habits by eating with others. Engaging them in food preparation enhances knowledge of food and promotes intake at meals.

Although the rate of growth is slow and steady during the preschool years, the child may have periods of **food jags** (eating only a few foods for several days or weeks) and greater or lesser intake. Parents should be advised to assess food intake over a 1- or 2-week period rather than at each meal to obtain a more accurate impression of total intake. Food jags can be handled by providing the desired food along with other foods to foster choice. The child who chooses not to eat at snack time or mealtime should not be given other foods in between. The child will become hungry and get accustomed to eating when food is provided. Three meals and two or three snacks daily are the norm. Fruit juice should be limited to 8 to 12 ounces daily, and begin teaching the "5-a-day" program that supports having five servings of fruits/vegetables each day.

The preschool period is a good time to continue encouraging good dental habits. Children can begin to brush their own teeth with parental supervision and help to reach all tooth surfaces. Fluoride supplements should be used when the water supply is not fluoridated. If the child has not yet visited a dentist, the first dental visit should be scheduled so the child can become accustomed to the routine of dental care.

School Age

The school-age years are a period of gradual growth when energy requirements remain at a steady level, although at some point during these years most children experience a preadolescent growth spurt. Girls may begin a growth spurt by 10 or 11 years, and boys a year or so later. Nutritional needs increase dramatically with this spurt, with large numbers of calories and increased amounts of other nutrients required (see Appendix G ⊘ for Dietary Reference Intakes).

School-age children are increasingly responsible for preparing snacks, lunches, and even some other meals. These years are a good time to teach children how to choose nutritious foods and plan a well-balanced meal. Because school-age children operate at the concrete level of cognitive thought, nutrition teaching is best presented by using pictures, samples of foods, videotapes, handouts, and hands-on experience.

School-age children often prefer the types of food eaten at home and may be resistant to new food items. A hospitalized child may refuse to eat, slowing the recuperative process. Nurses should encourage family members to bring favorite foods from home that meet nutritional requirements. This can be especially helpful when the hospital serves food only from the dominant cultural group. A child accustomed to a diet of rice, tofu, and vegetables may not enjoy a hospital meal of hamburger and fries. By school-age, food has become strongly associated with social interaction, so it is beneficial to have children eat together or to invite family members to take the child off the unit to eat or to bring in food from home and eat with the child. Many hospitals allow children to plan a pizza night or sponsor other events to encourage eating in a social atmosphere.

Most children consume at least one meal daily in school. While children may bring lunches to school, most participate in school lunch programs, and perhaps school breakfast programs. Nurses should become familiar with the policies of school districts in their areas for providing foods, snacks, and reduced-price food to students in need. During the past decade, many school systems in the United States have allowed vending machines for carbonated sweetened beverages and snacks to be installed in public schools. Part of the profits from these machines has enabled revenue-strapped school districts to enhance their incomes. However, schools are increasingly challenged about the presence of the machines, especially in light of the growing problem of overweight among youth. Some school districts have now limited the number of machines or the hours during which they can be used by students, and some have removed all sweetened beverages from vending machines. Nurses are able to provide information for districts about the problems of obesity and the need for healthy foods for youth. *Healthy People 2020* provides information about the importance of healthy diets and establishes goals for each developmental phase (USDHHS, 2011).

The opening quote in this chapter is from the mother of Joey, a young boy with cerebral palsy who has a gastrostomy feeding tube to assist him in ingestion of adequate nutrients. Joey is attending school and the teacher has been taught to administer his tube feedings. Nurses often assist families who have children with special needs to integrate them into the school environment. How might the nurse plan for Joey to participate in school lunchtime with peers? Since he can eat some soft foods

Healthy People 2020 Goals Weblink

by mouth, what types of foods are commonly available at school that he might be able to enjoy?

The loss of the first deciduous teeth and the eruption of permanent teeth usually occur at about 6 years, or at the beginning of the school-age period. Of the 32 permanent teeth, 22 to 26 erupt by age 12 years, and the remaining molars follow in the teenage years. See Chapter 34 for the typical sequence of tooth eruption and Chapter 36 for dental care needs during childhood. The school-age child should be closely monitored to ensure that brushing and flossing are adequate, that fluoride is taken if the water supply is not fluoridated, that dental care is obtained to provide for examination of teeth and alignment, and that loose teeth are identified before surgery or sports participation.

Adolescence

Most adolescents need well over 2000 calories daily to support the growth spurt, and some adolescent boys require nearly 3000 or more calories daily. When teenagers are active in a variety of sports, these requirements increase further. Because adolescents prepare much of their own food and often eat with friends, they need to be taught about good nutrition. Developing a diet that includes a large number of calories, meets vitamin and mineral requirements, and is acceptable to the teen may be a challenge.

The pregnant adolescent has even more challenging nutrient requirements. See Chapter 13 for details about needs during pregnancy. An adolescent who is hospitalized and does not like the hospital lunch might ask a friend who visits to bring a soft drink and chips; however, the teen may be receptive to offers of juice and pizza, a more nutritious meal. Small improvements should be viewed positively because they may lead to further changes. See *Evidence-Based Practice: Adolescents and Nutritional Choices.*

Fast food represents a significant intake for many adolescents. It is commonly high in fat, calories, and sodium while being low in essential nutrients such as calcium, folic acid, riboflavin, vitamins A and C, and fiber. Many schools are redesigning cafeterias and food programs to entice more teens to eat at school rather than nearby fast-food restaurants. Adding fruits and salads and allowing choice can enhance quality of food intake. School nurses play a vital role in helping to tailor a healthy school nutrition program and teaching teens about the healthiest choices at their favorite fast-food restaurants.

Peer group influence is important to teens, so group sessions in which adolescents eat lunch together can provide a forum for influencing food habits. What other methods might encourage positive nutritional habits among teens?

NUTRITIONAL ASSESSMENT

What is the best indication that a child's nutrition is adequate? Which data collection methods provide the most accurate information about a child's dietary intake? The nurse plays an important role in assessing the diets of children and in seeking additional evaluation from dietitians and nutritionists in complex situations.

Evidence-Based Practice Adolescents and Nutritional Choices

Clinical Question
Adolescents are largely independent in their food choices. They often eat "on the run" and are influenced by peers and the media. At the same time, rates of obesity are on an escalating upward trajectory. Nurses need to understand and apply evidence-based practices for influencing eating behaviors in adolescents.

The Evidence
The HEALTHY study found that a middle school–based intervention program resulted in significant positive changes in students' fruit and water intake (Siega-Riz et al., 2011). Another middle school program with young adolescents, the TEAMS study, asked parents, youth, and school officials to identify barriers to health and solutions for healthier environments. Students had knowledge deficits but identified low access to healthy foods and busy schedules as barriers, while teachers tended to believe parents frequently did not provide healthy food options and parents identified teens' preferences for unhealthy foods as an important barrier (Power, Bindler, Goetz, et al., 2010). School boards are instrumental in establishing school wellness policies (Agron, Berends, Ellis, et al., 2010). Achieving healthy weight by adolescents should include nutrition and activity teaching, technology-based approaches, and peer modeling (Ayliffe & Glanville, 2010). The community can be engaged in healthy weight goals by introducing measures to monitor weight, nutrition, and activity at all health visits. One tool called Passport to Health was developed and implemented successfully by nurse practitioners in a pediatric practice setting (Vaczy, Seaman, Peterson-Sweeney, et al., 2011).

Best Practice
Child and adolescent eating patterns set an important example for life. Family eating patterns, school setting, and community influences must all be examined to identify risk and protective factors in the adolescent diet. Barriers to adolescent healthy eating include lack of accurate information, availability of "junk food" snacks, lack of parental involvement in the lives of teens, peer influence, and media messages about food consumption.

Clinical Reasoning
1. What developmental stages of the adolescent provide both challenges to healthy eating and ability to make wise food choices?
2. Construct a list of questions about family food patterns that will help you identify risk and protective factors of the family.
3. Visit a local high school and then travel 1/2 mile in each direction from the school. Record the number of fast food restaurants, billboards about foods, and any other food-related resources or media. Watch 2 hours of television at 3–5 p.m., when adolescents frequently arrive home. Record the number of food-related messages, what types of foods are advertised, and other observations.
4. How can you integrate knowledge about adolescent nutrition into your potential role as a school nurse at a high school?

Activity | Critical Thinking: Fast Food Analysis | Video | Nutritional Status

Physical and Behavioral Measurement

Growth Measurement

A common method of evaluating the adequacy of diet is measurement of growth. **Anthropometric measurement** is the term used to refer to assessment of various parts of the body. Anthropometry of young children commonly includes weight, length, and head circumference. Standing height is substituted for length once the child can stand. Head circumference, also known as occipital-frontal circumference (OFC), is measured during infancy, and into early years when there are growth concerns. Additional measurements that may be included in special circumstances include chest circumference, mid-upper arm circumference, and skinfold measurement at sites such as triceps, abdomen, and subscapular regions. Grids are available for each measurement and assist in providing a thorough nutritional assessment when weight and height are abnormally high or low. Skills 9–1 through 9–6 in the accompanying *Clinical Skills Manual* SKILLS present techniques for accurate measurement of weight, length, height, chest circumference, and head circumference.

After collecting the measurements, the nurse plots them on the appropriate standardized growth curves for weight, length to height, head circumference, and body mass index (Figure 33–6 ●). **Body mass index (BMI)** is a calculation based on the child's weight and height, or length, and is calculated as kilograms of weight per square meter of height. This is a useful calculation for determining if the child's height and weight are in proportion and identifies which percentile the child falls in for each measurement. Children normally fall between the 10th and 90th percentiles. A measurement below the 10th percentile, especially for BMI, may indicate undernutrition, while one over the 90th percentile can indicate overnutrition. However, it is important to look at the differences between measurements.

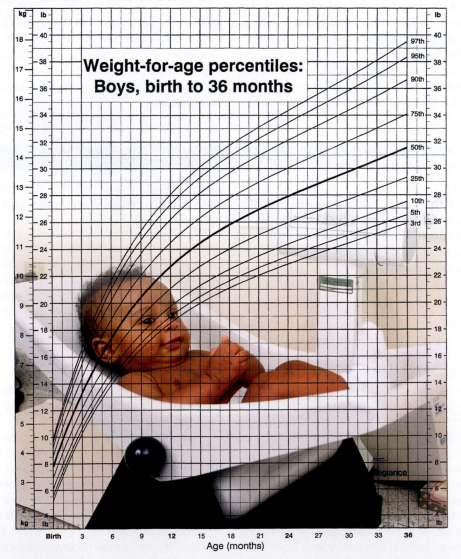

● **Figure 33–6** Plotting measurements on the growth curve. The nurse accurately measures the child and then places height and weight on appropriate growth grids for the child's age and gender.

An infant in the 90th percentile for length, weight, and head circumference is proportional and may be a naturally large baby. On the other hand, a child who is consistently in the 10th percentile for all measurements, but is growing steadily and is at a normal development level, may simply be a small child. Much cultural and individual variation exists in size. See Appendix C 🔗 for standardized growth curves by gender and age for infants, children, and adolescents. See www.nursing.pearsonhighered.com to find out more about the growth curves and a course in accurate assessment techniques. Visit the Centers for Disease Control and Prevention website (www.cdc.gov) to find specialized growth grids for children with conditions such as Down syndrome.

The nurse should plot measurements on the same growth curve with earlier percentiles for the child. When measurements follow the same percentile over time, growth is generally normal for the child and nutrition is likely adequate. However, a sudden or sustained change in percentile may indicate a chronic disorder, emotional difficulty, or a nutritional intake problem. Further assessment of physical status and dietary intake will be needed.

Additional Physical Measurements

Many observations from the physical assessment provide clues to nutritional status. Dietary intake can affect every body system, and a combination of certain symptoms may suggest specific nutritional problems. Some common physical manifestations of nutritional status are outlined in Table 33–3.

Laboratory measurements can provide useful information when nutritional status is questionable. Some common studies include hematocrit and hemoglobin, serum glucose and fasting insulin, lipids and lipoproteins, and liver and renal function studies. Adding some further measurements such as chest circumference and skinfolds (measurement of fat at certain body sites such as triceps, scapular, and abdominal areas) may also be useful (Lee & Nieman, 2010).

Dietary Intake

The nurse should obtain detailed information about the child's dietary intake when there is a potential for nutritional deficiency due to disease, knowledge deficit, or socioeconomic status. The mother's dietary intake during pregnancy may provide information about the child's nutritional state and it can be assessed for pertinent information. After the information is collected, the

Table 33–3   Clinical Manifestations of Dietary Deficiencies/Excesses

Nutrient	Deficiency Manifestation	Excess Manifestation
Vitamin A	Night blindness Skin dryness and scaling	Headache Drowsiness Hepatomegaly Vomiting and diarrhea
Vitamin C	Abnormal hair (coiled shape) Skin abnormalities (dermatitis and lesions) Purpura Bleeding gums Joint tenderness Sudden heart failure	Usually none—excess is excreted in urine
Vitamin D	Rib deformity Bowed legs	Drowsiness
B vitamins	Weakness Decreased deep tendon reflexes Dermatitis	Usually none—excess is excreted in urine
Protein	Hepatomegaly Edema Scant, depigmented hair	Kidney failure
Carbohydrate	Emaciation Decreased energy Retarded growth and development	Overweight
Iron	Lethargy Slowed growth and developmental progression Pallor	Vomiting, diarrhea, abdominal pain Pallor Cyanosis Drowsiness Shock

dietary intake should be compared to the recommended levels for a child of that age and gender (see Figure 33–1 for the U.S. MyPlate food guide; see Appendix G 🔗 for Recommended Dietary Allowances). The 24-hour recall of intake, a food frequency questionnaire, and a dietary screening history (Tables 33–4 and 33–5) provide a good overview of the infant's or child's intake and eating patterns. A food diary provides precise information about the child's food intake.

Twenty-Four-Hour Recall of Food Intake

The 24-hour diet recall is frequently used to assess the adequacy of the diet. People can generally remember their intake in the past day so results are fairly accurate, it is easy to gather the data and analyze results, and only a few minutes are needed. The nurse should ask the parent or child to list all foods eaten during the past 24 hours (Figure 33–7 ●). It is usually helpful to ask for a description of activities in the last day, then start with the most

Table 33–4	Dietary Screening History for Infants

Overview Questions

What was the infant's birth weight?
At what age did the birth weight double and triple?
Was the infant premature?
Does the infant have any feeding problems such as difficulty sucking and swallowing, spitting up, fatigue, or fussiness?

If Infant Is Breastfed

How long does the baby nurse at each breast?
What is the usual schedule for breastfeeding?
Does the baby also take any milk or formula? Amount and frequency? What type?

If Infant Is Formula Fed

What formula is used? Is it iron fortified?
How is it prepared?
Do you hold or prop the bottle for feedings?
How much formula is taken at each feeding?
How many bottles are taken each day?
Does the baby take a bottle to bed for naps or nighttime? What is in the bottle?

If Infant Is Fed Other Foods

At what age did the baby start eating other foods?

Cereal	Finger foods
Fruit/juices	Meats
Vegetables	Other protein sources

Do you use commercial baby food or make your own?
Does the baby eat any table foods?
How often does the baby take solid foods?
How is the baby's appetite?
Do you have any concerns about the baby's feeding habits?
Does the baby take a vitamin supplement? Fluoride?
Have there been any allergic reactions to foods? Which ones?

Does the baby spit up frequently?
Have there been any rashes?

What types of stools does the baby have? Frequency? Consistency?

Table 33–5	Dietary Screening History for Children

What types of food or beverage does the child especially like?
What foods or beverages does the child dislike?
What is the child's typical eating schedule? Meals and snacks?
Does the child eat with the family or at separate times?
　　Where does the child eat each meal?
Who prepares the food for the family?
　　What methods of cooking are used? Baking? Frying? Broiling? Grilling?
　　What ethnic foods are commonly eaten?
Does the family eat in a restaurant frequently? What type?
　　What type of food does the child usually order?
Is the child on a special diet?
Does the child need to be fed, feed himself or herself, need assistance eating, or need any adaptive devices for eating?
What is the child's appetite like?
Does the child take any vitamin supplements (iron, fluoride)?
Does the child have any allergies? What types of symptoms?
What types of regular exercise does the child get?
Are there any concerns about the child's eating habits?

- Food preparation methods, including adding fats to cook, removal or retention of fats on meats

- Vitamins and supplements, types and doses

- Whether the intake is typical (in situations such as illness or vacation, intake may be different than usual)

Once the 24-hour recall is obtained, the nurse needs to analyze the intake by first doing a quick check to compare servings of various food types with the U.S. MyPlate food guide, as described earlier. Next the nurse should do a detailed analysis to compute calories, carbohydrate, protein, and fat intake and compare them to recommended amounts. All major vitamins and minerals are also computed and comparisons made to the DRIs. This computation may be done by hand, using a book of nutrients in common foods, or may be done on the computer. Several computer programs are available, and the federal government

recent event and move backwards, integrating food intake into the daily schedule. For example, the nurse might begin by saying, "You mentioned you got up early to come to the clinic today. What did Sam eat at home before you left? Did he have a snack as you traveled here or after you arrived?" While asking about the foods eaten, the nurse should inquire specifically about the following:

- All meals and snacks

- Amounts of each food item consumed (having various size measuring cups, bowls, and plates available so accurate amounts can be indicated is helpful)

- Types of specific foods used, such as whole milk versus nonfat or 2%, brand names of cereals, specific types of margarine or butter

- Additives used, such as condiments, table salt, spices, milk to mix formula

● **Figure 33–7** Twenty-four-hour diet recall. The nurse is interviewing a child about foods eaten in the last day. Note the models of food and dishes for accurate assessment of serving sizes.

has a website that provides intake levels and comparisons to the RDAs. It may be useful to compute a personal 24-hour recall or that of a child in the clinical setting with the Healthy Eating Index.

Food Frequency Questionnaire

Food frequency questionnaires are available that can be easily administered to parents or children. Usually they ask about how often certain types of foods are eaten in a specified period such as a week. Long questionnaires can evaluate a total diet, while short ones focus on specific items such as fruit and vegetable intake. A short questionnaire about milk intake or fruit and vegetable intake may be helpful before planning a teaching project on nutrition to a class of school-age children. Knowing their usual intake of a food item can provide helpful information for planning the project. See www.nursing.pearsonhighered.com for one example of questions from a food frequency questionnaire.

Dietary Screening History

The nurse should ask the parent about the infant's or child's eating habits using the questions listed in Tables 33–4 and 33–5. Responses provide information about the family's eating habits and food beliefs beyond that collected on a 24-hour dietary recall or food frequency questionnaire.

Food Diary

Parents are asked to keep a food diary when the child has a nutrition problem or disorder that requires dietary management, such as malnutrition, obesity, or diabetes. All meals and snacks, with food preparation method and quantities eaten over a 1- to 7-day period, are recorded. Eating patterns change significantly for holidays or family gatherings, so parents should be asked to select typical days for the food diary or to record specific events affecting food intake. Including one weekday and one weekend day may be helpful. Parents need to be reminded of all the places children might have eaten, such as the childcare center, school, friends' houses, or neighbors. Food diaries can provide a great deal of helpful information, but they take time and motivation to complete well (Lee & Nieman, 2010). The nurse should be sure instructions are complete and that the form has a place to record amounts, preparation, events occurring, and where food was

---

Developing Cultural Competence
Dietary Intake Varies Among Cultures

Each culture has eating practices that influence dietary intake. It is important to understand the foods commonly eaten by each cultural group and their contribution to the total nutrition of the child. Depending on the populations nurses work with, they may need to ask about intake of freshly caught fish or wild game such as pheasants and elk. Home-prepared sausages and cheese may be part of diets. Berries and garden produce might be eaten. Foods from ethnic markets may include spices, dried mushrooms, and other products. Some groups do not eat meat or specific types of meats. Using open-ended questions when gathering data will increase the likelihood of obtaining an accurate evaluation of diet.

---

eaten. The nurse or parent may need to obtain the school lunch menu and talk with the school lunch personnel to add accurate school intake. The nurse completes the nutritional assessment indicated for a child and may consult with or refer the family to a dietitian or nutritionist for additional assessment and teaching.

Weblink | USDA Healthy Eating Index

COMMON NUTRITIONAL CONCERNS

Childhood Hunger

Although most Americans live in a land of plenty, significant numbers of children periodically experience hunger. **Food security** is access at all times to enough nourishment for an active, healthy life. In contrast, **food insecurity** indicates an inability to acquire or consume adequate quality or quantity of foods in socially acceptable ways, or the uncertainty that one will be able to do so; about 20% of U.S. children live in households that periodically experience food insecurity (U.S. Department of Agriculture, 2011).

The major cause of hunger in children is poverty, and since one in five children is poor, their families may be unable to provide sustainable nutrition at all times (Children's Defense Fund, 2010). Many single-income families have a head of household moving into the workforce, so incomes are often not sufficient to provide for family food needs (see Chapter 1 for a description of Temporary Assistance for Needy Families). Families may be ineligible for food assistance programs even though they cannot afford enough food for all their members. Children with special nutritional needs are at particular risk since it may be more costly to buy and prepare formula or foods for a child with allergies, diabetes, or an immune disorder.

Children with insufficient dietary intake are at risk for a wide array of health problems. They may become anemic; have a high rate of infectious disease due to lowered immune response; have slowed developmental maturation, delayed or stunted physical growth, and learning disorders; and be at greater risk of overweight, cardiovascular disease, and diabetes in adulthood (AAP Committee on Nutrition, 2009). Subsequently, the national and individual cost of childhood hunger is great.

Nurses are well positioned to evaluate families for food insecurity in a variety of hospital, clinic, school, and home settings. In addition to the assessment of the individual child's nutritional status, further questions can determine families with potential problems. Nurses should administer a screening tool to identify risk in families (Table 33–6). Most parents go without food themselves in order to feed their children, so food insecurity may not have directly affected all children. However, anxiety over providing food can be very stressful for families, and diet quality deteriorates as insecurity increases. If families have experienced food insecurity or may be likely to at some time, nurses should be sure to provide them with access to community agencies and programs that can help. What resources are available locally to help families with food insecurity?

Overweight and Obesity

The current incidence of overweight children in the United States is epidemic and is associated with a wide array of health

Table 33–6	Food Insecurity Screening

1. Does your household ever run out of money to buy food to make a meal?
2. Do you or members of your household ever eat less than you feel you should because there is not enough money for food?
3. Do you or members of your household ever cut the size of meals or skip meals because there is not enough money for food?
4. Do your children ever eat less than you feel they should because there is not enough money for food?
5. Do you ever cut the size of your children's meals or do they skip meals because there is not enough money for food?
6. Do your children ever say they are hungry because there is not enough food in the house?
7. Do you ever rely on a limited number of foods to feed your children because you are running out of money to buy foods for a meal?
8. Do any of your children ever go to bed hungry because there is not enough money to buy food?

Scoring: 5–8 yes responses = hungry; 1–4 yes responses = risk of hunger. From Washington State Department of Health.

problems, such as type 2 diabetes, stroke, gallbladder disease, arthritis, cardiovascular disease, sleep disturbances, hypertension, dyslipidemia, respiratory problems, certain cancers, interference with physical activity, social stigma, discrimination, depression, and low self-esteem (Centers for Disease Control and Prevention [CDC], 2011b). A historic high of 17% of children and adolescents are at or above the 95th percentile for BMI (obese) and

Teaching Highlights Community Resources for Food

Supplemental Nutrition Assistance Program (SNAP)—Eligibility based on household size and income; refer students and those with low incomes, especially when they have young children; education services often available

Child Nutrition Programs—School lunch, breakfast, and milk programs; free and lowered cost meals in schools; assist parents to apply

Special Child Programs—Summer programs, Head Start, childcare centers, and homeless children programs may provide nutritional support in some communities

Women, Infants, and Children (WIC)—Supplemental foods and nutrition education to pregnant, breastfeeding, and postpartum women and to their young children; assessment of child growth often included

Nutrition Education and Training Program—Nutrition education for teachers and school food service personnel

Community Services—May include food banks, field gleaning (collecting produce from farmers' fields that will not be sold due to excess or small blemishes), community gardens, and other programs

Find out what services are available to provide food and nutrition education in your community. Make a list to use in clinical settings with families.

about the same amount fall from the 85th to 94th percentiles for BMI (overweight), designating about one third of U.S. youth as overweight or obese (CDC, 2011b).

Many reasons are cited for the increase in overweight children. The number of calories consumed is not increasing, but children tend to exercise less, particularly in daily life. They infrequently walk or ride bikes, either because of the convenience of driving or due to unsafe neighborhoods. Television viewing is very high among youth; movies, Internet, computer games, social networking, and cell phones are further examples of media commonly used by youth. Children spend over 7 hours daily on such media (Strasburger, Jordan, & Donnerstein, 2010). Inactive pursuits do not require high caloric energy, leading to an imbalance in intake and demand for calories. Additionally television viewing is often accompanied by ingestion of high-calorie foods and subjects children to food marketing of unhealthy foods.

The percentage of calories from fat consumed in the United States is among the highest in the world. Although no more than 25% to 35% of calories should come from total dietary fat, and no more than 10% from saturated fat, about 35% of calories consumed in the United States are supplied by fat and over 11% by saturated fat (USDHHS, 2011). Most fats should be supplied from polyunsaturated and monounsaturated fatty acids, but current diets contain low amounts of those fats and high amounts of trans-fatty acids (USDHHS, 2011). The high rate of dietary fat is related to the amount of fast food consumed, and influenced by snacking as well.

Goals of nursing management are to prevent new cases of overweight, identify children who are overweight, and to support youth and families to establish healthy lifestyles that promote weight loss and maintenance of recommended weight. Perform assessment of height, weight, and BMI. Measure blood pressure and determine whether it is within normal limits. Evaluate amount of screen/social activities, sedentary behavior, and physical activity levels.

Nurses can help parents and children build good nutritional and exercise habits throughout life, thus decreasing the incidence of overweight and its attendant health risks. Parents should be advised that television viewing should be limited to a maximum of 2 hours daily, and that a television and video games should not be placed in children's bedrooms. Daily exercise routines of 30 to 60 minutes can be included in most families. Aim to meet the current recommendation of 60 minutes daily for children with some activity including muscle strengthening and flexibility. Also, nurses should teach about the MyPlate food guide and its integration into a healthy life. Healthy snacks include fruits, vegetables, grains, and nuts. "Super sizing" fast foods and eating out often should be avoided.

Risks for poor health often cluster together in individuals and families. Nurses need to be alert for situations in which parents are overweight and children have elevated blood pressure, exercise infrequently, or are in upper percentiles for weight, BMI, or skinfold measurements. Be alert for early menarche, which can help identify overweight girls who need intervention for obesity prevention. The presence of risk factors necessitates further dietary and risk assessment so that a management plan can be implemented. Visit www.nursing.pearsonhighered.com

Nursing Care Plan   **The Child Who Is Overweight**

Intervention	Rationale	Expected Outcome

1. Nursing Diagnosis: *Nutrition, Imbalanced: More than Body Requirements* related to excessive intake in comparison to metabolic needs (NANDA-I © 2012)

Intervention	Rationale	Expected Outcome
NIC Priority Intervention: *Weight reduction assistance:* Facilitating loss of weight and body fat		**NOC Suggested Outcome:** *Weight control:* Personal actions resulting in achievement and maintenance of optimum body weight for health

Goal: The child will demonstrate adequate intake of all nutrients without excessive energy intake.

Intervention	Rationale	Expected Outcome
■ Perform thorough nutritional assessment of child.	■ Assessment assists in identification of dietary risks and strengths as well as health conditions related to nutrition.	■ Child meets all dietary requirements while achieving weight and body mass index goal.
■ Share results of assessment with child and family by showing weight, height, and body mass index grids.	■ Many families do not consider their child overweight. Concrete information about the child's size in comparison with recommendations assists in establishing the importance of weight management.	
■ Assess access to sufficient nutritious foods for the family at all times.	■ Food insecurity promotes inadequate intake alternating with excess intake of high-calorie foods.	
■ Identify with the child and family 2–3 target areas to begin weight management. Examples might include: ● Having fast food only once weekly ● Switching to low-fat dairy products ● Keeping two more fresh fruits and vegetables in the house and two less snack foods	■ Changing dietary patterns drastically is difficult and may lead to giving up the attempt at weight management. Partnering with the family to set goals enhances chances of success.	
■ Integrate nutrition information into each visit. Examples of topics include: ● Dietary requirements for age group ● Effects of simple sugar and fat intake on weight ● Beneficial effects of fruits, vegetables, whole grains, and nonfat dairy ● Reading food labels ● Healthy choices in fast-food restaurants ● Calculation of fat content of foods	■ Nutrition information is best learned in an ongoing program.	
■ Use growth grids to help child and family establish a weight reduction or maintenance goal.	■ Goals motivate families to achieve desired health behaviors. The goal for a young child may be weight maintenance so that as the child grows in height, the correct proportion is reached, while weight reduction may be needed for older children or youth who are very obese.	

2. Nursing Diagnosis: *Coping: Family, Readiness for Enhanced,* related to need to foster health of family member (NANDA-I © 2012)

Intervention	Rationale	Expected Outcome
NIC Priority Intervention: *Health system guidance:* Facilitating child's use of appropriate nutrition and health services to foster weight control		**NOC Suggested Outcome:** *Health-promoting behavior:* Actions to promote, sustain, and increase wellness

Goal: The family will assist child to manage stressors and to develop new strategies to support weight control goals.

Intervention	Rationale	Expected Outcome
■ Include key family members in some of the counseling sessions with the child who is overweight.	■ Key members of the family are those who purchase foods, provide support for the child, and participate in decisions about health.	■ Child expresses satisfaction with family understanding and support of weight.
■ Encourage the family to eat together at least once daily if possible or to increase number of meals eaten together weekly.	■ The family is an important support system in weight loss programs. Eating as a family or in a social situation can provide a chance to promote healthy foods; intake is generally lower fat and calorie than when eating alone.	

(continued)

Nursing Care Plan   The Child Who Is Overweight—continued

Intervention	Rationale	Expected Outcome
■ Seek a resource for the child to be monitored about twice monthly; this may be a healthcare provider office, nutritionist, school nurse, or other person.	■ The resource provides opportunity to monitor the child's progress and to offer support, additional information, and problem-solving techniques.	

---

3. Nursing Diagnosis: *Activity Intolerance* related to sedentary lifestyle (NANDA-I © 2012)

NIC Priority Intervention:		NOC Suggested Outcome:
Exercise promotion: Facilitating regular exercise to maintain and increase endurance and energy use		*Endurance:* Extent that energy enables the child to sustain activity

Goal: The child will demonstrate activity tolerance by adequate oxygenation, respiratory effort, and ability to speak during brisk walking, biking, or other activity.

■ Establish daily exercise routine beginning with 15–30 minutes daily of walking.	■ Starting with brief amounts of exercise makes the child feel comfortable and enhances potential for success.	■ Child demonstrates ability to engage in moderate activity for 60 minutes with minimal respiratory discomfort.
■ Gradually increase activity over 1–2 months until 60 minutes of daily exercise is maintained.	■ Gradual increase as the cardiovascular and respiratory systems adapt is generally comfortable for children; 60 minutes of moderate activity daily is recommended for children.	
■ Use activities enjoyed by the child and suggest options as necessary; refer the family to community resources such as swimming pools, organized sports, and biking groups.	■ Activities the child enjoys will be more likely to remain in usual activity patterns; exercising with others in groups increases motivation.	
■ Have families plan at least 1–2 activities they can do together weekly.	■ This fosters family relationships and provides support and motivation for the child.	
■ Limit screen activities to a maximum of 2 hours daily. Have child keep a log of hours of television, video games, computer, and other similar activities. Tell child never to snack while doing screen activities.	■ Increased use of screen activities is related to poor dietary habits and increased sedentary behaviors and excess weight.	
■ Ask about use of tobacco in children in fifth grade or higher. Inquire about exposure to environmental tobacco smoke at all ages. Perform teaching to discourage tobacco use or offer cessation programs as needed.	■ Most adults who smoke began the habit in childhood; middle school years are the most common age for smoking initiation. Smoking by others in the household can be harmful to children. Smoking decreases respiratory reserves and worsens several cardiovascular disease risks.	

---

4. Nursing Diagnosis: *Self-Esteem, Chronic Low,* related to weight (NANDA-I © 2012)

NIC Priority Intervention:		NOC Suggested Outcome:
Self-esteem enhancement: Assisting the child to increase personal judgment of self-worth		*Quality of life and self-esteem:* Expressed satisfaction with life circumstances and positive judgment of self-worth

Goal: The child expresses positive perception of self-worth and confidence in ability to deal with issues related to weight.

■ Facilitate development of a positive outlook by exposing child to others who have been successful with weight loss.	■ Increases motivation and feelings of self-efficacy.	■ Child speaks positively about accomplishments in weight control management.
■ Praise child for weight loss, weight maintenance, increased physical activity, and other achievements. Help the child establish rewards for meeting goals, such as purchase of new clothing.	■ Enhances judgment of self-worth and pride in accomplishments.	
■ Partner with parents so that they understand the value of praise and never label the child using derogatory words such as "fat."	■ Family members are usually the most intimate support system for the child.	

for information that will be helpful to families in the clinical setting. See resources such as "Helping Your Overweight Child" and "Take Charge of Your Health: A Teenager's Guide to Better Health" (http://win.niddk.nih.gov/publications).

Consult the *Nursing Care Plan* in this chapter for further interventions appropriate for the child who is overweight.

Food Safety

Every year in the United States, about 48 million people (1 in 6) contract food-borne illnesses. Some cases are quite mild, whereas others can be very severe. About 72,000 people are hospitalized and over 1680 die from these illnesses (CDC, 2011c). Children are at greater risk of severe illness and death from food and water due to their immature gastrointestinal and immune systems. Children who are immunocompromised are at even greater risk. The most common pathogens are *Campylobacter, Salmonella, Shigella, Cryptosporidium, Listeria, Yersinia,* and *Escherichia coli* (CDC, 2011c). Worldwide over 3 million people die of illness related to unsafe drinking water each year, and most of those deaths are among children.

Foodborne illness transmission is associated with food preparation and storage practices, lack of adequate training of retail employees about foods and hygiene, and increasing amounts and types of foods being imported from other countries. Some examples of contaminated foods in the past few years include undercooked hamburger meat, cross-contamination of salad bar items from meats, unpasteurized apple cider, green onions, raw spinach,

 Growth and Development

Numerous research studies have found a positive relationship between body mass index and early menarche in girls. Additional factors contributing to early menarche may be exposure to environmental endocrine-disrupting chemicals such as phthalates, phytoestrogens, and polychlorinated biphenyls, and the effects of chronic stress (Walvoord, 2010). Early weight monitoring and careful physical assessment are important. The nurse should remain alert for signs of breast development in fourth- or fifth-grade students and early menarche in grade 6. Such youth may already be overweight and should receive obesity prevention interventions as well as counseling for management of body changes.

prepackaged salad and delicatessen meat, berries, and sprouts. While most infected persons experience acute diarrhea, some can develop complications such as hemolytic uremic syndrome (Chapter 53 🔗) or thrombocytic purpura (Chapter 50 🔗). Health personnel should integrate teaching regularly so that families can decrease risks of food-borne illness. Recommend that families avoid consumption of unpasteurized milk, raw or undercooked oysters, raw or undercooked eggs, raw or undercooked ground beef, and undercooked poultry (CDC, 2011c). Check the information regarding outbreaks at www.foodsafety.org.

Food may carry products other than microorganisms that can be harmful. An example is mercury, which may be concentrated in certain types of fish. This metal can cause harm to the developing nervous system of fetuses, infants, and young children when consumed regularly. The U.S. Food and Drug Administration (FDA) and Environmental Protection Agency (EPA) note that fish are an important part of a healthy diet, but that certain recommendations should be followed to lower the risk of experiencing mercury's detrimental effects. Women who may become pregnant, are pregnant or breastfeeding, and young children should:

- Eliminate shellfish, shark, swordfish, king mackerel, and tilefish from the diet.

- Eat up to 12 ounces (two average meals) a week of a variety of low-mercury fish, such as shrimp, canned light tuna, salmon, pollock, and catfish. Albacore or white tuna has more mercury than light tuna, so limit white tuna to one meal weekly.

Check for local advisories about the safety of fish caught in local waters. In the absence of advice, up to 6 ounces (one meal) weekly may be eaten from local waters. Do not eat other fish during that week (U.S. Food and Drug Administration, 2011).

Common Dietary Deficiencies

Dietary deficiencies can occur in children and some are common in selected populations. While children can have deficits in nearly any nutrient, a number of nutrient deficits are more common in childhood. Limitations in the food supply or patterns of dietary intake cause most deficiencies, while children with certain disease processes, such as metabolic diseases, may have difficulty absorbing or using nutrients ingested. (See Chapter 54 🔗 for a discussion of inborn errors of metabolism.) The nutrient deficiencies of a population are a result of genetic factors, characteristics of the food supply, and intake patterns of particular groups.

Iron

Newborns have a store of iron obtained from their mothers in the uterus if the maternal nutritional state was satisfactory and the baby was of normal gestational age. Breast milk contains little iron, but the iron it does contain has high bioavailability. However, by 4 to 6 months of age, the baby's iron stores begin to decrease and a dietary source of iron must be added. Enriched rice cereal is commonly used to meet these initial iron needs. In babies who do not have adequate stores or do not take in enough iron, **anemia**, or a reduction in the number of red blood cells, can result (Figure 33–8 ●). Feeding cow's milk during infancy can also cause anemia by irritating the gut and leading to small but consistent loss of blood from the gastrointestinal tract; cow milk should not be fed in the first year of life. When formulas are used, they should be iron fortified to help avoid iron-deficiency anemia. Iron-fortified infant cereals are a good source of the mineral.

Adolescent females comprise another group commonly deficient in iron. Their deficiency is related to loss of blood in menses, metabolic need of the growth spurt, and poor dietary balance due to sporadic dieting. Further discussion of the symptoms and treatment of iron-deficiency anemia can be found in Chapter 50 ●. Encourage intake of good iron sources such as meats, eggs, dried fruits, and iron-fortified cereal.

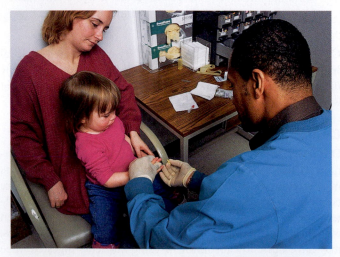

● **Figure 33–8** Screening for anemia. Most Head Start centers participate in screening programs to identify children at risk for anemia.

Calcium

Calcium is an essential nutrient for bone development during childhood and adolescence. An increased intake of soda pop and fruit juices is related to a decrease in calcium intake, especially among adolescents. During the adolescent growth spurt, almost 40% of the adult bone mass is accumulated (AAP Committee on Nutrition, 2009). Inadequate intake puts the person at risk for osteoporosis later in life since it is not possible to make up for earlier deficits. Although genetic variables account for some of the influence on adult bone mass, increasing calcium intake has been shown to promote bone formation. While the recommended daily intake for adolescents is 1300 mg, the average intake for adolescent males is 1145 mg and for females is only 700 to 850 mg (only half of the recommended level) (AAP Committee on Nutrition, 2009). Nurses should encourage foods such as milk and milk products, egg yolks, grains, legumes, nuts, and fruit juice with added calcium.

Adolescents at highest risk for impaired bone development include female athletes and others who diet to a great degree to maintain slimness. Teens who exercise excessively may manifest the "female athlete triad" of disordered eating that leads to excessive thinness, excessive exercise, and amenorrhea (Greydanus, Omar, & Pratt, 2010). A high rate of fractures and osteomalacia can result, in addition to an extreme risk of osteoporosis in adulthood (Ackerman & Misra, 2011). Asking about menstrual patterns as well as exercise and diet can be combined with physical measurements of height and weight to obtain pertinent information about the teen athlete. See the discussion of the eating disorders anorexia nervosa and bulimia nervosa later in this chapter.

Vitamin D

Vitamin D is needed for bone mineralization. Vitamin D deficiencies were once believed to be rare; however, an increase in cases of vitamin D–deficient rickets has recently been observed. Although vitamin D can be synthesized in the skin upon exposure to sunlight, the amount of sunlight needed for manufacture is variable and determined by the amount of skin exposed, the color of the skin, the latitude, and time of the year (Wagner, Greer, Section on Breastfeeding, et al., 2008). Due to this variability and the small amount of vitamin D in breast milk, it is now recommended that all infants from birth to 6 months receive a minimum intake of 400 International Units daily. All persons 6 months and older should receive 600 International Units daily (Ross, Taylor, Yaktine, et al., 2011). This vitamin is needed to enhance absorption of calcium, so a lack of vitamin D can contribute to calcium deficiency as well. When rickets is suspected, laboratory studies should include serum calcium, phosphorus, 25-OH vitamin D, alkaline phosphatase, parathyroid hormone, and hematocrit. Radiographs of extremities should be taken (LeFevre, 2010). Encourage parents to discuss vitamin D intake with the care provider at health promotion visits so proper intake can be ensured.

Folic Acid

Epidemiologic evidence has linked increasing maternal folic acid (the most common form of folate in the human body) intake with decreased incidence of neural tube defects such as

Drug Guide Iron

Overview of Action

Iron is a necessary component of hemoglobin and is therefore essential in the oxygen transfer carried out by red blood cells. It is used in microcytic and hypochromic anemia, which result from iron deficiency. Supplements are frequently used during pregnancy when intake often does not meet iron needs, and in infants with decreased iron stores, such as with small-for-gestational-age and premature infants.

Route, Dosage, Frequency

Ferrous fumarate: 3 mg/kg/day PO elemental iron
Ferrous gluconate: 8 mg/kg/day PO—over 2 years elemental iron
Ferrous sulfate: 5 mg/kg/day PO elemental iron
Ferrous sulfate dried: 160 mg/day PO elemental iron
Iron dextran: up to 25 mg/day (under 5 kg weight); up to 50 mg/day (5–10 kg weight); up to 100 mg/day (over 10 kg)—IM, IV

RDAs for Iron

7–12 months: 11 mg
1–3 years: 7 mg
4–8 years: 10 mg
9–13 years: 8 mg
14–18 years: males 11 mg; females 15 mg
Pregnancy: 27 mg
Lactation: 9–10 mg

Nursing Considerations

- Obtain a diet history; be alert for elements that can decrease iron absorption, such as low-calcium or high-phosphate diet, infection, or decreased GI acid; teach food sources of iron.
- Watch for signs of deficiency in infants after 4–6 months of age when maternal iron stores are depleted (earlier in premature infants).
- A CBC including hematocrit, hemoglobin, and reticulocytes is done to establish iron-deficiency anemia; monitor during treatment.

- Teach that oral preparation is taken between meals unless GI distress occurs; liquid forms are taken using a straw and water to decrease chance of teeth staining.
- Dairy products, eggs, whole grains, tea, and coffee decrease iron absorption and should not be taken at the same time as iron.

PO Administration

- Milligram doses of various forms of iron are not equivalent; rather, the amount of elemental iron in various preparations is important.
- Administration with a snack decreases absorption but is often recommended to lessen GI irritation.
- Accompanying iron with vitamin C may enhance iron absorption.
- Liquid preparations should be given with fluid, such as juice, and by a dropper or straw because they can stain teeth.

IM Administration

- Do not mix with other medications.
- Give in the upper outer buttock; therefore, this form is used only in older children and adults.
- Change needle after drawing up iron. Use long needle and Z-track injection technique. Permanent tissue staining can occur if not deep IM. Aspirate after inserting needle and inject slowly.

IV Administration

- Give undiluted and do not mix with other medications.
- Do not use the multidose bottle (latter only for IM injection).
- A small test dose is administered and, if no reaction occurs, the remainder of the dose is slowly infused over 1–6 hours. Verify dose with another nurse and follow prescriber instructions carefully. Flush vein after infusion with normal saline.
- Epinephrine 1:1000 is available for parenteral administration. Watch for hypersensitivity.

Source: Data from information in Bindler, R. M., & Howry, L. B. (2005). *Pediatric drug guide.* Upper Saddle River, NJ: Prentice Hall Health.

---

spina bifida in offspring. Folate levels are low among adolescents, putting them at particular risk of birth defects when they have babies (AAP Committee on Nutrition, 2009). The FDA approved fortification of cereals and breads with folate to decrease the population risk of related congenital anomalies. All women ages 15 to 45 years should consume 0.4 mg of folic acid daily, and pregnant women should consume 0.6 mg. In addition to cereals and breads, other good sources of folate include spinach, avocado, green leafy vegetables, beans and peas, liver, and fruits such as oranges and grapefruits.

Protein-Energy Malnutrition

Although the micronutrient deficiencies described previously are the most common problems in developed countries, macronutrient deficiencies are the most common nutritional problems worldwide. While kwashiorkor indicates protein deficiency, and marasmus is a lack of energy-producing calories, both deficiencies often occur together and are referred to as protein-energy malnutrition (PEM). Protein deficiency manifests with edema, leading to the large abdomens and rounded faces seen in severely

malnourished children. Other symptoms include scant, depigmented hair, skin changes, and decreased serum proteins. It can occur following severe diarrhea or other infection in susceptible children. Caloric deficiency results in emaciation, decreased energy levels, and retarded development (see Table 33–3). PEM may occur when a child is weaned in order for the mother to provide breast milk to a new baby. Adoptees and immigrants to developed countries sometimes manifest with at least mild PEM, so careful nutritional assessment is needed to provide adequate nutrition.

Celiac Disease

Celiac disease, or gluten-sensitive enteropathy, is a chronic malabsorption syndrome (van Koppen, Schweizer, Csizmadia, et al., 2009). About 1 in 133 persons have celiac disease. It is more common among members of the same family and in children with Down syndrome or Turner syndrome (National Institute of Diabetes and Digestive and Kidney Disease [NIDDK], 2012).

Celiac disease is an immunologic disorder characterized by intolerance for gluten, a protein found in wheat, barley, rye, and

American Celiac Society Weblink

Celiac Sprue Association Weblink

Gluten Intolerance Group Weblink

oats. Inability to digest glutenin and gliadin (protein fractions) results in the accumulation of the amino acid glutamine, which is toxic to mucosal cells in the intestine. Damage to the villi ultimately impairs the absorptive process in the small intestine.

In the early stages, celiac disease affects fat absorption, resulting in excretion of large quantities of fat in the stools (steatorrhea). Stools are greasy, foul smelling, frothy, and excessive. As changes in the villi continue, the absorption of protein, carbohydrates, calcium, iron, folate, and vitamins A, D, E, K, and B_{12} becomes impaired.

Symptoms usually occur when solid foods containing gluten are introduced to the child's diet (generally between 6 months to 2 years of age), although celiac disease is sometimes first diagnosed in adulthood. The classic features of celiac disease in infancy include chronic diarrhea, growth impairment, and abdominal distention. The child also demonstrates poor appetite, lack of energy, and muscle wasting with hypotonia. Atypical features are present in children diagnosed with delayed onset celiac disease around 5 to 7 years of age. Symptoms include nausea, vomiting, recurrent abdominal pain, bloating, tooth enamel defects, and aphthous ulcers (Rashid, Zarkadas, Anca, et al., 2011). Other symptoms may include delayed growth, iron deficiency, and abnormal liver function tests.

Diagnosis is confirmed through measurement of fecal fat content, duodenal biopsy, and improvement with removal of gluten products from the diet. Serum screening tests for IgA antiendomysial antibodies and IgA antitissue transglutaminase antibodies are commonly used in diagnosis (Garcia-Manzanares & Lucendo, 2011; NIDDK, 2012).

Management of the disease involves total exclusion of gluten from the diet. This gluten-free diet is a lifetime treatment. Barley, wheat, and rye are completely eliminated; oat products are sometimes tolerated. Symptoms generally improve within a few days to weeks. Supplementation with fat-soluble vitamins, vitamin B_{12}, folic acid, calcium, and iron may be needed, depending on results of serum testing (Daitch & Epperson, 2011).

The intestinal villi return to normal in about 6 months. Growth should improve steadily, and height and weight should reach normal range within 1 year.

Nursing Management

Nursing care focuses on supporting the parents in maintaining a gluten-free diet for the child. Thoroughly explain the disease process to the parents. Emphasize the necessity of following a gluten-free diet. Help parents to understand that celiac disease requires lifelong dietary modifications that should not be discontinued when the child is symptom-free. Discontinuation of the diet places the child at risk for growth retardation and the development of GI cancers in adulthood. All children with celiac disease should be seen by a dietitian several times during childhood. Nutritional assessment and continued teaching to maintain a gluten-free diet take place at these visits. Dietary management is made difficult by hidden gluten in many prepared foods, such as chocolate candy, prepared meats, ice cream, soups, condiments, and food starch.

An infant or toddler's diet is easily monitored at home. When the child enters school, however, ensuring adherence to dietary restrictions becomes more difficult. In addition to easily identified gluten-based foods, such as bread, cake, doughnuts, cookies, and crackers, the child must also avoid processed foods that contain gluten as a filler. School-age children and adolescents are often tempted to eat these foods, especially when among peers. Emphasize the need for compliance while meeting the child's developmental needs.

The child's special dietary needs can place a financial burden on the family. Parents need to purchase prepared rice or corn flour products or make their own bread and bakery products. Advise parents that getting a dietary prescription enables them to deduct the cost of these ingredients and commercially prepared products as a medical expense.

Because the entire family must adapt to the diet, parents and siblings need support and management skills. For information and support, refer parents and children to several organizations, including the American Celiac Society, the Celiac Sprue Association/United States of America, and the Gluten Intolerance Group.

Expected outcomes of nursing care include the following:

- The child maintains adequate nutrition to support growth and development needs.

- The child achieves growth and developmental milestones appropriate for age.

- The child and family understand the dietary restrictions and appropriately plan meals.

Feeding and Eating Disorders

Deficiencies in food intake related to available nutrients and safety of the food supply were discussed in the previous section. In addition to these issues of availability, nutrient intake is affected by psychologic issues of individuals as well. Disorders of food intake span the entire developmental spectrum and can affect pregnant women, young children, and adolescents. Some of the most common feeding and eating disorders are discussed in the following sections.

Colic

Colic is a feeding disorder characterized by paroxysmal abdominal pain and severe crying. The crying generally lasts at least 3 hours and occurs at least 3 day per week. Crying episodes peak around 6 weeks of age and generally resolve by 3 to 4 months of age (Holt, Wooldridge, Story, et al., 2011). The etiology of colic is unknown. Proposed causes include feeding too rapidly and swallowing large amounts of air.

Characteristically the infant cries loudly and continuously, often for several hours. The infant's face may become flushed. The abdomen is distended and tense. Often the infant draws up the legs and clenches the hands. Episodes occur at the same time each day, usually in the late afternoon or early evening. Crying may stop only when the child is completely exhausted or after passage of flatus or stool.

The symptoms initially may resemble intestinal obstruction or peritoneal infection. These conditions must be ruled out along with sensitivity to formula. Treatment is supportive;

no general medical consensus exists on effective treatments or interventions for colic. Some healthcare providers recommend medications such as simethicone (Mylicon) drops. Some recommend formula change to a soy formula or an elemental formula such as Pregestimil.

Nursing care requires a thorough history of the infant's diet and daily schedule and the events surrounding episodes of colicky behavior. Assessment of the infant's feeding patterns and diet includes type, frequency, and amount of feeding (if breastfeeding, maternal diet history) and frequency of burping. Inquire about onset, duration, and characteristics of cry during colic episodes. Ask the parents what measures are used to relieve crying and their effectiveness.

When possible, observe the feeding method. Parents of infants with colic are often tired and frustrated. They require frequent reassurance that they are not to blame for the infant's condition. Suggest ways of alleviating some of the infant's symptoms and discomfort. These include using a front-carrying sling, swaddling, playing soothing music, using a pacifier, or giving a warm bath or massage of the abdomen. The breastfeeding mother should avoid gas-producing foods and the infant should be burped frequently during feedings. An important consideration is the significant impact of colic on families. Colic can place extreme stress and fatigue on the family. Active support and counseling for the mother and other family members is essential (Moore, 2009).

Pica

Pica is an eating disorder characterized by ingestion of nonfood items or food items consumed in abnormal quantities or forms. Examples of ingested items include starch, peeling paint, paper, soil components, flour, and coffee grounds. Clinical manifestations include zinc and iron deficiencies as well as symptoms of lead or other heavy metal poisoning (see Chapter 43 🔗) if these substances are contained in peeling paint or other ingested material. Pica most commonly manifests in pregnancy when women have abnormal cravings for nonfood products, and this can seriously impair the developing fetus (see Chapter 14 🔗 for more information). Some children also ingest abnormal amounts of nonfood items and fail to take in adequate nutrients from food. Treatment for children involves removing access to the substances, ensuring an adequate and nutritious diet, and treating any dietary deficiencies noted.

Feeding Disorder of Infancy and Early Childhood (Failure to Thrive)

Feeding disorder of infancy and early childhood, or failure to thrive (FTT), describes a syndrome in which infants or young children fail to eat enough food to be adequately nourished. This disorder accounts for 5% to 10% of pediatric hospitalizations in children under 1 year of age, and many more children are managed in community settings (Kliegman, Stanton, St. Geme, et al., 2011).

Etiology and Pathophysiology. The cause of FTT can be organic, as in congenital acquired immunodeficiency syndrome (AIDS) (see Chapter 49 🔗), inborn errors of metabolism (see Chapter 54 🔗), congenital heart defect (see Chapter 48 🔗), neurologic disease (see Chapter 55 🔗), and esophageal reflux

(see Chapter 52 🔗). However, most cases of FTT have no organic cause. FTT resulting from nonorganic causes is called *feeding disorder of infancy or early childhood.*

Infants and children whose parents or caretakers experience poverty, depression, substance abuse, intellectual disability, or psychosis are at risk for this disorder. Parents may be socially and emotionally isolated, or may lack knowledge of infant nutritional and nurturing needs. A reciprocal interaction pattern may exist in which the parent does not offer enough food or is not responsive to the infant's hunger cues, and the infant is irritable, not soothed, and does not give clear cues about hunger. Parental neglect is a contributor to the condition. Preterm and small-for-gestational-age babies more commonly have eating disorders (AAP Committee on Nutrition, 2009; Bryant-Waugh, Markham, Kriepe, et al., 2010).

Clinical Manifestations. The characteristics of this feeding disorder are persistent failure to eat adequately with no weight gain or with weight loss in a child under 6 years of age that is not associated with other medical conditions or mental disorders, and is not caused by lack of or unavailability of food. Weight is generally below the 5th percentile, and weight-for-length is less than 80% of ideal weight (AAP Committee on Nutrition, 2009; Bryant-Waugh et al., 2010). Infants with feeding disorder refuse food, may have erratic sleep patterns, are irritable and difficult to soothe, and are often developmentally delayed (Figure 33–9 ●).

Clinical Therapy. A thorough history and physical examination are needed to rule out any chronic physical illness. The infant or child may be hospitalized so that healthcare providers can establish a routine for feeding and sleeping. The goals of treatment are to provide adequate caloric and nutritional intake, promote normal growth and development, and assist parents in developing feeding routines and responding to the infant's cues of physical and psychologic hunger. Interprofessional teams that include nutrition teaching, home visits, parenting skills information, and other support are most successful (Cole & Lanham, 2011).

● **Figure 33–9** Feeding disorder of infancy or failure to thrive (FTT). Infants with failure to thrive may not look severely malnourished, but they fall well below the expected weight and height norms for their age. This infant, who appears to be about 4 months old, is actually 8 months old. He has been hospitalized for feeding disorder of infancy.

NURSING MANAGEMENT *For the Child with Failure to Thrive*

Nursing Assessment and Diagnosis

Nursing assessment of the child is essential for establishing the best intervention plan for a child with FTT. Documenting accurate weight and height each time any child is seen for health care provides an important record of growth patterns over time. This helps identify the child with an eating disorder. The child's activity level, developmental milestones, and interaction patterns provide important information. When feeding the child, observe how the child indicates hunger or satiety, the ability of the child to be soothed, and general interaction patterns such as eye contact, touch, and "cuddliness."

Ask parents about stresses in their lives; these may prevent appropriate interaction with the child. Asking about the pregnancy and birth can elicit information about early disturbances in the child–parent relationship. Are there other children in the family and have eating problems occurred with them? Observe the child and parent behaviors while they feed the child; cues given by each person and interactional modes such as rocking, singing, talking, and body postures are important.

Some of the nursing diagnoses pertinent for the young child with an eating disorder include the following (NANDA-I © 2012):

- *Nutrition, Imbalanced: Less than Body Requirements* related to inability to ingest proper amounts of food
- *Growth and Development, Delayed,* related to inadequate food intake
- *Parenting, Risk for Impaired,* related to lack of knowledge about the child's nutritional needs
- *Fatigue* related to malnutrition

Planning and Implementation

Nursing care centers on performing a thorough history and physical assessment, observing parent–child interactions during feeding times, and providing necessary teaching to enable parents to respond appropriately to their child's needs. The child is often hospitalized initially and evaluated for potential organic causes while staff members feed the child. Tube feedings may be needed temporarily until normal intake can be ensured. Accurate weights, nutritional assessments, and developmental evaluation should be done to see if the child grows more normally. Additional diagnostic tests may be carried out at this time to rule out organic causes of poor growth.

Once a diagnosis of nonorganic failure to thrive is confirmed, parents become involved in feeding the child. Observations of

---

Developing Cultural Competence
Height and Weight Growth Standards

Each child should maintain a height and weight growth pattern similar to the population standard. Asian American children may normally be below the 5th percentile on growth charts and not have an eating disorder. Suspect an eating disorder when the infant or child falls one standard deviation below his or her own curve and either fails to gain weight or loses weight over several months.

---

feeding and continued careful physical assessments are needed. Carefully record the child's intake at each meal or feeding. Teach parents how to understand and respond to the child's cues of hunger and satiety. Teach them to hold, rock, and touch the infant during feedings and establish eye contact with infants and older children.

Upon discharge, referral to an agency that can continue monitoring of the home situation is needed. This provides an opportunity to observe feeding during a home visit and evaluate stresses and behavior patterns among family members. Frequent growth measurement and development must be ensured so the child is adequately nourished. Parents may need referral to community resources to help them manage stressful situations in their lives and to enhance their parenting skills.

Evaluation

Expected outcomes of nursing care include the following:

- Adequate growth and normal development of the infant is achieved.
- An improved parent–child relationship is established.

Anorexia Nervosa

Anorexia nervosa is a potentially life-threatening eating disorder that occurs primarily in teenage girls and young women. An estimated 5% of young women and 1% of young men in the United States are affected by anorexia nervosa or a related eating disorder (AAP Committee on Nutrition, 2009). The typical patient is white and from a middle- to upper-middle-class family. Age at onset varies from 12 years onward but with an average age of 19 years (National Institute of Mental Health [NIMH], 2010a).

Etiology and Pathophysiology.   Many causes are believed to contribute to the onset of anorexia. Cultural overemphasis on thinness may contribute to the excessive concern with dieting, body image, and fear of becoming fat that is experienced by many adolescents. Chemical changes have been found in the brain and blood of individuals with anorexia, leading to theories about a biologic cause. Often a significant life stress, loss, or change precedes the onset of anorexia. Stress hormones are commonly elevated in adolescents with anorexia, and immune system function may be disturbed.

Many experts view family issues as contributory to anorexia. Intrafamilial conflicts and dysfunctional family patterns may occur when parents are overly controlling and perfectionistic. The adolescent's eating behaviors may be an attempt to exercise independence and resolve internal psychologic conflicts.

The adolescent may engage in lengthy and vigorous exercise (up to 4 hours daily) to prevent weight gain. Laxatives or diuretics may be used to induce weight loss. As the disorder progresses, the adolescent perceives the ever-thinner body as becoming more beautiful. Youths may share weight loss techniques with friends who are anorectic and search out Internet sites that are positive about anorexia. The body responds to the abnormal eating behaviors as if starvation were occurring. Leukopenia, electrolyte imbalance, and hypoglycemia develop as a result of PEM. Once the body mass decreases below a critical level, menstruation ceases.

Clinical Manifestations.   Adolescents with anorexia are characterized by extreme weight loss accompanied by a preoccupation with weight and food, excessive compulsive exercising, peculiar patterns of eating and handling food, and distorted body image. They may prepare elaborate meals for others but eat only low-calorie foods. Characteristically, the fear of becoming fat does not decrease with continued weight loss. Accompanying signs and symptoms of depression, crying spells, feelings of isolation and loneliness, and suicidal thoughts and feelings are common. The disorder is often associated with mental illness such as obsessive-compulsive disorder, anxiety disorders (see Chapter 56 ⊘), and history of abuse.

Physical findings include cold intolerance, dizziness, constipation, abdominal discomfort, bloating, irregular menses, and malnutrition (Figure 33–10 ●). Hypothalamic suppression can lead to disturbances of gynecologic function, osteoporosis, decreased bone density, and fractures. Lanugo (fine, downy body hair) may be present. Fluid and electrolyte imbalances, especially potassium imbalances, are common. The child or adolescent is usually energetic despite significant weight loss. Extreme weight loss often leads to cardiac arrhythmias (bradycardia).

Clinical Therapy. Diagnosis is based on a comprehensive history, physical examination revealing characteristic clinical manifestations, and the criteria listed in Table 33–7. Diagnostic tests commonly include hematocrit and hemoglobin, serum electrolytes, and serum vitamins and vitamin precursors. Bone density examination for females with lengthy amenorrhea is recommended (AAP Committee on Nutrition, 2009).

The goal of treatment is to address the physiologic problems associated with malnutrition, as well as the behavioral and cognitive components of the disorder. A firm focus is placed on reaching a targeted weight with a gradual weight gain of 0.1 to 0.2 kg/day (0.25 to 0.5 lb/day). Weight gain of 1–2 pounds/week is a realistic goal (Treasure, Claudino, & Zucker, 2010). Enteral feedings or total parenteral nutrition (TPN) may be necessary to replace lost fluid, protein, and nutrients, although the adolescent often perceives these feedings as a punitive measure.

Individual treatment and family therapy are used to address dysfunctional family patterns and assist the family to accept and deal with the adolescent as an independent and less-than-perfect individual (Brewerton & Costin, 2011; Fisher, Hetrick, & Rushford, 2010; Lock, 2011). Family involvement is crucial to effect a lasting change in the adolescent. Nurses, psychologists, family therapists, and dietitians commonly partner to plan and implement therapy.

Long-term outpatient treatment, in either an individual or a group setting, is frequently necessary. Counseling that engages

● **Figure 33–10** Anorexia nervosa. Note the loss of subcutaneous tissue in the back, arms, and pelvis.
Source: Sally Greenhill/Alamy

Table 33–7	*DSM-5* Diagnostic Criteria for Anorexia Nervosa

A. Restriction of energy intake relative to requirements, leading to a significantly low body weight in the context of age, sex, developmental trajectory, and physical health. *Significantly low weight* is defined as a weight that is less than minimally normal or, for children and adolescents, less than that minimally expected.

B. Intense fear of gaining weight or of becoming fat, or persistent behavior that interferes with weight gain, even though at a significantly low weight.

C. Disturbance in the way in which one's body weight or shape is experienced, undue influence of body weight or shape on self-evaluation, or persistent lack of recognition of the seriousness of the current low body weight.

Specify whether:

■ *Restricting type:* During the last 3 months, the individual has not engaged in recurrent episodes of binge eating or purging behavior (i.e., self-induced vomiting or the misuse of laxatives, diuretics, or enemas). This subtype describes presentations in which weight loss is accomplished primarily through dieting, fasting, and/or excessive exercise.

■ *Binge-eating/purging type:* During the last 3 months, the individual has engaged in recurrent episodes of binge eating or purging behavior (i.e., self-induced vomiting or the misuse of laxatives, diuretics, or enemas).

Specify if:

■ *In partial remission:* After full criteria for anorexia nervosa were previously met, Criterion A (low body weight) has not been met for a sustained period, but either Criterion B (intense fear of gaining weight or becoming fat or behavior that interferes with weight gain) or Criterion C (disturbances in self-perception of weight and shape) is still met.

■ *In full remission:* After full criteria for anorexia nervosa were previously met, none of the criteria have been met for a sustained period of time.

Specify current severity:
The minimum level of severity is based, for adults, on current body mass index (BMI) (see below) or, for children and adolescents, on BMI percentile. The ranges below are derived from World Health Organization categories for thinness in adults; for children and adolescents, corresponding BMI percentiles should be used. The level of severity may be increased to reflect clinical symptoms, the degree of functional disability, and the need for supervision.

■ *Mild:* BMI ≥ 17 kg/m2
■ *Moderate:* BMI 16–16.99 kg/m^2
■ *Severe:* BMI 15–15.99 kg/m^2
■ *Extreme:* BMI < 15 kg/m^2

Source: Used with permission from American Psychiatric Association. (2013). *Diagnostic and statistical manual of mental disorders* (5th ed.). Washington, DC: Author. Copyright © 2013 American Psychiatric Association.

self-help techniques may be continued for 2 to 3 years to ensure that weight gain and self-image are maintained. Antidepressant drugs such as imipramine (Tofranil) or desipramine (Norpramin) may be prescribed for coexisting conditions such as depression, anxiety, or obsessive-compulsive disorders. However, they are not generally useful in primary treatment of the disorder (Flament, Bissada, & Spettique, 2011).

Indications for hospitalization include loss of 25% to 30% of body weight or being at 85% or less of healthy weight, fluid and electrolyte imbalances, cardiac arrhythmias, hypotension, or the need to provide a more intense period of therapy if outpatient treatment fails to produce improvement. Behavior modification techniques are used extensively in combination with counseling and other methods in the care of the hospitalized adolescent with anorexia.

NURSING MANAGEMENT *For the Child with Anorexia Nervosa*

Nursing Assessment and Diagnosis

Obtain a thorough individual and family history. Ask about usual eating patterns, daily caloric intake, exercise patterns, and menstrual history. Ask about medication use; include prescription, nonprescription, and herbal products. Is there a family history of eating disorders? Assess for signs of malnutrition. Obtain height and weight measurements and compare with norms for the general population. Because the patient with anorexia often wears layers of clothes when being weighed, strive to obtain an accurate measurement. Mid-upper arm circumference, skinfold thickness, waist-to-hip ratio, and body composition measurement may all be obtained (Mattar, Godart, Melchior, et al., 2011).

Nursing diagnoses for the adolescent with anorexia nervosa include the following (NANDA-I © 2012):

- *Nutrition, Imbalanced: Less than Body Requirements* related to inadequate food intake
- *Fluid Volume: Deficient, Risk for,* related to inadequate fluid intake or fluid volume loss from overuse of laxatives and diuretics
- *Body Temperature, Imbalanced, Risk for,* related to excessive weight loss and absence of subcutaneous fat
- *Constipation* related to inadequate food intake and overuse of laxatives
- *Body Image, Disturbed,* related to distorted perception of body size and shape
- *Self-Esteem, Chronic Low,* related to dysfunctional family dynamics
- *Coping: Family, Compromised,* related to parental tendency to be overly controlling and perfectionistic

Planning and Implementation

Nursing care centers on meeting nutritional and fluid needs, preventing complications, administering medications, supporting psychologic interventions, and providing referral to appropriate resources. Specific treatment measures vary depending on physical complications, length and degree of illness, emotional symptoms accompanying the disorder, and family dynamics. Resistance to treatment is common, and nurses who care for adolescents with anorexia must deal with their own feelings of frustration and anger.

Provide Psychologic Support

Care for the adolescent with anorexia necessarily includes psychologic support as an important component. The nurse will refer the family to a specialist who can counsel and recommend further treatment. Families of a youth with anorexia should be involved in support groups and should also receive information about the condition and the youth's plan of care. The adolescent is often treated with individual counseling and encouragement to participate is needed. Interventions that improve self-concept and lead to a realistic body image are needed. They may include encouragement for participation in sports, praise for participation in the treatment plan, and immediate referral for relapses as treatment progresses.

Meet Nutritional and Fluid Needs

Monitor nutritional and fluid intake, encourage consumption of food, and observe eating behaviors at mealtime. Elimination patterns may be altered as a result of increased intake during hospitalization. Monitor for possible problems, including abdominal distention, constipation, or diarrhea. Daily monitoring of serum electrolytes is necessary.

If TPN is administered, watch for complications such as circulatory overload, hyperglycemia, or hypoglycemia. Use strict aseptic technique when changing tubing or dressings.

Administer Medications

Monitor vital signs if the adolescent is receiving antidepressants. Watch for signs of hypertension and tachycardia. Administer medications after meals because it helps to prevent gastric irritation. Be alert for substance abuse. People with anorexia often use excess laxatives or products such as ephedra (also known as ma huang) to induce weight loss. Changes in the central nervous system, vital signs, and other findings may indicate over-the-counter or herbal drug use.

Provide Referral to Appropriate Resources

Refer parents and other family members to the American Anorexia and Bulimia Association, National Eating Disorders Organization, and National Association of Anorexia Nervosa & Associated Disorders for further information about the disorder and a list of support groups in their area.

Evaluation

Expected outcomes for nursing care include recommended level of weight gain, maintenance of adequate fluid volume and balanced electrolytes, maintenance of normal blood pressure and heart rhythm, beginning of positive sense of self-esteem, intake of nutritionally balanced diet, and use of psychologic counseling to understand the disorder.

Bulimia Nervosa

Bulimia nervosa is an eating disorder characterized by **binge eating** (a compulsion to consume large quantities of food in a short period of time). Usually the episodes of bingeing are followed by various methods of weight control (purging), such as self-induced vomiting, large doses of laxatives or diuretics, or a combination of methods. Bulimia affects 1% of the general population, with prevalence in young women about 3 times that in men (NIMH, 2010b). Like anorexia, it affects mainly adolescent girls and young women who are white and in the higher socioeconomic classes (AAP Committee on Nutrition, 2009). The disorder usually begins in middle to late adolescence at an average age of 20 years.

Etiology and Pathophysiology. Causes of bulimia nervosa are similar to those of anorexia nervosa: sensitivity to social pressure for thinness, body image difficulties, and long-standing dysfunctional family patterns. Families may be chaotic and distant, rather than overinvolved as with the person who has anorexia. Many individuals with bulimia experience depression. It is not clear whether the depression is a cause or a result of the individual's inability to control the bingeing and purging cycles. An adolescent with bulimia often binges after any stressful event.

Bingeing usually occurs in secret for several hours until the individual is stopped by abdominal discomfort, by another person, or by vomiting. At first, the episodes of binge eating are pleasurable. Immediately following the binge episode, however, feelings of guilt, shame, anger, depression, and fear of loss of control and weight gain arise. As these feelings intensify, the adolescent with bulimia becomes increasingly anxious. This usually initiates the purge behaviors.

Purging eliminates the discomfort from bloating and also prevents weight gain. This relieves the feelings of depression and guilt, but only temporarily. Adolescents with bulimia commonly practice the binge–purge cycle many times a day, losing their ability to respond to normal cues of hunger and satiety.

Clinical Manifestations.   Bulimia is often a "silent" disorder since it is easily concealed from healthcare providers and families. Only about 6% of those with the condition are believed to receive treatment. Adolescents with bulimia are preoccupied with body shape, size, and weight. They may appear overweight or thin and usually report a wide range of average body weight over the years. Physical findings depend on the degree of purging, starvation, dehydration, and electrolyte disturbance. Erosion of tooth enamel, increased dental caries, and gum recession, which result from vomiting of gastric acids, are common findings. The back of a hand can have calluses from inducing vomiting. Abdominal distention is often seen. Esophageal tears and esophagitis may also occur.

Clinical Therapy.   A comprehensive history is necessary because most adolescents with bulimia appear normal in weight or only slightly underweight. Diagnostic tests include hematocrit, hemoglobin, and serum electrolytes; they may identify signs of altered electrolyte and hematologic status. Lowered potassium levels are related to repetitive vomiting since gastric contents have a high potassium level. The diagnosis is confirmed by the presence of specific criteria (Table 33–8).

Treatment includes management of physiologic problems and cognitive-behavior therapy. Medications, such as fluoxetine 60 mg/day for adolescents, may be prescribed (Hay & Claudino, 2011). Management involves a variety of healthcare providers such as physicians, nurses, and therapists. Behavior modification focuses on modifying the dysfunctional eating patterns and restoring normal patterns. Until the episodes of bingeing and purging are under control, feelings of discouragement and hopelessness prevail. Thus, the focus early in treatment is on initiating an immediate behavioral change. Once initial interventions have been successful, group therapy sessions work well for people with anorexia or bulimia. Specific treatment measures may include the following:

- Educating the adolescent about good nutrition (including food choices and caloric content)

- Encouraging the adolescent to keep a log or food journal and assisting the adolescent to make connections between emotional states, stress, and the impulse to binge or purge

- Setting up a daily dietary routine of three meals and three snacks a day (using the same foods for each meal and snack every day to change misconceptions about the weight-gaining potential of certain foods and to decrease anxiety about what food must be eaten at the next meal)

Table 33–8 · DSM-5 Diagnostic Criteria for Bulimia Nervosa

A. Recurrent episodes of binge eating. An episode of binge eating is characterized by both of the following:
- Eating, in a discrete period of time (e.g., within any 2-hour period), an amount of food that is definitely larger than what most individuals would eat in a similar period of time under similar circumstances.
- A sense of lack of control over eating during the episode (e.g., a feeling that one cannot stop eating or control what or how much one is eating).

B. Recurrent inappropriate compensatory behaviors in order to prevent weight gain, such as self-induced vomiting; misuse of laxatives, diuretics, or other medications; fasting; or excessive exercise.

C. The binge eating and inappropriate compensatory behaviors both occur, on average, at least once a week for 3 months.

D. Self-evaluation is unduly influenced by body shape and weight.

E. The disturbance does not occur exclusively during episodes of anorexia nervosa.

Specify if:
- *In partial remission:* After full criteria for bulimia nervosa were previously met, some, but not all, of the criteria have been met for a sustained period of time.
- *In full remission:* After full criteria for bulimia nervosa were previously met, none of the criteria have been met for a sustained period of time.

Specify current severity:
The minimum level of severity is based on the frequency of inappropriate compensatory behaviors (see below). The level of severity may be increased to reflect other symptoms and the degree of functional disability.
- *Mild:* An average of 1–3 episodes of inappropriate compensatory behaviors per week.
- *Moderate:* An average of 4–7 episodes of inappropriate compensatory behaviors per week.
- *Severe:* An average of 8–13 episodes of inappropriate compensatory behaviors per week.
- *Extreme:* An average of 14 or more episodes of inappropriate compensatory behaviors per week.

Source: Used with permission from American Psychiatric Association. (2013). *Diagnostic and statistical manual of mental disorders* (5th ed.). Washington, DC: Author. Copyright © 2013 American Psychiatric Association.

Once these initial measures have been taken, the underlying psychosocial issues are explored. The goals of therapy are to provide the adolescent with bulimia with adaptive coping skills and to improve self-esteem.

Most adolescents with bulimia do not require hospitalization. Serious abnormalities in fluid and electrolyte levels caused by uncontrollable cycles of bingeing and vomiting, accompanied by depression or suicidal activity, are indications of the need for hospitalization. The prognosis is good with long-term therapy.

NURSING MANAGEMENT *For the Child with Bulimia Nervosa*

Nursing Assessment and Diagnosis

Obtain a thorough individual and family history, including daily dietary intake and weight fluctuations. Inquire about problems such as abdominal pain or distention, which may indicate an abnormal eating or elimination pattern. Assess the oral mucosa for signs of damage to tooth enamel caused by purging; examine hands for evidence of vomiting-induced calluses.

Following are nursing diagnoses that may be appropriate for the adolescent with bulimia nervosa (NANDA-I © 2012):

- *Nutrition, Imbalanced: Less than or More than Body Requirements* related to disordered food intake
- *Fluid Volume, Deficient, Risk for,* related to fluid volume loss
- *Mucous Membrane: Oral, Impaired,* related to chemical effects of vomited gastric acids
- *Knowledge, Deficient (Adolescent),* related to health risks of excessive use of laxatives and diuretics
- *Anxiety* related to discomfort with weight and eating patterns
- *Self-Esteem, Chronic Low,* related to dysfunctional family dynamics
- *Coping, Ineffective,* related to life stressors

Planning and Implementation

Nursing care includes monitoring nutritional intake and elimination patterns, preventing complications, and providing appropriate referrals.

During hospitalization the patient should keep a food diary. Be alert to the adolescent who hides, gives away, or discards food from the tray or who exits to use the bathroom after meals. The adolescent should be monitored for at least 30 minutes after meals by remaining in a central area in the company of the nurse or other responsible individuals. Withdrawal from laxatives and diuretics is managed with careful observation for alterations in fluid and electrolyte status. Cardiac monitoring may be necessary if potassium levels are seriously altered. Esophageal tearing or esophagitis is treated to promote mucosal healing. Medications such as antidepressants may be administered. Encourage continuation of group and other therapy sessions.

Adolescents with bulimia and their families can be referred to organizations such as those listed earlier in the section on anorexia for assistance and information about the disorder.

Evaluation

Expected outcomes for nursing care for the adolescent with bulimia include healthy mucous membranes and skin, adequate intake of fluids and food, balanced food intake, maintenance of normal weight, adequate support and healthy psychologic balance, and absence of bingeing and purging.

Food Reactions

Food reaction encompasses any adverse reaction to foods or substances ingested in foods. The most common food reaction is **food intolerance**, an abnormal physiologic response to a food that is not immunoglobulin E (IgE)-mediated. Examples include indigestion or flatulence upon eating certain foods, a sweating reaction to some spices, rhinitis, and hives with urticaria (Mansoor & Sharma, 2011). See the discussion of lactose intolerance that follows. Milk and grain products are common causes of food intolerance. Chemical additives, antibiotics, preservatives, and food colorings also can cause food sensitivity reactions.

The most serious type of reaction is **food allergy**, an IgE-mediated reaction that is potentially systemic, characteristically

rapid in onset, and may be manifested as swelling of the lips, mouth, uvula or glottis, generalized urticaria, and in severe reactions, anaphylaxis. Food allergies are the most common cause of anaphylaxis and are more prevalent in children with a family history of allergic reactions to various substances and foods (**atopy**). The foods that most commonly cause allergy are fish, shellfish, peanuts, tree nuts, eggs, soy, wheat, corn, strawberries, and cow's milk products. About 0.6% of children have an allergy to peanuts, and the incidence has increased in the past two decades (National Institute of Allergy and Infectious Diseases [NIAID], 2011). A majority of the 150 deaths from food allergies that occur annually in the United States are due to peanut allergy.

Children who have both food allergy and asthma are most at risk of death from anaphylaxis due to a food allergy. Allergic individuals need to be aware of hidden substances in prepared foods. For example, the child allergic to nuts will experience a reaction to a food if nut extracts are used in its preparation. Note that certain foods can cause either allergy or intolerance so accurate diagnosis is needed. An example is cow's milk, which can cause an allergy with IgE-mediated systemic reaction, or an intolerance from gastrointestinal response to milk proteins (diarrhea, vomiting, abdominal pain) as a result of lack of the enzyme lactase in the gastrointestinal tract.

Delayed hypersensitivity reactions are attributed to digestive products of food and require a thorough diet history over several days to identify the offending food. These reactions are more difficult to diagnose, since the reaction can occur up to 24 hours after ingestion of the food. There may also be biphasic reactions that occur 1 to 30 hours after an initial anaphylaxis. Such reactions can be severe and life threatening. Therefore every child with a food allergy who ingests the allergen should be promptly treated with epinephrine and transported to an emergency facility for further management and monitoring.

Diagnostic tests to identify suspected food allergies include measurement of serum IgE levels, scratch tests, and the **radioallergosorbent test (RAST)**, in which radioimmunoassay measures IgE antibodies to specific allergens. (See Chapter 49 🔗 for further information about these tests.) In cases of past allergic response, the food is absolutely avoided. In food intolerance, a diet diary is kept, noting date, type of foods eaten, and reaction, if any. Foods should be eaten singly for several days to determine whether they cause a reaction.

Treatment consists of eliminating the offending foods from the child's diet. Collaborative care involving the child, parents, school, and healthcare providers is needed to ensure that the child with food allergies does not get exposed to the offending allergen, and that all children with food reactions can avoid contact with foods to which they are allergic or intolerant. When the child is exposed to the food, epinephrine should be administered and transport to a treatment center should be immediate. Treatment in the hospital may include additional measures as needed such as bronchodilators, antihistamines, and oxygen therapy (NIAID, 2011).

Nursing Management

Prevention is the first step. Instruct parents of infants to introduce new foods at a rate of not more than one new food every 3 to 5 days. If food intolerance is noted, the causative food can be easily identified. Discuss any changes in diet or preparation of formula. Reassure parents that the child's symptoms will disappear when the offending foods are removed from the diet.

Be alert for skin, respiratory, and other characteristic manifestations of food allergy in children. Immediately call 9-1-1 for care. All such cases should be referred to an allergist for diagnosis. If an allergy is identified, help the family to identify and remove the offending foods. Emphasize the importance of reading food labels for hidden foods that can trigger an allergic response. The child, family, school, and other settings should be prepared at all times for immediate response to food allergy.

SAFETY ALERT!

Children with food allergies should wear an alert bracelet and carry emergency medication such as an EpiPen. Nurses in schools and offices must instruct families, schoolteachers, and others about the child's allergy and what to do in case of accidental ingestion of the food product. Assist them to set up prevention and emergency treatment plans.

Refer the family to the Food Allergy Network. Recognize that food allergies can be stressful for children and families, as they worry about exposure in daily life.

The child with food intolerance needs to avoid the food to ensure comfort and an absence of the annoying symptoms associated with it. Although, unlike with an allergic reaction, intolerance is not life threatening, the family needs to learn about hidden sources of the food product so that it can be avoided and alternative foods can be suggested for their use.

Lactose Intolerance

Lactose intolerance is the inability to digest lactose, a disaccharide found in milk and other dairy products. It results from a congenital or acquired deficiency of the enzyme lactase. Congenital lactase deficiency of infancy is a rare disorder. Lactose intolerance is considered a biologic norm, occurring in 80% to 100% of African Americans, Native Americans, and Asian Americans (AAP Committee on Nutrition, 2009).

Abdominal pain, flatulence, and diarrhea occur shortly after birth when the infant is unable to hydrolyze lactose. Diarrhea develops rapidly after the child ingests milk and milk products. Some children are able to tolerate small ingestions of lactose but have symptoms when larger amounts are consumed. Incidence of lactose intolerance increases with advancing age throughout childhood.

Diagnosis is based on a thorough history and a hydrogen breath test, which measures the amount of hydrogen left after fermentation of unabsorbed carbohydrates. Implementing a lactose-free diet for a period of time may eliminate the symptoms, thus confirming the diagnosis. Treatment for infants includes switching to lactose-free formula. For older children, eliminating lactose-containing foods is recommended. Lactase enzyme tablets can be added to milk or sprinkled on foods to aid digestion.

Nursing Management

Nursing care is primarily supportive. Carefully explain dietary modifications to parents and discuss alternative sources of calcium. Discuss the need for supplementation of calcium and vitamin D to prevent deficiencies. Teach families how to read food labels to find hidden sources of lactose. For example, milk solids may be found in breads, cakes, candies, salad dressings, margarine, and processed food. Suggest lactase tablets for children who want to eat some dairy products.

NUTRITIONAL SUPPORT

Sports Nutrition and Ergogenic Agents

Regular physical activity should be encouraged for all children, with at least 60 minutes of activity recommended daily. However, during vigorous or prolonged exercise, or during hot weather, child and adolescent athletes may have special nutritional needs. A well-balanced diet, reflective of recommended foods, is needed. A wide variety of fresh fruits and vegetables, grains, and complex carbohydrates usually provides for adequate caloric intake. When the child is hungry, extra calories should come from the food groups listed here, rather than from increased intake of fat. When the child or teen is very active, sports bars or drinks can provide the additional needed calories in a nutritionally balanced manner. As always, the height, weight, and BMI percentiles are the best assurance that the child is growing adequately over time. Adequate energy to perform the sport as well as be attentive and productive at school and for other activities should also be considered (Molinero & Marquez, 2009; Rodriguez, DiMarco, Langley, et al., 2009).

Water should be increased during activity both to minimize chance of dehydration and also to maximize performance. About 1 hour before vigorous exercise, the child should drink 1 to 2 glasses (8 to 16 ounces) of water and should repeat the same amount of fluid just before the exercise begins. Young children may not feel thirsty and should be encouraged to drink 6 to 12 ounces of fluid every 15 to 20 minutes during exercise (AAP Committee on Nutrition, 2009). Water is usually the best replacement, but during extended exercise, sports drinks may be a good alternative for some of the fluid intake. More water is needed after activity. Weight loss of 1 pound indicates a loss of about 1/2 quart of fluid. The nurse should be sure the child takes in fluid to replace all losses.

Some common nutrients that may be deficient in all teens, but even more often in the athlete, are calcium and iron. The increased blood volume common in the well-conditioned person necessitates greater intake. Calcium-rich foods such as milk products and dark green vegetables, and iron-rich foods such as meats and grains, can guard against deficiencies. While many adolescents believe that they need extra protein during athletic season, most Americans eat adequate protein to meet even the increased needs of sports. On the other hand, the vegetarian child or adolescent may need help to plan a diet with adequate protein.

Many teens take a wide variety of dietary supplements, believing that they act as **ergogenic aids**, or products that enhance performance during sports by influencing energy, alertness, or body composition. Most of the claims of these products are unproven, and their safety has not usually been investigated, especially in the young. Effects on youth whose bodies are still developing are particularly unknown and the risks are high for permanent interference with some normal growth patterns.

Weblink

Food Allergy Network

Case Study: Vegetarian Teens: Plan a 2-Day Menu

Activity

Offer guidance and help the family and teen investigate claims before choosing to use a product. If youths use supplements, they should be instructed about doses, desired effects, and potential side effects of supplements. Some sports and coaches may encourage small size and dieting, or encourage use of dietary supplements to increase weight and muscle. Children and adolescents in activities such as ballet, wrestling, track or running, and horse racing may have health risks associated with inconsistent or inadequate intake.

Approximately 3.3% of U.S. high school students (4.3% of males and 2.2% of females) report taking illegal anabolic steroids; up to 6.5% in some communities report use (CDC, 2010). These products can have a wide array of side effects. They may stop growth of long bones, lead to endocrine imbalance, and cause increased tendon rupture. They are also illegal in sporting events. Andro and DHEA are steroidal hormones used by some athletes. They can cause masculinization of females, disruption of glucose balance, insulin sensitivity, dyslipidemia, and aggressive behavior (Lumia & McGinnis, 2010).

Some common amino acid nutritional supplements include creatine, carnitine, and glutamine. Although the side effects of these substances are minimal, their possible enhancement of performance is temporary and outcomes of long-term use are unknown. Increasing protein intake to meet needs during periods of high activity is a better alternative. Creatine has been studied more than most supplements; it is made by the body and is present in many protein sources. Supplemental creatine increases the creatine level in muscle and may help to increase performance in short bursts of activity, while not affecting endurance sports. The increase in muscle mass that can occur is actually due to water and is lost quickly when the supplement is discontinued.

Minerals such as chromium, iron, and calcium are used by some youths. Ask about the athlete's social group and whether ergogenic aids are used; this is a strong predictor of adoption and is reason for additional counseling (Goulet, Valois, Buist, et al., 2010). The nurse should ask careful and sensitive questions such as "Many athletes take supplements to aid in performance in sports. What supplements do you take or are you considering?" Information should be provided to enhance the youth's understanding of nutrition and sports performance. Generally, a balanced diet with adequate carbohydrate, protein, and fat will meet the needs of most athletes and lead to maximal sport performance. School nurses can work with physical education teachers and coaches to plan appropriate programs for youth to prevent use of ergogenic aids.

Health-Related Conditions

Many health conditions influence the child's nutritional state. Conversely, the child's nutritional state can influence the state of health. See *Pathophysiology Illustrated* for examples of some common conditions that influence nutritional needs. These conditions are discussed in various chapters throughout the text. Discuss with classmates how to adjust normal nutritional assessment and teaching due to the presence of a healthcare concern. Which conditions influence absorption of nutrients? Which cause changes in nutritional intake requirements? Some children benefit from special dietary aids, such as eating utensils and cups

Academy of Nutrition and Dietetics

Weblink

Complementary Care Herbs, Probiotics, and Prebiotics

Many families use food products to promote health and treat diseases. These include herbal products that may be acquired from health food stores or the Internet. Herbs are not tested nor regulated by the government, so amounts of ingredients are often not known. Ask families about what herbal products they use regularly or to treat disease. Learn about the herbs and any research that has been conducted with children.

Another type of food product is a **probiotic**, a food supplement containing a live microorganism that alters the balance of gut microflora, thereby providing a health benefit. Common probiotics include *Lactobacillus* and *Bifidobacterium*, which are commonly found in the human gastrointestinal tract, are enhanced by eating yogurt with live cultures, and may be helpful in treating diarrhea or atopic dermatitis. Daily intake of pasteurized yogurt with live cultures can safely be encouraged for children.

A **prebiotic** is a nondigestable food ingredient that can stimulate growth or activity of probiotic bacteria (Thomas, Greer, & Committee on Nutrition, 2010). For example, oligosaccharides enhance proliferation of the beneficial *Bifidobacterium*.

Inquire about the family's treatment of common childhood disorders. Include questions about food and nutritional supplements at all well-child visits. Provide information for the family as needed.

that are easy to grasp. Therapists can evaluate and make recommendations about devices that can assist the child at meals.

Vegetarianism

Some families choose to eat vegetarian diets and can be helped and encouraged in their endeavors. Several variations in intake occur. **Vegetarians** eat no poultry, meat, or fish. Lacto-ovovegetarians eat eggs and dairy products, whereas lactovegetarians eat dairy products but not eggs. In contrast, **vegans** are strict vegetarians and eat no animal products. When someone says he or she is vegetarian, it is best if the nurse asks specific questions about what the individual will and will not eat.

The vegetarian diet is healthy, easy to follow, and may even provide extra health benefits (American Dietetic Association, 2009). Some deficiencies may exist; assessment and planning can ensure that they do not develop. Vegans should be sure to include adequate dietary vitamins D and B_{12}, zinc, iron, calories, protein, and fat. Completing a 24-hour diet recall for pregnant or lactating women and vegetarian children, with analysis for RDAs, can be helpful. The nurse should be sure to routinely assess growth and other nutritional measures, as well as provide ideas of various foods to meet nutritional needs and perform other general nutritional teaching. When a vegetarian child is hospitalized, the nurse should plan with the nutrition department and the child's family to meet intake needs.

Enteral Therapy

Enteral therapy is a form of nutritional support provided when a child cannot take in enough food orally to sustain health. Since it

Growth and Development

When a pregnant teen follows a vegetarian diet, she needs additional help to encourage adequate nutrition. A 24-hour or 2-day diet diary helps identify nutritional needs. Consider additional pregnancy needs for energy, protein, omega 3 fatty acids, iron, vitamin D, and calcium; note that vitamin B$_{12}$ is recommended as a supplement. Use the vegetarian food guide available through the American Dietetic Association.

● **Figure 33–11** Enteral therapy. This child has returned to school following surgery. Due to cerebral palsy, he has difficulty chewing and swallowing food. The school nurse has taught his teacher to safely administer some enteral feedings during school hours.

is the closest form of nutritional support to the natural method of eating, it has the least untoward effects and greatest rate of success. Some children who use enteral therapy are those with cerebral palsy or other neurologic conditions that lead to weakness of the throat and mouth, those with neoplasm or immune dysfunction, and those in acute states of recovery from accidents or illness (Figure 33–11 ●).

Although a tube can be inserted into the nasal opening and placed through the esophagus into the stomach (nasogastric tube), a tube surgically placed into the stomach through an abdominal opening, a jejunal or gastric tube, is preferred for long-term use. As long as the child can absorb and use nutrients, enteral therapy can be successful in providing calories and

essential nutrients. Commercially prepared formulas are available, and specially formulated solutions can be adapted for children with specific dietary needs. Nursing care includes care of the gastrostomy tube and entry site to prevent infection and skin breakdown. Ensure that a nasogastric tube is correctly placed before each tube feeding. For both nasogastric and gastric feedings an empty syringe is often used to check residuals or the amount of fluid not absorbed since the previous feeding. Teach families enteral feeding techniques when they will perform the process at home and arrange for periodic evaluation of technique. Perform regular nutritional assessments. See Chapter 52 ✑ for suggestions on management of nursing care during tube feedings. See also Skill 16–3 in the accompanying *Clinical Skills Manual* SKILLS.

Total Parenteral Nutrition (TPN)

Total parenteral nutrition (TPN) makes it possible to provide intravenous nutritional support for people who cannot eat or are unable to absorb nutrients from the intestinal tract in a normal manner and are at risk of severe malnutrition. Examples of children who benefit from this method of nutrition are those with congenital malformation of the gastrointestinal tract, brain injury, or severe burns; it may also be used for support after bone marrow transplant, sepsis, or other critical conditions.

A catheter is inserted so that a sterile nutrition solution is infused directly into the bloodstream. A central venous catheter is used to promote safe infusion. Fluids usually contain glucose; electrolytes such as sodium, potassium, calcium, magnesium, phosphate, and chloride; vitamins; and proteins. Lipid emulsions are another type of TPN used in some children. Meticulous care is needed, whether in the hospital or at home, to ensure safe TPN infusion and treatment. The nurse performs initial assessment, ongoing evaluation, and monitoring of treatment; verifies the solution type and rate of administration; ensures that solution storage recommendations are followed; and administers the solutions in the hospital or other settings. See Skill 12–7 for the protocols for TPN management in the *Clinical Skills Manual* SKILLS.

Video | Administering a Gavage/Tube Feeding

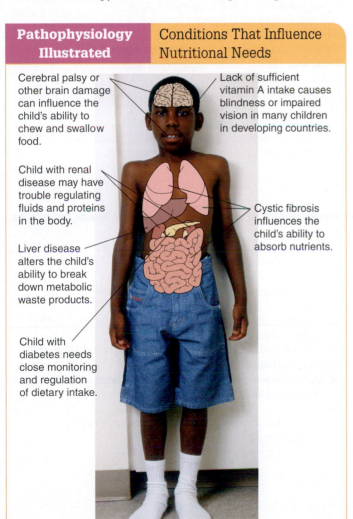

| **Pathophysiology Illustrated** | Conditions That Influence Nutritional Needs |

Cerebral palsy or other brain damage can influence the child's ability to chew and swallow food.

Lack of sufficient vitamin A intake causes blindness or impaired vision in many children in developing countries.

Child with renal disease may have trouble regulating fluids and proteins in the body.

Cystic fibrosis influences the child's ability to absorb nutrients.

Liver disease alters the child's ability to break down metabolic waste products.

Child with diabetes needs close monitoring and regulation of dietary intake.

Clinical Reasoning   The Child with Special Nutritional Needs

Joey was diagnosed with cerebral palsy early in life. He is now 11 years old and has recently been enrolled in school. Part of the healthcare plan being implemented in the school involves fostering a positive nutritional state. Joey has limited ability to swallow, related to muscle weakness of cerebral palsy, and is therefore unable to ingest enough calories by mouth to ensure his optimal growth and development. Joey had a feeding tube inserted into his stomach at an early age and receives some of his nutrition by this method.

The school nurse has met with Joey's parents and his home health nurse to learn about the amount and type of tube feedings he receives,

as well as the texture of oral feedings he can manage. The nurse will plan the feeding schedule at school to facilitate adequate nutrition in that setting. In addition, careful ongoing nutritional assessment will be needed to evaluate if Joey is getting the calories and other nutrients he needs for growth and development. The school nurse is also educating the classroom teachers and other school personnel about Joey's unique nutritional requirements.

How will you organize Joey's care and educate teachers and other staff if you are the case manager for his integration within the school system? *See www.nursing.pearsonhighered.com for possible responses.*

Critical Concept Review

LEARNING OUTCOME 33.1: Discuss major nutritional concepts pertaining to the growth and development of children.

Infancy:
1. Increased need for calories because of:
   - Rapid physical growth.
   - Increased physical activity.
2. Proper nutrition is needed for development of the nervous system and organs.
3. Should receive only breast milk or formula until tongue thrust has decreased and infant can sit well.
4. No cow's milk until 1 year of age.
5. Food introduction principles are needed by parents.

Toddlerhood:
1. Development of physiologic anorexia.
2. Amount of milk and fruit juice should be limited so child will eat nutritious solid food.
3. Should begin to learn to eat in social situations.

Preschool:
1. Should begin to help with simple food preparation.
2. May exhibit extreme food preferences (food jag).
3. Emphasize brushing of teeth and first dental visit.

School age:
1. Time of gradual growth with preadolescent growth spurt.
2. Increased need for calories during growth spurt.
3. May be resistant to trying new foods.
4. Expect loss of first deciduous teeth and eruption of permanent teeth.

Adolescence:
1. Need for increased calories during growth spurt.
2. Increased physical activity (such as sports) will increase caloric needs.
3. Encourage balanced intake and minimize fast foods.

LEARNING OUTCOME 33.2: Describe and plan nursing interventions to meet nutritional needs for all age groups from infancy through adolescence.

Infancy:
1. Encourage breastfeeding, if possible.
2. Assist mother to continue to breastfeed the hospitalized infant.
3. Discuss feeding during each contact with the mother.
4. To decrease occurrence of dental caries, teach parents that infant should not be given a bottle at bedtime.
5. Teach beginning dental care.
6. Supplemental foods begin with rice cereal and progress to vegetables and then fruit.
7. Begin use of cup for liquids at 8–9 months of age.

Toddlerhood:
1. Encourage parents to provide health foods that are easily eaten:
   - Small portions.
   - Place 1 tablespoon of food per year of age on child's plate.
2. Limit milk to 1 quart per day.
3. Limit fruit juice to 6 ounces per day.
4. Parents should establish mealtime rules.

Preschool:
1. Encourage parents to use meal preparation as time for teaching about proper nutrition and kitchen safety.
2. Limit fruit juice to 12 ounces per day.
3. Encourage parents to limit fast food to once per week.

School age:
1. Present nutritional teaching to child by using pictures and providing hands-on experiences.
2. Encourage families to bring food from home for the hospitalized child.
3. Allow hospitalized children to eat together.
4. Become knowledgeable concerning nutritional assistance available to the child and family.

Adolescence:
1. Encourage teen to drink fruit juice in place of soft drinks.
2. Provide healthy choices of food for teen.
3. Allow peer interaction during meals, if possible.

LEARNING OUTCOME 33.3: Integrate methods of nutritional assessment into nursing care of infants, children, and adolescents.

Nutritional assessments include:

1. Growth measurements:
   - Height (length).
   - Weight.
   - Head circumference.
   - Skinfold measurement.
2. Body mass index.
3. Laboratory tests:
   - Hemoglobin and hematocrit.
   - Lipid profile.
   - Liver function.
   - Renal function.
   - Serum glucose.
4. Mother's dietary intake during pregnancy.
5. 24-hour food recall.
6. Food frequency questionnaire.
7. Food diary.

LEARNING OUTCOME 33.4: Identify and explain common nutritional problems of children.

Common nutritional problems include:

1. Hunger due to poverty.
2. Obesity.
3. Foodborne illness.
4. Celiac disease.
5. Eating disorders.
6. Food allergy and intolerance.
7. Dietary deficiencies.

LEARNING OUTCOME 33.5: Develop nursing interventions for children with nutritional disorders.

1. Assessment:
   - Obtain individual and family history.
   - Obtain accurate height and weight.
   - Observe eating behaviors.
   - Investigate use of prescription and OTC medications.
2. Planning and implementation:
   - Monitor nutritional and fluid intake.
   - Encourage nutritious food consumption.
   - Monitor elimination pattern.
   - Administer medications as needed.
3. Evaluation:
   - Promote adequate food and fluid to establish healthy nutritional lifestyle.
   - Encourage positive self-esteem.

Clinical Reasoning in Action

A mother is seeing the pediatric nurse practitioner you are working with for her son Jonathan's 3-month, well-baby checkup at the local community health clinic. The baby is in the 90th percentile for weight and in the 50th percentile for length and is fed Similac formula with iron. According to the medical history, Jonathan had respiratory syncytial virus (RSV) when he was 1 month old and there are smokers in the house (see Chapter 47 🔗 for more information on RSV). The nurse practitioner has asked you to educate the mother about feeding her 3-month-old baby. The mother has raised concerns that the baby is not sleeping through the night and the baby's grandmother has suggested adding cereal to his bottle at night to help him sleep. Jonathan has met all developmental milestones and has not yet developed teeth.

1. What type of advice can you give the mother about adding cereal to the bottle?
2. Why is rice cereal recommended as the first food to introduce when Jonathan is able to start solid foods?
3. What is the reason only iron-fortified formula or breast milk is recommended the entire first year of life for Jonathan, rather than cow's milk?
4. Based on Jonathan's length and weight percentiles on the growth chart, his mother wonders if he should be put on a "diet." What would be the appropriate response to her concern?

See www.nursing.pearsonhighered.com for possible responses.

References

Ackerman, K. E., & Misra, M. (2011). Bone health and the female athlete triad in adolescent athletes. *Physician Sportsmedicine, 39*, 131–141.

Agron, P., Berends, V., Ellis, K., & Gonzalez, M. (2010). School wellness policies: Perceptions, barriers, and needs among school leaders and wellness advocates. *Journal of School Health, 80*, 527–535.

American Academy of Pediatrics (AAP). (2011). *Fruit juice and your child's diet*. Retrieved from http://www.healthychildren.org

American Academy of Pediatrics (AAP) Committee on Nutrition. (2009). *Pediatric nutrition handbook* (6th ed.). Elk Grove Village, IL: American Academy of Pediatrics.

American Academy of Pediatrics (AAP) Section on Breastfeeding. (2012). Breastfeeding and the use of human milk. *Pediatrics, 129*, e827–e841.

American Dietetic Association. (2009). *Vegetarian diets*. Retrieved from www.eatright.org/About/Content/aspx?id=8357&terms=Vegetarian%20diet

Ayliffe, B., & Glanville, N. T. (2010). Achieving healthy body weight in teenagers: Evidence-based practice guidelines for community nutrition interventions. *Canadian Journal of Dietetic Practice and Research, 71*, 378–386.

Bindler, R. M., & Howry, L. B. (2005). *Pediatric drug guide*. Upper Saddle River, NJ: Prentice Hall-Health.

Brewerton, T. D., & Costin, C. (2011). Long-term outcome of residential treatment for anorexia nervosa and bulimia nervosa. *Eating Disorders, 19*, 132–144.

Bryant-Waugh, R., Markham, L., Kriepe, R. E., & Walsh, B. T. (2010). Feeding and eating disorders of childhood. *International Journal of Eating Disorders, 43*, 98–111.

Centers for Disease Control and Prevention (CDC). (2010). Youth risk behavior surveillance—United States, 2009. *Morbidity and Mortality Weekly Report, 59* (SS-5), 1–146.

Centers for Disease Control and Prevention (CDC). (2011a). *Breastfeeding among U.S. children born 1999–2007* (CDC National Immunization Survey). Retrieved from http://www.cdc.ov/breastfeeding/data/NIS_data

Centers for Disease Control and Prevention (CDC). (2011b). *Overweight and obesity*. Retrieved from http://www.cdc.gov/obesity/childhood/data.html

Centers for Disease Control and Prevention (CDC). (2011c). *2011 estimates of foodborne illness in the United States*. Retrieved from http://www.cdc.gov/Features/dsFoodborneEstimates

Children's Defense Fund. (2010). *The state of America's children*. Washington, DC: Author.

Cloherty, J. P., Eichenwald, E. C., & Stark, A. R. (2012). *Manual for neonatal care* (7th ed.). Philadelphia, PA: Lippincott Williams & Wilkins.

Cole, S. Z., & Lanham, J. S. (2011). Failure to thrive: An update. *American Family Physician, 83*, 829–834.

Daitch, L., & Epperson, J. N. (2011). Celiac disease. *Clinician Reviews, 21*(4), 49–55.

Fisher, C. A., Hetrick, S. E., & Rushford, N. (2010). Family therapy for anorexia nervosa. *Cochrane Database Systematic Review, 14*(4), CD004780.

Flament, M. F., Bissada, H., & Spettique, W. (2011). Evidence-based pharmacotherapy of eating disorders. *International Journal of Neuropsychopharmacology, 15*, 189–207.

Garcia-Manzanares, A., & Lucendo, A. J. (2011). Nutritional and dietary aspects of celiac disease. *Nutrition in Clinical Practice, 26*, 163–173.

Goulet, C., Valois, P., Buist, A., & Cote, M. (2010). Predictors of the use of performance-enhancing substances by young athletes. *Clinical Journal of Sport Medicine, 20*, 243–248.

Greydanus, D. E., Omar, H., & Pratt, H. D. (2010). The adolescent female athlete: Current concepts and conundrums. *Pediatric Clinics of North America, 57*, 697–718.

Hagan, J. F., Shaw, J. S., & Duncan, P. M. (2008). *Bright futures: Guidelines for health supervision of infants, children and adolescents* (3rd ed.). Elk Grove Village, IL: American Academy of Pediatrics.

Hay, P. J., & Claudino, A. M. (2011). Clinical psychopharmacology of eating disorders: A research update. *International Journal of Neuropsychopharmacology, 15*, 209–222.

Holt, K., Wooldridge, N., Story, M., & Sofka, D. (2011). *Bright futures nutrition* (3rd ed.). Elk Grove Village, IL: American Academy of Pediatrics.

Institute of Medicine. (2011). *Dietary reference intakes: Calcium and vitamin D*. Washington, DC: National Academies Press.

Kliegman, R. M., Stanton, B., St. Geme, J., Schor, N., & Behrman, R. E. (2011). *Nelson textbook of pediatrics* (19th ed.). Philadelphia, PA: Elsevier Saunders.

Lawrence, R. A., & Lawrence, R. M. (2011). *Breastfeeding: A guide for the medical profession* (7th ed.). Philadelphia, PA: Mosby.

Lee, R. D., & Nieman, D. C. (2010). *Nutrition assessment* (5th ed.). Boston, MA: McGraw-Hill.

LeFevre, M. K. (2010). Rickets: A preventable growth delay. *Journal of Pediatric Health Care, 24*, 408–412.

Lock, J. (2011). Evaluation of family treatment models for eating disorders. *Current Opinion in Psychiatry, 24*, 274–279.

Lumia, A. R., & McGinnis, M. Y. (2010). Impact of anabolic androgenic steroids on adolescent males. *Physiology & Behavior, 100*, 199–204.

Mansoor, D. K., & Sharma, H. P. (2011). Clinical presentations of food allergy. *Pediatric Clinics of North America, 58*, 315–326.

Mattar, L., Godart, N., Melchior, J. C., & Pichard, C. (2011). Anorexia nervosa and nutrition assessment: Contribution of body composition measurements. *Nutrition Research Reviews, 24*, 39–45.

Molinero, O., & Marquez, S. (2009). Use of nutritional supplements in sports: Risks, knowledge, and behavioural-related factors. *Hospital Nutrition, 24*, 128–134.

Moore, D. J. (2009). Inflaming the debate on infant colic. *Journal of Pediatrics, 155*, 772–773.

National Institute of Allergy and Infectious Diseases (NIAID). (2011). *Guidelines for diagnosis and management of food allergy in the United States*. Washington, DC: U.S. Department of Health and Human Services.

National Institute of Diabetes and Digestive and Kidney Diseases (NIDDK). (2012). *Celiac disease*. Retrieved from http://digestive.niddk.nih.gov/ddiseases/pubs/celiac

National Institute of Mental Health (NIMH). (2010a). *Eating disorders among adults—Anorexia nervosa*. Retrieved from http://www.nimh.nih.gov/statistics/1EAT_ADULT_ANX.shtml

National Institute of Mental Health (NIMH). (2010b). *Eating disorders among adults—Bulimia nervosa*. Retrieved from http://www.nimh.nih.gov/statistics/1EAT_ADULT_RBUL.shtml

Power, T. G., Bindler, R. C., Goetz, S., & Daratha, K. B. (2010). Obesity prevention in early adolescence: Student, parent, and teacher views. *Journal of School Health, 80*, 13–19.

Rashid, M., Zarkadas, M., Anca, A., & Limeback, H. (2011). Oral manifestations of celiac disease: A clinical guide for dentists. *Journal of the Canadian Dental Association, 77*, b39.

Riordan, J., & Wambach, K. (2010). *Breastfeeding and human lactation* (4th ed.). Boston, MA: Jones & Bartlett.

Rodriguez, N. R., DiMarco, N. M., Langley, S., American Dietetic Association, Dietitians of Canada, & American College of Sports Medicine. (2009). Position of the American Dietetic Association, Dietitians of Canada, and the American College of Sports Medicine: Nutrition and athletic performance. *Journal of the American Dietetic Association, 109*, 509–527.

Ross, A. C., Taylor, C. L., Yaktine, A. L., & Del Valle, H. B. (Eds.). (2011). *Dietary reference intakes for calcium and vitamin D*. Washington, DC: Institute of Medicine.

Siega-Riz, A. M., El Ghormli, L., Mobley, C., Gillis, B., Stadler, D., Hartstein, J., . . . HEALTHY Study Group. (2011). The effects of the HEALTHY study intervention on middle school student dietary intakes. *International Journal of Behavioral Nutrition and Physical Activity, 8*, 7.

Strasburger, V. C., Jordan, A. B., & Donnerstein, E. (2010). Health effects of media on children and adolescents. *Pediatrics, 125*, 756–767.

Thomas, D. W., Greer, F. R., & Committee on Nutrition. (2010). Probiotics and prebiotics in pediatrics. *Pediatrics, 126*, 1217–1231.

Treasure, J., Claudino, A. M., & Zucker, N. (2010). Eating disorders. *Lancet, 375*, 583–593.

U.S. Department of Agriculture. (2011). *Food security in the United States*. Retrieved from http://www.ers.usda.gov/Briefing/FoodSecurity/stats_graphs.htm

U.S. Department of Health and Human Services. (2011). *Healthy People 2020*. Retrieved from http://healthypeople.gov/2020/topicsobjectives2020/pdfs/nutritionandweight.pdf

U.S. Food and Drug Administration. (2011). *What you need to know about mercury in fish and shellfish*. Retrieved from http://www.fda.gov/Food/FoodSafety

Vaczy, E., Seaman, B., Peterson-Sweeney, K., & Hondorf, C. (2011). Passport to health: An innovative tool to enhance healthy lifestyle choices. *Journal of Pediatric Health Care, 25*, 31–37.

Van Koppen, E. J., Schweizer, J. J., Csizmadia, C. G., Krom, Y., Hylkema, H. B., van Geel, A. M., . . . Mearin, M. L. (2009). Long-term health and quality-of-life consequences of mass screening for childhood celiac disease: A 10-year follow-up study. *Pediatrics, 123*, e582–e588.

Wagner, C. L., Greer, F. R., Section on Breastfeeding, & Committee on Nutrition (2008). Prevention of rickets and vitamin D deficiency in infants, children, and adolescents. *Pediatrics, 122*, 1142–1152.

Walvoord, E. C. (2010). The timing of puberty: Is it changing? Does it matter? *Journal of Adolescent Health, 47*, 433–439.

Pediatric Assessment

I was scared when we brought Aliyah to the hospital. She looked help-less, afraid, and sick. The nurses and doctors took over when we got to the hospital, and I felt better because they seemed to know what to do. —Father of Aliyah, 6 months old

Ryan McVay/Getty Images

LEARNING OUTCOMES

34.1   Describe the elements of a health history for infants and children of different ages.

34.2   Apply communication strategies to improve the quality of historical data collected.

34.3   Demonstrate strategies to gain cooperation of a young child for assessment.

34.4   Describe the differences in sequence of the physical assessment for infants, children, and adolescents.

34.5   Modify physical assessment techniques according to the age and developmental stage of the child.

34.6   List five normal variations in pediatric physical findings (such as a Mongolian spot in an infant) found during a physical assessment.

34.7   Evaluate the growth pattern of an infant or child.

34.8   Distinguish between expected and unexpected physical signs to identify at least five signs that require urgent nursing intervention.

How do examination techniques vary by the age of the child? How does the nurse encourage infants and toddlers to cooperate with the examination? This chapter provides an overview of pediatric assessment, including history taking and examination techniques geared to the unique needs of pediatric patients. Strategies for obtaining the child's history are presented first. The remainder of the chapter then outlines a systematic process for physical examination of the child.

ANATOMIC AND PHYSIOLOGIC CHARACTERISTICS OF INFANTS AND CHILDREN

Children and infants are not only smaller than adults but also significantly different physiologically. Knowledge of pediatric anatomic and physiologic differences will aid in recognizing normal variations found during the physical examination. It also assists with understanding the different physiologic responses children have to illness and injury. The illustration in *As Children Grow: Children Are Not Just Small Adults* provides an overview of important anatomic and physiologic differences between children and adults.

OBTAINING THE CHILD'S HISTORY

Communication Strategies

The health history interview is a very personal conversation with a parent, caretaker, or adolescent during which private concerns and feelings are shared. Try to ensure that both parties clearly understand this exchange of information and that it is an effective communication with the parent or the child. Effective communication is difficult to accomplish because parents and children often do not correctly interpret what the nurse says, just as the nurse may not understand completely what the parent or child says. People's interpretation of information is based on their life experiences, culture, and education.

Strategies to Build Rapport with the Family

When obtaining the history, make sure the parents understand the purpose of the interview and that the information will be used appropriately. To develop rapport, demonstrate interest in and concern for the child and family during the interview. This rapport forms the foundation for the collaborative relationship between the nurse and parent that will lead to the best nursing care for the child. The following strategies help to establish rapport with the child's family during the nursing history:

- *Introduce yourself* (name, title or position, and role in caring for the child). To demonstrate respect, ask all family members present what name they prefer you to use when talking with them.

- *Explain the purpose of the interview* and why the nursing history is different from the information collected by other health professionals. For example, "Nurses use this information to plan nursing care best suited for your child."

- *Provide privacy* and remove as many distractions as possible during the interview. If the patient's room does not offer privacy, attempt to find a vacant patient room or lounge. Assure the parents and the child that the information provided during the assessment is protected under the Health Insurance Portability and Accountability Act (HIPAA), a federal law that requires written consent to be provided before health information can be shared with healthcare providers outside the facility.

- *Direct the focus of the interview* with open-ended questions. Open-ended questions are useful to initiate the interview, develop a rapport, and understand the parent's perceptions of the child's problem. For example, "What

As Children Grow | Children Are Not Just Small Adults

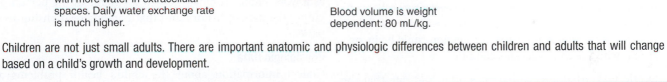

Body surface area large for weight, making infants susceptible to hypothermia.

All brain cells present at birth; myelinization and further development of nerve fibers occur during first year.

Anterior fontanelle and open sutures palpable up to about 18 months. Posterior fontanelle closes between 2 and 3 months.

Head proportionately larger, making child susceptible to head injury.

Tongue large relative to small nasal and oral airway passages.

Higher metabolic rate, higher oxygen needs, higher caloric needs.

Short, narrow trachea in children under 5 years makes them susceptible to foreign body obstruction.

Until puberty, percentage of cartilage in ribs is higher, making them more flexible and compliant.

Until late school age and adolescence, cardiac output is rate dependent not stroke volume dependent, making heart rate more rapid.

Until about 10 years, there is a faster respiratory rate, fewer and smaller alveoli, and less lung volume. Tidal volume is proportional to weight (7 to 10 mL/kg).

Abdomen offers poor protection for the liver and spleen, making them susceptible to trauma.

Up to about 4 or 5 years, diaphragm is primary breathing muscle. CO_2 is not effectively expired when child is distressed, making child susceptible to metabolic acidosis.

Until 12 to 18 months of age, kidneys do not concentrate urine effectively and do not exert optimal control over electrolyte secretion and absorption.

Until puberty, bones are soft and more easily bent and fractured.

Muscles lack tone, power, and coordination during infancy. Muscles are 25% of weight in infants versus 40% in adults.

Until later school age, proportion of body weight in water is larger, with more water in extracellular spaces. Daily water exchange rate is much higher.

Blood volume is weight dependent: 80 mL/kg.

Children are not just small adults. There are important anatomic and physiologic differences between children and adults that will change based on a child's growth and development.

---

problems led to Roberto's admission to the hospital?" Use close-ended questions or directing statements to clarify information or to obtain detailed information. For example, "How high was Tommy's fever this morning?"

■ *Ask one question at a time* so that the parent or child understands what piece of information is desired and so that it is clear which question the parent is answering. "Does any member of your family have diabetes, heart disease, or sickle cell disease?" is a multiple question. Ask about each disease separately to ensure the most accurate response.

■ *Involve the child in the interview* by asking age-appropriate questions. Young children can be asked, "What is your doll's name?" or "Where does it hurt?" Demonstrating an interest in the child initiates development of rapport with both child and parents. Ask older children and teens questions about their illness or injury. Offer them an opportunity to privately discuss their major concerns when their parents are not present.

■ *Be honest with the child* when answering questions or when giving information about what will happen. Children need to learn that they can trust their nurse.

■ *Choose the language style best understood by the parent and child.* Commonly used phrases or medical terms may have different meanings to different people. To improve communication, ask the parents or child questions to ensure that their understanding of a phrase or term is correct. For example, "You used the term *hyperactivity*. Tell me what this behavior means to you."

■ *Use an interpreter to improve communication when not fluent in the family's primary language.* Avoid using a family member for history taking to ensure patient and family confidentiality.

Careful Listening

Complete attention is necessary to "hear" and accurately interpret information the parents and child give during the nursing history. While carefully listening to the information provided, pay attention to how it is expressed, and observe behavior during the interaction.

- Does the parent hesitate or avoid answering certain questions?

- Pay attention to the parent's attitude or tone of voice when the child's problems are discussed. Determine if it is consistent with the seriousness of the child's problem. The tone of voice can reveal anxiety, anger, or lack of concern.

- Be alert to any underlying themes. For example, the parent who talks about the child's diagnosis, but repeatedly refers to the impact of the illness on the family's finances or on meeting the needs of other family members, is requesting that these issues be addressed.

- Observe the parent's *nonverbal* behavior (posture, gestures, body movements, eye contact, and facial expression) for consistency with the words and tone of voice used. Is the parent interested in and appropriately concerned about the child's condition? Behaviors such as sitting up straight, making eye contact, and appearing apprehensive reflect appropriate concern for the child. Physical withdrawal, failure to make eye contact, or a happy expression could be inconsistent with the child's serious condition.

Subtle nonverbal and verbal cues often indicate that the parent has not provided complete information about the child's problem. Observe for behaviors such as avoiding eye contact, change in voice pitch, or hesitation when responding to a question. Being supportive and asking clarifying questions encourage further description or the expression of information that is difficult for the parent or child to share. For example, "It sounds like that was a very difficult experience. How did Lily react?"

Encourage parents to share information, even if it is private or sensitive, especially when it influences nursing care planning. Often parents avoid sharing some information because they want to make a good impression, or they do not understand the value of the missing information. If parents hesitate to share information, briefly explain why the question was asked—for example, to make their child's hospital experience more pleasant or to begin planning for the child's discharge and home care. Silence is common in some Asian and Native American groups as they attempt to form responses to questions.

In some cases the parent may become too agitated, upset, or angry to continue responding to questions. When the information is not needed immediately, move on to another portion of the history to determine whether the parent is able to respond to other questions. Depending on the emotional status of the parent, it may be appropriate to collect the remaining information later.

Data to Be Collected

Nurses collect and organize health, medical, and personal-social history to plan a child's nursing care. The health status, psychosocial, and developmental data are organized to help develop the nursing diagnoses and the nursing care plan.

Patient Information

Obtain the child's name and nickname, age, sex, and ethnic origin. The child's birth date, race, religion, address, and phone number can be obtained from the admission form. Ask the parent for an emergency contact address and phone number, as well as a work phone number. Record the name of the person providing the patient history and that person's relationship to the patient.

Physiologic Data

Collect information about the child's health problems and diseases chronologically in a format similar to the traditional medical history.

Chief Complaint.   Identify the child's primary problem or reason for hospital admission or visit to a healthcare setting, stated in the parent's or child's exact words.

History of Present Illness or Injury.   Obtain a detailed description of the current health problem that includes the characteristics in Table 34–1. Each problem is described separately.

Past History.   This more detailed description of the child's prior health problems includes all major past illnesses and injuries. Identify all major illnesses, including common communicable diseases. Identify major injuries, their cause or mechanism, and their severity. Obtain information about each prior surgery, its purpose, and if the surgery required overnight hospitalization. For all hospitalizations, identify the reason and length of stay. Identify the circumstances for any prior transfusion (blood or blood products), type of transfusion, and reaction. Obtain information about each specific diagnosis, treatment, outcome, complication or residual problem, and the child's reaction to the event.

Table 34–1	History of Present Illness or Injury
Characteristic	**Defining Variables**
Onset	Sudden or gradual, previous episodes, date and time began
Type of symptom	Pain, itching, cough, vomiting, runny nose, diarrhea, rash, etc.
Location	Generalized or localized—be anatomically precise
Duration	Continuous or episodic symptoms, length of episodes
Severity	Effect on daily activities (e.g., interrupted sleep, decreased appetite, unable to attend school)
Influencing factors	What relieves or worsens symptoms, what precipitated the problem, recent exposure to infection or allergen
Past evaluation for the problem	Laboratory studies, physician's office or hospital where done, results of past examinations
Previous and current treatment	Prescribed and over-the-counter drugs used, complementary therapies (e.g., heat, ice, rest), response to treatments

Table 34–2	Birth History
Prenatal condition	■ Mother's age, health during pregnancy, prenatal care, weight gained, special diet, use of alcohol or drugs, expected date of birth ■ Details of illnesses, radiograph or sonogram findings, hospitalizations, medications, complications, and their timing during pregnancy ■ Prior obstetric history
Intrapartum—description of birth	■ Site of birth (hospital, home, birthing center) ■ Labor induced or spontaneous, time/duration or rupture of membranes, length of labor, color of amniotic fluid, complications ■ Vaginal or cesarean birth, forceps or suction used, vertex or breech position ■ Length of pregnancy (weeks), single or multiple birth
Condition of baby at birth	■ Birth weight, Apgar score, cried immediately ■ Need for incubator, resuscitation, oxygen, ventilator ■ Any abnormalities detected, meconium staining
Postnatal condition	■ Difficulties in the nursery—feeding, respiratory problems, jaundice, cyanosis, rashes, seizures ■ Length of hospital stay, special nursery, home with mother ■ Breastfed or bottle-fed, weight lost/gained in hospital ■ Medical care needed in first week—readmission to hospital

Use the guidelines in Table 34–2 to obtain a *birth history* when the child's present problem may be related to problems during the pregnancy, birth, and newborn care.

Current Health Status. Obtain a detailed description of each aspect of the child's typical health status.

- *Health maintenance*—child's primary care provider, dentist, and other healthcare providers, timing of last visit to each.

- *Medications*—prescribed and over-the-counter medications (oral, topical, injectable) used daily or frequently for fever, colds, coughs, and rashes. Ask about the use of herbs, plants, teas, or other complementary therapies.

- *Allergies*—to food, medication, animals, insect bites, or other exposures, and the type of reaction (e.g., respiratory difficulty, rash, hives, itching).

- *Immunizations*—review dates immunizations were received. Ask about any unexpected reactions. Inquire about the reason if not up to date. (See Chapter 44 🔗 for the recommended immunization schedule.)

- *Safety measures used*—car restraint system, window guards, medication storage, sports protective gear, smoke detectors, bicycle helmet, firearm storage, water safety, and others.

- *Activities and exercise*—usual play and/or sports activities; physical mobility and limitations, adaptive equipment used.

- *Nutrition*—formula-fed or breastfed; if breastfed, for how long, type and amount of daily formula and other liquid intake; when solid foods were introduced; enrollment in the special nutrition program for Women, Infants, and Children (WIC). Contrast food intake to the appropriate intake for age and weight (see Chapter 33 🔗).

- *Sleep*—infant sleep position, length and timing of naps and nighttime sleep; nightmares or night terrors, snoring, other sleep disturbances; where the child sleeps; bedtime rituals.

Familial and Hereditary Diseases. Collect data about familial and hereditary diseases for three generations of family members, including the parents, grandparents, aunts, uncles, cousins, child, and siblings, using information listed in Table 34–3. Collect information about the health status of each parent. Record information in either a family genogram or pedigree (see Chapter 7 🔗) or a narrative format.

Review of Systems. Collect a comprehensive overview of the child's health during the review of systems using the guidelines

Table 34–3	Familial or Hereditary Diseases
Infectious diseases	Tuberculosis, HIV, hepatitis, herpes
Heart disease	Heart defects, myocardial infarctions, hypertension, dyslipidemia, sudden childhood deaths
Allergic disorders	Eczema, hay fever
Eye disorders	Glaucoma, cataracts, vision loss
Ear disorders	Hearing loss, unusual shape or position of ears
Hematologic disorders	Sickle cell disease, thalassemia, G6PD deficiency, hemophilia
Respiratory disorders	Cystic fibrosis, asthma
Cancer	Retinoblastoma, cancer with early age of onset
Endocrine disorders	Diabetes mellitus type 1 and 2, hypothyroidism, hyperthyroidism, Turner syndrome
Brain disorders	Intellectual disability, epilepsy, psychiatric disorders
Musculoskeletal disorders	Muscular dystrophy, scoliosis, spina bifida
Gastrointestinal disorders	Pyloric stenosis, ulcers, colitis, celiac disease, polycystic kidneys
Metabolic disorders	Phenylketonuria, galactosemia, maple syrup urine disease, Tay-Sachs disease
Problem pregnancies	Repeated miscarriages, stillbirths
Learning problems	Attention deficit disorder, Down syndrome, Fragile X syndrome

from Table 34–4. Additional signs and symptoms associated with the child's condition may be identified, as well as other problems with no direct relationship to the child's health problem that could potentially impact nursing care or home care. For example, asking about allergies may reveal a latex allergy that requires the use of nonlatex supplies and preparation for allergic reactions. For each problem, obtain the treatment, outcomes, residual problems, and age at time of onset.

Psychosocial Data

Obtain information about family composition to establish a socioeconomic and sociologic context for planning the child's care in the hospital, community, and at home.

- *Family composition*—family members living in the home, their relationship to the child, marital status of parents or other family structure, and people helping to care for the child

- *Financial resources*—household members employed, family income, healthcare resources (e.g., private insurance, Medicaid, Child Health Insurance Program [CHIP]), and other resources (food stamps, Temporary Assistance for Needy Families [TANF], or WIC)

- *Home environment*—housing description (condition, potential lead exposure, safe play area); city or well water; sanitation; and availability of electricity, heat, and refrigeration

- *Community environment*—neighborhood description; safety, playgrounds, transportation, and access to shopping; school or childcare arrangements

- *Family or lifestyle changes*—for example, unemployment, relocations, or divorce; how the child and family members have coped

Newborns.   The psychosocial history for parents of newborns should focus on readiness to care for the newborn at home. Inquire about support for the parent in the initial postpartum period, safe transport, and a home environment that provides heat, refrigeration, and safe water supplies.

Children.   Information about the child's daily routines, psychosocial data, and other living patterns should focus on issues that have an impact on the quality of daily living (Table 34–5).

Adolescents.   The psychosocial history for adolescents should focus on critical areas in their lives that may contribute to a less than optimal environment for normal growth and development. Key topics that should be addressed are included in the HEEADSSS screening tool (Brown, 2011):

- Home environment
- Education and employment
- Eating
- Activities
- Drugs (substance abuse)
- Sexuality
- Suicidal thoughts
- Safety, savagery (exposure to violence)

Developmental Status

Information about the child's motor, cognitive, language, and social development will help to plan nursing care. Ask the parent about the child's milestones and current fine and gross motor skills. Obtain the age at which the child first used words appropriately and the current words used or language ability. Actual assessment of the child with the Denver II Developmental Test or a parent questionnaire may also be used to collect this information. For children in school, ask about academic performance to assess cognitive development. Ask the parent about the child's manner of interaction with other children, family members, and strangers. For adolescents, ask about school performance and activities indicating development of independence and autonomy. (See Chapter 32 🔗 for developmental assessment guidelines.)

Table 34–4	Review of Systems

Body Systems	Examples of Problems to Identify
General	General growth pattern, overall health status, ability to keep up with other children or tires easily with feeding or activity, fever, sleep patterns Allergies, type of reaction (hives, rash, respiratory difficulty, swelling, nausea), seasonal or with each exposure
Skin and lymph	Rashes, dry skin, itching, changes in skin color or texture, new lesions, tendency for bruising, swollen or tender lymph glands
Hair and nails	Hair loss, changes in color or texture, use of dye or chemicals on hair Abnormalities of nail growth or color
Head	Headaches, concern about size of head
Eyes	Vision problems, squinting, crossed eyes, lazy eye, wears glasses; eye infections, redness, tearing, burning, rubbing, swelling eyelids
Ears	Ear infections, frequent discharge from ears, or tubes in ears Hearing loss (no response to loud noises or questions, inattentiveness, date of last hearing test), hearing aids or cochlear implant
Nose and sinuses	Nosebleeds, nasal congestion, colds with runny nose, seasonal symptoms, sinus pain or infections Nasal obstruction, difficulty breathing, snoring at night
Mouth and throat	Mouth breathing, difficulty swallowing, lesions, sore throats, strep infections, mouth odor Tooth eruption, cavities, braces, orthodontic devices Voice change, hoarseness, speech problems
Cardiac and hematologic	Heart murmur, anemia, hypertension, cyanosis, edema, rheumatic fever, chest pain, bruises easily, easily tires with exercise
Chest and respiratory	Trouble breathing, choking episodes, cough, wheezing, cyanosis; exposure to tuberculosis, bronchiolitis, bronchitis, other infections
Gastrointestinal	Bowel movements, frequency, color, consistency, discomfort; constipation or diarrhea; abdominal pain; bleeding from rectum; flatulence Usual appetite; nausea or vomiting
Urinary	Frequency, urgency, dysuria, foul-smelling urine, dribbling, strength of urinary stream, undescended testicles Toilet trained—age when day and night dryness attained, enuresis
Reproductive 　Female 　Male 　Both	For pubescent children Menses onset, amount, duration, frequency, discomfort, problems; vaginal discharge, breast development Puberty onset, emissions, erections, pain or discharge from penis, swelling or pain in testicles Sexual activity, use of contraception, sexually transmitted infections
Musculoskeletal	Weakness, clumsiness, poor coordination, balance, tremors, abnormal gait, painful muscles or joints, swelling or redness of joints, fractures
Neurologic	Seizures, fainting spells, dizziness, numbness, brain injury or concussion; problems with articulation Memory or learning problems, attention span, hyperactivity

Developmental Approach to the Examination

The sequence and approach to the examination vary by age, but the techniques are the same for all ages (Table 34–6). Provide a comfortable atmosphere for the examination with privacy so that modesty is respected. Explain the procedures as you begin to perform them. In young children, a foot-to-head sequence is often used so that the least distressing parts of the examination are completed first. In older cooperative children, the head-to-toe approach is generally used. Experienced examiners often vary the sequence, such as by auscultating the lungs, heart, and abdomen when an infant or toddler is asleep or quiet.

Newborns and Infants Under 6 Months of Age

Infants are among the easiest children to examine, as they do not resist the examination procedure. Keep the parent present to provide comfort and security for the infant during the examination by feeding, using a pacifier, cuddling, or changing the diaper to keep the infant calm and quiet. Distraction such as rocking or clicking noises may help when the infant begins to get distressed.

Table 34–5	Daily Living Patterns
Role relationships	■ Family relationships/alterations in family process ■ Social and peer relationships and inter-actions, child care, preschool, school, clubs, sports groups
Self-perception/self-concept	■ Personal identity and role identity ■ Self-esteem, body image, presence of nonvisible disorder such as a brain injury
Coping/stress tolerance	■ Temperament, coping behaviors ■ Discipline methods used ■ Any substance abuse
Values and beliefs	■ Part of a spiritual group or faith community ■ Any foods, drinks, or medical interven-tions prohibited according to spiritual beliefs, special food preparation ■ Personal values/beliefs
Home care provided for child's condition	■ Resources needed/available, respite care available ■ Knowledge and skills of parents, other family members
Sensory/perceptual problems	■ Adaptations to daily living for any sensory loss (vision, hearing, cognitive, or motor)

Table 34–6	Examination Techniques
Technique	**Description**
Inspection	Purposeful observation of the child's physical features and behaviors during the entire physical examination. Physical feature characteristics include size, shape, color, movement, position, and location. Adequate lighting is essential. Detection of odors is also a part of the inspection.
Palpation	Use of touch to identify characteristics of the skin, internal organs, and masses. Characteristics include texture, moistness, tenderness, tempera-ture, position, shape, consistency, and mobility of masses and organs. The palmar surface of the fingers and the fingertip pads are used for deter-mining position, size, consistency, and masses. The ulnar surface of the hand is best for detect-ing vibrations.
Auscultation	Listening to sounds produced by the airway, lungs, stomach, heart, and blood vessels to iden-tify their characteristics. Auscultation is usually performed with a stethoscope to enhance the sounds heard in the chest and abdomen. Speech is also assessed during auscultation.
Percussion	Striking the surface of the body, either directly or indirectly, to set up vibrations that reveal the den-sity of underlying tissues and borders of internal organs in the chest and abdomen. As the density of the tissue increases, the percussion tone becomes quieter. The tone over air is the loudest, and the tone over solid areas is soft.

Note: Standard precautions are used during the physical examination. Perform good hand hygiene before contact with the child and wear gloves for any contact with mucous membranes and body fluids.

Observe the infant for general level of activity, overall mood, and responsiveness to handling.

Be flexible with the sequence of the examination, taking advantage of times when the infant is quiet or asleep to auscul-tate lung, heart, and abdominal sounds. If the infant continues to be quiet or can be quieted with a pacifier, palpate the abdomen while the muscles are relaxed. The remainder of the examination can proceed in a head-to-toe sequence. Portions of the examina-tion that may disturb the infant, such as the examination of the hips, should be performed last.

Infants over 6 Months of Age

Because of developing separation and stranger anxiety, it is often best to examine the infant and toddler on the parent's lap and then held against the parent's chest for some steps, such as the ear examination (Figure 34–1 ●). The infant will not object to having clothing removed, but make sure the room is warm for the infant's comfort. Observe the infant's general level of activity, mood, and responsiveness to handling by the parent.

Smile and talk soothingly to the infant during the proce-dure. Use toys to distract the older infant. Use a pacifier or bottle to quiet the child when necessary. Because the infant may be fearful of being touched by a stranger, begin with the feet and hands before moving to the trunk. However, take advantage of opportunities to listen to heart, lung, and abdominal sounds when the infant is sleeping or quiet.

● **Figure 34–1** Facilitating physical examination cooperation. Infants and toddlers are often fearful of separation from the parent. With the legs of the nurse and mother put together knee-to-knee, this infant has a surface to lie on that facilitates the abdominal examination.

Toddlers

Toddlers may be active, curious, shy, cautious, or slow to warm up. Because of stranger anxiety, keep toddlers with their parents, often examining them on the parent's lap. For invasive procedures (ear and mouth exam) the parent can hold the child close to the chest with legs between the parent's legs. Attempt to reduce the child's anxiety by demonstrating the use of instruments on the parent or security object. The cranial nerve assessment or developmental assessment can be used as a method to gain cooperation for other procedures.

Avoid asking the child if you can perform a part of the examination as the typical response will be "no." Rather, tell the child what you will do at each step of the examination, using a confident voice that expects cooperation. When a choice is possible, let the child have some control. For example, let the toddler choose which ear to examine first or to stand or sit for a certain part of the examination. Much of the neurologic and musculoskeletal assessment is performed by observing the child play and walk around in the examining room. Begin the examination by touching the feet and then moving gradually toward the body and head. Use instruments to examine the ears, eyes, and mouth last as they often cause anxiety.

Preschoolers

Assess the willingness of the child to be separated from the parent. Younger children may prefer to be examined on the parent's lap, while older children will be comfortable on the examining table. Most children are willing to undress, but leave the underpants on until conducting the genital examination. Most preschoolers are cooperative during the physical examination. Some children will prefer to have the head, eyes, ears, and mouth examined first while others will prefer to postpone them to the end.

Allow the child to touch and play with the equipment. Give simple explanations about the assessment procedures, and offer choice when there is one during the examination. Use distraction to gain cooperation during the examination, such as asking the child to count, name colors, or talk about a favorite activity. Give positive feedback when the child cooperates.

School-Age Children

School-age children willingly cooperate and want to be helpful during the examination, so have them sit on the examining table. Anticipate the development of modesty in school-age children and offer a patient gown to cover the underwear. Let the older school-age child determine if the examination will be conducted in privacy or with the parent or siblings present.

A head-to-toe sequence can be used in this age group. Demonstrate how the instruments are used and let the child handle them if they wish. During the examination, explain what you are doing and why. Offer as many choices as possible to help the child feel empowered. The examination is a good opportunity to teach the child about how the body works, such as letting the child listen to heart and breath sounds.

Adolescents

Protect the adolescent's modesty by providing a private place to undress and put on the patient gown, and then during the examination by covering the parts of the body not being assessed. Examine the adolescent in the head-to-toe sequence as used for adults. Perform the examination in private without parent or siblings unless the adolescent specifically requests the parent's presence. Provide a chaperone (preferably the same sex as the patient) during the examination when the parent or accompanying adult is not present.

Adolescents often have a lot of concerns regarding their developing bodies. When appropriate, provide reassurance about the normal progression of secondary sexual characteristic development and what further changes to expect.

GENERAL APPRAISAL

The examination begins upon first meeting the child (Figure 34–2 ●). Observe the child's general appearance and behavior. The child should appear well nourished and well developed. Infants and young children are often fearful and seek reassurance from their parents. Is the child encouraged to speak? Is the child appropriately reassured or supported by the parent? The child should feel secure with the parent and perceive permission to interact with the nurse.

Measure the infant's weight, length, and head circumference. (See Skills 9–1 through 9–5 in the *Clinical Skills Manual* SKILLS .) After the child is 2 years of age and can stand, measure the child's height rather than length. Accurate measurement is important as medication dosages and fluids are based on weight. Growth measurements are then plotted on growth charts throughout childhood to assure health or to identify the impact of disease on the child. (See the growth charts for all ages of boys and girls in Appendix C ● .) See www.nursing.pearsonhighered.com for links to special growth curves for children with Down syndrome, Turner syndrome, and children adopted from other countries.

● **Figure 34–2** Examination of the child begins from the first contact. Observe the behavior of the child and the tone the parent uses when talking with the child. Does the child appear well nourished? Does the child appear secure with the parent?

Once the weight and height of children have been measured, calculate the body mass index (BMI) (see Chapter 33 🔗). The BMI is a formula used to assess total body fat and nutritional status. For children it helps determine if their height and weight are proportional for their age. Visit the Centers for Disease Control and Prevention website and enter the child's height and weight for an automatic calculation of the BMI. A BMI for age under the 5th percentile indicates the child is underweight. The child is at risk for overweight when the BMI for age is greater than the 85th percentile, and the child is overweight when the BMI is greater than the 95th percentile.

Take the child's temperature, heart rate, respiratory rate, and blood pressure (see Skills 9–8 through 9–15 in the *Clinical Skills Manual* SKILLS).

ASSESSING SKIN AND HAIR CHARACTERISTICS

Examination of the skin requires good lighting to detect variations in skin color and to identify lesions. Daylight is preferred when available. Rather than inspecting the entire skin surface of the child at one time, examine the skin simultaneously with other body systems as each region of the body is exposed. Follow standard precautions by wearing gloves when palpating mucous membranes, open wounds, and lesions.

Inspection of the Skin

Skin Color

The color of the child's skin usually has an even distribution. Check for color variations—such as increased or decreased pigmentation, pallor, mottling, bruises, erythema, cyanosis, or jaundice—that may be associated with local or generalized conditions. Some variations in skin color are common and normal, such as freckles found in the white population and hyperpigmented patches (Mongolian spots) found on infants with dark skin. (See Chapter 25 🔗 for more information on newborn skin.)

Ecchymosis or bruising is common on the knees, shins, and lower arms as children stumble and fall. Bruises are uncommon in infants under 9 months of age without known medical conditions (Harris, 2010). Bruises found on other parts of the child's body, especially in various stages of healing, should raise a suspicion of child abuse (see Chapter 43 🔗). Bruises go through several skin color changes (red, purple, black, blue, yellow, green, and brown) as the body breaks down hemoglobin and blood cells over several days before returning to normal skin color. Note any tattoos or body piercings.

When a skin color abnormality is suspected, inspect the buccal mucosa and tongue to confirm the color change. This is

---

Developing Cultural Competence
Skin Tone Differences

The palms of the hands and soles of the feet are often lighter than the rest of the skin surface in darker-skinned children. In addition, their lips may appear slightly bluish.

---

important in darker-skinned children because the mucous membranes are usually pink, regardless of skin color. Press the gums lightly for 1 to 2 seconds. Any residual color, such as that seen in jaundice or cyanosis, is more easily detected in blanched skin. Generalized cyanosis is associated with respiratory and cardiac disorders. Jaundice is associated with liver disorders.

Palpation of the Skin

Lightly touch or stroke the skin surface to palpate the skin and to evaluate the following characteristics:

- *Temperature*—normally feels cool to the touch when the wrist or dorsum of the hand is placed against the child's skin. Excessively warm skin may indicate the presence of fever or inflammation, whereas abnormally cool skin may be a sign of shock or cold exposure.

- *Texture*—soft, smooth skin over the entire body. Identify any areas of roughness, thickening, or **induration** (area of extra firmness with a distinct border). Abnormalities in texture are associated with endocrine disorders, chronic irritation, and inflammation.

- *Moistness*—normally dry to the touch, but may feel slightly damp when the child has been exercising or crying. Excessive sweating without exertion is associated with a fever or with an uncorrected congenital heart defect.

- *Resilience*—taut, elastic, and mobile because of the balanced distribution of intracellular and extracellular fluids. To evaluate skin turgor, pinch a small amount of skin on the abdomen between the thumb and forefinger, release the skin, and watch the speed of recoil (Figure 34–3 ●). Skin with good turgor rapidly returns to its previous contour. Skin with poor turgor tents or takes longer to resume its original contour. Poor skin turgor is commonly associated with dehydration.

If **edema**, an accumulation of excess fluid in the interstitial spaces, is present, the skin feels doughy or boggy. To test for the degree of edema present, press for 5 seconds against a bone beneath the area of puffy skin, release the pressure, and observe how rapidly the indentation disappears. If the indentation

● **Figure 34–3** Tenting of the skin is associated with poor skin turgor. Assess skin turgor on the abdomen, forearm, or thigh. Skin with normal turgor will return to a flat position quickly.

disappears rapidly, the edema is "nonpitting." Slow disappearance of the indentation indicates "pitting" edema, which is commonly associated with kidney or heart disorders.

Capillary Refill Time

One technique to evaluate the adequacy of tissue *perfusion* (oxygen circulating to the tissues) is the capillary refill time (Figures 34–4*A* and *B* •). The capillary refill time is normally less than 2 seconds. When the time is prolonged, assess the child for dehydration, hypovolemic shock, or a physical constriction such as a cast or bandage that is too tight.

Skin Lesions

Skin lesions usually indicate an abnormal skin condition. Characteristics such as location, size, type of lesion, pattern, and discharge, if present, provide clues about the cause of the condition. Inspect and palpate the isolated or generalized skin color abnormalities, elevations, lesions, or injuries to describe all characteristics present.

Primary lesions (such as macules, papules, and vesicles) are often the skin's initial response to injury or infection. Hyperpigmented patches (Mongolian spots) and freckles are normal findings also classified as primary lesions. The illustrations in

A

B

• **Figure 34–4** Capillary refill technique. *A,* Press against the palmar tip of a finger, toe, or over a bony surface (e.g., jaw) for 2 to 3 seconds until the skin is blanched. *B,* Quickly release the pressure and count the number of seconds it takes for the color or blood to return to the veins. A capillary refill time of greater than 2 seconds could be related to dehydration, shock, or constriction around a limb such as a tight bandage or cast.

Pathophysiology Illustrated on page 890 describe common primary lesions. Secondary lesions (such as scars, ulcers, and fissures) are the result of irritation, infection, and delayed healing of primary lesions (see Table 58–1, *Common Secondary Skin Lesions and Associated Conditions*, in Chapter 58 ●).

Primary lesions often appear in common patterns that help distinguish between lesions.

- *Annular*—circular, begins in center and spreads to periphery (e.g., ringworm); when annular lesions run together they are polycyclic
- *Linear*—in a row or stripe (e.g., poison ivy)
- *Herpetiform*—grouped or clustered (e.g., herpes, chicken pox)
- *Reticulated*—networked or lace-like (e.g., parvovirus B19)

Inspection of the Hair

Inspect the scalp hair for color, distribution, and cleanliness. The hair shafts should be evenly colored, shiny, and either curly or straight. Variation in hair color not caused by bleaching or coloring may be associated with a nutritional deficiency. Normally, hair is distributed evenly over the scalp. Investigate areas of hair loss. Hair loss in a child may result from tight braids or skin lesions such as ringworm. (See Chapter 58 ● for information about fungal infections.) Notice any unusual hair growth patterns. An unusually low hairline on the neck or forehead may be associated with a congenital disorder such as hypothyroidism.

Children are frequently exposed to head lice. Inspect the individual hair shafts for small nits (lice eggs) that adhere to the hair (see Chapter 58 ●). None should be present.

Observe the distribution of body hair as other skin surfaces are exposed during examination. Fine hair covers most areas of the body. Body hair in unexpected places should be noted. For example, a tuft of hair at the base of the spine often indicates a spinal defect.

Note the age at which pubic and axillary hair develops in the child. Pubic hair begins to develop in children between 8 and 12 years of age, and axillary hair develops about 6 months later. (See Figures 34–29 and 34–30 later in this chapter.) Facial hair is noted in boys shortly after axillary hair develops. Development at an unusually young age is associated with precocious puberty.

Palpation of the Hair

Palpate the hair shafts for texture. Hair should feel soft or silky with fine or thick shafts. Endocrine conditions such as hypothyroidism may result in coarse, brittle hair. Part the hair in various spots over the head to inspect and palpate the scalp for crusting or other lesions. If lesions are present, describe them using the characteristics presented in *Pathophysiology Illustrated*.

> ### Developing Cultural Competence
> #### Hair Characteristics
>
> Hair varies by genetic origin. Children of African origin often have hair that can appear curly, wavy, or coiled, and this hair breaks easily. Children of Asian origin have hair that is coarse and straight. Children of Caucasian origin have hair with fine to medium coarseness that is straight or wavy.

Pathophysiology Illustrated | Common Primary Skin Lesions and Associated Conditions

Lesion name: Macule
Description: Flat, nonpalpable, diameter less than 1 cm (½ in.)
Example: Freckle, rubella, rubeola, petechiae

Lesion name: Patch
Description: Macule, diameter greater than 1 cm (½ in.)
Example: Vitiligo, Mongolian spot

Lesion name: Papule
Description: Elevated, firm, diameter less than 1 cm (½ in.)
Example: Warts, pigmented nevi

Lesion name: Nodule
Description: Elevated, firm, deeper in dermis than papule, diameter 1–2 cm (½–1 in.)
Example: Erythema nodosum

Lesion name: Tumor
Description: Elevated, solid, diameter greater than 2 cm (1 in.)
Example: Neoplasm, hemangioma

Lesion name: Vesicle
Description: Elevated, filled with fluid, diameter less than 1 cm (½ in.)
Example: Early chicken pox, herpes simplex

Lesion name: Pustule
Description: Vesicle filled with purulent fluid
Example: Impetigo, acne

Lesion name: Bulla
Description: Vesicle diameter greater than 1 cm (½ in.)
Example: Burn blister

Lesion name: Wheal
Description: Irregular elevated solid area of edematous skin
Example: Urticaria, insect bite

ASSESSING THE HEAD FOR SKULL CHARACTERISTICS AND FACIAL FEATURES

Inspection of the Head and Face

During early childhood the skull's sutures expand to allow for brain growth. Infants and young children normally have a rounded skull with a prominent occipital area. The shape of the head changes during childhood, and the occipital area becomes less prominent. An abnormal skull shape can result from premature closure of the sutures.

The head circumference of infants and young children is routinely measured until 2 to 3 years of age to ensure that adequate growth for brain development has occurred. The *Clinical Skills Manual* SKILLS describes the proper technique (see Skill 9–5). A larger-than-normal head is associated with hydrocephalus, and a smaller-than-normal head suggests microcephaly.

Inspect the child's face for symmetry when the child is resting, smiling, talking, and crying (Figure 34–5 ●). Significant asymmetry may result from paralysis of trigeminal or facial nerves (cranial nerves V or VII), in utero positioning, and swelling from infection, allergy, or trauma.

Next inspect the face for unusual facial features such as coarseness, wide eye spacing, or disproportionate size. Tremors, tics, and twitching of facial muscles are often associated with seizures.

Palpation of the Skull

Palpate the skull in infants and young children to assess the sutures and fontanelles and to detect soft bones (see *As Children Grow: Sutures*).

Sutures

Use your fingerpads to palpate each suture line. The edge of each bone in the suture line can be felt, but normally there is no separation of the two bones. If additional bone edges are felt, a skull fracture may be present.

Fontanelles

At the intersection of the sutures, palpate the anterior and posterior fontanelles. The fontanelle should feel flat and firm inside the bony edges. The anterior fontanelle is normally smaller than 5 cm (2 in.) in diameter at 6 months of age and then becomes progressively smaller. It closes between 12 and 18 months of age. The posterior fontanelle closes between 2 and 3 months of age.

● **Figure 34–5** Inspecting for facial symmetry. Draw an imaginary line down the middle of the face over the nose and compare the features on each side. Significant asymmetry may be caused by paralysis of cranial nerve V or VII, in utero positioning, or swelling from infection, allergy, or trauma.

As Children Grow | Sutures

The sutures are fibrous connections between bones of the skull that have not yet ossified. The fontanelles are formed at the intersection of these sutures where bone has not yet formed. Fontanelles are covered by tough membranous tissue that protects the brain. The posterior fontanelle closes between 2 and 3 months. The anterior fontanelle and sutures are palpable up to the age of 18 months. The suture lines of the skull are seldom palpated after 2 years of age. After that time the sutures rarely separate.

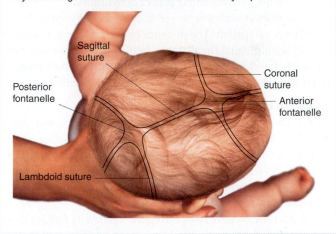

A tense fontanelle, bulging above the margin of the skull when the child is sitting, is an indication of increased intracranial pressure. A soft fontanelle, sunken below the margin of the skull, is associated with dehydration.

ASSESSING EYE STRUCTURES, FUNCTION, AND VISION

Equipment needed for this examination includes an ophthalmoscope, vision chart, penlight, small toy, and an index card or paper cup.

Inspection of the External Eye Structures

Inspect the external eye structures, including the eyeballs, eyelids, and eye muscles. Test the function of cranial nerves II, III, IV, and VI, which innervate the eye structures.

Eye Size and Spacing

Inspect the eyes and surrounding tissues simultaneously when examining facial features (Figure 34–6 ●). The eyes should be the same size but not unusually large or small. Observe for eye

Animation 3D Eye

● **Figure 34–6** External structures of the eye. Notice that the light reflex is at the same location on each eye.

● **Figure 34–7** Inspecting for palpebral slant. Draw an imaginary line across the medial canthi and extend it to each side of the face to identify the slant of the palpebral fissures. When the line crosses the lateral canthi, the palpebral fissures are horizontal and no slant is present. When the lateral canthi fall above the imaginary line, the eyes have an upward slant. A downward slant is present when the lateral canthi fall below the imaginary line. Look at Figures 34–6, 34–8, and 34–11. Which type of eye slant do these children have? Are epicanthal folds present?

bulging, which can be identified by retracted eyelids, or for a sunken appearance. Bulging may be associated with a tumor, and a sunken appearance may reflect dehydration.

Next inspect the eyes to see if they are appropriately distanced from each other. The distance between the inner canthi of the eyes should equal the distance between the inner and outer canthi of the child's eye (Hummel, 2011). **Hypertelorism**, or widely spaced eyes, can be a normal variation in children.

Eyelids and Eyelashes

Inspect the eyelids for color, size, position, mobility, and condition of the eyelashes. Eyelids should be the same color as surrounding facial skin and free of swelling or inflammation along the edges. Sebaceous glands that look like yellow striations are often present near the hair follicles. Eyelashes curl away from the eye to prevent irritation of the conjunctivae.

Inspect the conjunctivae lining the eyelids by pulling down the lower lid and then everting the upper lid. The conjunctivae should be pink and glossy. No redness or excess tearing should be present.

When the eyes are open, inspect the level at which the upper and lower lids cross the eye. Each lid normally covers part of the iris but not any portion of the pupil. The lids should also close completely over the iris and cornea. *Ptosis,* drooping of the lid over the pupil, is often associated with injury to the oculomotor nerve, cranial nerve III. *Sunset sign,* in which the sclera is seen between the upper lid and the iris, may indicate retracted eyelids or hydrocephalus.

Inspect the eyes for the palpebral slant (Figure 34–7 ●). The eyelids of most people open horizontally. An upward slant is a normal finding in Asian children; however, children with Down syndrome also often have an upward slant (Figure 34–8 ●). A downward slant is seen in some children as a normal variation. Children of Asian descent often have an extra fold of skin, known as the **epicanthal fold**, covering all or part of the lacrimal caruncle of the medial canthus of the eye.

Eye Color

Inspect the color of each sclera, iris, and bulbar conjunctiva. The sclera is normally white or ivory in darker-skinned children. Sclerae of another color suggest the presence of an underlying

● **Figure 34–8** The eyes of this boy with Down syndrome show an upward slant.

disease. For example, yellow sclerae indicate jaundice. Typically the iris is blue or light colored at birth and becomes pigmented within 6 months. Rarely the irises are different colors due to autosomal dominant inheritance (Tuli, Kockler, Kelly, et al., 2010). Inspect the iris for the presence of *Brushfield spots,* white specks in a linear pattern around the iris circumference, which are often associated with Down syndrome. The bulbar conjunctivae, which cover the sclera to the edge of the cornea, are normally clear. Redness can indicate eyestrain, allergies, or irritation.

Pupils

Inspect the size and shape of the pupils. Normally the pupils are round, clear, and equal in size. Some children have a **coloboma**, a keyhole-shaped pupil caused by a notch in the iris. This sign can indicate that the child has other congenital anomalies.

To test the pupillary response to light, shine a bright light into one eye. A brisk constriction of both the pupil exposed to direct light and the other pupil (consensual response) is a normal finding.

To test pupillary response to accommodation, ask the child to look first at a near object (e.g., a toy) and then at a distant object (e.g., a picture on the wall). The expected response is pupil constriction with near objects and pupil dilation with distant objects. These procedures test cranial nerve II.

Assessment of the Eye Muscles

It is important to detect *strabismus*, a muscle imbalance that makes the eyes look crossed, which can cause vision impairment if uncorrected. Use the following procedures to detect a muscle imbalance:

- *Extraocular movements.* Seat the child at eye level to evaluate the extraocular movements. Hold a toy or penlight 30 cm (12 in.) from the child's eyes and move it through the six cardinal fields of gaze. Make sure the child's eyes move rather than the head. Both eyes should move together, tracking the object. This procedure tests the oculomotor, trochlear, and abducens nerves (cranial nerves III, IV, and VI, respectively) (Figure 34–9 ●).

- *Corneal light reflex.* To test the corneal light reflex, shine a light on the child's nose, midway between the eyes. Identify the location where the light is reflected on the cornea of each eye.

● **Figure 34–9** Assessing extraocular movements. Have the child sit at your eye level. Hold a toy or penlight about 30 cm (12 in.) from the child's eyes and move it through the six cardinal fields of gaze. Both eyes should move together, tracking the object. This procedure tests cranial nerves III, IV, and VI.

The light reflection is normally symmetric, at the same spot on each cornea (see Figure 34–6). An asymmetric corneal light reflex after 6 months of age indicates a muscle imbalance.

- *Cover–uncover test.* This test can be used only for older, cooperative children, starting at about 5 years of age. See Figure 34–10 ● for the technique. Perform the procedure for both eyes. Because the eyes work together, no obvious movement of either eye is expected. Eye movement indicates a muscle imbalance.

A Right, uncovered eye is weaker.

B Left, covered eye is weaker.

● **Figure 34–10** Cover–uncover test. With the child at your eye level, ask the child to look at a picture on the wall. *A,* Cover one eye with an index card or paper cup and simultaneously watch for any movement of the uncovered eye. If the uncovered eye jumps to fixate on the picture, it has a muscle weakness. *B,* Remove the cover from the eye and simultaneously watch the eye that was covered for any movement to fixate on the picture. If the eye has a muscle weakness, it drifts to a relaxed position once covered.

Animation   Otoscope Examination

Vision Assessment

Because vision is such an important sense for learning, assessment is essential to detect any serious problems. Vision is evaluated using an age-appropriate vision test, but no simple method exists. Photo screening or an autorefractor may be used to assess vision in some preschool and school-age children. See Skill 9–18 in the *Clinical Skills Manual* SKILLS .

Infants and Toddlers

When the infant's eyes are open, test the blink reflex by moving your hand quickly toward the infant's eyes. A quick blink is the normal response. An absent blink reflex can indicate that the infant is blind.

To test an infant's ability to visually track an object, hold a light or toy about 15 cm (6 in.) from the infant's eyes. When the infant has fixated on or is staring at the object, move it slowly to each side. The infant should follow the object with the eyes and by moving the head. Once an infant has developed skills to reach for and then pick up objects, observe play behavior to evaluate vision. Children under 3 years of age should be able to easily find and pick up small pieces of food.

Standardized Vision Charts

Standardized vision charts can be used to test vision when the child can understand directions and cooperate, usually at about 3 or 4 years of age. The HOTV, Snellen E, and Picture charts are used to test visual acuity of preschool-age children just as the Snellen Letter chart is used for school-age children and adolescents. For all screening tools used to test far vision, make sure the child is the appropriate distance from the chart, usually 10 or 20 feet. Cover one eye so each eye is evaluated separately before testing them together. See Skills 9–16 and 9–17 in the *Clinical Skills Manual* SKILLS for the use of these charts.

Inspection of the Internal Eye Structures

The funduscopic examination with an ophthalmoscope allows the structures of the internal eye—the retina, optic disc, arteries and veins, and macula—to be examined. This examination is most often performed by experienced examiners. To assist the examiner, darken the room so the child's pupils dilate. Encourage cooperation by explaining the procedure to the child. Have a picture on the wall or have the parent or assistant hold a toy for the child to stare at so that the child's eye will remain open.

Red Reflex

A penlight or the light of an ophthalmoscope can be used to assess the **red reflex**, the orange-red glow of the vascular retina as the light travels through the cornea, aqueous humor, lens, and vitreous humor to the retina. Shine the light at both eyes from a distance of 45 cm (18 in.). The red reflexes should be an orange-red glow that is symmetric and uniform in shape and color. Black spots or opacities within the red reflex are abnormal and may indicate congenital cataracts, hemorrhage, or corneal scars. A white reflex is associated with a tumor or retinoblastoma (see Chapter 46 🔗).

ASSESSING THE EAR STRUCTURES AND HEARING

Equipment needed for this examination includes an otoscope, noisemakers (bell, rattle, tissue paper), and a 500- to 1000-Hz tuning fork.

Inspection of the External Ear Structures

The position and characteristics of the *pinna*, the external ear, are inspected as a continuation of the head and eye examination. See Figure 34–11 ● to determine if the pinna is considered "low set," which is often associated with congenital renal disorders.

Inspect the pinna for any malformation. The pinna should be completely formed, with an open auditory canal. Next, inspect

> ### ⬤ Clinical Tip
>
> Criteria for referral for further vision evaluation include:
>
> - Ages 3 to 12 months—failure to fix on an object and follow
> - Ages 3 and 4 years—20/50 or less in either eye
> - Age 5 years—20/40 or less in either eye
> - Age 6 years—20/30 or less in either eye
> - A difference in vision between the eyes of two lines or more on the Snellen eye chart, for example, 20/20 in one eye and 20/40 in the other eye, even when one eye is within the expected range
> - Any problems with ocular alignment
> - Any other indication of vision impairment, regardless of acuity
>
> Data from American Academy of Ophthalmology, Pediatric Ophthalmology/Strabismus Panel. (2007). *Preferred Practice Pattern® Guidelines. Pediatric eye evaluations*. San Francisco, CA: Author. Retrieved from http://one.aao.org/ce/practiceguidelines/ppp_content.aspx?cid=621682dc-7871-4351-830e-545b1273d84c.

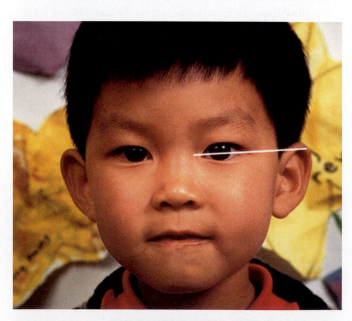

● **Figure 34–11** To evaluate the placement of the external ears, draw an imaginary line through the medial and lateral canthi of the eye toward the ear. This line normally passes through the upper portion of the pinna. The pinna is considered "low set" when the top lies completely below the imaginary line. Low-set ears are often associated with renal disorders.

the tissue around the pinna for abnormalities. A pit or hole in front of the auditory canal may indicate the presence of a sinus. If the one pinna protrudes outward, there may be swelling behind the ear, a sign of infection in the mastoid process of the temporal bone of the skull.

Inspect the external auditory canal for any discharge. A foul-smelling, purulent discharge may indicate the presence of a foreign body or an infection in the external canal. Clear fluid or a blood-tinged discharge may indicate a cerebrospinal fluid leak associated with a basilar skull fracture.

Inspection of the Tympanic Membrane

Examination of the tympanic membrane is important in infants and young children because they are prone to otitis media, a middle ear infection. To examine the auditory canal and tympanic membrane, use an otoscope, an instrument with a magnifying lens, bright light, and speculum. Choose the largest ear speculum that fits into the auditory canal to form a seal for testing the movement of the tympanic membrane and to reduce the risk for injury to the auditory canal if the child moves suddenly.

Toddlers and young children often resist having their ears inspected with the otoscope because of past painful experiences, so postpone this until the end of the assessment for this age group. Use simple explanations to prepare the child. Let the child play with the otoscope or demonstrate how it is used on the parent or a doll. Figure 34–12 ● illustrates one method of human restraint for an uncooperative toddler or preschool child. See also Skill 7–3 in the *Clinical Skills Manual* SKILLS .

To begin using the otoscope, hold the handle in the palm of the hand closest to the child's face. If using a pneumatic squeeze

● **Figure 34–13** To straighten the auditory canal, pull the pinna back and up for children over 3 years of age. Pull the pinna down and back for children under 3 years of age.

bulb, hold it between the index finger and the handle. When the child is cooperative, rest the back of the hand holding the otoscope against the child's head to stabilize it. The other hand is used to pull the pinna back and either up or down, whichever position straightens the auditory canal and provides the best view of the tympanic membrane (Figure 34–13 ●).

Slowly insert the speculum into the auditory canal, inspecting the walls for signs of irritation, discharge, or a foreign body. The walls of the auditory canal are normally pink, and some cerumen is present. Children often put beads, peas, or other small objects into their ears. If the auditory canal is obstructed by cerumen or a foreign body, warm water irrigation can be used to clean the canal.

SAFETY ALERT!
Never irrigate the ear canal if any discharge is present in the auditory canal, as the tympanic membrane may be ruptured. Water could enter the middle ear and potentially worsen the infection.

The tympanic membrane, which separates the outer ear from the middle ear, is usually pearly gray and translucent. It reflects light, and the bones (ossicles) in the middle ear are normally visible (Figure 34–14 ●). When the auditory canal is sealed and the pneumatic attachment is squeezed and released, the tympanic membrane normally moves in and out in response to the positive and negative pressure applied. Table 34–7 lists the abnormal findings during examination of the tympanic membranes. See Figures 46–4 and 46–5 🖉 for the tympanic membrane appearance when acute otitis media and otitis media with effusion are present.

Hearing Assessment

Hearing evaluation is important in children of all ages because hearing is essential for normal speech development and learning. Hearing loss may occur at any time during early childhood as the result of birth trauma, frequent otitis media, meningitis, or antibiotics that damage cranial nerve VIII. Hearing loss may also be associated with congenital anomalies and genetic syndromes.

● **Figure 34–12** Inspecting the tympanic membrane. To restrain an uncooperative child, place the child on the parent's lap with the child's head and chest held firmly against the parent's chest. Keep your hands free to hold the otoscope and position the external ear.

External
auditory canal

Pinna (auricle)

Malleus

Handle
of malleus

Incus

Normal tympanic membrane

Handle
of malleus

Umbo

Semicircular canals

Facial and
vestibulocochlear
nerves

Cochlea

Oval window

Round window

Eustachian tube

Tympanic
membrane

Umbo

Stapes
and foot plate

● **Figure 34–14** The tympanic membrane normally has a triangular light reflex with the base on the nasal side pointing toward the center. The bony landmarks, the umbo and handle of malleus, are seen through the tympanic membrane.

The hearing of newborns is evaluated at birth, and hearing is evaluated throughout childhood.

Evaluate hearing by observing the child's responses to various auditory stimuli using age-appropriate methods. Use hearing and speech articulation milestones as an initial hearing screen. When a hearing deficiency is suspected as a result of screening, refer the child for audiometry or tympanometry. *Audiometry* is a screening procedure using air conduction that measures hearing for pure-tone frequencies and loudness. The high- and low-pitch sounds are presented through earphones and are used to test different sound frequencies and the loudness needed to hear each sound. Hearing loss is determined when the child needs

higher-than-normal decibels (louder sound) to hear a tone. *Tympanometry* is a test to estimate the pressure in the middle ear, and it is an indirect measure of tympanic membrane movement. See Skills 9–19 and 9–20 in the *Clinical Skills Manual* SKILLS .

Infants and Toddlers

Select noisemakers with different frequencies that will attract the child's attention, such as a rattle, bell, and tissue paper. Ask the parent or an assistant to entertain the infant with a quiet toy, such as a teddy bear. Stand behind the infant, about 60 cm (2 feet) away from the infant's ear but outside the infant's field of vision, and make a soft sound with the noisemaker. Have the parent or

Table 34–7	Unexpected Findings on Examination of the Tympanic Membrane and Their Associated Conditions	
Characteristics	**Tympanic Membrane Unexpected Findings**	**Associated Conditions**
Color	Redness	Infection in middle ear
	Slight redness	Prolonged crying
	Amber	Serous fluid in middle ear
	Deep red or blue	Blood in middle ear
Light reflex	Absent	Bulging tympanic membrane, infection in middle ear
	Distorted, loss of triangular shape	Retracted tympanic membrane, serous fluid in middle ear
Bony landmarks	Extra prominent	Retracted tympanic membrane, serous fluid in middle ear
Movement	No movement	Infection or fluid in middle ear
	Excessive movement	Healed perforation

Growth and Development   Indicators of Hearing Loss

Infant:
- No startle reaction to loud noises.
- Does not turn toward sounds by 4 months of age.
- Babbles as a young infant but does not keep babbling or develop speech sounds after 6 months of age.

Young child:
- No speech by 2 years of age.
- Inability to follow age-appropriate directions, such as "Bring me the block."
- Speech sounds are not distinct at appropriate ages.

assistant observe the child for any of the following responses when the noisemaker is used: widening the eyes, briefly stopping all activity to listen, or turning the head toward the sound. Repeat the test in the other ear and with the other noisemakers.

Preschool and Older Children

Use whispered words to evaluate the hearing of children over 3 years of age. Position your head about 30 cm (12 in.) away from the child's ear, but out of the range of vision so the child cannot read your lips. Use words easily recognized by the child, such as *Mickey Mouse*, *hot dog*, and *Popsicle*, and ask the child to repeat the words. Repeat the test with different words in the opposite ear. The child should correctly repeat the whispered words. If the child will not repeat the whispered words, use a whisper to ask the child to point to different body parts or objects. Remember to stay out of the child's line of sight so lip reading is not possible. The child should point to the correct body part each time.

Bone and Air Conduction of Sound

A tuning fork may be used to evaluate the hearing of school-age children who can follow directions. Hold the stem and lightly tap the tines of the tuning fork to begin the vibration. Avoid touching the vibrating tines, which will dampen the sound. Test bone conduction by placing the handle of the tuning fork on the child's skull. Test air conduction by holding the vibrating tines close to the child's ear (Figure 34–15 ●).

- *Weber test:* Place the vibrating tuning fork on top of the child's skull in the midline. Ask the child to say where the sound is heard best, either in both ears equally or in one ear. The sound should be heard equally in both ears. If the

sound is heard better in one ear (lateralized to affected ear), conductive hearing loss may be present.

- *Rinne test:* Place the vibrating tuning fork handle on the mastoid process behind an ear. Ask the child to say when the sound is no longer heard. Immediately move the tuning fork, holding the vibrating tines about 2.5 to 5 cm (1 to 2 in.) from the same ear. Again, ask the child to say when the sound is no longer heard. The child normally hears the air-conducted sound twice as long as the bone-conducted sound. Repeat the Rinne test on the other ear. When the sound is heard longer by bone conduction than air conduction, the affected ear may have conductive hearing loss. When sound is heard longer by air conduction than bone conduction, but less than twice as long, the affected ear may have sensorineural hearing loss.

ASSESSING THE NOSE AND SINUSES FOR AIRWAY PATENCY AND DISCHARGE

An otoscope with a nasal speculum or a penlight is needed for this examination.

Inspection of the External Nose

Examine the external nose characteristics and placement on the face during the assessment of the facial features. Inspect the external nose for size, shape, symmetry, midline placement on the face, and for the presence of unusual characteristics. For example,

A   B   C

● **Figure 34–15** Testing bone and air conduction. *A,* Weber test. Place vibrating tuning fork on midline of the child's head. *B,* Rinne test, step 1. Place vibrating tuning fork on mastoid process. *C,* Rinne test, step 2. Reposition still vibrating tines between 2.5 and 5 cm (1 and 2 in.) from ear.

a crease across the nose between the cartilage and bone is often caused by the allergic child's wiping an itchy nose upward with a hand. **Nasal flaring**, widening of the nares with breathing, is a sign of respiratory distress and should not be present.

The nose should be proportional in size to other facial features, have symmetric nasolabial folds, and be positioned in the middle of the face. Asymmetry of the nasolabial folds may be associated with injury to the facial nerve (cranial nerve VII). A flattened nasal bridge is the expected finding in Asian and black children but may also be seen in children with Down syndrome. A saddle-shaped nose is associated with congenital defects such as cleft palate.

Palpation of the External Nose

When a deformity is noted, gently palpate the nose to detect any pain or break in contour. No tenderness or masses are expected. Pain and a contour deviation are usually the result of trauma.

Nasal Patency

The child's airway must be patent to ensure adequate oxygenation. To test for nasal patency, occlude one nostril and observe the child's effort to breathe through the open nostril with the mouth closed. Repeat on the other nostril. Breathing should be noiseless and effortless.

If the child struggles to breathe, a nasal obstruction may be present. Nasal obstruction may be caused by a foreign body, congenital defect, dry mucus, discharge, polyp, or trauma. Young children commonly place objects up their nose, and unilateral nasal flaring is a sign of such an obstruction.

Assessment of Smell

The olfactory nerve (cranial nerve I) can be tested in school-age children and adolescents, but it is rarely done. When testing smell, choose scents the child will easily recognize such as orange, chocolate, peanut butter, and mint. When the child's eyes are closed, occlude one nostril and hold the scent under the nose. Ask the child to take a deep sniff and identify the scent. Alternate odors between the nares. The child can normally identify common scents.

Inspection of the Internal Nose

Inspect the internal nose for color of the mucous membranes and the presence of any discharge, swelling, lesions, or other abnormalities. Use a bright light, such as an otoscope light or penlight. For infants and young children, push the tip of the nose upward and shine the light at the end of the nose. The nasal speculum of the otoscope can be used in older children (Figure 34–16 ●). Avoid touching the septum of the nose with the speculum to prevent injury.

 Growth and Development

Infants under 6 months of age will not automatically open their mouths to breathe when their nose is occluded, such as by mucus.

● **Figure 34–16** Technique for examining the nose.

Mucous Membranes and Nasal Septum

The mucous membranes should be dark pink and glistening. A film of clear discharge may also be present. Turbinates, if visible, should be the same color as the mucous membranes and have a firm consistency. When the turbinates are pale or bluish gray, the child may have allergies. A polyp, a rounded mass projecting from the turbinate, is also associated with allergies.

The nasal septum should be straight without perforations, bleeding, or crusting. Crusting will be noted over the site of a nosebleed.

Discharge

Observe for the presence of nasal discharge, noting if it is unilateral or bilateral. Nasal discharge is not a normal finding unless the child is crying. Discharge may be watery, mucoid, purulent, or bloody. A foul-smelling discharge in only one nostril is often associated with a foreign body. Table 34–8 lists conditions associated with nasal discharge.

Inspection of the Sinuses

The sinuses are air-filled spaces that develop during childhood. See the illustration in *As Children Grow: Sinus Development.* Inspect the face for any puffiness and swelling around one or

Table 34–8	Nasal Discharge Characteristics and Associated Conditions
Discharge Description	**Associated Condition**
Watery	
Clear, bilateral	Allergy
Serous, unilateral	Spinal fluid from a basilar skull fracture
Mucoid or purulent	
Bilateral	Upper respiratory infection
Unilateral	Foreign body
Bloody	Nosebleed, trauma

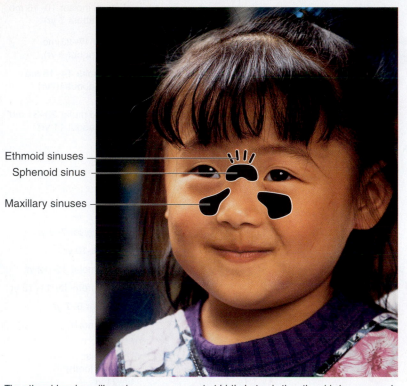

Ethmoid sinuses

Sphenoid sinus

Maxillary sinuses

The ethmoid and maxillary sinuses are present at birth, but only the ethmoid sinuses are air filled at that time. The maxillary sinuses become air filled by 4 years of age. The sphenoid sinuses are present by 5 years of age. The frontal sinuses form at about 7 to 8 years of age but are not completely developed until adolescence (Pappas & Hendly, 2011).

Lips

Inspect the lips for color, shape, symmetry, moisture, and lesions. The lips are normally symmetric without drying, cracking, or other lesions. Lip color is normally pink in white children and more bluish in darker-skinned children. Pale, cyanotic, or cherry-red lips indicate poor tissue perfusion caused by various conditions. Note any clefts or edema.

SAFETY ALERT!

Avoid examining the mouth if there are signs of respiratory distress, high fever, drooling, and intense apprehension. These may be signs of epiglottitis. Inspecting the mouth may trigger a total airway obstruction. (See Table 47–3 in Chapter 47 🕘 for more information.)

Teeth

Inspect and count the child's teeth. The timing of tooth eruption is often genetically determined, but it occurs in a regular sequence. See Figure 34–18 ● for the typical sequence of tooth eruption for both deciduous and permanent teeth.

Inspect the condition of the teeth, look for loose teeth, and note any spaces where teeth are missing. Note any dental care, braces, or orthodontic appliances. Compare empty tooth spaces with the child's developmental stage of tooth eruption. Once the permanent teeth have erupted, none should be missing. Teeth are

both eyes; normally, neither is present. To palpate over the maxillary sinuses, press up under both zygomatic arches with the thumbs. To palpate the ethmoid sinuses, press up against the bone above both eyes with the thumbs. No swelling or tenderness is expected. Tenderness may indicate sinusitis. Sinus infections can occasionally occur in young children.

ASSESSING THE MOUTH AND THROAT FOR COLOR, FUNCTION, AND SIGNS OF ABNORMAL CONDITIONS

Equipment needed to examine the mouth and throat includes a tongue blade and penlight. Wear gloves when examining the mouth.

Inspection of the Mouth

Young children often need coaxing and simple explanations before they will cooperate with the mouth and throat examination. Most children readily show their teeth. If the child resists by clenching the teeth, gently separate them with a tongue blade. Mouth structures for inspection are illustrated in Figure 34–17 ●.

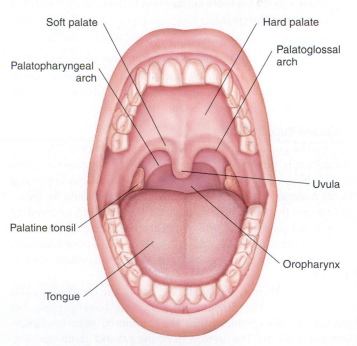

Soft palate

Hard palate

Palatopharyngeal arch

Palatoglossal arch

Uvula

Palatine tonsil

Oropharynx

Tongue

● **Figure 34–17** The structures of the mouth.

● **Figure 34–18** Typical sequence of tooth eruption for both deciduous and permanent teeth. The bottom deciduous teeth are shed before upper teeth, and bottom permanent teeth erupt first as well.

normally white, without a flattened, mottled, or pitted appearance. Discolorations on the crown of a tooth may indicate caries. Discolorations on the tooth surface may be associated with some medications or fluorosis.

Mouth Odors

During inspection of the teeth, be alert to any abnormal odors that may indicate problems such as diabetic ketoacidosis, infection, or poor hygiene. Be alert for alcohol odors in older children that could signal substance abuse.

Gums and Buccal Mucosa

Inspect the gums for color and adherence to the teeth. The gums are normally pink, with a stippled or dotted appearance. Use a tongue blade to help visualize the gums around the upper and lower molars. No raised or receding gum areas should be apparent around the teeth. When inflammation, swelling, or bleeding is observed, palpate the gums to detect tenderness. Inflammation and tenderness are associated with infection and poor nutrition. Hyperplasia may be associated with some medications, such as phenytoin.

Inspect the mucous membrane lining the cheeks for color and moisture. The mucous membrane is usually pink, but patches of hyperpigmentation are commonly seen in darker-skinned children. The *Stensen duct*, the parotid gland opening, is opposite the upper second molar bilaterally. Normally pink,

the duct opening becomes red when the child is infected with mumps. Small pink sucking pads can be present in infants. No areas of redness, swelling, or ulcerative lesions should be present.

Tongue

Inspect the tongue for color, moisture, size, tremors, and lesions. The child's tongue is normally pink and moist, without a coating, and it fits easily into the mouth. A protuberant tongue is associated with various genetic conditions, such as Down syndrome. A pattern of gray, irregular borders that form a design (geographic tongue) is often normal, but it may be associated with fever, allergies, or drug reactions. Tremors are abnormal. A white adherent coating on an infant's tongue may be caused by thrush, a *Candida* infection (see Chapter 58 ❷).

Observe the mobility of the tongue by asking the child to touch the gums above the upper teeth with the tongue. This tongue movement is adequate to enunciate all speech sounds clearly. Ask the child to stick out the tongue and lift it so the underside of the tongue and the floor of the mouth can be inspected.

Palate

Inspect the hard and soft palate to detect any clefts or masses or an unusually high arch. The palate is normally pink, dome shaped, and has no cleft. The uvula hangs freely from the soft palate. A high-arched palate can be associated with sucking difficulties in young infants.

Palpation of the Mouth Structures

Using gloves, palpate any masses seen in the mouth to determine their characteristics, such as size, shape, firmness, and tenderness. No masses should be found.

To assess the tongue's strength, while simultaneously testing the hypoglossal nerve (cranial nerve XII), place your index finger against the child's cheek and ask the child to push against your finger with the tongue. Some pressure against the finger is normally felt.

To palpate the palate, insert your gloved little finger, with the fingerpad upward, into the mouth. While the infant sucks against your finger, palpate the entire palate. This procedure also tests the strength of the sucking reflex, innervated by the hypoglossal nerve (cranial nerve XII). No clefts should be palpated.

Inspection of the Throat

Use a flashlight to inspect the throat for color, swelling, lesions, and the condition of the tonsils. Ask the child to open the mouth wide and stick out the tongue. Use a tongue blade, if needed, to visualize the posterior pharynx. Moistening the tongue blade may decrease the child's tendency to gag. The throat is normally pink without lesions, drainage, or swelling. The epiglottis lies behind the tongue and is normally pink like the rest of the buccal mucosa. Swelling or bulging in the posterior pharynx may be associated with a peritonsillar abscess (see Chapter 46 🔴).

During childhood the tonsils are large in proportion to the size of the pharynx because lymphoid tissue grows fastest in early childhood. The tonsils should be pink without exudate, but crypts (fissures) may be present as a result of prior infections. The size of the tonsils can be graded as indicated in the *Pathophysiology Illustrated: Tonsil Size with Infection* diagram.

When using a tongue blade to see the throat and tonsils, the gag reflex may be triggered. A symmetric rising movement of the uvula should be observed as the child gags. The gag reflex is not often specifically tested in children.

ASSESSING THE NECK FOR CHARACTERISTICS, RANGE OF MOTION, AND LYMPH NODES

Inspection of the Neck

Inspect the neck for size, symmetry, swelling, and any abnormalities such as *webbing*, an extra fold of skin on each side of the neck. A short neck with skinfolds is normal for infants.

Pathophysiology Illustrated	Tonsil Size with Infection

Tonsil size can be graded from 1+ to 4+ in relation to how much of the airway is obstructed. Tonsil size of 1+ and 2+ is normal. Tonsil size of 3+ is common with infections such as strep throat. Tonsils that "kiss" or nearly touch each other (4+) significantly reduce the size of the airway.

1+   2+

3+   4+

The neck is normally symmetric without swelling. Swelling may be caused by local infections such as mumps or a congenital defect. The neck lengthens between 3 and 4 years of age. Webbing is commonly associated with Turner syndrome (see Chapter 54 🔗).

Infants develop head control by 2 months of age. By this age an infant can lift the head up and look around when lying on the stomach. A lack of head control can result from neurologic injury, such as an anoxic episode.

Palpation of the Neck

Face the child and use your fingerpads to simultaneously palpate both sides of the neck for lymph nodes, as well as the trachea and thyroid.

Lymph Nodes

To palpate the lymph nodes, slide your fingerpads gently over the lymph node chains in the head and neck. One sequence is to palpate the lymph nodes in the occipital area, around the ears, under the jaw, and then the cervical chain in the neck (Figure 34–19 ●). Firm, clearly defined, nontender, movable lymph nodes up to 1 cm (½ in.) in diameter are common in young children. Enlarged, firm, warm, tender lymph nodes indicate a local infection.

Trachea

To palpate the trachea, place your thumb and forefinger on each side of the trachea near the chin and slowly slide down the trachea to determine its position and to detect the presence of any masses. The trachea is normally in the midline of the neck. It is difficult to palpate in children less than 3 years of age because of their short necks. Any shift to the right or left of midline may indicate a tumor or a collapsed lung.

Thyroid

As the fingers slide over the trachea in the lower neck, attempt to feel the isthmus of the thyroid, a band of glandular tissue crossing over the trachea. The lobes of the thyroid wrap behind the trachea and are normally covered by the sternocleidomastoid muscle. Because of the anatomic position of the thyroid, its lobes are not usually palpable in the child unless they are enlarged.

Range of Motion Assessment

To test the neck's range of motion, ask the child to touch the chin to each shoulder and to the chest and then to look at the ceiling. Move a light or toy in all four directions when assessing infants. Children should freely move the neck and head in all four directions without pain.

When the child is unable to move the head voluntarily in all directions, passively move the child's neck through the expected range of motion. Limited horizontal range of motion may be a sign of *torticollis,* persistent head tilting. Torticollis results from a birth injury to the sternocleidomastoid muscle or from unilateral vision or hearing impairment. Pain with flexion of the neck toward the chest (Brudzinski's sign) may indicate meningitis (see Chapter 55 🔗).

ASSESSING THE CHEST FOR SHAPE, MOVEMENT, RESPIRATORY EFFORT, AND LUNG FUNCTION

Examination of the chest includes the following procedures: inspecting the size and shape of the chest, palpating chest movement that occurs during respiration, observing the effort of breathing, and auscultating breath sounds. A stethoscope is needed.

● **Figure 34–19** Palpating the lymph nodes. The neck is palpated for enlarged lymph nodes around the ears, under the jaw, in the occipital area, and in the cervical chain of the neck.

Maxillary —
Buccal —
Sublingual —
Submandibular   Supraclavicular

Anterior auricular
Posterior auricular
Occipital
Superficial cervical
Tonsillar
Posterior cervical
Superior deep cervical

Inspection of the Chest

The chest skeleton provides most of the landmarks used to describe the location of findings during examination of the chest, lungs, and heart. The intercostal spaces are the horizontal markers. The sternum and spine are the vertical landmarks. When both a horizontal and a vertical landmark are used, the location of findings can be precisely described on the right or left side of the patient's chest (Figures 34–20 ● and 34–21 ●). The distance between the finding and the center of the sternum (midsternal line) or the spinal line can be measured with a ruler.

Position the child on the parent's lap or on the examining table with all clothing above the waist removed to inspect the chest. The thoracic muscles and subcutaneous tissue are less developed in children than in adolescents and adults, so the chest wall is thinner and the rib cage is more prominent unless obesity is present.

Size and Shape of the Chest

Inspect the chest for any irregularities in shape. In infants, the chest is rounded with the anteroposterior diameter approximately equal to the lateral diameter. By 2 years of age, the chest becomes more oval with growth, and the lateral diameter is greater than the anteroposterior diameter. If a child over 2 years of age has a rounded chest, a chronic obstructive lung condition such as asthma or cystic fibrosis may be present.

Chest circumference may be a useful measurement for comparison with the head circumference if the growth of either the head or chest is of concern. Measure the chest at the nipple line. The head and chest circumferences are expected to be approximately equal until 1 year of age when the chest circumference begins to surpass head circumference.

An abnormal chest shape may result from structural deformities, such as pectus carinatum and pectus excavatum (Figure 34–22 ●). Scoliosis, curvature of the spine, causes a lateral deviation of the chest (see Chapter 57 ⊘). A shield-shaped chest, unusually broad with widely spaced nipples, may be associated with Turner syndrome (see Chapter 54 ⊘).

Chest Movement and Respiratory Effort

The diaphragm is the primary muscle used for ventilation in infants and young children. As the thoracic muscles develop, they become primarily responsible for ventilation. Chest movement with breathing is normally symmetric bilaterally. On inspiration the chest and abdomen should rise simultaneously and fall on expiration. The chest movement of infants and young children is less pronounced than the abdominal movement. Asymmetric chest rise is associated with a collapsed lung.

The thoracic muscles serve as accessory respiratory muscles in infants and young children. When the child has a condition that causes a partial airway obstruction, the accessory muscles

Clavicle
Angle of Louis
Rib 2
Sternum
Intercostal space 5
Xiphoid process

Atlas
Axis
T1
Clavicle
Scapula
T12

A

B

● **Figure 34–20** Landmarks of the chest. Intercostal spaces and ribs are numbered to describe the location of findings. *A,* To determine the rib number on the anterior chest, palpate down from the top of the sternum until a horizontal ridge, the angle of Louis, is felt. Directly to the right and left of that ridge is the second rib. The second intercostal space is immediately below the second rib. Ribs 3–12 and the corresponding intercostal spaces can be counted as the fingers move toward the abdomen. *B,* To determine the rib number on the posterior chest, find the protruding spinal process of the seventh cervical vertebra at the shoulder level. The next spinal process belongs to the first thoracic vertebra, which attaches to the first rib.

● **Figure 34–21** Vertical landmarks of the chest. The sternum and spine are the vertical landmarks used to describe the anatomic location of findings. Imaginary vertical lines, parallel to the midsternal and spinal lines, are used to further describe the location of findings. The midclavicular line is through the middle of the clavicle. The midaxillary line is through the middle of the axilla. The scapular line is through the bottom angle of the scapula. *A,* Anterior vertical landmarks. *B,* Posterior vertical landmarks.

● **Figure 34–22** Abnormal chest shape. In pectus carinatum (pigeon chest) the sternum protrudes, increasing the anteroposterior diameter. In pectus excavatum (funnel chest) the lower portion of the sternum is depressed, decreasing the anteroposterior diameter. *A,* Pectus excavatum. *B,* Pectus carinatum.

are used for inspiration and retractions are seen. **Retractions**, visible depression of tissue between the ribs of the chest wall with each inspiration, indicate an increased work of breathing and often respiratory distress (see *Pathophysiology Illustrated: Retraction Sites* in Chapter 47 ●).

Respiratory Rate

Because infants and young children use the diaphragm as the primary breathing muscle, observe or feel the rise and fall of the abdomen to count the respiratory rate in children under age 6 years. Table 34–9 gives the normal respiratory rates for each age group.

Table 34–9	Normal Respiratory Rate Ranges by Age
Age	**Respiratory Rate per Minute**
Newborn	30–55
1 year	25–40
3 years	20–30
6 years	16–22
10 years	16–20
17 years	12–20

 Growth and Development   Respiratory Rate

Infants and children have a faster respiratory rate than adults because of their higher metabolic rate and oxygen requirement. Young children are also unable to increase the depth of respirations because the intercostal muscles are inadequately developed to lift the chest wall and increase intrathoracic volume (Chameides, Samson, Schexnayder, et al., 2011, p. 42).

To get the most accurate reading of a young infant's respiratory rate, wait until the baby is sleeping or resting quietly. Use the stethoscope to auscultate the rate or place your hand on the abdomen. Count the number of breaths for an entire minute, because newborns and young infants can have irregular respirations.

Tachypnea, an increased respiratory rate, occurs in response to excitement, fear, respiratory distress, fever, and other conditions that increase oxygen needs. A sustained respiratory rate higher than normal for age is an important sign of respiratory distress. The child is at risk for developing hypoxemia if treatment is not started. An abnormally slow respiratory rate occurs in response to respiratory failure.

Palpation of the Chest

Palpation is used to evaluate chest movement, respiratory effort, deformities of the chest wall, and tactile fremitus.

Chest Wall

To palpate the chest motion with respiration, place your palms and outspread fingers on each side of the child's chest. Confirm the bilateral symmetry of chest motion. Use your fingerpads to palpate any depressions, bulges, or unusual chest wall shape that might indicate abnormal findings such as tenderness, cysts, other growths, crepitus, or fractures. None should be found. **Crepitus**, a crinkly sensation palpated on the chest surface, is caused by air escaping into the subcutaneous tissues. It often indicates a serious injury to the upper or lower airway.

Tactile Fremitus

To palpate **tactile fremitus**, vibrations produced by crying and talking, place the palms of your hands on each side of the chest.

Ask the child to repeat a series of words or numbers, such as *puppy dog*, *kitty cat*, or *ice cream*. As the child repeats the words, move your hands systematically over the anterior and posterior chest, comparing the quality of vibrations side to side. The vibration or tingling sensation is normally palpated over the entire chest. Decreased sensations indicate that air is trapped in the lungs, as occurs with asthma.

Auscultation of the Chest

Auscultate the chest with a stethoscope to assess the quality and characteristics of breath sounds, to identify abnormal breath sounds, and to evaluate vocal resonance. Use an infant or pediatric stethoscope when available to help localize any unexpected breath sounds. Use the stethoscope diaphragm because it transmits the high-pitched breath sounds better.

Breath Sounds

Evaluate the quality and characteristics of breath sounds over the entire chest, comparing sounds between the sides. Select a routine sequence for auscultating the entire chest so assessment of all lobes of the lungs will be consistently performed. Figure 34–23 ● shows one suggested chest auscultation sequence. Listen to an entire inspiratory and expiratory phase at each spot on the chest before moving to the next site.

Three types of normal breath sounds are usually heard when the chest is auscultated. *Vesicular breath sounds* are low-pitched, swishing, soft, short expiratory sounds. They are usually heard in older children but not in infants and young children. *Bronchovesicular breath sounds* are medium-pitched, hollow, blowing sounds heard equally on inspiration and expiration in all age groups. The location of these sounds on the chest is related to the child's developmental status. *Bronchial/tracheal breath sounds* are hollow and higher pitched than vesicular breath sounds.

Breath sounds normally have equal intensity, pitch, and rhythm bilaterally. Absent or diminished breath sounds may indicate a pneumothorax or airway obstruction.

 Growth and Development
Auscultating Breath Sounds

Auscultation of breath sounds is difficult when an infant is crying. If the infant continues to cry after giving a pacifier, bottle, or toy, all is not lost. At the end of each cry the infant takes a deep breath, which you can use to assess breath sounds, vocal resonance, and tactile fremitus.

Encourage toddlers and preschoolers to take deep breaths by blowing a pinwheel or piece of tissue off of your hand. This may enhance auscultation of subtle wheezes that occur at the end of expiration.

When trying to encourage the child to breathe normally while auscultating the chest, use suggestive language to increase cooperation: "You certainly are good at breathing slowly. Have you been practicing?" The child will often deepen and slow the breathing pattern as you praise the effort.

ANTERIOR

A

POSTERIOR

B

● **Figure 34–23** One sequence for auscultation of the chest.

Clinical Tip

Infants and young children have a thin chest wall because of immature muscle development. The breath sounds of one lung are heard over the entire chest. It takes practice to accurately identify absent or diminished breath sounds in infants and young children. Because the distance between the lungs is greatest at the apices and midaxillary areas in young children, these sites are best for identifying absent or diminished breath sounds. Carefully auscultate, comparing the quality of breath sounds heard bilaterally.

Vocal Resonance

Auscultate to evaluate **vocal resonance**, that is how well voice sounds are transmitted over the chest. Have the child repeat a series of words, such as *apple*, *banana*, and *cereal*. Use the stethoscope to auscultate the chest, comparing the quality of sounds from side to side and over the entire chest. Voice sounds, with words and syllables muffled and indistinct, are normally heard throughout the chest.

   If voice sounds are absent or more muffled than usual, an airway obstruction condition such as asthma may be present. When a lung consolidation condition such as pneumonia is present, the vocal resonance quality changes in characteristic ways. **Whispered pectoriloquy** is present when syllables are heard distinctly in a whisper. **Bronchophony** is the increased intensity and clarity of sounds while the words remain indistinct. **Egophony** is the transmission of the "eee" sound as a nasal "ay" sound.

Abnormal Breath Sounds

Abnormal breath sounds, also called adventitious sounds, generally indicate disease. Examples of abnormal breath sounds are crackles, rhonchi, and **wheezing** (a noise resulting from the passage of air through mucus or fluids in a narrowed lower airway). To further assess abnormal breath sounds, identify the following:

■ Location, for example, side of body and lung lobe(s)

■ Presence during part or entire phase of inspiration or expiration

■ Change in character or disappearance when the child coughs or changes position

It takes practice to routinely identify these adventitious sounds. Table 34–10 describes adventitious sounds.

Abnormal Voice Sounds

Observing the quality of the voice and other audible sounds is also important during an examination of the lungs. *Stridor* is a noise resulting from air moving through a narrowed trachea and larynx; it is associated with croup. A cough is a reflexive clearing of the airway associated with a respiratory infection. Hoarseness is associated with inflammation of the larynx.

Percussion of the Chest

Percussion of the chest may be performed by an experienced examiner to assess the resonance of the lungs and size of underlying organs, such as the heart. Radiograph examination is commonly used for this evaluation.

Table 34–10	Description of Selected Adventitious Sounds and Their Cause	
Type	**Description**	**Cause**
Fine crackles	High-pitched, discrete, noncontinuous sound heard at end of inspiration; does not clear with coughing *(Rub pieces of hair together beside your ear to duplicate the sound.)*	Air passing through watery secretions in the smaller airways (alveoli and bronchioles)
Sibilant rhonchi (wheezing)	Musical, squeaking, or hissing noise usually heard continuously during inspiration or expiration, but generally louder on expiration; does not clear with coughing	Air passing through mucus or fluids in a narrowed lower airway (bronchioles) as with asthma
Sonorous rhonchi (coarse crackles)	Coarse, low-pitched sound like a snore, heard during inspiration or expiration; may clear with coughing	Air passing through thick secretions that partially obstruct the larger bronchi and trachea

Clinical Reasoning Assessing a Child with Bronchiolitis

Aliyah, 6 months old, is brought by her mother and father to the emergency room. She is an emergency admission from the local pediatrician's office with a diagnosis of bronchiolitis. As Aliyah's nurse, you are responsible for assessing her condition after she arrives on the pediatric nursing unit.

What procedures are used to perform a physical examination on a 6-month-old? Identify all the components of the physical assessment used to detect signs of respiratory difficulty.
See www.nursing.pearsonhighered.com for possible responses.

ASSESSING THE BREASTS

Inspection of the Breasts

The nipples of prepubertal boys and girls are symmetrically located near the midclavicular line at the fourth to sixth ribs. The areola is normally round and more darkly pigmented than the surrounding skin. Inspect the anterior chest for other dark spots that may indicate *supernumerary nipples*, small, undeveloped nipples and areola that may be mistaken for moles. Their presence may be associated with congenital renal or cardiac anomalies.

See the later section in this chapter for a discussion of pubertal development.

Palpation of the Breasts

Prepubertal boys and girls have no palpable breast tissue. Palpate the developing breasts of adolescent females for abnormal masses or hard nodules. With the girl lying down, use a concentric or vertical stripe pattern covering all areas of each breast, including the axilla, areola, and the nipple. Gently squeeze the nipples for discharge. Breast tissue normally feels dense, firm, and elastic. Any mass needs further evaluation.

The majority of boys have *gynecomastia*, unilateral or bilateral breast enlargement during adolescence. It is often most noticeable around 14 years of age and commonly disappears by the time of full sexual maturity. Palpate the tissue to differentiate actual breast tissue from fatty tissue in the pectoral area, and to detect any masses.

ASSESSING THE HEART FOR HEART SOUNDS AND FUNCTION

A stethoscope and sphygmomanometer are needed to assess the heart.

Inspection of the Precordium

Begin the heart examination by inspecting the precordium, or anterior chest. Place the child in reclining or semi-Fowler's position, either on the parent's lap or on the examining table. Inspect the shape and symmetry of the anterior chest from the front and side views. Asymmetry and bulging of the left side of the chest wall may indicate an enlarged heart. Observe for any chest movement associated with the heart's contraction. A *heave*, an obvious lifting of the chest wall during contraction, may indicate an enlarged heart.

Palpation of the Precordium

Lightly place the surface of your fingers together on the chest wall to systematically palpate the precordium for any pulsations, heaves, or vibrations. Palpating with minimal pressure increases the chance of detecting abnormal findings.

The **apical impulse**, the point of maximum intensity, is located where the left ventricle taps the chest wall during contraction. The apical impulse is sometimes seen on the anterior chest wall of thin children, but it is normally felt as a slight tap against one fingertip. Use the topographic landmarks of the chest to describe its location (see Figures 34–20 and 34–21).

 Growth and Development

The location of the apical impulse changes as the child's rib cage grows. In children under 7 years old, it is located in the fourth intercostal space just medial to the left midclavicular line. In children over 7 years old, it is located in the fifth intercostal space at the left midclavicular line.

Any other sensation palpated is usually abnormal. A *lift* is the sensation of the heart lifting up against the chest wall. It may be associated with an enlarged heart or a heart contracting with extra force. A *thrill* is a rushing vibration that feels like a cat's purr. It is caused by turbulent blood flow from a defective heart valve and a heart murmur. If present, the thrill is palpated in the right or left second intercostal space. To describe a thrill's location, use the topographic landmarks of the chest (see Figures 34–20 and 34–21) and estimate the diameter of the thrill palpated.

Heart Rate and Rhythm

The apical heart rate can be counted at the site of the apical impulse (Skill 9–8 SKILLS) either by palpation or by auscultation. Count the apical rate for 1 minute in infants and in children who have an irregular rhythm. The brachial or radial pulse rate should be the same as the ausculted apical heart rate. Table 34–11 gives normal heart rates in children of different ages.

Listen carefully to the heart rate rhythm. Children often have a normal cycle of irregular rhythm associated with respiration called *sinus arrhythmia* in which the child's heart rate is faster on inspiration and slower on expiration. When any rhythm irregularity is detected, ask the child to take a breath and hold it while you listen to the heart rate. The rhythm should become regular during inspiration and expiration. Other rhythm irregularities are abnormal (see Chapter 48).

Auscultation of the Heart

Auscultation is used to count the apical pulse, to assess the characteristics of the heart sounds, and to detect abnormal heart sounds. Use the bell of the stethoscope to detect these lower pitched sounds.

Auscultate the heart with the child in both sitting and reclining positions. Differences in heart sounds caused by a change in the child's position or by a change in the position of the heart near the chest wall can then be detected. If differences in heart sounds are detected with a position change, place the child in the left lateral recumbent position and auscultate again.

Differentiation of Heart Sounds

Heart sounds result from the closure of the valves and vibration or turbulence of blood produced by that valve closure. Two primary sounds, S_1 and S_2, are heard when the chest is auscultated.

The first heart sound, S_1, is produced by closure of the tricuspid and mitral valves at the beginning of ventricular contraction. The two valves close almost simultaneously, so only one sound is normally heard.

The second heart sound, S_2, is produced by the closure of the aortic and pulmonic valves. Once blood has reached the pulmonic and aortic arteries, the valves close to prevent leakage back into the ventricles during diastole. The timing of the valve closure varies with respirations. Sometimes S_2 is heard as a single sound and at other times as a split sound, that is, two sounds heard a fraction of a second apart.

Sound is easily transmitted in liquid, and it travels best in the direction of blood flow. Auscultate heart sounds at specific areas on the chest wall in the direction of blood flow, just beyond the valve (Figure 34–24 ●). The sounds produced by the heart valves or blood turbulence are heard throughout the chest in thin infants and children. Both S_1 and S_2 can be heard in all listening areas.

Auscultate heart sounds for quality (distinct versus muffled) and intensity (loud versus soft). First, distinguish between S_1 and S_2 in each listening area. Heart sounds are usually distinct and crisp in children because of their thin chest wall. Muffled or indistinct sounds may indicate a heart defect or congestive heart failure. Document the area where heart sounds are heard the best. Table 34–12 and Figure 34–24 review the location where each sound is normally best heard for assessment of quality and intensity. If the child has a potential murmur, auscultate the heart in the sitting, reclining, and left lateral recumbent positions to detect any differences associated with position change.

Splitting of the Heart Sounds

After distinguishing the first and second heart sounds, try to detect *physiologic splitting*, the split S_2 that is heard more often after the child takes a deep breath. More blood returns to the right ventricle, causing the pulmonic valve to close a fraction of a second later than the aortic valve. Auscultate over the pulmonic area while the child breathes normally and then while the child takes a deep breath. Splitting is normally more easily detected after a deep breath. The splitting returns to a single sound with

Table 34–11	Normal Heart Rates for Children of Different Ages	
Age	Heart Rate Range (beats/min)	Average Heart Rate (beats/min)
Newborns	100–170	120
Infants to 2 years	80–130	110
2–6 years	70–120	100
6–10 years	70–110	90
10–16 years	60–100	85

Second left interspace

Second right interspace

Aortic valve

Mitral valve

Tricuspid valve

Pulmonic valve

Third left interspace

Fourth left interspace

Fifth left interspace (apex)

● **Figure 34–24** Auscultating heart sounds. Sound travels in the direction of blood flow. Rather than listen for heart sounds over each heart valve, auscultate heart sounds at specific areas on the chest wall away from the valve itself. These areas are named for the valve producing the sound. *Aortic*: second right intercostal space near the sternum. *Pulmonic*: second left intercostal space near the sternum. *Tricuspid*: fifth right or left intercostal space near the sternum. *Mitral* (apical): in infants—third or fourth intercostal space, just left of the left midclavicular line; in children—fifth intercostal space at the left midclavicular line.

Table 34–12	Listening Sites for Auscultation of the Quality and Intensity of Heart Sounds	
Heart Sound	**Sites Where Best Heard**	**Sites Where Heard Softly**
S_1	Apex of the heart Tricuspid area Mitral area	Base of the heart Aortic area Pulmonic area
S_2	Base of the heart Aortic area Pulmonic area	Apex of the heart Tricuspid area Mitral area
Physiologic splitting	Pulmonic area	
S_3	Mitral area	

regular breathing. If splitting does not vary with normal and deep respirations, it is called *fixed splitting*, an abnormal finding associated with an atrial septal defect in the heart.

Third Heart Sound

A third heart sound, S_3, is occasionally heard in children as a normal finding. The S_3 heart sound is caused when blood rushes through the mitral valve and splashes into the left ventricle. It is heard in diastole, just after S_2. It is distinguished from a split S_2 because it is louder in the mitral area than in the pulmonic area.

Murmurs

Occasionally, abnormal heart sounds are auscultated. These sounds are produced by blood passing through a defective valve, great vessel, or other heart structure. Some murmurs are benign or innocent, whereas others may indicate a congenital heart defect. Consult an experienced examiner to distinguish between murmurs.

To hear murmurs in children takes practice. Often, murmurs must be very loud to be detected. For softer murmurs, normal heart sounds must be distinguished before an extra sound is

recognized. When a murmur is detected, define the characteristics of the extra sound, including:

- *Intensity.* How loud is it? Can a thrill also be palpated?
- *Location.* Where is the murmur the loudest? Identify the listening area and precise topographic landmarks. Is the child sitting or lying down? Do the murmur characteristics change when the child changes position?
- *Radiation or transmission.* Is the sound transmitted over a larger than expected area of the chest, to the axilla, or to the back?
- *Timing.* Is the murmur heard best after S_1 or S_2? Is it heard during the entire phase between S_1 and S_2?
- *Quality.* Describe what the murmur sounds like—for example, machinelike, musical, or blowing.

Venous Hum

A venous hum is a continuous low-pitched hum heard throughout the cardiac cycle caused by turbulent blood flow in the internal jugular veins. Auscultate over the supraclavicular fossa above the middle of the clavicle or over the upper

 Clinical Tip

Following are guidelines for grading the intensity of a murmur:

Intensity	Description
Grade I	Barely heard in a quiet room
Grade II	Quiet, but clearly heard
Grade III	Moderately loud; no thrill palpated
Grade IV	Loud; a thrill is usually palpated
Grade V	Very loud, heard when the stethoscope is barely on the chest wall; a thrill is easily palpated
Grade VI	Heard without the stethoscope in direct contact with the chest wall; a thrill is palpated

anterior chest with the bell of the stethoscope. A venous hum is heard as a continuous low-pitched hum throughout the cardiac cycle. It is heard louder during diastole and does not change with respirations. It may be quieted when the child turns the neck, lies down, or when the jugular vein is occluded. A venous hum may be associated with anemia, but it has no pathologic significance.

Completing the Heart Examination

A complete assessment of cardiac function also includes palpating the pulses, measuring the blood pressure, and evaluating signs from other systems.

Palpation of the Pulses

Palpate the characteristics of the pulses in the extremities to assess the circulation. The technique and sites for palpating the pulse are the same as those used for adults. Evaluate the pulsation for rate, regularity of rhythm, and strength in each extremity and compare your findings bilaterally. Palpate the femoral arteries, which should be as strong as the brachial pulsations. A weaker femoral pulse is associated with coarctation of the aorta.

Blood Pressure

To assess the blood pressure, wait until the child has been seated and quiet for 3 to 5 minutes. To obtain the most accurate reading, select an appropriately sized cuff for the extremity used. Use the right arm consistently as this arm was used for development of blood pressure standards. See Skill 9–10 in the *Clinical Skills Manual* SKILLS for the technique for obtaining the blood pressure in children.

With the cuff snugly wrapped around the arm, hold the arm with the antecubital fossa at the level of the heart. Use the bell of the stethoscope to hear softer Korotkoff sounds. The systolic reading is the onset of Korotkoff sounds. The diastolic reading is the fifth Korotkoff sound (Lande, 2011).

Measure the blood pressure twice and average the two readings. Compare the systolic and diastolic readings with the standard blood pressure values by age, gender, and height percentile in Appendix D 🖉. A blood pressure value at the 50th percentile for the child's age, gender, and height percentile is considered the midpoint of the normal blood pressure range. A systolic or diastolic reading at or above the 95th percentile indicates hypertension.

In any child in which there is a concern about a heart condition, obtain a blood pressure reading in both an arm and a leg and compare the readings. The blood pressure in the leg should be 10 to 20 mm Hg higher than the arm reading (Bernstein, 2011). If the reading in the leg is lower than that in the arm, coarctation of the aorta may be present.

 Growth and Development

Infants have a low systolic blood pressure, and detecting the distal pulses is often difficult. Use the brachial artery in the arms and the popliteal or femoral artery in the legs to evaluate the pulses. The radial and distal tibial pulses are normally palpated easily in older children.

Other Signs

Skin color, capillary refill, and respiratory distress are additional elements of a complete heart examination. Cyanosis is most commonly associated with a congenital heart defect in children. A capillary refill time of greater than 2 seconds indicates poor perfusion of the tissues. Signs of respiratory distress (tachypnea, flaring, and retractions) may be associated with the child's attempts to compensate for hypoxemia caused by a congenital heart defect.

ASSESSING THE ABDOMEN FOR SHAPE, BOWEL SOUNDS, AND UNDERLYING ORGANS

The location of underlying organs and structures of the abdomen must be considered when the abdomen is examined. The abdomen is commonly divided by imaginary lines into quadrants for the purpose of identifying underlying structures (Figure 34–25 ●). A stethoscope is needed to examine the abdomen. Perform inspection and auscultation before palpation and percussion because touching the abdomen may change the characteristics of bowel sounds.

Inspection of the Abdomen

Begin the examination of the abdomen by inspecting the shape and contour, condition of the umbilicus and rectus muscle, and abdominal movement. Inspect the shape of the abdomen from the front and side with good lighting to identify an abnormal contour. The child's abdomen is normally symmetric and rounded or flat when the child is supine. A scaphoid or sunken abdomen is abnormal and may indicate dehydration.

See Chapter 25 🖉 for guidelines to assess the newborn's umbilical stump. After the stump falls off, inspect the umbilicus

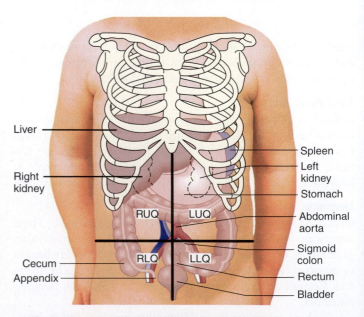

● **Figure 34–25** Topographic landmarks of the abdomen. The abdomen is commonly divided by imaginary lines into quadrants for the purpose of identifying underlying structures.

for continued drainage, which may indicate an infection or a granuloma. Inspect the umbilicus in infants and toddlers because these children often have an *umbilical hernia*, a protrusion of abdominal contents through an open umbilical muscle ring.

Inspect the abdominal wall for any depression or bulging at midline above or below the umbilicus, indicating separation of the rectus abdominis muscles. The depression may be up to 5 cm (2 in.) wide. Measure the width of the separation to monitor change over time. As abdominal muscle strength develops, the separation usually becomes less prominent. However, the splitting may persist if congenital muscle weakness is present.

Abdominal Movement

Infants and children up to 6 years of age breathe with the diaphragm. The abdomen rises simultaneously with the chest during inspiration and falls with expiration. Other abdominal movements such as peristaltic waves are abnormal. *Peristaltic waves* are visible rhythmic contractions of the intestinal wall smooth muscle, which moves food through the digestive tract. Their presence generally indicates an intestinal obstruction, such as pyloric stenosis (see Chapter 52).

Auscultation of the Abdomen

To evaluate bowel sounds, auscultate the abdomen with the diaphragm of the stethoscope. Bowel sounds normally occur every 10 to 30 seconds. They have a high-pitched, tinkling, metallic quality. Loud gurgling (borborygmi) is heard when the child is hungry. Listen in each quadrant long enough to hear at least one bowel sound. Before determining that bowel sounds are absent, auscultate at least 5 minutes in each quadrant. Absence of bowel sounds may indicate peritonitis or a paralytic ileus. Hyperactive bowel sounds may indicate gastroenteritis or a bowel obstruction.

Next auscultate over the abdominal aorta and the renal arteries for a vascular hum or murmur. No murmur should be heard. A murmur may indicate a narrowed or defective artery.

Percussion of the Abdomen

Indirect percussion is often used by experienced examiners to evaluate borders and sizes of abdominal organs and masses while the child is supine. To perform indirect percussion, lay the middle finger of your nondominant hand on the child's abdomen, keeping other fingers off the abdomen. With a spring-like motion, use the fingertip from the other hand to tap the finger on the abdomen. Listen for the tone to detect underlying structures. Dullness is found over the liver, spleen, and full bladder. Tympany is found over the stomach or the intestines when an obstruction is present. Tympany may be found over areas beyond the stomach in infants because of air swallowing. A resonant tone may be heard over other areas.

Palpation of the Abdomen

Both light and deep palpation are used to examine the abdomen's organs and to detect any masses. *Light palpation* evaluates the tenseness of the abdomen (how soft or hard it is), the liver, the presence of any tenderness or masses, and any defects in the abdominal wall. *Deep palpation* detects masses, defines their shape and consistency, and identifies tenderness in the abdomen.

Growth and Development
Abdominal Assessment

Infants and toddlers often feel more secure for the abdominal assessment when lying supine across both the parent's and the examiner's laps. A bottle, pacifier, or toy may distract the child and improve cooperation for the examination.

When examining the child, use suggestive words to help the child relax the abdomen. "How soft will your tummy get when my hand feels it? Does it get softer than this? Yes. See, it softens as you breathe out. Will it also be softer here?" In this way, the child learns to relax the abdomen and is challenged to do it better.

When children are ticklish, use a firm touch and do not pretend to tickle the child at any point in the examination. Alternatively, put the child's hand on the abdomen and place your hand over the child's. Let your fingertips slide over to touch the abdomen. The child has a sense of being in control, and you may be able to palpate directly.

Older children may need distraction, especially when abdominal tenderness and guarding are present. Have the child perform a task that requires some concentration, such as pressing the hands together or pulling locked hands apart.

To make the most accurate interpretation, perform the abdominal examination when the child is calm and cooperative. To begin palpation, position the child supine with knees flexed. Stand beside the child and place your warmed fingertips across the child's abdomen. Organs and other masses are more easily palpated when the abdominal wall is relaxed. Watch the child's face during palpation for a grimace or constriction of the pupils, which indicates pain.

Light Palpation

For light palpation, use a superficial, gentle touch that slightly depresses the abdomen. Usually the abdomen feels soft and no tenderness is detected. Palpate any bulging along the abdominal wall, especially along the rectus muscle and umbilical ring, which could indicate a hernia. If an umbilical hernia is present, measure the diameter of the muscular ring, rather than the protrusion. The muscle ring normally becomes smaller and closes by 4 years of age.

Locate and lightly palpate the lower liver edge. Place the fingerpads in the right midclavicular line at the level of the umbilicus and move the fingers closer to the costal margin with each expiration. As the liver edge descends with inspiration, a flat, narrow ridge is usually felt. The liver edge is normally palpated 2 to 3 cm (1 in.) below the right costal margin in infants and toddlers, but it may not be palpated in older children. If the liver edge is more than 3 cm (1 in.) below the right costal margin, the liver is enlarged, possibly due to congestive heart failure or hepatic disease.

Deep Palpation

To perform deep palpation, press the fingers of one hand (for small children) or two hands (for older children) more deeply into the abdomen. Because the abdominal muscles are most relaxed when the child takes a deep breath, ask the child to take regular deep breaths when palpating each area of the abdomen.

The spleen tip may be felt at the left costal margin in the midclavicular line when the child takes a deep breath. The spleen is enlarged if it is easily palpated below the left costal margin. The kidneys are in a deep layer of abdominal muscles and intestines, and they are rarely palpated except in newborns. A tubular mass commonly palpated in the lower left or right quadrant is often an intestine filled with feces. A distended bladder is often palpated as a firm, central, dome-shaped mass above the symphysis pubis in young children.

SAFETY ALERT!

If an enlarged kidney or mass is detected during abdominal palpation, do not continue to palpate the kidney. Notify the primary care provider immediately. The mass could be a Wilms' tumor.

Assessment of the Inguinal Area

The inguinal area is inspected and palpated during the abdominal examination to detect enlarged lymph nodes or masses. The femoral pulse, a part of the heart examination, may be assessed simultaneously with the abdominal examination.

Inspect the inguinal area for any change in contour, comparing sides. A small bulging noted over the femoral canal in girls may be associated with a femoral hernia. A bulging in the inguinal area in boys may be associated with an inguinal hernia.

Palpate the inguinal area for lymph nodes and other masses. Small lymph nodes, less than 1 cm (½ in.) in diameter, are often present in the inguinal area because of minor injuries on the legs. Any tenderness, heat, or inflammation in these palpated lymph nodes could be associated with a local infection.

ASSESSING THE GENITAL AND PERINEAL AREAS FOR EXTERNAL STRUCTURAL ABNORMALITIES

Nurses may perform an external genital examination or assist another healthcare provider. In younger children the genital and perineal examination is performed immediately after assessment of the abdomen. Gloves, lubricant, and a penlight are needed for the examination.

Examination of the genitalia and perineal area can cause stress in children because they sense their privacy has been invaded. To make young children feel more secure, position them on the parent's lap with their legs spread apart. Children can also be positioned on the examining table with their knees flexed and the legs spread apart like a frog.

Inspection of the Female External Genitalia

Inspect the external genitalia of girls for color, size, and symmetry of the mons pubis, labia, urethra, and vaginal opening (Figure 34–26 ●). Simultaneously look for any abnormal findings such as swelling, inflammation, masses, lacerations, or discharge.

Inspect the mons pubis for pubic hair and its characteristics. See pages 914–915 for guidelines to assess the stage of pubic hair development.

The labia minora are usually thin and pale in preadolescent girls but become dark pink and moist after puberty. In young infants the labia minora may be fused and cover the structures in the vestibule. These adhesions may need to be separated.

Use the thumb and forefinger of one gloved hand to separate the labia minora for viewing structures in the vestibule. Inspect the vestibule for lesions. No lesions or signs of inflammation are expected around the urethral or vaginal opening. Redness and excoriation are often associated with an irritant such as bubble bath. The hymen is just inside the vaginal opening. In preadolescents it is usually a thin membrane with a crescent-shaped opening. The vaginal opening is usually about 1 cm (½ in.) in adolescents when the hymen is intact. Sexually active adolescents may have a vaginal opening with irregular edges.

Preadolescent girls do not normally have a vaginal discharge. Adolescents often have a clear discharge without a foul odor. Menses generally begin approximately 2 years after breast bud development. A foul-smelling discharge in preschool-age children may be associated with a foreign body. Various organisms may cause a vaginal infection in older children.

 ### Clinical Tip

Preschool-age children are often taught that strangers are not permitted to touch their "private parts." When a child this age actively resists examination of the genital area, ask the parent to tell the child you have permission to look at and touch these parts of the body. You may wish to reinforce the teaching by saying the nurse or doctor can look only when the parent is in the room.

Some children develop modesty during the preschool period. Briefly explain what you need to examine and why. Then calmly and efficiently examine the child.

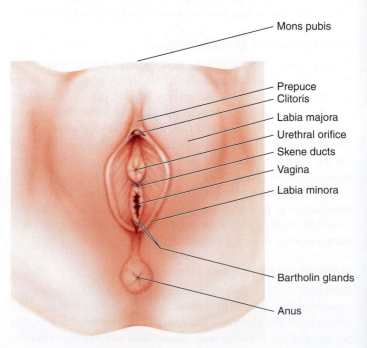

Mons pubis
Prepuce
Clitoris
Labia majora
Urethral orifice
Skene ducts
Vagina
Labia minora
Bartholin glands
Anus

● **Figure 34–26** Anatomic structures of the female genital and perineal area.

An internal vaginal examination is indicated when abnormal findings such as a vaginal discharge or trauma to the external structures is noted. An experienced examiner should perform the vaginal examination of the child.

Palpation of the Female Genitalia

Palpate the vaginal opening with a finger of your free, gloved hand. The Bartholin and Skene glands are not usually palpable. If such glands are palpated in preadolescent children, this indicates enlargement because of an infection such as gonorrhea.

Inspection of the Male Genitalia

Inspect the male genitalia for the structural and pubertal development of the penis, scrotum, and testicles. Have boys sit with their legs crossed in front of them. This position puts pressure on the abdominal wall to push the testicles into the scrotum. See pages 914–915 for guidelines to assess the staging of pubic hair and external genital development.

Penis

Inspect the penis for size, foreskin, hygiene, and position of the urethral meatus. The length of the nonerect penis in the newborn is normally 2 to 3 cm (1 in.). The penis enlarges in length and breadth during childhood and puberty. The penis is normally straight. A downward bowing of the penis may be caused by a *chordee*, a fibrous band of tissue associated with hypospadias.

When the penis is circumcised, the glans penis is exposed, and it is normally clean and smooth without inflammation or ulceration. The urethral meatus is a slit-shaped opening near the tip of the glans. No discharge should be present. If the penis is not circumcised, a foreskin opening large enough for a good urinary stream is normal, even when the foreskin does not fully retract, a common finding in boys between 3 and 6 years of age. To inspect the glans penis of an uncircumcised boy, the foreskin is gently retracted by the child, parent, or examiner. Avoid forcible retraction of the foreskin to prevent damage to the tissues and the formation of adhesions between the foreskin and glans. Evaluate the degree of foreskin retraction and the meatal location and size. It is usually possible to visualize the meatus.

Location of the urethral meatus at another site on the penis is abnormal, indicating hypospadias or epispadias (see Chapter 53 🔗). A round, pinpoint urethral meatus may indicate meatal stenosis. *Phimosis* is the presence of an abnormal ring of tissue distal to the glans that prevents retraction of the foreskin to allow visualization of the meatus. Erythema and edema of the glans (*balanitis*) may result from an infection or trauma.

Inspect the urinary stream. The stream is normally strong without dribbling.

Scrotum

Inspect the scrotum for size, symmetry, presence of the testicles, and any abnormalities. The scrotum is normally loose and pendulous with rugae, or wrinkles. The scrotum of infants often appears large in comparison to the penis. A small, undeveloped scrotum that has no rugae indicates undescended testicles. Enlargement or swelling of the scrotum is abnormal. It may indicate an inguinal hernia, hydrocele, torsion of the spermatic cord, or testicular inflammation. A deep cleft in the scrotum may indicate ambiguous genitalia.

Palpation of the Male Genitalia

Palpate the shaft of the penis for nodules and masses. None should be present.

Palpate the scrotum for the presence of the testicles. Make sure your hands are warm to avoid stimulating the cremasteric reflex that causes the testicles to retract. Place your index finger and thumb over both inguinal canals on each side of the penis. This keeps the testicles from retracting into the abdomen (Figure 34–27 ●).

Gently palpate each testicle with only enough pressure to identify the shape and size. The testicles are normally smooth and equal in size. They are approximately 1 to 1.5 cm (½ in.) in diameter until puberty, when they increase in size. A hard, enlarged, painless testicle may indicate a tumor.

If a testicle is not palpated in the scrotum, the examiner palpates the inguinal canal for a soft mass. When the testicle is found in the inguinal canal, an experienced examiner may try to move it to the scrotum to palpate the size and shape. The testicle is descendable when it can be moved into the scrotum. An undescended testicle is one that does not descend into the scrotum or cannot be palpated in the inguinal canal.

Palpate the length of the spermatic cord between the thumb and forefinger from the testicle to the inguinal canal. It normally feels solid and smooth. No tenderness is expected.

When bulging or swelling of the scrotum is present, palpate the scrotum to identify the characteristics of the mass. Try to determine whether the mass is unilateral or bilateral. An experienced examiner may try to reduce the mass by pushing it back through the external inguinal ring and then distinguishes between a reducible inguinal hernia, hydrocele, and an incarcerated hernia.

● **Figure 34–27** Palpating the scrotum for descended testicles and spermatic cords. Note the position of the index finger over the inguinal canal to keep the testicle in the scrotum.

Anus and Rectum

When the child is supine or prone, inspect the anus for sphincter control and any abnormal findings such as inflammation, fissures, or lesions. The external sphincter is usually closed. Inflammation and scratch marks around the anus may be associated with pinworms. A protrusion from the rectum may be associated with a rectal wall prolapse or a hemorrhoid.

Lightly touching the anal opening should stimulate an anal contraction or "wink." Absence of a contraction may indicate the presence of a lower spinal cord lesion. Passage of meconium by newborns indicates a patent anus.

A rectal examination is not routinely performed on children. It is indicated for symptoms of intra-abdominal, rectal, bowel, or stool abnormalities. Only an experienced examiner should perform a rectal examination. To reduce anxiety associated with this examination, distract the child with an age-appropriate toy or discussion when assisting with this procedure. Let the child know that the lubricant might feel cold. As the examiner's finger is positioned, help the child to relax the sphincter by "pushing out the poop."

ASSESSING PUBERTAL DEVELOPMENT AND SEXUAL MATURATION

The age of onset of secondary sexual characteristics can vary with race and ethnicity, environmental conditions, geographic location, and nutrition. For example, in the United States, black females and males have an earlier onset of secondary sexual characteristics than white females and males (Susman, Houts, Steinberg, et al., 2010). A higher body mass index appears to contribute to earlier development of puberty in females, but not in males (Walvoord, 2010).

Females

Breast development in girls usually precedes other pubertal changes. Figure 34–28 ● shows the Tanner stages of breast development. *Thelarche* or breast budding is the first stage of pubertal development in the majority of girls, indicating breast Tanner stage II. Breast tissue is seen and palpated below a slightly enlarging areola (1 cm in diameter of palpable glandular tissue) (Hermann-Giddens, Bourdony, Dowshen, et al., 2011). While breast budding normally occurs between 9 and 14 years of age, breast development may begin as early as 6 years in black girls and 7 years in white girls. Breast development before these ages is abnormal and needs further evaluation (Biro et al., 2010).

Inspect the adolescent's breasts while she is sitting to determine the stage of development. A girl's breasts often develop at different rates and appear asymmetric.

During the genital examination, observe for pubic hair development. Preadolescent girls have no pubic hair. Initial pubic hair is lightly pigmented, sparse, and straight along the labia majora. Figure 34–29 ● illustrates the normal stages of female pubic hair development. Breast development usually precedes pubic hair development. The presence of pubic hair before 8 years of age is unusual and may indicate premature pubertal development.

Stage I

Stage II

Stage III

Stage IV

Stage V

● Figure 34–28 Normal stages of breast development.

Males

Initial signs of pubertal development in males are enlargement of the testicles and thinning of the scrotum. Straight, downy pubic hair first appears at the base of the penis 6 months later. The hair becomes darker, dense, and curly, extending over the pubic area in a diamond pattern by the completion of puberty.

● **Figure 34–29** The stages of female pubic hair development with sexual maturation. In stage 2, soft downy hair along the labia majora is an indication that sexual maturation is beginning. Hair grows progressively coarse and curly as development proceeds.

● **Figure 34–30** The stages of male pubic hair and external genital development with sexual maturation.

The presence of pubic hair before 9 years of age may be an indication of premature pubertal development. Delayed onset of testicular enlargement after 14 years of age needs evaluation. Penile enlargement generally follows testicular enlargement about 1 year later in genitalia Tanner stage 3. Stages of pubic hair and external genital development follow a standard pattern, as seen in Figure 34–30 ●.

Sexual Maturity Rating

The sexual maturity rating (SMR) is an average of the breast and pubic hair Tanner stages in females and of the genital and pubic hair Tanner stages in males. The rating is a number between 2 and 5, as stage 1 is prepubertal. The SMR is then related to other physiologic events that happen during puberty.

Compare the stage of the child's secondary sexual characteristics with information in Table 34–13.

In females, menarche generally occurs in SMR 4 or breast stage 3 to 4. While the mean age of stage 2 breast development has lowered for females over time, the age at menarche has

remained fairly constant, between 12 and 13 years (Walvoord, 2010). The peak height velocity usually occurs before menarche at a mean age of 11.5 years.

In males, ejaculation usually occurs at SMR 3, with semen noted between SMR 3 and 4. The peak height velocity usually occurs in SMR 4 or genital stage 4 to 5, at about 13.5 years of age.

ASSESSING THE MUSCULOSKELETAL SYSTEM FOR BONE AND JOINT STRUCTURE, MOVEMENT, AND MUSCLE STRENGTH

Inspection of the Bones, Muscles, and Joints

Inspect and compare the arms and then the legs for differences in alignment, contour, skinfolds, length, and deformities. The extremities normally have equal length, circumference, and

Table 34-13	Sexual Maturity Timeline
Gender and Development Categories	**Time Span and Developmental Changes**
Female	
Breast development	Over 4 to 4.5 years, proceeding from stage 2 to 5
Pubic hair development	Over 4 to 4.5 years, usually initiated after breast development
Onset of menstruation	At about breast stage 4 (see Figure 34–28)
Growth spurt	Over 5 years, height velocity increases soon after stage 2 with peak height velocity between breast and pubic hair stages 3 and 4 (see Figures 34–28 and 34–29)
Male	
Genital (penis and testes) development	Over 4.5 years, proceeding from stage 2 to 5; testicular development precedes growth of the penis (see Figure 34–30)
Pubic hair development	Over 3.5 years
Facial and axillary hair	Begins about 2 years after pubic hair development begins
Voice change	Greatest change between genital stages 3 and 4
Onset of ejaculation	At about genital stage 3
Growth spurt	Over 4 to 5 years, greatest height velocity is in the first 2 to 3 years with peak height velocity between genital and pubic hair stages 3 and 4 (see Figure 34–30)

Source: Data from Hermann-Giddens, M. E., Bourdony, C. J., Dowshen, S. A., & Reiter, E. O. (2011). *Assessment of sexual maturity stages in girls and boys.* Elk Grove Village, IL: American Academy of Pediatrics; Fonseca, H, & Greydanus, D. E. (2007). Sexuality in the child, teen, and young adult: Concepts for the clinician. *Primary Care Clinics in Office Practice, 34,* 275–292; Susman, E. J., Houts, R. M., Steinberg, L., Belsky, J., Cauffman, E., De Hart, G., . . . Eunice Kennedy Shriver NICHD Early Child Care Research Network. (2010). Longitudinal development of secondary sexual characteristics in girls and boys between ages 9½ and 15½ years. *Archives of Pediatric and Adolescent Medicine, 164*(2), 166–173.

numbers of skinfolds bilaterally. Extra skinfolds and a larger circumference may indicate a shorter extremity.

Inspect and compare the joints bilaterally for size, discoloration, and ease of voluntary movement. Joints are normally the same color as surrounding skin, with no sign of swelling. Children should voluntarily flex and extend joints during normal activities without pain. Redness, swelling, and pain with movement may indicate injury or infection.

Palpation of the Bones, Muscles, and Joints

Palpate the bones and muscles in each extremity for muscle tone, masses, or tenderness. Muscles normally feel firm, and bony masses are not normally present. Doughy muscles may indicate poor muscle tone. Rigid muscles, or hypertonia, may be associated with an active seizure or cerebral palsy. A mass over a long bone may indicate a recent fracture or a bone tumor.

Palpate each joint and surrounding muscles to detect any swelling, masses, heat, or tenderness. None is expected when the joint is palpated. Tenderness, heat, swelling, and redness can result from injury or a chronic joint inflammation such as juvenile idiopathic arthritis.

Range of Motion and Muscle Strength Assessment

Range of Motion

Observe the child during typical play activities, such as reaching for objects, climbing, and walking, to assess range of motion of all major joints. Children spontaneously move their joints through the full normal range of motion with play activities when no pain is present. Limited range of motion may indicate injury, inflammation of a joint, or a muscle abnormality.

When a joint is suspected of having limited active range of motion, perform passive range of motion. Flex and extend, abduct and adduct, or rotate the affected joint cautiously to avoid causing extra pain. Full range of motion without pain is normal. Limitations in movement may indicate injury, inflammation, or malformation. Increased passive range of motion may indicate muscle weakness.

Muscle Strength

Observe the child's ability to climb onto an examining table, throw a ball, clap the hands, or move around on the bed. The child's ability to perform age-appropriate play activities indicates good muscle tone and strength. Attainment of age-appropriate motor development is another indicator of good muscle strength (Table 34–14).

To assess the strength of specific muscles in the extremities, engage the child in some games. Compare muscle strength bilaterally to identify muscle weakness. For example, the child squeezes the examiner's fingers tightly with each hand; pushes against and pulls the examiner's hands with his or her hands, lower legs, and feet; and resists extension of a flexed elbow or knee. Children normally have good muscle strength bilaterally. Unilateral muscle weakness may be associated with a nerve injury. Bilateral muscle weakness may result from hypoxemia or a congenital disorder such as Down syndrome. Asymmetric weakness may be associated with conditions such as cerebral palsy.

When generalized muscle weakness is suspected in a preschool- or school-age child, ask the child to stand up from the supine position. Children are normally able to rise to a standing position without using their arms as levers. Children who push their body upright using their arms and hands may have generalized muscle weakness, known as a positive Gowers' sign. This may indicate muscular dystrophy (see Chapter 57 ⊘).

Table 34–14	Selected Gross Motor Milestones for Age

Gross Motor Milestones	Average Age Attained
Rolls over from prone to supine position	7 months
Sits without support	6 months
Pulls self to standing position	10 months
Creeps or crawls	10 months
Walks alone	12 months
Climbs on furniture	24 months
Walks up stairs, one step at a time	24 months
Rides tricycle	36 months

Source: Data from Zitelli, B. J., McIntire, S. J., & Nowalk, A. J. (2012). *Atlas of pediatric physical diagnosis* (6th ed.). Philadelphia, PA: Elsevier Saunders; Feigelman, S. (2011a). The first year. In R. M. Kliegman, B. F. Stanton, J. W. St. Geme, N. F. Schor, & R. E. Behrman, *Nelson textbook of pediatrics* (19th ed., pp. 26–31). Philadelphia, PA: Elsevier Saunders; Feigelman, S. (2011b). The second year. In R. M. Kliegman, B.F. Stanton, J. W. St. Geme, N. F. Schor, & R. E. Behrman, *Nelson textbook of pediatrics* (19th ed., pp. 31–33). Philadelphia, PA: Elsevier Saunders.

Posture and Spinal Alignment

Posture

Inspect the child's posture when standing from a front, side, and back view. The shoulders and hips are normally level. The head is held erect without a tilt, and the shoulder contour is symmetric. After beginning to walk, young children often have a pot-bellied stance because of lumbar lordosis. The spine has normal thoracic convex and lumbar concave curves after 6 years of age. Table 34–15 describes normal posture and spinal curvature development.

Spinal Alignment

Assess the school-age child and adolescent for *scoliosis*, a lateral spine curvature. Stand behind the child, observing the height of

● **Figure 34–31** Evaluating spinal alignment. Does this child have legs of different lengths or scoliosis? Look at the level of the iliac crests and shoulders to see if they are level. See the more prominent crease at the waist on the right side? This child could have scoliosis.

the shoulders and hips (Figure 34–31 ●). Ask the child to bend forward slowly at the waist, with the head and arms toward the floor. No lateral curve should be present in either position. The ribs normally stay flat bilaterally. The lumbar concave curve should flatten with forward flexion (Figure 34–32 ●). A lateral curve to the spine or a one-sided rib hump is an indication of scoliosis (see Chapter 57 🔗).

Table 34–15	Normal Development of Posture and Spinal Curves

Age	Posture and Spinal Curves
2–3 months	Holds head erect when held upright; thoracic kyphosis when sitting.
6–8 months	Sits without support; spine is straight.
10–15 months	Walks independently; straight spine.
Toddler	Protruding abdomen; lumbar lordosis.
School-age child	Height of shoulders and hips is level; balanced thoracic convex and lumbar concave curves.

● **Figure 34–32** Inspection of the spine for scoliosis. Ask the child to slowly bend forward at the waist with arms extended toward the floor. Run your forefinger down the spinal processes, palpating each vertebra for a change in alignment. A lateral curve to the spine or a one-sided rib hump is an indication of scoliosis.

● **Figure 34–33** Transverse crease on palmar surface of the hand is associated with Down syndrome.

Source: NMSB/Custom Medical Stock Photo, Inc.

Inspection of the Upper Extremities

The alignment of the arms is normally straight, with a minimal angle at the elbows, where the bones articulate.

Count the fingers. Extra finger digits (*polydactyly*) or webbed fingers (*syndactyly*) are abnormal. Inspect the creases on the palmar surface of each hand. Multiple creases across the palm are normal. A single transverse crease across the entire palm of the hand is associated with Down syndrome (Figure 34–33 ●).

Inspect the nails for size, shape, and color. Nails are normally convex, smooth, and pink. **Clubbing**, widening of the nailbed with an increased angle between the proximal nail fold and nail, is abnormal (see Figure 48–3 in Chapter 48 ●). Clubbing is associated with chronic respiratory and cardiac conditions.

Inspection of the Lower Extremities

Assess the hips of newborns and young infants for dislocation or subluxation. First inspect and compare the number of skinfolds on the upper legs. An uneven number of skinfolds may indicate a hip dislocation or difference in leg length. Then check for Allis' sign, a difference in knee height symmetry (Figure 34–34 ●). The

● **Figure 34–34** Checking knee height symmetry. Flex the infant's hips and knees so the heels are as close to the buttocks as possible. Place the feet flat on the examining table. The knees are usually the same height. A difference in knee height (Allis' sign) is an indicator of hip dislocation.

Source: Used with permission International Hip Dysplasia Institute.

Ortolani-Barlow maneuver is used to assess an infant's hips for dislocation or subluxation. (See Figure 25–36 in Chapter 25 ●.)

View the child from behind and observe as the child stands on one leg and then the other. The iliac crests should stay level. If the iliac crest on the lifted leg appears lower, the hip abductor muscles on the weight-bearing side are weak, known as Trendelenburg sign.

Legs and Feet

Inspect the alignment of the legs with the child standing. After a child is 4 years of age, the alignment of the long bones is straight, with minimal angle at the knees and feet where the bones articulate. Assess alignment of the lower extremities in infants and toddlers to ensure that normal changes are occurring. To evaluate the toddler with bowlegs, have the child stand on a firm surface. Measure the distance between the knees when the child's ankles are together. No more than 1.5 in. (3.5 cm) between the knees is normal. See Figure 34–35 ● for assessment of knock-knees.

Inspect the feet for alignment, the presence of all toes, and any deformities. The weight-bearing line of the feet is usually in alignment with the legs. Many newborns have a flexible forefoot inversion (*metatarsus adductus*) that results from uterine positioning. Any fixed deformity is abnormal.

Inspect the feet for the presence of an arch when the child is standing. Children up to 3 years of age normally have a fat pad over the arch, giving the appearance of flat feet. Older children

● Growth and Development Leg Alignment

Infants are often born with a twisting of the tibia caused by positioning in utero (tibial torsion). The infant's toes turn in as a result of the tibial torsion. Toddlers go through a skeletal alignment sequence of bowlegs (genu varum) and knock-knees (genu valgum) before the legs assume a straight alignment.

● **Figure 34–35** To evaluate the child with knock-knees, have the child stand on a firm surface. Measure the distance between the ankles when the child stands with the knees together. The normal distance is not more than 2 in. (5 cm) between the ankles.

normally have a longitudinal arch. The arch is usually seen when the child stands on tiptoe or is sitting. Inspect the nails of the feet as for the hands.

ASSESSING THE NERVOUS SYSTEM

The nervous system is assessed for cognitive function, balance, coordination, cranial nerve function, sensation, and reflexes. Equipment needed for this examination includes a reflex hammer, cotton balls, a penlight, and tongue blades.

Cognitive Function

Observe the child's behavior, facial expressions, gestures, communication skills, activity level, and level of consciousness to assess cognitive functioning. Match the neurologic examination to the child's stage of development. For example, cognitive function is evaluated much differently in infants than in older children because infants cannot use words to communicate.

Behavior

The alertness of infants and children is indicated by their behavior. Infants and toddlers are curious but seek the security of the parent, either by clinging or by making frequent eye contact. Older children are often anxious and watch the examiner's actions. Lack of interest in assessment or treatment procedures may indicate a serious illness. Excessive activity or an unusually short attention span may be associated with an attention deficit hyperactivity disorder.

Communication Skills

Speech, language development, and social skills provide good clues to cognitive functioning. Listen to speech articulation and words used, comparing the child's performance with standards of social development and expected language development for age (Table 34–16). Toddlers can normally follow simple directions such as "Show me your mouth." By 3 years of age, the child's speech should be easily understood. Delay in language and social skill development may be associated with cognitive disability or hearing loss.

Memory

Immediate, recent, and remote memory can be tested in children starting at approximately 4 years of age. Immediate memory can be tested by asking the child to repeat a series of words or numbers, such as the names of favorite characters from a book, television show, or movie. Children can remember more words or numbers with age: three words or numbers at age 4 years, four words or numbers at age 5 years, and five words or numbers at age 6 years.

To evaluate recent memory, ask the child to remember a special name or object. Then 5 to 10 minutes later during the

Table 34–16	Expected Language Development for Age
Language Milestones	**Age Attained**
Babbles speech-like sounds, including *p*, *b*, and *m*	4–6 months
Has 1–2 words like *mama*, *dada*, *bye-bye*	12 months
Increases words each month; two-word combinations (e.g., "Where baby?" and "Want cookie")	1–2 years
Two- to three-word sentences to ask for things or talk about things; large vocabulary; speech understood by family members	2–3 years
Sentences may have four or more words; speech understood by most people	3–4 years
Says most sounds correctly except a few like *l, s, r, v, z, ch, sh, th*; tells stories and uses same grammar as rest of family	4–5 years

Source: Data from American Speech and Language Association. (2011). *How does your child hear and talk?* Retrieved from http://www.asha.org/public/speech/development/chart.htm.

examination, have the child recall the name or object. To evaluate remote memory, ask the child to repeat his or her address or birth date or a nursery rhyme. By 5 or 6 years of age, children are normally able to recall this information without difficulty.

Level of Consciousness

When approaching the infant or child, observe his or her level of consciousness and activity, including facial expressions, gestures, and interaction. Children are normally alert, and sleeping children arouse easily. The child who cannot be awakened is unconscious. A lowered level of consciousness may be associated with a number of neurologic conditions such as a brain injury, seizure, infection, or brain tumor.

Cerebellar Function

Observe the young child at play to assess coordination and balance. Development of fine motor skills in infants and preschool children provides clues to cerebellar function.

Balance

Observe the child's balance during play activities such as walking, standing on one foot, and hopping. See Table 34–17 for

Table 34–17	Expected Balance Development for Age
Balance Milestones	**Age Attained**
Stands without support briefly	12 months
Walks alone well	15 months
Walks backwards	2 years
Balances on 1 foot momentarily	3 years
Hops on 1 foot	4 years

Clinical Tip

The neurologic examination provides an opportunity to develop rapport with the child. Many of the procedures can be presented as games that young children enjoy. You can assess cognitive function by how well the child follows directions for tests of strength and coordination. As the assessment proceeds, the child develops trust and may be more cooperative with examination of other body systems.

● **Figure 34–36** Romberg procedure. Ask the child to stand with feet together and eyes closed. Protect the child from falling by standing close. Preschool-age children may extend their arms to maintain balance, but older children can normally stand with their arms at their sides. Leaning or falling to one side is abnormal and indicates poor balance.

Table 34–18	Expected Fine Motor Development for Age

Fine Motor Milestones	Average Age Attained
Transfers objects between hands	5–6 months
Thumb finger grasp	8 months
Scribbles with crayon or pencil	13 months
Builds two-block tower	15 months
Feeds self	18 months
Builds six-block tower	22 months

Source: Data from Zitelli, B. J., McIntire, S. J., & Nowalk, A. J. (2012). *Atlas of pediatric physical diagnosis* (6th ed.). Philadelphia, PA: Elsevier Saunders; Feigelman, S. (2011a). The first year. In R. M. Kliegman, B. F. Stanton, J. W. St. Geme, N. F. Schor, & R. E. Behrman, *Nelson textbook of pediatrics* (19th ed., pp. 26–31). Philadelphia, PA: Elsevier Saunders; Feigelman, S. (2011b). The second year. In R. M. Kliegman, B. F. Stanton, J. W. St. Geme, N. F. Schor, & R. E. Behrman, *Nelson textbook of pediatrics* (19th ed., pp. 31–33). Philadelphia, PA: Elsevier Saunders.

expected balance milestones for age. The Romberg procedure can also be used to test balance in children over 3 years of age (Figure 34–36 ●). Once balance and other motor skills are attained, children do not normally stumble or fall when tested. Poor balance may indicate cerebellar dysfunction or an inner ear disturbance.

Coordination

Tests of coordination assess the smoothness and accuracy of movement. Development of fine motor skills can be used to assess coordination in young children (Table 34–18). After 6 years of age, the tests for adults (finger-to-nose, finger-to-finger, heel-to-shin, and alternating motion) can be used (Figure 34–37 ●). Jerky movements or inaccurate pointing (past pointing) indicate poor coordination, which can be associated with delayed development or a cerebellar lesion.

Gait

A normal gait requires intact bones and joints, muscle strength, coordination, and balance. Inspect the walking child from both the front and rear views. The iliac crests are normally level during walking, and no limp is expected. Toddlers beginning to walk have a wide-based gait and limited balance, and eventually gain more balance and a more narrow-based gait.

A limp may indicate injury or joint disease. Staggering or falling may indicate cerebellar ataxia. Scissoring, in which the thighs tend to cross forward over each other with each step, may be associated with cerebral palsy or other spastic conditions.

Cranial Nerve Function

To assess the cranial nerves in infants and young children, modify the procedures used to assess school-age children and adults (Table 34–19 on page 922). Abnormalities of cranial nerves may be associated with compression due to an injury, tumor, or infection in the brain.

Sensory Function

To assess sensory function, compare the responses of the body to various types of stimulation. Bilateral equal responses are normal. Loss of sensation may indicate a brain or spinal cord lesion. Withdrawal responses to painful procedures indicate normal sensory function in an infant.

To test *superficial tactile sensation*, stroke the skin on the lower leg or arm with a cotton ball or a finger while the child's eyes are closed. Cooperative children over 2 years of age can normally point to the location touched.

To test *superficial pain sensation*, ask the child to close the eyes, and touch the child in various places on each arm and leg. Alternate the sharp and dull ends of a broken tongue blade or a paper clip. Children over 4 years of age can normally distinguish between a sharp and dull sensation each time. To improve the child's accuracy with the test, let the child practice describing the difference between the sharp and dull stimulation.

An inability to identify superficial touch and pain sensation may indicate sensory loss. Identify the extent of sensory loss, such as all areas below the knee. Other sensory function tests (temperature, vibratory, deep pressure pain, and position sense) are performed when sensory loss is found. Refer to other texts for a description of these procedures.

● **Figure 34–37** Tests of coordination. *A, Finger-to-nose test.* Ask the child to close the eyes and touch his or her nose, alternating the index fingers of the hands. *B, Finger-to-finger test.* Ask the child to alternately touch his or her nose and your index finger with his or her index finger. Move your hand to several positions within the child's reach to test pointing accuracy. Repeat the test with the child's other hand. *C, Heel-to-shin test.* Ask the child to rub his or her leg from the knee to the ankle with the heel of the other foot. Repeat the test with the other foot. This test is normally performed without hesitation or inappropriate placement of the foot. *D, Rapid alternating motion test.* Ask the child to rapidly rotate his or her wrist so the palm and dorsum of the hand alternately pat the thigh. Repeat the test with the other hand. Hesitating movements are abnormal. Mirroring movements of the hand not being tested indicate a delay in coordination skill refinement.

Common Newborn Reflexes

Evaluate the movement and posture of newborns and young infants by the Moro, palmar grasp, plantar grasp, placing, stepping, and tonic neck newborn reflexes. These reflexes appear and disappear at expected intervals in the first few months of life as the central nervous system develops. Movements are normally equal bilaterally. An asymmetric response may indicate a serious neurologic problem on the less responsive side. (See Table 25–4, *Common Newborn Reflexes*, in Chapter 25 ⊘ for more information.)

Superficial and Deep Tendon Reflexes

Evaluate the superficial and deep tendon reflexes to assess the function of specific segments of the spine.

Superficial Reflexes

Assess superficial reflexes by stroking a specific area of the body. The plantar reflex, testing spine levels L4 to S2, is routinely evaluated in children (Figure 34–38 ●). The cremasteric reflex is assessed in boys by stroking the inner thigh of each leg. The testicle and scrotum on the stroked side normally rise.

Deep Tendon Reflexes

To assess the deep tendon reflexes, tap a tendon near specific joints with a reflex hammer (or with the index finger for infants), comparing responses bilaterally. Inspect for movement in the associated joint and palpate the strength of the expected muscle contraction. The numeric scoring of deep tendon reflexes is as follows:

Grade	Response Interpretation
0	No response
1+	Slow, minimal response
2+	Expected response, active
3+	More active or pronounced than expected
4+	Hyperactive, clonus may be present

Table 34–20 (on page 923) provides guidelines for assessment of the biceps, triceps, brachioradialis, patellar, and Achilles deep tendon reflexes. The best response to deep tendon reflex testing is achieved when the child is relaxed or distracted. Making the child focus on another set of muscles may provide a more accurate

Table 34–19	Age-Specific Procedures for Assessment of Cranial Nerves in Infants and Children
Cranial Nerve[a]	**Assessment Procedure and Normal Findings[b]**
I Olfactory	Infant: Not tested. Child: Not routinely tested. Give familiar odors to child to sniff, one naris at a time. *Identifies odors such as orange, peanut butter, and chocolate.*
II Optic	Infant: Shine a bright light in eyes. *A quick blink reflex and dorsal head flexion indicate light perception.* Child: Test vision and visual fields if cooperative. *Visual acuity appropriate for age.*
(III Oculomotor) (IV Trochlear) (VI Abducens)	Infant: Shine a penlight at the eyes and move it side to side. *Focuses on and tracks the light to each side.* Child: Move an object through the six cardinal points of gaze. *Tracks object through all fields of gaze.* All ages: Inspect eyelids for drooping. Inspect pupillary response to light. *Eyelids do not droop and pupils are equal size and briskly respond to light.*
V Trigeminal	Infant: Stimulate the rooting and sucking reflex. *Turns head toward stimulation at side of mouth and sucking has good strength and pattern.* Child: Observe the child chewing a cracker. Touch forehead and cheeks with cotton ball when eyes are closed. *Bilateral jaw strength is good. Child points to location touched by cotton ball.*
VII Facial	All ages: Observe facial expressions when crying, smiling, frowning, etc. *Facial features stay symmetric bilaterally.*
VIII Acoustic	Infant: Produce a loud sound near the head. *Blinks in response to sound, moves head toward sound or freezes position.* Child: Use a noisemaker near each ear or whisper words to be repeated. *Turns head toward sound and repeats words correctly.*
(IX Glossopharyngeal) (X Vagus)	Infant: Observe swallowing during feeding. *Good swallowing pattern.* All ages: Elicit gag reflex. *Gags with stimulation.*
XI Spinal accessory	Infant: Not tested. Child: Ask child to raise the shoulders and turn the head side to side against resistance. *Good strength in neck and shoulders.*
XII Hypoglossal	Infant: Observe feeding. *Sucking and swallowing are coordinated.* Child: Tell the child to stick out the tongue. Listen to speech. *Tongue is midline with no tremors. Words are clearly articulated.*

[a]Bracketed nerves are tested together.
[b]Italic text indicates normal findings.

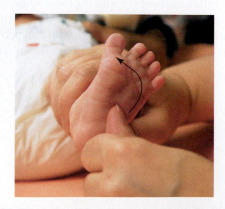

● **Figure 34–38** To assess the plantar reflex, stroke the bottom of the infant's or child's foot in the direction of the arrow. Watch the toes for plantar flexion or the *Babinski response*, fanning, and dorsiflexion of the big toe. The Babinski response is normal in children under 2 years of age. Plantar flexion of the toes is the normal response in older children. A Babinski response in children over 2 years of age can indicate neurologic disease.

response. When testing the reflexes on the lower legs, have the child press his or her hands together or try to pull them apart when gripped together. Responses are normally symmetric bilaterally. The absence of a response is associated with decreased muscle tone and strength. Hyperactive responses are associated with muscle spasticity.

ANALYZING DATA FROM THE PHYSICAL EXAMINATION

Once the physical examination has been completed, group any abnormal findings for each system with those of other systems. Use clinical judgment to identify common patterns of physiologic responses associated with health conditions. Individual abnormal physiologic responses are also the basis of many nursing diagnoses. Be sure to record all findings from the physical assessment legibly, in detail, and in the format approved by your institution.

Table 34–20   Assessment of Deep Tendon Reflexes and the Associated Spinal Segment Tested

Deep Tendon Reflex	Technique and Normal Findings*	Spine Segment Tested
Biceps	Flex the child's arm at the elbow, and place your thumb over the biceps tendon in the antecubital fossa. Tap your thumb. *Elbow flexes as the biceps muscle contracts.*	C5 and C6
Triceps	With the child's arm flexed, tap the triceps tendon above the elbow. *Elbow extends as the triceps muscle contracts.*	C6, C7, and C8
Brachioradialis	Lay the child's arm with the thumb upright over your arm. Tap the brachioradial tendon 2.5 cm (1 in.) above the wrist. *Forearm pronates (palm facing downward) and elbow flexes.*	C5 and C6

(continued)

Table 34–20	Assessment of Deep Tendon Reflexes and the Associated Spinal Segment Tested—continued	

Deep Tendon Reflex	Technique and Normal Findings*	Spine Segment Tested
Patellar 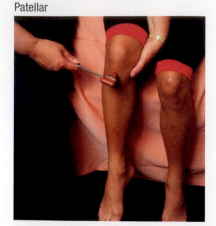	Flex the child's knees, and when the legs are relaxed, tap the patellar tendon just below the knee. *Knee extends (knee jerk) as the quadriceps muscle contracts.*	L2, L3, and L4
Achilles	While the child's legs are flexed, support the foot and tap the Achilles tendon. *Plantar flexion (ankle jerk) as the gastrocnemius muscle contracts.*	S1 and S2

*Italic text indicates normal findings.

Critical Concept Review

LEARNING OUTCOME 34.1: Describe the elements of a health history for infants and children of different ages.

Historical data to collect includes:
1. Chief complaint.
2. History of the present illness or injury.
3. Past history.
4. Current health status.
5. Review of systems.
6. Family history.
7. Psychosocial data.
8. Developmental data.

LEARNING OUTCOME 34.2: Apply communication strategies to improve the quality of historical data collected.

1. Introduce self, including purpose of interview.
2. Provide privacy, including confirmation of confidentiality.
3. Use open-ended questions.
4. Ask one question at a time.
5. Direct the question to the child when appropriate.
6. Be honest with the child and family.
7. Obtain feedback from parents to confirm understanding.

LEARNING OUTCOME 34.3: Demonstrate strategies to gain cooperation of a young child for assessment.

1. Allow the young child to stay in caretaker's lap for most of the examination.
2. Allow the young child to hold and examine any equipment before it is used on the child.
3. Make a game out of tests for muscle strength, coordination, and developmental assessment.

LEARNING OUTCOME 34.4: Describe the differences in sequence of the physical assessment for infants, children, and adolescents.

1. Be flexible in the examination sequence to assess the heart, lungs, and abdomen when the infant is quiet or asleep.
2. Any procedures causing anxiety (examination of throat and ears) should be delayed until the end of the physical assessment of toddlers and young children.
3. Physical examination of the school-age child should proceed in a head-to-toe fashion, with the exception of the genitalia examination (should be done last).
4. The physical examination of the adolescent may be completed without the presence of the parent, especially the examination of the genitalia.

LEARNING OUTCOME 34.5: Modify physical assessment techniques according to the age and developmental stage of the child.

Infants and toddlers:
1. Head circumference is required until age 2 years.
2. Palpate fontanelles until closure.
3. Assess vision and hearing response with the use of toys and familiar objects.
4. Perform the examination with the infant and toddler on the lap of the caregiver and use distraction.

Preschooler:
1. Ask young child to show teeth to begin assessment of the mouth and throat.

2. Use words or names easily recognized to assess hearing and memory.
3. Use play and activities to assess muscle strength and coordination.
4. Males should sit with knees crossed to assess genitalia.

Adolescent:
1. Ask if the adolescent wishes the parent to be present, and if not have a chaperone of the same gender present.
2. Assess stage of breast and pubic hair development in females. Assess stage of genital and pubic hair development in males.

LEARNING OUTCOME 34.6: List five normal variations in pediatric physical findings (such as a Mongolian spot in an infant) found during a physical assessment.

1. Epicanthal folds of the eyes.
2. Sucking pads in mouth of infant.
3. Rounded chest in infants.
4. Breath sounds heard over entire chest in infant.
5. Splitting of second heart sound that varies with breathing.
6. Abdominal movement with breathing.
7. Bowlegs and knock-knees.
8. Pubertal development.

LEARNING OUTCOME 34.7: Evaluate the growth pattern of an infant or child.

1. Weigh the child, taking two measurements and averaging them.
2. Measure the infant's length or child's height.
3. Measure the infant's head circumference (up to age 2 to 3 years).
4. Plot the child's current measurement on a growth curve appropriate for age and gender that has prior measurements plotted.
5. Identify the percentile in which weight, length, or height and head circumference fall. Determine if the plotted prior measurements indicate steady expected growth or a change in percentile that reflects poor growth or faster growth than expected for age.
6. Plot the infant's weight for length or calculate and plot the child's body mass index to determine if the child's weight is appropriate for height.

LEARNING OUTCOME 34.8: Distinguish between expected and unexpected physical signs to identify at least five signs that require urgent nursing intervention.

1. Altered level of consciousness.
2. Bradycardia.
3. Tachypnea (greater than 60 breaths per minute).
4. Pain.
5. Signs of dehydration (no tears, dry mucous membranes, doughy skin turgor, sunken fontanelle, increased urine concentration).
6. Stridor.
7. Retractions.
8. Cyanosis.

Clinical Reasoning in Action

It is a relatively calm night in the children's hospital emergency department when a 6-month-old infant named Colby is brought in by emergency personnel from an automobile crash. Colby was buckled in his infant, rear-facing, car safety seat, riding with his parents when another car rear-ended them. The parents were not hurt and did not need to go to the hospital.

The father immediately called 911 on his cell phone after the crash. When the ambulance arrived at the emergency room, the EMT gave you this report. Colby was alert and quiet in his father's arms when the ambulance arrived on the scene, and he did not have any obvious signs of trauma. Colby and his father were brought to the hospital to make sure Colby did not sustain any injuries from the crash. His vital signs are as follows: temperature—98.9°F, respirations—32, pulse—110, and blood pressure—85/39. Colby is in no apparent distress. His pupils are equal, round, and reactive to light. His anterior fontanelle is flat, and he has equal movements of extremities.

His breath sounds are clear and equal bilaterally. His heart sounds have a regular rate and rhythm without murmur. He voided around 2 hours ago, before the accident.

1. The fontanelles are an important body part to examine in infants and toddlers. In the scenario with Colby, it can give an indication of increased intracranial pressure related to a brain injury. Describe the placement of the fontanelles, and when they should close and no longer be palpated. Why is the head more likely to sustain injury in an infant like Colby versus an adult?

2. After reviewing the scenario, what can you tell the parents about Colby's vital signs at this time? What is the difference between adult vital signs and Colby's vital signs?

3. Describe what structures in the chest and abdominal area of Colby's body would be of concern after being in this automobile crash.

4. If a heart murmur were to be found on examination of Colby, what would be the five ways to describe it?

See www.nursing.pearsonhighered.com for possible responses.

References

American Academy of Ophthalmology Pediatric Ophthalmology/Strabismus Panel. (2007). *Preferred Practice Pattern® Guidelines. Pediatric eye evaluations.* San Francisco, CA: Author. Retrieved from http://one.aao.org/ce/practiceguidelines/ppp_content.aspx?cid=621682dc-7871-4351-830e-545b1273d84c

American Speech and Language Association. (2011). *How does your child hear and talk?* Retrieved from http://www.asha.org/public/speech/development/chart.htm

Bernstein, D. (2011). Coarctation of the aorta. In R. M. Kliegman, B. F. Stanton, J. W. St. Geme, N. F. Schor, & R. E. Behrman, *Nelson textbook of pediatrics* (19th ed., pp. 1567–1570). Philadelphia, PA: Elsevier Saunders.

Biro, F. M., Galvez, M. P., Greenspan, L. C., Succop, P. A., Vangeepuram, M., Pinney, S. M., . . . Wolff, K. S. (2010). Pubertal assessment method and baseline characteristics in a mixed longitudinal study of girls. *Pediatrics, 126*(3), e583–e590.

Brown, N. (2011). Adolescent medicine. In M. M. Tschudy & K. M. Arcara (Eds.), *The Harriet Lane handbook* (19th ed., pp. 118–135). St. Louis, MO: Elsevier.

Chameides, L., Samson, R. A., Schexnayder, S. M., & Hazinski, M. F. (Eds.). (2011). *Pediatric advanced life support: Provider manual.* Dallas, TX: American Heart Association.

Feigelman, S. (2011a). The first year. In R. M. Kliegman, B. F. Stanton, J. W. St. Geme, N. F. Schor, & R. E. Behrman, *Nelson textbook of pediatrics* (19th ed., pp. 26–31). Philadelphia, PA: Elsevier Saunders.

Feigelman, S. (2011b). The second year. In R. M. Kliegman, B. F. Stanton, J. W. St. Geme, N. F. Schor, & R. E. Behrman, *Nelson textbook of pediatrics* (19th ed., pp. 31–33). Philadelphia, PA: Elsevier Saunders.

Fonseca, H., & Greydanus, D. E. (2007). Sexuality in the child, teen, and young adult: Concepts for the clinician. *Primary Care Clinics in Office Practice, 34*, 275–292.

Harris, T. S. (2010). Bruises in children: Normal or child abuse? *Journal of Pediatric Health Care, 24*(4), 216–221.

Hermann-Giddens, M. E., Bourdony, C. J., Dowshen, S. A., & Reiter, E. O. (2011). *Assessment of sexual maturity stages in girls and boys.* Elk Grove Village, IL: American Academy of Pediatrics.

Hummel, P. (2011). Newborn assessment. In E. M. Chiocca, *Advanced pediatric assessment* (pp. 199–229). Philadelphia, PA: Wolters Kluwer Lippincott Williams & Wilkins.

Lande, M. B. (2011). Systemic hypertension. In R. M. Kliegman, B. F. Stanton, J. W. St. Geme, N. F. Schor, & R. E. Behrman, *Nelson textbook of pediatrics* (19th ed., pp. 1639–1647). Philadelphia, PA: Elsevier Saunders.

Pappas, D. E., & Hendly, J. O. (2011). Sinusitis. In R. M. Kliegman, B. F. Stanton, J. W. St. Geme, N. F. Schor, & R. E. Behrman, *Nelson textbook of pediatrics* (19th ed., pp. 1436–1438). Philadelphia, PA: Elsevier Saunders.

Purnell, L. D. (2009). *Guide to culturally competent care* (2nd ed.). Philadelphia, PA: Davis.

Susman, E. J., Houts, R. M., Steinberg, L., Belsky, J., Cauffman, E., De Hart, G., . . . Eunice Kennedy Shriver NICHD Early Child Care Research Network. (2010). Longitudinal development of secondary sexual characteristics in girls and boys between ages 9½ and 15½ years. *Archives of Pediatric and Adolescent Medicine, 164*(2), 166–173.

Tuli, S. S., Kockler, V., Kelly, M. N., & Tuli, S. Y. (2010). What's your diagnosis? Heterochromia iridis. *Consultant for Pediatricians, 9*(11), 405–406.

Walvoord, E. C. (2010). The timing of puberty: Is it changing? Does it matter? *Journal of Adolescent Health, 47*(5), 433–439.

Zitelli, B. J., McIntire, S. J., & Nowalk, A. J. (2012). *Atlas of pediatric physical diagnosis* (6th ed.). Philadelphia, PA: Elsevier Saunders.

Pearson Nursing Student Resources Find additional review materials at: **nursing.pearsonhighered.com**

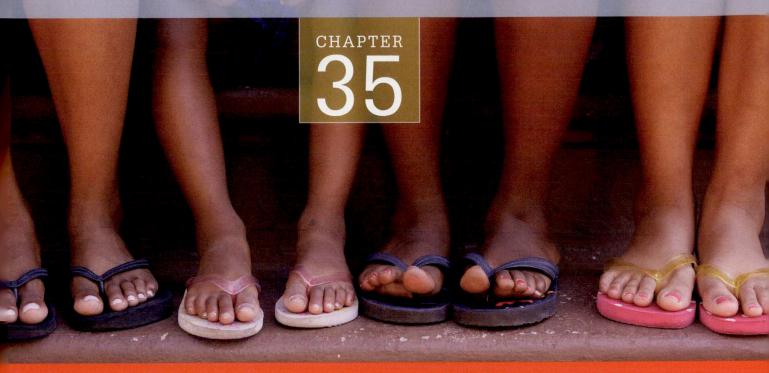

Health Promotion and Maintenance: General Concepts, the Newborn, and the Infant

Mommy was really glad to go see the nurse today. She brought our baby and me. Grandma said that they would give us a card that would help us buy food. I'm glad because I'm tired of eating peanut butter. Mommy said we could get some milk and juice, and even some chicken. —Melody, age 4, sister of 7-month-old Amanda

Roger Charity/Getty Images

LEARNING OUTCOMES

35.1   Define health promotion and health maintenance.

35.2   Describe how health promotion and health maintenance are facilitated by partnering with families during health supervision visits.

35.3   Describe the components of a health supervision visit.

35.4   Analyze the nurse's role in providing health promotion and health maintenance for the newborn and infant.

35.5   Perform the general observations made of infants and their families as they come to the pediatric healthcare home for health supervision visits.

35.6   Synthesize the areas of assessment and intervention for health supervision visits of newborns and infants: growth and developmental surveillance, nutrition, physical activity, oral health, mental and spiritual health, family and social relations, disease prevention strategies, and injury prevention strategies.

35.7   Plan health promotion and health maintenance strategies employed during health supervision visits of newborns and infants.

35.8   Recognize the importance of family in newborn and infant health care, and include family assessment in each health supervision visit.

35.9   Integrate pertinent mental health care into health supervision visits for newborns and infants.

35.10   Evaluate data about the family and other social relationships to promote and maintain health of newborns and infants.

927

A major goal of *Healthy People 2020* is to help individuals attain long, healthy lives free of preventable disease, disability, injury, and premature death across all life stages (U.S. Department of Health and Human Services, 2011). The concepts of health promotion and health maintenance provide for nursing interventions that contribute to meeting these goals. Many students in health professions begin their studies with a strong interest in the care of ill individuals. However, as time progresses, they learn that "well" people need care also. They need teaching to improve diet, reduce stress, and obtain immunizations. They may seek information about how to exercise properly or ensure a safe environment for their children. These examples of care and teaching are components of health promotion and health maintenance.

Nursing is a holistic profession that examines and works with all aspects of the lives of individuals, and has a strong focus on family and community as well. Nurses are uniquely positioned to provide health promotion and health maintenance activities, and indeed these activities should be a part of each encounter with families. What is the difference between health promotion and health maintenance? When should nurses engage in activities that focus on health? How are these activities integrated into health supervision visits for the infant and young child? How do nurses partner with other healthcare professionals to offer comprehensive health services in settings accessible to parents and young children? How can nurses help children and their families to maximize length and quality of life? These are some of the questions that will be explored in this chapter, with specific activities that target families with newborns, infants, and young children.

GENERAL CONCEPTS

To understand health promotion and health maintenance, it is important to develop a definition of health. The World Health Organization (WHO) defines **health** as a state of complete physical, mental, and social well-being and not merely the absence of disease and infirmity (WHO, 2010). Others view the quality of "complete well-being" as impossible to attain, and therefore have further developed the concept to apply to persons with health challenges as well as those who are "healthy." Health in this expanded view is dynamic, changing, and unfolding; it is the realization of a state of actualization or potential (Pender, Murdaugh, & Parsons, 2011). This basic human right is necessary for the development of societies.

Health promotion refers to activities that increase well-being and enhance wellness or health (Pender et al., 2011). These activities lead to actualization of positive health potential for all individuals, even those with chronic or acute conditions. Examples include providing information and resources in order to:

- Enhance good nutrition at each developmental stage.
- Integrate physical activity into the child's daily events.
- Provide adequate housing.
- Promote oral health.
- Foster positive personality development.

Health promotion is concerned with development of strategies that seek to foster conditions that allow populations to be healthy and to make healthy choices (WHO, 2011). Nurses engage in health promotion by partnering with children and families to promote family strengths in the areas of lifestyles, social development, coping, and family interactions. They also provide **anticipatory guidance** for families because they understand the child's upcoming developmental stages, and they teach families how to provide an environment that helps children achieve the milestones of each stage. This concept is explored more fully later in this chapter.

Health maintenance (or health protection) refers to activities that preserve an individual's present state of health and that prevent disease or injury occurrence. Examples of these activities include conducting developmental screening or surveillance to identify early deviations from normal development, providing immunizations to prevent illnesses, and teaching about common childhood safety hazards. Health maintenance activities are commonly preventive in nature, and terminology common to community or public health nursing explains the levels and aims of preventive actions. Prevention levels are identified as primary prevention, secondary prevention, and tertiary prevention (Table 35–1).

While it is clear that health promotion and health maintenance activities are closely linked and often overlap, there are some differences. Health maintenance focuses on known potential health risks and seeks to prevent them or to identify them early so that intervention can occur. Health promotion looks at the strengths and goals of individuals, families, and populations, and seeks to use them to assist in reaching higher levels of wellness. It involves partnerships with the family as health goals are set, and with other health professionals and resources to provide for meeting a family's goals. Nurses apply both health promotion and health maintenance concepts when providing health care, recognizing that the concepts overlap. Health promotion and health maintenance are integrated into healthcare visits for children, with the care provider applying both knowledge of health maintenance concepts and adding information the family has identified that will assist in increasing health or wellness (health promotion). These activities commonly take place at "well-child" or health supervision visits.

Health supervision for children is the provision of services that focus on disease and injury prevention (health maintenance), growth and developmental surveillance, and health promotion at key intervals during the child's life. What health promotion and health maintenance activities are parts of health supervision visits? How can these activities be integrated into all settings where care is provided for children? What are the recommended times for health visits to occur and what care is provided at certain times? How can health supervision visits be organized to accomplish the goals of the family and health professionals? These and other questions will be answered in this section and the following section focused on nursing management.

All children need a medical home, where accessible, continuous, and coordinated health supervision is provided during the developmental years. Accessibility refers to both financial and geographic access; continuous indicates that the care is ongoing with consistent care providers; coordination refers to the need for communication among health professionals to provide for the needs of the child. A medical home or **pediatric healthcare home** is therefore the site where comprehensive, continuous, culturally sensitive, coordinated, and compassionate health care is provided by a pediatric healthcare professional focused on the overall well-being of children and families (National Association of Pediatric Nurse Associates and Practitioners [NAPNAP], 2009). When a family has an established partnership with a care provider, family-centered health services can be provided based on the family's risks and protective factors. These services may be provided in physicians' offices, community health clinics, the home, schools, childcare centers, shelters, or mobile vans (Figure 35–1 ●). The U.S. Department of Health and Human Services, the American Academy of Pediatrics (AAP), and the American Medical Association have developed national guidelines for preventive healthcare services for infants, children, and adolescents. NAPNAP supports the list of comprehensive services of a pediatric healthcare home identified by the AAP (2010a).

The health supervision visit is individualized to the family and child. Standardized screenings and examinations are included, and time is provided for the family's specific concerns and questions about the child's health. Nurses play an integral part in these comprehensive visits, and they partner with other healthcare providers to accomplish health supervision.

Table 35–1	Levels of Preventive Health Maintenance Activities	
Level	**Description**	**Examples of Nursing Actions**
Primary prevention	Activities that decrease opportunity for illness or injury	Giving immunizations Teaching about car safety seats
Secondary prevention	Early diagnosis and treatment of a condition to lessen its severity	Developmental screening Vision and hearing screening
Tertiary prevention	Restoration to optimal function	Rehabilitation activities for child after a car crash

Source: Data from Murray, R. B., Zentner, J. P., & Yakimo, R. (2009). *Health promotion strategies through the life span* (8th ed.). Upper Saddle River, NJ: Pearson Prentice Hall.

Clinical Tip

The American Academy of Pediatrics and the National Association of Pediatric Nurse Associates and Practitioners concur that a pediatric healthcare home should offer the following:

- Family-centered care and trusting partnership
- Sharing of unbiased and clear information
- Provision of primary care to include acute and chronic care, breastfeeding promotion, immunizations, growth and development, screenings, healthcare supervision, and counseling about health, nutrition, safety, parenting, and psychosocial issues
- Continuously accessible care
- Continuity of care
- Provision of compassionate, developmentally appropriate, and culturally competent care
- Referral to early intervention and child care
- Coordination of services and collaboration of professionals
- Maintenance of a comprehensive central record
- Referral to specialists as needed

Source: Data from American Academy of Pediatrics. (2008). *The National Center for Medical Home Initiatives for Children with Special Needs.* Retrieved from http://www.medicalhomeinfo.org/training/index.html; National Association of Pediatric Nurse Practitioners (NAPNAP). (2009). NAPNAP position statement on the pediatric health care/medical home. *Journal of Pediatric Health Care, 23*(3), 23A–24A.

● **Figure 35–1** Delivery of health promotion services. *A,* A nurse is providing a health supervision visit in the child's home after discharge from the hospital for an acute illness. *B,* A nurse is providing information to a child visiting a mobile healthcare van.

A tracking system in the pediatric healthcare home site helps to identify appropriate health supervision activities for each child at every visit. Most often computers are used to list appropriate topics for visits at specific ages. If a child misses a visit, the family can be contacted by phone and encouraged to come in for the recommended care. A family may be called if their child is lacking some immunizations. Recognizing that not all families get into the healthcare home for each recommended visit, every health encounter, including an episodic illness visit or care for a chronic illness, is a potential time to complete health promotion and health maintenance activities. For example, immunizations may sometimes be given during a visit for an acute condition such as otitis media (ear infection) if the child has missed a prior health supervision visit. Even when children are

seen in hospitals, emergency departments, or other settings, it is important to ask about their pediatric healthcare home and when the last visit occurred. Identify children who need basic health supervision services and provide them or refer to other settings for meeting these needs at another time.

Nurses play an important role in managing health supervision visits. Depending on the setting, the nurse may provide all services or support other care providers by obtaining an updated health history, screening for diseases and other conditions, conducting a developmental assessment, and providing immunizations, anticipatory guidance, and health education. Nurses in all settings are instrumental in identifying children who need health supervision and are not obtaining recommended care (Figure 35–2 ●).

● **Figure 35–2** Identifying children who need health care. The nurse plays many roles in providing health promotion and health maintenance for children. *A,* Data are collected from the time a nurse calls the child and family to the examination room and during the history-taking phase. The nurse asks questions while observing the child's behaviors and the relationship between parent and child. The nurse also performs screening tests, including blood pressure, tuberculosis, vision and hearing, and developmental screening. *B,* Interventions that include teaching may take place. *C,* A nurse may administer immunizations as parents watch and assist by holding the child. Nurses also play important roles in teaching families information to enhance health.

While health supervision visits can address many health-related topics, there is generally a limited time in which to engage a child or family. The nurse needs to direct the encounters and have some ideas for pertinent agendas. *Bright Futures* booklets provide guidance about how the nurse can manage health supervision visits. Six concepts should be integrated into care (Hagan, Shaw, & Duncan, 2008):

1. The care provider *builds effective partnerships* with the family. A **partnership** is a relationship in which participants join together to ensure healthcare delivery in a way that recognizes the critical roles and contributions of each partner in promoting health and preventing illness. The partners in child health include the child, family, health professionals, and the community.

2. The nurse *fosters family-centered communication* by showing interest in the child and family, and effectively conveying information and understanding.

3. The nurse *focuses on health promotion and health maintenance topics during visits*, recognizing that families may not initiate these discussions.

4. The nurse *manages time well* to enable health promotion topics to be addressed during visits. This includes reviewing the child's health record and selecting topics pertinent to the child's age and the family's situation.

5. The nurse *educates the family during "teachable moments."* Large teaching plans are not always needed; children and families often learn best when presented with small bits of information based on the parent's questions or the nurse's observations.

6. The nurse *becomes an advocate for child health issues.* When an issue arises while caring for a child, seek additional data from various sources, talk with others, and strategize how the problem could be solved.

COMPONENTS OF HEALTH PROMOTION/HEALTH MAINTENANCE VISITS

The nurse identifies and addresses pertinent topics for health promotion and health maintenance during health supervision visits. Nurses also apply their knowledge of areas that need to be addressed with an infant or child of a particular age, and then make general observations of the child and family to identify additional topics for discussion. While categories to consider vary depending on the age of the child, the family's particular needs, and community resources, there are some common topics that generally require attention. Often, nurses start with the topics described as follows, integrating general observations as the visit progresses, and further identifying assessment areas needed in particular situations.

Pediatric nurses make *general observations* of infants and their families whenever they encounter them. Nurses who are observant during the health supervision visit have many opportunities for assessing the family. These general observations begin when the family is called in and welcomed by the nurse to the facility. They continue as the infant or child is weighed and measured, and throughout the visit. Nurses observe the physical contact between the child and other family members, the developmental tasks displayed by the child, and parental level of stress or ease in conducting childcare activities.

Growth and developmental surveillance provides important clues about the child's condition and environment. The child's height, weight, and body mass index are calculated at each health supervision visit, and results are placed on percentile charts (see Chapter 32 🔗 and Chapter 33 🔗 for more information). Parents are given the information in written form and it is interpreted for them. A thorough physical assessment is performed to ensure the child is growing as expected and has no abnormal or unexplained physical findings (see Chapter 34 🔗). **Developmental surveillance** is a flexible, continuous process of skilled observations that provides data about the child's capabilities, allows for early identification of any neurologic problems, and helps to verify that the home environment is stimulating. Early development is important to later health and it must be evaluated consistently and systematically during healthcare visits (AAP, 2010a). Information may be collected from several sources, for instance, a questionnaire that the parent completes, questions asked during the interview, or observation of the child during the visit. Parents can also be interviewed to identify any developmental concerns they may have about the child or adolescent. When talking with parents, review physical, social, and communication milestones for infants, young children, older children, or adolescents. Detailed milestones for each age group are found in Chapter 32 🔗. Standardized developmental questionnaires are effective for developmental surveillance of most children, especially when time for health supervision visits is limited. Screening tests should be administered at the 9-, 18-, and the 24- or 30-month visits (Lipkin, 2011). A commonly used test is the Denver II, which can be applied as a developmental chart, like a growth curve, to monitor the child's developmental progress (Figure 35–3 ● and Figure 35–4 ●). When performing developmental screening with the Denver II or any other standardized screening tools, nurses make sure all directions are followed by:

- Choosing the proper test for the child's age and desired information
- Reading directions thoroughly or using specific training tools available
- Practicing as needed until proficient with the test
- Calculating the infant's or child's age correctly, especially if premature
- Attempting to develop rapport with the infant or child to get the best performance
- Following directions for administration of items; in some cases, parents can be asked if a child demonstrates specific skills at home, especially if the child is not willing to perform an item during testing
- Noting the behavior and cooperativeness of the child during the screening process
- Analyzing the findings using the test instructions to make the correct interpretation

A

B

C

D

● **Figure 35–3** The Denver II assessment. Follow all directions for performing the Denver II assessment and for interpreting responses. Develop rapport with the child and approach the assessment as fun. This often helps the child participate more actively during the entire Denver II assessment. *A,* The mother reports personal-social tasks the child has performed. The 6-month-old girl is able to perform the following age-appropriate behaviors: *B,* Look for yarn and follow it 180 degrees; *C,* bang two cubes together; *D,* sit without support.

Failure to perform an item in a single domain does not mean the child has failed the test (see *Developing Cultural Competence: English as a Second Language and Developmental Testing*). The child should be reevaluated at a future visit. Schedule the appointment at a time of day when the child is awake and rested. Provide parents with guidance on specific methods for stimulating the child. Failure of multiple items within one domain or across multiple domains is of greatest concern. When poor development patterns in one or more domains are revealed, referral for diagnostic developmental assessment is needed.

Nutrition evaluation is a vital part of each health supervision visit. It makes important contributions to general health and fosters growth and development. Include observations and screening relevant to nutritional intake at each health supervision visit. Eating proper foods for age and activity ensures that children have the energy for proper growth, physical activity, cognition, and immune function. Nutrition is closely linked to both health promotion and health maintenance. See Chapter 33 🔗 for detailed nutritional assessments

Developing Cultural Competence
English as a Second Language and Developmental Testing

Children who have recently come from other countries and even some born in this country who live in families from minority ethnic groups may have difficulty with some items on developmental tests. For example, children who are not skilled in the English language may not understand some instructions or be able to answer questions about definitions of words. When parents do not speak English as a primary language and the examiner uses English, common terms might be misinterpreted. Parents might not understand what is meant if you ask, "Does your baby have a mobile over the crib at home?" or "Is she starting to be afraid of strangers?" How can you be alert for language differences and become sensitive to miscommunication?

for each age group. Find out what questions parents have about feeding their children. Use the information gathered to provide both health promotion and health maintenance interventions.

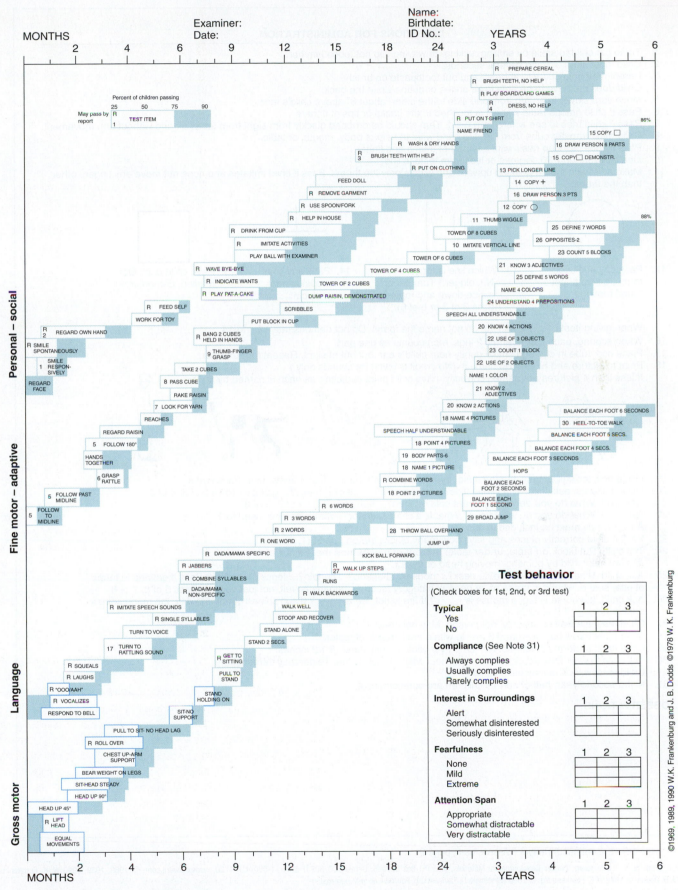

Figure 35–4 Denver II Assessment, page 1.

DIRECTIONS FOR ADMINISTRATION

1. Try to get child to smile by smiling, talking, or waving. Do not touch him/her.
2. Child must stare at hand several seconds.
3. Parent may help guide toothbrush and put toothpaste on brush.
4. Child does not have to be able to tie shoes or button/zip in the back.
5. Move yarn slowly in an arc from one side to the other, about 8" above child's face.
6. Pass if child grasps rattle when it is touched to the backs or tips of fingers.
7. Pass if child tries to see where yarn went. Yarn should be dropped quickly from sight from tester's hand without arm movement.
8. Child must transfer cube from hand to hand without help of body, mouth, or table.
9. Pass if child picks up raisin with any part of thumb and finger.
10. Line can vary only 30 degrees or less from tester's line.
11. Make a fist with thumb pointing upward and wiggle only the thumb. Pass if child imitates and does not move any fingers other than the thumb.

12. Pass any enclosed form. Fail continuous round motions.
13. Which line is longer? (Not bigger.) Turn paper upside down and repeat. (pass 3 of 3 or 5 of 6).
14. Pass any lines crossing near midpoint.
15. Have child copy first. If failed, demonstrate.

When giving items 12, 14, and 15, do not name the forms. Do not demonstrate 12 and 14.

16. When scoring, each pair (2 arms, 2 legs, etc.) counts as one part.
17. Place one cube in cup and shake gently near child's ear, but out of sight. Repeat for other ear.
18. Point to picture and have child name it. (No credit is given for sounds only.)
    If less than 4 pictures are named correctly, have child point to picture as each is named by tester.

19. Using doll, tell child: Show me the nose, eyes, ears, mouth, hands, feet, tummy, hair. Pass 6 of 8.
20. Using pictures, ask child: Which one flies?... says meow?... talks?... barks?... gallops? Pass 2 of 5, 4 of 5.
21. Ask child: What do you do when you are cold?... tired?... hungry? Pass 2 of 3, 3 of 3.
22. Ask child: What do you do with a cup? What is a chair used for? What is a pencil used for?
    Action words must be included in answers.
23. Pass if child correctly places <u>and</u> says how many blocks are on paper. (1, 5).
24. Tell child: Put block **on** table; **under** table: **in front of** me, **behind** me. Pass 4 of 4.
    (Do not help child by pointing, moving head or eyes.)
25. Ask child: What is a ball?... lake?... desk?... house?... banana?... curtain?... fence?... ceiling? Pass if defined in terms of use, shape, what it is made of, or general category (such as banana is fruit, not just yellow). Pass 5 of 8, 7 of 8.
26. Ask child: If a horse is big, a mouse is_____? If fire is hot, ice is_____? If sun shines during the day, the moon shines during the ____? Pass 2 of 3.
27. Child may use wall or rail only, not person. May not crawl.
28. Child must throw ball overhand 3 feet to within arm's reach of tester.
29. Child must perform standing broad jump over width of test sheet (8 1/2 inches).
30. Tell child to walk forward, ⊂○⊃⊂○⊃⊂○⊃ → heel within 1 inch of toe. Tester may demonstrate.
    Child must walk 4 consecutive steps.
31. In the second year, half of normal children are non-compliant.

OBSERVATIONS:

● **Figure 35–4** (continued) Denver II Assessment, page 2 .

Source: From W. K. Frankenburg, Denver Developmental Materials, Inc., PO Box 371075, Denver, CO 80237-5075, 1-800-419-4729, www.denverii.com. © 1969, 1989, 1990 W. K. Frankenburg and J. B. Dodds. © 1978 W. K. Frankenburg. © 2009 Wilhelmine R. Frankenburg. Reproduced with permission.

Physical activity provides many physical and psychologic health benefits. However, there is a growing disparity between recommendations and reality among most children. Research by the Centers for Disease Control and Prevention (CDC) has identified that about 23% of children from 9 to 13 years report no free-time physical activity. When schools do not offer daily physical education, many children have no regular activity. Participation in physical activity declines as youth get older, and females are considerably less active than males (CDC, 2010b). Inquire about activities the child prefers and amount of time for activity during the day. As the child grows older, include questions about sedentary activities such as number of hours spent watching television or playing computer games. See if the child plays sports at school or in the community. Ask about activities in a typical day to measure amount of activity. Once the nurse gathers data about physical activity, interventions are implemented to enhance activity patterns.

Although *oral health* may seem to require the knowledge of a specialist, it has many implications that relate to general health care. Oral health is important because teeth assist in language development, impacted or infected teeth lead to systemic illness, and teeth are related to positive self-image formation. Dental caries is the most common chronic disease of children. Many youth in the United States are affected by tooth decay and pain that interfere with activities of daily living such as eating, sleeping, attending school, and speaking (CDC, 2011a, 2011b). The nurse applies health promotion to dental health by teaching about oral care and access to dental visits. Health maintenance activities relate to prevention of caries and illness related to dental disease.

Mental and spiritual health are important concepts to address in health promotion and health maintenance visits. Parents can be encouraged to keep a record of mental health issues to bring to health supervision visits. This helps them understand that the healthcare professional is willing to partner with them to assist in dealing with mental health. Suggest topics such as child and parental mood, child temperament, stresses and ways that family members manage stress, or sleep patterns. Make notes in the record as a reminder of questions to ask at the next visit. The child and family are both observed for appropriateness of affect and mood. Be alert for signs of depression, stress, anxiety, and child abuse or neglect. The nurse establishes both health promotion and health maintenance goals related to child and family mental health. Health promotion goals relate to adequate resources to meet family challenges and protective factors such as involvement in extended family and the community. Teaching stress reduction techniques such as meditation, relaxation, and imagery, as well as providing resources for yoga or other techniques, is helpful. Health maintenance goals relate to prevention of mental health problems. Examples include providing resources when domestic violence occurs, or referring cases of suspected child abuse or neglect. The **spiritual dimension** is a connection with a greater power than that in the self, and guides a person to strive for inspiration, respect, meaning, and purpose in life (Murray, Zentner, & Yakimo, 2009). Spiritual health is seen in the large context as those entities that provide meaning in life. For some, this may be membership in a faith-based group; for others it may be feeling part of a society with a purpose of greater good, or setting goals for the future. Ask about the family's meaningful activities. Provide links to faith-based groups as needed.

The *relationships* that a child establishes with others begin at birth. The first and most important set of relationships develops with the family. The mother, father, siblings, and perhaps extended family are the contexts in which the baby learns to relate with others. With growth the world widens to encompass other children, friends of the family, peers, school, and the larger community network. Analyzing the child's relationships at all ages provides important clues to social interactions. From the moment the family is called in from a waiting area, be alert for clues to family interactions. Likewise, other social interactions are important to evaluate. Does the young infant interact in an age-appropriate manner with the healthcare provider or other children in the area? Ask the parents questions about family and social interactions. Once assessment has taken place, establish goals and interventions related to family and social relationships.

Disease prevention strategies focus mainly on health maintenance, or prevention of disease. Some health disruptions can be detected early and treatment for the condition can begin. **Screening** is a procedure used to detect the possible presence of a health condition before symptoms are apparent. It is usually conducted on large groups of individuals at risk for a condition and represents the secondary level of prevention (Figure 35–5 ●). Most screening tests are not diagnostic by themselves but are followed by further diagnostic tests if the screening result is positive. Once a screening test identifies the existence of a health condition, early intervention can begin, with the goal of reducing the severity or complications of the condition (secondary prevention). Another way to prevent diseases is to immunize children against common communicable diseases (primary prevention). See Chapter 44 ● for the complete list of childhood immunizations and schedules for administration.

Developing Cultural Competence
Unmet Dental Needs

Over one half of children from homes with low incomes have not received dental care in the past year; twice as many have unmet dental needs when compared to children in homes with adequate finances (Child Trends, 2011). Hispanic children, children with disabilities, and children with parents who are poor, have a low educational level, or lack health insurance are also more likely to have unmet dental needs (Child Trends, 2011; Tanski, Garfunkel, Duncan, et al., 2010). All children in the Medicaid program are eligible for dental coverage through the Early and Periodic Screening, Diagnostic, and Treatment (EPSDT) program. Private and public clinics in many communities provide low-cost or free care for families with limited financial resources. Many families do not realize their children could receive these services. Find out what resources are available in your state and community, and refer as needed. See Chapter 1 ● for further description of programs mentioned here.

Activity · Case Study: Domestic Violence

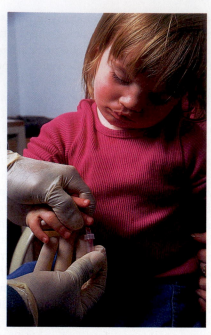

● **Figure 35–5** Blood screening test. This young child is having a blood screening test to detect iron deficiency anemia. Children are often screened for adequate levels of iron in later infancy and during toddlerhood.

Most childhood mortality and hospitalization is related to injury (CDC, 2010a) (see Chapter 1 🔗 for more information). Therefore, it is important for the nurse to integrate *injury prevention* strategies in all health supervision visits. The family is constantly challenged to maintain a safe environment as the child grows older, reaches more advanced developmental levels, is exposed to a widening world outside of the family, and has less supervision. Safety teaching should be integrated with developmental progression. Asking parents to bring their questions about safety to each visit can be a good starting point for discussion. The nurse considers knowledge about the age of the child and information from the health supervision visit to plan health maintenance interventions related to injury. Teaching is performed, resources are made available, and parents and children who have experienced injury are invited to present their experiences.

Many other topics might be discussed during health supervision visits. They may relate to either health maintenance activities designed to preserve health, or health promotion activities designed to enhance or improve the state of wellness. Topics include extended family members and their role in the child's life, cultural variations or inclusion, or development of moral values and ethical behaviors.

HEALTH PROMOTION AND MAINTENANCE OF THE NEWBORN AND INFANT

The month following delivery is a time of huge transition for the new mother and her family. Not only is the mother coping with hormonal shifts and a **postpartum** (after giving birth) body, but

roles and relationships are also changing. The role of the nurse is to assess knowledge about self-care and newborn care, teach health promotion and maintenance activities, promote parental confidence in newborn caregiving, and facilitate a partnership among healthcare professionals and the family.

Infancy is a major life transition for the baby and parents. The infant accomplishes phenomenal physical growth and many developmental milestones while the family adapts to the addition of a new member and establishes new goals for each of its existing members. Infant health supervision visits are very important to support the health of the baby and the family unit. These visits begin after the newborn period, at about 1 month of age. This is the time when parents establish an ongoing partnership with a healthcare provider. A "medical home" or "pediatric healthcare home" is identified to serve the baby's health needs. The goals of health supervision visits are to identify and address the health promotion and health maintenance needs of the infant.

Facilitating breastfeeding, helping parents to understand their newborn's and infant's temperament, and employing strategies to ensure adequate sleep by the baby and parents are examples of health promotion activities. Health maintenance activities focus on disease and injury prevention. Some examples of these interventions include administering immunizations and teaching about infant car seats.

An established relationship with a healthcare provider and agency is important so that trust develops and the family will feel comfortable about turning to the professionals for information and guidance as the baby grows. Nurses play a vital role in welcoming new families into office and clinic settings, establishing rapport, and applying principles of communication so that trust and positive partnerships develop between providers and families. Infancy is a time when the child grows in physical, psychologic, and cognitive ways; health supervision visits play a key role in fostering healthy growth and development. When should the infant be seen for health supervision visits? What are key components of these visits? How can the nurse best assess and intervene to ensure the infant's health and safety? These are some of the questions that will be answered in this section of the chapter.

Early Contacts with the Family

Most obstetric care providers encourage the expectant mother to choose her newborn's care provider prior to the baby's birth (see *Clinical Reasoning: Choosing the Newborn's Care Provider*). Pediatric care providers usually welcome a short office visit, sometimes at no charge, to allow the expectant mother and care provider to assess their compatibility prior to initiating the care provider relationship. Many pediatric care providers provide written information to expectant parents, explaining their professional philosophy of care as well as information about services.

Health promotion and maintenance for the newborn begin during the stay in the hospital or birthing center (see Chapters 26, 27, and 28 🔗). On discharge, referral may be indicated to a lactation consultant or follow-up healthcare visit. The hospital length of stay for a healthy mother and newborn after term delivery is short, approximately 48 hours for a vaginal birth and 72 to 96 hours for an uncomplicated cesarean birth. Discharge of the mother and baby should only occur after appropriate growth is confirmed and a thorough physical examination shows normal results. There should be time to identify any problems and to make certain that the family can care for the newborn at home, and ideally the mother and newborn should be discharged together (AAP, 2010b, 2011). For newborns discharged between 48 and 72 hours of age, the first follow-up healthcare visit should occur by 5 days of age. The purpose of this visit is to ensure that the newborn is continuing to progress normally and that no previously undiscovered problems have surfaced. At this initial contact, the nurse promotes maternal confidence in caregiving and offers education and anticipatory guidance. Careful assessments are made for hyperbilirubinemia, feeding problems, or other abnormalities. Further visits are established as needed from 5 days to 1 month; the first scheduled health supervision of infancy is at 1 month of age.

Health promotion and maintenance for infancy occur in a series of health supervision visits during the first year of life. Schedules vary among facilities, but a common pattern includes visits at about 1 month, 2 months, 4 months, 6 months, 9 months, and 1 year of age. In addition, most children have some episodic illnesses such as gastrointestinal illness or otitis media and visit the facility at other times for treatment of these illnesses. A few children have chronic or serious healthcare problems during the first year, and have extensive contact with the healthcare home and other services.

During these first visits, assess the family for protective factors and risks. Protective factors might include knowledge level of infant needs, support from family and friends, and the mother's good health and nutritional state during pregnancy. Risk factors could include limited financial resources, lack of preparation for the baby, and illness or other stress among family members. Ask about how the family traveled to the visit, and if convenient times and transportation are available. Lack of access during times the family is not at work and other health system barriers sometimes interfere with attendance at health supervision visits. Knowledge of risk factors will shape the nursing interventions during the first health supervision in infancy. The nurse applies health promotion principles by building on strengths and fosters health maintenance by intervening to minimize risks.

General Observations

When the family comes to the clinic or office for care with a newborn or infant, general observations should begin at first contact (Figure 35–6 ●). Welcome the family warmly to

● **Figure 35–6** General observations. The nurse begins assessment of the infant's family when they are seen in the waiting room and called in for care. What observations can you make of the infant's general appearance? Developmental accomplishments? Interaction of parents with the baby?

the facility and comment on the baby. Ask how the family is doing with the baby and how the adjustment is going. Be alert for signs of fatigue or depression in the parents, as these can occur when caring for an infant and can interfere with bonding and positive transition. Look for clues about cultural orientation. The nurse gathers information in order to assess the needs of the family, to invite discussion, to validate positive parenting efforts, and to promote partnership between the family and the healthcare team. Upon entering the examination room, it is helpful to explain the plans for the visit, such as "I will weigh and measure Sarah now and show you how she is growing. Then I'll ask a few questions about her eating, sleeping, and other things. Then the nurse practitioner will be in to do Sarah's physical examination. Do you have any questions as we start? Will you undress Sarah now so we can weigh her accurately?"

Growth and Developmental Surveillance

Assessment of growth and development begins at birth and continues in newborn and infant health promotion and maintenance visits. (See Chapter 32 ⊘ for important background/theoretical information about growth and development.) Note the posture, flexion, reflexes, and physical attributes that help evaluate gestational age. Physical growth and meeting of developmental milestones provide important information about infants. The baby is measured for accurate length, weight, and head circumference (Figure 35–7 ●). (See the *Clinical Skills Manual* SKILLS and Chapter 34 ⊘ for detailed information about the physical examination.) The measurements should be placed on growth grids and interpreted. Parents enjoy seeing how the baby is progressing and are usually eager to learn about the child's weight gain and growth percentiles. Be alert for an infant who demonstrates a change in percentile range. For example, if the baby was in the 75th percentile for length and

Clinical Reasoning Choosing the Newborn's Care Provider

Parents are encouraged to visit the pediatric healthcare home before the baby is born. This will help the parents decide if the healthcare provider offers the type of care they want for their infant. Prepare a list of questions that parents could ask during a visit to the provider they are interested in interviewing. Be sure this list addresses the availability of healthcare providers, frequency of well-child supervision, cost and insurance information, and other pertinent topics.

See www.nursing.pearsonhighered.com for possible responses.

● **Figure 35–7** Measuring physical growth. Weighing and measuring length during health supervision visits provides important information about the child's nutrition and general development. This young infant was measured and then while the parents dressed the child the nurse placed the findings on the growth grid.

weight at birth, but has fallen to below the 50th percentile for weight, additional assessment of the baby's feedings is needed. Likewise, if the head circumference is much lower or higher than the length and weight percentiles, further neurologic and developmental assessment should be done.

Growth measurement is followed by a physical assessment. The nurse may complete parts of the assessment, with the remainder performed by the physician, nurse practitioner, or other primary care provider. The assessment evaluates each body system, with particular attention paid to the heart, skin, musculoskeletal system, abdomen, and neurologic status. See Chapter 25 ● for assessment of the newborn and Chapter 34 ● for a thorough discussion of physical assessment throughout infancy and childhood.

Developmental surveillance is integrated into each infant healthcare visit by observing developmental milestones in the infant. (See Chapter 32 ● for a summary of milestones expected at different ages.) When there is no opportunity to observe a skill directly, ask parents about whether the infant performs the skill (see *Developing Cultural Competence: Cultural Influences on Developmental Tests*). In addition to direct observation, parents

Developing Cultural Competence
Cultural Influences on Developmental Tests

Be alert for differences in cultural practices and beliefs that may influence developmental milestones. For example, if a child is kept on a cradleboard for much of the time, the baby may be slow in learning to crawl. This baby may progress directly to standing by furniture without demonstrating as much creeping or crawling as other infants. If an item such as "waves good-bye" or "plays patty-cake" represents a practice not common in another culture, the child may not have had exposure to the skill. Be alert for cultural variations, allow the child time to learn a developmental skill, and retest during future healthcare visits.

are usually requested to fill in a form that asks questions about common developmental tasks. Review the results and determine if additional questions should be asked. Signs of **developmental delay**—a delay in mastering functions, such as motor coordination and behavioral skills—in a full-term infant usually merit immediate investigation by a pediatrician, pediatric developmental specialist, pediatric neurologist, or a multidisciplinary team of professionals. Parents require additional emotional support, clear and honest communication, and resources to cope with the stress of this situation.

The nurse establishes health promotion and maintenance interventions related to growth and development assessment data. Anticipatory guidance related to development is a major component of health promotion. The nurse anticipates the next milestones the infant will be meeting, and recommends ways for the parents to support the infant in progression. Some health promotion activities include:

■ Teach about introducing foods that will foster growth.

■ Encourage use of toys and activities that will assist in meeting the next developmental milestones.

■ Demonstrate gross and fine motor skills that the infant has achieved.

■ Demonstrate to parents how the child will focus on their faces and mimic their vocal sounds.

Other interventions are focused on health maintenance or disease and injury prevention. Safety hazards and ways to avoid them are discussed, and parents are given brochures, website addresses, or videotapes to enhance injury prevention information. Can you outline additional health promotion and health maintenance interventions that relate to the newborn's and infant's growth and development?

Nutrition

The importance of nutrition during the newborn period and the first year of life cannot be overestimated. The baby will triple his or her birth weight by 1 year of age and has a great need for nutritional balance. From the first sips of breast milk or formula as a newborn, to eating the family meal at 1 year of age, the fast progression of nutritional intake patterns is obvious. See Chapter 26 ● for details about the importance of breastfeeding and Chapter 33 ● for a thorough description of nutritional needs for the infant.

During each visit the nurse seeks to learn what the baby is eating, and whether the family has any questions or concerns related to intake (Hagan et al., 2008). Open-ended questions are a good way to begin, with more specific questions inserted after the parent's perceptions are known. Breastfeeding is encouraged and supported during the newborn and infancy periods with information about safe formula feeding provided when the family has chosen that method of feeding. Once the baby is in the second half of the first year, food patterns of the family become more important. Consider childcare settings as well.

Observations from other portions of the visit can provide clues about additional questions to ask. If an infant has not gained weight as expected and has fallen into a lower weight percentile, more specific analysis of intake is needed. Ask for a recall of the baby's intake in the previous day. When the baby does not meet developmental milestones on schedule or is lethargic, intake may be inadequate for age. In these cases support may be needed to ensure adequate intake; a thorough description of feeding may be the first step in analyzing the problem and planning interventions. When the child's ability to take in nutrients or the parent's ability to feed the baby is questioned, an observation of a feeding might take place, either at the healthcare setting or during a home visit.

Additional nutritional assessment measures are used at certain points in the first year. A hematocrit or hemoglobin is generally performed between 9 and 12 months of age. Lead screening may be needed in certain population groups (see Chapter 43 🔗 for more information). Food security screening can be used when appropriate (see Chapter 33 🔗) (AAP Committee on Nutrition, 2009). Each visit includes nutritional teaching about important items. The topics for discussion vary according to age group. See Table 35–2 for suggested teaching topics at specific ages. Desired outcomes for nutrition in infancy include adequate growth, normal nutritional assessment findings, and knowledge by parents of the nutritional needs of the infant.

Physical Activity

Muscle development begins early in fetal life. The flexed position of the newborn demonstrates development of the flexor muscles and relaxation of the extensor muscles. This flexed position protects the newborn, conserves energy by reducing movement, and reduces heat loss. During the first month of life, the newborn gradually "unfolds" and the body straightens. Movements begin to change from reflexive to purposeful.

Physical activity is needed for adequate development of fine and gross motor skills in infancy. Unlike other times of life, the focus is on providing only the opportunities for activity, without a need to focus on motivation. As long as infants are meeting developmental milestones and have a stimulating environment that provides opportunity for fine and gross motor activity, they will use their motor skills, thus enhancing their performance. Time should be provided each day for the infant to reach for objects, freely exercise legs and arms, and increasingly use head control.

Table 35–2	Nutrition Teaching for Health Promotion and Health Maintenance Visits	
Age	**Nutrition Teaching**	
Newborn	Support breastfeeding efforts. Teach correct formula types and preparation if used. Teach burping and rate of feeding information.	Encourage families to view feedings as social interactions; emphasize importance of holding the infant and not propping bottles.
1 month	Continue teaching listed above. Offer support for breastfeeding and reinforce that breast milk is the only intake needed by infants at this age.	
2 months	Continue teaching listed above. Review fluid needs of infants. Reinforce food safety for partially used bottles of breast milk or formula. Use warm water for heating bottles rather than microwave to avoid burning.	Warn against feeding honey in the first year of life due to risk of botulism. Begin daily cleaning of infant gums. Provide information about any supplements needed (for example, iron for premature infant; continuation of 400 International Units/day of vitamin D for all infants).
4 months	Continue teaching listed above. Discuss introduction of first foods between 4 and 6 months, and surveillance for symptoms of allergy or intolerance.	Discuss changing food patterns such as increasing amounts and decreasing numbers of daily milk feedings.
6 months	Continue teaching listed above. Reinforce proper introduction of new foods, to include rice cereal, vegetables, and fruits. Discuss any unusual food reactions observed. Introduce cup for drinking. Introduce soft finger foods.	Serve juice only in a cup and limit to no more than 6 ounces daily. Caution about common choking foods and items. Provide information about fluoride supplement if water supply is not fluoridated.
9 months	Continue teaching listed above. If mother does not continue to breastfeed, teach family to use iron-fortified formula for the first year of life. Encourage self-feeding of finger foods, integrating common foods for the family.	Introduce source of protein such as tofu, cheese, mashed beans, and slivers of meats.
12 months	Continue teaching listed above. Support mother who wishes to continue breastfeeding beyond 1 year of age.	Encourage cups for all feedings other than breast.

Playing with parents or others and being surrounded by toys and other stimulating items will encourage motor behavior in all body parts. Ask the parents for a description of the infant's typical day and listen for these types of play periods. While infants should sleep on their backs, they need supervised play periods when they are awake that are spent on the stomach. This encourages developmental skills and lessens flattening of the back of the head from excessive positioning on back (Koren, Reece, Kahn-D'Angelo, et al., 2010). Observe the physical skills of the infant (see Chapter 32 🔗) for motor developmental norms, ask questions about play periods provided, and compose a list of the family protective factors and risk factors in this area. Table 35–3 lists some risk and protective factors related to physical activity of newborns and infants.

Based on the results of assessment and using the concept of anticipatory guidance, the nurse plans appropriate teaching for health promotion. Health maintenance deals with prevention of physical development delays. Examples of nursing activities are teaching parents to allow the arms and legs of infants to be outside of covers for some period each day to enhance movement, and suggesting toys that encourage attention and movement, such as mobiles and music boxes. The nurse evaluates the success of interventions by the child's progression in physical activity milestones at each health supervision visit. Adequate parental understanding of the importance of physical activity and the means of supporting the child's activities is an important outcome of care.

Oral Health

The first teeth begin to erupt about midway during infancy. Two front teeth are common at about 6 months of age. However, even before this, parents lay the foundation for good oral health. The mother's intake during pregnancy and breastfeeding is essential to ensuring adequate availability of calcium and other nutrients that will be used as the infant's teeth develop. The nurse in child health supervision settings ensures that the infant has adequate intake of these nutrients via breastfeeding and other foods. A dietary recall of the mother's intake, as well as the infant's, is one way of assessing for nutrients. When the water supply is not fluoridated, inquire about use of fluoride drops.

Help the family establish healthy dental habits. The parents should wipe the infant's gums with soft moist gauze once or twice daily. This helps to clean residues of food from the gums and gets the infant accustomed to having something wiping the gums, a practice that may assist when toothbrushing begins. Families are also cautioned to avoid having the infant breastfeed when sleeping, to avoid use of bottles in bed, and not to allow the infant to drink at will from a bottle during the day. These practices are linked to **early childhood caries** (see Chapter 33 🔗) and can lead to tooth decay. Nurses assess for the presence of teeth and whether patterns are similar to those expected (see Chapter 34 🔗 for additional information). It is wise to ask if the infant has had any difficulty with teeth eruption. Many infants have increased crying and disrupted sleep when teething. Suggest comfort measures such as offering cool beverages and safe "teething toys" for the infant. The American Academy of Pediatric Dentistry recommends an oral examination within 6 months of the eruption of the first tooth and no later than 12 months of age (CDC, 2011a).

Mental and Spiritual Health

The infant's mental health is related to early experiences, inborn characteristics such as temperament and resilience, and relationships with caregivers. The first year of life provides many opportunities for the infant to develop positive mental health; interventions during this important period can enhance the child's future mental status.

One way to evaluate mental health is to look carefully at the growth and development surveillance data that were described earlier. Children who feel secure and have nurturing environments usually grow as expected and perform milestones at usual times. Slow growth and delayed development are sometimes related to feeding disorders of infancy and early childhood (see Chapter 33 🔗). In these cases a disturbed relationship with the primary caregiver influences the psychologic state of the infant and results in decreased food intake. Another way to assess mental health is to observe the child and parent interacting. Does the parent hold the newborn securely and does the infant cuddle and settle in to the parent's arms? (See Figure 35–8 ●.) Is there eye contact between parent and infant? Does the parent appear comfortable in holding and comforting the newborn? These interactions indicate bonding or positive attachment.

Table 35–3	Risk and Protective Factors Regarding Physical Activity in the Newborn and Infancy Periods
Risk Factors	**Protective Factors**
■ Premature birth ■ Delayed developmental milestones ■ Limited stimulation by family or other care providers ■ Lack of knowledge by family about infant's physical activity needs ■ Limited community resources for families with infants	■ Meets developmental milestones at expected ages ■ Has contact with parents, siblings, and others for significant time each day ■ A supportive environment with room to play safely; stimulating surroundings ■ Physically active family ■ Family knowledge about infant's physical activity needs ■ Community programs that promote physical activity in infants and information for families

Source: Data from Hagan, J. F., Shaw, J. S., & Duncan, P. M. (Eds.). (2008). *Bright futures: Guidelines for health supervision of infants, children, and adolescents* (3rd ed.). Elk Grove Village, IL: American Academy of Pediatrics.

● **Figure 35–8** Assessing mental health. Interactions between the parent and infant provide clues to mental health. Do the adult and child appear comfortable with each other? Is eye contact and vocalization present? Are their bodies soft and relaxed or tense?

During the first year, the infant learns to identify the primary caregivers; beginning at about 6 months of age, infants may cry or protest when another person holds them. This is called **stranger anxiety** and indicates expected attachment to parents. Similarly, infants in the second half of the first year of life may exhibit **separation anxiety** by inconsolable crying and other signs of distress when parents are not present. These behaviors are normal, demonstrate healthy attachment to primary caregivers, and indicate mental health. Help parents to recognize them as expected occurrences. Provide ideas of how to deal with this behavior. The parents can remain in sight and talk to the baby during health supervision examinations. They should be encouraged to hold and comfort the baby after painful procedures like immunizations. Once the infant has experienced that the parent leaves and returns, security in the care of others can emerge.

Another important indication of infant mental health is the ability to comfort oneself. **Self-regulation** is the process of dealing with feelings, learning to soothe self, and focusing on activities for increasing periods of time. Newborns learn how to comfort and calm themselves. Ask parents if the newborn or infant sucks a finger, softly rocks, or otherwise comforts self when distressed. Some infants prefer to be alone and quiet when tired or distressed; others calm better when held, rocked, or placed in an infant swing. Help the parents to identify and reinforce the baby's methods of self-soothing, and teach swaddling and rocking techniques. Self-regulation is needed by the baby when learning to go to sleep while tired and agitated. Nurses use health promotion principles to teach about sleep patterns in infants, and implement health maintenance when partnering with families to deal with problem sleep behaviors that lead to infant and parent fatigue (see *As Children Grow: Infant Sleep Patterns* and *Evidence-Based Practice: Infant Sleep*).

The newborn enters a family with spiritual strengths and limitations. The nurse assesses the family and provides additional resources when needed. Although the infant is not mature enough to understand the family's spiritual framework, the atmosphere in the family that relates to nurturing, valuing children, providing a safe and secure environment, and recognizing mental balance is conveyed readily to the infant. The infant's social and psychologic health are closely related to these factors. Assess the family's meaningful activities and practices and engagement in faith-based practices. Ask if they have needs or desires for referrals in the community such as to an organized religious body or other meaningful activities.

Many of the nurse's interventions are aimed at healthy mental health development in the infant. Health promotion activities focus on teaching parents the needs of infants for security and interaction. Suggest healthy sleep patterns starting with the newborn visit and explain how they can be achieved. Teach self-regulation skills so that the parents can help the infant become quiet and calm. Health maintenance seeks to identify infants with disruptions in mental health status, often manifested by growth or interaction abnormalities. When the infant has disturbed sleep patterns or difficulty calming self when upset, or the parents do not interpret infant cues related to hunger or discomfort, the nurse plans interventions to help prevent further problems. An expected outcome for these activities is the reestablishment of expected growth and development and age-appropriate interactions of the infant with others.

Relationships

Family adaptation to a new baby begins in pregnancy, and evidence of initial family adaptation to pregnancy may be predictive of future parental coping (Hagan et al., 2008). Upon birth, the family is the primary site where the infant learns to interact with other people. Therefore, family dynamics must be examined during health supervision visits. Strengths and needs of the family are identified during psychosocial screening. Some factors in the mental health of the parents directly affect the atmosphere in the home, and the resulting health of the newborn and infant. Depression in parents or other family members is an important condition that has the potential to influence the infant's health. (See Chapter 31 for information about risks in the postpartum family.) Interactions with parents who are depressed will be altered; caretaking, both physical and emotional, can be impaired. Another challenge to the mental health of families and the infants in these families is that of domestic violence, a situation in which parents or adult care providers commit violent acts toward one another. Child abuse or maltreatment is another risk that occurs in some families with infants. This problem is a serious issue that causes disturbed mental status in the baby. See Chapter 43 for a detailed description of child abuse and its effect on infants and older children. Suspected child abuse must be reported to legal authorities in order to protect children.

The infant's social interactions both within and outside the family display unbelievable growth in the first year. The role of the nurse related to infant social interactions in health supervision visits is to evaluate the social skills of the infant, learn what parents have noticed about the baby's temperament and how

Evidence-Based Practice   Infant Sleep

Clinical Question

Many babies have limited sleeping periods during the night, and their night awakenings disturb parents' sleep. Parents may have busy days and be unable to nap and, hence, possibly not be able to perform at a safe and productive level during the day. Parental stress and depression are associated with frequent child awakenings, and strategies are needed to assist them in supporting the infant's sleep.

The Evidence

Sleep of the infant is an important concern for many parents, but there is little research-based evidence about what strategies really improve infant sleep. A study of 314 twin pairs found that most sleep disturbances in early childhood are linked to environmental factors, and thus behavioral interventions with parents are suggested for altering infant sleep patterns (Brescianini, Volzone, Fagnani, et al., 2011). Consistent with these findings, a study evaluating 170 parents for knowledge of child sleep found that most parents could not answer the majority of questions correctly. The researchers suggested that evaluating parental knowledge and teaching about developmental progression of sleep patterns should occur during health visits (Schreck & Richdale, 2011).

A cross-cultural study found that parents from predominantly Asian countries were more likely to identify sleep disturbance in their children than those from countries with a majority of white parents. These findings suggest that information is needed about cultural differences in sleep expectations of parents (Sadeh, Mindell, & Rivera, 2011).

Best Practice

This evidence-based practice provides implications for nursing care. Ask parents of young newborns to record the infant sleep patterns. As the infant nears 3 to 4 months of age, patterns should demonstrate few night wakenings and feedings. Teach parents about how to minimize stimulation and interaction at night. Provide opportunities to review results at future health supervision visits, or offer telephone or other support to parents.

Clinical Reasoning

What reasons might working parents have for responding eagerly and interacting with an infant who awakens at night? Do you think there are other reasons why infants awake at night? What clues help you to decide if an infant sleep problem exists?

---

it fits with their lives, and make suggestions for positive social development. Desired outcomes for the infant include establishment of close relationships with parents and other family members, a stimulating home environment that is responsive to the baby's temperament, and developmental progression in social interactions.

Disease Prevention Strategies

Disease prevention in the newborn period includes metabolic screening, hearing screening, eye examination, immunization, prevention of environmental smoke exposure, sudden infant death syndrome (SIDS) risk reduction, formula safety, minimizing exposure to disease, and hand hygiene for the family.

Infants are prone to many infectious diseases, especially once passive immunity from the mother wanes at about 6 months of age (see Chapter 44 and Chapter 49). Recommended immunizations are administered on schedule to provide protection from some diseases. Recommended immunizations for newborn and infancy are listed in Table 35–4. Further details on immunizations can be found in Chapter 44 . Instruct parents about upcoming immunizations and when the infant should be seen again. Be sure the parent understands the risks and benefits of each immunization. Answer their questions truthfully, and have resources on hand such as brochures and videotapes for interested parents.

During each health supervision visit in infancy, the nurse performs recommended screenings and counsels the parents about why such screenings are important. Vision and hearing screenings are consistently performed. Screenings for anemia and lead poisoning are added at particular times or with certain groups. Families with certain genetic diseases such as sickle cell

disease or cystic fibrosis may choose to have screening for the infant so that supportive care can begin early if the child has the disease. Parents benefit from teaching about common diseases and conditions of young children and measures for their prevention. Ask about secondhand smoke (environmental tobacco smoke) and encourage smoking parents to quit. Teach parents to put infants to sleep on their backs to assist in lowering the chance of SIDS (see Chapter 47 for a thorough discussion of SIDS). Be sure parents have a phone number to call when they have questions about conditions or whether the baby should be

---

As Children Grow   Infant Sleep Patterns

Newborn
16–20 hours daily

1–3 months
10–16 hours of sleep daily in about five sleep periods of 30 minutes to 4 hours; sleep spans day and night hours

3–6 months
14–15 hours of sleep daily with a longer sleep at night plus two to three naps daily

6–12 months
12–14 hours of sleep daily with a longer sleep at night plus one to two naps daily

Source: Data from Murray, R. B., Zentner, J. P., & Yakimo, R. (2009). *Health promotion strategies through the life span* (8th ed.). Upper Saddle River, NJ: Pearson Prentice Hall.

Table 35–4	Routine Immunizations Recommended During Newborn and Infancy Periods
Immunization	**Age Recommended**
Hepatitis B	At birth (1st dose) 1–2 months (2nd dose) 6–18 months (3rd dose)
Hepatitis A	12 months (1st dose) 18 months or at least 6 months after 1st dose (2nd dose)
Diphtheria, tetanus, pertussis	2, 4, and 6 months (3 doses)
Rotavirus	2 and 4 months (2 doses) **OR** 2, 4, and 6 months (3 doses) (The requirement of 2 or 3 doses is related to which of the two available vaccines is used.)
Haemophilus influenzae type b	2, 4, and 6 months (3 doses; 3rd dose is not needed if PRP-OMP [Pedvax HIB or Comvax] is used for primary series)
Inactivated poliovirus	2, 4, and 6–18 months (3 doses)
Pneumococcal	2, 4, and 6 months (3 doses)
Influenza	Annually from 6 months

Teaching Highlights When to Contact the Healthcare Provider

Instruct parents to contact a provider if the child has:

- Rectal temperature ≥ 38.0°C (100.4°F)
- Seizure
- Skin rash, purplish spots, petechiae
- Change in activity or behavior that makes the parent uncomfortable
- Unusual irritability, lethargy
- Failure to eat
- Vomiting
- Diarrhea
- Dehydration
- Cough

Data from Hagan, J. G., Shaw, J. S., & Duncan, P. M. (Eds.). (2008). Bright futures: Guidelines for health supervision of infants, children, and adolescents (3rd ed.). Elk Grove Village, IL: American Academy of Pediatrics.

seen by the healthcare provider (see *Teaching Highlights: When to Contact the Healthcare Provider*). Desired outcomes for disease prevention strategies include adequate management of health problems, integration of immunization and other preventive measures into care of the infant, and family understanding of preventive measures recommended for infants.

Injury Prevention Strategies

New parents are sometimes unaware of sources of potential injury for the newborn. Some aspects of injury prevention are pertinent to the newborn's immediate care and other topics promote discussion and provide opportunities for anticipatory guidance during all of infancy. In the immediate newborn period, the nurse should assess the parents' knowledge of injury prevention strategies, and promote healthy and safe behaviors. Injury prevention strategies include proper and consistent use of an infant car seat, and strategies to prevent falls, burns, choking, drowning, and suffocation.

During the first year of life, injury becomes an increasingly common cause of mortality. Strategies must be included in every health supervision visit to lower the risk of injury. Nurses should never assume that parents understand how to insert an infant car seat correctly or what types of toys and foods can lead to choking. Know the most common hazards at each age and teach parents methods of avoiding them (Tables 35–5 and 35–6).

Begin the conversation by asking parents what safety hazards they are aware of in the child's environment. Use this information as the starting point for discussion. Give positive feedback for their awareness of hazards and measures they have taken to

prevent them. Consider using a home assessment survey that assists parents in identifying hazards that may be present in their homes. When infants visit friends, relatives, or neighbors, they may be exposed to other hazardous situations. Grandparents may not have a home that is "baby-proofed" and the infant could have access to electrical cords, machinery, medicines, or other hazards. Help the parents to evaluate the childcare home or center. Focus on car safety since this is a frequent cause of injury for infants. Provide brochures and other types of information about recommendations. Refer every family for a car seat examination at a certified examination center. Provide resources for car seats if the family is not able to afford one. Discuss other possible safety hazards such as extensions on the parent's bicycle and use of baby strollers in areas where cars are present.

NURSING MANAGEMENT *For the Health Promotion and Maintenance of the Newborn and Infant*

Nursing Assessment and Diagnosis

The nurse working in clinics, offices, and other settings that offer primary care for newborns and infants should be skillful in assessing health promotion and health maintenance. The infant's growth, developmental level, general physical health, and mental/social health are assessed. Family interactions and other settings where the infant spends time are evaluated for risks and protective factors that influence the child's development. Assess the health of siblings and patterns of integrating the infant into the rest of the family. Particular attention is directed at assessment of risk for diseases and injuries. The data-gathering phase always provides parents with the opportunity to ask questions and relay concerns. Further assessment may need to be directed at these areas.

Based on the assessment data, the nurse establishes nursing diagnoses that become the basis for nursing interventions. Both areas of strength and need are included; often the family's strengths can be used to further promote health. Nursing

Table 35–5	Injury Prevention in Infancy	
Hazard	**Development Characteristics**	**Preventive Measures**
Falls	Mobility increases in first year of life, progressing from squirming movements to crawling, rolling, and standing.	Do not leave the newborn or infant unsecured in infant seat, even in newborn period. Do not place on high surfaces such as tables or beds unless holding child. *(A)* Once mobile by crawling, keep doors to stairways closed or use gates. Standing walkers have led to many injuries and are not recommended.
Burns	Infant is dependent on caretakers for environmental control. The second half of the first year is marked by crawling and increased mobility. Objects are explored by touching and placing in mouth.	Check temperature of bath water and food/liquids for drinking. Cover electrical outlets. Supervise infant so that play with electrical cords cannot occur.
Motor vehicle crashes	Infant is dependent on caretakers for placement in car. On impact with another motor vehicle, an infant held on a lap acts as a torpedo.	Use only approved restraint systems (according to federal motor vehicle safety standards). The seat must be used for every trip, even if very short. The seat must be properly buckled to the car's lap belt system. *(B)*
Drowning	Infant cannot swim and is unable to lift head.	Never leave a newborn or infant alone in a bath of even 2.5 cm (1 in.) of water. Supervise when in water even when a life preserver is worn. Supervision should be provided by adults, not older children. Flotation devices such as arm inflatables are not certified life preservers.
Poisoning	Newborns and infants are dependent on caretakers to keep harmful substances out of reach.	Keep medicines out of reach. Teach proper dosage and administration of medicines to parents. Cleaning products and other harmful substances should not be stored where the infant can reach them. Remove plants from play areas. Have poison control center number by telephone.
Choking	The second half of infancy is marked by exploratory reaching and mouthing of objects. Infant explores objects by placing them in the mouth. *(C)*	Avoid foods that commonly cause choking. Keep small toys away from infants, especially toys labeled "not intended for use by those under 3 years."
Suffocation	The newborn and young infant have minimal head control and may be unable to move if vomiting or having difficulty breathing.	Position newborn and infant on back for sleep. *(D)* Do not place pillows, stuffed toys, or other objects near head. Do not use plastic in crib. Avoid latex balloons. Co-sleeping with the parent is discouraged due to danger of suffocation. Sleep with the baby near but not in the parental bed.
Strangulation	Infant is able to get head into railings or crib slats but cannot remove it.	Be sure older cribs have slats spaced 6 cm (2⅜ in.) or less apart. The mattress must fit tightly against the crib rails.

A Never leave infant unsecured or on high surface.

B Always use approved restraint system. Place infant in rear-facing seat in back seat of car.

C Explores objects with mouth.

D Place infant on back for sleeping; keep toys clear.

Table 35–6	Injury Prevention Topics by Age	

Age	Injury Prevention	Teaching Topics
Birth–1 month	Use car safety seat approved for the infant; install as directed in rear-facing direction in the back seat. Put baby to sleep on back. Avoid loose bedding and toys in crib; avoid clothes and blankets with loose strings and do not tie a pacifier around the neck or with a string. Avoid tobacco use in the environment. Provide adult supervision of the baby at all times by trusted individuals. Test bath water temperature and never leave the baby alone in the bath.	Never place baby on high object such as counter, table, or bed; always keep one hand on the baby during activities like diaper changes to prevent falling. Wash hands correctly and often. Avoid contact with persons with communicable diseases. Have smoke alarms and avoid fire hazards. Learn infant CPR and airway obstruction removal. Never shake the baby. Have plans for emergency care.
2 months	Follow the above. Use only recommended playpens or cribs and keep sides up. Avoid moldy environments. Keep baby toys cleaned.	Avoid exposure to direct sunlight for the baby. Keep sharp and small objects out of baby's environment. Keep hot water heater lower than 120°F. Review emergency plan with all care providers.
4 months	Follow the above. Get all poisonous substances out of baby's view and reach; install locks to keep them inaccessible.	Do not use latex balloons or plastic bags near the baby.
6 months	Follow the above. Use only a car seat approved for the weight of the child and always use the seat in rear-facing position in the back seat. Empty containers of water immediately after use; be sure pools or other bodies of water are locked and not accessible to baby. Use sunscreen, hat, and long sleeves when baby is in the sun. Keep heavy and sharp objects out of reach; check that all poisons are locked away including in homes visited; keep pet food and cosmetics out of reach.	Do not drink hot liquids or eat soup while holding the baby. Have poison control number by phones and programmed into cell phones. Be alert for dangers of hot curling irons and other appliances. Have electrical cords out of reach and not hanging down. Have home and environment checked for lead hazards. Lower infant crib mattress if still in upper position. Install gates and guards on stairs and windows. Never use an infant walker.
9 months	Follow the above. Crawl on the floor and look for hazards at baby's eye level. Pad sharp corners on tables and other furniture.	Watch for tables, chairs, and other devices the baby may use for climbing to unsafe places.
12 months	Follow the above. Keep the infant in a rear-facing car seat until 2 years of age; place in back seat and never in front seat with a passenger air bag; have installation checked for safety. Start teaching the child to wash hands frequently, demonstrating and washing with the child. Provide own personal items such as clothing and blankets to childcare providers; wash often. Change batteries in home smoke alarms and check system.	Turn handles to back of stove; use back rather than front burners; watch for hot liquids. Check care provider setting for safety hazards. Remember that responsible adults should always supervise your infant, not other children. Peruse home once again for hazards now that the child is more active, climbing, and walking. Check playgrounds for hazards and always supervise the child in a playground.

Source: Data from Hagan, J. G., Shaw, J. S., & Duncan, P. M. (Eds.). (2008). *Bright futures: Guidelines for health supervision of infants, children, and adolescents* (3rd ed.). Elk Grove Village, IL: American Academy of Pediatrics.

diagnoses established during a health supervision visit of an infant might include the following (NANDA-I © 2012):

- *Breastfeeding, Readiness for Enhanced,* related to the mother's confidence and knowledge

- *Breastfeeding, Interrupted,* related to the mother's resumption of employment outside the home

- *Coping: Family, Compromised,* related to recent role changes

- *Attachment, Risk for Impaired (Parent/Child),* related to anxiety associated with parenting role

- *Sleep Pattern, Disturbed (Infant),* related to frequently changing sleep routines and cycles

- *Skin Integrity, Impaired (Infant),* related to developmental factors

- *Infection, Risk for (Infant),* related to inadequate acquired immunity

- *Injury, Risk for (Infant),* related to design of environment

- *Growth and Development, Delayed,* related to parental substance abuse

Planning and Implementation

The nurse plays a vital role in successful health promotion and health maintenance activities. The newborn period is essential for building a relationship between parents and healthcare professionals that sets the stage for the months and years to come. Explain to the parents what procedures are being performed and their purpose. Encourage them to ask questions and share their perceptions of the infant's personality, development, and other traits. This will enhance their understanding that healthcare involves a partnership between them and the care providers. It will lead to trust that promotes their ability to share concerns honestly. The first year of the baby's life is a key time for establishing a trusting relationship with health professionals.

Recognize the importance of data provided by simple assessments such as length and weight. Analyze all findings to learn if the child is developing as expected. Much of the visit is spent in teaching parents about topics such as safety measures, providing anticipatory guidance related to development, assisting with integration of the newborn into the family, and relaying resources for support of the family in the community, on the Internet, or in other areas. Parenting classes, childcare facilities, and family planning resources are examples of common parental needs. Perform recommended physical and developmental assessment, administer screening tests, and give immunizations. Be sure parents understand the need for tests and treatments, and relay the results of tests to them.

Nurses who work in hospitals, emergency services, and other facilities are an important link in health supervision. Ask where and how often the child is seen for care. Check immunization schedules to be sure they are up to date. When the child is not being seen regularly, find out if the family does not know the importance of these visits or lacks resources to obtain the necessary care. Refer them to resources as needed so that they can identify a pediatric healthcare home. Some agencies that provide health supervision are equipped to perform home visits on a regular basis or in case of special need. When nurses make regular home visits to families with many risk factors, health outcomes are improved. Seeing the family in the natural setting enables the nurse to tailor interventions to the specific situation. Nutrition, safety, and other teaching is more effective when it matches the family's needs. For example, showing how to set up a stimulating environment with safe materials, even if toys are limited, is an effective nursing strategy. Ensure that home visits are performed whenever appropriate and available, either through the pediatric healthcare home or other community agency.

Before the family leaves the facility, be sure they have the next appointment scheduled. Summarize content of the present visit, emphasizing the family's strengths and the baby's newly acquired developmental skills. Sensitively list any areas that require work in the coming weeks, such as "baby-proofing" the home or encouraging the infant to reach for objects. Provide a journal or notebook in which the parents can record the infant's development and write down questions to ask during future visits. Suggest possible topics for the parents to think about, and provide books, brochures, and other printed material.

Evaluation

Expected outcomes of nursing care for the infant and family in health promotion and health maintenance include the following:

- Parents state common safety hazards at the infant's present and upcoming ages.
- The newborn and infant demonstrate normal patterns of growth and progression in developmental milestones.
- The newborn and infant remain free of disease and injury.
- The newborn and infant are well adjusted, showing positive response to the environment and interactions with significant others.

Critical Concept Review

LEARNING OUTCOME 35.1: Define health promotion and health maintenance.

1. Health promotion:
   - Activities that increase well-being and enhance wellness or health.

2. Health maintenance:
   - Activities that preserve an individual's present state of health and prevent disease or injury occurrence.

LEARNING OUTCOME 35.2: Describe how health promotion and health maintenance are facilitated by partnering with families during health supervision visits.

1. Health promotion and health maintenance are integrated into healthcare visits.

2. Care provider adds identified information gathered at the visit which the nurse can then use to direct the activities.

LEARNING OUTCOME 35.3: Describe the components of a health supervision visit.

1. Assessment of:
   - Growth and development.
   - Amount and type of physical activity.
   - Oral health.
   - Nutrition.
   - Mental and spiritual health.
   - Relationships.
2. Conduct disease and injury prevention screenings.

LEARNING OUTCOME 35.4: Analyze the nurse's role in providing health promotion and health maintenance for the newborn and infant.

1. Build effective partnerships with families.
2. Foster family-centered communication.
3. Address health promotion and health maintenance needs.
4. Manage time to provide for health promotion during routine healthcare visits.
5. Educate during the family's teachable moments.
6. Advocate for children and their families.

LEARNING OUTCOME 35.5: Perform the general observations made of infants and their families as they come to the pediatric healthcare home for health supervision visits.

1. Do child and parent have close physical contact, eye contact, and vocalization during visit?
2. Do parents appear relaxed or stressed?
3. Does child behave as expected for age and situation?
4. Is parent able to effectively handle child being seen as well as any siblings present?
5. Does the baby respond to eye contact, movements, and vocalizations by the nurse?

LEARNING OUTCOME 35.6: Synthesize the areas of assessment and intervention for health supervision visits of newborns and infants: growth and developmental surveillance, nutrition, physical activity, oral health, mental and spiritual health, family and social relations, disease prevention strategies, and injury prevention strategies.

1. Growth and development:
   - Obtain length, weight, and head circumference.
   - Observe and interview family to determine if infant is reaching appropriate developmental milestones.
2. Nutrition:
   - Determine type of infant feeding family is using.
   - Instruct family concerning appropriate nutrition for infant's age.
3. Physical activity:
   - Assess daily routines and infant's ability to participate.
   - Provide instruction concerning appropriate toys.
4. Oral health:
   - Inspect infant's mouth.
   - Instruct parents concerning importance of toothbrushing.
5. Mental and spiritual health:
   - Instruct family concerning expected stranger anxiety and separation anxiety.
   - Explain need for infant to develop self-regulating (self-comforting) behaviors.
6. Family and social relations:
   - Encourage parents to play daily with infant and take a break when infant care becomes frustrating.
7. Disease prevention strategies:
   - Administer necessary immunizations.
   - Instruct parents concerning when to call the physician.
8. Injury prevention strategies:
   - Instruct parents in proper use of car seats and prevention of falls.

LEARNING OUTCOME 35.7: Plan health promotion and health maintenance strategies employed during health supervision visits of newborns and infants.

1. Explain procedures and the purpose of these procedures.
2. Encourage parents to ask questions and share general perceptions of the child.

LEARNING OUTCOME 35.8: Recognize the importance of family in newborn and infant health care, and include family assessment in each health supervision visit.

1. Health supervision visits begin with collaborative planning with the family.
2. Each visit should include:
   - Interview with family concerning developmental status of the child.
   - Observation of family interaction.
   - Discussion of parental concerns.

LEARNING OUTCOME 35.9: Integrate pertinent mental health care into health supervision visits for newborns and infants.

1. Mental health issues to be addressed include:
   - Assessment of occurrence of common problems such as nightmares and temper tantrums.
   - Explanation of the promotion of positive self-esteem.
   - Guidance in assisting infant in self-regulating behaviors.
   - Explanation of emergence of methods to assist child in handling daily stressors.
   - Instruction in normal developmental tasks such as toilet training.

LEARNING OUTCOME 35.10: Evaluate data about the family and other social relationships to promote and maintain health of newborns and infants.

1. Health promotion and maintenance activities related to social relationships focus on:
   - Increasing social skills with the people in the child's environment.
   - Successful management of temperament characteristics.
   - Adjusting to time away from home.
   - Improving language and communication skills.

Clinical Reasoning in Action

Sahil is a 6-month-old boy who is brought to the clinic by his mother, Clarisse, and his grandmother, who just moved into the home to help Clarisse. Sahil's father recently needed to leave the country on a prolonged work assignment. Clarisse is very nervous about being the main adult responsible for Sahil since her husband's departure. As you assess Sahil you find that he is smiling readily, is able to sit on his own with little support, and has length and weight at the 50th percentiles. His mother told you that she is breastfeeding and has been feeding Sahil some table food such as rice and tofu. She has returned to work so the grandmother will provide care during the day while Clarisse is at work. You review the immunization record and find that several immunizations are due at today's visit.

1. As Clarisse returns to work, Sahil will likely be consuming less breast milk and have more table foods and formula added to the diet. What questions will you ask Clarisse and Sahil's grandmother to evaluate their knowledge of dietary recommendations for infants? Compose a teaching plan that is appropriate for integration of increasing types of food into the diet of a 6-month-old child.

2. What immunizations are generally needed for 6-month-old infants? When should Sahil return for his next immunizations?

3. You have identified that Clarisse needs support and socialization with other young mothers. How will you locate community resources that are helpful to young families? Decide what parenting information would be helpful to build Clarisse's confidence in caring for Sahil without her husband present. Suggest some ways that she, Sahil, and the father can communicate with each other regularly.

4. The major health problem for infants is related to safety hazards. Sahil is becoming more mobile and curious. Write a teaching plan that includes topics and specific teaching requirements at his age.

See www.nursing.pearsonhighered.com for possible responses.

References

American Academy of Pediatrics (AAP). (2008). *The National Center for Medical Home Initiatives for Children with Special Needs.* Retrieved from http://www.medicalhomeinfo.org/training/index.html

American Academy of Pediatrics (AAP). (2010a). *Integrating surveillance and screening with the medical home.* Retrieved from http://www.medicalhomeinfo.org/downloads/pdfs/Integsurveil.pdf

American Academy of Pediatrics (AAP). (2010b). Policy statement: Hospital stay for healthy term newborns. *Pediatrics, 125*(2), 405–409. doi:10.1542/peds.2009-3119

American Academy of Pediatrics (AAP). (2011). *Where we stand: Newborn discharge from hospital.* Retrieved from http://www.healthychildren.org/English/ages-stages/prenatal/delivery-beyond/pages

American Academy of Pediatrics (AAP) Committee on Nutrition. (2009). *Pediatric nutrition handbook* (6th ed.). Elk Grove Village, IL: Author.

Brescianini, S., Volzone, A., Fagnani, C., Patriarca, B., Grimaldi, V., Lanni, R., . . . Stazi, J. A. (2011). Genetic and environmental factors shape infant sleep patterns: A study of 18-month-old twins. *Pediatrics, 127*, e1296. doi:10.1542/peds.2010-0858

Centers for Disease Control and Prevention (CDC). (2010a). *Causes of death by age group.* Retrieved from http://www.cdc.gov/injury/wisaars/leadingcauses.html

Centers for Disease Control and Prevention (CDC). (2010b). Youth risk behavior surveillance—United States, 2009. *Morbidity and Mortality Weekly Report, 59*(SS-5), 1–148.

Centers for Disease Control and Prevention (CDC). (2011a). *Caries experience and untreated tooth decay.* Retrieved from http://apps.nccd.cdc.gov/nohss/IndicatorV.asp?Indicator=2,3

Centers for Disease Control and Prevention (CDC). (2011b). *Oral health.* Retrieved from http://www.cdc.gov/chronicdisease/resources/publications/AAG/doh.htm

Child Trends. (2011). *Unmet dental needs.* Retrieved from http://www.childtrendsdatabank.org/?q=node/77

Hagan, J. G., Shaw, J. S., & Duncan, P. M. (Eds.). (2008). *Bright futures: Guidelines for health supervision of infants, children, and adolescents* (3rd ed.). Elk Grove Village, IL: American Academy of Pediatrics.

Koren, A., Reece, S. M., Kahn-D'Angelo, L., & Medeiros, D. (2010). Parental information and provider practices related to tummy time and back to sleep. *Journal of Pediatric Health Care, 24*(4), 222–230. doi:10.1016/j.pedhc.2009.05.002

Lipkin, P. H. (2011). Developmental and behavioral surveillance and screening within the medical home. In R. G. Voight (Ed.), *Developmental and behavioral pediatrics* (pp. 69–92). Elk Grove Village, IL: American Academy of Pediatrics.

Murray, R. B., Zentner, J. P., & Yakimo, R. (2009). *Health promotion strategies through the life span* (8th ed.). Upper Saddle River, NJ: Pearson Prentice Hall.

National Association of Pediatric Nurse Associates and Practitioners (NAPNAP). (2009). *NAPNAP position statement on pediatric healthcare/medical home: Key issues on delivery, reimbursement, and leadership.*

Retrieved from http://www.napnap.org/Docs/PediatricHealthcare.pdf

Pender, N. J., Murdaugh, C. L., & Parsons, M. A. (2011). *Health promotion in nursing practice* (6th ed.). Upper Saddle River, NJ: Pearson Prentice Hall.

Sadeh, A., Mindell, J., & Rivera, L. (2011). "My child has a sleep problem": A cross-cultural comparison of parental definitions. *Sleep Medicine, 12*(5), 478–482.

Schreck, K. A., & Richdale, A. L. (2011). Knowledge of childhood sleep: A possible variable in under or misdiagnosis of childhood sleep problems. *Journal of Sleep Research, 20*, 589–597. doi:10.1111/j.1365-2869.2011.00922.x

Tanski, S., Garfunkel, L. C., Duncan, P. M., & Weitzman, M. (2010). *Performing preventive services: A Bright Futures book.* Elk Grove Village, IL: American Academy of Pediatrics.

U.S. Department of Health and Human Services. (2011). *Healthy People 2020. The vision, mission, and goals of Healthy People 2020.* Retrieved from http://www.healthypeople.gov/2020/Consortium/HP2020Framework.pdf

World Health Organization (WHO). (2010). *Health promotion.* Retrieved from http://www.who.int/topics/health_promotion/en

World Health Organization (WHO). (2011). *Health promotion: 7th global conference on health promotion.* Retrieved from http://www.who.int/healthpromotion/conferences/7gchp/en

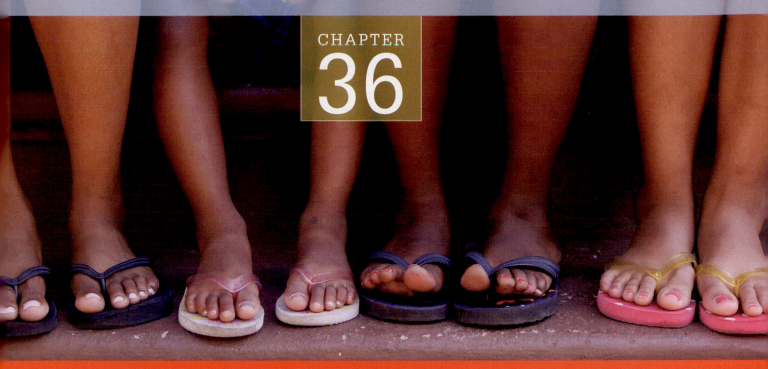

36

Health Promotion and Maintenance: The Toddler, the Preschooler, and the School-Age Child

Our school nurse is really great. She answers our questions about diabetes without making us feel like we're different than other kids. We can keep equipment like syringes in her office and she helps us to program our insulin pumps. —Jessalyn, 11 years old, child with diabetes

Mel Curtis/Getty Images

LEARNING OUTCOMES

36.1 Describe the areas of assessment and intervention for health supervision visits for children: growth and developmental surveillance, nutrition, physical activity, oral health, mental and spiritual health, family and social relations, disease prevention strategies, and injury prevention strategies.

36.2 State components of self-concept for preschool and school-age children.

36.3 Plan health promotion and health maintenance strategies employed during health supervision visits of children.

36.4 Discuss the importance of family in child health care, and include family assessment in each health supervision visit.

36.5 Integrate pertinent mental health care into health supervision visits for children.

36.6 Examine data about the family and other social relationships to prioritize interventions and to maintain health of children.

HEALTH PROMOTION AND MAINTENANCE: THE TODDLER AND PRESCHOOLER

The years following infancy are challenging for parents as the child grows and acquires new developmental skills. The child progresses from the first tentative steps and words at a year of age through the "terrible twos" of toddlerhood and into preschool age when over half of children attend some type of education program, have developed effective verbal communication, and acquire many gross and fine motor skills (Child Trends, 2012). Toddler and preschool ages are often grouped as "young childhood," since the family remains the primary system within which the child interacts. Care providers address common health concerns such as nutrition, sleep, and growing independence. Facing consistent changes in development, parents rely on the pediatric healthcare home (medical home) for advice and information. Regular visits are recommended at 12, 15, and 18 months, and at about 2, 3, 4, and 5 years of age. Nurses apply concepts of anticipatory guidance during visits for health promotion and health maintenance to assist parents in the transitions they face.

Health supervision of young children applies:

1. *Assessment*, including screening tests, evaluations, and observations
2. *Education*, including anticipatory guidance about coming developmental tasks
3. *Intervention*, including parent counseling, home visits when appropriate, and scheduling of future visits
4. *Care coordination* among resources serving the family

General Observations

The relationship with the family should be established as a partnership in care of the child. If, however, the family is new to this healthcare home, reach out to welcome family members warmly and express interest in them as individuals and parents. Families may feel uncomfortable in healthcare settings, and it is important to establish positive rapport so they will be able to ask questions and bring up concerns about the child.

While calling the toddler in from the waiting room, it is wise to recall the child just 1 year before. It is amazing that this young child is now able to walk in, even if with a bit of help. Watch for the child's desire for independence or signs of continuing reliance on the parent. By preschool age, the child is totally independent in walking and usually engages in conversations easily. After welcoming the preschool child warmly, assess the child's social skills and motor activities. Direct greetings or questions to the child to evaluate stranger anxiety and ability to understand simple commands or questions. What verbal skills are observed? Observe the child's general appearance, nutrition, and state of health.

Health supervision visits are adapted for older toddlers and preschoolers to include observations of parental discipline and interaction style. Does the parent respond to the child's questions? Were age-appropriate toys or activities brought to the visit to help occupy the child while waiting? Is the child alert and observant of the environment?

Growth and Developmental Surveillance

An essential assessment integrated into the visit is measurement of growth. Weight and length are measured and compared to expected patterns of growth. Once the child can stand upright to be measured, sometime between 2 and 3 years of age, charts for standing height rather than recumbent length are used. Body mass index (BMI) is first calculated at 2 years of age and provides information about the relationship of height and weight (see Chapter 33 ⊘ for additional information). Head circumference is usually measured until 1 to 2 years of age. (Consult growth grids in Appendix C ⊘.)

Growth continues to be a primary way of evaluating the child's nutritional status. It may also provide clues about conditions that have not yet been evaluated such as endocrine, cardiac, or other disorders. Depending on the results of growth measurements, the nurse may gather additional data. For a child under the 5th percentile for weight or BMI, detailed recording of nutritional intake should begin. Laboratory studies such as hematocrit and hemoglobin can be performed. Patterns of family growth can be examined. What size are the parents and siblings? Ask if the child has had any illness or hospitalization. For children above the 85th percentile for BMI, detailed dietary intake and physical activity history should be taken.

The physical assessment is performed, with some parts conducted by the nurse and others by the primary care provider such as a physician or nurse practitioner. See Chapter 34 🔗 for a thorough discussion of physical examination. The order of the examination and the approaches to the child are particularly important at this age. Leave intrusive procedures such as ear and eye examinations and visualization of genitalia until the end of the examination. Integrate techniques such as allowing the child to play with the stethoscope, asking the child to "blow out" the light from the otoscope, or having the child make a game of pushing the legs against the examiner to measure symmetry of strength (Figure 36–1 ●). Preschoolers are generally interested in their bodies, and teaching about parts of the examination is helpful. During the physical examination, ask the parents pertinent questions. Consider the young child's expected developmental milestones (see information in Chapter 32 🔗) and ask questions related to these milestones. Developmental surveillance is integrated throughout the visit as you observe the child's fine motor, gross motor, language, and social skills. Developmental screening or testing is performed; also ask if the child has had developmental testing done at a childcare agency or another site.

Nurses generally have in-depth knowledge of child development, through growth and development courses and pediatric nursing curricula, and are thus well positioned to address parental concerns related to child development. Development is the key organizing principle of early childhood health care.

Developmental screening and services should be integrated within healthcare, childcare, and school settings, to include the multiple sites common for young children (Halfon, Larson, & Russ, 2010). Topics pertinent at health supervision visits of young children include sleep patterns, discipline techniques, toilet training, learning and reading practices, communication, and parental issues and questions. Many children, especially by preschool age, are attending a childcare center (Child Trends, 2012). Ask about the experience and whether developmental skills are a focus of activity. Ask if the parent is pleased with the childcare experience or needs further resources.

Health promotion growth and development issues for toddlers and preschoolers are addressed at each visit. Some common examples include:

■ Explaining growth patterns and what is expected in the months ahead

■ Providing toys that encourage development of the coming developmental milestones

■ Showing parents the child's developmental progression on a screening tool

Likewise, health maintenance activities are included in health supervision visits, with the primary purpose being prevention of disease and injury. Specific examples are included throughout the chapter, but some general areas addressed are:

■ Connecting developmental skills with risks for injury such as drowning and motor vehicle crashes

■ Recognizing the possibility of exposure to infectious diseases as the child begins a childcare experience and addressing recognition of and treatments for common diseases

Expected outcomes for the child include normal growth and development patterns for motor, language, and social skills; parental knowledge of stimulating activities for the child;

A

B

● **Figure 36–1** Examining the toddler or preschooler. The approach to examination of the toddler or preschooler is important in order to elicit cooperation. *A,* The toddler may accept parts of the examination best when seated on the parent's lap as shown in this photo of a boy with his father. *B,* The preschooler likes the opportunity to touch and become comfortable with equipment used or, in this case, holds a doll that receives the same examinations as the child.

awareness of the family about risks to growth and development; and healthy body systems for the child.

Nutrition

The child's nutritional status continues to play an important part in promoting health and preventing health disruptions during toddler and preschooler years. Good nutrition fosters normal growth patterns, promotes developmental progression, and helps prevent disorders such as anemia, tooth decay, and immune dysfunction. Eating takes on an increasingly social dimension during early childhood as children interact more with adults and other children at mealtimes. See Chapter 33 for further information about nutritional needs and challenges.

For toddlers, questions for the family focus on introduction of foods, the child's eating patterns, and transition from breast or bottle to other liquids. The toddler often consumes small amounts of foods, and parents consequently worry about the change in appetite. Showing them that the child is growing normally can help allay their anxiety about this common developmental variation. Preschoolers increasingly interact with others during food preparation and meal consumption. Questions focus on the child's likes and dislikes for particular foods, behavior at the table, and establishment of healthy family eating patterns. Ask how often the family eats out, especially at fast-food restaurants. When parents are busy and older siblings are in activities, both toddlers and preschoolers may be eating foods such as french fries or milk shakes several times weekly. Suggest

alternative approaches to the busy lifestyle, such as bringing fresh fruit slices along when an older sibling is at a sporting event, keeping a cooler in the car to maintain cool items, and limiting fast-food meals to no more than one or two weekly. Obtain nutritional information about common fast-food options in your community and share these with parents. Assist them to make healthy choices when eating out. Encourage the family to set times when they all eat together, even if only a few times weekly. If children help with preparations for this family meal, and then eat together, nutritional knowledge and intake can be positively enhanced. When the child is in a childcare center or home, encourage the parents to find out what food is provided for the child in that setting.

During the toddler and preschool years, children are gaining much more independence about food choices and patterns of eating. At the same time, their eating patterns depend mainly on the family, so assessment should involve the entire family unit (see *Developing Cultural Competence: Family Nutrition*). Parents can benefit from receiving information about nutrition for young children (Table 36–1).

Health promotion interventions include actions such as supporting breastfeeding for young toddlers and being sure preschoolers have a role in selecting foods for healthy snacks. Parental education is influential in shaping their young child's diet and should be integrated into all visits (Holt, Wooldridge, Story, et al., 2011). Important health promotion teaching includes the concept of "5 a day," or ensuring five servings of fruits and

Table 36–1	Nutrition Teaching for Health Promotion and Health Maintenance Visits	
Age	**Nutrition Teaching**	
1 year	Support mother who continues to breastfeed. Wean child from bottle by substituting cup. If beginning to use cow's milk, use whole milk (may change to 2% at 2 years of age). Limit juice to 4–6 ounces daily; offer water several times daily; use plain water and avoid flavored water or sugared/electrolyte drinks. Encourage safety measures—use high chair with strap, secure child and use caution in grocery carts, do not allow foods to be eaten in car. Provide information on choking and airway obstruction removal training.	Provide food and water safety guidelines (see Chapter 33). Be sure all major food groups have been introduced. Limit high-fat and high-sugar foods. Review amounts of food commonly consumed and frequency of feedings. Review use of fluoride if water supply is not fluoridated.
2 years	Ask if the mother is still breastfeeding and support the decision to continue or to wean child, as she desires. Encourage total removal of bottle if still in use. Ensure that all foods common to family have been offered. Offer child-sized eating utensils. Child can change to low-fat or skim milk if family desires. Limit milk to 2–3 servings daily.	Teach parents methods for dealing with temper tantrums over food—make food available at meal and snack times only, do not force intake, offer a variety of foods. Teach that child may have days of very low intake due to slowing growth rate.
3 years	Most children are weaned from breastfeeding and drink 1% or 2% milk. Teach normal intake and decreasing number of snacks. Engage child in food preparation and pouring liquids from small pitcher. Recognize that food jags (periods when only 1 or 2 foods are eaten) are common.	Recognize importance of social nature of eating; expect child to sit for a short period at meals with family. Meals and snacks should not be eaten while watching television.
4 years	Encourage involving child in snack selection and preparation. Start to teach food groups and importance of nutrition for the body.	Alter intake as appropriate depending on weight and BMI. Dairy products consumed should all be low or reduced fat.

Weblink

National Association for Sport and Physical Education (NASPE)

Developing Cultural Competence
Family Nutrition

Each family integrates their own cultural backgrounds and past experiences into food preparation and choices. Ask what foods are common in the child's cultural group and help the family learn when to introduce each food. For example, rice may be a first food for an Asian baby, rather than rice cereal. Be sure the child also takes in adequate iron sources in the first foods offered. Tofu or bean paste may be a common protein source in some diets. A Native American child may eat fish or wild game, along with berries and roots. Ask and learn about each family's cultural patterns. Learn what you can about cultural groups in your community. Encourage the family to offer the young child their usual foods, as long as they meet needs for requirements, are prepared with minimal salt and seasoning, and are soft enough to avoid choking. Perform diet recalls and analyses to check for any specific teaching needs in all families.

● **Figure 36–2** This toddler enjoys motor activity that uses large muscle groups. The preschooler begins to spend increasing amounts of time in coordination of both small and large muscle mass. List several physical activities that you can suggest for the parents of children in each of these age groups.

vegetables in the daily diet (American Academy of Pediatrics [AAP] Committee on Nutrition, 2009). Likewise, "3 a day of dairy" encourages families to provide at least three servings of dairy for children every day. Nurses and parents partner together to ensure that the young child establishes healthy eating habits at home and in other daily settings. Health maintenance activities focus primarily on disease and injury prevention, with examples of feeding practices that do not include common choking foods, and limiting daily fruit juice intake to prevent dental caries and excessive caloric intake. Desired outcomes related to nutrition include meeting normal growth and development milestones, maintaining a recommended weight, increasing understanding of healthy food patterns, and preventing nutrition-related disorders.

Physical Activity

The toddler and preschooler consistently show gains in fine and gross motor abilities. They move around independently and have more physical activity away from the home base. They commonly visit parks, swim, attend childcare centers, and help with some household tasks. These activities are important, both because they assist the child to continue to develop motor skills and because they limit the amount of time spent in sedentary behavior. The toddler and preschool years are an important time for setting the habits for physical activity during all of childhood.

During toddler years the main emphasis is on providing experiences that encourage further motor development. The child needs to walk, run, hop, push and pull objects, and throw balls. Motor activity is a major component in all playtimes, and activities should engage the child's large and small muscle groups. The National Association for Sport and Physical Education (NASPE) has established recommendations for toddlers and preschoolers: a minimum of 60 minutes per day of unstructured physical activity, a minimum of 60 minutes per day of structured physical activity, and a maximum of 60 minutes of sedentary behavior at any one time exclusive of sleep (Beets, Bornstein, Dowda, et al.,

2011; Centers for Disease Control and Prevention [CDC], 2010a, 2011) (Figure 36–2 ●).

By the preschool years, coordination becomes increasingly important. Physical activity is important for all children, including those with developmental disabilities. The preschooler learns to balance, walk on one foot, skip, and throw and catch with greater accuracy. **Kinesthesia**, or the sense of one's body position and movement, develops during these years. Eye–hand coordination improves at the same time that visual acuity matures. The social component plays an important role as children learn to engage in games and activities cooperatively with others.

The nurse applies the concept of resilience by identifying both risk and protective factors related to physical activity (Table 36–2). The assessment becomes the basis for nursing interventions, both to reinforce positive physical activity and to make recommendations for changes where needed.

Both children and adults are commonly overweight and sedentary in today's society, so emphasis on physical activity should be a part of each health supervision visit. Nurses and parents are partners in planning activities for the young child; patterns set in motion at this early age will continue into the rest of childhood and into adulthood. Suggestions for the family may include setting guidelines to limit television and other screen activities to a maximum of 2 hours daily in order to facilitate adequate physical activity time. Children should not have television and computers in their bedrooms. Health promotion teaching imparts to parents the benefits of activity, such as a healthy immune and cardiovascular system, positive self-concept of the child, and the child's learning of important motor skills. Health maintenance teaching focuses on disease prevention, such as avoidance of overweight, and injury prevention, with use of protective gear for sports.

Table 36–2	Risk and Protective Factors Regarding Physical Activity in Toddlerhood and Preschool
Risk Factors	**Protective Factors**
■ Developmental delay ■ Slow development of social skills	■ Expected developmental progression
■ Limited stimulation by family or other care providers ■ Limited social time with other children ■ Long work hours by parents	■ Easily engages socially with others ■ Regular contact with other young children
■ Reluctance to try new physical activity ■ Limited access to balls, slides, balance beams, tricycles, and other materials that foster physical activity ■ Adequate safety gear for activities is not available	■ Eagerness to try new physical activity ■ Access to balls, slides, balance beams, tricycles, and other materials that foster physical activity ■ Adequate safety gear that properly fits child is available
■ Parents who have little physical activity on a daily basis ■ Lack of knowledge by family about child's physical activity needs	■ Family members engage in daily physical activity ■ Family members spend time in physical activity with child ■ Family understands motor developmental milestones and importance of physical activity in childhood
■ Television or other screen activities are engaged in for more than 2 hours daily	■ Television and other screen activities are limited to no more than 2 hours daily
■ Limited community resources for child care and physical activity ■ Unsafe neighborhood and lack of lawns, parks, and other facilities	■ Neighborhood contains access to child care that integrates physical activity ■ Neighborhood is safe, and contains lawns, parks, and other facilities

Making the Pacifier Decision

Video

Expected outcomes of health promotion and health supervision related to physical activity are daily inclusion of at least 60 minutes of activity into life patterns, normal developmental progression of the musculoskeletal system, growth in coordination, and appropriate balance between dietary intake and physical activity so that normal weight is maintained.

Oral Health

The early childhood years play an important part in the child's future oral health, and yet dental care remains one of the most preventable and common unmet healthcare needs for children in developed countries. Dental caries have increased in the 2- to 5-year-old age group from 19% in the 1988–1994 survey to 24% in the most recent National Health and Nutrition Examination Survey (CDC, 2009). **Early childhood caries (ECC)** is defined as one or more decayed, missing, or filled tooth surfaces in a child 71 months of age or younger (National Maternal and Child Oral Health Resource Center, 2010). This condition is promoted by inadequate preventive care, which can include diet, brushing, feeding habits, and lack of dental care. ECC is serious because young children with the condition are more likely to have continuing dental problems that can influence speech, cause pain, and delay development. Teaching prevention at an early age is key to preventing the problem.

The nurse assists the family to ensure oral health for the young child. By 1 year of age, the child should have made a first visit to the dentist. By about 2 years of age, the toddler has a full set of 20 primary teeth, called **deciduous teeth**, that will be lost during childhood, beginning at about 6 years. Evaluate these teeth for condition and number. They help to maintain space for the permanent teeth, foster positive eating habits, and

are needed for language development. Inquire about how the family cleans the teeth and, if the child has any dental decay, ask them to demonstrate their daily care. At the end of preschool, the first of the deciduous teeth are lost, an important developmental event for most children.

By 2 to 4 years of age, young children have discontinued pacifiers and thumbsucking. These habits are harmful when permanent teeth begin erupting around 6 years (American Dental Association [ADA], 2011). Parents should be instructed to gradually remove the pacifier by 1 to 2 years of age. Many young children continue to thumbsuck, which is a comforting and reassuring habit. Usually the child who is 2 to 4 years old is ready to discontinue thumbsucking, and parents can promote this process by praising the child for not sucking, helping the child to find alternative sources of comfort such as rubbing a blanket, putting a sock on the hand at nap or nighttime to serve as a reminder, and working with the preschooler to identify the reward when no thumbsucking is seen for a week or more (ADA, 2011).

Based on the results of the assessment of the child's teeth, observation of language skills, and answers to questions directed at parents, plan interventions that will foster maintenance of oral health, thus preventing dental disease. (See Chapter 46 ✪ for emergency treatment of dental injury.) These may include referral to low-cost dental clinics, provision of toothbrush and toothpaste, demonstration to the parents and young child about proper brushing technique, and teaching about limiting sweet snacks and drinks. A dental visit will assist in identifying children at moderate or high risk of dental caries; for these children, a "smear" of fluoridated toothpaste should be used for brushing, and in 2 to 5 year olds, a pea-size amount of fluoridated toothpaste can be used. For other children, nonfluoridated toothpaste is used (American Academy of Pediatric Dentistry [AAPD], 2012a). Remember to positively reinforce health promotion practices such as good oral hygiene for toddlers and preschoolers who brush, visit the dentist, and are careful to limit intake of sweets. Desired outcomes for oral health are eruption of a normal set of deciduous teeth, regular dental care, nutrition and hygiene practices that foster dental health, and knowledge of child and parent about oral health.

Mental and Spiritual Health

The family plays a key role in fostering a positive self-image and setting the stage for the young child's mental health. As the family is called in for the visit, begin an assessment of the family's methods of influencing mental health. Observe communication and interactions in the family and the child's ability to interact with healthcare providers. Ask for a description of a typical day or what the child has recently begun to do. The child's sense of self and mental status are related to new accomplishments. Inquire about toilet training, tooth brushing, choosing clothes and getting dressed, using crayons, or other developmental tasks.

Toddlers and preschoolers use **self-regulation** (the ability to soothe and comfort the self) to control anger, excessive desires for objects or foods, and other nonsocial behaviors. To assist the child in developing the ability to control and regulate self, parents often use discipline techniques. Ask about how the parent deals with the child who is having a temper tantrum or showing other undesirable behaviors. Reinforce positive ways of helping the child set limits for self and make suggestions when parents need assistance (see *Teaching Highlights: Positive Discipline*). The goal of discipline is to help the child develop a sense of right and wrong, and to learn acceptable ways of dealing with other people.

Adequate sleep and rest are needed for children to master self-regulation. Most toddlers have established regular sleeping patterns with occasional night awakenings. They sleep about 10 to 12 hours at night with one or two daytime naps (Murray, Zentner, & Yakimo, 2009). Parents have usually learned to establish clear routines such as reading a story, rubbing a back, and then leaving the child alone. Occasionally parents who work during the day may feel guilty about putting the child to sleep. Help them to spend quality time with the child after arriving home, and then to establish clear sleeping expectations. Transitional objects such as blankets or toys are important for the toddler and can be used during childcare experiences to provide comfort and help maintain normal routines. Some families prefer to have children sleep in the bed with parents. Advise against this pattern, but if this is the parents' decision, be sure they are aware of safety hazards such as suffocation in excessive bedding, injury related to falling between headboard and frame, parental smoking that could lead to a fire, or parental deep sleeping or alcohol and drug use that can lead to such sound sleep that it is possible to roll onto and suffocate the child.

The preschooler sleeps about 9 to 11 hours and may have one or no naps each day (Murray et al., 2009). Some quiet playtime can be beneficial even for the preschooler who does not nap. At this age, some children begin to awaken at night and may need some assistance in falling back to sleep. **Nightmares** are frightening dreams that awaken the child, who is often crying and upset. Parents can reassure the child, rub the child's back, provide some repeat of a bedtime routine such as reading a story, and then allow the child to settle into sleep again. It is not advisable to bring children to the parental bed since they may start to awaken at night in order to continue this practice. **Night terrors** (or sleep terrors) are

---

Teaching Highlights Positive Discipline

First, provide structure that enhances the possibility of desirable behaviors:

- Limit rules to those that are essential. It will be easier to enforce a few important rules than many that are nonessential.
- Provide an environment where the child is mainly free to explore safely in order to avoid constant cautions. For example, have adequate play space for toddlers with limited fragile glassware in the usual daily environment. It is easier for the toddler to learn not to touch a few objects when adequate objects are provided for play.
- Spend time interacting with the child several times each day. Praise positive behaviors frequently. Preschoolers often like to have charts with stars to record picking up toys, helping a parent, and other positive behaviors. Once a certain number of stars is reached, a reward, such as stickers or an outing with the parent, is earned.

When the child shows undesirable behaviors:

- Use distraction as the first approach and praise the child for selecting the new activity suggested by the parent.
- Tell the child one time that the behavior is unsatisfactory and what will happen if the behavior persists.

- Separate the child from a setting in which behavior is undesirable. Place the child in "time-out," a separate place that is safe. Toddlers can be placed in a playpen or crib, while preschoolers are told to sit on a chair. One minute of time-out per year of age is a good length of time. Once time-out is over, provide a positive activity and move the child directly toward the activity.

When undesirable behaviors include other people, such as biting or hitting:

- Tell the child clearly that it is not okay to hurt another person. Encourage and role model proper language to explain feelings.
- Separate the child immediately from the situation and use time-out.
- If there are repeated episodes, be sure the child is getting adequate sleep and food, has opportunities for active play that releases energy, and has positive attention from many people in the environment. Be sensitive to stresses such as a recent trauma or a new sibling.
- Encourage the child to "use words" instead of hitting or biting. Until able to do so on their own, parents can model this behavior. "You feel like saying, 'I am really upset that you took my toy away.' Let's use words instead of hitting so your sister knows that."

Video | Temper Tantrums

characterized by a child who cries out, appears frightened, and has tachycardia and tachypnea. However, in contrast to nightmares, the child having a night terror is not fully awake and may appear disoriented (Murray et al., 2009). Parents should quietly talk to and comfort the child, allowing the child to return to sleep. The child has no recollection of these events the next morning.

The toddler gains more independence in many aspects of life such as mobility and speech. The control over toileting is another milestone that signals greater independence and can lead to a sense of self-control. Ask parents if the toddler has shown interest in toilet training and how they intend to work with the child to attain control over bowel and bladder. (See Chapter 32 🔴 for further discussion about toilet training.) Preschoolers are generally well trained for bowel and bladder with only occasional accidents. These should be treated with understanding rather than blame in order for healthy self-concept to develop.

Preschoolers are increasingly aware of gender and sexuality issues. They may ask questions about kissing, love, or their genitals. These questions should be truthfully answered, leaving the child with a positive sense of sexuality. Some exploration of genitals may occur, and children should be told simply that it is something that should occur in private, and then be offered other activities to engage them when with other people.

The family's spiritual orientation takes on additional meaning for the toddler and preschooler. They can participate in the family's faith-based practices, which enlarge their microsystem influences to include that of the religious group, thus reinforcing the child's learning about right and wrong. The nurse assesses the family's faith-based or spiritual beliefs and provides support for the family's approach, whether it is in established religious organizations or in the family's other meaningful activities.

Health promotion activities focus on development of a healthy self-concept in the toddler and young child by helping parents to set up successful play experiences, to praise the child for successes, to use effective limit-setting techniques, and to realize and appreciate the child's unique characteristics. Health maintenance seeks to avoid the poor self-image that can occur with constant criticism or expectations not in alignment with the toddler's or preschooler's developmental capabilities. Further examples of the family interactions that can influence the child's self-concept are provided in the following section on relationships.

Desired outcomes for the child related to mental and spiritual health include emergence of a positive self-esteem, ability to self-regulate behaviors, emergence of methods to handle daily stressors, and normal developmental progression in tasks such as toilet training and sleep.

Relationships

Family members are part of the microsystem for the toddler and preschooler and, as such, form a vital part of the child's environment. Families with members who handle stress well and have healthy lifestyle patterns offer security for the young child. When parents are stressed or depressed, the mental status of all family members can be affected. Ask how things are going for the family in general. Inquire about siblings and whether there are any issues of concern that might influence the toddler or preschooler. Illness or behavior problems in a sibling can decrease

the parent's ability to deal with other children. The focus on a sibling in need can be confusing to a toddler or preschooler. Be alert for signs of child abuse and for substance abuse in family members. Have the parents become separated or divorced? Is there a new stepparent?

During questions and observations, the nurse identifies family risk and protective factors. Reinforce strengths and provide services and referrals to deal with risks. Some strengths include the following:

- The family spends time together each day.
- Parents are proud of the child's accomplishments and knowledgeable about developmental progression.
- Childcare center personnel and family members interact regularly to plan consistent approaches for the toddler and preschooler.
- The teen mother of a toddler is enrolled in a high school continuation program with a childcare component.

Examples of risks to mental health include the following:

- Mother has been diagnosed with depression.
- Family member in home uses street drugs.
- Child awakens with night terrors.
- Child was recently in a serious car crash.
- Teen mother is estranged from own family and has few goals and resources.

Toddlers continue to grow in social abilities, while preschoolers demonstrate large strides in socializing with others. Expect that most toddlers will enjoy playing with other children, although they play "side by side" in a parallel manner and not cooperatively. They also engage in play with adults for short periods, such as throwing a ball. However, preschoolers begin to engage in activities that involve other children directly in cooperative play. They play "house" where one child plays the mother, and another the child. They engage in simple games where each plays a separate role. Their interactions with adults display similar maturity as they take on tasks such as setting the table for dinner or picking up books from the floor. Social skills involve getting along with others. Young children exhibit increasing skill in language development, a primary medium for social exchange. From just a few words at 1 year, the child has progressed to stating three-word sentences by 3 years of age. While all parts of speech are not in place, young children certainly have the ability to make needs and thoughts known. Assessment of language skills provides a mirror into this important means of socializing.

Successful social skills involve separating from the parent at times. During toddlerhood, most children spend some time away from parents. Initially they may be fearful and display crying, but gradually they learn to adapt to the new person and place. Preschoolers need to begin developing relationships with other adults and children in order to adapt to the school setting at about 5 years of age. Ask how many people the child has contact with each week and how they manage separation from the parent. Encourage parents to see separation as a skill the child is learning rather than something that is guilt producing for them.

When they leave the child in a secure setting, they should hug, provide a favorite object, and leave. Short periods initially will teach the child that the parent can be trusted to return.

Expected outcomes of health promotion and health maintenance activities with young children include increasing social skills with parents, siblings, and other children and adults; successful management of temperament characteristics; adjustment to time away from the home; and improving language/communication skills.

Disease Prevention Strategies

Toddlers and preschoolers commonly have 6 to 10 upper respiratory infections annually, so teaching good hygiene is a helpful preventive measure (Lucille Packard Children's Hospital, 2012). Some immunizations are given during this age period in order to complete a basic series. For the child who has not had all immunizations, extra visits to catch them up to recommended levels may be needed. At the end of the preschool period, a complete review of the immunization record is done so that any needed immunizations are administered before school entry. See Table 36–3 for immunizations recommended during toddlerhood and preschool (additional immunizations may be needed for children at high risk for certain diseases). Toddlers and preschoolers should be screened for health problems during health supervision visits, such as asthma, obesity, or other issues manifested by a review of body systems. Earlier visits may have failed to identify a problem due to the child's young age, so areas such as vision, hearing, and developmental milestones are always included.

Recognize that the environment is a powerful influence on the health of children. Ask if parents or others in the home smoke. Discourage this practice and describe the health implications for the child. Is the neighborhood generally safe? Is there toxicity exposure from air, water, or other mediums? Ask about lead exposure in the home (see Chapter 43 🔗 for more information). How much television and other screen time is common in the home? Older siblings who allow the preschooler to play violent video games or watch many hours of inappropriate television can affect the mental health of the young child. Do parents watch the evening news, even when it involves violence, in front of young children? Do they discuss television shows with the child?

Ask if the child has had any diseases, whether common ones such as a middle ear infection, or less common ones such as a serious respiratory infection. Has the child been diagnosed with a chronic disorder such as cystic fibrosis or hemophilia? How has that affected his or her general health and family functioning?

Desired outcomes for disease prevention include integration of a healthy lifestyle into the family's daily life, prompt treatment of acute diseases, and individualization of all health supervision topics for the child with a chronic condition or special healthcare need.

Injury Prevention Strategies

Injuries remain a common healthcare problem for children during the toddler and preschooler years. Toddlers' and preschoolers' mobility, physical skills, and lack of understanding of the presence of hazards put them at particular risk. In addition, children are sometimes left to play alone for short periods, and toddlers and preschoolers can quickly get into dangerous situations. Every healthcare visit needs to include an assessment of risks and teaching to prevent injuries. Tables 36–4 and 36–5 list injury hazards and his or her prevention during these age periods.

Ask parents what they think the most common hazards are for the age of the child, and add other hazards to their awareness. Car safety always needs reinforcing as the types of seats recommended change as the child matures. Children should be in a rear-facing car seat until at least age 2 years, and preferably until 4 years or when the child has reached the top height or weight limit allowed by the car seat manufacturer. From 4 to 7 years, a forward-facing car seat with a harness should be placed in the back seat. Once the child has outgrown the recommendations for height and weight for the forward-facing car seat, a booster seat in the back seat is recommended (AAP Committee on Injury, Violence, and Poison Prevention, 2011; National Highway Traffic Safety Administration, 2012).

Recommend that parents have their car seat checked by a child safety seat inspector. Give them the addresses of the closest inspection stations. These can be located by going through the National Highway Traffic Safety Administration

Table 36–3	Routine Immunizations Recommended During Toddlerhood and Preschool Age
Immunization	**Age Recommended**
Hepatitis B	6–18 months: Administer dose #3 if series not completed during infancy (usually doses #1 and #2 are administered in early infancy, with dose #3 from 6–18 months of age)
Hepatitis A	Series of 2 doses with first at 12 months and second at least 6 months later
Diphtheria, tetanus, acellular pertussis (DTaP)	15–18 months (#4) (first 3 administered in infancy) 4–6 years (#5)
Haemophilus influenzae type b	12–15 months (#4 or will be #3 for PRP-OMP type that requires only 3 doses for whole series) (first doses administered in infancy)
Inactivated poliovirus	4–6 years (#4) (first 3 doses administered in infancy)
Measles, mumps, rubella	12–15 months (#1)
Varicella	12–18 months (#1) 4–6 years (#2)
Pneumococcal	12–15 months (#4)
Influenza	Annually

Note: Schedule may need to be adapted if child did not receive all recommended immunizations during infancy. See Chapter 44 🔗 and the CDC and AAP websites for further information.

Table 36–4   Injury Prevention in Toddlerhood

	Hazard	Developmental Characteristics	Preventive Measures
	Falls	Gross motor skills improve: Toddler is able to move chairs to counters and can climb up ladders.	Supervise toddler closely. Provide safe climbing toys. Begin to teach acceptable places for climbing.
	Poisoning	Gross motor skills enable toddler to climb onto chairs and then cabinets. Medicines, cosmetics, and other poisonous substances are easily reached.	Keep medicines and other poisonous material locked away. Use child-resistant containers and cupboard closures. Post the Poison Control Center number (1-800-222-1222) by telephone and tape it on cell phones and program the cell phone with the number.
	Burns	Toddler is tall enough to reach stove top. Toddler can walk to fireplace and may reach into fire. Electrical cords may be placed in mouth.	Keep pot handles turned inward on stove. Do not burn fires without close supervision. Use a fire screen. Supervise child during play and keep electrical cords, power strips, and other hazards out of reach or covered securely.
	Drowning	Toddler can walk onto docks or pool decks. Toddler may stand on or climb seats on boat. Toddler may fall into buckets, toilets, and fish tanks and be unable to get top of body out.	Supervise any child near water. Swimming classes do not protect a toddler from drowning. Use child-resistant pool covers. Use approved child life jackets near water and on boats. Empty buckets when not in use.
	Motor vehicle crashes	Toddler may be able to undo seat belt, may resist using car seat, demonstrating characteristic negativism and autonomy.	Use approved safety seat only; toddler is not large enough to use car seat belts. Insist on safety seat use for all trips and position seat in rear seat of car. Verify that child is belted in properly before starting car. Keep the child in a rear-facing seat until at least 2 years of age and preferably longer, until achieving the highest weight or height recommended for the seat by the manufacturer; then a forward-facing car seat with harness should be used in the back seat.

Table 36–5   Injury Prevention in the Preschool Years

	Hazard	Developmental Characteristics	Preventive Measures
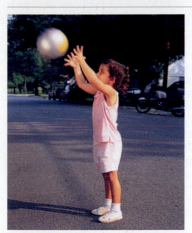	Motor vehicle crashes	By about 4–5 years, the child independently gets into car and puts on seat belt. Child may forget to belt up or may do so incorrectly.	Verify that child is belted in properly before starting car. Keep the child in a rear-facing seat secured in the back seat until at least 2 years of age and preferably longer, until achieving the highest weight or height recommended for the seat by the manufacturer. Forward-facing seats with harness placed in the back seat are used next. Once the child has outgrown the car seat a booster seat is used in the back seat.
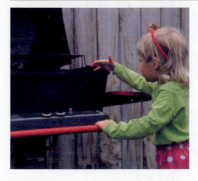	Motor vehicle and pedestrian accidents	Preschooler increasingly plays outside alone or with friends. Preschooler is unable to judge speed of moving car and assumes driver knows that he or she is present.	Teach child never to go into road. A safe, preferably enclosed, play yard is recommended. The child should be supervised by adults at all times.
	Drowning	Preschooler who has had swimming lessons may choose to go into a lake or pool.	Teach child never to go into water without an adult. Provide supervision whenever child is near water.
	Burns	Preschooler can understand the hazards of fire.	Teach child to stop, drop, and roll if clothes are on fire. Practice escapes from home are useful. A visit to a fire station can reinforce learning. Teach child how to call 9-1-1.
	Needlesticks in hospital and home	Preschooler can ambulate and is interested in new objects.	Keep needles out of reach. Remove from hospital unit immediately after use. Instruct families on safe disposal if a family member uses needles at home (for example, a family member with diabetes).
	Electrical injury in hospital and home	Preschooler is mobile and may trip over cords and equipment or may choose to examine them.	Avoid use of electrical cords if possible. Keep equipment out of major traffic areas. Cover any electrical outlets not being used for equipment. Monitor child closely.

(www.nhtsa.dot.gov). Check your particular state laws regulating car safety seats for children.

Other common and serious safety hazards are falls and drowning. In addition to providing general guidelines about safety, these most common injuries should be directly addressed. Children often fall down stairs, from counters where they have been placed or crawled, and from grocery carts. Drowning episodes occur when toddlers and preschoolers are not watched every moment while in the bathtub, near a pool or spa, at a lake or

ocean, or when they fall from boats without personal flotation devices on. While all young children should begin to take swimming lessons, this does not guarantee their safety around water. The American Academy of Pediatrics (2011c) recommends swimming lessons for all children by age 4 years and for children from 1 to 4 years if lessons are available and the parents believe the child is ready for lessons. Children also play with balls, and may follow them as they roll or are thrown into the street. Nursing interventions concentrate on relaying to parents the severity of the risk of falls, drowning, and other hazards for children. Teach them to be aware of the dangers and to avoid them, both at home and in other settings. Refer them to classes on first aid and cardiopulmonary resuscitation.

The child spends increasing time away from the parent. Childcare situations should provide the same supervision the child receives at home. Help parents to ask questions and feel confident in safety at other settings. For example, while parents may be cautious about gun safety at home, few of them inquire if a home the child is visiting has guns and how they are stored.

Preschool is a time when teaching can become directed both to the parents and to their children. Preschoolers are receptive to practicing street crossing and tricycle/bicycle riding skills. It may be helpful to have a place in the clinic or office where they can be taught basic skills such as hand washing or street crossing. Consider the time of year, climate, and geographic location and teach appropriately. Spring is often a good time to teach bicycle and water safety, while winter hazards may include teaching about the hazards of wood stoves or other heating devices. See Table 36–6 for further information about toddler and preschooler hazards and safety teaching needed.

SAFETY ALERT!

Young children die each year when they are left confined in parked vehicles. Occasionally children gain access to a vehicle and accidentally lock themselves inside. In most cases, however, parents leave a child unattended, either forgetting the child is in the car, or remembering but underestimating the danger of heat effects. Nurses can be effective in instructing families to keep cars locked so young children cannot gain access, and to never leave a child in a parked car, either in or out of a car seat, even for a few moments, no matter what the outside temperature (Safe Kids, 2011a).

Table 36–6	Disease and Injury Prevention Topics by Age

Age	Injury Prevention Teaching Topics	
15 months	Wash adult and toddler hands frequently. Clean toys with soap and water regularly. Provide child's own bedding for childcare setting and wash weekly. Use forward-facing car safety seat if child is 20 lb; install correctly and have installation checked; place in back seat and never in front seat with a passenger air bag. Empty containers of water immediately after use; be sure pools or other bodies of water are locked and not accessible. Use sunscreen, hat, and long sleeves in the sun. Keep heavy and sharp objects out of reach; check that all poisons are locked away including in homes visited; keep pet food and cosmetics out of reach.	Have poison control number by phones and taped onto and programmed into cell phones. Be alert for dangers of hot curling irons and other appliances. Have electrical cords out of reach and not hanging down. Keep water temperature no higher than 120–125°F. Have home environment checked for lead hazards; arrange for blood lead level testing when appropriate (see Chapter 43). Secure the child in shopping carts. Do not let child have access to alcoholic drinks. Remember that responsible adults should always supervise your child, not other children. Know CPR, airway obstruction removal, and other first aid.
18 months	Follow the above. Bolt heavy objects securely to the wall to prevent them from being pulled down (such as bookcases and televisions). Be cautious of the toddler near machinery in the yard, such as lawn mowers and farm equipment.	Use a helmet on the child when taking the child on the back of a bicycle. Check batteries in home smoke alarms, CO or radon monitors, and check system monthly; change batteries on a scheduled basis as recommended by manufacturer. Ask care providers about discipline methods; do not allow corporal punishment.
2–3 years	Follow the above. When the child is 40 lb, switch to a belt-positioning booster seat, using vehicle lap and shoulder belt; continue to place booster seat in rear seat of the car. Teach hand hygiene after toileting and other activities. Clean potty chair thoroughly. Keep guns unloaded and locked away in a different locked place than ammunition; have trigger locks installed.	Teach how to cross streets. Provide a helmet for riding tricycles. Check playgrounds for safety hazards and hard surfaces under equipment; ensure cushioned surface.
3–4 years	Follow the above. Do not let child play unsupervised.	Know CPR, airway obstruction removal, and other first aid for the child who has become a preschooler.
4–5 years	Follow the above. Continue teaching safety skills to the child. Continue supervising when near streets or water sources.	Teach safety around strangers (never go with a stranger; find a trusted person such as a parent or police).

Source: Data from Hagan, J. F., Shaw, J. S., & Duncan, P. M. (Eds.). (2008). *Bright futures: Guidelines for health supervision of infants, children, and adolescents* (3rd ed.). Elk Grove Village, IL: American Academy of Pediatrics.

Desired outcomes for the child are integration of safe practices into car restraints and other daily activities, progression through toddlerhood and preschool with no serious injuries, prompt care for minor injuries, and increasing understanding by child, parent, and other care providers of the common safety hazards at this age.

NURSING MANAGEMENT *For the Health Promotion and Maintenance of the Toddler and Preschooler*

Nursing Assessment and Diagnosis

Nurses partner with other healthcare professionals such as physicians, nurse practitioners, and speech therapists to assess health promotion and health maintenance status of young children. The toddler and preschool years are characterized by much developmental progression, and strategies need to be constantly adapted to meet the particular needs of the child and family. It is important to realize that the parents are partners in the care of the child and that every health supervision visit should address their questions and concerns. Their observations of the child are an invaluable part of the process. As the preschooler becomes more verbal, he or she becomes another partner in the healthcare team. Ask preschoolers what they want to learn, what questions they have about staying well, and other pertinent questions.

Toddlers and preschoolers are examined for growth, physical health status, and mental/social characteristics. Development is an area that many pediatricians feel ill prepared to address but which parents commonly want addressed. Additionally, developmental surveillance must occur at every healthcare visit, with standardized screening at 9, 18, and 24 to 30 months. Nurses are adept at describing normal developmental milestones, evaluating the progression of children, and using anticipatory guidance to address parental developmental concerns.

Based on a thorough assessment, the nurse will establish nursing diagnoses that are appropriate for the young child and family. Potential nursing diagnoses established during a health supervision of a toddler or preschooler might include the following (NANDA-I © 2012):

- *Anxiety* related to change of environment (new care provider)
- *Role Conflict, Parental,* related to lack of support from significant others
- *Growth and Development, Delayed,* related to lead exposure
- *Sleep Deprivation* related to nightmares and night terrors
- *Knowledge, Readiness for Enhanced,* related to parental desire for safety information
- *Skin Integrity, Impaired,* related to hyperthermia (sunburn)

Planning and Implementation

Based on the nursing diagnoses, the nurse works with other partners to plan strategies to meet the needs of the family. Explain that assessment questions are asked to provide a picture of the child that can be helpful in partnering with parents to plan health care. Reinforce the importance of the family coming to health supervision visits with their own list of issues. Work with other healthcare professionals to be sure all needs of a particular child and family are addressed.

Some teaching takes place as the examination occurs. Explain the height and weight measurements and what they mean. Relate them to questions about dietary intake and family food patterns. During the physical examination, insert information about common infections such as otitis media (middle ear infection) and share immunization information.

If the family has been reluctant to ask questions, reflect on the child's development. "Many children have trouble sleeping through the night; is that the case for Cassandra? What helps her to sleep? What is it like at her bedtime?" Developmental areas such as sleep, discipline, toilet training, and expected developmental milestones should be addressed. If the parents were provided in an earlier visit with a journal to record observations and questions, ask if they have brought it with them.

Health promotion activities are emphasized during the visit. Health promotion related to physical activity includes teaching about toys that encourage activity, such as balls, music, push toys, and tricycles. Review nutritional intake and encourage introduction of new foods, healthy snack and meal choices, and positive eating for busy families. Emphasize the importance of play to healthy child development. Provide ideas for incorporating free playtime each day. Apply concepts of anticipatory guidance as you address the child's approaching developmental progression. If the child will soon be toilet trained, provide information about possible approaches. If the child is learning to swim or has access to water, reinforce safety precautions near water. For the child going to a new childcare center, provide the parents with a list of questions they can ask the care provider, and tips to assist in the transition to a new setting.

Health maintenance activities are added to the visit as you give immunizations and screen for tuberculosis, lead screening, or problems with language, vision, or hearing. Provide instruction on use of nonprescription medications, including use of acetaminophen after immunizations. Precautions, safe dosing, and checking with the healthcare provider should be addressed. The focus of these activities is to prevent disease or to find it early before serious consequences arise. Whenever you find information that may indicate a problem, be sure to refer the child to the primary care provider, such as the physician or nurse practitioner. You may even recommend that another specialist, such as a speech pathologist or dentist, see the child. Other health maintenance activities that must be part of each visit with a toddler or preschooler involve teaching about common hazards and how to avoid them. Emergency care in case of injury is also helpful information for parents, so first aid classes can be recommended. Ask about daycare, preschool, or kindergarten attendance or future plans.

Conclude the visit with some words of praise about both the parent's and child's accomplishments. Schedule the date for the next visit. List any resources helpful to the family, including the clinic/office contact information and emergency services.

Teaching Highlights Toy and Playground Safety

Play is essential to the physical and cognitive growth of toddlers and preschoolers. However, toys can present hazards for young children, and parents need guidelines to follow when selecting toys. These include (Safe Kids, 2011c):

- Select toys intended for the age of the child, as indicated on the label. Some toys have small parts or can break into small parts, and should not be given to children younger than 3 years. They should not be too heavy for the child to manipulate them appropriately. Toys with strings, straps, or cords longer than 7 inches pose strangulation hazards.
- Assemble toys as directed and check them frequently for breakage; remove all packing materials before providing toys for the child.
- Do not use older repainted toys unless certain that paint used contained no lead.
- Select cloth toys that are nonflammable, flame resistant, or flame retardant. Avoid electrical and battery-powered toys in children younger than 8 years.
- Do not allow latex balloons and especially noninflated balloons to be used as toys.

Playgrounds provide a location for healthy development of children, but can also be responsible for child injuries. Home playgrounds are the sites of most playground injuries. Falls, strangulation, and head impacts are examples of frequent playground injuries. Some tips can be provided to parents (Safe Kids, 2011b):

- Surfaces should be composed of soft and loose material such as mulch or fine sand. The surface should be 12 inches deep and extend 6 feet around equipment.
- Equipment should not allow the child to be more than 5 feet off the surface.
- Strangulation poses a high risk so be sure to remove ties, ribbons, drawstrings, and other hanging items from clothing and play areas.
- Ensure that the equipment is intended for the age of the child. Separate playgrounds for young and older children are recommended.
- Consult the U.S. Consumer Product Safety Commission for playground equipment standards. Inspect equipment regularly.
- Always supervise the young child on a playground at all times.

Evaluation

Parents should be asked occasionally to evaluate the care they are receiving at the health promotion and health maintenance site. Use these comments to monitor and adjust procedures as needed. The expected outcomes for nursing care of the toddler and preschooler include the following:

- The child demonstrates normal patterns of growth and progression in developmental milestones.
- The child remains free of disease and injury.
- Parents relay satisfaction with the pediatric healthcare home.
- The child manifests positive physical, social, and emotional adjustment.

HEALTH PROMOTION AND MAINTENANCE: THE SCHOOL-AGE CHILD

The older childhood years span the time when most children enter kindergarten at about 5 years of age, and progress until about 12 to 13 years of age, when adolescence begins. Even though health promotion and health maintenance remain important during this time, less frequent visits to the pediatric healthcare home are recommended. In addition, most children are relatively healthy and need few immunizations, which may lead to only sporadic visits for care. Whenever older school-age children are seen in health care, even for illness or emergency care, it is wise to ask when the last "well-child" or health supervision visit was scheduled. Encourage the parents to make an appointment if the

child is due for a visit. Visits are generally recommended at about 5 years of age, when most children are going to kindergarten, and then at 6 years, 8 years, and 10, 11, and 12 years. The visits during this time will focus on monitoring physical and developmental changes, establishing good health habits related to important issues such as nutrition, physical activity, and mental health; learning the importance of avoiding tobacco, alcohol, and drugs; ensuring success in school, family, and extracurricular activities; and fostering good decision-making and problem-solving skills.

General Observations

The first school-age visit usually occurs just before entry into kindergarten. During this visit the child has a thorough examination to be certain that physical development is normal, developmental milestones have been met for fine and gross motor skills, school readiness is displayed in social skills and language, and final sets of basic immunizations are completed. The child is often excited about the visit because it is associated with beginning school; some anxiety is often felt, as it may be the first time the child is aware of getting "shots." As with earlier visits, the nurse's observations begin as the child is called in for the visit. It is wise to speak to the child first, introducing yourself and welcoming the child and parents to the office or clinic. Many children of this age actively participate in conversations, making teaching and gathering data easy. For children who are quiet or look to the parents, allow more time for them to get to know the personnel, directing most initial questions to parents. This may be the first visit where the child is old enough to be a partner in the healthcare visit. Establishing positive rapport with the child will be more likely to enhance efforts designed to teach about health. At the same time, family-centered care, or a partnership to include decision making jointly by the family and the health-care provider, is important for school-age health (Kuo, Houtrow, Arango, et al., 2011).

Notice whether the child brought a book, toy, or some other object to the visit. How are the parents interacting with the child? What types of speech tones are used? Is there mutual respect or are parents and child ignoring each other or having disagreements? The child should walk with symmetry and ease of movement, follow instructions about where to go and taking off shoes for weighing, and demonstrate clear language skills with parent or healthcare personnel.

By the time children come for visits at age 6 and 8 years, they are expected to be increasingly active in sports, school activities, music, or other interests. Look for clues about their interests as they arrive. Did they bring books or an iPod? What are the book topics or favorite types of music? Ask what they are doing during the summer or what their two favorite after-school activities entail. Have them describe a typical day to obtain clues about their life.

Some children do not commonly come to clinics, offices, or other settings for health supervision visits. School nurses or nurse practitioners in school-based clinics sometimes offer health promotion/health maintenance activities in the school setting. A major focus of school nurses is making the environment conducive to health for groups of children. School nurses may:

- Offer some parts of examination to individual children, such as growth and developmental surveillance.
- Conduct health screenings, such as vision, hearing, or scoliosis.
- Work with food service personnel and administration to improve meal and snack quality and minimize unhealthy choices in vending machines.
- Work with teachers to integrate concepts such as physical activity and self-esteem into classroom activities.

The nurse often links children with healthcare needs to other community services.

During health supervision visits, watch the parents' responses as children answer questions. Be alert for the parent who interrupts the child or constantly "corrects" what is said. Comments by the parent should involve praise of the child or looking to the child for opinions on certain topics. This indicates that a partnership is developing in the family and that family members work together and value each other. Direct some questions to the parents also. Ask if they came with specific questions or concerns that should be addressed. If the child has an individualized education or health plan (see Chapter 38 🔗), ask if the parent brought a copy, if the plan is still appropriate, or if it needs updating; facilitate a meeting with the school district about the plan if indicated. Allow the parent an opportunity to meet with the physician, nurse practitioner, or other professional in a private place and without the child present if desired. Be alert for family dynamics that can influence mental health status. Ask if there have been any important changes in the family and how they have influenced the child. During conversations, be alert for reports of separation, divorce, remarriages, ill parents or siblings or grandparents, recent or upcoming moves, parent job changes, substance abuse, incarceration of family members,

custody disputes, or other issues. Integrate a family history of diseases into the examination. Such topics can be followed up with further questions, as described later in the mental health section, to learn how they influence the child.

Growth and Developmental Surveillance

As the child comes into the health supervision site, take height and weight measurements. Be sure to have the child remove shoes and coats. Ask the child and parents if they know the child's current height and weight, and if they have any questions. Plot the percentiles for these measurements, calculate body mass index (BMI) and its percentile, and explain the meaning of these findings later in the visit. Recognize that children do not grow uniformly; they have periods of slow growth followed by fast spurts. Similar to earlier ages, watch for children who have changed channels on a growth grid, and for those above the 85th percentile or below the 5th percentile for body mass index, and gather additional nutritional data in these cases (see Chapter 33 🔗).

School-age children are learning about their bodies, and so should be active participants in the physical examination. Explain what you are doing and why. Carry out a head-to-toe examination, paying particular attention to systems and skills that influence performance in school, such as vision, hearing, muscular strength, and coordination. See Chapter 34 🔗 for detailed information about the physical examination. Remember to provide feedback about the findings; families appreciate knowing that the child's vision is normal and strength is well developed. Tell them what findings are normal as well as areas that may need more assessment or intervention. Inquire about the child's sleep patterns. During the examination, ask for a description of any illnesses the child has had. Children of school age are generally healthy, with only a few upper respiratory infections or other minor illnesses annually. Unusual complaints may indicate a need for further testing, as discussed in the disease prevention section later in this chapter.

School-age children frequently have minor injuries. These might include falls from bicycles, skin rashes from exposure to plants on a hiking trip, bruises from a ball sport, and other minor mishaps. Be alert for more serious problems that may indicate a need for additional detailed data gathering and teaching (see the injury prevention section later in this chapter for examples).

Developmental surveillance continues to be an important part of the examination for school-age children. Some milestones can be observed during the visit, while other information is obtained by report of parent and child. This information is combined with reports about school and other activities in order to establish that the child is developing as expected.

Desired outcomes for growth and developmental surveillance include normal progression with developmental tasks, absence of physical and psychosocial abnormalities or trauma, and integration of safe practices into daily life.

Nutrition

Key concepts related to nutrition in school-age children are independence and formation of habits that influence the future. First, children are increasingly independent in food choices. They usually have strong likes and dislikes for certain foods. They may arrive home from school each day to an empty house and prepare their own snacks. During school, they choose what to eat from the school lunch or the sack lunch sent by family. They may even have access to vending machines or sales of snacks during school hours. While independence in food choices is growing, the child is greatly influenced in those choices by friends and the media. Foods that may be rejected often include fresh vegetables and fruits, since they get little media attention, and friends may not prefer them.

At a time when the child chooses many of the foods in the daily diet, habits are being formed that will affect nutrition and health in general in the years to come. Good choices will help to promote health—to maintain weight at a recommended level, provide nutrients for adequate growth and activity, and prevent onset of some chronic diseases. Conversely, poor choices can lead to overweight and its accompanying problems, lack of adequate calcium and resultant osteoporosis, eating disorders, or lack of energy for brain growth and optimal performance in school. The patterns established during this period are often influential in later nutritional status. Knowledge about foods, family participation in good nutritional practices, and access to healthy foods can all be enhanced by nursing intervention during this critical formative period.

Continue to perform height and weight measurements, body mass index calculations, and examination of percentiles for growth grid measurements. Slow, steady growth is the norm during the early school-age years; it will be followed by a growth spurt when the child nears puberty.

During the visit, observations provide information about nutritional status. What is the condition of the nails, skin, and hair? What is the energy level and reported physical activity? Does the child look lean or overweight? As the child nears puberty, there may be an increase in fat stores as a preparation for the pubertal growth spurt. Integrate some questions for the parent and child into the visit that provide clues about diet. While observing the child and family and asking dietary questions, list risks and protective factors related to nutrition. Examples of protective factors include adequate access to nutritious foods, a family garden, and weight and height within normal limits; risk factors may include inadequate access to nutritious foods, excess intake of calories during television viewing, and lack of vegetables in the daily diet. Reinforce the positive practices of the family and inform the child of how food choices relate to energy level, school performance, and general health. Risk factors become the basis for teaching and planning with the family for necessary change. It is difficult to tackle several nutritional changes at one time, so concentrate on those most needing attention, and on those the family agrees are important. Provide information about healthy snacks to keep at home, ways to improve calcium intake, the importance of getting at least five fruit/vegetable servings daily, limitation of soda pop to one serving daily, and the importance of family meals (Figure 36–3 ●). Desired outcomes for health maintenance include absence of overweight and other potential chronic diseases, adequate intake of all nutrients, and increasing child and family knowledge about nutrition.

Physical Activity

Just as food choices during the school-age years are likely to influence the child's future nutrition, physical activity during these years is often crucial to development of lifelong exercise habits. During these years, the child who is physically active

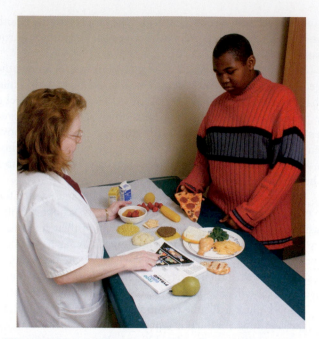

● **Figure 36–3** This school-age child is receiving teaching from the nurse about food choices. What benefit do the food models provide in this situation? What other teaching techniques can you suggest?

continues to refine skills such as eye–hand coordination, muscular strength, agility, and speed. Some children become skilled at ball sports such as basketball, football, soccer, or baseball. Others focus on gymnastics, wrestling, horseback riding, or hockey (Figure 36–4 ●). Some do not like team or organized

● **Figure 36–4** Everyone needs to be physically active. Some children participate in school sports. Others, such as these boys playing hockey, choose a sport that is available in the community. Other children prefer to walk, ride a bike, or engage in other more solitary activities. Determine what is enjoyable for a particular child and provide assistance in integrating desired activity into daily routines.

sports but choose rollerblading, skateboarding, skiing, or biking. Whatever the interest, it is important that children identify some physical activity and continue to develop motor skills. The benefits include socialization, positive sense of accomplishment and self-esteem, weight control, and increasing physical ability (Figure 36–5 ●). Children who do not have an activity of importance often fall behind their peers in agility and skill, making future attempts at an activity very difficult and less likely to be successful.

As in earlier periods in life, the nurse lists risk and protective factors related to school-age physical activity (Table 36–7). Families are often significant in promoting physical activity for children. Find out what the parents do for physical activity and how often. Do they attend a sports club after work or does the child see them engaging in exercise? Most families can include some walking, yard work, or other activity that is done together in order to engage the child. Do they walk to a neighbor's house or a nearby store rather than driving? Do they always take elevators, or choose the stairs in buildings? What is the activity level of siblings? When older siblings are involved in sports, the younger child often is encouraged to develop skills in the same sport.

● **Figure 36–5** Benefits of physical activity. School-age children often enjoy hikes with family, clubs, or other groups. What are the physical and mental health benefits from this activity?

Table 36–7	Risk and Protective Factors Regarding Physical Activity in School-Age Children

Risk Factors	Protective Factors
■ Developmental delay and special needs	■ Expected developmental skill level
■ Limited role modeling of daily physical activity by parents and other family members	■ Parents exercise daily and exercise with the child some of this time in a setting the child can see ■ Parents set expectation that everyone in family will choose a physical activity and engage in it regularly
■ Limited facilities in the neighborhood to encourage activity, such as parks, skateboard facilities, rinks, ball courts	■ Neighborhood provides access to parks, skateboard facilities, rinks, ball courts, and other facilities
■ Inadequate financial resources to join clubs or pay for organized sports	■ Family has adequate financial resources to pay for health club or organized sports
■ Safety gear for activities chosen is not available due to cost, or child is reluctant to use the gear	■ Recommended safety gear that properly fits child is available ■ The child understands importance of safety gear and accepts using such equipment
■ School cuts to physical education programs and recess	■ Schools provide physical education each day with a variety of offerings; student gets to choose and set goals for some activities ■ Schools schedule recess or physical activity breaks twice daily
■ School tryouts for sports that eliminate all but the best players in certain sports	■ Sports teams are leveled so that all students desiring to play a particular sport, such as soccer, are able to do so
■ Reluctance to try new activity	■ Willing to try new activities
■ Worry about competence and physical appearance	■ Feels self-confident in ability and physical appearance ■ Sets goals for learning physical skills
■ Television viewing or other screen activities for more than 2 hours daily	■ Television viewing and other screen activities are limited to no more than 2 hours daily

Source: Data from Hagan, J. F., Shaw, J. S., & Duncan, P. M. (Eds.). (2008). *Bright futures: Guidelines for health supervision of infants, children, and adolescents* (3rd ed.). Elk Grove Village, IL: American Academy of Pediatrics.

The child spends much of the day in school, and so this setting is important to consider. In an effort to conserve financial resources, some schools have decreased physical education (PE) programs. Children may not have regular PE classes, and there may be few standards of performance. In addition, many states and provinces have established tests and standards for performance in certain cognitive areas. In an attempt to increase teaching time to meet standards, some schools have cut out recess and other breaks. Some schools are located in unsafe areas and outside recreation is not advisable.

It is unrealistic to expect children to sit for long periods without physical activity, and such practice reinforces the poor habits of inadequate exercise among children. Schools that offer a variety of activities, including intramural (rather than only organized competitive) sports, are more likely to encourage a wide variety of children to be active. At least half of the recommended 60 minutes of daily vigorous physical activity should be provided in school, along with an adequate amount of unstructured playtime during recess (CDC, 2011). Nurses are influential members of school committees and can encourage the integration of activity in the school day. They may be able to serve on a school or community committee, informing other committee members of the benefits of exercise to enhance cognitive performance and general health. Teachers and school administrators can be supplied with models of successful school activity programs. Nurses can often be influential in finding community volunteers to work with teams of students. Student nurses, physical education students, senior citizens, and others in the community may be able to help young children play baseball, tennis, or soccer. Other volunteers may teach stretching or warm-up activities. Community partners such as businesses may provide protective gear or uniforms for school sports, especially if the business name can be displayed. In addition, schools can offer alternative activities that some children might prefer to traditional organized sports.

It is essential to consider physical activity for the child who has special healthcare needs. It may be difficult for schools to plan an activity for the child with cerebral palsy, visual impairment, or developmental delay. Search for other community resources and help the family to access them. There may be programs for children to ride horses, swim, ski, and engage in other physical activities. Search out the Special Olympics for children with disabilities. Imagine the thrill that awaits a child who has rarely moved quickly when riding a sled or sliding on skis.

To summarize, health promotion activities for the nurse include teaching about activities that parents can do with their children, becoming active in fostering physical education programs in schools, acting as a positive role model, and helping interested children to partner with community resources for activity. Health maintenance outcomes include encouragement for use of safety gear and correct techniques to prevent injury from sport participation.

Oral Health

Many changes occur in the mouth during the school-age years, necessitating periodic examination. At about 6 years of age, most children lose a tooth, usually in the front. Following that, all 20 of the deciduous or primary teeth will be lost, and the permanent teeth will simultaneously begin to erupt. See Chapter 34 ∂ for the schedule of deciduous tooth loss and permanent tooth eruption. In addition, the jaw line elongates and teeth move into new positions. Periodic dental visits focus on both the placement of teeth and oral hygiene.

During the health promotion visit, examine the teeth. Look to see how many deciduous and permanent teeth are present. Describe the child's oral hygiene. Ask how often the child brushes, flosses, and visits the dentist. The child should have learned how to brush and floss during preschool years and now be performing the skills independently. If dental caries or poor oral hygiene is apparent, ask the child to demonstrate brushing and flossing. Reinforce the need for brushing twice daily and flossing once daily. Provide toothpaste and toothbrushes as gifts during health supervision visits. Local dentists will often provide these supplies to encourage oral hygiene.

Dental visits are recommended every 6 months. If the child is not visiting on that schedule, ask if finances or transportation is an issue, if the family needs a referral to a dentist, or if there is some other reason. If caries or malocclusion is present, stress the need for a dental appointment soon. Inquire about use of fluoride if the water supply is not fluoridated. Ask if the child has had sealants applied to the permanent teeth; most dentists believe these will help to prevent future caries (AAPD, 2012b). Offer to help parents locate resources to assist with dental care expenses if needed. State and community programs are often available to assist families, and nurses should search out resources in their own communities and regions.

Many children have a high intake of sugared foods and snacks. If this is apparent from the nutritional assessment, discuss the importance of limiting these foods and brushing after their consumption. Frequent brushing is needed when the child has braces. Ask how they are caring for the braces and what the orthodontist has recommended.

The nurse's health promotion activities include positive reinforcement of good hygiene habits, and health maintenance involves teaching about the need for improved care and limiting food that furthers the formation of caries. Desired outcomes include proper oral hygiene, attendance at recommended dental visits, and absence of dental caries.

Clinical Reasoning   Dental Health

The family of 7-year-old Mario just moved to your city. You learn in a healthcare visit that Mario has never been to a dentist. You notice that several of his teeth are decayed. He has started to lose his primary teeth and has two permanent teeth in place. A dietary recall demonstrates that he drinks two to three sweetened beverages daily and likes to eat candy whenever possible.

Describe the daily dental hygiene that Mario should be practicing. Plan a teaching session for Mario and his parents. What other cues will you look for in his dietary recall in order to identify risk and protective factors for oral health? How will you locate resources in the community to recommend for the family so that Mario can receive dental care?

See www.nursing.pearsonhighered.com for possible responses.

Mental and Spiritual Health

Self-Esteem and Self-Concept

The school-age years are marked by the emergence of new cognitive skills and the development of self-esteem. **Self-esteem** reflects feelings of self-worth or value. **Self-concept** refers to evaluations of the self in certain specific areas, such as those related to academic achievement, athletic ability, physical appearance, and social interactions (Santrock, 2011). A child with a positive self-concept feels competent, is able to meet challenges, and applies lessons from successes and failures. Specific facets of self-concept include **body image**, the idea that one forms about one's body, and **sexuality**, the person's view of self as a sexual being. Together, self-concept and self-esteem include all of the cognitive, emotional, spiritual, sexual, and physical aspects of the individual.

The child who believes in his or her ability to face good times and bad has a lowered chance of mental illness such as depression, eating disorder, and anxiety. Parents are encouraged to evaluate and help to build the child's sense of self-esteem (see *Teaching Highlights: Evaluating and Fostering Self-Esteem*).

Many of the areas discussed already in this chapter provide clues to the child's self-concept. Does the child take part in sports or other physical activities? Such activity may reflect a positive self-concept and body image. However, if the child is forced to do these sports by parents and feels inadequate in their performance, these activities may promote a negative self-concept and body image. Ask about children's activities and how they feel about them. Do they enjoy them? How do they rate their performance?

Is the child increasingly independent and responsible for self? Success in achieving developmental milestones leads to a positive sense of self-esteem in the child. Parents are encouraged to evaluate and help to build the child's sense of self-esteem. A low sense of self-esteem is noted when the child states a disinterest in exercise, school clubs, and family activities. This can lead to loneliness, depression, and mental health problems such as eating disorders. When these feelings are noted during a health supervision visit, the nurse should recommend that the child see a counselor at school or another setting, and should recommend that parents be included in the sessions so that they can best help the child.

It is obvious that the family plays a critical part in the child's developing self-esteem and mental health. To understand the child, it is necessary to ask questions about and explore dynamics in the family. Several protective factors have been identified for families (U.S. Department of Health and Human Services, 2011):

- Nurturing bonds and attachment are formed.
- Parents have knowledge about parenting skills and child development.
- Parents demonstrate resilience by recognizing their own stress and enhancing their problem-solving abilities.
- Parents have a wide array of support systems to provide social connections.
- Caregivers are available who provide resources to meet basic needs, such as finances, housing, and food.

School-age children continue to develop their abilities to self-regulate activities and responses to situations. At this age the abilities to solve problems and assume more responsibility for self are important. Encourage parents to discuss issues with the child and to seek solutions together when appropriate. The child assumes more responsibility for assisting with meal preparation and home chores, coming home alone after school, and caring for younger siblings. Encourage the parents to praise the child for assuming more family responsibilities and recognize that the child will need some guidance when taking on new tasks.

Teaching Highlights Evaluating and Fostering Self-Esteem

Parents play an important part in fostering a child's self-esteem. The nurse can ask them to evaluate the child and provide suggestions about positive actions.

Evaluation Questions	Positive Actions
What does your child do well?	Build on the child's strengths and talents; affectionately point out the child's abilities.
How does your child respond to failure?	Assist the child to assess his or her own performance; help the child see lessons that mistakes can teach.
Does your child have close friends?	Arrange structured playtimes such as going to a movie or cooking with a friend.
How does your child respond to new challenges?	Give the child responsibilities at home; encourage your child to try new experiences; help the child feel a sense of control over outcomes.
How does your own personality compare to your child's?	Recognize differences in style; appreciate the unique qualities of each child; tailor expectations to the child and not to self or other children.
Are you setting reasonable and attainable expectations for your child?	Be a positive role model; establish goals for behaviors together.

Source: Data from *Developing your child's self-esteem*. (2011). Retrieved from http://kidshealth.org/parent/emotions/feelings/self_esteem.html.

Ask about and observe the family's relationships. Evaluate the effect of family interactions on the child. Model respectful interchanges by listening carefully to the child, as well as the parent. Gently speak directly to the child if parents answer for the child or seem to put him or her down. Provide brochures and examples of ways to show children their importance. Encourage both parents to come to child healthcare visits and support the involvement of both parents in childrearing. Ask about family stressors such as job changes, financial concerns, illness, substance abuse, and domestic violence. About one half of marriages end in divorce, so be prepared to offer suggestions to deal with this situation. Ask about and identify risk factors and protective factors. The child's strengths are used to assist the family functioning and will, in turn, give the child a sense of accomplishment. Some examples include the following:

- A child who is able to act independently can be given responsibility for parts of the home or family function, such as planning the menu for dinner two evenings weekly, caring for a family pet, or completing household chores.

- A creative child can be given the task of planning book readings and other activities for a younger sibling.

- A child with a talent for design can be asked to set the table for dinner guests.

Sexuality and Sexuality Education

The school-age child is developing a sense of body image and sexuality. Look at the child's appearance and dress. Some children may have poor posture, display a sense of insecurity, and seem uncomfortable with themselves. Others may dress as if they were much older, seem sophisticated, and are clearly assuming the role identification with their gender group. Ask the parents in a private setting what observations they have about the child's body image and sexuality. Inquire about friends in whom the child seems romantically or sexually interested, and whether the parent has concerns.

Questions related to sexuality will emerge during school years. They should be answered truthfully and fully. Even children who do not ask questions usually need information related to sexuality education. They may get information in school beginning in about fourth grade, but often still have misconceptions about the bodies of men and women, sexual intercourse, how babies are born, and other topics. Suggest that parents read books with their children that deal with these issues at a level children understand. If books are available at home, children will be likely to look at them and ask questions. They should be in the home from third grade on since many young girls have body changes as early as 9 or 10 years of age (see Chapter 34 🔗). This can often put both the parent and child at ease and open the door to discussion. Parents should be advised to talk with teachers to learn what is presented in school and be able to supplement and clarify this information. Having discussions at a young age will help lead to further discussion as the child gets older. Nurses often perform sexuality education in schools or work with school districts in establishing policies regarding sexuality education plans. Help the parents plan to discuss appropriate and inappropriate touch so that the child understands and states those who

can help in situations that lead to discomfort. (See Chapter 43 🔗 for a thorough discussion of child abuse.)

Suggest to parents that computers and other media provide information that can confuse children. Encourage them to watch movies with their children, engage in frank discussions related to sexuality observed, and answer questions truthfully. Children generally learn about topics such as sexual intercourse, homosexuality, and childbirth from school discussions and the media. It is better to learn from parents than from friends or the media. A few moments alone with parents and the child separately at healthcare visits may help to identify the concerns of each related to sexuality.

By about fourth to sixth grades, most girls have started to have prepubertal body changes and may have begun to menstruate. This is another opening for discussions about mature bodies of men and women and the transformation from childhood to greater maturity. Boys mature about 2 years later than girls. Without an event such as menstruation, parents may be less likely to start discussions with male children. Suggest that parents consciously begin conversations with boys periodically to explain changes they see in themselves and their peers. See Chapter 34 🔗 for further discussion of the body changes seen in the prepubertal period and during puberty.

Sleep

Sleep is important for children because it helps provide the energy they will need to perform well in school and other activities. They generally take charge of bedtime routines with reminders about the time to go to sleep, and they sleep through the night. Sleep time varies from 8 to 12 hours, depending on child and activity level. Busy schedules may interrupt this pattern, leading to irritability, lack of concentration, or even hyperactive behavior. Help children and families plan for healthy practices of **sleep hygiene**, or behaviors that foster a regular and sufficient sleep pattern, as well as daytime alertness (Mayo Clinic, 2009; Mindell, Meltzer, Carskadon, et al., 2009).

Sleepwalking and sleep talking sometimes occur at this age, but usually decrease as the child nears adolescence. Children who have stress at home, such as parental fighting, ill family members, or inadequate food or shelter, may not get enough sleep and fall asleep at school. Ask the child if he or she is falling asleep in class, and seek additional information about family stressors. This can lead to interventions such as recommending family counseling or referring to resources to obtain better housing or more stable food sources.

School

School is a major microsystem that influences the lives of children and plays a role in self-concept and mental health formation. The child is usually ready for kindergarten when:

- Communication and cognitive skills are sufficient to support learning.

- The child can successfully separate from parents.

- Experiences with other children show ability to make friends and regulate own behavior.

- The child can follow rules and directions (Hagan et al., 2008).

Teaching Highlights Sleep Hygiene

Nurses should inquire about the sleep patterns and amount of sleep that children receive. Ask if they are frequently tired or have trouble sleeping. Some simple behaviors help to promote sleep and are referred to as sleep hygiene. They include (Mayo Clinic, 2009; Mindell et al., 2009):

- Go to bed and get up at approximately the same time each day, including weekends.
- Follow a bedtime routine to prepare for sleep.
- Recognize that we do not "make up" sleep that is "lost" by sleeping in.
- Avoid caffeine, including tea, coffee, and carbonated beverages, for several hours before sleep.
- Avoid exposure to alcohol or tobacco for several hours before sleep.
- Gradually slow down activity about an hour or two before bedtime.
- Do not watch television, play games, text on the phone, or conduct other activities in the sleep location.
- Avoid naps in the late afternoon or evening.
- Darken the room for sleep.

Help parents learn ways that they can facilitate a healthy transition to school, such as ensuring good sleep and eating routines, reading with the child, showing interest in school activities, and finding a space in the home for the child's school-related work.

When examining a school-age child, ask for a description of a best friend. If the child is unable to provide this, isolation may be occurring. Inquire about what the three best and three worst things are about school. Children with low self-concepts often have trouble talking about and evaluating school. Find out where the child attends school, if the area is generally safe, and how the child gets to school. Encourage the parents to meet the child's teachers, to become active in school activities, and to be available to solve problems with school personnel when needed. Partner with the parents and child when interventions are needed. An office nurse may contact a school nurse when the child needs support in the school environment. This may occur if the child has become ill and missed school, has family stressors, does not get along well with a teacher, or has a condition such as attention deficit disorder. Identify the risk and protective factors in the school environment and plan interventions to support the child when risks are present.

Evaluating Mental Health and Spiritual Health

Certain mental health disorders are commonly seen during the school years. One example is anxiety problems that result in worries, fears, physical symptoms, stress, and sleep disorders without significantly impairing daily functioning. However, some anxiety disorders affect functioning and have more striking characteristics such as clinging, abdominal pain and headache, and refusal to attend school. Posttraumatic stress syndrome and depression may also be seen. See Chapter 56 🔗 for further description of these disorders. Anxiety disorder, posttraumatic stress, and depression should be referred to a mental health specialist for treatment. However, all children worry at times, and this type of anxiety can be helped by learning coping skills and relaxation techniques.

Spiritual health is the ability to develop a spiritual nature, including awareness of a life purpose or meaning, a sustaining power during times of stress, a feeling of harmony with the universe, and a sense of fulfillment (Murray et al., 2009; Pender, Murdaugh, & Parsons, 2011). School age is a time when children learn more about the people and the world around them, and begin to find their place in that world. Connection with faith-based groups assists some children and families in defining the purpose of life, while others may do so through social activity or a strong moral sense of responsibility. Ask children what brings happiness, how they help other people, or if they are members of a church, synagogue, or mosque. If families seem to have little purpose, parents are withdrawn or depressed, or the child has difficulty answering questions about meaningful activities, suggest methods of engagement in the community. Strategies might include providing contacts at local religious events, posting flyers about community events designed to bring unity to various cultural groups, or suggesting services needing volunteers in the community. Families who spend time together and find meaning in supporting each other nurture the spiritual health of their members. Suggest that every family plan a "family night" weekly when they play games, talk, eat, or engage in other activities together.

The nurse has an important role in fostering the mental and spiritual health of school-age children. Health promotion fosters the strengths of families and children, leading to healthy self-concept and positive self-esteem. Health maintenance seeks to prevent mental health disruptions. Be alert for risk factors in families since they represent the need for intervention. Expected outcomes for health promotion and health maintenance activities with school-age children include formation of a positive sense of self-esteem and healthy body image, use of coping skills to deal with stress, sleep patterns that meet needs for rest, and a growing purpose and meaning in life.

Relationships

Although the school-age child is gradually moving away from the family as the center of life, the family remains an important anchor. Ask about siblings, grandparents, and other extended family members. Sometimes these persons assist in the child's formation of a self-concept. Peers are increasingly important to the school-age child's self-identity. School age is a time of cooperative engagement with others. All children need to learn how to make and maintain friendships and work with others on projects and in recreation.

Inquire about the child's friends and activities at school. In private, ask parents if they are comfortable with the child's selection of friends. Find out if the parents facilitate friendships by allowing other children to come to the home and providing transportation as needed. When the child experiences a risk factor such as a move to a new town or school, role-play how to meet new children and how to make friends. If the child feels like an outcast or outsider among peers at school, explore how the family can create a safe and secure place for the child through extracurricular activities with children who have similar interests. When children are home schooled, the family should encourage social events and contacts after usual school hours.

Since peers are important to the school-age child, the child may feel pressure to appear like others, to fit in, and to do what others encourage. Although such pressures are often associated with teen years, they usually begin earlier, at least by 8 or 9 years of age. Ask children what kinds of things their friends try to get them to do that they know they should not do, or if friends have tried to get them to smoke. Middle school years are the most common age for beginning to smoke, so always ask if the child has tried smoking, being careful to do this when the parent is not present and the child is more likely to be honest. When parents are not in the room they may also tell you about other activities, such as playing with guns, trying alcohol or other substances, or other risky behavior. It is best to ask children what they do in these situations, what they want to do, and who they can talk to about these events. Offer information about the risks connected with behaviors that are described, and suggest people such as parents, teachers, counselors, or clergy who are possible resources. If the child's health is at risk, be sure to report the activity to the physician or other healthcare provider so that it can be pursued and the child's safety can be assured. Activities such as playing with firearms or visiting a friend whose parents are making methamphetamine, for example, place children in extreme danger.

Parents often need guidance to help them in setting limits for their school-age children. The child is becoming more independent but unacceptable behaviors must still be managed by successful discipline techniques. Some guidelines that can help families include talking calmly about behaviors that are unacceptable, using techniques such as natural consequences or withholding privileges, modeling, and suggesting stress relief such as physical activity (AAP, 2011b; Knox, 2010).

School age is often a time when children first experience violence in relationships with others. Some children are bullied, while others are the bullies. Anger and aggression can occur, and children may engage in violence with each other. Ask children to describe when they last had a disagreement with someone and how the problem was solved. Suggest people who can help, such as school nurses, teachers, and counselors, and be sure that children feel safe in schools, neighborhoods, and homes. Ask parents how they resolve arguments between children at home and what help they need to help children learn problem-solving skills. Find out what policies the local schools have to assist in decreasing harassment of and by children. Become active on school committees that help children learn how to solve problems peacefully and how to respond to episodes of violence. See Chapter 43 ⊘ for further discussion of violence in children and a detailed discussion of bullying.

The child's temperament (see Chapter 32 ⊘) still plays a part in response to situations and the ability to self-regulate. The "difficult" child may have trouble getting to sleep or being quiet in the classroom. Have parents plan more physical activity for this child. Teach the child that bedtime routines are helpful and that sitting near the front of the class can help with concentration. The "slow to warm up" child may need ideas about what to say when meeting new people. Parents can help the child prepare for a new school by visiting the school with the child, talking about it, and meeting with the teacher so that a warm welcome

can occur. The "easy" child is usually adaptable in most situations and is regular in activities. However, this child may object when other children interrupt, fail to take turns, or otherwise "break the rules" of behavior. They might need help to understand differences in temperament in order to be more tolerant of classmates and their behaviors. Often nurses in schools address the issue of individual differences by speaking with classes or small groups of children.

The nurse takes an active role in promoting the child's health by anticipating developmental issues and preparing the parents and child to deal with them. Health maintenance outcomes include prevention of problems such as bullying.

Disease Prevention Strategies

School-age children are generally healthy. The immune system is mature (see Chapter 49 ⊘), personal hygiene practices are more developed than at earlier ages, and immunizations are usually complete. Engage school-age children in active pursuit of their own health. Teach strategies that can enhance the prevention of diseases. Nurses in offices and schools can teach children how to wash hands effectively, how respiratory infections are transmitted, what can cause gastrointestinal illness, and how to best manage their own health problems (Figure 36–6 ●). Ask children in your settings what topics are of most interest to them and be prepared to suggest common areas of concern such as safety, skin care, athletics, and illnesses. Children can understand the connection between eating well and avoiding illness, maintaining normal weight and preventing type 2 diabetes, avoiding smoking to prevent cancer and other respiratory diseases, maintaining oral hygiene to promote oral health, and exercising to prevent hypertension.

School-age children are in the concrete stage of intellectual development, according to Piaget (see Chapter 32 ⊘). This means that teaching is most effective when opportunities are provided to touch, feel, and otherwise become actively engaged

● **Figure 36–6** School nurse's role in managing health problems. A student with diabetes is showing the school nurse how she programs her insulin pump. The nurse has partnered with nurses in the endocrinology office to learn about the type of pump the student is using. Such collaboration contributes to the monitoring and management of diabetes.

● **Figure 36–7** Concrete experiences for health teaching. This boy is learning about the effects of smoking on the body through the concrete experience of examining a model of the lungs. Why does this type of hands-on technique help school-age children to learn concepts?

in learning. When teaching about smoking, provide models of lungs and have the students breathe through a straw to demonstrate the effects of airway narrowing. These concrete activities will teach them concepts better than simple lecture or reading (Figure 36–7 ●). Concepts of health promotion tend to be abstract since they deal with supporting one's highest potential for wellness. Thus, it becomes even more important to provide concrete methods of learning.

Immunizations are generally up to date for school-age children. However, some children may have missed earlier doses due to illness or missed healthcare visits. Evaluate the immunization record to be sure it meets all recommendations. The most common immunization needs at this time include the following:

- Hepatitis B (whole series or a missed third dose)
- Hepatitis A (two doses if not previously administered)
- Polio, and measles-mumps-rubella (if booster doses of each were not given prior to school entry)
- Tetanus-diphtheria-acellular pertussis (Tdap) at the 11–12-year visit
- Varicella if not given earlier and the child has not had the disease
- Human papillomavirus (HPV) three-dose series at 9 years or older
- Meningococcal conjugate vaccine at 11 years with booster at 16 years
- Influenza annually
- Certain vaccines for children at high risk, such as meningococcal and pneumococcal (see Chapter 44 🔗 for further information on immunizations)

Screenings for health risks should occur during the visit. These include hearing and vision screening, blood pressure

monitoring, tuberculin skin test, and in some cases screening for hyperlipidemia and lead exposure. Unusual complaints may indicate a need for further testing. Examples include the following:

- Pain other than brief discomfort after an injury
- Headaches
- Bruising
- Lack of coordination
- Repeated infections
- Decreasing vision or hearing
- Problems or changes in school performance or behavior

Children who have an identified health problem or developmental disability may have additional needs for screening and for interventions to assist with health maintenance. For example, the child with cystic fibrosis will need information to reduce the risk of respiratory infection, and the child with diabetes may need additional blood studies. The child who has difficulty reading will need alternative approaches to teaching correct hand hygiene; demonstration with explanation may be the best approach. A family history of some diseases increases the child's risk and necessitates testing. For example, if a parent has had early cardiovascular disease (before age 55 years), a lipid profile should be performed on the child.

Inquire about any medications the child takes, including vitamins, fluoride, and nonprescription medications. Some families use complementary therapy for common conditions such as respiratory infections or gastrointestinal complaints. Complementary therapy is quite common in families where children have chronic conditions such as attention deficit hyperactivity disorder, autism, and skin conditions (Ben-Arye, Traube, Schachter, et al., 2011; Sibinga & Kemper, 2010).

Parents should receive explanations about the screening tests performed and the results obtained. Inform them about vision and hearing results. Send home or call about results of blood tests when available. Be sure they understand the findings and have resources to assist in preventing or treating the specific disease in their children. Have them call with questions about health problems the child develops, and provide information about lowering risks of diseases. Be sure that families know when to keep children home from school (elevated temperature, active vomiting or diarrhea, coughing up brown or green mucus). Assist schools in setting guidelines for management of infectious diseases in that setting. Contact the local county and state health department for infectious disease guidelines for schools. Desired outcomes for the school-age child include prevention of infectious diseases, prompt treatment for acute infections, and careful management of existing health conditions in order to maximize health potential.

Injury Prevention Strategies

Injuries are a common cause of morbidity and mortality among school-age children, and each health maintenance encounter should include injury prevention strategies. Children of this age have more independence and may be harmed by activities they engage in without adults present, such as playing with fire or firearms. They participate in many sports and other physical activities and may sustain related injuries. Some children unfortunately suffer from harm due to physical abuse or other forms of violence (see Chapter 43).

Many common injuries are preventable with simple use of protective gear and the following safety guidelines. About 10% of youth rarely or never wear seat belts in automobiles (CDC, 2010b). Certain groups of children are more at risk than others of not taking protective measures. Many children ride bicycles, but only a fraction of them use helmets. Strategies to make helmet use more attractive and to ensure correct wearing of helmets are needed (see *Evidence-Based Practice: Bicycle Helmet Effectiveness and Use*).

Identify youth engaging in risky activities and teach them safe practices. Join with schools and community groups to establish education programs. Provide information about adequate conditioning for sports in order to decrease chance of overuse

---

Developing Cultural Competence
Use of Safety Protection

There are marked differences in behaviors that influence unintentional injuries. Although about 8% of children rarely or never wear a seat belt in the car, black males are most at risk, with almost 13% not using seat belts. In addition, nearly 88% of youth who ride bicycles rarely or never wear a bicycle helmet, but the rates vary, with 92% of black and Hispanic youth not wearing helmets, while 86% of white youth do not wear bicycle helmets (CDC, 2012). How will you inquire about seat belt and bicycle helmet use in an open-ended manner during health promotion visits? Consider asking these questions:

- Where do you sit when you ride in the car?
- Who do you usually ride with?
- Are there seat belts? How often do you use them?
- Do you ride a bike?
- Do you have a bicycle helmet? How often do you wear the helmet?

Plan strategies to include all children and families, especially those at high risk of not using seat belts or bicycle helmets.

---

injury. Each visit should contain basic history questions related to injury prevention. Pursue topics that appear to indicate problems. Once information has been collected during the visit, plan two or three health maintenance topics that seem most important for injury prevention in the family. When there is a history of injury in the child, partner with the family to plan ways to avoid repeated harm. Table 36–8 lists some common injury hazards during the school years, and Table 36–9 offers suggestions for injury prevention teaching.

NURSING MANAGEMENT *For the Health Promotion and Maintenance of the School-Age Child*

Nursing Assessment and Diagnosis

Assessment of health promotion and health maintenance topics occurs in many settings with school-age children. They may be seen in offices, clinics, or other settings designed to provide such care. They may come for episodic care for a fracture or infection when health promotion and health maintenance can be easily integrated. They may be seen in the home or neighborhood center, and are frequently encountered by nurses in schools. Opportunities for assessment and intervention should be used whenever they occur. The individual child is examined, and the family, friends, school, and community are addressed. In addition these visits provide an opportunity to identify early and intervene for health-related problems that emerge or become apparent in school age.

Assessment can be considered on two levels with school-age children. Individual children may be assessed for height and weight, for immunization status, and for use of protective gear during sports. Populations of children may also be assessed since school age is the first time that large numbers of children are together in certain settings. The findings from such assessments will become the basis of an **individualized approach** or a **population-based approach** to health promotion and health maintenance. For example, nurses commonly measure height and weight, calculate body mass index for *individual* children seen in a clinic, share results with the family, and address appropriate teaching about weight control and nutritious intake.

Evidence-Based Practice Bicycle Helmet Effectiveness and Use

Clinical Question
About 900 children die of bicycle-related injuries annually in the United States. Children from 5 to 14 years old have the highest rate of bicycle injuries (CDC, 2010b). Although helmets can reduce injury, many times they are not worn or are worn incorrectly.

The Evidence
Wearing bicycle helmets is associated with higher household incomes, living in a state with a bicycle helmet law, younger ages, and having health insurance (Dellinger & Kresnow, 2010; Devoe, Tillotson, Wallace, et al., 2012). Many children wear a helmet incorrectly, most often positioning it too far back on the head (Hagel, Lee, Karkhaneh, et al., 2010).

Best Practice
Nurses should provide information about helmet use for bicycles and other vehicles. Engage children at community events and in schools. Inquire about helmet use at every healthcare visit. Reinforce proper fit and maintenance of helmets.

Clinical Reasoning
Where will you find information about helmet safety? What educational programs are available in your schools and communities? Are helmets made available for families that might not be able to buy them? How do you determine if a child is wearing a helmet correctly? Plan educational materials and programs for children who bicycle, ride skateboards, or use scooters.

Table 36–8	Injury Hazards in the School-Age Years

	Hazard	Developmental Characteristics	Preventive Measures
	Motor vehicle/ pedestrian/ biking crashes	Child plays outside; may follow ball into road; rides two-wheeler.	Teach child safe outside play, especially near streets. Reinforce use of bike helmet. Teach biking safety rules and provide safe places for riding.
	Firearms	Child may have been shown location of guns; is interested in showing them to friends.	Teach child never to touch guns without parent present. Guns should be kept unloaded and locked away. Guns and ammunition should be stored in different locations. Be sure guns have trigger locks.
	Burns	Child may perform experiments with flames or toxic substances.	Teach child what to do in case of fire or if toxic substances touch skin or eyes. Reinforce teaching about 9-1-1.
	Assault	Child may be left alone after school and may walk, bike, or take public transportation alone.	Provide telephone numbers of people to contact in case of an emergency or if child feels lonely. Leave child alone for brief periods initially, and evaluate child's success in managing time. Teach child not to accept rides from, talk to, or open doors to strangers. Teach child how to answer the phone.

In other settings, nurses may measure a *classroom* of children and use the collective data to plan appropriate interventions. If 40% of children in a school are classified as overweight by BMI percentile, much emphasis should be placed on teaching about dietary intake, physical activity, and the relationship of recommended weight levels to chronic disease risk. However, if only a small number of children are overweight, interventions may not be as extensive about this topic.

Nurses perform assessment of growth in school-age children, look for achievement of developmental tasks, assess physical and mental health, and assess social characteristics. Based on the assessment of the individual child or populations of children,

nursing diagnoses for children and families are established. Possible nursing diagnoses include the following (NANDA-I © 2012):

- *Growth and Development, Delayed,* related to abuse
- *Parenting, Impaired,* related to lack of knowledge about child health maintenance
- *Sleep Deprivation* related to sleep terrors
- *Violence: Other-Directed, Risk for,* related to history of witnessing family violence
- *Loneliness, Risk for,* related to long periods alone after school

Table 36–9	Injury Prevention Topics by Age	
Age	**Injury Prevention Teaching**	
5–8 years	Use a booster seat, properly positioned in the back seat of the car; once large enough for the vehicle seat belt, use both lap and shoulder belts. Never place a child in the front seat of a car with a passenger air bag. Restrain all children younger than 13 years in the rear seat. Be sure the child knows how to swim and works on these skills regularly. Protect the child with sunscreen when outside. Check smoke alarms and keep them functioning properly. Have an escape plan in case of fire in the home. Keep poisons, electrical appliances, and fire starters locked. Keep firearms unloaded and locked; store ammunition in a separate locked location; have trigger locks installed on guns; keep dangerous knives locked. Provide protective gear for bicycling and other activities and insist that it be worn. Teach safety precautions for bicycling and other activities.	Teach safety with strangers. Provide a list of people a child can approach if feeling threatened by touch or other experience. Choose care providers carefully; occasionally pick up child earlier than expected; ask about policies regarding discipline and do not leave child with someone who uses corporal punishment. Be sure the child knows emergency numbers, names, and plans. Review carefully any hazardous event that has occurred with the child and summarize what was done correctly and how response could be improved. Limit screen time to 2 hours daily; do not allow violent games or viewing. Review behavior with strangers regularly such as not getting in cars and not engaging in phone or Internet conversations.
8–10 years	Use car booster seat until child sits upright against back seat with bent knees over edge of seat; insist on use of lap and shoulder belts. Do not place child in front seat of car with a passenger air bag.	Do not allow child to operate power tools or machinery. Continue to reinforce other teaching described above, include child more fully, and expand responsibility to the child with increasing age.
10–12 years	Continue to reinforce teaching described above. Parents and child should attend class on cardiopulmonary resuscitation and airway obstruction removal.	Avoid high noise levels such as when listening to music through earphones.

Source: Data from Hagan, J. F., Shaw, J. S., & Duncan, P. M. (Eds.). (2008). *Bright futures: Guidelines for health supervision of infants, children, and adolescents* (3rd ed.). Elk Grove Village, IL: American Academy of Pediatrics.

Planning and Implementation

The nurse is instrumental in planning interventions to promote and maintain health in school-age children. These interventions may take place in offices, homes, or clinics with an individual child, or in schools and other community settings with groups of children.

When working with individuals, summarize the strengths and needs identified during the visit, and ask the child and family if they concur. Plan together with them to provide the needed information for topics developed during the visit. Be sure to emphasize those areas where the family excels. For example, positively reinforce use of car seat belts (see *Teaching Highlights: Car Safety for the School-Age Child*), use of protective sports gear, and being current with immunizations. Summarize the next expected developmental tasks, such as increasing independence and growing self-responsibility for choosing snacks and television shows. Then provide anticipatory guidance to assist with the child's growing independence. As peers are becoming more important, always focus some discussion on maintaining healthy social relationships through school peers, religious or community events, and sibling contacts.

Most families welcome a combination of discussion and reading material or pertinent websites for later exploration. Provide telephone numbers of resources for questions and community contacts. Tell the parents when the next health

Teaching Highlights Car Safety for the School-Age Child

Even though parents may have been diligent about car seat and seat belt use when children were younger, guidelines change and they need teaching about current requirements for the school-age child.

Recommendations include the following:

- The child should be kept in a rear-facing seat as long as possible. Generally by 4 years of age the child has outgrown the rear-facing seat and should be in a forward-facing car seat with a harness in the back seat. This type of seat is recommended for children 4–7 years of age.
- Once the child outgrows the largest height and weight recommended by the manufacturer for the forward-facing seat (usually by 8 years of age), a booster seat is used in the back seat.
- Once the child is large enough for the regular seat belt, the lap belt must lie snugly across the upper thighs and the shoulder belt should be snug across the shoulder and chest.
- Keep all children in the back seat until 13 years of age; this is the safest location for them in the car (AAP, 2011a; AAP Committee on Injury, Violence, and Poison Prevention, 2011; National Highway Traffic Safety Administration, 2012).

promotion/maintenance visit is recommended. If working with school children for episodic care, ask when the last health maintenance visit occurred. If a child is seen for health care after a bicycling accident, the family may be receptive to teaching about safety precautions. When the child is exposed to skin injuries, a review of the last tetanus booster may reevaluate health maintenance needs. Use every opportunity to work with individual children and insert appropriate health promotion/health maintenance topics.

When working with groups of children, health promotion focuses on known needs, interests, and risk areas. Nurses in school settings have used a variety of creative approaches to promote the health of youth. Nurses in schools can set up a program to train students in health topics; these students then become peer coaches or health advocates in working with other students. Another activity is evaluating the components of school health programs and making recommendations for additions as needed. In school settings, nurses have used a variety of creative approaches to promote the health of youth. Nurses in this setting can establish programs to train students in health topics; these students then become coaches or health advocates who can work with other students, especially those of younger ages. Nurses may also evaluate components of school health programs and offer recommendations for additions as needed. Bulletin boards, community newspapers, television, and community group membership may all be as effective as teaching in school classrooms. Stress reduction teaching should be provided on group and individual levels. Nurses can teach or assist in development of progressive relaxation, deep breathing, biofeedback, yoga, or meditation. Interventions will be most effective if they begin with an understanding of the population served.

Evaluation

Seek evaluation from parents during visits for care. Were their questions answered? Do they know where to turn for advice? Do they know when the child should be seen again for health promotion/maintenance?

The expected outcomes for nursing care of individual school-age children include the following:

- The child demonstrates normal patterns of growth and development.
- The child, family, and community provide a supportive and nurturing environment for the child.
- The child shows growing independence in directing own health promotion activities.

Expected outcomes of nursing care for groups of children include the following:

- The children identify lifestyle decisions that influence their health status.
- The school and community offer resources that help to lessen risk factors related to health and disease/injury prevention.

Critical Concept Review

LEARNING OUTCOME 36.1: Describe the areas of assessment and intervention for health supervision visits for children: growth and developmental surveillance, nutrition, physical activity, oral health, mental and spiritual health, family and social relations, disease prevention strategies, and injury prevention strategies.

1. Growth and development:
   - Obtain height and weight, and perform physical examination.
   - Observe the child and interview family to determine if the child is reaching appropriate developmental milestones.
2. Nutrition:
   - Evaluate family food patterns.
   - Instruct family concerning appropriate nutrition for the child's age.
3. Physical activity:
   - Assess daily physical activity and sedentary behavior.
   - Provide instruction concerning appropriate activities and the need for at least 60 minutes/day of structured physical activity.
4. Oral health:
   - Inspect the child's mouth and teeth.

- Instruct parents concerning importance of preventing early childhood caries, performing daily oral hygiene, and scheduling regular dental visits.
5. Mental and spiritual health:
   - Instruct family concerning sleep needs.
   - Explain need for the child to develop a positive self-concept.
6. Relationships:
   - Evaluate family strengths and needs.
   - Encourage the development of a widening social circle for the child.
7. Disease prevention strategies:
   - Administer necessary immunizations.
   - Evaluate presence of potential environmental toxins.
8. Injury prevention strategies:
   - Instruct parents in proper use of car seats and prevention of falls, poisoning, and drowning.

LEARNING OUTCOME 36.2: State components of self-concept for preschool and school-age children.

1. Self-concept refers to the evaluation of the self by the child.
2. Self-concept includes ideas about body image and sexuality.
3. Self-esteem reflects the child's feeling of self-worth or value.

LEARNING OUTCOME 36.3: Plan health promotion and health maintenance strategies employed during health supervision visits of children.

1. Summarize the strengths and needs (risk and protective factors) of the child and family based on assessment during the health supervision visit.
2. Establish a nursing diagnosis list appropriate for the child and family.
3. Use a variety of approaches such as discussion, web resources, and printed material to provide the information that children and families need regarding topics such as nutrition, physical activity, relationships, and safety.

LEARNING OUTCOME 36.4: Discuss the importance of family in child health care, and include family assessment in each health supervision visit.

1. Health supervision visits begin with collaborative planning with the family.
2. Each visit should include:
   - Interview with family concerning developmental status of the child.
   - Observation of family interaction.
   - Discussion of parental concerns.

LEARNING OUTCOME 36.5: Integrate pertinent mental health care into health supervision visits for children.

1. Mental health issues to be addressed include:
   - Assessment of occurrence of common problems such as nightmares and temper tantrums.
   - Explanation of the promotion of a positive self-image.

LEARNING OUTCOME 36.6: Examine data about the family and other social relationships to prioritize interventions and to maintain health of children.

1. Health promotion and maintenance activities related to social relationships focus on:
   - Increasing social skills with the people in the child's environment.
   - Successful management of temperament characteristics.
   - Adjusting to time away from home.
   - Improving language and communication skills.

Clinical Reasoning in Action

Quinton and his mother have come into the office for his 2-year-old well-child checkup. During the visit you learn that his mother stays home with him during the day and his father often works overtime. His only significant medical history incident was when he had stitches placed in his forehead for falling on the edge of a table when he was 15 months old. There is a family history of attention deficit disorder and Crohn's disease. His height is in the 75th percentile, weight is in the 50th percentile, and body mass index is between the 25th and 50th percentiles. His temperature is 98.9°F and his pulse is 80. He is described by his parents as a picky eater and tends to eat the same foods frequently. They also say he tends to eat well on some days and other days will hardly eat anything. On the days he is not eating well, his mother will often resort to giving him soda or a sugary snack just so he is "getting something." Quinton sleeps about 7 hours per night and his mother usually ends up sleeping with him because he continues to fight going to sleep after being put to bed. He does not have a regular bedtime or rest routine and he usually naps in the car during the day. His mother tells you that her only break during the day when she is at home with Quinton is when he is watching television in his bedroom, so he often watches 2 to 4 hours per day. Quinton has a soft stool every day and has not showed any interest in potty training at this time. He is developmentally able to go up and down stairs, kick a ball, scribble on paper, and is able to speak in three- to four-word sentences. During the visit at the office, it is obvious his parents have difficulty controlling him and frequently make threats and offer bribes to get him to behave properly. He starts screaming and kicking when his parents set limits on his behavior in the office and his parents say they are frequently exhausted and do not know what to do about his high energy level. They also are concerned because they feel like the discipline methods they have been using are not working, and he is getting into so many things in the home that they are concerned he may hurt himself. They have used spanking and time-outs, but they do not seem to improve his behavior. They think he may have some type of medical condition like attention deficit disorder considering it does run in their family.

1. At 2 years of age, a consistent routine will help a toddler behave more appropriately. What are some of the things you can tell Quinton's parents regarding his sleep and nutrition habits to help establish a better routine?
2. How can you advise Quinton's parents about positive approaches to disciplining him?
3. How can you advise Quinton's parents about disciplining him when it is needed?
4. What are some suggestions you can give Quinton's parents about handling his temper tantrums?

See www.nursing.pearsonhighered.com for possible responses.

References

American Academy of Pediatric Dentistry (AAPD). (2012a). *Guideline on infant oral health care (2012)*. Retrieved from http://www.aapd.org/assets/1/7/G_InfantOralHealthCare.pdf#xml=http://pr-dtsearch001.americaneagle.com/service/search.asp?cmd=pdfhits&DocId=574&Index=F%3a%5cdtSearch%5caapd%2eorg&HitCount=8&hits=44d+44e+47d+47e+743+744+102a+102b+&hc=337&req=fluoridated+toothpaste

American Academy of Pediatric Dentistry (AAPD). (2012b). *Policy on third-party reimbursement of fees related to dental sealants*. Retrieved from http://www.aapd.org/media/Policies_Guidelines/P_3rdPartSealants.pdf#xml=http://pr-dtsearch001.americaneagle.com/service/search.asp?cmd=pdfhits&DocId=330&Index=F%3a%5cdtSearch%5caapd%2eorg&HitCount=16&hits=18+46+57+11f+149+155+162+18e+1b6+1d2+207+228+246+269+2a8+2ca+&hc=314&req=sealants

American Academy of Pediatrics (AAP). (2011a). *Car safety seats*. Retrieved from http://www.healthychildren.org

American Academy of Pediatrics (AAP). (2011b). *Discipline*. Retrieved from http://www.healthychildren.org

American Academy of Pediatrics (AAP). (2011c). *Water safety and young children*. Retrieved from http://www.healthychildren.org/English/safety-prevention/at-play/Pages/Water-Safety-And-Young-Children.aspx

American Academy of Pediatrics (AAP) Committee on Injury, Violence, and Poison Prevention. (2011). Child passenger safety. *Pediatrics, 127*, 788–793.

American Academy of Pediatrics (AAP) Committee on Nutrition. (2009). *Pediatric nutrition handbook* (6th ed.). Elk Grove Village, IL: Author.

American Dental Association (ADA). (2011). *Thumbsucking*. Retrieved from http://www.ada.org/2977.aspx

Beets, M. W., Bornstein, D., Dowda, M., & Pate, R. R. (2011). Compliance with national guidelines for physical activity in U.S. preschoolers: Measurement and interpretation. *Pediatrics, 127*(4), 658–664.

Ben-Arye, E., Traube, Z., Schachter, L., Jaimi, M., Levy, M., Schiff, E., & Lev, E. (2011). Integrative pediatric care: Parents/attitudes toward communication of physicians and CAM practitioners. *Pediatrics, 127*(1), 384–395.

Centers for Disease Control and Prevention (CDC). (2009). Quick stats: Percentage of children ages 2–4 years who ever had caries in primary teeth, by race/ethnicity and sex—National Health and Nutrition Examination Survey, United States, 1988–1994 and 1999–2004. *Morbidity and Mortality Weekly Report, 58*(2), 34.

Centers for Disease Control and Prevention (CDC). (2010a). *Physical activity guidelines for Americans: Children and adolescents*. Retrieved from http://www.cdc.gov/HealthyYouth/physicalactivity/guidelines.htm

Centers for Disease Control and Prevention (CDC). (2010b). Youth risk behavior surveillance—United States, 2009. *Morbidity and Mortality Weekly Report, 59*(SS-5), 1–148.

Centers for Disease Control and Prevention (CDC). (2011). *How much physical activity do children need?* Retrieved from http://www.cdc.gov/physicalactivity/everyone/guidelines/children/html

Centers for Disease Control and Prevention (CDC). (2012). Youth risk behavior surveillance—United States, 2011. *Morbidity and Mortality Weekly Report, 61*(SS04), 1–162.

Child Trends. (2012). *Early childhood program enrollment*. Retrieved from http://www.childtrendsdatabank.org/?q=node/280

Dellinger, A. M., & Kresnow, M. J. (2010). Bicycle helmet use among children in the United States: The effects of legislation, personal and household factors. *Journal of Safety Research, 41*, 375–380.

Devoe, J. E., Tillotson, C. J., Wallace, L. S., Lesko, S. E., & Pandhi, H. (2012). Is health insurance enough? A usual source of care may be more important to ensure a child receives preventive health counseling. *Maternal and Child Health Journal, 16*, 306–315.

Hagan, J. F., Shaw, J. S., & Duncan, P. M. (2008). *Bright futures: Guidelines for health supervision of infants, children, and adolescents* (3rd ed.). Elk Grove Village, IL: American Academy of Pediatrics.

Hagel, B. E., Lee, R. S., Karkhaneh, M., Voaklander, D., & Rowe, B. H. (2010). Factors associated with incorrect bicycle helmet use. *Injury Prevention, 16*(3), 178–184.

Halfon, N., Larson, K., & Russ, S. (2010). Why social determinants? *Healthcare Quarterly, 14*, 8–20.

Holt, K., Wooldridge, N., Story, M., & Sofka, D. (2011). *Bright futures: Nutrition* (3rd ed.). Elk Grove Village, IL: American Academy of Pediatrics.

Knox, M. (2010). On hitting children: A review of corporal punishment in the United States. *Journal of Pediatric Health Care, 24*(2), 103–107.

Kuo, D. Z., Houtrow, A. J., Arango, P., Kuhlthau, K. A., Simmons, J. M., & Neff, J. M. (2011). Family-centered care: Current applications and future directions in pediatric health care. *Maternal Child Health Journal, 16*(2), 297–305.

Lucille Packard Children's Hospital. (2012). *Upper respiratory infection*. Retrieved from http://www.lpch.org/DiseaseHealthInfo/HealthLibrary/respire/uricold.html

Mayo Clinic. (2009). *Teen sleep: Why is your teen so tired?* Retrieved from http://www.mayoclinic.com/health/teens-health

Mindell, J. A., Meltzer, L. J., Carskadon, M. A., & Chervin, R. D. (2009). Developmental aspects of sleep hygiene: Findings from the 2004 National Sleep Foundation Sleep in America Poll. *Sleep Medicine, 10*(7), 771–779.

Murray, R. B., Zentner, J. P., & Yakimo, R. (2009). *Health promotion strategies through the life span* (8th ed.). Upper Saddle River, NJ: Pearson Prentice Hall.

National Highway Traffic Safety Administration. (2012). *Car seats and booster basics*. Retrieved from http://www.safercar.gov/parents/RightSeat.htm

National Maternal and Child Oral Health Resource Center. (2010). *Resource highlights: Focus on early childhood caries*. Retrieved from http://www.mchoralhealth.org/highlights/ecc.html

Pender, N. J., Murdaugh, C. L., & Parsons, M. A. (2011). *Health promotion in nursing practice* (6th ed.). Upper Saddle River, NJ: Pearson Prentice Hall.

Safe Kids. (2011a). *Never leave your child alone in a car*. Retrieved from http://www.safekids.org/safety-basics/safety-guide/kids-in-and-around-cars.html

Safe Kids. (2011b). *Playground safety fact sheet*. Retrieved from http://www.safekids.org/our-work/research/fact-sheets/playground-safety-fact-sheet.html

Safe Kids. (2011c). *Preventing injuries: At home, at play, and on the way*. Retrieved from http://www.safekids.org/our-work/research/fact-sheets/toy-safety-fact-sheet.html

Santrock, J. W. (2011). *Child development* (12th ed.). Boston, MA: McGraw-Hill.

Sibinga, E. M., & Kemper, K. J. (2010). Complementary, holistic, and integrative medicine: Meditation practices for pediatric health. *Pediatric Reviews, 31*(12), e91–103.

U.S. Department of Health and Human Services. (2011). *Strengthening families and communities*. Washington, DC: Author.

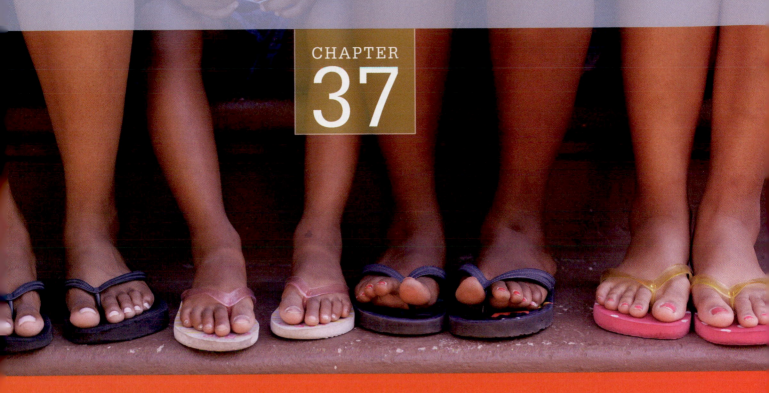

Health Promotion and Maintenance: The Adolescent

I know I should not be using chewing tobacco, but a lot of my friends use it, and I want to fit in with them. I would like to quit, but I really don't know how. —Jeremy, 16 years

LEARNING OUTCOMES

37.1 Identify the major health concerns of the adolescent years.

37.2 Describe the general observations made of adolescents and their families as they come to the pediatric healthcare home for health supervision visits.

37.3 Apply communication skills to interactions with adolescents and their families.

37.4 Apply assessment skills to plan data-gathering methods for nutrition, physical activity, and mental health status of youth.

37.5 Synthesize data from history and examination of the adolescent and family with knowledge of adolescent development to intervene with the adolescent and family during health supervision visits.

37.6 Plan with adolescents to help them integrate activities to promote health and to prevent disease and injury.

Adolescents are often seen only sporadically for health care, even though visits are recommended annually. They are usually healthy, may not need immunizations, and consequently do not often come for health care. If adolescents seek care for a minor illness, birth control, or a sports examination, the visit should be viewed as a health supervision opportunity.

While all components of the usual visit may not be performed, at least those parts most important are inserted into care. If time is limited, the nurse has to decide which topics to address during a healthcare visit. It is advisable to start with the topic of most interest to the teen and then to include injury prevention teaching, since injury is the greatest risk to teens. Health promotion topics such as dietary and exercise habits could be discussed if there is time.

Lifestyle behaviors are responsible for most of the preventable diseases, and all typically have origins in adolescent years, including sedentary lifestyle, unhealthy diet, tobacco and other substance use, and risk taking. Mental health assessment and teaching are other areas of prime importance. If the teen is at immediate risk, such as considering suicide in response to depression, this must be dealt with immediately by collaborating with a mental health specialist.

What general principles can guide programs to promote health in adolescents? Some researchers have analyzed theory application and approaches of programs, and others have suggested key elements of programs (see *Clinical Reasoning: Applying Theory to Plan for Adolescent Health*). Programs assist adolescents in taking on health promotion behaviors by fostering a sense of competence, promoting decision making, and increasing motivation for change toward healthy behaviors (Murray,

---

Clinical Reasoning Applying Theory to Plan for Adolescent Health

Several theories guide healthcare professionals in establishing health promotion programs for adolescents. These theories provide an organized approach to planning and suggest the strategies that will be most successful, based on the person's motivation and developmental age (Murray et al., 2009). One such theory that is commonly used in adolescent care is the social cognitive theory.

This theory was developed by Albert Bandura, whose work is described in Chapter 32 🔗, and is frequently used in health research (Bandura, 1986, 1997a, 1997b; Bricker et al., 2010; Connor, George, Gullo, et al., 2011). The key components of his theory involve **self-efficacy** (the person's belief in the ability to perform a behavior) and **outcome expectancy** (what the person expects to get from performing a certain behavior). Learning a new behavior occurs through **modeling**, or imitating the behavior of someone else. Bandura believes that individuals make decisions about health behaviors based on thoughts about the consequences and outcomes of those behaviors. The person's characteristics, such as self-efficacy and outcome expectancy, interact with the external environment and the behavioral choices available. All of these components together determine health behaviors, and all can be influenced to promote health.

When seeking to promote physical activity behaviors in youth, essential components include the following:

- Encourage the youth to believe they can perform the activity (self-efficacy).
- Point out the positive aspects of the behavior (outcome expectancy).
- Show the youth how to do the activity (modeling).
- Provide a physical setting and opportunity for performing the behavior (environment).
- Allow trial and error, choice in time, and extent of activity (behavioral choices).

Compose a teaching plan to encourage increased physical activity for a teen, using all components of the social cognitive theory. List the outcome measures or goals for the teaching, the interventions, and methods of evaluation.
See www.nursing.pearsonhighered.com for possible responses.

Zentner, & Yakimo, 2009). When establishing youth programs, whether with individual adolescents or with groups, the nurse includes evaluation of the effectiveness of the plan, and uses methods to expand and sustain successful approaches.

GENERAL OBSERVATIONS

The beginning of the visit with an adolescent can be an important time to gather information, just as it is with younger children. However, the observations you make will relate to the adolescent's more advanced stage of development.

Ideally the facility has a waiting area that is designed for adolescents. Teens often dislike waiting for health care with either young children or older adults. Teen waiting areas are popular because they provide a special place, thereby relaying that the adolescent is important, and can use video kiosks and other contemporary methods to impart health information while the teen waits (Figure 37–1 ●). As you call the adolescent back for care, observe if parents or friends are present, or if the teen is alone. Young adolescents often come with parents to the facility, and parents often then wait in the waiting room during the examination. If the young adolescent comes in for a special problem, such as a skin lesion or other health concern, the parent may accompany the adolescent into the examination room. If someone

● **Figure 37–1** Healthcare visit with a teen. Parents often accompany teens with a healthcare problem in for the examination. Provide an opportunity to see both the teen and parent privately and integrate general health promotion and health maintenance into the visit. What questions can you ask this teen? What teaching might be needed?

comes with the teen, it may be necessary to provide some private time by asking the other person to wait outside for a moment. Reassure parents that there will be time to talk with them about any of their concerns and questions, and provide them with an opportunity to ask questions and obtain information.

Some teens are comfortable in healthcare settings and actively engage in conversation, while others are nervous and will need more explanations and reassurance during the first steps of measurement and blood pressure. By adolescence, boys and girls should be assuming more of a partnership role in their own health care. As the visit begins, greet adolescents warmly, ask what concerns and questions they have, and ask for their opinions and reactions throughout the visit. This will show that their thoughts are important and that they play an important role in guiding the healthcare visits. When adolescents are visiting the same office or clinic that they came to during childhood, they usually know and feel comfortable with the care providers. If the setting is new to them, explain procedures and introduce personnel so they feel more at ease.

GROWTH AND DEVELOPMENTAL SURVEILLANCE

Adolescence spans several years, and growth and developmental issues vary throughout the period. For young adolescents, or those from about 12 to 13 years of age, growth measurement remains important. These youth are still growing, and use of percentile grids continues to be an important part of care. Growth should remain in the same percentile channel as during childhood, with girls reaching nearly adult height at this age, and boys still continuing to grow. As always, be alert for youth who have either increased or decreased percentiles, or are above the 85th percentile or below the 5th percentile for body mass index. They will need additional assessment of nutritional intake and physical activity.

By middle (14 to 16 years) and late adolescence (17 to 19 years), adult growth is nearly achieved, earlier for girls than boys. While measurement continues to be performed, nurses assess the BMI more carefully to be sure the height and weight indicate appropriate intake and exercise. Overweight at this age is likely to continue into adulthood, particularly if parents are overweight, so early intervention will be needed to decrease this potential. Other youth may have eating disorders and should be referred to a specialist for care. Children from homes without sufficient financial resources may be hungry and lack adequate food of high quality (known as *food insecurity*). Parents who were eligible for Women, Infants, and Children (WIC) Nutrition Program services when children were younger may not receive them once the child is an adolescent, so the increasing dietary intake needs of their teens cannot be met. If an adolescent is thin and has little energy, consider this possibility; administer a food security questionnaire such as the one provided by the U.S. Department of Agriculture (www.ers.usda.gov). Even the child who is overweight may live in a family with insufficient resources since foods with high fat and caloric content are often less expensive than those with greater nutrient value. For example, a "dollar menu" at a fast-food restaurant meets hunger needs faster and with less expense than a home-prepared meal of fresh fruits, vegetables, and grains. In addition, people who have experienced periods of hunger from inadequate food resources may overeat when food is available, a pattern that promotes weight gain.

Few options exist for measuring the developmental competence of adolescents, but observations and questions during care provide information about the meeting of developmental milestones. Key tasks for adolescents involve separating from the parents and establishing positive relationships with peers. The young teen may come to an appointment with a parent and still rely on that parent to answer some questions during the examination. However, middle and late teens should be increasingly able to come alone, answer questions themselves, and assume responsibility for healthcare decisions. Offer older teens the option of coming into the room alone, stating, "Your mom can wait here and we can come and get her later. Does that sound all right?" During time with the adolescent, ask questions to learn about peer interactions and activities.

The adolescent may receive a physical examination from either the nurse practitioner or the physician. See Chapter 34 🔗 for components of the examination. Some particular parts of the examination to include for teens are scoliosis screening, sexual maturity rating (Tanner stages), breast exam, testicular exam, testing for sexually transmitted infections (among those sexually active), pelvic exam and pap smear (for sexually active females), annual hematocrit for anemia in menstruating adolescents, hearing screening (at 12, 15, and 18 years), annual blood pressure, lipid screening for those with family history of early heart disease or other risk factors, and tuberculosis screening for those in high-risk areas.

Most adolescents do not want their parents present during the examination, but occasionally will want a parent present for something like a first pelvic examination or a blood draw. Ask them their wishes in a confidential setting so they can freely make the choice. They also may choose to have a same-gender healthcare provider complete the genitourinary examination. Expected outcomes of care include screening and early identification for common health problems, normal patterns of growth, and meeting of developmental milestones.

NUTRITION

The young adolescent needs a well-balanced diet to support the growth of this period, and the late adolescent requires intake that supports physical activity and provides nutrients for metabolism and to promote the immune system. While nutritional intake is important, teens often do not eat well. They may be busy and do not want to plan meals, they like to eat foods that are popular with other teens (so high fat and sugar intake can be common), they may be dieting to achieve weight loss, and some do not have enough financial resources to access proper foods.

Combine the information from measurement of the adolescent with the answers to questions about diet to identify possible areas for intervention. Find out what questions the teen has about foods, diet, maintaining desired weight, and topics such as vegetarianism or supplements to enhance athletic performance. See Chapter 33 🔗 for further detail about these special nutritional topics. Health promotion plans focus on practices

that lead to healthy growth and development. They may include teaching about:

- Getting five fruits and vegetables daily
- Including whole-grain products to replace refined products whenever possible
- The importance of eating three meals each day, including breakfast and lunch
- Eating together as a family several times weekly, which enhances quality food intake
- How to plan menus and prepare foods for balanced intake

Health maintenance plans center on those practices that prevent disease, including:

- Limiting refined sugar and high-fat intake (such as soft drinks and fried foods) to maintain weight at recommended level
- Including two to three servings of dairy products daily to enhance bone formation and decrease chance of osteoporosis as an adult
- Using resources for treatment of eating disorders if they are identified

While much of nutrition teaching should be aimed directly at the adolescent, parents are also included. They can be effective contributors to healthy intake by providing plenty of fruits and vegetables for snacks, having foods attractively prepared and ready for consumption when the teen is hungry, planning several meals together as a family each week, encouraging milk or other forms of calcium intake, and setting a good example for food intake. Help parents to identify the youth with an eating disorder and provide resources for intervention in these cases. Consider as well the teen with a baby. The adolescent who is pregnant or breastfeeding has even more need for nutritional teaching and may need financial resources to access sufficient food (see Chapter 13 🔗). How can the nurse combine in the teaching plan the growth and developmental needs of an adolescent with those of her new baby?

PHYSICAL ACTIVITY

Many adolescents suffer from the effects of inadequate physical activity. As children get older and enter the teenage years, physical activity decreases, particularly in girls. Sixty minutes daily of moderate or vigorous activity is recommended for teens, but 23% do not get this level of exercise even 1 day a week (Eaton et al., 2010). Only about 29% of adolescents report daily vigorous activity each day of the week (Eaton et al., 2012). The percentage is lower among some groups, with only 28% of females reporting that level of activity. Only about 31% of teens in 12th grade report exercise (Eaton et al., 2010). At a time when teens are not very active as a group, physical education requirements in school are also decreasing. Only 28% of 12th-grade students regularly attend a physical education class (Eaton et al., 2012). Physical activity levels must therefore be assessed at each health supervision visit or in other contacts with adolescents. Apply resilience theory as discussed in Chapter 32 🔗, and assess youth, family, and community for risk and protective factors regarding physical activity (Table 37–1).

Table 37-1	Risk and Protective Factors Regarding Physical Activity in Adolescence

Risk Factors	Protective Factors
■ Lives in rural or other isolated setting with little opportunity for contact with other teens ■ Lives in urban area that is unsafe or provides little opportunity for outside physical activity ■ Presence of neighborhood hazards and unsafe areas ■ Lack of neighborhood programs for physical activity promotion	■ Has opportunities for participation in physical activity at home, at school, and in the community ■ School provides daily physical education classes ■ Neighborhood and community provide physical activity options ■ Has many friends living close who participate in physical activity ■ Public policies maintain parks, green spaces, biking trails, playgrounds
■ Has a developmental disability that impairs physical movement	■ Programs are available for adolescents with developmental disabilities or other healthcare needs
■ Does not like physical activity	■ Likes physical activity
■ Has a pattern and history of low activity levels ■ Is overweight ■ Does not feel competent in most sports	■ Has exercised during all of childhood, often with parents
■ Limited financial resources to pay registration fees or buy protective gear for sports	■ Availability of financial and other resources for sports gear and protective equipment
■ Family members who have little physical activity ■ Parents who are not active in school sports and committees ■ Parents who do not like physical activity and have had low levels while their teen was growing up ■ Parents who have little time or facilities for exercise, or always exercise at a club—out of view of their family	■ Parents participate in regular physical activity and encourage the adolescent to do so also ■ Youth and parents agree to a limit of 2 hours daily of screen time
■ Lack of youth and parent knowledge about physical activity needs and benefits	■ Knowledgeable about benefits of activity; committed to maintaining exercise patterns

Source: Data from Hagan, J. F., Shaw, J. S., & Duncan, P. M. (Eds.). (2008). *Bright futures: Guidelines for health supervision of infants, children, and adolescents* (3rd ed.). Elk Grove Village, IL: American Academy of Pediatrics.

● **Figure 37–2** Teen use of safety measures. This teen girl is an avid "boarder." How can you encourage and praise her for this activity? What clues do you have that she is using adequate safety measures?

for wrestling, running, or other sports. Integrate nutritional teaching that includes the importance of adequate intake for sports performance. Other athletes use nutritional supplements to enhance performance. While most are not harmful, few have proven benefits and their cost is not warranted. Some may actually be harmful to adolescents, such as prolonged use of creatinine and any use of steroids.

Other youth have very little physical activity and feel incompetent in performing many sports. Work with them to find at least one thing they can do on a daily basis—walking their dog in the neighborhood, riding a bike to the store, using stairs instead of elevators when possible, parking on the far side of the school lot and walking farther, swimming at a club their parents belong to or at a local YMCA or YWCA, or saving money to take lessons for something they have always dreamed of doing, such as horseback riding or golf. The community health nurse can form interest groups at schools and community centers that provide an outlet for adolescents who cannot "make the team" for school sports. Encourage parents and adolescents to set goals together to integrate some physical activity daily.

What risk and protective factors for physical activity exist in your community? Go to www.activelivingbydesign.org to examine the positive effect community planning can have on its members' exercise levels.

The nurse's activities for health promotion concentrate on teaching the health and mental benefits of physical activity such as increased energy, weight control, and a feeling of control and success. Health maintenance focuses on viewing physical activity as a method to prevent disease such as cardiovascular disease and diabetes. Youth who have family members with these diseases or meet adults who have them are more likely to

Some youth have established regular physical activity programs, and their behaviors should be encouraged (Figure 37–2 ●). Be alert for adolescents who exercise but have other health problems. Some athletes try to eat very little to remain a certain weight understand the importance of their own activity. Desired outcomes include maintenance of weight within recommended level, daily exercise of 60 minutes, and establishment of lifetime exercise routines.

ORAL HEALTH

Continued dental care during the adolescent years can ensure oral health. The recommendations remain the same as those for young children. The adolescent should floss daily, brush twice daily with a small amount of fluoridated toothpaste, and visit a dental care provider every 6 months. By about 14 years of age, those adolescents who do not have fluoridated water and have been taking fluoride can stop this supplement. Even the molars have been formed by that age so fluoride tablets are no longer needed. Continue to examine the condition of the teeth and the number of erupted permanent teeth present. Be alert for any unusual growths and ulcers in the mouth and refer for care as needed.

Unavailability of dental insurance for the adolescent is a potential concern. The teen whose family does not have dental insurance needs referrals for care to affordable resources. Dental specialists clean off plaque that has formed, apply sealants to erupting molars, examine the teeth for caries, and perform restorative care. Certain groups are more at risk for inadequate dental care (see *Developing Cultural Competence: Dental Care*). When working with these populations, nurses can question access to care and make recommendations that foster regular checkups.

Evaluate risk factors for threats to oral health such as tobacco use, particularly chewing tobacco (see quote from Jeremy in the chapter-opening scenario). A risk for oral injury exists with engagement in certain sports. Ask about physical activity and recommend that a mouth guard be worn if the youth engages in hockey, football, or some other sports. Some teens may wish to whiten the teeth or obtain orthodontia to improve appearance. The nurse can help the youth and parents to find resources for needed care.

Developing Cultural Competence
Dental Care

Analysis of several national surveys, such as the National Center for Health Statistics and the National Health Interview Survey, shows marked disparity in oral health. The major factor in disparity of dental care is lack of dental insurance. While 49% of youth from families without insurance did not have a dental visit in the previous year and 27% of them had unmet dental needs, only 17% of youth from families with insurance lacked a previous year visit and only 4% had unmet dental needs. People without dental insurance commonly are poor. In these families, 21% of children have unmet dental needs in contrast with 4% in families living above the poverty level. Hispanic youth are most at risk; 11% have unmet dental needs (Child Trends, 2010).

When working with adolescent populations from groups at high risk for lack of dental coverage or high incidence of caries, include dental assessment in health supervision visits, and have resources for care readily available to carry out referrals as needed.

Expected outcomes for oral health include dental visits twice annually, daily positive oral health habits, absence of risk factors for poor oral health or injury, and obtaining recommended follow-up care for problems.

MENTAL AND SPIRITUAL HEALTH

Adolescents have many challenges to their mental health and need support to emerge from adolescence with mental and spiritual strengths. Mental health topics must be addressed at each health supervision opportunity to promote mental health among teens. Mental health is closely linked to developmental tasks such as growing independence, formation of close relationships with peers, becoming confident in accomplishments, and setting goals for the future. Some chronic mental health disorders such as schizophrenia can emerge during adolescence, so mental health screening is important to perform with this age group.

As during other developmental stages, the self-concept continues to evolve, influencing how the adolescent reacts to the environment. Self-regulation—making decisions to govern oneself—becomes critically important. Self-esteem, or a positive feeling about the self, is key to meeting life's challenges. Ask what the teen is proud of and has accomplished and what disappointments have occurred as well. Provide resources to deal with disappointments and praise the teen's accomplishments.

The adolescent's self-esteem is connected to perception of body image. Factors such as early or late maturation, overweight or underweight, or the role of the media can influence the teen's body image. A healthy image includes the realization that the body has positive and less positive attributes and that the individual can influence the body by healthy eating and physical activity. Be alert for the teen whose wish for a different body leads to eating disorders and excessive exercise or intake of nutritional supplements.

Sexuality involves both body changes that signal mature sexual development, and the mental concept of oneself as a sexual being. Body changes and mental concepts do not necessarily mature at the same time, and adolescents may not be ready for sexual maturity; decisions about sexual behavior are not necessarily equivalent to achieving sexual maturation. Most young adolescent girls have begun menstruating, and by early to middle adolescence, boys are having nocturnal emissions and ejaculations. Ask teens if they have received information about puberty, body changes, and sexuality. Tell young adolescents that most teens have questions and that they may ask about any areas of interest, including contraception and sexually transmitted infections. Ask older adolescents directly if they have had sexual intercourse and if so, what they are doing to protect against pregnancy and sexually transmitted infections. Provide support for adolescents who have decided not to have sexual intercourse, encouraging them to continue this plan, telling them that sexual feelings are normal, but that decisions about sexual intercourse are their right and privilege. Ask if the adolescent has ever experienced unwanted pressure for intercourse and if there has been help and support to deal with the situation. Intimate partner violence, date rape, and other trauma signals a need for referral to a mental health specialist. See Chapter 43 🔗 for further information.

Ask if teens have confusion about their sexuality. If teens have self-identified as homosexual, let them know they are welcome and ask about decisions regarding sexual practices, reinforcing the need for protection against sexually transmitted infections. Provide community resources to support gay or lesbian teens so that they can develop a social group in which they feel comfortable. Some adolescents are seen for health care at the time they become sexually active. Use this opportunity to reinforce and correct prior knowledge about the body and protection against pregnancy and sexually transmitted infections.

Most adolescents still need discipline or guidance from parents at certain times. Rather than a constant battle over daily events, it is best if there are just a few important rules that parents have to enforce only rarely. When working with parents, nurses can assist them to set useful boundaries for teens and offer resources such as parenting groups and websites for assistance.

Sleep is necessary for anyone to function safely and at a level of one's potential. Unfortunately, many youth do not get the sleep needed for healthy functioning. Teens have an increased need for sleep due to their growth rates and activity levels. At the same time, their internal clocks change, making it more difficult to get to sleep at the usual time. It is thought that a decrease in secretion of melatonin occurs, so the teen does not feel tired in the late evening. However, they often do not have the number of hours of sleep needed by the time they wake up for school or work. The problem may be worsened if the student participates in sports or other activities. They may need to get to school before normal starting hours for music, sports, or other activities, or perhaps stay late into the evening for practices. Some adolescents then work weekends or evenings as well. And of course social activities usually fill much of their time. Although about 9 hours of sleep is needed, most adolescents get about 6 hours (Mayo Clinic, 2009). The effects of sleep deprivation can be serious. Teens cannot perform to their potential

in school or at work. Many parents state that adolescents are moody and difficult to communicate with when they are tired. There may be a connection between lack of sleep and substance abuse, and teens commonly use caffeinated beverages to stay awake. Some people tend to eat more when they are tired, and get less physical activity. Perhaps one of the most serious consequences deals with the danger of driving while sleepy; this is a common cause of accidents. Ask adolescents about what time they go to bed, when they awaken, and whether they are frequently tired. Provide suggestions for regular sleep schedules, avoiding caffeine products in the evening, making screen technology unavailable during sleep time, and planning a day of relaxation into every week.

School plays an increasingly important role in adolescent mental health. Peer support, meaningful activities, and a forum for learning time management and other skills are all provided by school. At the same time, some youth stress because of inability to fit in, worry about grades and their futures, and violent or unsupportive school situations. Discuss the elements of school that adolescents like and those they do not like. Determine what support is available in the schools. Ask the adolescent about future plans and how those are influencing choices for courses and friends in school.

Temperament or personality type characteristics continue into adolescence and generally do not change from earlier years. For example, the active infant and young child is usually an active teenager. The slow-to-warm-up baby may be the adolescent who needs more time to adjust to a new school or teachers. If the adolescent or parent has trouble with personality characteristics, it may be helpful to talk about these traits, help them to establish a positive sense about the attributes, and discuss ways to adapt the environment as needed. For example, parents should not expect a slow-to-warm-up teen to be interested in running for a class office. Someone with irregular sleep and eating habits will find it difficult to have a job at a set time and will need to set alarms and other reminders.

Spirituality offers comfort and support for the adolescent. Being a member of a teen group in a faith-based home can offer a peer group with similar values and bring meaning to life. Some adolescents reject the faith of their parents and seek a different group; others seek to leave religious practices totally while others become more committed to them. Ask them if they have the resources they need to bring meaning to their lives; provide them if needed. Realize that participation in community food kitchens, raising money for causes, and other activities also provide meaning for many adolescents (Figure 37–3 ●).

The nurse actively promotes the mental health of youth by understanding their developmental needs and providing information and resources. Gentle guidance and active partnership with youth help to provide the resources to ensure healthy self-concept, sexuality, and personality development. While most teenagers have many protective factors that can be identified and fostered, a few have risks that can harm mental health. It is important to identify the risks, and to use health maintenance techniques to lessen the risk factors. Depression and substance use are two common risks to mental health. Depression is discussed in Chapter 56 🔗 and substance abuse is discussed in Chapter 43 🔗.

Clinical Tip

The nurse who works with adolescents dealing with sexuality issues may find that the values of some teens are very different from one's personal values. How do you react when a teen decides to have sexual intercourse or has become pregnant? Can you help teens to make wise decisions without telling them what they should do?

It is important for adolescents to learn the significance of sexual intercourse and the meaning of close relationships. Teaching them early about this will enable them to respect others at the time they do have intimate relations. Respect is also the key to working with teens. Nurses should treat them with respect, expecting them to consider options and make wise decisions. Nurses who cannot work with certain groups of teens because of moral values differing from their own have the obligation to refer the teens for care to resources where they can receive the information and services they are requesting.

● **Figure 37–3** Spiritual health for teens. Teens often become associated with causes. This helps them to feel part of a social group and also provides opportunities for examining belief systems and making decisions about meaningful activities.

Source: Jeff Greenberg/Alamy

See the quick checklists in Table 37–2 to help in identifying these problems during health supervision visits.

Although health promotion and health maintenance activities commonly occur in office or clinic settings, there are many other settings where nurses work with adolescents, and mental health activities are often integrated into these settings. Consider offering health promotion/maintenance wherever students might be found. Some nontraditional settings include correctional facilities, school-based health centers, and programs for pregnant teens. Adolescents in these facilities can benefit from services to improve diet, physical activity, and lifestyle behaviors that influence mental health.

The desired outcomes for mental and spiritual health promotion and maintenance include meaningful activities in the adolescent's life, emerging independence, good choices about lifestyle behaviors, and development of successful coping skills.

Table 37–2	**Signs of Depression and Substance Abuse**
Depression	**Substance Abuse**
Changes in appetite and weight	Changes in school performance, sleep, and appetite
Changes in sleep schedules and patterns	Unusual behavior, such as getting into trouble at school
Changes in school performance	
Physical complaints	Accidents and other unexplained events
Loss of interest and pleasure in usual activities and friends	Lack of responsibility for actions
Depression, irritability, poor concentration	Increased mood changes
	Inability to set goals
Feelings of worthlessness, helplessness	A variety of physical changes depending on the substance used
Thoughts of death or suicide	

Adapted from Tanski, S., Garfunkel, L. C., Duncan, P. M., & Weitzman, M. (2011) Performing preventive services. Elk Grove Village, Il: American Academy of Pediatrics.

RELATIONSHIPS

Adolescents form stronger bonds with friends than at any time earlier in development; at the same time they need their parents for guidance and reassurance as they become more independent. As teenagers strive for independence, they frequently strike out at parents, test limits, and have conflicts with parents. Interactions in the family provide consistent and important ties at the same time that social interactions become a central part of life. Health promotion helps teens to form strong friendships with peers and to continue to value and participate in the family. It helps parents to understand the developmental needs and their role in establishing a new type of relationship with the emerging young adult in the family. Partnerships with care providers are important to help families work together to achieve these outcomes.

When adolescents are seen for healthcare visits, assess relationships with others. Provide time alone with both the adolescent and the parents (if they are present) so that everyone has time to talk freely and to ask questions. Some areas already discussed, such as school performance and activities, provide information about the adolescent's friends and how time is spent. Ask teens to describe their best friends and what they do together. Ask parents their opinions of the youth's friends. Inquire about the youth's roles in the family. Does the teen have jobs and responsibilities? What freedom is allowed? What are relationships like with siblings and extended family members such as grandparents and cousins? What activities are done together as a family? Are there differences in the teen's and the parents' answers to these questions? What are the teen's and parents' desires for how the family unit functions?

Provide an opportunity to talk with the teen alone about issues such as domestic violence. Is the youth abused or is there violence between adults in the family? Are there stressors such as lack of sufficient finances, an ill parent, or a lost job? How have these occurrences affected the adolescent? Minor adjustments can be helped by discussion, whereas some major problems will need referral to mental health specialists.

In their relationships with peers, adolescents often have many of the same issues that emerge with parents. They may have disagreements with friends or feel hurt by things that are said or done. Ask teens about how things are going with friends and what problems they have. Talk about negotiating, joining groups to form new friendships, and the importance of respecting and not making fun of others. Give them strategies for living up to their own standards even when friends are enticing them to do other things. Suggest that having friends one can trust and who have the same ideals can be very supportive and fun in adolescent years. Expected outcomes are the formation of strong relationships both within and outside of the family, along with independence in decision making.

DISEASE PREVENTION STRATEGIES

Teenagers typically do not have many diseases and most are minor illnesses like respiratory and gastrointestinal illness. However, there are some diseases that occur and nurses must always be aware of signs of potential disease. Some common health issues that are described throughout this book include the following:

- Acne and skin infections (see Chapter 58 🔗)
- Body piercing and tattooing (see Chapter 43 🔗)
- Sports overuse injuries (see Chapter 57 🔗)
- Constipation and diarrhea (see Chapter 52 🔗)

Other observations may signal more serious health concerns and need to be referred for further evaluation. Examples include the following:

- Scoliosis (see Chapter 57 🔗)
- Anemia (see Chapter 50 🔗)
- Excessive tiredness (see Chapter 51 🔗)
- Bruising (see Chapter 50 🔗)
- Depression, suicidal thoughts, other mental health issues (see Chapter 56 🔗)
- Sexually transmitted infections (see Chapter 53 🔗)
- Eating disorder (see Chapter 43 🔗)
- Abuse or severe bullying (see Chapter 43 🔗)

Several screening tests should be performed during health supervision visits with adolescents, including vision, hearing, smoking, depression, stress, alcohol or other substance use, blood pressure, urinalysis, sexually transmitted infection risk, and in some cases pap smears and breast examinations. Screening tests with abnormal results require follow-up and intervention. For example, if the adolescent is anemic, iron tablets may be needed and teaching about high-iron foods should be done. Vision impairment requires referral to an eye specialist. Presence of sexually transmitted infections requires teaching and medication treatment. History of sexual activity will guide the nurse to tests that should be included in the examination (see *Clinical Tip*).

The adolescent should receive extensive information about ways to protect health and prevent disease. The hazardous outcomes of smoking are discussed, and smoking cessation programs are encouraged for smokers. Unprotected sexual activity is presented as a serious health threat. Use of sunscreens to prevent burns and future skin cancer is encouraged. Females are taught breast self-exam, and males are taught testicular exam. For youth who are overweight and sedentary, the possible outcomes such as type 2 diabetes and cardiovascular disease are mentioned. While it would not be advisable to threaten or frighten an adolescent with descriptions of diseases, an understanding of the potential serious outcomes can be motivators for behavior change.

In addition to teaching to prevent disease, the nurse also administers any needed immunizations. Many adolescents have not had immunizations since about school entry time, so their record should be carefully reviewed (see Chapter 44 🔗). When checking the adolescent's record, consider the following questions about some common immunizations that are needed:

- **When was the last tetanus-diphtheria (Td) booster?**
  It is recommended every 10 years if no wounds have required an update in the interim. If the child received

Clinical Tip

Sexually active teens should be screened annually for the following:

- Chlamydia
- Gonorrhea
- Trichomoniasis
- Human papillomavirus
- Herpes simplex virus
- Bacterial vaginosis
- Human immunodeficiency virus

Individuals should be screened for syphilis and HIV/AIDS if requesting testing or meeting any of these criteria:

- History of sexually transmitted infection
- More than one sexual partner in past 6 months
- Intravenous drug use
- Sexual intercourse with a partner at risk
- Sex in exchange for drugs or money
- Homelessness
- Males—sex with other males
- Syphilis—residence in areas where disease is prevalent

See Chapter 53 🔗 for further information on screening procedures.

Source: Data from Hagan, J. F., Shaw, J. S., & Shaw, P. M. (2008). *Bright futures: Guidelines for health supervision of infants, children, and adolescents* (3rd ed.). Elk Grove Village, IL: American Academy of Pediatrics.

it at age 5 years, a booster is needed at 15 years. A Tdap (tetanus-diphtheria-acellular pertussis) booster is given, with the preferred age of 11–12 years. If a dose of Td was given during adolescence, wait for at least 5 years, and administer one dose of Tdap.

- **Was a second measles-mumps-rubella administered?** A second dose may not have been routine when teens were younger so they may need it now.
- **Is hepatitis A common in your state?** If so, the teen needs to get that vaccine.
- **Has the youth had hepatitis B vaccine?** This is important for all youth, and some may not have received it as infants.
- **Did the youth have a documented history of varicella disease?** If not, two doses of the vaccine are needed.
- **Has the youth received meningococcal vaccine?** Meningococcal vaccine is now recommended for all youth.
- **Have the adolescent female and male received the human papillomavirus vaccine?** Human papillomavirus vaccine (3-dose series) is recommended for females and males from 11 to 12 years, or for those 13 to 26 years not previously immunized. The vaccine can be given as early as 9 years of age.
- **Has the youth received the annual influenza vaccine?** Annual influenza vaccine is now recommended for all children and adolescents.

The results of health screening are shared with the teen and with the parent as appropriate. Teaching and other interventions for

Activity | Case Study: Immunization Update

disease prevention are examples of health maintenance activities. Expected outcomes are increasing knowledge of common diseases and methods of prevention among teen and parent, use of screening tests by the healthcare provider, and use of the healthcare home by the adolescent for treatment of diseases.

INJURY PREVENTION STRATEGIES

Injury is the greatest health hazard for adolescents, so injury prevention must be integrated into every health contact with youth. The major hazard is automobile crashes (see Chapter 1 🔗). Many teens learn to drive and have a license by 16 years of age. They often transport friends, get distracted by social interactions in the car, have little experience about what to do if a car slides or has mechanical problems, may drink and drive, talk or text on cell phones while driving, and are often tired when driving (Figure 37–4 ●). Many states have instituted graduated driving licensing to help decrease some risks. Know the graduated driver license laws in your state and reinforce them with youth and families. Driving should always be presented as a privilege and a responsibility. Suggest that parents consider enforcing serious consequences such as losing the ability to drive for a time after any infraction. Because of the great risk of injury and death from motor vehicle crashes, ask at each health visit if the teen drives, rides with other teens, what rules parents have established about driving, and whether the teen ever drinks and drives or rides with someone who does. Reinforce the need to wear a lap and shoulder belt at all times and to never drink and drive.

SAFETY ALERT!

Major risk factors for teen drivers include inexperience (especially vulnerable time is the first 6 months of driving), transporting other teens, night driving, non-use of seat belt, and distractions such as texting and playing music. Graduated driver licensing is an approach used to decrease motor vehicle crashes among novice teen drivers. The CDC recommends that no learners' permits be allowed before 16 years of age, that permits must be held for at least 6 months, that driving from 10 p.m. to 5 a.m. not be allowed except with adult chaperone, that other youth not be transported, and that regular licenses (without youth restrictions) not be allowed until 18 years of age. Zero-tolerance policies for drinking, texting or cell phone use, and non-use of seat belts should be enforced (Centers for Disease Control and Prevention [CDC], 2010). How can nurses be active in political discussions to promote graduated driver licensing and support parents of novice teen drivers?

Youth are at risk for injury with other motorized vehicles. Motorcycles, four-wheelers, boats, jet skis, farm machinery, and tools are other sources of injury. Ask about the youth's exposure to various machines and teach about avoiding alcohol and drug use, and safety gear and precautions to be used. Every health visit should include other questions that help to identify a wide variety of injury hazards. Be sure to discuss and provide written material to perform injury prevention teaching. Such measures are important health maintenance activities (Table 37–3 and Table 37–4). Desired outcomes for nursing care include absence of serious injury, the ability to state sources of risk for injury, and emergency plans for assistance when engaging in any risky activities.

● **Figure 37–4** Injury prevention for teens. Adolescents often drive motorized vehicles and may be at risk for injury if not properly prepared or protected. What teaching and experience do these youth need for safe enjoyment of the experience of driving and riding with friends? Do schools in your area offer driver education classes? What are the state requirements for youth driver licensure?

Source: © UpperCut Images/Alamy

NURSING MANAGEMENT *For the Health Promotion and Maintenance of the Adolescent*

Nursing Assessment and Diagnosis

Nurses assess adolescents in a variety of settings, including offices, clinics, schools, homes, correctional facilities, extended care facilities, sports-related facilities, and family planning clinics. A wide array of health concerns should be included in these assessments:

- Measurement of growth
- Presence of any unusual findings on physical examination
- Lifestyle choices related to dietary intake, physical activity, and oral hygiene
- Assessment of mental status, family interactions, and social connections with peers
- Any risky behaviors the adolescent engages in such as smoking, unprotected sexual relations, alcohol or drug use, or unsafe driving practices

The people and organizations around the adolescent such as family, school, and neighborhood are all assessed. Remember to list both risks and protective factors. The protective factors can be used during implementation to enhance the youth's resilience.

Based on a thorough assessment, you will establish nursing diagnoses that are appropriate for the adolescent and family. Some possible nursing diagnoses might include the following (NANDA-I © 2012):

- *Rape-Trauma Syndrome* related to date rape
- *Dentition, Impaired,* related to ineffective oral hygiene

Table 37–3	Injury Prevention in Adolescence

	Hazard	Developmental Characteristics	Preventive Measures
	Motor vehicle crashes	Adolescents learn to drive, enjoy new independence, and often feel invulnerable.	Insist on driver's education classes. Enforce rules about safe driving. Seat belts should be used for every trip. Discourage drug and alcohol use. Get treatment for teenagers who are known substance abusers.
	Sporting injuries	Adolescents may participate in physically challenging sports such as soccer, gymnastics, or football. They may be allowed to drive motorboats.	Encourage use of protective sporting gear. Teach safe boating practices. Perform teaching related to hazards of drug and alcohol use, especially when using motorized equipment.
	Drowning	Adolescents overestimate endurance when swimming. They take risks diving.	Encourage swimming only with friends. Reinforce rules and teach them about risks.

- ***Nutrition, Imbalanced: More Than Body Requirements,*** related to lack of basic nutritional knowledge and obesity in both parents
- ***Nutrition, Readiness for Enhanced,*** related to increasing interest in nutritional knowledge
- ***Sleep Pattern, Disturbed,*** related to frequently changing sleep–wake schedule
- ***Self-Esteem, Situational Low,*** related to situational crisis of friends making fun of adolescent

Planning and Implementation

Whatever the setting, the nurse partners with the adolescent, the parents, and other persons such as teachers or school counselors to plan appropriate goals and related interventions. Nurses work with individual adolescents in offices, schools, and other settings, and often work with groups of adolescents to perform teaching. Apply communication skills that are effective with teens, such as listening to concerns, allowing for discussion, and bringing in peers who have had experiences related to the topic being discussed.

Many nursing interventions involve teaching, so it is wise to develop a number of resources for working with teens. Consult the resources on this textbook's companion website, and visit agencies in your community to gather appropriate materials. Teaching topics should be directed both at health promotion (providing information to enhance the adolescent's state of health) and health maintenance (sharing tips about how to avoid disease and injury). A good starting point is to have the adolescent identify a personal health goal and begin teaching there. In addition to teaching, direct care is provided when administering immunizations, performing vision screening, and examining the spine and posture for scoliosis.

One of the challenges during health supervision for adolescents is including the right mix of teen and parent decision making and involvement. It is again important to apply communication skills by tactfully allowing time for both parent and adolescent to be seen alone. Realize that health supervision provides support and information for parents, such as useful discipline techniques, recognition of common parental feelings about teens, and the need for growing independence by their youth. When providing teaching to groups of teens in schools, there may be policies about what needs to be sent home to parents. For topics such as sexually transmitted infections or substance use, some schools require that an outline be sent home for parents

Weblink   The National Institute for Occupational Safety and Health

Table 37–4	**Injury Prevention Topics for Adolescents**
Topic	**Teaching**
Driving	Always wear seat and shoulder belts. Do not drink alcohol or take drugs and drive or ride with others who do. Do not talk or text on a cell phone as you drive. Do not drive when you are tired. Drive with parents or other adults for several months in winter driving conditions if you live where there is snow, ice, or heavy rains. Keep your car in good repair.
Sun	Wear sunscreen. Limit direct exposure to the sun, especially early in the summer when the skin is most sensitive to burns. This can be achieved by wearing sunscreen, hats, and clothing that prevent sunburns.
Machinery	Learn how to use power tools correctly. Always have someone near when you use tools or machinery.
Emergency care	Learn first aid, CPR, and airway obstruction removal.
Water safety	Learn to swim well. If you supervise younger children near water, never leave them alone, even for a minute.
Fires	Do not play with fire. Follow guidelines to avoid igniting gasoline. Test smoke alarms in your house every 6 months and change batteries annually.
Firearms	Know and follow rules to keep firearms locked, with ammunition locked in a separate place. Never take out a gun to show a friend unless your parent is also present. Take firearm safety classes if you hunt or target shoot.
Hearing	Avoid loud music especially for long periods and through ear phones.
Sports	Wear protective gear recommended for your sport.
Abuse	Report any abuse to an adult you trust. Date with other couples whenever possible and report date rape. Do not drink or take drugs.

Data from Hagan, J. F., Shaw, J. S., & Duncan, P. M. (2008). *Bright futures: Guidelines for health supervision of infants, children and adolescents* (3rd ed.). Elk Grove Village, IL: American Academy of Pediatrics.

Evidence-Based Practice   Farm Injury and Hazards

Clinical Question

Injury is common in communities where children live and work on farms. More than 23,000 farm injuries occur annually in the United States among youth, and over 100 youth victims die (Zaloshnja, Miller, & Lee, 2011). Most injuries occur on weekends during the spring or summer. Before lunch and late afternoon are common times of the day for injury, likely due to being tired at those times.

The Evidence

Farms contain a number of hazards and commonly employ youth. Machinery is a major cause of injury; other examples of hazards include electric currents, bodies of water, grain storage, and actions of large animals. Nearly half of the injuries occur on beef cattle farms (CDC, 2011; Zaloshnja et al., 2011). Exposure to pesticides and other environmental elements also influences youths' health. Nine percent of youth from ages 16 to 19 years working on farms have been diagnosed with asthma and 8% have had an asthma attack in the last year; nearly 10% of those who drive tractors have had a recent asthma attack (Syamlal & Mazurek, 2008). Most farms are in rural areas located far from emergency medical facilities. One study found that training high school students on farms in first aid and safety was one effective strategy to lower injury rates and provide emergency care (Carruth et al., 2010).

Best Practice

Nurses should work with families from rural areas to help them plan to promote safety for children on the farm. Realize that many rural families seek health care in urban areas, so even the nurse who works in a city may see rural families in the agency. Encourage parents to consult the North American Guidelines for Children's Agricultural Tasks (www.nagcat.org/nagcat/) to match the child's physical and mental abilities with the tasks on a farm. Then suggest that parents supervise children in farm tasks, know first aid to follow for injuries, realize that serious accidents can occur, have a cell phone to call for help, and know what facilities are available for phone advice and for emergency rescue. Help families plan ahead to keep rural children safe.

Clinical Reasoning

What items would you include on a checklist for parents of children on a farm? How might pesticides or other chemicals used on a farm injure youth who work near them? Plan educational materials and programs for families that live on farms.

---

to read. Parents may call with questions about content and approach, or some may choose to attend the presentation. To create an effective presentation, the nurse must partner with the school administration, teachers, parents, and others. The ability to collaborate successfully with many individuals and agencies is an important skill for the nurse.

Wherever adolescents are seen, whether in offices or other private settings, schools, correction facilities, or other places with groups present, it is important to leave information about how to contact the nurse or another care provider. Provide brochures, referral numbers, names, and emails related to the topics discussed. Encourage annual visits for health supervision and suggest a variety of places to obtain this care. For example, if a youth will soon graduate from high school, find out if he or she will be working or attending college and provide links to health insurance or care providers in the new location.

Evaluation

Expected outcomes for care of adolescents and their families during health promotion and health maintenance include the following:

- Normal growth patterns and healthy weight are maintained.

- The adolescent is physically active for 60 minutes daily.
- Debris and plaque are absent on dental surfaces.
- The adolescent establishes a positive self-concept.
- The adolescent establishes positive relationships with peers, family members, teachers, and others.
- Healthy lifestyle habits are maintained that promote prevention of disease and injury.

Critical Concept Review

LEARNING OUTCOME 37.1: Identify the major health concerns of the adolescent years.

1. School performance.
2. Sexual issues.
3. Body image issues.
4. The need for independence.

LEARNING OUTCOME 37.2: Describe the general observations made of adolescents and their families as they come to the pediatric healthcare home for health supervision visits.

1. Teen waiting areas.
2. Presence of parents.
3. Teen conversation.

LEARNING OUTCOME 37.3: Apply communication skills to interactions with adolescents and their families.

1. Assist parents to understand that the adolescent is striving to be independent.
2. Reassure adolescent that the parent is trying to provide guidance during a confusing time of life.
3. Encourage parents to reward positive behaviors.
4. Encourage adolescent to discuss specific issues rather than global subjects.

LEARNING OUTCOME 37.4: Apply assessment skills to plan data-gathering methods for nutrition, physical activity, and mental health status of youth.

1. Nutrition:
   - Discuss weight changes since last healthcare visit.
   - Discuss usual meal routines and favorite foods.
2. Physical activity:
   - Question adolescent regarding participation in sports, including amount of practice.
   - Discuss other forms of physical activity engaged in daily or weekly.
3. Mental health status:
   - Assess adolescent's perception of accomplishments and disappointments in life.
   - Ask adolescent about sexual activity.

LEARNING OUTCOME 37.5: Synthesize data from history and examination of the adolescent and family with knowledge of adolescent development to intervene with the adolescent and family during health supervision visits.

1. Partner with the adolescent, parents, and others to plan care.
2. Apply communication skills effective with teens.
3. Develop resources in order to apply effective teaching with adolescents.

LEARNING OUTCOME 37.6: Plan with adolescents to help them integrate activities to promote health and to prevent disease and injury.

1. Screening tests:
   - Scoliosis.
   - Mental health status.
   - Anemia.
   - Sexually transmitted infections.
2. Review immunization status.
3. Review information concerning need for sun protection.
4. Discuss birth control and prevention of sexually transmitted infections.
5. Discuss safe driving practices:
   - Use seat belts.
   - Do not drink and drive.
6. Discuss prevention of common sports injuries.

Clinical Reasoning in Action

Tammy is a 13-year-old coming into the office for her yearly checkup and she has never been in the hospital or had surgery. She is a good student and is excited to start seventh grade next year. She has not had any immunizations since going into kindergarten. Tammy arrives with her mother, with whom she lives; she has no contact with her biologic father. Her mother decides to stay in the waiting room, but did note on the written history form that there is a family history of high cholesterol and heart disease in family members under 50 years old. Tammy's mother is a single parent working full time with two other children at home. Tammy's body mass index is in the 85th percentile and she passed her hearing and vision tests. Her blood pressure is 115/70 and her urinalysis shows blood, but Tammy has her menses today. Tammy has a period every month and menarche started at 10 years old. Her menses lasts 5 to 7 days and she denies experiencing cramping or excessively heavy menses. Tammy enjoys being a member of the volleyball team and is involved in a church youth group. She does not get to spend much time with her friends because she watches her two younger siblings in the afternoons while her mother is at work. When her mother is away, she admits to sitting and playing video games or watching TV most of the day. Tammy says she has had a boyfriend, but denies sexual activity. She also denies any experimentation with substance use.

1. What vaccines is Tammy due for at this age if she has not already had them?

2. A dietary assessment demonstrates that Tammy frequently skips meals and eats fast food almost daily. What are some of the suggestions you can give Tammy to improve her nutritional status?

3. What are some of the injury prevention topics you can discuss with Tammy?

4. Based on the additional information you collected about Tammy, what are some of the areas of recommended health teaching?

5. Develop a concept map for Tammy that includes all of the health promotion areas important to all youth, such as nutrition, oral health, physical activity, social interactions, family relationships, and disease/injury prevention. How can her development be enhanced to draw on strengths and improve areas of need? What part does the healthcare provider play in promoting her health?

See www.nursing.pearsonhighered.com for possible responses and an interactive template for a concept map.

References

American Academy of Child & Adolescent Psychiatry. (2010). *Depression and substance abuse.* Retrieved from www.aacap.org

Bandura, A. (1986). *Social foundations of thought and actions: A social cognitive theory.* Englewood Cliffs, NJ: Prentice Hall.

Bandura, A. (1997a). *Self-efficacy in changing societies.* New York, NY: Cambridge University.

Bandura, A. (1997b). *Self-efficacy: The exercise of control.* New York, NY: Freeman.

Bricker, J. B., Liu, J., Constock, B. A., Peterson, A. V., Kealey, K. A., & Marek, P. M. (2010). Social cognitive mediators of adolescent smoking cessation: Results from a large randomized intervention trial. *Psychology of Addictive Behaviors, 24*(3), 436–445.

Carruth, A. K., Pryor, S., Cormier, C., Bateman, A., Matzke, B., & Gilmore, K. (2010). Evaluation of a school-based train-the-trainer intervention program to teach first aid and risk reduction among high school students. *Journal of School Health, 80*(9), 453–460.

Centers for Disease Control and Prevention (CDC). (2010). *Policy impact—Teen driver safety.* Retrieved from http://www.cdc.gov/motorvehiclesafety/teenbrief

Centers for Disease Control and Prevention (CDC). (2011). *Agricultural safety.* Retrieved from http://www.cdc.gov/niosh/topics/aginjury

Child Trends. (2010). *Unmet dental needs.* Retrieved from http://www.childtrendsdatabank.org/?q=node/282

Connor, J. P., George, S. M., Gullo, M. J., Kelly, A. B., & Young, R. M. (2011). A prospective study of alcohol expectancies and self-efficacy as predictors of young adolescent alcohol misuse. *Alcohol and Alcoholism, 46*(2), 161–169.

Eaton, D. K., Kann, L., Kinchen, S., Shanklin, S., Ross, J., Hawkins, J., . . . Wechsler, H. (2010). Youth risk behavior surveillance—United States, 2009. *Morbidity and Mortality Weekly Report, 59*(SS-5), 1–146.

Eaton, D. K., Kann, L., Kinchen, S., Shanklin, S., Flint, K. H., Hawkins, J., . . . Wechsler, H. (2012). Youth risk behavior surveillance—United States, 2011. *Morbidity and Mortality Weekly Report, 61*(SS04), 1–162.

Hagan, J. F., Shaw, J. S., & Duncan, P. M. (Eds.). (2008). *Bright futures: Guidelines for health supervision of infants, children, and adolescents* (3rd ed.). Elk Grove Village, IL: American Academy of Pediatrics.

Mayo Clinic. (2009). *Teen sleep: Why is your teen so tired?* Retrieved from http://www.mayoclinic.com/health/teens-health

Murray, R. B., Zentner, J. P., & Yakimo, R. (2009). *Health promotion strategies through the life span* (8th ed.). Upper Saddle River, NJ: Pearson Prentice Hall.

Syamlal, G., & Mazurek, J. M. (2008). Prevalence of asthma among youth on Hispanic-operated farms in the United States. *Journal of Agromedicine, 13*(3), 155–160.

Zaloshnja, E., Miller, T. R., & Lee, B. C. (2011). Incidence and cost of nonfatal farm injuries, United States, 2001–2006. *Journal of Agromedicine, 16*(1), 6–18.

Family Assessment and Concepts of Nursing Care in the Community

Sometimes Jessica's asthma attacks really frighten me because she struggles so hard to breathe. She has a lot of trouble with asthma in the summertime with all the heat. I'm afraid to let her play outside with her friends for fear that she will have another attack. I'd really like to know how to keep Jessica's asthma under control. —Mother of Jessica, 8 years old

Ryan McVay/Getty Images

LEARNING OUTCOMES

38.1   Contrast the categories of family strengths that help families cope with stressors.

38.2   Summarize the advantages of using a family assessment tool.

38.3   Assemble a list of family support services that might be available in a community.

38.4   Discuss the community healthcare settings where nurses provide health services to children.

38.5   Compare the roles of the nurse in each identified healthcare setting.

38.6   Summarize the special developmental needs of children to consider in disaster preparedness planning.

C hildren receive most of their health care in community settings. Depending on the community, healthcare resources, and age of the child, this care may be provided in a variety of settings. When providing health care to the child and family, it is important for the nurse to assess the family's strengths, be aware of community resources, and help families manage the complex health care that is often provided in the home.

FAMILY ASSESSMENT

A **family** is defined as two or more individuals who are joined together by marriage, birth, or adoption and live together (U.S. Census Bureau, 2010). A family may also be a self-identified group of two or more persons joined together through the sharing of resources and emotional closeness. Families are guided by a common set of values or beliefs about the worth and importance of certain ideas and traditions. Each family and its members are unique in their strengths and their responses to complex and often conflicting demands for time and attention.

Children and families live within a variety of home environments, and interactions within those settings directly or indirectly influence behaviors and learning. Because of these environmental influences on the family, it is important to consider the relationship of the family with the social networks within the community.

Nurses must be able to assess family strengths and support mechanisms, to identify strategies for **coping** (the use of learned behavioral and cognitive strategies to manage or relieve perceived stress), and to determine when families have overextended their resources and need additional support. In some cases nurses can provide the additional support needed, and at other times referral to other health professionals and community resources is appropriate to address the family's needs.

Family Stressors

Family stress theory focuses on the family's response to unexpected or unplanned events, which can be very disruptive for the family (Kaakinen & Hanson, 2010). Family stressors come from many sources, such as work demands, school issues, extended family demands, the desire to achieve quality family time, and community roles. Many families live in a stressed state due to inadequate finances, healthcare concerns, relationship challenges, and other pressures. Most families have developed coping strategies to deal with daily routine stressors (completion of household chores, homework, etc.).

Nonroutine stressors (such as surgery or the birth of a child) and unexpected events (accidents or emergency department visits) are often more stressful because the family has not had time to review resources and prepare a response. A child's illness or injury affects every member of the family. Family members respond to this stress, sometimes in a way that changes interactions among family members and with the environment. Identify how families respond to the stress of a child's illness or injury so that nursing interventions include support that may reduce the impact on the entire family.

Family Strengths

Family strengths are the relationships and processes that support and protect families and family members during times of adversity and change (Moore, Whitney, & Kinukawa, 2009). Nurses can identify and use a family's strengths when problem solving within the family (Wright & Leahey, 2009, p. 151). Strengths that enable families to develop and adapt to stressors include (Leske & Brasel, 2010):

- Family member and individual resources, such as finances, education, and prior experiences
- Supportive patterns of communication and problem solving
- Coping strategies to maintain family relationships and emotional stability